THE Nursing Profession

OCT   2001

THE Nursing Profession

Tomorrow and Beyond

Norma L. Chaska *Editor*

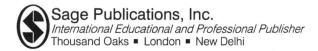

Sage Publications, Inc.
International Educational and Professional Publisher
Thousand Oaks ▪ London ▪ New Delhi

The author gratefully acknowledges the kind permission of Henry Holt and Co. to reprint excerpts from "The Road Not Taken," from *The Poetry of Robert Frost,* edited by Edward Connery Lathem. Copyright © Henry Holt and Co., Publishers, New York, 1969.

For information:

Sage Publications, Inc.
2455 Teller Road
Thousand Oaks, California 91320
E-mail: order@sagepub.com

Sage Publications Ltd.
6 Bonhill Street
London EC2A 4PU
United Kingdom

Sage Publications India Pvt. Ltd.
M-32 Market
Greater Kailash I
New Delhi 110 048 India

Printed in the United States of America

Library of Congress Cataloging-in-Publication Data

Main entry under title:

The nursing profession: Tomorrow and beyond / edited by
Norma L. Chaska.
p.   cm.
Includes bibliographical references and index.
ISBN 0-7619-1943-0 (cloth: alk. paper)
1. Nursing.   2. Nursing—Forecasting.
I. Chaska, Norma L.
RT82 .N8687   2000
610.73–dc21   00-009517

Printed on acid-free paper.

01   02   03   04   05   06   07   7   6   5   4   3   2

Acquisition Editors:	Rolf Janke/Dan Ruth
Editorial Assistant:	Heidi Van Middlesworth
Production Editor:	Sanford Robinson
Production Services:	Books By Design, Inc.
Cover Designer:	Ravi Balasuriya

IN MEMORY OF

my parents

James and Edna

and

Wolcott Dean Baird

DEDICATED TO

J. C.

and

Lieutenant Colonel (Retired) Shirley M. Chaska Baird, EdD

sister, friend, and mentor throughout my
professional career

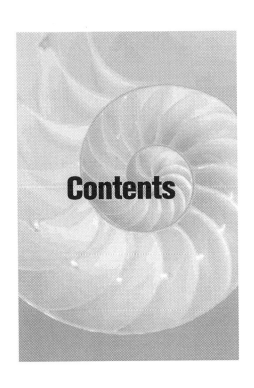

Contents

Part II: NURSING EDUCATION

Part III: NURSING THEORY

Part IV: NURSING RESEARCH

Part V: NURSING PRACTICE

Part VI: NURSING ADMINISTRATION—SERVICE

Part VII: NURSING ADMINISTRATION—ACADEMIC

Part VIII: THE FUTURE OF NURSING

Part IX: SUMMARY

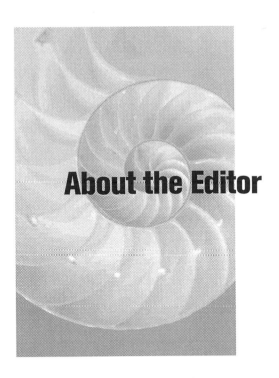

About the Editor

NORMA L. CHASKA, PhD, RN, FAAN, is a leader in nursing education and nursing administration. Currently, she is a consultant for academic administration in universities.

Her educational preparation includes a diploma in nursing from St. Marys School of Nursing, Saint Marys Hospital, Rochester, Minnesota; a bachelor of science in nursing (BSN) degree from the School of Nursing, The Catholic University of America, Washington, DC; a master of science (MS) degree from the School of Nursing, Boston University; and a doctor of philosophy (PhD) degree in sociology from Boston University. Prior to her graduate education, she held numerous clinical and administrative positions in most every specialized area of nursing for a total of 15 years of experience in nursing practice. Upon earning her doctoral degree she was on the staff of the Mayo Clinic, Rochester, Minnesota, for $2^1/2$ years conducting patient and health care research.

Dr. Chaska has had 22 years of significant experience in nursing education and academic administration. She has held faculty positions at Boston University, the University of Minnesota, and at the School of Nursing, Indiana University, Indianapolis, and in the Department of Sociology, School of Liberal Arts, Indiana University–Purdue University at Indianapolis (IUPUI); faculty and administrative positions at the University of Illinois, College of Nursing in Chicago; the School of Nursing, Medical College of Georgia in Augusta, and most recently as Professor and Dean of the School of Nursing at the University of San Francisco, San Francisco.

Dr. Chaska is widely sought as a consultant for academic administration in universities and for nursing education programs. She has served on national research and nursing education review teams for funding of proposals submitted for nursing research and nursing education programs. She has been active in numerous professional organizations. She was elected to Sigma Theta Tau International in 1963, elected as a Fellow in the American

Academy of Nursing in 1978, Sigma Xi Scientific Research Society in 1978, and listed in *Who's Who of World's Women* in 1983. She has been awarded numerous other faculty and service honors.

Throughout her academic career, Dr. Chaska has drawn extensively on her clinical experience in service and research settings. This background is also reflected in her numerous presentations, publications, and consultations. The underlying theme that frequently is cited as a quote in her many presentations and speeches is as follows:

> I shall pass through this world but once. Any good therefore that I can do let me do it now, for I shall not pass this way again.
>
> Source Unknown

A major concern in all her work is the evolution of nursing as a profession. This concern is most evident in her four texts: *The Nursing Profession: Views Through the Mist,* McGraw-Hill, 1978; *The Nursing Profession: A Time to Speak,* McGraw-Hill, 1983; *The Nursing Profession: Turning Points,* C.V. Mosby, 1990; and her latest book, *The Nursing Profession: Tomorrow and Beyond,* Sage, 2001. The *Views Through the Mist* textbook was the first nursing issues type of book ever published. The *Time to Speak* book received the *American Journal of Nursing* Book of the Year Award in 1983 for Nursing Education and Nursing Administration, and the *Turning Points* volume received that same award in 1990.

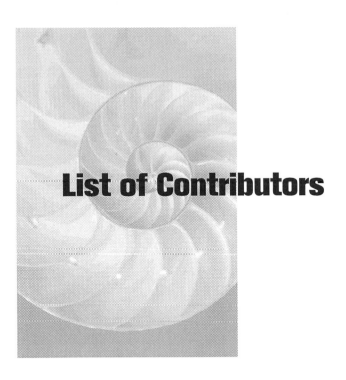

List of Contributors

THE NURSING PROFESSION: Tomorrow and Beyond (2001)
Editor: Norma L. Chaska, Sage Publications, Inc., Thousand Oaks, CA

Jacqueline Agnew, PhD, RN, FAAN
Associate Professor and Director
Occupational Health Nursing Program, Department of Environmental Health Science
    and Division of Occupational Health
School of Hygiene and Public Health, Johns Hopkins University
Baltimore, MD

Judith W. Alexander, PhD, RN, CNAA
Associate Professor
Department of Family and Community Health Nursing
College of Nursing, University of South Carolina
Columbia, SC

Carole A. Anderson, PhD, RN, FAAN
Dean and Professor
College of Nursing, Ohio State University
Columbus, OH

Ida M. Androwich, PhD, RNC, FAAN
Associate Professor
Community, Mental Health and Administrative Nursing
Marcella Niehoff School of Nursing, Loyola University
Chicago, IL

Sara E. Barger, DPA, MN, RN, FAAN
Dean and Professor
Capstone College of Nursing, University of Alabama
Tuscaloosa, AL

Diane M. Billings, EdD, RN, FAAN
Associate Dean for Teaching, Learning, and Information Resources
School of Nursing, Indiana University
Indianapolis, IN

Diana L. Biordi, PhD, RN, FAAN
Professor and Assistant Dean
School of Nursing, Kent State University
Kent, OH

Donna L. Boland, PhD, RN
Associate Professor and Associate Dean for Undergraduate Programs
School of Nursing, Indiana University
Indianapolis, IN

Mary G. Bourbonniere, MSN, RN
Doctoral Candidate
School of Nursing, University of Pennsylvania
Philadelphia, PA

Peter I. Buerhaus, PhD, MS, RN, FAAN
Associate Dean for Research and Valere Potter Professor
School of Nursing, Vanderbilt University
Nashville, TN

Jacquelyn C. Campbell, PhD, RN, FAAN
Associate Dean for the PhD Programs and Research and
    Anna D. Wolf Endowed Professor
School of Nursing, Johns Hopkins University
Baltimore, MD

Michael A. Carter, DNSc, RN, FAAN
Dean and Professor
College of Nursing, University of Tennessee–Memphis
Memphis, TN

Norma L. Chaska, PhD, RN, FAAN
Consultant
Academic Administration for Universities and Editor
San Francisco, CA

Peggy L. Chinn, PhD, RN, FAAN
Professor
School of Nursing, University of Connecticut
Storrs, CT

Euisoo Choi, MSN, RN
Project Officer
Primary and Secondary Prevention Program
Hornsby Ku-ring-gai Ryde
Division of General Practice
Wahroonga, Sydney, Australia

Margaret M. Conger, EdD, RN, CM
Professor
Department of Nursing, Northern Arizona University
Flagstaff, AZ

Inge B. Corless, PhD, RN, FAAN
Professor
Graduate Program in Nursing, MGH Institute of Health Professions at
   Massachusetts General Hospital
Boston, MA

Anne J. Davis, PhD, DSC (H), RN, FAAN
Professor Emerita
School of Nursing, University of California–San Francisco
San Francisco, CA

Professor
Nagano College of Nursing, Komagane City
Nagano, Japan

Carol Deets, EdD, RN
Professor and Associate Dean for Research and Director of the Doctoral Program
College of Nursing and Health, University of Cincinnati
Cincinnati, OH

Jacqueline A. Dienemann, PhD, RN, CNAA, FAAN
Clinical Associate Professor
School of Nursing, Georgetown University
Washington, DC

Joanne M. Disch, PhD, RN, FAAN
Professor of Nursing
Director, Katharine J. Densforth International Center for
   Nursing Leadership
Katherine R. and C. Walton Lillehei Chair of Nursing Leadership
School of Nursing, University of Minnesota
Minneapolis, MN

Eleanor Donnelly, PhD, RN
Professor
Department of Environments for Health
School of Nursing, Indiana University
Indianapolis, IN

Shirley L. Dooling, EdD, RN
Professor and Dean Emerita
Marcella Niehoff School of Nursing, Loyola University–Chicago
Chicago, IL

Virginia J. Duffy, PhD, RN, CS, NP
Advanced Practice Registered Nurse–PMH
Owner: PsychSense, A Mental Health Education & Consulting Company
Co-Owner: Health Answers–Health Consultation On Line
Rochester, NY

Jacqueline Fawcett, PhD, RN, FAAN
Professor Emerita
School of Nursing, University of Pennsylvania
Philadelphia, PA

Professor

Geraldene Felton, EdD, RN, FAAN
Professor and Dean Emerita
College of Nursing, The University of Iowa
Iowa City, IA

Executive Director
National League for Nursing Accrediting Commission
New York, NY

Anastasia Fisher, DNSc, RN
Postdoctoral Scholar
Department of Psychosocial and Community Health
School of Nursing, University of Washington
Seattle, WA

Mary L. Fisher, PhD, RN, CNAA
Associate Professor
Department of Environments for Health
School of Nursing, Indiana University
Indianapolis, IN

Joyce J. Fitzpatrick, PhD, MBA, RN, FAAN
Professor, Endowed Chair and Dean Emerita
Frances Payne Bolton School of Nursing, Case Western University
Cleveland, OH

Editor
Nursing and Health Care Perspectives, National League for Nursing
New York, NY

Juanita W. Fleming, PhD, RN, FAAN
Special Assistant to the President for Academic Affairs
University of Kentucky
Lexington, KY

Marilyn E. Flood, PhD, RN
Associate Dean, Academic Programs
School of Nursing, University of California–San Francisco
San Francisco, CA

Robin Dawn Froman, PhD, RN, FAAN
Professor, Associate Dean for Research, and Director for the Office for
    Nursing Research and Scholarship
School of Nursing, University of Texas Medical Branch
Galveston, TX

Barbara C. Gaines, EdD, RN
Consultant for Curriculum Development and Evaluation and Professor Emerita
School of Nursing, Oregon Health Sciences University
Portland, OR

Rose M. Gerber, PhD, RN
Associate Professor Emerita
College of Nursing, The University of Arizona
Tucson, AZ

Patricia A. Grady, PhD, RN, FAAN
Director
National Institute of Nursing Research, National Institutes of Health
Department of Health and Human Services
Bethesda, MD

Mikel L. Gray, PhD, RN, CUNP, CCCN, FAAN
Nurse Practitioner
Department of Urology, University of Virginia
Charlottsville, VA

Associate Professor
School of Nursing, University of Virginia Health Sciences Center
Charlottsville, VA

Hurdis M. Griffith, PhD, RN, FAAN
Dean and Professor
College of Nursing, Rutgers, The State University of New Jersey
Newark, NJ

Sheila A. Haas, PhD, RN
Professor and Dean
Marcella Niehoff School of Nursing, Loyola University–Chicago
Chicago, IL

Barbara Habermann, PhD, RN
Postdoctoral Scholar
Department of Family and Child Nursing
School of Nursing, University of Washington
Seattle, WA

Assistant Professor
School of Nursing, University of Alabama–Birmingham
Birmingham, AL

Sally Brosz Hardin, PhD, RN, FAAN
Professor and Director
PhD Nursing Program
Barnes College of Nursing, University of Missouri–St. Louis
St. Louis, MO

Bevely J. Hays, PhD, RN
Associate Professor
College of Nursing, University of Nebraska
Omaha, NE

Janet Heinrich, DrPH, RN, FAAN
Associate Director
Health Finance and Public Health, U.S. General Accounting Office
Washington, DC

Sharon E. Hoffman, PhD, MBA, RN, FAAN
Senior Vice President for Academic Affairs
Spalding University
Louisville, KY

Linda Hollinger-Smith, PhD, RN
Assistant Dean for External Affairs and Associate Professor
College of Nursing, Rush University
Chicago, IL

Director of Nursing
Rush Primary Care Institute, Rush-Presbyterian–St. Luke's Medical Center
Chicago, IL

Eun-Ok Im, PhD, MPH, CNS, RN
Assistant Professor
School of Nursing, University of Wisconsin–Milwaukee
Milwaukee, WI

Jean F. Jenkins, PhD, MSN, RN
Clinical Nurse Specialist and Consultant for the National Cancer Institute,
    National Institutes of Health
Department of Health and Human Services, Public Health Service
Bethesda, MD

Cheryl B. Jones, PhD, RN, CNAA
Associate Professor
School of Nursing, University of North Carolina–Chapel Hill
Chapel Hill, NC

Dorothy A. Jones, EdD, RN, FAAN
Professor
Adult Health Department
School of Nursing, Boston College
Chestnut Hill, MA

Nurse Scientist
Massachusetts General Hospital
Boston, MA

Rebecca A. Patronis Jones, DNS, RN, CNAA
Director and Professor
School of Nursing & Health Sciences, Texas A&M University–Corpus Christi
Corpus Christi, TX

Charlie Jones-Dickson, EdD, RN, FAAN
Professor
School of Nursing, University of Alabama–Birmingham
Birmingham, AL

Christine E. Kasper, PhD, RN, FAAN, FACSM
M. Adelaide Nutting Chair, Professor and Director of Doctoral Programs
School of Nursing, Johns Hopkins University
Baltimore, MD

Sarah B. Keating, EdD, RN, C-PNP, FAAN
Former Dean and Professor Emerita
Samuel Merritt–Saint Mary's Intercollegiate Nursing Program
Oakland, CA

Karlene M. Kerfoot, PhD, RN, CNAA, FAAN
Senior Vice President for Nursing and Patient Care Services and
    Chief Nurse Executive and Associate Dean, Nursing Practice
School of Nursing, Indiana University
Indianapolis, IN

Clarian Health Partners, Inc.
Methodist–UI–Riley
Indianapolis, IN

Shake Ketefian, EdD, RN, FAAN
Professor and Director of Doctoral and Postdoctoral Studies and
    Director of International Affairs
School of Nursing, University of Michigan
Ann Arbor, MI

Hesook Suzie Kim, PhD, RN
Professor
College of Nursing, University of Rhode Island
Kingston, RI

Professor II
Institute of Nursing Science, Faculty of Medicine, University of Oslo
Oslo, Norway

JoEllen Koerner, PhD, RN, FAAN
President
Global Nursing Academy
Boulder, CO

Beverly Kopala, PhD, RN
Associate Professor
Marcella Niehoff School of Nursing, Loyola University–Chicago
Chicago, IL

Mary Jo Kreitzer, PhD, RN
Director
Center for Spirituality and Healing
Academic Health Center, University of Minnesota
Minneapolis, MN

Phyllis Beck Kritek, PhD, RN, FAAN
Florence Thelma Hall Distinguished Professor of Nursing
School of Nursing, University of Texas Medical Branch
Galveston, TX

Lois A. Lane, JD, MSN, RNCS
Former Associate Dean of Service Innovation
Assistant Clinical Professor
School of Nursing, Indiana University
Indianapolis, IN

PhD Student-Health Care Ethics, Saint Louis University
Saint Louis, MO

Ramon Lavandero, MA, MSN, RN
Director of Development and Strategic Alliances
American Association of Critical-Care Nurses
Aliso Viejo, CA

Elizabeth R. Lenz, PhD, RN, FAAN
Anna C. Maxwell Professor of Nursing Research and Associate Dean
    for Research and Doctoral Studies
School of Nursing, Columbia University
New York, NY

Andrea R. Lindell, DNSc, RN
Dean and Schmidlapp Professor of Nursing
College of Nursing and Health

Associate Senior Vice President for Interdisciplinary Education
University of Cincinnati Medical Center
Cincinnati, OH

Carol A. Lindeman, PhD, RN, FAAN
Dean and Professor Emeritus
School of Nursing, Oregon Health Sciences University
Portland, OR

Ada M. Lindsey, PhD, RN, FAAN
Dean and Professor
College of Nursing, University of Nebraska Medical Center
Omaha, NE

Marilyn Loen, PhD, RN
Professor
Department of Nursing, Metropolitan State University
St. Paul, MN

Carol O. Long, PhD, RN
Assistant Professor
College of Nursing, Arizona State University
Tempe, AZ

Kathleen M. McCauley, PhD, RN, CS, FAAN
Associate Professor of Cardiovascular Nursing and Acting Associate Dean and
    Director of Undergraduate Studies
School of Nursing, University of Pennsylvania

Cardiovascular Clinical Specialist
Hospital of the University of Pennsylvania
Philadelphia, PA

Maureen P. McCausland, DNSc, RN, FAAN
Chief Nursing Executive
University of Pennsylvania Health System

Professor of Nursing Administration and Associate Dean for Nursing Practice
School of Nursing, University of Pennsylvania
Philadelphia, PA

Margaret L. McClure, EdD, RN, FAAN
Professor
New York University
New York, NY

Mary Ann McDermott, PhD, RN, FAAN
Professor
Department of Maternal–Child Nursing
Marcella Niehoff School of Nursing, Loyola University–Chicago

Director
Center for Faith and Mission, Loyola University–Chicago
Chicago, IL

Elizabeth A. McFarlane, DNSc, RN, FAAN
Associate Professor
School of Nursing, The Catholic University of America
Washington, DC

Afaf I. Meleis, PhD, Dr. PS (Hon), RN, FAAN
Professor
Department of Community Health Systems
School of Nursing, University of California–San Francisco
San Francisco, CA

Kenneth P. Miller, PhD, RN, CFNP, FAAN
Professor and Associate Dean for Research and Clinical Scholarship
College of Nursing, University of New Mexico, Health Sciences Center
Albuquerque, NM

Betty M. Neuman, PhD, RN, FAAN
Independent International Consultant
Watertown, OH

Amy A. Nichols, EdD, RN
Associate Professor
School of Nursing, San Francisco State University
San Francisco, CA

Steven V. Owen, PhD
Professor
School of Nursing and Department of Preventive Medicine and Community Health

Senior Statistician
Office of Biostatistics, University of Texas Medical Branch
Galveston, TX

Craig Paterson, LLB, MA
PhD Candidate–Health Care Ethics and Adjunct Faculty
Department of Philosophy, Saint Louis University
Saint Louis, MO

Shannon E. Perry, PhD, RN, FAAN
Professor and Director
School of Nursing, San Francisco State University
San Francisco, CA

Daniel J. Pesut, PhD, RN, CS, FAAN
Professor and Chairperson
Department of Environments for Health
School of Nursing, Indiana University
Indianapolis, IN

SueEllen Pinkerton, PhD, RN, FAAN
Senior Vice President and CNO
Shands Health Care, Shands Jacksonville
Jacksonville, FL

Timothy P. Porter-O'Grady, EdD, PhD, RN, FAAN
Senior Partner
Tim Porter-O'Grady, Inc.
Atlanta, GA

Carol H. Pullen, EdD, RN
Associate Professor and Assistant Dean
Rural Nursing Education
College of Nursing, University of Nebraska
Omaha, NE

Larry Purnell, PhD, RN, FAAN
Professor
College of Health and Nursing Sciences, University of Delaware
Newark, DE

Richard W. Redman, PhD, RN
Professor and Associate Dean
School of Nursing, University of Colorado Health Sciences Center
Denver, CO

Andrea Renwanz-Boyle, DNSc, RN
Associate Professor
School of Nursing, San Francisco State University
San Francisco, CA

Karen R. Robinson, PhD, RN, FAAN
Associate Director for Clinical Operations
Veterans Affairs Medical Center
Fargo, ND

Mary Ann Schroeder, PhD, RN, FAAN
Senior Data Analyst
Harris Methodist Health System
Fort Worth, TX

Elizabeth F. Sefcik, PhD, RN, CS
Professor and School Nurse Coordinator
School of Nursing & Health Sciences, Texas A&M University–Corpus Christi
Corpus Christi, TX

Joan L. F. Shaver, PhD, RN, FAAN
Dean and Professor
College of Nursing, University of Illinois–Chicago
Chicago, IL

Grayce M. Sills, PhD, RN, FAAN
Professor Emerita
College of Nursing, Ohio State University
Columbus, OH

Mariah Snyder, PhD, RN, FAAN
Professor
School of Nursing, University of Minnesota
Minneapolis, MN

Kathleen R. Stevens, EdD, RN, FAAN
Professor, School of Nursing
Director, Academic Center for Evidence-Based Nursing
The University of Texas Health Science Center at San Antonio
San Antonio, TX

Editor, *Online Journal of Knowledge Synthesis for Nursing*

Eileen M. Sullivan-Marx, PhD, RN, FAAN
Assistant Professor
School of Nursing, University of Pennsylvania
Philadelphia, PA

Katherine A. Thomas, MN, RN
Executive Director
Texas Board of Nurse Examiners
Austin, TX

Sandra P. Thomas, PhD, RN, FAAN
Professor and Director
PhD Program in Nursing
College of Nursing, University of Tennessee
Knoxville, TN

Patricia E. Thompson, EdD, RN
President
Sigma Theta Tau International

Associate Professor and Associate Dean for Baccalaureate Education
College of Nursing, University of Arkansas for Medical Sciences
Little Rock, AR

Marita G. Titler, PhD, RN, FAAN
Director of Research, Quality, and Outcomes Management
Department of Nursing Services and Patient Care, University of Iowa
  Hospital and Clinics
Iowa City, IA

Catherine M. Todero, PhD, RN
Associate Professor and Associate Dean of Undergraduate Programs

Project Director, UNMC–Cosmopolitan Mobile Nursing Center
College of Nursing, University of Nebraska Medical Center
Omaha, NE

Mary Wakefield, PhD, RN, FAAN
Professor and Director
Center for Health Policy, Research and Ethics
College of Nursing and Health Sciences, George Mason University
Fairfax, VA

Jean M. Watson, PhD, RN, HNC, FAAN
Former Dean and Distinguished Professor of Nursing–Scoville-Murchinson
    Endowed Chair in Caring Science
School of Nursing, University of Colorado Health Sciences Center
Denver, CO

Elizabeth E. Weiner, PhD, RN, FAAN
Professor of Nursing; Director, Center for Academic Technologies;
    Acting Associate Director, Academic Information Technology Services
College of Nursing and Health, University of Cincinnati Medical Center
Cincinnati, OH

Rosalee C. Yeaworth, PhD, RN, FAAN
Professor Emerita and Dean Emerita
College of Nursing, University of Nebraska
Omaha, NE

Carolyn J. Yocom, PhD, RN, FAAN
Associate Professor
College of Nursing, Rutgers, The State University of New Jersey
Newark, NJ

Lani Zimmerman, PhD, RN
Associate Professor and Chair
Adult Health and Illness Department
College of Nursing, University of Nebraska Medical Center
Omaha, NE

Writing the Introduction for the Book

Margretta M. Styles, EdD, RN, FAAN
Professor Emerita and Former Dean
School of Nursing, University of California–San Francisco
San Francisco, CA

Past President, American Nurses Association, International Council
    of Nurses, and American Nurses Credentialing Center

Currently, Consultant, ANCC

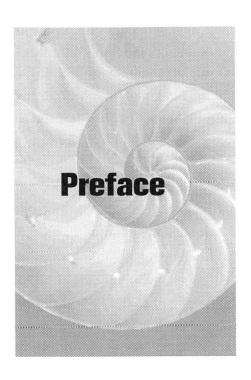

Preface

Two roads diverged in a yellow wood,
And sorry I could not travel both
And be one traveler, long I stood
And looked down one as far as I could
To where it bent in the undergrowth;

Then took the other, as just as fair,
And having perhaps the better claim,
Because it was grassy and wanted wear;
Though as for that the passing there
Had worn them really about the same,

And both that morning equally lay
In leaves no step had trodden black.
Oh, I kept the first for another day!
Yet knowing how way leads on to way,
I doubted if I should ever come back.

I shall be telling this with a sigh
Somewhere ages and ages hence:
Two roads diverged in a wood, and I—
I took the one less traveled by,
And that has made all the difference.

Robert Frost (1916/1993, p. 1)

The poem, *The Road Not Taken,* by Robert Frost illustrates the predominant theme throughout this volume—that there are various paths that nursing as a profession can take. Nursing as a profession always has had choices to make regarding directions for the future. But for the 21st century, options abound. So too do the challenges. Following the leadership provided by the contributing authors in this volume—through the roads of professionalization, education, theory, practice, administration, and the future—professionals will be enabled to choose "paths" that make a difference.

The purpose of this book is to provide an in-depth global scope and study of nursing as a profession. Specifically, its aim is to project patterns of thought and considerations about the state of nursing now and far beyond into the future of the 21st century. You will find perspectives that are challenging, disconcerting, and refreshing. The content should cause you to reflect, consider, and dialogue regarding the various paths presented. Then, positioning to move forward on a path can occur.

This book is a companion to *The Nursing Profession: Views Through The Mist,* 1978, and *The Nursing Profession: A Time to Speak,* 1983, both published by McGraw-Hill; and *The Nursing Profession: Turning Points,* published by C. V. Mosby in 1990. The text, *The Nursing Profession: Views Through The Mist,* 1978, was the first nursing issues type of textbook ever published. The second and third texts were recipients of the American Journal of Nursing Book of the Year Award for 1983 and 1990, respectively. This year 2001 volume is similar in format to the 1990 text.

For each book, persistent effort was made to provide original writing by nurse authors who represent diverse disciplines in their doctoral preparation. Thus this volume contains 78 *original* chapters by 105 contributing authors. All 78 *primary* authors for the chapters are doctorally prepared, representing the disciplines of nursing, sociology, psychology, anthropology, philosophy, education, and law. All coauthors are doctorally prepared with exception of four who are master's prepared or doctoral candidates. Twenty of the 105 contributing authors also were authors in either *Views Through The Mist, A Time To Speak,* or *Turning Points.* Eighty-five of the contributors are new to this volume. Two of the authors have appeared in all four textbooks. The contributors represent all geographic regions of the United States and include one person in Japan, one in Norway, and another in Australia, who currently are employed professionally in those countries. The contributors are recognized leaders in the profession of nursing. Sixty-four of the contributing authors are elected Fellows of the American Academy of Nursing.

Nine Parts comprise this book: Professionalization, Nursing Education, Nursing Theory, Nursing Research, Nursing Practice, Nursing Administration—Service, Nursing Administration—Academic, The Future of Nursing, and Summary. An Introduction that leads off

with lines from Robert Frost's poem provides the opening for each Part. You are encouraged to reflect on the poet's lines for their relevance to the content of the chapters in each Part. Each chapter has a Concluding Statement by the author(s) and ends with Editor's Questions for Discussion.

The Summary Part consists of a final chapter, Paths to Make a Difference. In this chapter, I highlight particular points of the contributing authors. I then trace the predominant patterns and themes introduced in the chapters and Parts. I identify paths that the authors have projected to make a difference for the profession in the future far beyond. The Concluding Statement includes a synthesis of these paths that, if followed—I believe—will make a difference.

By reading the volume, reflecting on the questions, and positing possible answers, you should be able to gain a comprehensive perspective of the profession. The questions should be of value to practitioners, graduate and undergraduate students, faculty, and administrators alike. Consequently, you as a responsible or aspiring professional may contribute to unification of the profession and attainment of personal and the profession's goals. In so doing, it seems appropriate to heed the words of Ursula K. LeGuin: "It is good to have an end to journey towards; but it is the journey that matters, in the end" (1969, p. 220).

■ Acknowledgments

This volume owes its existence to significant shared interest and concern for nursing on the part of the contributing authors, who had the difficult task of addressing complex subjects in nursing within the confines of minimal pages. Their patience and good will in responding to stringent deadlines are gratefully appreciated. Shirley Dooling particularly warrants special recognition. Though ill, she insisted on completing her portion of the chapter for which she was responsible. Shirley passed away February 19, 2000.

Appreciation is extended to numerous colleagues and friends who advocated completion of this fourth book and provided a strong support network. Particularly, Sister M. Ann O'Brien, PBVM; Phyllis Beck Kritek, PhD, RN, FAAN; and Richard K. Grosboll, Esq., are acknowledged in gratitude for paving the road and illuminating the path toward developing this book. I am most indebted to my sister Shirley M. Chaska Baird, EdD, RD, for her invaluable comments and supportive suggestions related to the total manuscript. In addition, I am most grateful for the support of my sister, Marjorie, and brothers, James and Willard—and their spouses: Paul, Vivian, and Jill; my nephews and nieces—Benjamin, Paula, Allan, Peggy, Judy, Angela, Edna, Susan, Jeffrey, James, and Amy and their spouses: Dave, Randy, Dirk, Bill, Scot, Steve, Susan, Kelly, and Cornel; and my great nephews and great nieces—Ryan, Kelly, Katie, Mark, Travis, Nathan, Alyssa, Christopher, Krista, Britta, Joseph, and Bea Louise. Whereas the elders have long traveled successfully on the road of life and the middle generation is well established on unique paths, it is the youngest cohorts of the family whom we expect will choose distinctive roads. I particularly thank these great-nephews and great-nieces who have provided love, support, and entertainment in ways exceptional to each of them. Without this close family network, this volume would not have been possible.

Finally, I would be remiss if I did not acknowledge my special feline family Pepper-

mint Pete and Peppermint Pattie. They faithfully wagged their furry tails in my face *early* each morning to "get to work" and diligently guarded me at the computer on my desk, lest I take too many "breaks." While lying on top of a stack of papers, they occasionally voiced their approval or disapproval of my work. Unfortunately, though they tried to assist in typing on occasion, their prancing across the keys caused too many errors. But without them, this book could never have been completed!

I am most grateful to Julianne Tolson, Internet Applications Specialist, San Francisco State University, who tutored me in the computer machinations that sometimes are overwhelming. Her expert technical support prevented innumerable crises.

I extend special appreciation to Dan Ruth, Acquisition Editor, Sage Publications, Inc., for initially encouraging me to edit this volume and to Rolf Janke, Editorial Director, and Sanford Robinson, Senior Production Editor, for their sustained support and encouragement. I thank Leticia Gutierrez, Contracts Coordinator, for her development and management of contracts for all participants in this volume. I am particularly grateful to Michele Lingre, Books Marketing Manager, for her interest, advice, and development of marketing materials, and to Heidi Van Middlesworth, Editorial Assistant, for her counsel in the production of this volume. My association with all at Sage Publications, Inc., is valued highly.

Norma L. Chaska

■ References

Frost, Robert. (1916/1993). The road not taken. In Robert Frost, *The road not taken and other poems* (p. 1). New York: Dover Publications, Inc. Originally published by Henry Holt and Company (1916).

Le Guin, U. K. (1969). *The left hand of darkness.* New York: Ace Books.

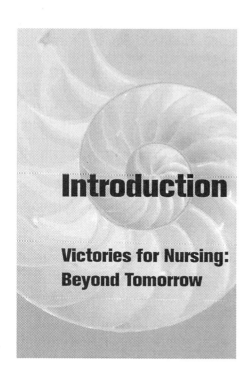

Introduction

Victories for Nursing:
Beyond Tomorrow

The Nursing Profession: Tomorrow and Beyond! Much is promised in that title. And much is delivered in these pages.

In reviewing the manuscript, I was impressed by the credentials and diverse expertise of the authors, awed by their knowledge and insight, caught up in the sweeping scope of topics, and impelled by the currents of the future—and was reminded of one of the most powerful moments of my career.

In the summer of 1995, as President of the International Council of Nurses, I was privileged to address an audience of Greek dignitaries and nurses from all over the world at sunset in an ancient outdoor theater at the foot of the Acropolis in Athens. Against such a backdrop, on a stage where legendary Greek philosophers had spoken, it was for me a moment of great challenge. I stretched my vision to its limits, raised my arms in V configuration, and exhorted those sitting on the

grassy, stone steps to anticipate and celebrate *seven ultimate victories for nursing:*

■ I. Education: The Foundation of All Nursing

Victory will be declared and celebrated the day that every nation has accepted that, as a minimum standard, nurses will be prepared comparably to other professions.

■ II. Practice: The Purpose of the Profession

Victory will be declared and celebrated the day that all countries have established regulatory and health care systems enabling nurses to practice autonomously to the full extent of their substantial and expanding capabilities and to be properly accountable for that practice.

■ *III. Research: The Source of Knowledge for Nursing Practice*

Victory will be declared and celebrated the day that nurses everywhere contribute to, access, and conscientiously utilize growing libraries of nursing research findings.

■ *IV. Management: An Essential for Influence and Accountability*

Victory will be declared and celebrated the day that, in all health care settings, well-qualified and equipped nurse executives are responsible and accountable for all nursing care and for all nursing personnel and that nurses are optimally positioned within the highest echelons of health care systems.

■ *V. Socioeconomic Welfare: An Incentive and Reward, an Entitlement for Respected Professionals*

Victory will be declared and celebrated the day that nurses receive the same salaries and benefits as other professionals with equivalent preparation, value, and responsibilities.

■ *VI. Ethics: The Conscience of Nursing*

Victory will be declared and celebrated when all nurses are skilled in identifying and analyzing ethical issues, when all nurses speak out on behalf of patients who are unable to be advocates for themselves, and when nurses are recognized in all circles where ethical problems and issues are addressed.

■ *VII. Policy: The Might of Nursing*

Victory will be declared and celebrated the day that a nurse, backed by a unified and respected profession, first occupies the position of Director-General of the World Health Organization.

I concluded that evening in Athens on a high note by asserting that these victories should be anticipated by the profession, victories to be achieved through the minute by minute, day by day personal victories of nurses everywhere.

Why did I choose to speak of victories for a profession absorbed in its own development? Because I have been strongly influenced by the views of my husband, a clergyman, that prayers should be affirmative, not beseeching God to do something, but rather thanking God that it shall be done. We must have a vision and then move confidently and inexorably toward its achievement.

This volume reminds me of that moment in three respects. First, there is acknowledgment herein of the many sectors in which nursing must strive and succeed—socialization, education, theory, research, practice, administration, ethics, economics, regulation, workplace advocacy, organizational development, and health care policy. These sectors are linked, and therefore each is critical; to fail in some is to weaken others.

Second, the themes of *Tomorrow and Beyond* and choosing the right paths to victory resonated that evening and pervade the rich discourse nourished within these covers. Writings such as these, widely disseminated and utilized, help us to see the challenges, to view the choices, and to select the paths—the means toward the desired future. These chapters, these leaders point the way. They do so principally by stimulating forward thinking and posing provocative questions for discussion.

Third, that occasion in the ancient Greek theater comes to mind because it focused on anticipated victories, the goals. To select the paths, we must know the destination. We may dispute the particular victories posed that evening. We must not dispute, however, the need for each of us to have such a vision. Early in the reading of this book—to reap its benefits to the fullest—you must begin to articulate your own ultimate goals for the profession.

The final chapter, Paths to Make a Difference, should inspire you to hope that nursing will achieve the victories so reachable by the paths chosen and mapped by the authors. Each of you—administrator, practitioner, faculty member, graduate student, or undergraduate student alike will help make it all possible through individual acts and personal victories.

Margretta Madden Styles, EdD, RN, FAAN

Professor Emerita and Former Dean
School of Nursing, University of California
San Francisco, CA

Past President, American Nurses Association,
International Council of Nurses, and
American Nurses Credentialing Center

Currently, Consultant, ANCC

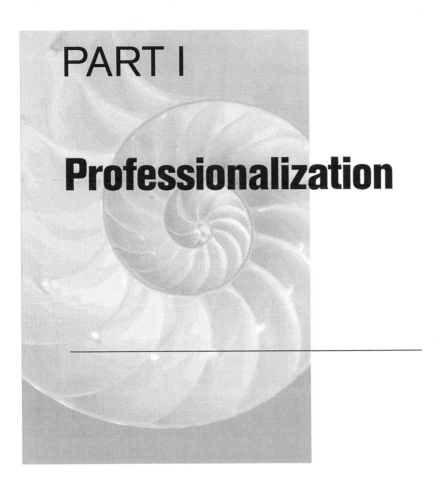

PART I

Professionalization

"... And be one traveler, long I stood ..."

One line in particular from Robert Frost's poem "The Road Not Taken" offers two clear goals for the profession: unification and endurance. To be "one traveler," a profession needs to be one and the professional person must be "whole." Further, the "traveler" is obliged to show those distinctive qualities throughout the life of the profession and length of the travelers' practice. In this manner the profession will advance and the practitioner will thrive.

The roads to professionalism are diverse. The first part of this volume manifests the foundation for the profession of nursing and its practitioners. Attributes characterizing the profession and requisites for practitioners are explored, and dominant concerns are addressed. While reading, reflect on the altruistic values and identity of the profession that may be captured for unification of the profession. Consider strategies for the 21st century positioning of nursing as a profession.

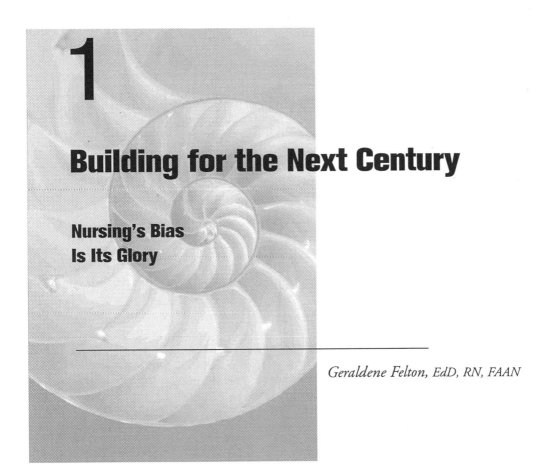

1

Building for the Next Century

Nursing's Bias Is Its Glory

Geraldene Felton, EdD, RN, FAAN

A *Wall Street Journal* (Anderson, 1998) editorial bemoaned the current crisis in nursing—fewer trainees entering the profession, poor pay, low morale, patient neglect, and fragmentary care. Anderson argued that we are witnessing a crisis in professionalism—brought on by the movement away from hospital apprenticeship training in its "climate of seriousness, calm, modesty, purpose, and emphasis on purpose—to university education with the emphasis on theory, expertise, managerialism, and loyalty to knowledge replacing duty to vocation" (p. A22). The conclusion to be drawn is that in this process true professionalism of nursing has been seriously damaged (as it has been in law, medicine, teaching, and other professions). Anderson maintains that what has been lost are the virtues of purpose, quiet formality, and a community of people with likeminded character espoused by Florence Nightingale. The *Wall Street Journal* editorial ends with the sentence: "The late 20th century has tried to have professions without virtue, and it has not worked" (p. A22).

Traditional characteristics are associated with any discipline called a profession. There is

The author owes a debt of gratitude to Mrs. Linda Whitaker, RN, for her interest and enthusiasm, her perceptions of the obvious, and her constructive criticism. All helped clarify nursing "commonness."

general agreement that a profession (Begun & Lippincott, 1993)

- provides society with an essential service that directly benefits the recipients of that service;

- provides an identifiable service that requires mastery of a body of knowledge and judgment so special and mysterious that the layman cannot practice it safely;

- has a body of specialized knowledge and a defined scope of practice;

- has a trust relationship with society that includes recognition, status, and privilege in exchange for the provision of defined services and unrestricted access to services;

- has a particular culture (commitment and investment, informal/formal networks, language, symbols, norms, beliefs, and a shared consciousness) and is part of a community that shares common goals, or expects disagreement of flourish in civility, and treatment of each other with respect;

- requires members to receive an intense, systematic, and lengthy education within a system of higher education, as well as familiarity with society's institutions, particularly its systems of laws, its historical roots, and its values, ideals, roles, and privileges;

- has a system of organization and regulation by a professional society that controls entry into the discipline and maintains standards of practice; and

- has community sanctions in the form of a license that serves as a social contract with society

■ *Background*

Nursing obviously meets the definition of *profession*. The question is whether nursing, as a profession, is without virtue! After all, if people were asked, there would be little disagreement that nurses (and other health care providers, as well) are biased in favor of quality assurance and discipline—specific successful performance.

In defining the nursing identity, we say that, among the important characteristics that graduates have acquired, are

- technical and interpersonal competencies that are important to performance after graduation and that are likely to endure;

- high-level communication and computation skills and technological literacy that enable the graduate to gain and apply new knowledge and skills as needed;

- ability to arrive at informed clinical judgments—that is, to define problems, gather and evaluate information related to those problems, and develop solutions to manage multiple problems effectively;

- ability to function in a diverse community, including knowledge of different cultural and economic contexts; and

- a range of attitudes and dispositions including self-awareness, empathy, and flexibility and adaptability.

Moreover, the best nurses demonstrate all these competencies in addressing specific problems in complex, real-world settings and conditions in which the development of workable solutions are required.

By most accounts, the improvement of health and health care lies in improving the education of health professionals. That includes sharpening clinical decision-making and clinical skills, enforcement of and adherence to accepted principles of scientific research and statistical analysis, knowledge of cost and resource management, interrelationships among processes of care delivery—as well as ability to work in teams and to learn to use ideas and methods of continuous improvement to influence human health care quality and value as part of lifelong professional development and practice. To this end, any health occupation that aspires to full professional recognition must understand certain essentials. These include legal and organizational processes that clearly demarcate a profession from another type of vocational grouping and development of an identity and a title around particular knowledge, skills, and competencies for a domain of practice. Each health profession has a cluster of practices and relationships arising from its functions at a given time and place. Each has work that is defensible, a scientific base, and a unique and internally coherent clinical component that permits rational choice by informed consumers (Felton, 1998).

These attributes give each discipline a reasonable claim for distinction and access to unprecedented linkages within and outside the profession. Linkages instill the spirit of shared experience by focusing on the well-being of people. And, as is appropriate, education paves the way for new patterns in professional life and institutional practices that inevitably evolve as information technology frees practitioners from the constraints of time, distance, and bricks and mortar.

Further, if a profession is to be preserved from becoming just an association of health care workers, work must begin and end on the fundamental values that define the professional. Education (specifically modeling by nurse educators and nurse executives), perhaps more than any other institution affecting the profession, is in a position to form these values initially and reinforce them throughout a person's professional life because characteristic ways of professional thinking, acting, and feeling are first formed in professional education. However, to be able to struggle with the question of values, professionals must develop their own clarity about values. Without such clarity graduates are not likely to emerge with any predictable sense of direction or of obligations that guide professional life, responsibility, change, and engagement in principled debate. Finally, there is a curious illogic in not believing there are economies of scale that enhance the hallmarks of a profession: dignity, decency, understanding, sensitivity, compassion, clarity of vision, and concern about values.

■ American Health Care

American health care is in the throes of two great and wrenching transitions. The first—a shift to health maintenance organizations (HMOs) and for-profit managed care corporations—is well known. But to most people the second may come as a total surprise. It is the systematic attempt to make physicians, nurses, hospitals, and other health care organizations practice consistently on the basis of the best scientific evidence—that is to set up systems to measure the quality of what they do, analyze outcomes to determine what really works, and then share that information with patients and the public. It is a process without a convenient label, but it can be summed up in the phrase "doing the right thing and doing the right thing right."

Science is the organized systematic enterprise that gathers knowledge about the world and condenses that knowledge into testable laws and principles. Diagnostic features of science that distinguish it from pseudoscience are, first, repeatability—the same phenomenon is sought again, preferably by independent investigation, and the interpretation given to it is confirmed or discarded by means of novel analysis and experimentation. The second diagnostic feature of science is economy—scientists attempt to abstract the information obtained into a form that is both simplest and aesthetically most pleasing (called *elegance*) while yielding the largest amount of information with the least amount of effort. The third diagnostic feature of science is mensuration—if something can be properly measured using universally accepted methods, generalizations about it are unambiguous. The fourth diagnostic feature of science is heuristics—the best science stimulates further discovery, often in unpredictable new directions, and the new knowledge provides an additional test of the original principles that led to its discovery. The fifth and final characteristic of science is consilience—the explanations of different phenomena most likely to survive are those that can be connected and proven to be consistent with one another.

As the work comes together, the scientist also thinks about the audience to whom the science will be reported, most often planning to publish the results in a reputable, peer-reviewed journal. One of the strictures of the scientific ethos is that a discovery does not exist until it is properly reviewed and in print.

Moreover, because scientific and technological advances evolve at a different pace (usually more quickly) than social, moral, and legal consensus, professionals must foster public discourse on ethical, moral, and legal dilemmas in health care, the service delivery system, difficult choices in resource allocation, and the limits of medical care. Too seldom are these issues discussed in nursing circles. Nonetheless, the implications of choices associated with such dilemmas need professional discussion, broad public discussion, and some attempt at consensus.

Embittered Workers

During the past few years, as employers have become more aggressive in their attempts to redefine relationships, labor confrontations and disputes have exploded among higher paid, highly skilled occupational groups—basketball superstars; FedEx pilots; ABC off-camera employees; registered nurses; salaried staff physicians, residents, interns; postresidency attending physicians in municipal hospitals; and private physician practitioners. At a time when many believe that unions are for blue collar workers only, not professionals, how does a group of white collar, college-educated professionals become something many of them thought they would never be—card-carrying, button-wearing, solidarity song-singing members of organized labor? Obviously, some union stereotypes may no longer apply.

For nurses, the story will sound familiar. Restructuring and downsizing by many employers were modeled on production-line actions that were insulting and potentially dangerous. Long-time staffers found themselves having to reapply for their jobs and suffering pay cuts or transfers to less amenable positions. The pace at work went from busy to harried. Some nurses found themselves inadequately trained to perform some of their new assignments. The amount of time that nurses had with patients and their families was shrinking. And they felt powerless to do anything about it. Because today's workers and professionals have invested so much of themselves in their jobs, an uncertain work environment is deeply unsettling. Moreover, there used to be an implicit agreement—a social contract—that workers who did a good job would be employed as long as a company was doing well. That this contract no longer exists may be one of the few things on which both business and labor leaders today can agree. Many are embittered to a surprising degree and the very real losses in productivity caused by their feelings of regret, envy, frustration, betrayal, isolation, and lack of respect for direct care delivery, constitute continuing unresolved problems in the workplace.

Common Observations About Collective Bargaining Among Professionals

It is the nature of being professional to want productive discourse, mutual respect, and engagement in creative thinking. When management crosses a line, nurses and physicians throughout the country have been willing to walk the line. They have raised their voices on issues that cut straight to the heart of professionalism, such as the ability to practice safe and quality patient care, engage in collaborative problem solving, and to receive sustenance and guidance from management.

The decision to strike is never made lightly, especially in an unfavorable health care climate, discontent over managed care, and the perception of mean spiritedness. Nurses and other professionals agonize over the impact on their patients, families, and careers. Issues that are verbalized relate to (a) staffing; (b) respect; (c) input into decision-making; (d) patient and provider safety; (e) equipment; (f) cost containment; (g) refusal of physicians to accept lower reimbursement rates ordered by a managed-care organization; (h) dismissal of physicians involved in a union drive (or insubordination or both); (i) pressure for making HMOs liable if they overrule the physician and patients are hurt as a result; (j) wages, benefits, hours, and working conditions; (k) stepped-up restrictions imposed by hospitals and managed-care organizations; (l) increased competition that has prompted many hospitals to substitute unlicensed caregivers for registered nurses (RNs) at a time when patients generally are more acutely ill and in greater need of skilled care; (m) such hazards as adverse occurrences, medication errors, and cuts in service; and (n) movement toward a tiered health care system.

Physicians' Independent Practitioner Associations (IPAs)

To skirt the antitrust barrier, many physicians are forming physicians' Independent Practitioner Associations (IPAs), which essentially are large group practices that allow physicians to bargain with HMOs. These groups are often likened to unions, allowing physicians to act as collective units to negotiate contracts with health insurance companies and giving them more leverage at the bargaining table. But, unlike doctors' unions, these associations do not limit doctors to membership in only one association, and doctors who disagree with the terms of a contract signed by an association can disregard the agreement and make their own deals.

According to Feldstein (1996); Isaacs, Sandy, and Schroeder (1997); and Bauer (1998), administrators of national umbrella groups for such associations estimate that there are more than 3,000 IPAs throughout the country. They maintain that they want to give physicians back the ability to ensure delivery of the kind of care patients need. They remind HMOs that they are insurance companies, not providers, and in some cases, they have won significant concessions (e.g., restored power to make referrals without company approval). The 9,000-member Committee of Interns and Residents, the nation's oldest doctors' union, which was founded in 1957 in New York City, merged with the 1.3-million-member Service Employees International Union in 1997. And the Union of American Physicians and Dentists, a 26-year-old, 5,000-member organization based in Oakland, California, joined in 1997 with the 1.3-million-member American Federation of State, County and Municipal Employees (AFSCME). The Office and Professional Employees International Union now comprises 10,000 U.S. podiatrists and 2,000 medical doctors from the University Physicians Group of Long Island. And the AMA wants a piece of the action. It is warning its 700,000 doctor members not to sign up with other groups, believing it to be preferable for physicians to form independent bargaining units not affiliated with traditional trade unions and therefore less likely to have to engage in a strike or any other tactic that interferes with patient care. Many doctors share the AMA's fears about strikes by physicians. Such strikes are rare, but they have occurred—for the most part in New York City in 1981, 1990, 1991, and 1997.

The number of physicians in unions is expected to grow by 15% or more each year. The Henry J. Kaiser Family Foundation (1997) estimates that 35,000 doctors, or 5% of the nation's physicians, belong to unions—up from about 25,000 in 1996. As with IPAs, an important incentive for physicians in private practice to join unions is to give themselves more power when they negotiate with HMOs. What all this ferment shows is that, when physicians, nurses, and other professionals dig beneath the surface of a complicated topic, they often learn that their ideological preconceptions are unrealistic.

■ Some Solutions

Past and Present

Nurses are situated in the present—between the past and a future they have yet to make. A fundamental challenge is providing everyone in the United States with access to high-quality, affordable health care. Compounding everything else are key issues that need nursing input and broad public debate. Such dialogue is particularly needed on the limits on societal resources for the provision of health care services and the need to allocate among competing priorities. Feldstein (1996) and Cunningham and Kemper (1998) believe that these issues of social injustice are not well understood. They maintain that there is both income inequality and loss of the safety net.

Income Inequality

Substantial evidence exists that the nature of technology in an information-intensive era is stacked in favor of workers with college-level verbal and math skills. That leaves at least half the workforce behind. In the United States, the richest country in history, a fifth of its children live in poverty. That this has taken place when the national unemployment rate has fallen to less than 4% raises the question: What will happen when the next recession strikes?

Facts indicate that nearly 20% of U.S. households possess no net wealth (the value of their liabilities, such as mortgage debt, offsets the value of assets), nor negative net wealth (their liabilities exceed their assets). The bottom 40% of households control a meager 0.2% of total wealth. By contrast, the wealthiest 1% of households control nearly 40% of the total wealth. This income disparity leads directly to inequality in health services and health care.

Loss of the Safety Net

Millions of adults have dropped out of the labor force because they cannot afford to replace their employee government-paid health insurance plan with a private policy. Nor can they afford day care for their young children. The percentage of the population without health insurance has risen to about 16% and is nudging higher. An ominous trend is that workers are increasingly turning down offers by employers for insurance because employees cannot afford to pay the premiums. The economy has turned quickly and viciously against unskilled workers, leaving many families adrift. Investing in training can help offset rising inequality.

America's largest generation, the baby boomers, were children of an America that had only recently created social insurance programs. Bringing so many children into the world was an act of faith by families who believed that citizens would honor their obligations to each other, across lines of class and generation. With increasing life expectancies and declining birthrates, almost one in four people in the developed world will be 65 or older by 2030. And, in the United States, the outlays for just five programs—Social Security, Medicare, Medicaid, and federal civilian and military pensions—are projected to exceed total federal revenues by 2030 (Pearson, 1998; Safriet, 1998).

HMO Treatment

Herzlinger (1997), analyzing data from the American Association of Health Plans, concluded that managed care plans are entrenched in the economy, enrolling 6% of the population. But activists maintain that managed care has lost its luster as an industry and as the answer to the nation's health care needs. Choose your side. Needless to say, managed care has so far served as a different way to pay for medical care, not a better way to provide it. Its savings to large employers have been real, contributing significantly to the current economic boom, but savings are likely to prove temporary with coverage becoming more difficult to provide or coverage even being dropped. Nor can HMOs track the quality of care provided. Meanwhile, lawmakers face demands for consumer protection from those impatient with the restrictions of managed care. Despite the passage of several laws intended to expand coverage incrementally, the number of Americans without insurance has risen steadily each year since 1987 (an average of 1 million a year) and now exceeds 41 million, or roughly one sixth the population (KPMG Peat Marwick, 1997). In 1997 Congress created a Children's Health Insurance Program to finance health care for low-income children (Title 21, Section 4901, Part of the Balanced Budget Act of 1997, P.L. 105-33). Congress had cleared for the president's signature the Health Insurance Portability and Accountability Act of 1996, known in the press as the Kassebaum–Kennedy bill, a law to make insurance more readily available to millions of people who change their jobs or lose them (P.L. 104-191). But several problems have arisen (Baker & Wheeler, 1998; Feldstein, 1996; Isaacs & Knickman, 1997).

- Federal and state officials say that insurance companies have found ways to skirt the Kassebaum–Kennedy law by shunning people with medical problems or by charging them high premiums. The law does not limit what insurers can charge.

- Sweeping changes in federal welfare policy may inadvertently increase the number of uninsured children, offsetting some of the expected gains in coverage from the new Children's Health Insurance Program.

- The federal government has struggled to carry out its duties under these new laws. Federal officials had assumed that states would quickly adopt the standards established by Kassebaum–Kennedy, but that has not happened. Moreover, while a Senate committee has drafted a patients' health care bill of rights, the measure does not have the components favored in the nursing community and by many Democrats.

- Enrolling participants in HMOs has failed to deliver expected savings. Moreover, the practice of managed care—with doctors, clinics, and hospitals working together with HMOs to control patient care—is breaking down in rural areas. For many of the poor, access to care has become more difficult. For many others, eligibility has become harder to establish and to hold.

Nursing Self-Awareness and Self-Regulation

Does nursing still have the vitality and drive to help overcome the many divisions among the various disciplinary interests in health care? Can a new forward-looking message be found? How does nursing define reality and the realization that its practice is at risk of being delegated to less than professional status (Lindeke & Block, 1998)?

Sometimes this kind of thinking turns out to be something more, some glimpse of life that expands like those Japanese paper balls that, upon being dropped in water, bloom like a flower and the flower is so marvelous that you cannot believe that all you saw was a paper ball and a glass of water. With skillful handling, the flower story turns out to be distinctly "something more"—getting to know and reveal nursing by multiple explorations of subjects: flowers, nursing, history, ecology, the fascination of an obsession, or figuring out how people find order and contentment and a sense of purpose in the universe by fixing their sights on one thing or one belief or one desire. In point of fact, vision and philosophy are not nursing's most important challenges. Brute persistence in *business* and *strategy* is; *productivity* is; our definition of *culture* is.

Unfortunately, in a time of great upheaval in health care and education, anxiety soars as we wonder about the security of our positions and ability to practice or to manage as we have done in the past. We feel immature, and the tendency to blame others—administrators, managed care, professional organizations, and colleagues—is at an all-time high. Psychiatrists who consult with individuals, couples, and families report on the apparently innate tendency of each of us to blame others for our situation. Husbands and wives point a finger at each other, citing need for the spouse to change. At work, we blame a colleague or supervisor for our misery and discomfort. We are blind to the fact that we cannot change others—we can only change ourselves. And yet as we defend (and often with good reason) why the other person needs to change (and likewise our partner or colleague), we perpetuate a guaranteed status quo—that nothing will change. Only by taking responsibility for our part of the problem, can we contribute to lessening the chaos in relationships and allow change to occur.

An individual's ability to begin seeing his or her contribution to the problem in a marriage or at work that allows the person to remain in the relationship. Otherwise, the person takes on the role of victim and can do nothing about changing his or her behavior or the behavior of others. Others will respond to a person's change in behavior and recognize a difference, thus potentially effecting change in the relationship, work system, or institution. In the end, however, maturity is about taking responsibility for oneself, articulating a clear vision of beliefs, and acting on well-thought-out principles. The words "we can only change ourselves and not others" continue to reverberate and to challenge us.

What this also means is that we must look carefully at what other people are doing and try to understand their behavior in context before we judge it. It means that other people may not share our desires or our perceptions. It also means that we have to recognize the arbitrary nature of our own choices and be willing to reexamine them by learning about the choices that other people have made. Solving problems depends on putting them in categories, and the categories we use are cultural, not universal.

Understanding culture will help build cross-disciplinary teams that are accountable for the quality, appropriateness, and outcomes of care delivery. It enhances the capacity of an organization to perform by embracing the concept that all types of health professionals should be expected and permitted to perform every useful service for which they are appropriately trained and credentialed. Restricting any health professional from doing what his or her training and documented skills safely allow violates the central tenet of professionalism—the subordination of self-interest in the service of the patient and the community.

In reality, it is very hard to hold individual areas of responsibility and the organization together in these times of turmoil, change, and chaos. We are often left with the feeling that things are falling apart and flying out of control. We feel the lack of the "glue" that transforms problems of low morale, and impotence, and fear, into positive attributes of commitment, caring, and dedication to the mission of the organization. All the while, leaders ache for all to have a true sense of connection to people in the organization and to the organization's goals.

The last point addresses two other elements of culture as a sense of community and the outcome of how people relate to one another. Some call these elements sociability and solidarity. Sociability is a measure of friendliness; solidarity is a measure of the community's ability to pursue shared objectives quickly and efficiently.

Sociability requires compatible people, frequent casual gatherings, reduced formality, limited hierarchical differences, consistent demonstrations of caring, keeping people aware of the competition, creating a sense of urgency, stimulating the will to win with incentive systems, and encouraging commitment to shared corporate goals. Building solidarity and sociability means (a) leveraging each worker's critical knowledge, intellectual skills, and accumulated experience in the organization; (b) willingness to labor long and intensively because the group is involved in matters of great significance; (c) high aspirations and optimism about being a part of a lively, high-achieving, dedicated group; (d) spontaneity, intellectual intensity, valuing truth and seeking it, open exchange, and willingness to share information; and (e) high affiliation with the organization and its mission.

Creating What Could Be: Differentiated Practice

I do not agree that correct chatter is preferable to the yawning abyss of avoidance and denial that passes for differences in nursing educational programs in the United States today. With nursing and public interests in mind, we must have the courage to grapple with substantial issues of differentiation—and with the painful truth of differentiated practice (Boston, 1990).

The concept of differentiated nursing practice describes a system of sorting roles, functions, and work of registered nurses according to education, clinical experience, and defined competence and decision-making required by different client needs and settings in which nursing is practiced. This concept calls for matching skills and core competencies needed in nursing practice, the best set of educational experiences and care that results in these skills and core competencies, and distinctive accreditation policies. Accreditation policies must demand active participation in developing, measuring, and promoting educational outcomes for different practice domains and core competencies at each level along a continuum of nursing practice. Nursing has tired itself out with an endless loop of debate on entry into practice. It has confused the consumer and angered and frustrated the nurse. This confusion and anger have been exploited by administrators at all levels. And yet the marketplace wants nurses willing to give direct care. That is what Anderson (1998) is really wailing about—we have lost something along the way.

Problems that persist in health care demand nursing solutions, and nursing can offer coherence amid the commotion and expertise in managing and solving complex care problems (Bauer, 1998). Nursing can provide such solutions when nursing identity is formed by a combination of skills, knowledge, attitudes, competencies, and clinical decision-making abilities. However, the emerging health care market will value highly the services provided by nurses and others only as they make a contribution to outcomes. These outcomes include: (a) controlling or lowering costs; (b) enhancing consumer satisfaction; (c) improving quality of outcomes in promotion of health for all age groups as well as competency in personal care; (d) prevention of health problems that endanger productivity; (e) ability to cope and life satisfaction; (f) reduction of the impact of health problems on individuals and families; and (g) assistance in the diagnosis and treatment of illness.

The next key is *opportunism,* which may seem a bit peculiar because the word generally has a pejorative connotation. In the context of career, however, it is meant to suggest seizing and even making opportunities for growth and development. Becoming and remaining marketable means that a person must be constantly learning, as the need to broaden and deepen knowledge and skills is never-ending, which includes gaining an education and developing a positive attitude toward lifelong learning.

Another key to success is one with which everyone is familiar but which too often is underrated: that of interpersonal competence. It is astounding how much this single factor figures in the careers of individuals at all levels. Nursing in most settings is a group effort, not a solo practice, and the ability of people to work well with others is a serious and valued asset. Individuals who contribute on an interpersonal level are generally positive, constructive, and productive; and they are generous with their talents and treat their colleagues with respect (Balik, 1998; Fralic, 1998; O'Neil, 1998).

A final essential key to success is integrity— a steadfast adherence to a strict ethical code. Integrity means that the individual has internalized his or her value orientation to such an extent that is operational in daily life, and more important, forms a cohesive whole. The ethical code for nursing has long been a guiding force for the profession's principles and practices. Through painful experience we have learned that, no matter the cost, some things cannot be compromised (e.g., meeting professional obligations).

Anderson (1998) has it wrong. All helping professions are not "without virtue." The concept of what is a professional has been and is working in nursing, even as we accept the subtext that nursing's weaknesses can pose as big a challenge to the discipline as its strengths. Further, even if a need is being met today, data must be made available to decision makers to show how changing demographics, increasing numbers of uninsured, escalating need for primary care, and other changing conditions will produce a greater demand for nursing services 5 years or 10 years in the future.

To discuss differentiated practice intelligently, we need to assess complex issues and show commitment to principle and skill in getting things done by diplomacy, insight, persuasiveness, a sense of timing and nursing's relevance to the mission of the systems of care that are emerging. Fagin (1999) maintains:

> Ignoring the scientific knowledge, professional judgment, and interpersonal and technical skills integral to nurses' clinical expertise can lead to dangerous outcomes for patients. The health of our health care system depends on nurses. To demean, diminish, or eliminate them puts the entire system in jeopardy. (p. E22)

■ Finding a Comfort Zone

The choice of a profession that leads to a career is a very personal decision. The most endearing and enduring quality of nursing is that it is not always glamorous, even as easing suffering and pain can be intoxicating. Moreover, in addition to money, factors such as intellectual challenge, prestige, employment opportunities, job stability, geographic location, time for leisure, and a desire to help others or to benefit society are often involved. However, what nursing has been and must continue to be is at heart an altruistic profession.

Nursing is a reality-based profession in a hyped, virtual-reality world. Choosing nursing is an act of faith and belief that unselfish attention to the welfare of others is inherent in the privilege of being a nurse. Sticking with nursing requires some old-fashioned virtues— courage, stamina, and the unshakable belief that the person is doing something important. This is not to say that financial return and security are unimportant. Yet the essential character of the profession is jeopardized if financial self-interest becomes the primary issue of concern to nurses or students contemplating a nursing career. To lose sight of just how fortunate nurses are to have a profession in which we do well for ourselves by doing well for others reflects a puzzling loss of perspective. Thus the many health reform initiatives being introduced require vigilance and attention to maintaining the special qualities of the nursing profession, rather than a narrow focus on financial returns and incentives.

The notion of what makes a life paves the way for the lessons about the complexity of what fills it. A special quality is to see a larger picture than the daily events of life. The first key to what probably makes that more important today than ever before is the development and maintenance of a "career" concept as a guide to a professional life. The career concept may be defined as a series of systematic, progressive, related states that are hierarchically arranged and through which an individual passes in order to reach an occupational goal. This definition implies a prolonged, even a lifetime, commitment to moving toward that goal.

■ Concluding Statement

One of the basic steps in taking a long view of one's professional life is to assess one's talents. The idea of talent appears to be one that we too often neglect. All of us have different aptitudes and abilities. Some of us are better than others at certain aspects of life—art, writing, singing, working with machinery, or even listening. The wonderful thing about nursing is that the profession needs people with a variety of talents. Witness the widely divergent aptitudes required in such areas as the operating room, neonatal intensive care unit, public health, hospice, legislative offices, and occupational health nursing. There really is something for almost everyone. What this means is that after a person has considered his or her talents there is need to assess and periodically reassess the market for those talents and be conversant with the language of business. Health care is changing rapidly, and keeping up with the direction of those changes and dealing with them will continue to require flexibility and adaptability. What will be constant is a career within the profession. However, unlike their predecessors, most nurses today will probably not work for one or two organizations—or even necessarily stay within one specialty. Instead, they will move more frequently, building one experience on another. This is how nurses can look to the future and pursue their mission with fierce determination that gives everything they do a singular coherence.

Professionalism is in fact compendious. Anderson (1998) calls for a renewed sense of purpose. Few jobs in today's marketplace call for purpose. Even fewer are important. So, it may be that we have the bases covered for when the pendulum swings the other way!

■ References

Anderson, D. (1998, October 29). Work without virtue, on the decline of professionalism. *Wall Street Journal,* p. A22.

Baker, L. C., & Wheeler, S. K. (1998). Managed care and technology diffusion: The case of MRI. *Health Affairs, 17* (September/October), 195–207.

Balik, B. (1998). The impact of managed care and integrated delivery systems on registered nurse education and practice. In E. O'Neil & J. Coffman (Eds.), *Strategies for the future of nursing* (pp. 41–63). San Francisco: Jossey-Bass.

Bauer, J. C. (1998). *Not what the doctor ordered* (2nd ed.). New York: McGraw-Hill.

Begun, J. W., & Lippincott, R. C. (1993). *Strategic adaptation in the health professions.* San Francisco: Jossey-Bass.

Boston, C. (1990). Differentiated practice: An introduction. In C. Boston (Ed.), *Current issues and perspectives on differentiated practice* (pp. 1–3). Chicago: American Hospital Association and American Organization of Nurse Executives.

Children's Health Insurance Program, Title 21, Section 4901 of the Balanced Budget Act of 1997, P.L. 105–33, August 5, 1997, *U.S. Statutes at Large* (Volume III, pp. 251–788). Washington, DC: U.S. Government Printing Office.

Cunningham, P. J., & Kemper, P. (1998, September 9). Ability to obtain medical care for the uninsured. *The Journal of the American Medical Association,* 921–927.

Fagin, C. M. (1999, March 16). Essay: Nurses, patients and managed care. *New York Times,* p. E22.

Feldstein, P. J. (1996). *The politics of health legislation: An economic perspective* (2nd ed.). Chicago: Health Administration Press.

Felton, G. (1998). Politicization of health profession regulation. *Advanced Practice Nursing, 4*(3), 14–23.

Fralic, M. F. (1998). How is demand for registered nurses in hospital settings changing? In E. O'Neil & J. Coffman (Eds.), *Strategies for the future of nursing* (pp. 64–86). San Francisco: Jossey-Bass.

Health Insurance Portability and Accountability Act of 1996, P.L. 104–191, August 21, 1996. *U.S. Statutes at Large* (Volume 110, pp. 1936–2104). Washington, DC: U.S. Government Printing Office.

Henry J. Kaiser Family Foundation. (1997). *Medicaid facts: Medicaid and managed care.* Washington, DC: Kaiser Commission on the Future of Medicaid.

Herzlinger, R. (1997). *Market-driven health care.* Reading, MA: Perseus.

Isaacs, S. L., & Knickman, J. R. (Eds.). (1997). *To improve health and health care: The Robert Wood Johnson Foundation anthology.* San Francisco: Jossey-Bass.

Isaacs, S. L., Sandy, L. G., & Schroeder, S. A. (1997). Improving the health care workforce: Perspectives from twenty-four years' experience. In S. L. Isaacs, L. G. Sandy, & S. A. Schroeder (Eds.), *To improve health and health care: The Robert Wood Johnson Foundation anthology* (pp. 21–52). San Francisco: Jossey-Bass.

KPMG Peat Marwick. (1997, June). *Health Benefits.* Washington, DC: Author.

Lindeke, L. L., & Block, D. E. (1998). Monitoring professional integrity in the midst of interdisciplinary collaboration. *Nursing Outlook, 46,* 213–218.

O'Neil, E. (1998). Nursing in the next century. In E. O'Neil & J. Coffman (Eds.), *Strategies for the future of nursing* (pp. 211–224). San Francisco: Jossey-Bass.

Pearson, L. J. (1998). Annual update of how each state stands on legislative issues affecting advanced nursing practice. *The Nurse Practitioner, 23*(1), 14–66.

Safriet, B. J. (1998). Still spending dollars, still searching for sense: Advanced practice nursing in an era of regulating and economic turmoil. *Advanced Practice Nursing Quarterly, 4*(3), 24–33.

■ *Editor's Questions for Discussion*

Is there a crisis regarding professionalism in nursing? How does Felton refute the *Wall Street Journal* editorial? Are the helping professions "without virtue"? What virtue is present in the profession of nursing? Provide examples to illustrate your beliefs. What values should nurses, as health professionals, develop? How might these values be nurtured in education programs? How might values be assessed prior to entry into a professional nursing program and on completion of a program? What special qualities exist in nursing as a profession?

What significant issues does the profession of nursing need to address when professionals become members of organized labor? What impact does managed care have on professionalism and the quality of care provided by nurses? How can the profession of nursing influence the various disciplinary interests in health care? What effect has managed care had on nursing practice and the profession of nursing? What type of health reform issues does nursing need to be alert for and respond to as a profession? What is nursing's definition of health culture? How responsible is the profession of nursing for the health culture today? To what extent may nursing have contributed to the chaos in health care relationships today? How can positive change in such relationships occur?

What issues in nursing education programs are being avoided or denied? How might issues be directly acknowledged and resolved? Propose and discuss educational outcomes for different practice domains and core competencies at each level of nursing practice.

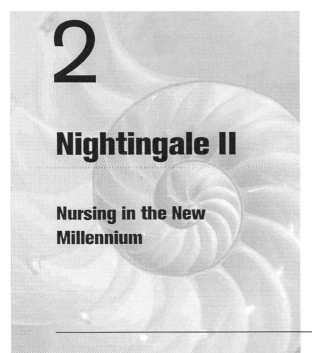

2

Nightingale II

Nursing in the New Millennium

JoEllen Koerner, PhD, RN, FAAN

Just as Vatican II redefined the Catholic Church, changes sweeping the globe are redefining the meaning of health and the role of the healing disciplines. At the turn of the 20th century, Florence Nightingale predicted that a new nursing paradigm would emerge by the year 2000 because of improvements in technology, pharmacology, and medical science. She called for nurses with a social imagination and a social conscience (Dolan, 1969, pp. 32, 42). At the turn of the 21st century, a small but growing coterie of professional practitioners is emerging with these qualities. This group also is calling for social action on behalf of the people it is privileged to serve. Nightingale II has been launched!

■ *Nursing Transformation versus Nursing Transition*

We stand on the eve of a new millennium and new world view. Nurses are scientists. We have been operating on the basis of a traditional mechanical science model for the past 300 years (Wilbur, 1996). In this model, every system (personal, family, and organization) is viewed as a well-oiled machine in which discrete parts are managed and controlled, measured and counted, and predicted and produced. Nursing tools for this scientific viewpoint reflect a blend of the problem-oriented approach to patient symptoms (the

I gratefully acknowledge my collaborator, Louise Woerner, who is an expert in business and entrepreneurship and contributed equally to the chapter.

nursing process) and care planning, emerging from a belief that "the nurse is the expert." In true behavioristic styling from the 1960s through the 1980s, nurses viewed health as bio-psycho-social balance. Each part of the person was measured by examination and testing, adjusted through medications and technology, and monitored and controlled by a plan of care created by the "expert practitioner" on behalf of the person served. If the client did not remain on the regimen of care, that person was judged to be noncompliant by the all-knowing professional.

This model worked well when information was available only to the expert and illness was caused by external factors such as coal dust and pneumococci. But suddenly we face the era foretold by Nightingale. The information age and the Internet have made health information available to all. Eighty percent of all illness is related to lifestyle. In fact, risk behavior will replace the AIDS epidemic as the biggest health hazard in the 21st century (Botelho, 1999). Once individuals have acquired a chronic disorder such as diabetes or cancer, they are a careerist. They live with the disease for the rest of their lives. Suddenly, the incentive to manage risk behaviors and minimize disability motivate people to become more actively involved in their own health activities. Changes in the locus of control, power, and decision-making are altering the entire health care landscape.

Science is changing, and in those changes lie the blueprints for Nightingale II. We now see systems (personal, family, organizational community, and ecosystems) as *living systems* (Capra, 1996). Instead of defining elements of the universe as light or matter, we now acknowledge that everything starts as pure energy. How the energy comes together depends on the environment or context and the relationships within it. Thus things are no longer seen as a particle or a wave ("either-or" dualistic thinking) but as matter that changes with its environment ("this and that" thinking). A molecule of water at the North Pole is a particle; at the Equator, it becomes a wave.

Reflecting the quantum view, nurse theorist Martha Rogers (1994) observed that "health is person–environment balance" (p. 4). Today's practitioner knows that the person cannot be treated in isolation but must be considered in the context of family and living circumstances. Whole-person strategies, including capacity enhancement for the entire family, are essential for sustained health and well-being.

Today, nurses practice in both scientific paradigms, as are patients who seek various types of care. Richness in the nursing profession is the diversity within the practice *if it is matched with the desires and needs of the patient, as expressed by the patient.* Though all people are equal, they do not all need equal care. "One-size-fits-all" nursing is the most blatant form of discrimination. Nightingale observed that "diseases are not individuals arranged in classes, like cats and dogs, but conditions growing out of one another" (Dolan, 1969, p. 32). A social conscience seeks to keep the person and need central. A social imagination can cocreate with the person what is needed, transcending a total reliance on diagnosis and predetermined pathways and protocols. Those tools should serve as a foundation from which to improvise an appropriate plan of care in the moment. Finally, social action calls for nursing to facilitate the person, family, community, and ecosystem to enhance their capacity for health and wholeness in a rapidly changing world.

■ Redefining Health

Alvin Toffler in *The Third Wave* (1980) predicted the emergence of a health care "prosumer," the merging of the producers of goods and services with the consumers of goods and services. Toffler noted that the marketization of our economy, which he refers to as the Second

Wave, puts distance between producer and consumer. This distance is changed again with the development of new products and services that can be used by the individual.

Small changes can be indicative of what lies ahead, even though their significance may not be noted at the moment. The first home pregnancy test kit, popularized in the 1970s in Europe, was an early indicator of consumer-driven health (Toffler, 1980). In less than 10 years, millions of women were self-testing for pregnancy, eliminating the need for physicians and laboratories. The deprofessionalization of health continues as technology enables nonprofessionals to perform tasks that previously required a professional. The Internet and the media in general now disseminate health science and information to nonprofessional audiences. Entrepreneurs are moving innovation into the hands of the individual without going through governmental and political systems, which previously slowed progress (Toffler, 1995). Herein lies the fertile soil for Nightingale II.

Transitions in Nursing Practice

Nursing practice has a proud tradition of whole-person strategies and has incorporated the community into this practice. The community is where nurses engage imaginatively. They can be spokespeople for the health care consumer, acting as the social conscience for the health care system. This role, however, must be approached in a nonjudgmental and empowering way, explaining and facilitating a new paradigm and new science, not lamenting the change from old processes of care delivery.

The image of a New York City Visiting Nurse climbing over rooftops to see people in the community certainly evokes the vision of a nurse with a social conscience and a social imagination in the early part of the 20th century. Why then is what Nightingale called for a transformation and not a transition? Is it not simply "back to the future"?

During the 1940s through the 1970s, nursing curricula and nursing practice focused on hospital-based care, with technology serving as a target of training. Nursing followed medicine, focusing on disease and specialty areas of care. As this transition occurred, nurses moved away from the social context of the individual and the whole person to the context of the disease process within an institutional setting. The payor also began to play a stronger role in health care, starting with the government's establishment of health insurance programs such as Medicare (and to a lesser degree Medicaid) and provisions such as Title III of the Older Americans Act of 1965, as amended. This development shifted attention to the rules of the payor, in essence establishing another customer for health care services—the payor customer—who became increasingly demanding. We could never imagine an individual health care consumer saying, "If it isn't documented, it didn't happen," but that was the quality standard established by the payor customer. The organizing principle of care became the payor and financial constraints rather than the person or society and its most pressing needs. The result of this influence was the shift in focus of care from the individual to the paper record and to "allowable" care, creating another focus overtaking patient need.

Transition Consequences

These transitions moved nursing away from imagination and conscience, possibly as Nightingale had anticipated. The result was sufficiently serious that in 1999, for the first time, pharmacists passed nurses as the most respected health care professional (American Organization of Nurse Executives [AONE], 1999). Nurses who long had held the position of preferred health care communicator were again second to pharmacists.

We now have more centralized models of health care delivery. The progression began with individually based care at the beginning of the 20th century to institutionally based care at mid century to mega-systems involving payors, institutions, and deliverers of care at the century's end. Unable to work with the individual on a whole-person basis, in the context of family and community, nurses narrowed their perspective. Unfortunately, nursing did not redefine "community" to mean the hospital community and all areas of practice and administration that affect patient care, but focused more and more tightly on the individual patient and the patient's relationship with the nurse. In a struggle for autonomy and authority, the profession entered the "this is my patient, and I am their nurse" mind-set.

The consequence of this narrowing of focus was that the nurse became more and more separate from other areas of health care delivery, with a territorial boundary set up around the nurse and the patient. As a result, nurses have not emerged as key leaders in health care, even though they are recognized as individuals with the most knowledge about patient care. In fact, nurses are not sitting at the table where health care delivery is being designed, partly because they are seen as "too strong advocates for nursing" and as individuals who cannot see the "community" (Health Care Resources [HCR], 1997, p. 6).

This mental model must be transformed. Nightingale II calls for nursing to re-member community with respect and mutual regard, even given its diversity and complexity. Getting back on track, transcending our victim mentality, and returning to our roots—armed with all the rich lessons from our recent experience—will facilitate the health agenda of our society.

■ Redefining Professional Nursing

The shift in world view toward expanding awareness of the environment, prevention, and self-determination is under way in the entire field of health care. According to the *Medical World News* (1998)

> self-care—the idea that people can and should be more medically self-reliant—is a fast rolling new bandwagon. . . Across the land, ordinary people are learning to handle stethoscopes and blood pressure cuffs, administer breast self-examinations and Pap smears, even carry out elementary surgical procedures. . . . This rush to treat one's own problems . . . reflects a substantial change in our values, in our definition of illness, and in our perception of body and self. (p. 10)

This willing movement from consumer of health to provider of self-care has incalculable ramifications.

Nurses are at the forefront of rethinking the relationships between the human family and all other forms of life and between nurses and those they are privileged to serve. Some nurses are reweaving the roles of community, public health education, families, and individuals, showing them how to share responsibilities for healthier life styles, healthier cities, economics, and societies. Expert nurses, in partnership with entrepreneurs, agencies, and consumers are restructuring the current hierarchical, bureaucratic medical–industrial complex, which is geared toward high-tech crisis interventions. These nurses are creating social health models with a more decentralized, human-scale, affordable system based on cooperation and cocreation, wellness, and overall quality of life.

On a global scale, health is a universally desired goal. In most societies, it is aligned closely with (a) goals of human development, (b) social well-being, (c) satisfaction of basic needs, (d) meaningful work, and (e) spiritual meaning and significance in life. To meet these needs at home and abroad, assumptions and beliefs for the profession must be grounded in living organic systems principles. Environmental philosopher Max Oelschlaeger (1991) observed that this complex and dynamic world view is based on different assumptions. He states that the domination of nature and women are linked. The earth is our nurturing home and should be nurtured in return. Culture–nature, human–nonhuman, and male–female are not superior–inferior pairs. Masculine concepts, values, and institutions are hurtful to the earth. Nursing comes out of the feminine paradigm and holds the balance needed for the evolving health care debate.

Balance is desperately needed as specialization and fragmentation have reached classic proportions. The debate over means, money, and institutional rivalries among providers overshadow society and its health care needs. Economics has emerged as the predominant social science, transcending public sector policymaking and private sector market interactions. Economist Hazel Henderson (1998) identified the following principles of living systems essential to new structures and models in holistic care:

1. interconnectedness at every system level;

2. redistribution and recycling of all elements and structures;

3. heterarchy, intercommunication between networks, mutual causality, and self-organization;

4. complementarity, beyond either/or dichotomous logics and zero sum games;

5. uncertainty, moving from static, mechanical models to living dynamic systems;

6. change as fundamental. (p. 37)

Nightingale as a Model

How does nursing incorporate these principles when re-membering community? An answer lies in closer examination of the patterns lived and modeled by Florence Nightingale. On the one hand, she thought of nature

as God's laws; statistical formulation of these laws were her passion—"statistics reveal the character of God" (Cook, 1913/1942, p. 480). On the other hand, her God was a spirit—"a living thought, feeling, purpose, residing in a conscious being" (Cook, 1913/1942, p. 206). She understood herself to be a mystical experience of good, as well as a statistical recorder of the results of God's laws. She was living the fullness of the paradox and dialectic of "being."

Physicist David Bohm saw her example as a form of "process science" (1990, p. xvii). In this approach, we start with a multidimensional view of the whole, rather than starting with the primary parts of the phenomenon being explored. From this viewpoint the whole is primary and the parts secondary. This undivided, multidimensional wholeness recognizes a flow of energy called the "holomovement." We come to understand that the explicate order of our lived experience unfolds from the implicate order contained in that underlying flow of energy (Bohm, 1990).

Nightingale would tell us that both views have their place in a material and a spiritual universe; in health care, we must attend to both. Thus we must take the best of mechanical science with us, expanding it to include the holistic view of a living, interacting system. If we accept this assertion, we first would have a new consciousness of the universe and our place in it. As a living, undivided, and interacting organism, we are one part—an equal part—with all other parts. This consciousness would foster cooperation among disciplines, incorporating the patient as partner and paraprofessionals and family members as equal players on the team.

Second, we would understand that any individual action is interconnected. This awareness would increase our sense of responsibility and accountability, calling all to a high ethical plane. Concern for the whole would supersede individual needs and goals. The resulting synergy through sharing and pooling of resources and activities toward common ends would create a field of abundance. Thus the nursing agenda must include consideration of the community and the macro-level environment as clients.

The Community as Client

During the AONE Consumer Health Summit in Washington, DC, in 1997, 150 consumer groups spoke with the nursing community. Consumer advocate Charles Inlander, president of Peoples Medical Society, inquired from the floor:

> Nurses, where are you? For so long, you have advocated for us at the bedside, helping us navigate the hospital and clinic. But where are you in the community? At this time I can get insurance to pay for my leg amputation, but cannot get health education that would prevent the loss of the leg. We need some of you in the halls of social policy to help translate the issues of the aggregate into a language that others can understand. (AONE, 1997)

When the community is our client, we will address some of the issues that foster disease: poverty, safety, clean water, and homelessness. This use of nursing resources is more efficient than providing care for an individual in end-stage disease from an environmental hazard. By making the planet our client, we move toward global nursing action. What we do in our country has great implications for the rest of the world. An understanding of these links will give us a global connection that will assist with activities around the agenda for Healthy People 2000.

To empower the profession, we need to transform our holistic beliefs about health, healing, and caring. By fostering and facilitating relationships, individually through our associations and in partnership with other concerned organizations, we will enter into the larger global, social, economic, and political environment to address health-related concerns.

Nursing Leadership

New leadership is needed for this work. Leadership Development in Nursing Initiative: Customer Perspective was prepared for the University of Illinois at Chicago, College of Nursing (HCR, 1997). The survey reported on the ideas of corporate leaders for increasing nursing leadership and for changing nursing education. About half the respondents thought that, for nurses to enhance their leadership in traditional or formal positions of authority, nursing curricula would have to be changed to incorporate more courses in which analytical and critical skills are taught and decision-making ability is developed. The other half believed that nurses had the needed knowledge base, but were weak in the application of that knowledge outside the clinical setting. Or, as it was further explained by one respondent, nurses must learn to think through issues from multiple perspectives, beyond patient care to patient satisfaction, patient retention, cost of care, and so forth.

■ Promotion of Wellness in Health Care

According to Sheila A. Ryan, PhD, RN, FAAN (1998), health care in the future will be a continuum of care, not an inpatient setting. It will focus on maintaining and promoting wellness, instead of treating illness; it will be accountable for the health of a defined population, instead of care for individual patients; it will have a value-added services emphasis on primary care, health promotion, and ongoing health management of chronic illness instead of community products. The new capability from a hospital systems perspective will focus on covered lives instead of a share of admissions, on care provided at the appropriate level instead of trying to fill hospital beds. The hospital will manage a network of services instead of an organization and will manage a market instead of a department and actively manage and improve quality instead of coordinating services.

Dr. Ryan believes that there will be three stages of managed care. Stage I will be *event driven cost avoidance,* with the primary objective of reducing hospitalization after illness commences and the secondary objective of slowing specialty physician use. Stage II will be *value improvement,* with the principal objective of controlling resource intensity and the secondary objective of improving consumer satisfaction. Stage III will be *health improvement,* with a primary objective of improving health status, using population-based strategies, and a secondary objective of reducing health services costs.

Dr. Ryan also comments on what she believes to be the competencies needed in the 21st century: (a) multidisciplinary collaboration; (b) community-based practice, especially health promotion and disease prevention; (c) clinical outcomes research supported by research on quality, cost, and access; and (d) informatics, with practice, research, and learning components.

The Wisconsin Network for Health Policy Research reports that 70% of illness is preventable.

> As managed care becomes more pervasive—89% of employers now offer some form—it's getting harder for companies to cut health costs further. . . . Now the only way to find additional savings is to make your employees more healthy. . . . According to the health care consulting firm Hewitt Associates, 39% of all employers surveyed used a financial incentive or penalty to encourage healthier behavior among their workers . . . in 1997, . . . up from 14% in 1992. (Jaffe, 1998, pp. B1-2)

*Nursing Leadership in
Health Promotion*

Nola Pender (1997) has stated that many elements of nurses' professional expertise are applicable to health promotion and make nurses highly qualified to lead needed health promotion activities. They include holistic assessment, patient teaching, anticipatory guidance, family dynamics, care delivery in context, coordination of multiple services work with vulnerable groups, life span perspective, behavioral change, innovative use of limited resources, and impact of health policies on clients.

Pender also observed that health promotion and preventive care are best delivered by a collaborative team of health professionals with complementary skills that offer the consumer quality care at a reasonable cost. What is needed, according to Pender, are

- alternative pathways mapped to change behavior and maintain change,

- outcome measures to determine effects of health promotion and prevention on health trajectories,

- processes to assist clients in developing health promotion paths and track their performance, and

- use of informatics in health promotion.

If nursing is to move beyond illness care to a stronger emphasis on health, it may be time to consider clinical experiences focused on health. Working in schools, day care centers, and centers for successful aging as primary care sites before rotations in secondary and tertiary care centers would give the professional a framework of health from which to draw, as opposed to a framework of the most acute pathology.

■ Redefining the Role of the Person as Consumer

Health information has moved from the exclusively professional channels of information, such as the *New England Journal of Medicine* and the *Journal of the American*

Medical Association (*JAMA*), to the general literature in the form of articles in the newspaper or on the Internet. Because the physician and other health care professionals are no longer information gatekeepers, the public can become active in the decision-making process, thus strengthening its role as a health care "prosumer."

Role for Nursing

Supporting the health care "prosumer" is an obvious role for nursing. Fundamental skills of nursing are teaching and self-care. These skills simply need to be transformed into the context of serving as a guide and educator, to teach people how to validate information and strategies. To do so, nursing education must focus less on the task to be performed in a given situation and more on how to determine ways to approach a health concern.

Jeremy Nobel of Harvard reports that 60% of all doctors' office visits are without medical benefit. Why are those people there? For peace of mind, a role that should be filled by a nurse. Assuring individuals or showing them how to track their conditions (through processes such as interactive surveillance and longitudinal profiling) save time for physicians who want to practice in new ways and create patient empowerment through nurses who can use technology in innovative strategies.

Another factor favoring nursing leadership is the increasing skepticism on the part of the health care consumer about the motivations for certain recommendations from the physician, the insurer, or the health system. This distrust has occurred as many health providers have become business people (professional corporations) instead of service-oriented professionals. Some doctors own laboratories, and others are recipients of incentives for certain referral patterns; information about these relationships has slowly become generally known. Educated consumers are taking it upon themselves to consider their health care strategies; they no longer believe that the doctor has their best interests in mind.

Positioning of Nurses

The change to health care prosumption provides an excellent opportunity for the nurse to be the "honest broker" in the health care system for the individual. Nurses are trusted; they have not been part of various incentive programs that affect decisions about the delivery of care. As a result, nurses are well positioned to interpret the information that abounds and help the individual sort credible, science-based or evidence-based practices from other strategies. This circumstance places an added responsibility on the nurse of the 21st century. With the proliferation of professional journal and news articles, knowing how to evaluate the quality of an article has become more important than simply reading and accepting it. Thus the nurse will move away from a role as a chronicler and reporter of information to that of interpreter and evaluator.

■ Evaluating and Selecting Complementary Strategies

Survey research conducted by Dr. David Eisenberg and colleagues documents the growth in absolute usage of complementary therapies in the United States between 1990 and 1997. His research further determined that complementary medicine is now taught in the majority of U.S. schools of medicine (Eisenberg et al., 1998). My own anecdotal experience in Rochester is that—although the University of Rochester Medical School rotates residents through the Equipoise Center of America, LLC, wellness center and teaches students interventions such as acupuncture—this situation is not true of any of the nursing schools in Rochester. The possible exception is therapeutic touch, a type of energy medicine.

As we move to a more global society, there will be an increased need for a knowledge of "complementary" or "alternative" medicine. The use of these modalities is high in Asian countries. According to Eisenberg and colleagues, public opinion polls and consumers' association surveys suggest high prevalence rates throughout Europe and the United Kingdom. Almost one half of Australians use alternative therapies (Eisenberg et al., 1998, p. 1569). In 1997, the Group on Educational Affairs of the Association of American Medical Colleges (AAMC) announced formation of the Special Interest Group in Alternative and Complementary Medicine (Muehsam, 1997).

The findings in the survey research of Eisenberg and his colleagues (1998) could have been anticipated through an understanding of Alvin Toffler's *The Third Wave* in which Toffler described life in a new culture—characterized by change and diversity—the integration of nature, time, and space. He described this new culture in terms of holism, which is basic to many types of complementary medicine and certainly to integrative medicine (Toffler, 1980). Nurses need to rethink quickly their practice and retool their areas of expertise in light of these rapidly emerging, nonlinear trends. A transformation is needed.

■ Arrangement of Human Capital

Health care is a trillion-dollar industry, representing about 14% of the U.S. gross domestic product—more than is spent on durable goods, food, or housing. General Motors, Ford Motor Co., and Chrysler Corp. combined spent $6.7 billion for health care in 1996, more than they spent on all the steel that goes into their vehicles (Woerner, 1998).

The growing role of human capital in corporate wealth is causing employers to weigh into the health care equation, as is the high cost of health care to companies. Woerner (1998) observed that the new environment of global competitiveness will drive health care change. Thinking of health care as a major cost factor in the competitive marketplace requires a new perspective. Because health care is in the middle of this new competitiveness, experiencing change internally and being driven externally by more change at the same time is both awkward and extremely challenging. Other industries have come through such dramatic shifts successfully (e.g., banking and the airlines), and health care will also.

Change is resulting in more cost-effective, higher-quality health care. Examples include births, home care, and technology. Nurses are superbly qualified to succeed in this environment. Although they are well-positioned to recommend strategies to improve the delivery of health care, nurses must learn to use their skills in new ways. The competencies necessary for success, according to Ryan (1998), are (a) analytical ability and critical thinking skills applied outside the clinical setting, (b) increased congruity between the leadership styles of health care organizations and the predominant leadership styles of the nurses within them, and (c) more inclusive and partnering style across disciplines. Nurses should evaluate their own strengths in these areas and embark on strategies to refresh themselves, where required.

■ The Future

The National Institutes of Health reports that four health risk behaviors account for a million deaths annually—nearly one half all deaths in the United States—tobacco use, alcohol use, physical inactivity, and poor diet. Nursing of the future needs to focus on risk behaviors with the same vigor and vigilance we focus on disease management. We need to move beyond focusing exclusively on the person and disease by encompassing the whole person, family, and environment as an integrated entity. We need to re-member community with the same enlarged view: Within the hospital, the community is the cadre of providers, departments, and support services; within the larger community, it is all people in their varied states of health. Wherever there are people, nursing has an opportunity to support health and well-being in partnership with others, including social service agencies, protection agencies, and educational and recreational services. Through cooperation and cocreation, a synergy will be formed that can transform the total well-being of society. Alone, nursing cannot do it. Without nursing, it cannot be done.

■ Concluding Statement

These are our viewpoints, not yours. We invite you to assess your own beliefs about health, your mental models of nursing, patients and families, professionals and layworkers, payors and administrators, and government and regulation. You are encouraged to identify the relationships among them and their relationship to your own work. Assess your own ideology, values, and dreams about the nursing profession within the context of your own life and the environment in which you live. Look at your practice from the framework and vantage points of other ideas and examples. Then you will know if moving into the 21st century will be, for you, a transition or a transformation.

■ References

American Organization of Nurse Executives (AONE). (1997, March). *Consumer summit*. Washington, DC.

American Organization of Nurse Executives (AONE). (1999, March). *Nursing leadership for the new millennium forum*. Charlotte, NC.

Bohm, D. (1990). *Wholeness and the implicate order*. London: Routledge & Kegan Paul.

Botelho, R. (1995). Motivating change in health behavior. *Primary Care, 22*, 565–589.

Capra, F. (1996). *The web of life: A new scientific understanding of living systems*. New York: Anchor Books, Doubleday.

Cook, Sir Edward. (1913, reissued 1942). *The life of Florence Nightingale*. New York: Macmillan.

Dolan, M. (1969). *Notes on nursing . . . What it is and what it is not*. (Nightingale, as cited in Dolan, pp. 32, 42). Ontario, Canada: Dover.

Eisenberg, D. M., Davis, R. B., Ettner, S. L., Appel, S., Wilkey, S., Van Rompay, M., & Kessler, R. C. (1998). Trends in alternative medicine use in the United States, 1990–1997. *Journal of the American Medical Association, 280*(18), 1569–1575.

Health Care Resources (HCR). (1997). *Leadership development in nursing initiative: A customer perspective*. Unpublished report for the University of Illinois, Chicago. Rochester, NY: HCR.

Henderson, H. (1998). *Building a win–win world: Life beyond global economic warfare*. San Francisco: Berrett-Koehler.

Jaffe, G. (1998, February 3). Corporate carrots, sticks cut health bills. *Wall Street Journal*, pp. B1–B2.

Muehsam, P. (1997, Spring). Alternative and complementary medicine special interest group. *GEA Correspondent*, 10.

Oelschlaeger, M. (1991). *The idea of wilderness: From prehistory to the age of ecology.* London: Harrison & Sons.

Pender, N. (1997). *The multidimensions of health promotion.* Unpublished presentation at Health Care Resources (HCR), Rochester, NY.

Rogers, M. (1994). Nursing science evolves. In M. Madrid & E. Barrett (Eds.), *Rogers' scientific art of nursing practice* (pp. 1–9). New York: National League for Nursing.

Ryan, S. (1998). *Education and partnerships in the global community.* Unpublished presentation at Health Care Resources (HCR), Rochester, NY.

Selfcare is new healthcare bandwagon. (1998, September 10). *Medical World News,* 10.

Toffler, A. (1980). *The third wave.* New York: William Morrow and Company.

Toffler, A. (1995). *Creating a new civilization: The politics of the third wave.* Atlanta: Turner Publishing.

Wilbur, K. (1996). *A brief history of everything.* Boston: Shambhala.

Woerner, L. (1998). *Health care: Whose business is it?* Unpublished speech by Health Care Resources (HCR) for Rochester Institute of Technology Executive MBA Discussion Group, April 3, Rochester, NY.

■ Editor's Questions for Discussion

What are the implications of Koerner's discussion about "living systems" for chapters in the Nursing Practice Part? Identify and discuss transitions in nursing practice. What have been the effects of those transitions on nursing practice? Why is what Nightingale calls for a transformation and not a transition? How is Koerner's "returning to our roots" message similar to Felton's plea (Chapter 1)? How may professional relationships between nurses be affected if the "narrow focus" by nurses is transformed as described by Koerner? How can nursing apply the principles identified by Henderson in working with one another? What changes are essential in the profession for nursing to function as a cooperative unit moving toward global nursing action?

Provide examples of nurses "creating" social health models. Provide examples of how nurses may include science with the holistic view of a system in providing care. How may nurses appreciate that individual actions are interconnected?

How can nursing programs promote a global community perspective in health? What student learning activities and experiences will transform focus from a narrow disease framework to health and wellness? How may the role of nursing be merged with that of "prosumer" (uniting provider and consumer)? What transformation in nursing and delivery systems is necessary for "health care prosumption" to occur? How realistic is it to promote and effect transformation? How might resistance to change be reduced?

3

A New Approach to the Regulation of Nursing Practice

Mutual Recognition

Carolyn J. Yocom, PhD, RN, FAAN
Katherine A. Thomas, MN, RN

Revolutionary changes have occurred during the past 10 years that have had a direct impact on the delivery of nursing services. Changes having the greatest impact, from a regulatory perspective, are those that have occurred within health care delivery systems and telecommunications. The dominate corporate structure of health care delivery systems has long been characterized by single site, sole purpose institutions, such as an individual hospital providing only acute care services, or free-standing home health care

At the time this chapter was written Dr. Yocom was Director of Research Services—National Council of State Boards of Nursing.

The authors would like to acknowledge that this chapter is based on the work and input of multiple groups and individuals. Included are boards of nursing, National Council's Board of Directors, former and current members of the APRN Coordinating Task Force, Multistate Regulation Task Force, Multistate Regulation Workgroups (Alternative Programs, Discipline, Fiscal, Operations, Trial by Distance), Multistate Board Attorney Comment Group, Nursing Regulation Task Force, Mutual Recognition Interim Compact Administrators Group, Mutual Recognition Master Plan Coordinating Group, and former and current National Council staff members Jennifer Bosma, Carolyn Hutcherson, Vickie Sheets, and Susan Williamson.

The conclusions and positions stated in this chapter are consistent with those of the National Council of State Boards of Nursing.

agencies. Now evolving are integrated systems comprising multisite and multiservice corporations, partnerships, and alliances. Additionally, service areas of health care provider institutions have expanded from local geographic areas to regional and multistate areas. Several institutions have enlarged their networks to include diverse locations within the United States. For example, The Mayo Clinic of Rochester, Minnesota, has formed the Mayo Health System, a partnership with other institutions serving areas in Minnesota, Iowa, and Wisconsin. The system also has affiliates in Scottsdale, Arizona, and Jacksonville, Florida.

■ Emerging Access for Nursing Services

Involvement of nurses in postdischarge management of patients in acute care hospitals also has expanded greatly within the past decade. Further, enlarged geographic service areas of health care delivery systems steadily increase the likelihood that a nurse may be providing in-hospital and postdischarge services to an individual residing in another state. Likewise, nurses employed in home health care agencies, especially those located close to state borders or those working for managed care companies, find themselves in similar circumstances. Such nurses can no longer assume that patients and families with whom they interact are from one of the surrounding communities within their state's geographic borders.

Advances in telecommunications technology and its application to health care delivery also have contributed to the emergence of multistate nursing practice as a regulatory issue. An ever-increasing job market for nurses is created throughout the United States by modern conditions. These circumstances include availability of telephone triage centers, health care consumers' desires for instant access to assistance and information, and expanded use of tele-

phonic communication systems by health service delivery and management companies.

According to the *Wall Street Journal* (Telephone Triage, 1997), 24-hour telephone nursing service was available to 2 million Americans in 1990, 35 million Americans in 1997, and projected to be available to more than 100 million Americans by 2001. In most cases, these telehealth services operate nationwide as a benefit to enrollees of private and public health benefit plans.

Use of more advanced telecommunications systems also has been introduced. In Home Health Services (IHHS), affiliated with Newton Memorial Hospital, Newton, New Jersey, has implemented the use of telenursing technology for patients in need of intensive monitoring and teaching in their homes. As announced on its Web page, IHHP's system

operates over regular telephone lines and consists of patient units and a central nurses station. The patient units are equipped with a blood pressure and pulse apparatus, a telephonic stethoscope and an ancillary lens for close-up views. The nurse and the patient can see each other on a color video telephone screen. This telenursing technology can be used in combination with face-to-face home visits, and will capture vital signs and heart and lung sounds, schedule daily events and teach patients and their caregiver self-care techniques while remotely managing the plan of care. (In Home Health Services, 1999)

Implementation of this system and others like it will only increase the public's access to nursing care that is unconstrained by state borders.

■ The Regulatory Dilemma

State nurse licensing systems have worked effectively for nearly 100 years to regulate the practice of nursing within the states' geographic boundaries. However, evolution of integrated health care systems, increased mobility of nurses, and modern communication technologies have substantially altered the way nursing is practiced. An estimated 12% of all nurses now hold more than one state license (Evelyn Moses, DHHS, Division of Nursing, personal communication, 1998). Of greater concern is the unknown number of nurses who are practicing in multiple states who may not have appropriate licenses in all the states.

Origins of the current nurse licensure system began in 1903 when the first boards of nursing were established in North Carolina, Virginia, and New York (Goodnow, 1929; National Council of State Boards of Nursing [NCSBN], 1999). Impetus for their development was public concern about the quality of nursing education and inability of the public to distinguish between safe and unsafe practitioners (Waddle, 1979). Subsequently, efforts of early nursing leaders, including Isabel Hampton Robb, Sophia Palmer, and Lavinia Dock, were instrumental in gaining introduction and passage of legislation establishing the first boards (Goodnow, 1929; Shannon, 1975).

Authority for states to control and license health professionals is vested in the Tenth Amendment to the Constitution. The ability of each state to adopt laws to protect the health, safety, and general welfare of its citizens falls under police powers reserved to states (United States Constitution, Amendment X; *Dent v. West Virginia,* 1888). The state's interest in protecting the public relates directly to assurance that those whom it authorizes to practice the profession possess the minimal, essential competence required for their practice to be safe and effective.

Today all 50 states, the District of Columbia, and U.S. territories of American Samoa, Commonwealth of the Northern Marianas, Guam, Puerto Rico, and the Virgin Islands regulate nursing practice. Each board of nursing has a legislative mandate (i.e., a Nurse Practice Act [NPA]) to protect the health and safety of its state's citizens as related to delivery of nursing services. An NPA describes powers and duties of a board of nursing, levels of licensure, criteria for initial licensure and license renewal, legal scope of practice, grounds for disciplinary action against a licensee, and disciplinary remedies that it may impose. Five states have separate boards of nursing for registered and licensed practical or vocational nurses. Although each of the 61 NPAs evolved independently during the 20th century, criteria for initial licensure and license renewal for practical and vocational nurses (LPN/LVNs) and for registered nurses (RNs) from state to state have converged as a consequence of the passage of time and evolution of nursing practice. The same cannot be said for advanced practice registered nurses (APRNs). Four APRN groups govern practice by nurse anesthetists, nurse practitioners, nurse midwives, and clinical nurse specialists. Interstate differences in licensure, criteria for authority to practice, and legal scopes of practice for each APRN group are the result of their more recent emergence as separate entities within regulated health professions groups and political forces at work through the legislative process.

Multistate Practice

Within the current regulatory system, the privilege of practicing nursing within the boundaries of a specific state can only be granted by that state's board of nursing. Therefore, if a nurse licensed in one state desires to practice in another, that nurse must apply for licensure in the other state. A nurse licensed in State A and practicing in State B without a license can have serious ramifications. The board of nursing in State A has no legal authority to allow the nurse to practice in State B. However, the board of nursing in State B has no authority to address complaints lodged by citizens or employers in State B about the practice of the nurse, who is licensed only in State

A. Therefore citizens in State B have no legal recourse against the nurse or the states.

The nurse desiring to practice legally in multiple states must, under the current system, seek licensure in each individual state. This process—licensure by endorsement—requires that the candidate for licensure must at minimum complete an application, pay a fee, and request the original state of licensure to verify that the candidate graduated from a state-approved nursing education program and passed the licensure examination. In addition, the original state of licensure and possibly all other states of current and past licensure must be requested to verify licensure status (active, inactive, or disciplined). Each request for verification must be accompanied by payment of the appropriate fee to the responding board of nursing. Several states also require endorsement applicants to provide an official transcript or other document verifying completion of the basic nursing education program. This process is time consuming, costly, and duplicative—on the part of both the nurse and the licensing boards—especially if the nurse seeks licensure by endorsement in several states.

Not all nurses engaged in interstate practice comply with this requirement. Whether by design, ignorance of the law, or lack of awareness of being engaged in interstate practice, this failure places the public at risk and without legal recourse. The state in which the nurse practiced without a license has no legal authority to take action against the license issued by another state. A licensing board's ability to investigate a licensee's alleged malpractice in another state is also hampered because it has no subpoena power outside its own borders.

License Discipline

Boards of nursing have authority to remove from or limit practice of licensed individuals for unethical or unsafe behavior that has the potential for harm or has resulted in actual harm to a recipient of nursing services. Each board has jurisdiction only over its own licensees and can take action to deal with infractions of the NPA that have occurred within boundaries of its state. Disciplinary action and grounds for discipline are communicated to the National Council of State Boards of Nursing for inclusion in its Disciplinary Tracking Service (DTS). If a nurse is licensed in more than one state, notification to boards of nursing in all other states of licensure is accomplished in one of two ways: directly by the state taking disciplinary action or indirectly via monthly DTS reports circulated by the National Council, a service provided to its membership. The National Council has had a disciplinary databank for more than 15 years.

To reduce risk of its citizens' exposure to unsafe or unethical practice, many boards have the authority to impose disciplinary action against one of its licensees when disciplinary action has been taken by another state board under which the individual holds a license. However, due to restrictions contained in each state's administrative law, most boards of nursing currently are prohibited from communicating alleged malpractice, misconduct, or investigatory information to other boards until disciplinary action, if warranted, is imposed. From the time a complaint is filed until its final resolution, several months to more than a year may ensue. Meanwhile, that nurse may continue to practice in any other state of licensure, with boards in those states remaining unaware of investigation and pending disciplinary action.

Weaknesses in the current system—relating to lack of jurisdiction, restricted communication until disciplinary action has been taken in another state, and unlicensed practice—expose the public to risk. However, requiring a nurse repeatedly to demonstrate eligibility for licensure in each state of practice creates unnecessary barriers to nurse mobility and can delay a nurse's entry into the workforce if delays in application processing occur. This restriction limits the public's access to qualified providers.

■ A Regulatory Solution to the Dilemma: Mutual Recognition

Consideration of changes occurring in health care and delivery of nursing services led the National Council of State Boards of Nursing to evaluate the strengths and weaknesses of the current regulatory system and to consider alternative regulatory models (NCSBN, 1997a). As a result, the National Council adopted a policy goal—simplification of governmental processes and removal of regulatory barriers—and expects to achieve it to increase access to safe nursing care. The vision statement guiding the National Council, as it considered models that could support multistate regulatory modes, was "a state nursing license, recognized nationally and enforced locally" (NCSBN, 1997a, p. 2). Continuation of authority for regulating nursing practice at the state level was envisioned. Therefore a mechanism was needed to allow states to permit a nurse licensed in another state to practice legally within their boundaries. Thus citizens affected by a nurse's practice would be protected regardless of where the citizen or provider was located.

Supporting Data

Subsequently, extensive data collection and analysis was initiated by the National Council. Outcomes of this endeavor further supported the need for a multistate nursing regulation model (NCSBN, 1997a). A survey of 6,000 nurses revealed that 17% of the respondents held more than one license and that 8% (10% of RNs and 7% of LPNs or LVNs) had worked in more than 1 state (and in as many as 50 states) during the previous 12 months. Not all those working in multiple states reported holding more than one license (NCSBN, 1997a).

Based on the vision statement, problems associated with the existing system and features of a desired system, the National Council identified, described, and analyzed a continuum of regulatory models. Serious consideration was given various versions, including current licensure processes, mutual recognition, fast endorsement, single state licensure with a multistate option, reciprocity, corporate credentialing, single state or multistate option, multistate license with state "carve out," multistate license, and federal license. Pros and cons of each model from the perspective of various stakeholders—including licensees, boards of nursing, employers and consumers—were identified.

The outcome of this evaluation revealed that a Mutual Recognition (MR) model of nursing regulation would best fulfill the policy goal and vision and address shortcomings of the current licensure system. In this appraisal, the MR model was compared to regulatory processes now in place that address initial licensure, practice across states, changes to a new state of licensure (e.g., endorsement), license renewal, issues regarding lapsed or reentry or reinstatement of licenses, and discipline. Analysis revealed that many current processes could still be used with some modifications. This finding is significant in that changing to an MR model would not require boards of nursing to redesign existing operational systems completely.

The Mutual Recognition Model

The MR model provides that a nurse is held accountable for practicing nursing within limits established by NPAs and rules and regulations in the state where that nurse provides nursing services to citizens of a state. This expectation does not differ from that which is in effect with the current regulatory model. A nurse licensed in multiple states is expected to know and practice within the limits established by NPA(s) and administrative rules in the state(s) of current practice.

The following general concepts underlie the MR model.

- Each state sets its own licensure requirements (note: uniform licensure requirements are not necessary for implementation of the MR model but remain an ultimate goal).

- States voluntarily enter into an agreement via interstate compact to legally recognize licenses issued by other states, regardless of differences in standards; a licensee may practice in any state participating in the agreement under the license issued by the licensee's state of residence.

- Practice across state lines is allowed, whether by physical presence or electronic means, unless the nurse is practicing under disciplinary or other monitoring agreement that restricts interstate practice. Thus a nurse will have only one license and one licensing record—in the state of residence—and only needs to renew this one license as long as the nurse remains a resident of the issuing state.

- A nurse who moves must immediately obtain a license in the new state of legal residence and must simultaneously relinquish the license issued by the former state of residence.

In August 1997, the membership of the National Council of State Boards of Nursing unanimously selected Mutual Recognition as the model for nursing regulation that would best facilitate multistate practice (NCSBN, 1997b). Compact language essential for implementation of the model was adopted by the National Council's membership in December 1997 (NCSBN, 1997c). This model language was further revised in November 1998 (NCSBN, 1998).

■ *Interstate Compact*

The mechanism to implement the MR model of nurse licensure is an interstate compact. An interstate compact is a legal agreement between two or more states for the purpose of remedying a particular problem of multistate concern. Interstate compacts enable states mutually to accomplish tasks that are within their realms but that require multistate action. An interstate compact enables states to accomplish what they could not do alone because of lack of control over the entire subject matter, lack of resources, or inability to share information.

Nearly 200 interstate compacts were in existence as of the early 1990s. These compacts govern a variety of areas—including natural resources, taxation, corrections, and health—and may be regional or national in character. Generally, interstate compacts are negotiated by organizations composed of state officials who have authority over a particular issue. These officials develop a compact that must then be enacted in identical form by each state legislature as a statute. One example of a compact that currently affects many individuals in the United States, the Drivers License Compact, has been entered into by most states. It allows an individual licensed to drive a car in one state to drive in any other state as long as the traffic laws in the second state are followed. If the driver is found guilty of breaking a traffic law in another state, the individual is subject to penalties in that state and most likely in the state that issued the license.

A compact is enforceable as a law and a contract, and it supersedes all other conflicting state statutes—whether enacted prior or subsequent to the compact. For a compact to be established, two or more states must adopt identical legislation that defines the compact and its role. States adopting a compact are referred to as *party* states. An existing compact may be modified with consent of the party states. Congressional approval of the MR interstate compact is not necessary because regulation of health professionals is within the realm of state authority.

Although the MR interstate compact is the mechanism that provides for practice across state lines, each state's NPA remains the authority for regulating nursing practice. Furthermore, the compact does not affect federal or state statutory authority concerning administrative procedures for rule making, discipline of licensees, or collective bargaining.

The general purposes of the MR interstate compact are to (a) facilitate the states' responsibility to protect the public's health and safety; (b) ensure and encourage the cooperation of party states in the areas of nurse regulation, investigation, and adverse actions; (c) promote compliance with the laws governing the practice of nursing in each state; and (d) invest all party states with the authority to hold a nurse accountable for meeting all state practice laws in the state in which the patient is located at the time care is rendered through the mutual recognition of party state licenses (NCSBN, 1998).

In implementing MR, the compact establishes relationships between party states in the areas of jurisdiction, discipline, information sharing, and compact administration (NCSBN, 1998).

Shared Jurisdiction

The compact establishes that a license to practice nursing as issued by a home state (i.e., a nurse's primary state of residence) to a resident in that state, will be recognized by each party state as authorizing a multistate licensure privilege to practice as a nurse within each of the party states. Every nurse practicing in a party state must comply with the state practice laws of the state in which the patient is located at the time care is rendered. The decision to require a nurse to be licensed in the state of residence, as opposed to the state of practice, was made for several reasons. The MR licensure model is similar to many other activities based on an individual's place of residence, including obtaining a driver's license, paying taxes, and voting. Because of the many employment settings in which nurses work, there is likely to be less confusion about where a nurse resides than about location of the nurse's primary state of practice. Finding a nurse in event of a complaint investigation would be more readily accomplished with a residence link than a practice or employment link. Confusion over how to define primary state of practice when nurses work in multiple states would create an administrative nightmare for boards of nursing. Furthermore, defining practice in the compact would supersede state definitions of practice and could change states' scopes of practice. This outcome was felt to be in direct opposition to the intent of state regulatory law and would render the primary practice site impossible to use (Hutcherson & Williamson, 1999).

Shared Discipline

To protect its citizens, both the home state and a party state other than home state, must be able to impose disciplinary action. Therefore boards of nursing in party states may, in accordance with state due process laws, limit or revoke the multistate licensure privilege of any nurse to practice within a party state and may take any other actions under applicable state laws necessary to protect the health and safety of their citizens. It is important to note that only the home state may take action (e.g., suspension, revocation, or placement on probation) against the licensee. In contrast, a remote state may take any action allowed by law except licensure actions. Examples of actions that a remote state could take would be to impose fines or limit, revoke, or suspend the privilege to practice within that state.

As in the current system, final disciplinary actions imposed by any party state are reportable to the National Council's DTS and thus to every board of nursing. Contrary to the current system, which prohibits sharing information about complaints and investigations prior to imposition of discipline, the compact authorizes party states to share information among themselves before action is taken. This process is applicable to cases in which there is evidence of grounds for a complaint, which, if proved true, would indicate more than minor infraction or that the nurse represents an immediate threat to public health and safety. Based on shared investigatory information, therefore, disciplinary action can occur simultaneously within the party states, according to each party state's due process procedures. Investigatory information will not be made available to nonparty states or to the public until disciplinary action, if warranted, is taken by a party state's board of nursing.

The compact does not override a party state's ability to allow nurse participation in an alternative program for chemical dependency or mental illness, in lieu of licensure action. Nor does it override the nonpublic nature of program participation if required by the party state's laws. Importantly, the compact does limit opportunity of impaired nurses to seek a "geographic cure" for their problems. Party state nurses who enter alternative programs are required to agree not to practice in any other party state during the term of the alternative program without prior authorization from such other party state.

Shared Information

A major support system essential to implementation of MR is establishment of a central licensee information system to support party states' needs for timely access to licensure and discipline information. Thus the interstate compact provides for a not-for-profit entity, composed of and controlled by state licensing boards, to maintain a system to collect, store, and share information on nurse licensure and enforcement activities related to nurse licensure laws. In collaboration with its membership, the National Council of State Boards of Nursing, a not-for-profit organization, has committed to enhancing its information systems to support implementation of the MR model. The information system, Nur*sys,* is a highly secure, closed system for use primarily by boards of nursing. Under current regulations, to comply with public information and privacy requirements, limited access to the data will be provided to employers and consumers. Investigatory information contributed by party states prior to final determination of discipline will be accessible only to those boards of nursing that are party to the interstate compact.

Establishment of Nur*sys* also facilitates licensure endorsement processes of all boards of nursing. When a nurse must apply for licensure by endorsement in a new party state due to change of residence, or a nurse in a nonparty state (i.e., not a member of interstate compact) desires to obtain a license in another nonparty state, information contained in Nur*sys* is provided. Such information includes original state of licensure, basic nursing education program, licensure examination passage, all states of licensure, and any history of license discipline. The information would be available instantly to the board in the new state, thus shortening the amount of time necessary to process an application.

Shared Administration of the Interstate Compact

Administration of the compact is provided through formation of a compact administrators group composed of the head of the nurse licensing authority in each party state. The compact administrators have authority to write rules and regulations implementing the compact. Proposed rules and regulations need to be reviewed in each party state according to procedures set forth in each state's administrative law. The compact administrator group reviews comments received from each state prior to finalizing the rules and regulations. A primary responsibility of the compact administrator in each party state is to make available information and documents such as licensure data, identifying information, investigatory information, and disclosable alternative program participation to compact administrators in each party state. Again, the intent is to assure the public's access to a competent nurse workforce.

■ *Implementation of the Mutual Recognition Interstate Compact*

Currently, the MR interstate compact only authorizes multistate practice of RNs, and LPNs/LVNs. As noted earlier, relative uniformity exists in licensure requirements and legal scopes of practice for RNs and LPNs/LVNs. Therefore, even though greater uniformity in licensure requirements is a goal, its lack is not an impediment to implementation of MR for these two levels of licensure.

As strategies for implementing MR were being developed, it became apparent that the model must be based on establishment of uniform requirements for legal recognition of advanced practice registered nurses (APRNs) by the states. Therefore inclusion of APRNs in the MR model will occur on a different timeline. A number of strategies are being implemented currently. Collaborating to address the unifor-

mity issue are a broad spectrum of nursing organizations representing various types of APRNs or with an interest in their education and practice. In the summer of 1999, uniform requirements for APRNs licensure and authority to practice were drafted by the National Council and participating organizations. Development of a mechanism to adopt and implement these requirements is under consideration.

Legislative activity to implement the compact began in early 1998 and continues. By mid 2000, the compact has been signed into law in Arkansas, Iowa, Maryland, Mississippi, Nebraska, North Carolina, South Dakota, Utah, and Wisconsin. Legislative consideration of the interstate compact currently is occurring in additional states. Other boards are expected to become members of the compact after the model is implemented effectively; the goal is for 100% participation. During the transition phase of implementation, both current regulatory schema and the MR model will be in effect. Nurses practicing in nonparty states will continue to be required to obtain licensure by endorsement in all states of practice. However, those living in a party state will have the privilege to practice in all party states.

■ *Concluding Statement*

Adoption of the Mutual Recognition interstate compact by all states will have a positive impact on nursing practice and the ability of boards of nursing to fulfill legislative mandates to protect the public's health and safety. Nurses will have greater mobility and legal authority to practice, under one license in any state. The public will have greater, faster access to nursing services and be assured that nurse licensees can be held legally accountable for their practice wherever it may occur.

■ References

Dent v. West Virginia, 129 U.S. 114 (1888).

Goodnow, M. (1929). *Outlines of nursing history.* Philadelphia: W. B. Saunders.

Hutcherson, C., & Williamson, S. (1999, May 31). Nursing Regulation for the New Millennium: The mutual recognition model. *Online Journal of Issues in Nursing* [On-line]. Available: http://www.nursingworld.org/ojin/topic9/topic9_2.htm.

In Home Health Services. (1999). *First in New Jersey in telenursing* [On-line]. Available: http://www.itsyourlife.com/telenurs.htm.

National Council of State Boards of Nursing. (1997a). Report of the Multistate Regulation Task Force. *Book of reports.* Chicago: Author, Tab 10-C, 1-42.

National Council of State Boards of Nursing. (1997b). *Boards of nursing adopt mutual recognition model* [On-line]. Available: http://www.ncsbn.org/search/accufacts/ newsreleases/nr970825.asp.

National Council of State Boards of Nursing. (1997c). *Boards of nursing approve proposed language for an interstate compact for a mutual recognition model of nursing regulation* [On-line]. Available: http://www.ncsbn.org/search//accufacts/ newsreleases/nr971216.asp.

National Council of State Boards of Nursing. (1998). *Revised approved interstate compact language* [On-line]. Available: http://ncsbn.org/files/msrtf/compact9811.pdf.

National Council of State Boards of Nursing. (1999). *Member Board Profiles—1998.* Chicago: Author.

Shannon, M. L. (1975). Nurses in American history. Our first four licensure laws. *American Journal of Nursing, 79,* 1327–1329.

Telephone Triage. (1997, February 4). *Wall Street Journal,* pp. A-1, A-6.

United States Constitution. *Amendment X.*

Waddle, F. (1979). Licensure achievements and limitations. In *The study of credentialing in nursing: A new approach. Volume II. Staff working papers* (pp. 126–164). Kansas City, MO: American Nurses Association.

■ Editor's Questions for Discussion

Discuss the effects on the nursing profession of multisite services in integrated systems that cross state boundaries. What is the difference between licensure by endorsement and mutual recognition? How do expectations differ between the two? How does mutual recognition help if a nurse must still obtain a license in the new state of legal residence should he or she move? Is that license then obtained by endorsement and not by mutual recognition? How do interstate compacts governing nursing licenses and driving licenses differ? What benefit results in requiring licensure in the state of residence rather than the state of practice? How is nursing license by a state different from compliance with the nursing practice laws in the state where a patient may be located? What effects may result in the difference between the two? Must nurses abide by state practice laws both in the state of residence and the state(s) where nursing services are provided? How should the council facilitate accurate understanding for nursing professionals and consumers of services about mutual recognition and licensure? How are confidentiality and issues pertaining to ethics regarding distribution of information protected and preserved in the mutual recognition model and endorsement of licensure?

What effect should multistate mutual recognition have on home health care? How do Yocom and Thomas' predictions support statements by Schroeder and Long (Chapter 47) and Hollinger-Smith (Chapter 45)? How do Yocom and Thomas' predictions support other means for nursing health care as promoted by McDermott (Chapter 49), Pullen (Chapter 50), Todero (Chapter 51), Duffy (Chapter 53), and Barger (Chapter 52)? How does Yocom and Thomas' chapter address concerns expressed by Gray (Chapter 42) regarding advanced nursing practice?

4

Continued Competence of the Nurse

A New Look at an Old Problem

Charlie Jones-Dickson, EdD, RN, FAAN

Few would disagree that most people regardless of culture have a short attention span. This trait is evidenced in the fact that newly identified problems receive considerable attention from policy makers for a short time, only to be replaced by other evolving problems. That ever-present process is manifested throughout the health care professions, and nursing is not an exception. Currently, unlicensed assistive personnel is a compelling licensure issue, but other crucial problems related to nursing practice exist and must be explored. For example, continued competence of the nurse has assumed a new level of importance as the new millennium begins. The changing landscape of health care is directly related to (a) increased demand for accountability, (b) performance measurement, (c) focus on consumers of care, (d) benchmarking, and (e) total quality management. All these phenomena suggest the need for assessing the nurse's ability to achieve desirable outcomes under varied circumstances. Likewise, the current world of advanced knowledge and technology, work redesign, changing regulatory requirements, cost containment, and other market forces in health care illuminate the need to strengthen ways of ensuring consumer protection (Finocchio, Dower, Blick, Gragnola, & Taskforce, 1998).

■ Historical Perspective of Competency Assurance

Historically, a number of widely disseminated documents have described the significance of competency and of the competent nurse. For example, the fifth statement of the Code for Nurses contains the phrase "the nurse maintains competence in nursing" (American Nurses Association [ANA], 1998, p. 1). Nursing's Social Policy Statement included a statement that considered the "competent nurse within the realm of a scope of practice that responded to the changing needs of society" (ANA, 1995). *The Standards of Clinical Nursing Practice,* 2nd ed. (ANA, 1998) included statements describing key indicators of competent practice. More than a century and a half ago, Florence Nightingale recognized the need for continuous updating of the nurse's knowledge when she wrote, "nurses have to learn new and improved methods in medicine, surgery and hygiene" (Florence Nightingale, 1859/ 1946). The Model Nursing Practice Act states that, "because practice in the health care delivery system, in general, and in the delivery of nursing service in particular, continuously change, it is essential that nurses maintain a degree of nursing competency which assures the public safe and effective care" (National Council of State Boards [NCSBN], 1996, p. 22). A common aspect of the Joint Commission on Accreditation of Healthcare Organizations (JCAHO) is the inclusion of management of human resources standards that concentrate on staff "qualifications, competencies, orientation and inservice education and performance evaluation" (Patterson, 1998, p. 13). Similarly, the standards place accountability on organizational leaders for measures that "assess competence and its maintenance and improvement" (Patterson, 1998, p. 13).

According to a Citizen Advocacy Center (CAC) report almost two decades ago, the National Organization for Competence Assurance disseminated guidelines on continuing competence that stated:

> Continuing competence assurance is necessary. . . . Health care technology is advancing too fast for a certificate of competence earned at the beginning of one's career to constitute proof of competence many years later. Demonstrations of continuing competence are as reasonable and necessary as are required demonstrations of entry-level competence. (Swankin, 1995, p. 1)

In concert with this earlier recommendation, nearly a decade ago the PEW Health Professions Commission Task Force on Health Care Workforce Regulation noted that the endeavors of the regulatory boards must include

> assessing the continued competence of practitioners, a much more difficult task at which many professional license bodies have done very little, other than requiring attendance at continuing education courses. There should be more attention to assessing the actual practice performance of licensees using quality assurance techniques and evaluation of consumer and professional criticisms about licenses. (Swankin, 1995, p. 1)

In today's changing health care environment, employers, consumers, and regulators are seeking assurances that health care providers are maintaining competence as evidenced during initial licensure. Very few individuals, if any, have written as much as Benjamin Shimberg, CAC board chair, about failure of regulatory boards to assess the continuing competence of the individuals they license. Shimberg has expressed astonishment about the fact that regulatory boards have failed to determine little additional information about its licensees. In fact, Shimberg concludes that most boards simply maintain the address of the licensee and therefore erroneously conclude that such information validates the fact that the licensee is still alive and practicing during annual or biennial license renewal. Therefore a licensee may practice for two or three decades with no determination of the quality of professional services delivered to the public. Further, there is no likelihood that the regulatory board will contact the licensee unless the licensee is subject to disciplinary action (Swankin, 1995).

■ The Historical Impetus for Regulatory Boards

Historically, states generally have given authority and power to regulatory boards, under the Tenth Amendment of the Constitution of the United States. This vested power provides the impetus for each regulatory board to devise necessary strategies to protect the public from unqualified and unscrupulous practitioners. The board of nursing is the most direct link between the public and the practice of nursing in each individual state (Sheets, 1996). Thus boards of nursing, since the early years of the 20th century, have developed means of measuring competence for entry into practice via two avenues: (a) nursing education program approval in selected states; and (b) subjecting qualified applicants to an examination that tests minimal knowledge and application of knowledge to selected clinical situations.

Individual states have the responsibility for licensing nurses. However, after granting the nurse an initial license, most states never mandate that the nurse demonstrate continued competence through maintenance of the knowledge, skills, and abilities needed for nursing practice. Most citizens in the United States have come to enjoy a certain number of inalienable rights. Yet, the practice of nursing is postulated to be a privilege, not a right. Therefore to require nurses to demonstrate regularly their qualifications as a stipulation of having that privilege seems logical (Swankin, 1995).

■ New Impetus for Regulatory Boards

To date, no system has been established to measure continued competence for general nursing or for advanced practice nursing under a regulatory agency. The area of nursing regulation is experiencing pressure, from a variety of sources, to place additional emphasis on postentry competency. A number of factors are forcing the evolution of continued competency mechanisms. One important factor is that the number of disciplinary cases submitted to boards of nursing that constitute perceived incompetence in practice have increased considerably over the past decade.

The PEW Health Professions Commission Report (Finocchio et al., 1998) provides the most influential impetus for looking at regulatory boards and has strengthened consumer protection regulation. In essence, the Commission recommended that regulatory boards require that all health professionals, regardless of discipline, meet specific competency requirements throughout the duration of their careers. Such actions obviously are needed, in light of the recent findings pertaining to deaths associated with injuries from medical errors. The Institute of Medicine's report (National Academies News, 1999) presents the following conclusions. Reducing medical errors, one of the leading causes of death and injury, will require arduous changes throughout the nation's health care system. Each year costly medical errors kill an estimated 44,000 people to 98,000 people. Even at the lower level, medical errors kill more people each year than more devastating diseases such as breast cancer, AIDS, or automobile accidents. Also, the health care industry appears to be at least a decade behind other industries in matters pertaining to client safety. One way to ensure consumer safety is for regulatory bodies to implement periodic reexaminations of primary health care providers—including doctors, nurses, and other key primary care providers. The purpose of such reviews would be to ascertain the extent of competency-based skills and knowledge of safety-related practices of these practitioners.

Attorneys have entered the debate and collectively have noted that the primary role of nursing regulatory boards is to protect the consumer. They have also asserted that such protection should be aimed at detecting incompetence as a result of failure to meet a standard of care, rather then defining or measuring the nurse's competence. Reeves (1996) stated, "I believe that it is much easier to recognize incompetence than competence, and therefore, believe the disciplinary function should be emphasized more than it currently is" (p. 1). Similarly, Kobs (1997) noted that "in the absence of error, competence can be assumed. If a caregiver has been performing successfully and there have been no adverse outcomes there can be an assumption of competence" (p. 10). However, other individuals have questioned the methodology for measurement and determination of incompetence, particularly in light of the fact that elements of competence have not been appropriately defined, delineated, and measured. Mann (1999) believes that "a profile of the competent nurse can be assembled and used to facilitate model development" (p. 85). Mann further concludes that it is possible to develop a profile of the competent nurse through a systematic and rigorous study of the population of interest (e.g., consumers, practitioners, educators, organizations, regulatory boards, and so forth).

Continuing competence has been defined in a number of ways. For example, the College of Nurses of Ontario (CNO) proposed a definition of competence for nursing as follows:

> Competence means the integration of the professional attributes required for the performance of the scope of nursing in a given role or situation, and in accordance with the standards of practice.

> Professional attributes means knowledge, skills, judgment, self-concept (attitudes and values), trait and motives. (Campbell, 1998, p. 4)

The National Council of State Boards of Nursing (1996) has defined competence as "the application of knowledge and the interpersonal, decision making and psychomotor skills expected for the nurse's practice role within the context of public health safety and welfare" (p. 47).

■ Continued Competence–
Whose Responsibility?

According to Gross (1984), standards related to licensing of professionals should be designed to place major responsibility on individuals and less on regulation. More specifically, Gross noted that many individuals believe that there should be a mandate for a state to protect the public. Gross further noted that those who consume health care should rely more on themselves as personal advocates for safe and effective health care. In other words, Gross believes that individual consumers of health care should take on heightened degrees of responsibility to safeguard against medical errors.

Nursing care consumers in Alabama were asked who has the responsibility for determining that a nurse is competent to practice nursing. One of every four of the respondents believed that the "Nursing Board" is responsible for determining competency of a nurse who practices in Alabama (Mann, 1999). In this Alabama study, 19% of the respondents considered "supervisors"—including other nurses and doctors—to be the responsible parties for determining that a nurse is competent to practice nursing in Alabama, followed by "hospital," 9%, and "educational programs," 9% (Mann, 1999, p. 16). More than one of four indicated they did not really know who

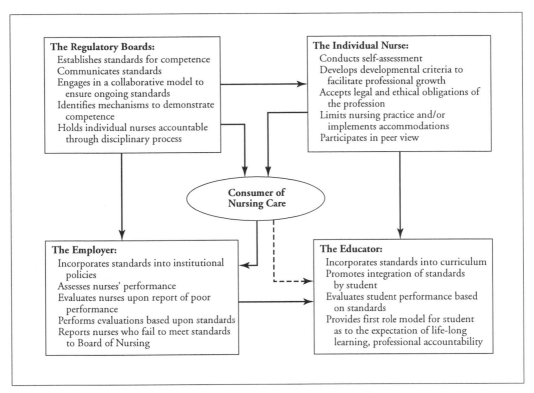

The Regulatory Boards:
    Establishes standards for competence
    Communicates standards
    Engages in a collaborative model to
        ensure ongoing standards
    Identifies mechanisms to demonstrate
        competence
    Holds individual nurses accountable
        through disciplinary process

The Individual Nurse:
    Conducts self-assessment
    Develops developmental criteria to
        facilitate professional growth
    Accepts legal and ethical obligations of
        the profession
    Limits nursing practice and/or
        implements accommodations
    Participates in peer view

Consumer of Nursing Care

The Employer:
    Incorporates standards into institutional
        policies
    Assesses nurses' performance
    Evaluates nurses upon report of poor
        performance
    Performs evaluations based upon standards
    Reports nurses who fail to meet standards
        to Board of Nursing

The Educator:
    Incorporates standards into curriculum
    Promotes integration of standards
        by student
    Evaluates student performance based
        on standards
    Provides first role model for student
        as to the expectation of life-long
        learning, professional accountability

Figure 4.1   Competence Accountability.

was responsible for determining that a nurse is competent to practice nursing in Alabama.

The NCSBN (1996) has described continued competence of the nurse as a joint responsibility. Similarly, major accountability for attaining, maintaining, and enhancing competence rests with the licensee. Accountability also rests with the licensee's employer, educational program, nursing board, and the discipline of nursing. Figure 4.1 clearly depicts how collaboration among these major entities will facilitate competence assurance.

■ Continued Competency: A State Responsibility

While ensuring continued competence of nurses upon entry into practice has continued as a major effort, nursing boards have also expanded efforts to ensure competency of

nurses throughout their careers. In Nebraska, the Board of Nursing, Nursing Association, and the Licensed Practical Nurse Association developed a strategic initiative to fulfill education, practice, and consumer demands of nursing. This leadership group believed that it was crucial to facilitate consensus, foster communication, and develop political awareness in the nursing community prior to creating a continued competence model for Nebraska.

The nurse leadership group also included in its strategic plan an initiative to "define initial, new role and continued role competencies for nursing" and to synthesize "core competencies for RNs and LPNs" (Burbach & Exstrom, 1999, p. 11).

In concert with recommendations from other states and upon recommendation of the Texas Nurses Association, the Texas State Board of Nursing supported legislation to "develop, monitor, and evaluate pilot programs to ascertain the effectiveness of mechanisms for assuring maintenance of clinical competency by registered nurses" (NCSBN, 1998b, p. 183).

The Oklahoma Board of Nursing, in an effort to protect Oklahoma's consumers, appointed a task force and gave it the responsibility for developing recommendations to verify continued competence in the practice of nursing. The task force recommended implementation of a "professional practice profile." The nursing board and Oklahoma's nurses believe that the plan will provide consumer documentation of "the nurses" continued competence to practice, provide direction for future practice related learning and or career development" and support license renewal. Likewise, the Board believes that "the professional practice profile showcases an individual's achievements and ascribes value to everyday activities and experiences" (NCSBN, 1998a, p. 187).

The Alabama Board of Nursing has considered various ideas and perspectives within nursing about regulation of practice in the interest of public protection. However, the Board acknowledged that any plan to ensure continued competence should also recognize public and consumer concerns. Accordingly, a four-phase research project was authorized to determine perceptions of consumers, licensees, educators, and representatives of selected organizations regarding competence in nursing.

Nursing competence is an evolving regulatory mandate in Kentucky. The Kentucky Board of Nursing (KBN) developed a position paper entitled "Accountability and Responsibility of Licensees to Assure Nursing Competency in February 1997" (McGuire, Stanhope, & Weisenbeck, 1998). This document proposed a regulatory model for demonstrating continuing competence and stimulated discussion and examination of critical issues. Major tenets of the model suggest that every nurse is answerable for continued competence. The Kentucky Board surveyed licensed nurses to

identify skills and abilities essential for nursing practice in the 21st century. This projected postentry competence model could mandate maintenance of a file or portfolio to illustrate evidence of professional competence (McGuire, Stanhope, & Weisenbeck, 1998).

■ Continued Competency: Impetus for Change from Vested Stakeholders

Regulatory boards are investigating requirements for postentry competency. Several models of ensuring practitioners' competence are evolving. These models will raise issues regarding costs, feasibility, and even the validity of employing structural models to determine competency-based nursing practice. Germane to the nursing regulatory boards' investigations and decision-making are the 11 policy issues raised by the Citizen Advocacy Center (CAC). Exploration of these policy issues will assist regulatory boards in their quests for models to ensure that practitioners are competent throughout their careers. Table 4.1 lists the essential questions that merit examination.

Important guidance is contained in comments offered by the National Council of State Boards of Nursing relative to competence assurance mechanisms. It noted that nursing regulatory boards should be "looking for an APPLE" in approaches to assuring competence. More specifically, the Council has stated that these models should be "*administratively* feasible, *publicly* credible, *professionally* acceptable, *legally* defensible, and *economically* feasible" (NCSBN, 1996, p. 2).

■ Competency and Legal Issues

Toni Massaro, attorney for National Council of State Boards of Nursing (Massaro, personal communication, 1987), responded to an

---

TABLE 4.1 Essential Questions for Regulatory Boards in Consideration of Models for Examination of Competency

---

1. What techniques should be employed to evaluate continuing competence?

2. Should practitioners be given the option of demonstrating continuing competence by a variety of approved techniques, or should licensing boards specify the one or ones to be utilized?

3. How frequently should licensees be required to demonstrate competence?

4. Should all licensees, or only those whose performance causes the licensing board to question their competence, be required periodically to demonstrate their continuing competence? If the latter, what criteria (markers) should apply?

5. What relationship, if any, should exist between licensing board continuing competence requirements and those of specialty certification boards? On what basis might licensing recognize and accept the findings of specialty boards?

6. Is recertification a de facto limited license? If so, is it fair or good policy to grant a general license to first-time licensees but only a limited license at the time of recertification?

7. What needs to be done to ensure that a recertification system meets the required legal standards of fairness, reliability, accuracy, and nondiscrimination?

8. How should continuing education needs assessment be accomplished? Are all methods equally viable?

9. Who should pay the costs of recertification? Licensees? The state? What is affordable?

10. What rules of confidentiality should apply to recertification information? What information should be provided to the public concerning the results of assessments?

11. What is the legal status of a licensee who cannot meet recertification standards? Should the licensee be given a period of time to upgrade his or her skills? If so, how long? What is the legal status of a license during this interim period? Is the fact that the licensee has not been recertified public information?

NCSBN inquiry regarding the legal implications of alternative state-imposed regulatory schemes to govern continued competency. He outlined legal principles to guide regulatory boards in selecting a regulation approach, as listed in Table 4.2.

In addition, Massaro stated that the United States Constitution limits the state's authority to regulate the professions in two ways. First, the regulatory scheme must bear a rational relationship to a valid stated purpose. Second, the regulatory scheme must provide a person who is denied the right to practice the profession—or a specialty within that profession—certain procedural rights, such as notice and an opportunity to be heard about the denial.

■ Continuing Education

Mandatory continuing education is the method some nursing regulatory boards have selected to deal with demonstration of continuing competence by its licensees. Thirty-two of the 61 member boards of the National Council of State Boards of Nursing have mandatory continuing education for relicensure. Four of those 32 jurisdictions have mandatory continuing education for advanced practice only. In 29 jurisdictions, continuing education also is used for reinstatement of a license. Continuing education by subject matter is required as part of licensure maintenance in five jurisdictions. For example, Florida requires evidence of continuing educa-

---

TABLE 4.2   Legal Principles for Guiding Regulatory Boards in Selecting a Regulation Approach

---

- First, the more restrictive a regulatory scheme is on the right to practice nursing, the more vulnerable that regulatory scheme becomes to legal challenges on constitutional grounds, and to resistance from the profession. As such, the objective basis for increased regulation should be clear and documented.

- Second, the more subjective the regulatory requirements are (e.g., peer review versus an objective written examination), the more vulnerable the requirements are to charges of unlawful arbitrariness, discrimination or unreasonableness. Correlatively, subjective requirements must be accompanied by greater procedural mechanisms, to protect against unfairness or discrimination. These procedures, which may include evidentiary hearings, involve time and money.

- Third, increased regulation of the profession may have anti-competitive effects. Special licensure, relicensure, certification or other restrictions on the right to practice nursing will create a special group of nurses who have either met the qualifications, or have been "grandfathered" in. This group may be able to charge higher rates for their special services, or may enjoy an advantage in the employment market generally. Increased regulation also may extend the time necessary for individuals to enter the new field and reduce access to the field. These anti-competitive effects may violate the federal antitrust laws, 15 U. S. C. § 1 (1975), unless the regulation is expressly authorized and actively supervised by the state. This means that the state legislature must expressly authorize any regulation that restrains competition and must participate actively in establishing the terms of the regulation, and in monitoring and enforcing the regulation. The state cannot safely delegate general authority to the state board members to adopt regulations with anti-competitive effects; nor can the board cede its regulatory authority to private entities. In either situation, a court might conclude that the regulatory scheme violated the antitrust laws and enjoin enforcement of the regulations, or award money damages.

(Reprinted from Direct Communication to the State Boards of Nursing, Toni Massaro, 1987, pp. 1–2)

---

tion in HIV/AIDS and domestic violence for all relicensures (NCSBN, 1998b).

In 1994, after 12 years of mandatory continuing education, the Colorado Board of Nursing abolished such a requirement. The Board's action was not due to lack of support for continuing education by individual licensees, but rather to lack of support for continuing education being tied to license renewal (Colorado Board of Nursing [CBN], 1994).

Challenges against the effectiveness of continuing education as means of ensuring competence have become intertwined with other national concerns about competent practice, competency of practitioners, and the role of regulatory agencies in ensuring public protection. The PEW Commission believes that most professionals concur with its assessment that nursing competence diminishes following initial licensure and that continuing education does not ensure competence (Finocchio et al., 1998).

An important issue regarding use of continuing education as an indicator of continued competence is its significance to the nurse's scope of practice. To ensure practice competency, educational experience should be structured to enhance or further knowledge, skills, and abilities that are within the nurse's present or future scope of practice (NCSBN, 1996). A similar concern with continuing education is that assessment of outcome is generally limited to attainment of theoretical knowledge or technical skills. Continuing education evaluation generally does not measure the extent to which recently obtained knowledge, skills, and abilities are applied in the nurses' work setting. Therefore continued competence in the nurse's work setting is clearly not guaranteed through the obtainment of continuing education units (NCSBN, 1996). Other alternatives actually may prove to be more beneficial in determining competency-based nursing practice after initial licensure (e.g., retesting).

■ *Retesting*

Anthony Zara, NCSBN Director of Testing, in discussion of the logic of testing as a continued competence evaluation method, asserted that,

> although not stated explicitly, the logic of requiring licensure candidates to pass an entry-level examination is that the regulatory board needs some objective evidence that the candidate can demonstrate the requisite knowledge, skills, and abilities, necessary to practice safely prior to licensure. (Zara, 1997, p. 1)

Similarly, Zara warns that "the regulatory boards' need for independent evidence of competence for entry-level candidates logically leads to the need for that same evidence for licensure renewal" (Zara, 1997, p. 3). Likewise, he endorsed a flexible continued competency testing design, including a test in the focused area of practice, concentrating on what the nurse genuinely needs to know to provide safe and effective care. Zara's proposal would entail use of specialist licenses with a designated practice area and demonstration of suitable accountability. His idea of mandatory postentry testing merits consideration because it would provide nursing regulatory boards with a consistent licensure requirement. Similarly, Reeves (1996) noted that many individuals overlook the fact that, whereas almost all regulated professionals qualify for and are issued generic licenses, they tend to specialize in practice. He also raised the question: "What would be the point of imposing a generic continuing competency exam on a . . . psychiatric nurse?" In contrast to Zara's contentions, Reeves raised

five significant questions regarding testing for continued competence.

1. How could a board funded almost completely by the proceeds of license renewal fees afford legally defensible competency exams?

2. What about the vested property rights of a professional license?

3. Should those property rights be taken away through a hopelessly flawed reexamination process?

4. How much litigation would occur when significant numbers of experienced professionals lose licenses in this process?

5. What is the point of giving exams if no one fails? (Reeves, 1996, p. 6)

Reeves also admonished regulators to try to envision the political commotion that would occur if experienced and ethical providers lost their licenses for reasons other then unethical or illegal conduct. He also considered the fiscal impact of competency exams, noting the tremendous amount of tax dollars required—for constructing and staffing educational facilities that train health care professionals—which would be lost for each professional who lost a license due to a flawed reexamination.

■ *Concluding Statement*

The issue of validating continued competency of practicing nurses is of paramount concern. In the latter part of the 20th century, considerable debate centered on issues of competency-based practice. Advocates for continuing education units, as a mandatory requirement for relicensure, pitted their rationale against advocates for retesting or other methods (e.g., portfolio review). Issues continue to surface regarding competency-based practice, but the recent Institute of Medicine's report (National Academies News, 1999) concerning the number of medical errors occurring yearly in the U.S. health care system underscores the need for some reliable method of validating continued safe practice. Competence is definable and measurable. Continued competence in the practice of nursing can be observed directly through a number of viable assessment modes, including testing and retesting, professional portfolios, employer review, peer review, certification and recertification, and the like.

Regardless of the method of assessment used to measure continued competence, which is bound to be complex, the process itself must be based on valid, reliable, and legally defensible standards. The challenge for the new millennium is to find an adequate middle ground that ensures public safety on the one hand and provides a reasonable degree of stability and autonomy to nursing practitioners on the other hand.

■ References

American Nurses Association. (1985). *Code for nurses with interpretive statements.* Kansas City, MO: Author.

American Nurses Association. (1995). *Nursing's social policy statement.* Washington, DC: American Nurses Publishing.

American Nurses Association. (1998). *Standards of clinical nursing practice* (2nd ed.). Washington, DC: American Nurses Publishing.

Burbach, V., & Exstrom, S. (1999). Continued competence in Nebraska: Process and progress. *Issues, 20*(2), 1, 5, 9, 11.

Campbell, B. (1998, May). *Consultation report on competence assessment.* College of Nurses of Ontario. Canada: Toronto, Ontario.

Citizen Advocacy Center. (1997). *Continued professional competence: Can we assure it?* Washington, DC: Author.

Colorado Board of Nursing. (1994). *Press release/continuing education.* Denver: Author.

Finocchio, L., Dower, C., Blick N., Gragnola, C., & the Taskforce on Health Care Workforce Regulation. (Eds.). (1998). *Strengthening consumer protection: Priorities for health care workforce regulation.* San Francisco: PEW Health Professions Commission.

Gross, S. (1984). *Of foxes and hen houses: Licensing and the health professions.* Westport, CT: Quorum Books.

Kobs, A. (1997). Competence: The shot heard around the nursing world. *Nursing Management, 28*(2), 10–13.

Mann, J. (1999). *Assessment of nursing competency in Alabama.* Montgomery, AL: Alabama Board of Nursing.

McGuire, C., Stanhope, M., & Weisenbeck, S. (1998). Nursing competence— An evolving regulatory issue in Kentucky. *Nursing Administration Quarterly, 23*(1), 24–28.

National Academies News. (1999). *Preventing death and injuries from medical errors requires dramatic, system wide change.* (Press release). Author.

National Council of State Boards of Nursing. (1996). *Assuring competence: A regulatory responsibility.* Chicago: Author.

National Council of State Boards of Nursing. (1998a). *Member boards profile.* Chicago: Author.

National Council of State Boards of Nursing. (1998b). *1998 Concurrent educational research sessions.* Chicago: Author.

Nightingale, F. (1859/1946). *Notes in nursing: What it is and what it is not.* Philadelphia: Lippincott.

Patterson, C. (1998). The current health care environment and the Joint Commission's Agenda for Change. *Issues, 19*(3), 12–13.

Reeves, R. (1996). *A response to the recommendations of PEW Health Professions Commission Task Force on Regulation.* Montgomery: Alabama Board of Nursing.

Sheets, V. (1996, July). *Public protection or professional self-preservation* [On-line]. Available: http://www.ncsbn.org/files/online/publicpro.html.

Swankin, D.A. (1995). *The role of licensing in assuring the continued competence of health care professionals: A resource guide.* Washington, DC: Citizens Advocacy Center.

Zara, A. (1997). *Perspectives on continued competence: Retesting for competence.* Paper presented at National Council State Board of Nursing, Area Meeting. Chicago: Author.

■ *Editor's Questions for Discussion*

Discuss the relationships between the content presented by Yocom and Thomas (Chapter 3) and that presented by Jones-Dickson. What information has been obtained from consumer groups regarding criteria for competency in nursing practice? What assurance is there in relicensure that quality care is being provided? How can competency standards be developed and enforced? How effective has mandatory continuing education been to ensure competency? What evidence exists regarding relationships between mandatory continuing education and competency?

Discuss the issues concerning measurement of competency. How can regulatory boards come to agree on approaches for developing models to measure competency? Respond to each of the questions in Table 4.1 regarding the development of models. How may consensus be reached by regulatory boards, consumers, and professional associations regarding responses to those questions?

Discuss alternatives for determining competency after initial licensure. Debate the pros and cons of retesting for competency in licensure renewal. How could consistency be developed in such retesting for those who have specialized in practice? Address each of the questions posed by Reeves (1996) concerning testing for continued competence. How could professional organizations and associations join with regulatory boards to address continued competency measurement and needs? Suggest strategies for resolving the continued competency debate and issues.

5

Professional Nursing

Issues and Ethics

Beverly Kopala, PhD, RN

E thical conflicts are numerous and are encountered every day in nursing practice. Some conflicts clearly challenge core beliefs about what ought to be done. Others have a moral component that may go unrecognized. Although many ethical conflicts can be examined and dealt with thoughtfully over time, others allow little time for reflection. In either case, professionals must make the best decisions they can, based on the information and resources available to them at the time. In this chapter, I address ethical issues and struggles for nurses in various areas of practice.

■ The Nurse as Person and Professional

When something has value, it is important to the individual, group, organization, society, or to all of these. Personal, professional, organizational, and societal values shape a person's choices and behavior. Personal values, influenced by family, friends, culture, religion, education, experiences and other factors, account for differing viewpoints about what ought to be done when an ethical conflict arises.

Professional values such as integrity, altruism, autonomy, respect for human dignity, and social justice (American Association of Colleges of Nursing [AACN], 1998) are learned and reinforced in educational and practice settings. A person with moral integrity has a commitment to moral principles, values, or norms and defends them when they are threatened. A nurse's integrity is expressed in actions that are congruent with the nursing's code of ethics and professional standards. According to the preamble of the American Nurses Association (ANA) *Code for Nurses With Interpretive Statements* (1985), nurses base their clinical judgments on consequences and on universal moral principles, including autonomy, beneficence, nonmaleficence, veracity, confidentiality, fidelity, and justice as fairness.

A health care organization's values are expressed in its philosophy, mission statement, and policies. To minimize moral distress, it is important that nurses select a work environment in which organizational values and the nurse's personal and professional values do not conflict frequently. Societal values are evident in societal policies, laws, and the rights that society chooses to grant to its members. Members of the society expect that nurses will strive for the individual's well-being and the welfare of society.

As individuals and professionals, nurses have duties or obligations to others. Nurses have duties to patients and their families, other health care providers, employers, and to society. Nurses also have duties to themselves and their families. Sometimes, these duties conflict.

When values, principles, or duties conflict, a moral choice is required. Sometimes, the choice is easy and made effortlessly, out of habit. At other times, the decision is difficult. Regardless of potential difficulties, nurses must act ethically in their roles as educators, researchers, practitioners, and administrators, and in their relationships with and responsibilities to others, whether at the individual, organizational, societal, or global level.

■ Nursing Education

An examination of recent nursing practice literature reveals that minimal attention has been given to numerous ethical issues arising for students, faculty, nursing staff, and administrators within and outside schools of nursing. As a result, nurses generally are not aware of conflicts encountered in this area. Yet, recognizing and resolving issues in nursing education is as important as it is in practice settings.

Classroom and Clinical Issues

Questions of academic dishonesty arise in the classroom and clinical setting. Cheating on examinations, falsifying data on patients' charts, and lying about making home visits are several examples of such dishonesty. These unprofessional behaviors erode trust and can jeopardize patient safety if the health care provider lacks requisite knowledge, provides incorrect information on which crucial treatment decisions are made, or fails to make indicated assessments. To help faculty foster expected professional values and support personal and professional integrity, students may be asked to abide by an honor code or sign an academic integrity statement. Adherence to such a code can create conflicts and distress for students. Although they have agreed to report dishonest or otherwise inappropriate actions, students may find themselves required to report a friend's behavior and may fear retaliation for reporting someone or an incident.

If society is to have adequate numbers of nurses and benefit from their knowledge and skills, the learning laboratory cannot remain solely within the school of nursing. Patients, their families, various agencies, and agency employees must also be involved in students' education.

Although questions about students and licensed professionals "practicing" on patients have been raised, patients generally benefit from contact with students. However, burdens also are associated with this involvement. For example, early in their professional education, nursing students require more time to complete a task and use more resources than seasoned practitioners. Preoperative or pain medication may be delayed because of difficulties in calculating dosages or manipulating syringes and vials. In addition, equipment may be contaminated or otherwise unnecessarily wasted while a student is still learning a procedure. Resources are costly and finite; they must be used with care.

Different types of conflicts have been reported by students. Some are related to (a) rights of students, faculty, and employees; (b) personal, professional, and scientific integrity; (c) discrimination; (d) abuse of drugs and alcohol; (e) struggles surrounding: patients' rights and staff paternalism; (f) dying with dignity; (g) patient safety; (h) lack of adherence to advance directives; and (i) conflicts between or among nurses, clients, family, and physicians (Cobb, 1995).

Faculty and Administrators

Conflicts can surface in the teaching role. For example, curriculum vitae and letters of reference are required as part of the employment process. Although accuracy of this summary of a person's work is an expectation, there have been anecdotal reports—although rare—of falsification of credentials. Faculty members are frequently asked to write letters of reference for students, graduates, or peers seeking admission to graduate school or employment. When concerned about an individual's ability or performance, faculty must decide whether to write a letter of reference or not to do so. If deciding to provide the reference, faculty then must decide whether to write (a) a positive let-

ter focusing on abilities the person has demonstrated, (b) a noncommittal letter of recommendation, or (c) a letter containing information that will likely result in nonacceptance or nonemployment.

Students may recognize when a peer is having difficulty meeting course objectives but may not recognize that this failure can raise ethical issues for faculty. For example, a clinical faculty member who consistently spends extra time with one student who is exhibiting unsafe behaviors or having difficulty performing or prioritizing tasks, has less time available for other students. If supervision for the majority of students is decreased, the learning of students and oversight of patients may be adversely affected.

Conflicts of interest in academia also have been explored. Examples include faculty (a) coercing students to participate in research, (b) expecting authorship credit on student papers when faculty participation does not warrant it, (c) adopting a textbook in order to obtain a share of royalties, and (d) giving preferential treatment to students who are children of major contributors to the institution (Goldrick, Larson, & Lyons, 1995).

Administrators are not immune to ethical issues related to students, faculty, and clinical agencies. Administrators may find themselves criticized for decisions made, yet constrained from revealing the reasons for their actions because of confidentiality concerns. For example, a student may share personal information about illness, rape, divorce, abuse, suicidal thoughts, drug use, or some other personal problem and request that this information not be revealed to others. Such a situation may require withholding information from faculty who recognize a problem and seek the administrator's assistance. If the student encounters academic difficulty that may be linked to the personal situation, but does not share this with the supervising faculty member, the administrator must decide how to proceed.

Occasionally a faculty member may not be fulfilling contractual duties relating to supervision of students. Staff may find themselves taking on an unexpected or unwanted supervisory role, and administrators at the agency and school must deal with the situation.

■ Nursing Research

Institutional Review Boards (IRBs) were formed in response to societal concerns about exploitation of subjects such as those in the Willowbrook and the Tuskegee syphilis studies. These Boards focus on protecting the rights of human participants in proposed and ongoing federally funded biomedical and behavioral research and must grant approval before such research can proceed.

Research raises ethical issues associated with consent, harm, deception, privacy, and confidentiality (Punch, 1994). Among the principles underlying ethical conduct of research are autonomy, beneficence, nonmaleficence, justice, and veracity. Self-determination and respect for autonomy are evident in the right of a competent person to make decisions and have those decisions respected. Autonomy is the principle underlying informed consent or refusal.

According to Beauchamp and Childress (1994), informed consent for research involves competence, disclosure, understanding, voluntariness, and consent. Competence is a legal term that refers to an individual's ability to understand and make a decision about whether to authorize certain therapeutic interventions or participate in research. Material information, including the purpose and nature of the research, risks, benefits, and the right to withdraw at any time must be disclosed and adequately understood by the potential participant. Voluntariness connotes freedom from coercion and manipulation. The participant, or someone having legal authority to act on the participant's behalf, then gives informed consent or refuses to do so. Although good arguments can be made occasionally for nondisclosure, incorporating substantial deception into research makes its justification difficult.

Assent should be sought from children beginning at about 7 years of age. In general, a researcher should honor a child's refusal to participate, even if the child might be expected to consent if older (Jonsen, Siegler, & Winsdale, 1998).

Several categories of persons may be characterized as vulnerable. They include those who (a) lack decision-making capacity, such as infants, young children, the severely mentally ill, and severely disabled; (b) fear that their care will be compromised by refusal to participate in or withdrawal from the study; (c) are so desperate for some treatment that they will accept great risk; or (d) are motivated to participate solely for incentives offered. These vulnerable potential research participants must be protected from exploitation.

Researchers must attempt to minimize risks to research participants. The degree of risk, whether physical or psychological, is evaluated on the basis of likelihood and magnitude of harm. Minimal risk is no greater than that encountered in everyday life. Maximum risk is certain permanent damage or death. When the risk–benefit ratio is evaluated, potential benefits must exceed or be in proportion to the degree of risk to participants. When the degree of harm exceeds the potential benefit, the proposed research will be difficult to justify.

Therapeutic research offers the possibility of benefit to participants. Nontherapeutic research will yield knowledge and may benefit others in the future, but participants in the study are not expected to derive any direct benefit themselves. Whether children should be allowed to be participants in nontherapeutic research is subject to debate. Whether adults and children have a moral obligation to participate in research, if not for their own benefit but for benefit of others in the future, is also open to discussion.

Respect for privacy means that it is the participant who decides whether to reveal any information and, if so, what information is to be given to whom, when, and where. Measures must be in place to ensure that confidentiality of data (in oral, written, and electronic form) is maintained. Justice is achieved in fair and equitable distribution of benefits and risks to participants, who should not be overrepresented or underrepresented in terms of age, gender, ethnicity, and other characteristics.

In some facilities, participation in research is a condition of employment. Whether it is a requirement or not, nurses with a role in research studies, whether as principal investigators, coinvestigators, data collectors, or in some other capacity, are responsible for ethical conduct. Numerous resources, including research texts, are available to guide the process. In *Ethical Guidelines in the Conduct, Dissemination, and Implementation of Nursing Research,* Silva (1995) addresses relevant topics such as respecting autonomy and personhood, protecting privacy, promoting good and minimizing harm, distributing benefits and burdens in the selection of participants, dealing with scientific misconduct, and maximizing benefits and minimizing harm to animal subjects.

Research is conducted for the benefit of individuals and society. Although investigator misconduct in the form of data falsification, misappropriation of funds, or unauthorized research are occasionally reported, the vast majority of research studies are conducted with care, concern, and integrity.

■ Nursing Theory—Caring and the Ethics of Care

Caring is a way of being in the world, and nursing is a practice wherein caring is primary (Benner & Wrubel, 1989). As a concept central to professional nursing practice, caring "encompasses the nurse's empathy for and connection with the patient, as well as the ability to translate these affective characteristics into compassionate, sensitive, appropriate care" (AACN, 1998, p. 8). As the essence of nursing, care has moral and ethical dimensions, with the ethics of care guiding nursing knowledge and decision-making (Leininger, 1990). Watson's (1988) theory for nursing integrates human science and human care.

Care has four aspects—caring about another, taking care of another, caregiving, and care receiving—each of which, in turn, has a moral dimension (Tronto, 1993). An ethics of care demands that moral elements associated with each phase—attentiveness, assuming responsibility for care, competence, and responsiveness of the care-receiver to the care-giver—be integrated into a whole (Tronto, 1993). It is a whole that requires knowledge of the situation, its participants, and the care process. It also requires making judgments that must consider the social, political, and personal context (Tronto, 1993). According to Chambliss (1996), "caring not only describes what nurses do, but also what they believe they should do" (p. 63). The ethics of care is a less traditional, relationship-based approach to moral reasoning that has become closely linked with nursing. Instead of emphasizing rules, rights, or weighing of benefits and burdens, this approach focuses on engagement, context, and partiality.

All approaches to moral reasoning have shortcomings. It is suggested that the ethics of care may be (a) too vague, (b) exploitive of caregiver, (c) ineffectual in resolving ethical conflicts, (d) relativistic, (e) too partial, (f) too intense, (g) too focused on the nurse versus less on the patient, and (h) compromising of patient care if an emotional response is required (Crigger, 1997). Kuhse (1997), who examined caring from perspectives of nurses, women, and ethics, holds that care is a necessary though not sufficient basis for ethics and that "an adequate ethic needs justice as well as care" (p. x). According to Beauchamp and Childress (1994), ethics of care is a theory that is underdeveloped, but not necessarily incorrect.

■ Nursing Practice

According to the *Code for Nurses* (ANA, 1985), both consequences and universal moral principles provide bases for prescribing and justifying nursing actions. Several of these principles are used here as organizing concepts to address some of many possible conflicts encountered in nursing practice.

Capable adult decision-makers are expected to be able to exercise informed judgments and give informed consent or refusal of treatment, including life-sustaining treatment. Partially capable decision-makers may be able to make informed decisions only at certain times of day or about certain treatment plans versus others. Efforts to respect autonomy can be problematic when concerns about an individual's decision-making capacity arise. On occasion, health care providers may engage in paternalistic actions by attempting to override a competent patient's informed choice.

To be able to make informed choices, to be able to trust communications of health care providers, and for numerous other reasons, patients need truthful information. Deception occurs in situations where placebos are used, necessary information is withheld, or erroneous or misleading information is provided to the patient.

When persons who have expressed goals, values, and life plans are no longer capable of making decisions for themselves, substitute judgment is used. In this case, the surrogate decision maker considers these expressions of values, goals, and plans and attempts to decide as the patient would if he or she were capable of doing so. Choices should reflect the patient's values, not the surrogate's.

Surrogates are expected to make decisions in the best interests of patients who have never been autonomous or of persons who are no longer capable of making autonomous choices and have not expressed values that can guide a surrogate's decision. Parents, generally, are given authority to make decisions for a child because they are expected to have their child's best interests at heart; moreover, the child might be expected to develop values similar to those of the parents. Sometimes parents (or a surrogate) make a decision that does not appear to be in a patient's best interests. If it falls within the wide range of acceptable alternatives, that decision should be honored. However, if a decision seems egregious, or outside an acceptable range, health care providers are expected to protest it. One challenge may occur in a court of law, as sometimes happens when parents' religious practices preclude their child from receiving potentially life-saving treatment.

On occasion, a nurse may find it necessary to refuse to comply with a patient's or parent's morally justified request because doing so would compromise that nurse's core values. In this case, the nurse would need to follow institutional policy related to conscientious objection. Although transferring care of the patient to another nurse who does not have similar objections may be possible, abandoning the patient is not acceptable. Conscientious objection should be a rare occurrence. If it happens with any regularity, the nurse may need to seek employment elsewhere.

Nurses strive to do good for and avoid harming their patients. However, doing good may also bring with it risk of some harm. For example, negative side effects of chemotherapy accompany beneficial effects of treatment. Giving adequate amounts of medication to relieve a terminally ill patient's pain may accelerate the patient's death. Benefits of treatment must be weighed against potential harm or burdens. Sometimes, health care providers may find it difficult to understand a patient's decision that the benefits of treatment are not worth the actual or potential harms.

Issues of distributive justice often arise in relation to access to and allocation of scarce resources, such as organs for transplantation. However, a nurse's time and expertise also are resources that are rationed; some patients get more, others get less. When a different level of quality care is provided to patients who are large donors to the facility or when financial interests, gifts, honoraria, and the like influence use of products, devices, or clinical judgment, conflicts of interest in practice are evident (Goldrick, Larson, & Lyons, 1995) and issues of fairness arise.

Today, nurses in all practice settings are providing care for increasing numbers of patients while implementing cost containment strategies. The challenge for nursing lies in maintaining quality care for those affected by such measures.

■ Research and Nursing Practice

Researchers have explored ethical conflicts experienced by nurses in various settings. For example, 12 nurses caring for patients in acute, long-term, and home care settings reported concerns related to (a) truth-telling and withholding information, (b) access issues and inequalities of care, (c) conflict between professional and organizational values, and (d) reporting of broken rules (Gold, Chambers, & Dvorak, 1995). A group of 136 nurses attending an ethics session at a national oncology conference reported undertreatment of pain, truth-telling, and the right to refuse treatment as three ethical issues of greatest importance to them (Ferrell & Rivera, 1995). Approximately one third of 118 pediatric nurse practitioner respondents in ambulatory settings reported experiencing conflicts in the parent/child and practitioner relationship, including disagree-

ments with parents' decisions about treatment, protecting the child's rights, and confidentiality (Butz, Redman, Fry, & Kolodner, 1998). Research on ethical conflicts encountered in varied nurse practice settings or roles is summarized by Redman and Hill (1997).

■ Nursing Administration—Service

Nursing service administrators face ethical conflicts when attempting to balance needs and interests of patients, staff, and the health care organization. In one survey (Camunas, 1994), 315 nurse executive respondents identified three issues as foremost in presenting ethical dilemmas: (a) allocating and rationing scarce resources, (b) making decisions about staff level and mix, and (c) developing and maintaining care standards. Measures designed to preserve financial integrity of an institution also can create ethical concerns. For example, managed care threatens professional integrity and creates conflicts for nurse executives forced to choose between cutting costs and losing their jobs (Camunas, 1998).

When units are short-staffed, concerns about patient safety may be voiced to administrators. A nurse's behavior may suggest misuse of alcohol or drugs, perhaps with medications diverted for the nurse's use. Occasionally a nurse may threaten to reveal, to others outside the organization, a situation perceived as morally offensive and not being adequately addressed.

Keeping the patient foremost, advocating quality care, acting justly, challenging evolving policies and practices, and fostering integrity of the organization confront today's nurse administrator (Erlen, 1997). According to Camunas (1994), "the leadership that nurse administrators provide in the establishment and maintenance of an ethical climate can directly affect the quality of moral reasoning and ethical decision-making throughout the institution" (p. 45).

▪ Future of Nursing

For the profession to remain viable, it must attract new members and retain others. Just as nurses care for and about patients, they must care about other members of their profession. Such caring requires that seasoned nurses recognize difficulties inherent in being a recent graduate or a nurse new to a unit or type of practice and attempt to facilitate their transition.

For the profession to continue to progress, measures must be taken to ensure the safety of its members. To minimize risk, certain protective measures (e.g., blood and body fluid precautions) are required by law. However, these measures only protect against certain communicable diseases. There is increasing concern about the physical and psychological harm that may come to nurses delivering care in settings such as the patient's home and the emergency room. Nurses need to consider the magnitude of risk to themselves and their responsibility to patients in evaluating how to respond to threats to their own safety. Health care organizations need to establish policies and institute measures designed to protect staff from great risk of harm.

The future of nursing is closely linked to societal values that are expressed in public policy. Social, economic, and health policy decisions about access, resource allocation, and distribution of benefits and burdens reflect society's priorities. The values that society chooses to support will effect changes in the health care system and influence the types of practitioners needed (Sullivan, 1998b).

Nursing is challenged to have an increasingly international perspective. Johnstone (1998) holds that nursing ethics must have a global agenda and that bioethics has neglected ethical issues involving care of (a) the mentally ill; (b) children, partners, and elders who have been abused; (c) the homeless; (d) those living in poverty; (e) the disabled; and (f) other vulnerable populations throughout the world.

Nurses have the opportunity to respond to this challenge through practice, education, and research initiatives.

Change is a certainty. How nurses respond, as individuals and as a group—being proactive, reactive, or silent—will have an impact on future nursing practice. According to Sullivan, "As nurses and citizens of the world, we are creating the future by what we do or do not do today. The world of the 21st century is bound only by our imaginations, our values, and our resources" (1998a, p. 192).

▪ Resources

A variety of resources are available to nursing students and nurses facing ethically problematic situations. These include case conferences, ethics consults and committees and centers, the literature, education offerings, and the Internet. A major ANA site for accessing position statements and other information is http://www.nursingworld.org/ethics/.

Case conferences may involve patients and families, physicians, nurses, pastoral care representatives, ethics consultants, and others involved in care management. These conferences provide a forum for persons to express both similar and conflicting views and, perhaps, arrive at a plan or alternative that enables resolution of disagreements about what ought to be done. If no agreement is reached initially, those involved may become more aware of and, possibly, more sensitive to others' values, goals, and beliefs.

The ANA is attentive to ethical issues, and in 1990, it established a Center for Ethics and Human Rights. Center activities include (a) consultation with state associations, nurse educators, administrators, nurses, and others, including human rights organizations; (b) policy development related to health care and end of life issues, genetic advances, and diversity issues; and (c) ethics education and outreach.

The ANA *Code for Nurses With Interpretive Statements* (1985) document provides ethical guidelines for nursing practice. The Code currently is being reviewed and analyzed for possible revision. The ANA also publishes position statements such as (a) *Assisted Suicide* (1994a), (b) *Foregoing Medically Provided Nutrition and Hydration* (1995a), (c) *The Right to Accept or Reject an Assignment* (1995c), (d) *Risk Versus Responsibility in Providing Nursing Care* (1994b), and (e) *Promotion of Comfort and Relief of Pain in Dying Patients* (1995b). Position statements are designed to clarify the stance of the professional organization on an issue. In addition, state nurse's associations may have individuals or committees to assist with the resolution of ethical issues at the local level. Other specialty organizations also address ethical issues. For example, the Oncology Nursing Society (ONC) publishes positions statements such as *Endorsement of the American Nurse's Association Position Statement on Active Euthanasia and Assisted Suicide* (1997a), *Cancer Pain Management* (1998), and *The Use of Placebos for Pain Management in Patients With Cancer* (1997b). Additionally, *The Core Curriculum for Oncology Nursing* (Gwin & Richters, 1998) includes a section on ethics.

The Joint Commission on Accreditation of Healthcare Organizations (JCAHO) requires that organizations receiving its accreditation have a mechanism to handle ethical issues raised in the course of care delivery. These mechanisms are often found in policies that provide direction for obtaining an ethics consult or accessing an ethics committee and for handling cases of conscientious objection. The functions of these ethics committees include reviewing, consulting, and making recommendations to help resolve difficult cases.

Nursing literature is responsive to ethical issues in nursing practice, education, research, and administration. Many current nursing ethics texts are available, and professional journals routinely publish articles or columns addressing ethical issues or concerns. *Nursing Ethics,* an international journal, is devoted exclusively to the subject. In addition, a number of frameworks designed to guide ethical decision-making have been published. Some Internet sites allow nurses and others to obtain answers to questions about ethical practice. A number of computerized databases can be accessed to locate ethics research, reviews, and other literature, but Bioethicsline is specific to ethics literature. Ethics education also can take the form of ethics rounds, formal coursework, and continuing education offerings that can develop knowledge and skills for recognizing, reflecting on, and resolving ethical issues.

■ Concluding Statement

Ethical conflicts arise in all practice settings. The rapidity with which decisions must be made falls on a continuum. At one end of the continuum, a decision must be made immediately and with little time for reflection. On such occasions, a nurse attempts to make the best possible choice from available alternatives given the information at hand. At the other end of the continuum, considerable time is available to gather information, consult with others, and reflect on what should be done. Many decisions fall somewhere in between. Thus it is possible to take advantage of available resources even if, for those immediate decisions, resources are used later to examine a decision made or an action taken.

When an ethical dilemma has been resolved, the nurse should examine the choices made to determine if anything could or should have been done differently. Such reflection can help the decision maker when faced with a similar situation in the future. It may also help in anticipating and preventing some ethical conflicts from arising.

■ *References*

American Association of Colleges of Nursing. (1998). *The essentials of baccalaureate education for professional nursing practice.* Washington, DC: Author.

American Nurses Association. (1985). *Code for nurses with interpretive statements.* Kansas City, MO: Author.

American Nurses Association. (1994a). *Assisted suicide.* Washington, DC: Author.

American Nurses Association. (1994b). *Position statement on risk versus responsibility in providing nursing care.* Washington, DC: Author.

American Nurses Association. (1995a). *Position statement on foregoing medically provided nutrition and hydration.* Washington, DC: Author.

American Nurses Association. (1995b). *Position statement on promotion of comfort and relief of pain in dying patients.* Washington, DC: Author.

American Nurses Association. (1995c). *The right to accept or reject an assignment.* Washington, DC: Author.

Beauchamp, T. L., & Childress, J. F. (1994). *Principles of biomedical ethics* (4th ed.). New York: Oxford University Press.

Benner, P., & Wrubel, J. (1989). *The primacy of caring.* Menlo Park, CA: Addison-Wesley.

Butz, A. M., Redman, B. K., Fry, S. T., & Kolodner, K. (1998). Ethical conflicts experienced by certified pediatric nurse practitioners in ambulatory settings. *Journal of Pediatrics Health Care, 12*(4), 183–190.

Camunas, C. (1994). Ethical dilemmas of nurse executives: Part I. *Journal of Nursing Administration, 24*(7/8), 45–51.

Camunas, C. (1998). Managed care, professional integrity, and ethics. *Journal of Nursing Administration, 28*(3), 7–9.

Chambliss, D. F. (1996). *Beyond caring.* Chicago: University of Chicago Press.

Cobb, L. A. (1995). Editorial. Ethics most relevant. *Journal of Professional Nursing, 11*(5), 257–258.

Crigger, N. J. (1997). The trouble with caring: A review of eight arguments against an ethic of care. *Journal of Professional Nursing, 13*(4), 217–221.

Erlen, J. A. (1997). Ethical issues for nurse administrators in a changing environment with evolving roles. In S. Moorehead & D. G. Huber (Chair of Board) (Eds.), *Nursing roles: Evolving or recycled?* (pp. 15–28). Thousand Oaks, CA: Sage.

Ferrell, B. R., & Rivera, L. M. (1995). Ethical decision making in oncology. *Cancer Practice, 3,* 94–99.

Gold, C., Chambers, J., & Dvorak, E. M. (1995). Ethical dilemmas in the lived experience of nursing practice. *Nursing Ethics, 2*(2), 131–142.

Goldrick, B. A., Larson, E., & Lyons, D. (1995). Conflict of interest in academia. *Image: Journal of Nursing Scholarship, 27*(1), 65–69.

Gwin, R. R., & Richters, J. E. (1998). Selected ethical issues in cancer care. In J. K. Itano & K. N. Taoka (Eds.), *Core curriculum for oncology nursing* (3rd ed., pp. 741–745). Philadelphia: Saunders.

Johnstone, M. J. (1998). Advancing nursing ethics: Time to set a new global agenda? *International Nursing Review, 45*(2), 43.

Jonsen, A. R., Siegler, M., & Winslade, W. J. (1998). *Clinical ethics* (4th ed.). New York: McGraw-Hill.

Kuhse, H. (1997). *Caring: Nurses, women and ethics.* Malden, MA: Blackwell.

Leininger, M. M. (Ed.). (1990). *Ethical and moral dimensions of care.* Detroit: Wayne State University.

Oncology Nursing Society. (1997a). *Endorsement of the American Nurses Association position statement on active euthanasia and assisted suicide.* Pittsburgh: Author.

Oncology Nursing Society. (1997b). *The use of placebos for pain management in patients with cancer.* Pittsburgh: Author.

Oncology Nursing Society. (1998). *Cancer pain management.* Pittsburgh: Author.

Punch, M. (1994). Politics and ethics in qualitative research. In N. K. Denzin & Y. S. Lincoln (Eds.), *Handbook of qualitative research* (pp. 83–97). Thousand Oaks, CA: Sage.

Redman, B. K., & Hill, M. N. (1997). Studies of ethical conflicts reported by nursing practice settings or roles. *Western Journal of Nursing Research, 19,* 243–260.

Silva, M. C. (1995). *Ethical guidelines in the conduct, dissemination, and implementation of nursing research.* Washington, DC: American Nurses Association.

Sullivan, E. J. (1998a). The future: Imagine the possibilities, Part I—Society. (Editorial). *Journal of Professional Nursing, 14*(4), 191–192.

Sullivan, E. J. (1998b). The future: Imagine the possibilities, Part III—Nursing. (Editorial). *Journal of Professional Nursing, 14*(6), 317–318.

Tronto, J. C. (1993). *Moral boundaries.* New York: Routledge.

Watson, J. (1988). *Nursing: Human science and human care.* New York: National League for Nursing.

■ *Editor's Questions for Discussion*

How may a nurse determine whether her values match those of an organization prior to employment? How are values addressed in nursing education programs? Suggest strategies for preventing academic dishonesty.

Discuss the most common ethical issues in nursing education programs. What ethical issues arise in evaluating qualifications for students entering nursing programs? How should these issues be addressed and resolved? How is equity in grading processes and procedures assured? To what extent are faculty obligated to provide remedial opportunities to students to enable them to acquire clinical skills? What ethical issues are evident in admission, progression, and disqualification of students? How can standards, policies, and procedures prevent or resolve ethical situations?

Identify ethical issues pertaining to faculty appointment, reappointment, retention, promotion, tenure, and disqualification of faculty. How should these issues be anticipated and prevented or resolved when they arise, by whom, and at what level in university programs and by university administration? To what extent and to whom do obligations exist regarding reference letters? How should these obligations be met? What ethical obligations do search and screen committees have regarding employment of faculty and administrators?

Discuss ethical situations presented in conjunction with clinical agencies and experiences for students and faculty. How may conflict situations be anticipated and prevented and resolved when they do occur? What ethical obligations exist for nursing programs and clinical agencies concerning patients, faculty, and students? What processes are essential for students and faculty when conducting research in an agency?

Identify ethical issues that are also associated with legal situations as presented by Lane and Paterson (Chapter 7). What ethical situations may arise in expanded settings for health care, such as parishes, community health care, home health care, palliative care, primary care, rural health care, nursing centers, entrepreneurship, faculty practice, and genetics? Review all the chapters in the Nursing Practice Part of this book. What strategies may effectively resolve ethical issues in various settings discussed?

6

Ethics in International Nursing

Issues and Questions

Anne J. Davis, PhD, DSC, RN, FAAN

Ethics has been a central concern of modern nursing since the time of Florence Nightingale. It plays a role in the socialization of nursing students, in the development of important professional documents, and in the practice of clinical nursing. Development of ethics codes at national and international levels of nursing indicates the importance of nursing's values and ethics to society and to nurses themselves.

During the past 40 years in the Western world, health care ethics and nursing ethics have received renewed attention, which has led to much activity. Health care ethics activities also have been underway elsewhere but they are less known in the West due to lack of English language publications.

This chapter focuses on several interrelated issues: (a) impact of Western philosophical ethics on international nursing ethics; (b) values underlying these ethics and formal mechanisms, such as informed consent and advance directives; (c) whether ethical theories and mechanisms developed in the West should be used in international nursing; and (d) whether nursing can have an international ethics and, if so, what that might mean.

■ *Bioethics and Nursing Ethics in the West*

Western bioethics and nursing ethics can best be characterized as secular ethics that draws its knowledge base from Western moral philosophy. Bioethics and nursing ethics, as applied fields of study, take their content from moral philosophy and use it in research, clinical work, and policy development. In such places as the United States and Western Europe, this moral philosophy has a long history, beginning with the ancient Greek philosophers who raised fundamental questions about life. In philosophical dialogues over the centuries, Western moral philosophy placed emphasis on the individual as an important unit of concern and analysis.

Because of this emphasis, individual rights became a major focus that was later reinforced by the historical era, known as the Enlightenment. The values expressed in the Enlightenment framed both the American and French revolutions. The Bill of Rights and other U.S. national documents written by the founding fathers were greatly influenced by these values. This influence continues today in an America that has become ever more culturally diverse. This reality requires an examination of basic assumptions in the United States about the dominant ethics, the applied ethics in health care drawn from this dominant ethics, and the influence that American bioethics and nursing ethics have had globally. Bioethics has had a great influence on U.S. nursing ethics over the past 40 years, and together they have gone overseas.

In this discussion, I raise some questions about the ethical system in health care in the United States and also about exporting these ideas. This concentration on U.S. influence does not imply that other countries have had no influence on nursing ethics internationally. But certain factors have come together to create a powerful U.S. force of influence in global nursing, including nursing ethics (Davis, 1999).

Values and Ethics

Neither bioethics nor nursing ethics is value free. Nursing ethics, like nursing itself, comprises many values, some of which are unspoken and unacknowledged. In basic ways nursing concepts, including those in ethics, reflect the culture in which they are developed and used. In the United States, an idealized value of individualism and self reliance permeates the society, and this value most certainly has had an impact on nursing values and ethics (Davis, 1999).

What values and concepts specifically have driven U.S. nursing ethics? An early major influence in bioethics as well as in nursing ethics was the publication of a book focused on ethical principles and rules that could be applied in health care ethics (Beauchamp & Childress, 1979). These principles and rules are (a) patient autonomy, (b) do no harm, (c) do good, (d) justice, (e) truth-telling, and (f) promise-keeping. That book detailed various philosophical approaches to ethics and discussed individual rights and the common good. It also discussed ethics theory based on the act itself (means) and ethics theory that looks at consequences of the act (ends). From this and similar books, health care professionals began to think more about patient autonomy and the meanings of not doing harm.

Autonomy tended to be the most prominent ethical principle and driving force in bioethics and nursing ethics. Implementation of this principle led to several formal mechanisms, including informed consent, advanced directives, and the Patient Self-determination Act (P.L. 101–508, November 5, 1990). The value of self-determination underlies these mechanisms, enabling patients to exercise their autonomy. In the United States, a moral good is for individuals to make their own decisions. An independent, responsible adult is the valued cultural ideal. Informed consent for treatment or research participation enables the individual to have considerable impact on the patient's role or research subject. Advanced directives give people an opportunity to decide about their end-of-life care, whereas the patient self-determination act mandates that patients admitted to health care facilities be asked about their advanced directives.

A lesson for international nursing can be taken from an earlier study on ethnics and ethnicity undertaken in a U.S. West Coast city. Terminally ill cancer patients from four ethnic groups and their families were observed and interviewed over time to discover their major concerns and ethical decisions. Health professionals constructed a bioethically ideal patient as self-governing, future oriented, and willing to engage in frank discussions about difficult medical topics, including his or her own death. This constructed ideal patient matches the values underlying Western philosophical bioethics. But not all these patients and their families had been born into or socialized within U.S. culture, with its Western approach to end-of-life ethical questions and therefore were not "ideal" patients (Davis, 2000). Conflicts arose between staff and patients or family values and assumptions underlying health care ethics and the mechanisms for enforcing these values.

Virtues and the Ethics of Care

Although this research looked at end-of-life decisions from an ethical principle perspective, similar questions about virtues and ethics of care can also be raised. That is, could Western moral philosophical virtues be considered central to nursing practice in all cultures? For example in the United States, giving patients truthful information is a virtue. We tell the truth to patients because it is a virtuous thing to do and such information is necessary if patients are to be involved in the decisions about themselves. But is truthfulness considered a virtue in all cultures? And whereas the ethics of care may be central to nursing, what constitutes the essence of caring and does this essence represent a universal value that can and should be used in all cultures?

In an educational exercise in Japan, 90 undergraduate nursing students responded to a case study. In this case study, the older male patient lives with his eldest son and daughter-in-law and is now terminally ill with cancer. Family members, following the norm in Japan, are given the information by the physician and decide not to tell the patient his diagnosis and prognosis. After some time the patient, realizing that he is not getting any better, turns to the nurse and asks her to tell him what is wrong with him.

The students were asked what this nurse should do to be ethical. Most said that the nurse should not tell the patient the truth because the family knew the patient best and notions of obligations were involved. After attending a nursing ethics course that presented both Western ethics and Japanese ethics, the students responded to the same case study. Most of the responses were the same as in the previous exercise, but a few more students said that they would tell, and some said that they should tell but would not tell (Davis, Ota, Suzuki, & Maeda, 1999).

Western ethics in nursing did not make much of an impact on these students. Their cultural norms and values continue strong, and two Japanese cultural concepts are important for understanding these students' responses. Omagase means leaving every decision to others in your group and having a peaceful, relieved feeling of trust because they accept you unconditionally. The other concept and value, satsuru, means that people interact with tacit understanding so that talking about things is not necessary.

Given these cultural concepts, what ethics is used here and can Western ethics be considered a universal? If Japanese nurses do not use Western ethics in ethical decisions and behaviors, does this then allow Western nurses to view the Japanese (and others) as needing more knowledge and development in using Western, universal ethics? An attitude sometimes found in the West is that, if only people in other countries would learn and understand these universal (Western) ethics, they would be ethical. This may be viewed as a new or renewed type of colonialism by those who live in non-Western cultures.

Western Ethics as a Universal

The Western argument goes as follows. Standard Western bioethics and nursing ethics are derived from the morality shared in common by members of Western society. These ethics are held to transcend the divergent religions and metaphysical commitments of multiple moral communities in culturally diverse Western society. Thus standard bioethics and nursing ethics should apply to non-Western societies in which distinct particular moral communities exist (Davis, 1998b).

Two assumptions appear here: (a) a morality is shared by members of Western societies, and (b) this same morality is shared by members of non-Western societies. But it is problematic to take Western ethics as the universal standard of morality for nursing ethics and bioethics without much more deliberation than has occurred to date.

Such an attitude assumes that values everywhere are the same because values are the foundations of ethics. Values, basic to a given way of life, serve to give direction to life but are usually taken for granted; they are not always on a conscious level. Much of what goes into ethical decisions is unarticulated and remains as unspoken values (Davis, Aroskar, Liaschenko, & Drought, 1997). But are these values the same across diverse cultures either within a society or in different societies? Has a type of colonial thinking emerged in equating Western ethics with universal ethics?

Ethics and morality are a social enterprise and not just an invention or discovery of individuals or professional groups for their own guidance alone. Ethics is social in its origins, its sanctions, and its functions because we are born into a society that had developed and continues to maintain mores, laws, and ethical codes. This condition raises the fundamental question as to whether we actually have universal international ethics and human rights standards. Some argue that we do have universal ethics and standards. But then, how do we reconcile them with the reality of international cultural diversity (Davis, 1998a)?

In international nursing, at least two questions are basic: (a) Do all nurses everywhere value the same thing and in the same way? (b) Does international nursing really have universal ethics, or have Western ethics been used as if they constitute universal ethics? I address this issue of universal ethics and cultural pluralism in more detail later.

■ Codes of Ethics in Nursing

A code of ethics, one of the marks of a profession, serves to inform both members of a profession and the public about the profession's collective values. Many countries have their own nursing code of ethics, but others use the code developed by the International Council of Nurses (ICN). Some differences can be found between some of the national codes and the ICN Code. These different codes reflect the sociocultural setting in which they have been developed and in which nurses use them as guides in their practice.

An example of an important difference can be found in comparing the American Nurses Association (ANA) Code for Nurses with the ICN Code. In the ANA Code, the nurse is to have respect for human dignity and uniqueness of the client and to safeguard the client's right to privacy.

The ICN Code says that inherent in nursing is respect for life, dignity, and rights of man and that the nurse respects the beliefs, values, and customs of the individual. This section of these two codes sounds very similar, but in fact they differ. The ANA Code also has "The Interpretative Statements" that accompany the code, outlining ethical principles that underpin each section of the code. Developed within Western philosophy, these principles greatly value individualism. These principles, with their underlying values, may serve well as the bases for nursing ethics and bioethics in the United States. However, they may or may not be sufficient or appropriate to provide the bases for nursing ethics and bioethics in other, and especially very different, cultures. The people who wrote the ICN Code wisely left each section open for interpretation, making it possible for many cultures to use this code. The argument can be made that each culture has notions of right and wrong, good and bad, but what constitutes the content of these ethical concepts may differ.

All codes of ethics are open to interpretation, but those grounded in Western philosophical principles do have a specifically defined value base and delineated boundaries. Such a code can serve to guide professionals in the West, but it is not clear that the same code content would be useful in some other countries. For example, the Japan Nurses' Association code of ethics does not depend on ethical and legal notions of individual rights. Japan is an ancient culture where obligations—not rights—and the group—not the individual—are the value base of society. The attempt to import Western philosophical health care ethics into Japan has created difficulties (Davis, 1998c). It would be of interest to know whether the nurses in Japan who have the greatest difficulties with clinical ethical problems are those who have been socialized more into Western ways of thinking. The underlying question might be whether these nurses give greater credence to individual patient rights in a society where the group (in this case the family) has obligations and no patient has individual rights.

■ Theoretical Concerns in International Nursing Ethics

Some nurses practice with the ideals of cultural pluralism and ethical universals without realizing the potential for conflict. Some authorities on the subject state that universal human rights and ethics exist, but others say that they do not exist. Both positions affect the way we conceptualize international nursing ethics and also how we practice nursing ethics within a specific culture.

Cultural Relativism

Cultural relativism challenges the idea of universal ethics. Most of us are immediately attracted to the concept of cultural relativism because it seems anti-imperial and tolerant of differences and diversity while fostering the value of cultural egalitarianism. Cultural relativism makes two claims: (a) that each culture has a way of life that is of equal validity to all others, and (b) that ethical claims deriving outside a given culture have no validity within that culture. But cultural relativism cannot make a qualitative judgment and rank cultures as equal or unequal with regard to certain practices. They can only say that values derive endogenously, leading them to the position that moral judgments derived outside a culture being judged have no validity. However, to take this position makes ethics a slave to custom. The ethical "ought" can never transcend the cultural "is." The 19th century English philosopher John Stuart Mill called this the despotism of customs (Mill, 1977).

Cultural relativism sanctions as ethical the predominant opinion in any locality. Immediately the question arises: Which cultural morality or ethics is authoritative within a culture? Such authority comes from numerous sources within a culture, such as the majority, the elite, and ethnic, racial, or religious groups. This view of ethics could lead us to abandon a normative for a merely descriptive world view and could greatly hamper, if not destroy, the possibility for a dialogue on international ethics.

Universal Ethics

Having raised some potential problems with the relativism position of culture and ethics, let's now focus on the major issue with universal ethics. The position of universal ethics and human rights raises the basic question: Whose ethics and definition of human rights will be used to establish universal ethics and to describe and judge the greatly diverse cultures around the world?

Essentially, we have two main opposing concerns, namely, (a) the absolute right of cultural self-determination and (b) the right of the individual not to be subjected to a tradition or practice that might be harmful or even fatal. In an earlier paper, I cited the example of female circumcision, or what the World Health Organization (WHO) calls female genital mutilation, to raise these more theoretical issues in international ethics (Davis, 1998a).

To take the position that ethics and human rights are universal is not the same as saying that their understanding or interpretation is self-evident or immutable. Obviously, we cannot deny the various cultural contexts in which ethics and human rights are always embedded and played out in everyday life. But in order to have universal ethics, must all societies have the same content in their cultural values and ethics concepts?

Universal Ethics Across Cultures

In the final analysis we can take the relativism position, tolerating anything and everything because it occurs within a culture, and say that those outside the culture have nothing ethically valid to add. Or we can take the position that some actions and practices within a

culture are ethically wrong and violate universal ethical standards and human rights. To move beyond this confrontation between universalism and cultural relativism, perhaps we need to take the position that universal ethics does exist across cultures and therefore in international nursing. In taking this position, we need to proceed with great caution and awareness of the vast complexities and difficulties involved (Lane & Rubinstein, 1996).

We need full awareness of the attitudes we have, the language we employ, and the values behind them both. One of the very basic problems comes in use of Western ethics as the standard by which all else is developed and critiqued. English concepts in ethics, such as rights, autonomy, self-determination, and so forth, are value laden. These values and concepts may not be the same on the international level. For example, what does it mean to say the nurse acts as the patient's advocate? What does the nurse advocate for in a given clinical situation, and would this advocacy be the same if the nurse were in the United States, Israel, South Africa, Sweden, or Japan?

The previously mentioned educational exercise with Japanese students demonstrates that the cultural norm in Japan is not to give terminally ill patients information about their health status. Would we expect the nurse to view and act on this clinical situation in the same way regardless of the cultural norms and values of her or his country? If the nurse in Japan or another Asian country took action different from the ethical ideals of Western nursing ethics, would we in the West view that nurse as unethical? And if we did, how would we have arrived at this judgment? Would we be aware of the reasoning process and our underlying assumptions and values?

Each nurse lives in a society that has ideas of right and wrong, good and bad, but the content of these ideas differ. For example, in the United States, it is considered a good thing to tell terminally ill patients about their condition so that they can make autonomous decisions. Given the values and the ethical principle of autonomy, the nurse would advocate for information disclosure. But in Japan, a society where the group constitutes the basic unit of concern and analysis, it is considered a bad thing to tell patients about their terminal state.

The Japanese word for self (jibun) literally means self-part or part of the larger whole that consists of groups and relationships. Just as the individual is the lowest common denominator of society in the West, so the group (dantai) is in Japan. Here individual autonomy is inimical to group cohesion and harmony where the social fabric is that of mutual dependency, referred to as amae (Asai, 1996; Doi, 1985; Rosenberger, 1992). So the nurse in Japan would choose a different action to advocate for this patient. Deeply held cultural values support the differences in actions undertaken in the name of advocacy.

■ Ethics Theories in Nursing Ethics

All three ethics theories used in nursing ethics—virtue ethics, principle-based ethics, and the ethics of care—are grounded in values that may not be universal in their content. Surely, nursing in all countries values virtuous nurses, ethically principled nurses, and caring nurses. But which virtues? What principles and what do they mean? And what is the notion of caring in a specific society? By making this comment and asking these questions, we frame the discussion in the three ethical theories developed in the West. Are there other ways of thinking about nursing ethics? For example, could nursing have a theory of ethical obligation that might provide international nursing with another, more universal approach to ethics? Or perhaps nursing needs an entirely new way of theoretically thinking about nursing ethics. Nurses wedded to any or all of the ethical theories just discussed might have difficulty breaking out of their way of conceptualizing nursing ethics and may be limited in their ability to develop an international nursing ethics.

Based on the U.S. West Coast study on ethnics and ethnicity mentioned earlier, we can argue that, when people immigrate to another country, such as the United States, Sweden, or the United Kingdom, these new citizens should change their world view and values in order to live in the dominant culture with its laws and ethics. But what does such an argument do to the notions of respecting each person's culture? Are universal ethics and respect for cultural pluralism possible? The only positive answer to this question lies in an agreement that the content of our ethics—virtue, principles, and caring—must be broad enough to allow different interpretations. Although there are universals in ethics, there also are cultural differences in the meaning of the ethics concepts.

Having said this, the next logical question is: How far can this argument be pushed? For example, in two societies if health care professionals have the concept of "do no harm" but the societies define what "do no harm" means in very different ways, one group of health care professionals may seem very unethical to the health care professionals in the other society. Is this not relativism in ethics, and therefore can it not lead to the idea that anything is ethically justifiable because it fits culturally in that society? Then the question becomes: What, if any, limits would and should be placed on the behavior of others who seem to be unethical? Female circumcision is a case in point here. This practice, an ingrained part of many cultures in Africa and Southeast Asia, migrates with populations to cities where nurses and midwives participate in this practice. These health professionals argue that female circumcision is culturally necessary and better if they do this procedure rather than having it performed by the village healer (Davis, 1998a).

So we must ask: What do we mean when we say that we must respect cultural differences? Does this mean that we respect everything? Suppose that you are a midwife in the Western world and a mother brings her small daughter to you for circumcision. What would you do from an ethical perspective? What should you do? How would you ethically justify your decision? To what extent would you respect this integral part of this woman's culture? Suppose that you are a nurse midwife in Africa where female circumcision is culturally sanctioned. What should you do to be ethical if confronted by this mother? What would be the ethical basis of your decision? And would culture be a variable in your thinking? Should it be?

■ Concluding Statement

From these brief remarks on this complex topic, it is clear how much more deliberation in international nursing ethics must be undertaken in order to develop more fully a workable professional ethics that is truly international in scope. But how do we begin this needed work and what do we do with our individual values? Certainly we cannot and should not check them in some locker room until we have accomplished this work.

Do we assume that there can be international nursing ethics and if so, what could serve as the theoretical base of such ethics? Can we define in some detail the content of virtue ethics, ethical principles, ethical obligations, ethics of care, and other new approaches to nursing ethics? Or will these ethics need to be drawn for international nursing in very broad strokes, leaving much open for interpretation depending on the cultural context in which the nurse practices? Difficult questions but necessary ones that exist for the profession of nursing in all countries as well as internationally.

■ References

Asai, A. (1996). Barrier to informed consent in Japan. *Eubios Journal of Asian and International Bioethics, 6,* 91–93.

Beauchamp, T. L., & Childress, J. F. (1979). *Principles of biomedical ethics.* New York: Oxford University Press.

Davis, A. J. (1998a). Female genital mutilation: Some ethical questions. *Medicine and Law, 17,* 6–10.

Davis, A. J. (1998b). Development of nursing ethics: Are there universals? *International Nursing Review—Japanese Edition, 2,* 69–72. (In Japanese)

Davis, A. J. (1998c) Integrating nursing functions and ethics. *Proceedings of Japan Academy of Nursing Symposium,* 23–28. (In Japanese)

Davis, A. J. (1999). Global influence of American nursing: Some ethical issues. *Nursing Ethics, 6*(2), 118–125.

Davis, A. J. (2000). Bioethically constructed ideal dying patient in the U.S.A. *Medicine and Law 9,* 6–9.

Davis, A. J., Aroskar, M. A., Liaschenko, J., & Drought, T. S. (1997). *Ethical dilemmas and nursing practice.* Stamford, CT: Appleton & Lange.

Davis, A. J., Ota, K., Suzuki, M., & Maeda, J. (1999). Nursing students' response to a case study in ethics. *Nursing and Health Science Journal, 1,* 3–6 .

Doi, L. T. (1985). *The anatomy of dependency.* Tokyo: Kodansha International.

Lane, S. D., & Rubinstein, R. A. (1996, May–June). Judging the other: Responding to traditional female genital surgeries. *Hastings Center Report,* 31–40.

Mill, J. S. (1977). On liberty, In *Collected works of John Stuart Mill* (Vol. 18, Chapter 1, p. 3). Toronto: University of Toronto Press. (Originally published 1859), London: Longman, Roberts, & Greene.

Patient Self-determination Act of 1990. P.L. 101–508, November 5, 1990. Sections 4206 and 4751 of the *Omnibus Budget Reconciliation Act.*

Rosenberger, N. R. (Ed.). (1992). *Japanese sense of self.* New York: Cambridge University Press.

■ Editor's Questions for Discussion

Provide examples of ethnic differences in values that influence morality of a culture. Should standards of morality in a particular culture apply to all persons in that culture regardless of ethnic differences? May Western ethics be imposed as a universal? Does the profession of nursing expect nurses to apply Western ethics universally? What differences exist between the International Council of Nurses (ICN) Code of Ethics, the American Nurses Association (ANA) Code, and other national codes for nurses? Present arguments for the right of each culture to have ethical concepts that differ. What defined value base and delineated boundaries exist in the ANA and ICN Codes for Nurses. Does universal ethics exist across cultures and, if so, how, and to what extent?

What difficulties do nurses in the United States have in applying the ANA Code of Ethics? How might they be resolved? How does cultural relativism challenge the idea of universal ethics? How might cultural relativism be an ethics issue for nurses practicing in the United States? What ethical issues arise when a nurse becomes a patient advocate in a clinical situation? What reasoning process may the nurse use to arrive at ethical judgments? How can a reasoning process be taught? To what extent does a person's cultural and ethnic background influence ethical clinical reasoning? To what extent should a nurse's culture and ethnicity be utilized in ethical clinical decision-making? Is everything ethically justifiable if it fits culturally in a particular society? Address the questions raised by Davis and provide arguments and examples in your responses.

7

Legal Perspectives in Nursing Education

Lois A. Lane, JD, MSN, RNCS
Craig Paterson, LLB, MA

Professional nursing education has undergone an evolution in recent years: from a hospital-based training program, with a primary mission focused on service, to a university-based education program. Emphasis is now on academic standards and cultivation of teaching and research excellence. However, nursing as a profession, despite shifts in setting and standards, retains its primary devotion to service. Pursuing university-based education and the higher standards of professionalism that accompany higher education, should be seen (dissenting voices notwithstanding) as being complementary to that primary mission. Properly interpreted, the cultivation of rigorous but fair academic standards increases the level of service the pro-

fession can provide to the public in an era of ever increasing technological and organizational sophistication (Antrobus & Kitson, 1999).

Inevitably, faced with the need to adhere to high academic and clinical standards, nursing faculty need to know what legal, moral, and prudential duties are incumbent upon them. Those duties and responsibilities start from day one in the school of nursing. This chapter is designed to respond to this need by providing a "rough guide" to the existing legal terrain.

Within the context of a profession, questions of regulation and adherence to standards are never far away. Professional organizations publish standards and state licensing agencies promulgate rules that govern the practice of nursing in each state and stipulate educational criteria. Federal and state lawmaking bodies concern themselves with health and safety. Professional standards in nursing education do not exist in isolation, abstracted from the dynamics of change taking place in the wider arenas of health care delivery and academia. Health care delivery and academia constitute, so to speak, two major overlapping social systems that have a direct impact on nursing practice and education (McBride, 1999). In terms of the academic social system, universities are unambiguously shifting the focus of educational worth toward the four kinds of scholarship articulated by Boyer—discovery, integration, utilization, and teaching (mentioned in McBride, 1999, p. 116).

There can be little doubt that this shift in focus will continue to influence higher education, and schools of nursing cannot remain immune from the change. Having made the transition to university-based education, nursing education cannot hold back the tide of change that comes from being a part of this wider enterprise. Such transformation undoubtedly forces schools of nursing to work smarter and harder. Adaptability to the "signs of the times" is essential if nursing is to continue to be taken seriously as a full-fledged member of academe. More specifically, the priorities for nursing education in these "transformational times" should certainly include (though not be restricted to) the (a) cultivation of first-class leadership skills, (b) well-designed pedagogical and clinical processes, (c) diligent review of structure and content, and (d) resolute commitment to continuous quality improvement (Massy, 1996).

■ School of Nursing Mission and the Law

A good practical starting point for an institution committed to taking those challenges seri-

ously is the mission statement. A well-crafted mission statement can help motivate faculty toward the pursuit of excellence in teaching, research, and service. Further, it can assist the creation of standards needed to guide students toward the pursuit of high academic and clinical achievement. We are of the opinion that a commitment to the pursuit of excellence should be strongly encouraged within nursing education, and the mission statement of a school of nursing ought to reflect that commitment. The following mission statement, from Indiana University School of Nursing, without being abstractly idealistic, captures just such a commitment. It states that the mission of the School of Nursing is " . . . to improve the health of the citizens of Indiana, the nation and beyond by meeting society's need for effective nurses at different educational levels and by contributing to the body of knowledge that provides the basis for practice in a range of settings" (Indiana University, School of Nursing, 1999).

The law plays a significant part in the educational process, and a proper regard for the role of the law can help (although granted, can sometimes hinder) the mission of a school. However viewed, the law cannot simply be sidestepped or glossed over as an inconvenience when it is seen to conflict with other desirable goals. Legal questions in nursing education can emerge in a variety of ways and must be faced with due regard to the authority of legislatures and courts, whether they arise from contract, tort, or (on rare occasions) criminal law. In this regard, schools of nursing are not unique and need to tackle many of the same legal issues faced by other schools and departments. Typical shared issues involve academic performance, student grievances, disabilities, and so forth. Such shared concerns, however, do not negate the legal significance of some particular areas unique to the education of health professionals. Thus, for example, the mission of educating health professionals brings with it liability issues concerning the protection of the public from incompetent (physical and mental) student learners in clinical settings (Brent, 1997).

At this juncture, a significant caveat is in order: The "professional responsibility" of nursing faculty educators concerning the future conduct of students who have graduated cannot automatically be severed with the attainment of state licensure. Professional responsibility goes beyond strict legal obligation. Due regard for the law should not result in the opposite excess of adopting a "minimalist mentality" to problems. The incompetence of a licensed nurse who has graduated from a professional program does not "ordinarily" entail any legal liability on nursing faculty—due no doubt to the difficulty of demonstrating a causal connection between defective education and outcome. However, nursing faculty surely cannot be exempt from a certain share of the "moral" blame resulting from avoidable malpractice due, in part, to defective instruction.

This issue is no mere academic hobby horse, for, if recent Institute of Medicine reports are accurate concerning the incidence of many avoidable "medical errors," the nursing profession, as well as the medical profession, must take a long and hard look at the question of quality standards in educational outcome (Reed, Blegen, & Goode, 1998).

■ Internal Forum

Relationships that impose legal duties on a nursing school and its faculty exist within the university and outside the university. Within the university, relationships exist between the (a) school or department and the university administration, (b) school administration and its faculty, (c) faculty and other faculty (within the school or department and with other schools or departments), (d) faculty and student, and (e) student and administration.

Nursing Faculty

General Remarks

Nursing faculty at whatever level, instructor to full professor, represent the university as its employees. Within their scope of employment, their actions generate legally binding obligations on the school and university. Many of the policies and procedures that are written by the school and the university flow from these responsibilities. The university should go to considerable lengths to communicate to individual employees what their responsibilities are, and mechanisms should be put in place to protect itself from financial loss, whether that loss arises from breach of contract or tort. Effective communication and clear procedural guidelines are essential to minimize the possibility of legal action by employees and students alike.

Promotion and Tenure

In many universities, the processes of appointment, reappointment, promotion, tenure, and post-tenure review of nursing faculty are obscure. Those who make decisions are often not required to account for them. Procedures should be as well defined and objective as possible. Yet, the criteria employed for promotion and tenure are often vague and subjective. The courts are reluctant to interfere with what they essentially regard as an academic assessment by peers. The courts recognize that the evaluation of faculty is vital to the life and reputation of the institution. Thus, for the most part, courts generally eschew a review of evaluations of faculty academic performance or research and leave it to the institution to sort out. See, for example, *Dorsett v. Board of Trustees for State Colleges and Universities* (1991). The court stated here that " . . . we have neither the competence nor the resources to [. . .] micromanage the administration of thousands of state educational institutions" (p. 124).

Nursing Students

Admission Standards and Procedure

Now, more than ever, attempts are being made by schools of nursing to conform to the rigors of academia, as well as to the wider pressures of the profession toward baccalaureate degree entry. Nursing faculty should be cognizant of the need for admission standards that reflect the entry of students who are likely to progress and graduate with the ability to practice safe and effective clinical nursing. If admission standards are lowered to allow a diluted level of academic achievement, the result will likely be an unacceptably high rate of failure in licensure examinations, a continuing and unacceptable rate of "medical mistakes," and a larger amount of faculty resources spent on a smaller number of students. Ultimately, better students are then penalized by lack of faculty contact.

Some tools used to determine admission to schools of nursing include interview, grade point average score, and testing. If and when these tools are used to assess the admission of a potential student, the school must continuously evaluate the process to see whether the tools really do predict success (i.e., graduation and pass rates in licensure examinations).

Out of concern for procedural fairness, and the transparency of standards and techniques applied, the whole process needs to be documented in a way that outside reviewers and parties can see "how and why" decisions have been reached. Anything less could leave the school exposed to potential challenge on the grounds of unjust discriminatory practice.

The authors strongly recommend that admission and progression standards in schools of nursing not be lowered. For example, studies have documented that publicly educated students come to college "less proficient in basic academic skills" such as reading and math (Leon & Zareski, 1998). The answer in this case is for the school to arrange for remedial education, probationary admission, academic probation, and so forth to bring students up to the set standard for full-fledged entry, or continuance, in the program.

Disability Questions

The Americans with Disability Act (ADA) was passed to eliminate discrimination against people with disabilities. Titles II and III of the ADA and section 504 of the Rehabilitation Act of 1973 apply to colleges and universities. The ADA states that a "qualified disability" exists when an individual " . . . (a) [has] a physical or mental impairment that substantially limits one or more of the major life activities of such individual; (b) [has] a record of such an impairment; or (c) [is] regarded as having such an impairment." The ADA's definition of "qualified disability" is generally the same as the use of "handicap" in the Rehabilitation Act.

It is important to bear in mind that the ADA, by employing the terminology "qualified individual with a disability," intended that the statute should not cover every impaired person. Rather, the statute covers only individuals able to perform the essential functions of the job. In the educational setting, a qualified individual with a disability is one who fulfills the essential eligibility requirements of the school of nursing and who meets the essential eligibility requirements of the school with or without a modification of the school's policies and procedures to accommodate the disability. For a detailed example of essential abilities requirements specific to nursing students see Billings and Halstead (1998, p. 60).

Nursing faculty may need additional education to accommodate the learning needs of the student who is a qualified individual with a disability. Maintenance of standards is important (i.e., the "same degree of rigor" should be applied in terms of outcome). Lower outcome standards may negatively affect the disabled person. However, "reasonable accommodations" should be made to meet the legitimate needs of the disabled student, and these needs should be assessed on a case-by-case basis. Rhodes, Davis, and Odom (1999) state a useful "rule of thumb" for an admissions board when considering the issue of safety in clinical practice: " . . . safety depends on the nurse's ability to assimilate information and make appropriate decisions, not on the performance of physical tasks" (p. 50). Consequently, in evaluating a potential student, that evaluation should be "reasonably accommodated" (as required by the ADA) to reflect the person's knowledge, not the disability per se.

For a good example of the application of reasonable accommodation in the educational setting, see *Betts v. Rector & Visitors of Univ. of Va.* (1999). In this case, the Fourth Circuit Court reversed a district court decision and held that a medical student with short-term memory and reading speed problems was qualified under the ADA. It held that double time on examinations was a "reasonable accommodation" to meet essential eligibility requirements for continuing progress in the light of his disability.

Academic Evaluation and Progression

Evaluation is key to the progression of nursing students through the program. Procedures designed to implement evaluation should be as objective, measurable, and documentable as is reasonably possible. That is not to say that there is not value in the collection and assessment of subjective information. But in order to demonstrate to a third party (probably not a nurse) the validity of the evidence used to hold back or dismiss a student, the data must clearly warrant the action. Objective data are much easier to defend in that regard should questions of fairness concerning a decision emerge.

The following instance illustrates the clear need for good documentation and evaluation procedures by nursing faculty: A student's performance in one class may not fall to the level to warrant remedial action or dismissal, but pending other problems in the student's academic career, the individual course evaluation may provide evidence of a pattern of deficient performance. Good documentation serves the school well and allows faculty a high degree of confidence should any decisions be scrutinized. See for example, *Clements v. The County of Nassau* (1987). There a community college nursing student failed to maintain the requisite standards of sterilization required for the adequate performance of clinical procedures. Students could not proceed unless they had satisfactorily passed the clinical components of a course. Adequate opportunity was provided to rectify the inadequate performance of the student in question.

Clearly, dismissing a student from a nursing program can be devastating to the individual. The former student may have spent much time and money pursuing this educational path to a career. Such a decision should be undertaken only with good evidence. While nursing faculty often proceed with a heavy heart in matters of academic discipline, compassion for the student must be strongly tempered by the interests of patients, interests that form the very raison d'être of the profession. It is not uncommon for former students faced with the predicament of dismissal to consider a lawsuit against the school and university. The legal basis for such a lawsuit may include: (a) breach of contract—more likely in a private academic institution, (b) lack of due process, (c) discrimination, and (d) educational malpractice.

Basis for Lawsuits

Contract

Many preventive measures for avoiding potential lawsuits are available to nursing faculty simply by diligence in the pursuit of teaching excellence. Clear and consistent expectations are crucial for the guidance of students. It is important for nursing faculty to realize that students rely on documentation issued to them by the school. Such documentation should be reviewed and updated frequently to reflect changing circumstances. Attention should also be given to the question of consistency among documents. Faculty should be familiar with documents and abide by what they say. Often, however—when trouble arises—they have not done so. It is plain common sense that nursing faculty cannot apply standards fairly and impartially if they are not aware of them! Being armed with a good knowledge of policy and procedure, faculty should then explicitly hold students responsible for reading the documents and living up to the standards stated in those documents. A few examples of such documentation would be marketing brochures, advertisements, bulletins, student handbooks, and academic codes of conduct (Brent, 1997).

Additionally, a syllabus or course catalog may—in some instances—be seen as giving rise to contractual obligations, express or implied. See for example the case of *Southwell v. University of the Incarnate Word* (1998), concerning a private university's refusal to grant a baccalaureate degree to a nursing student. The Texas Court of Appeals stated that a court must look to the precise nature of the representations made in establishing whether or not a contract existed, and if so, its terms. Much will depend on the precise wording of the various documents and the circumstances surrounding issuance.

To avoid potential questions concerning breach of contract, some faculty go so far as to have students sign the syllabus and put disclaimers on the syllabus to say that changes may occur. However, faculty cannot have it both ways. If faculty place a disclaimer and enact changes, it follows that some degree of flexibility is required in the implementation of those changes. Needless to say, where possible, it is always better to discuss and reach consensual agreement on the nature of the changes being proposed. Nursing faculty should be willing to listen to student concerns and should respond to them with respect, even if it is not feasible to implement them.

Due Process and Academic Performance

Due process is a protection against arbitrary action provided by the United States Constitution. The 14th Amendment states, in part, that no " . . . State [shall] deprive any person of life, liberty or property, without due process of law." Public institutions, by a process of judicial interpretation, are included under the auspices of what is meant by "the State." As ruled by the Supreme Court in *Rendell-Baker v. Kohn* (1982), except in very unusual circumstances, due process does not apply to private institutions even though they may be receiving external funding from state or federal sources.

For the sake of brevity, we will take due process in this context to mean that a student shall have a fair procedural opportunity to know about and defend against dismissal or other disciplinary action by a public university. Hence fair procedures must be in place before disciplinary action can be undertaken. Poor or shoddy procedure is literally to surrender a major hostage to fortune. As found by a federal court of appeals in *Gaspar v. Bruton* (1975), since the powers exercised are of a "quasi-judicial" nature, they cannot be exercised arbitrarily. However, on the facts of the case, a practice nurse was not unfairly dismissed when various reviews of her performance were carried out, affording her ample opportunity to rectify her deficient performance.

To ensure a fair hearing, policies and procedures should reflect the quasi-judicial nature of the power being exercised. Not only should they exist, but those policies and procedure should also be carefully adhered to. The student has a right to defend the claims against him or her, and the student should have a right to question witnesses, the accuracy of evidence, and so forth. These policies and procedures can be very detailed and certainly become overwhelming for the ordinary faculty member who may rarely encounter them. Clear and concise documentation and specification of steps to be taken can be invaluable to a faculty member's comprehension. Additionally, we strongly suggest early recourse to key people knowledgeable in the area for advice. If in doubt, seek advice, is always good advice! The dean of a school or program is often an excellent source to be called upon for help. In cases of some complexity, the main university administration and even legal counsel may need to become involved.

It is common and entirely acceptable practice for the internal policies and procedures of an institution to afford students more due process procedure than is minimally required by law. The important point here is that if the institution does provide more protection than the minimum required by law, then the faculty and administration are legally obliged to follow those procedures. The courts, in general, will not interfere with the outcome of a process when proper procedures have been followed and have been exhausted by the student. Moreover, if a student goes to court without having attempted to utilize, to the full extent, the procedures available to him or her, the court is likely to refuse a hearing for the case.

A typical case is *Rossomando v. Board of Regents of the University of Nebraska* (1998). It involved dismissal of a student from a postgraduate orthodontics program on the grounds of poor academic performance, despite remedial help. The federal district court held that the dismissal of a student for academic reasons met with the requirements of due process if the student had prior notice of faculty dissatisfaction with performance, the possibility of dismissal, and the decision to dismiss the student was careful and deliberate.

Due Process and Student Misconduct

Students facing discipline at public universities receive constitutional protection, as the federal courts view the student's continued enrollment as a property interest immune from arbitrary state action. However, students facing discipline at private universities do not have that protection (being a nonstate entity), and any remedy would need to be of a contractual (or quasi-contractual) nature.

Most universities have policies and procedures that dictate how these issues should be handled by the faculty and administration. To avoid losing a lawsuit, the university must give the student due process. That is, the student must be treated fairly and not discriminated against, and the policy and procedure must be applied across the board to all students. The faculty role here is critical in being objective and documenting the incident, behavior, and proceedings. Well-crafted decision-making tools are indispensable to faculty faced with a misconduct action.

Student misconduct falls into several categories, and different categories of misconduct may be afforded different degrees of due process protection. All categories of misconduct should be defined and described in writing both for the benefit of nursing faculty and for the benefit of the student. Vague and complicated procedures may frustrate or defeat the goals that lie behind the desire to take disciplinary steps and may unwittingly allow students to abuse the system and progress in spite of misconduct. To meet requirements of due process, the policies and procedures used to judge a student's action must be "fair in the circumstances."

Two basic categories of student misconduct are (a) academic misconduct, and (b) personal misconduct. The following are examples of each category:

Academic misconduct—cheating; fabrication; plagiarism; interference (with the work or progress of another student); violation of course rules; and academic dishonesty.

Personal misconduct—false accusation against other students or faculty; release of computer passwords; physical or verbal abuse; damage to university property; failure to comply with university regulations; possession or distribution of illegal drugs; and possession of firearms against university regulation.

There is less latitude here than for due process relating to academic performance. The key difference lies in the potential for disgrace that attaches to a finding of wrongdoing in these cases. Thus, for example, when a school of nursing disciplines a student claiming that a student has altered a transcript, falsified a crucial admissions requirement, or cheated on a test or clinical demonstration, the student should be able to challenge that opinion through "cross examination" or the presentation of contrary testimony in an appropriate forum.

Here, the leading case is *Dixon v. Alabama State Board of Education* (1961), which forms the basis for due process considerations concerning misconduct and can be regarded as laying down minimally acceptable standards in this context: (a) the student should receive notice of the complaint, the grounds upon which it is based, and the nature of the specified action proposed; (b) the student should be provided with the facts and the names of those who give evidence concerning the complaint; (c) the student should be provided with a proper opportunity to rebut the complaint; (d)

the result of the process should be presented in a report open to the inspection of the student (pp. 158–159).

Discrimination

Discrimination represents a potentially wide class of action against the nursing school and university. We discussed discrimination concerning disability previously. Other areas of discrimination pertain to gender and race (although there are certainly other significant categories). In general, when taking measures against students for academic nonperformance or for academic or personal misconduct, faculty should follow the policies and procedures in ways that protect against the possibility of bias. It is crucial that allegations of favoritism and partiality in treatment be avoided. The clearest "rule of thumb" is to treat similar cases in a similar fashion, regardless of gender or race. However, attention to circumstances concerning "similarity" is important. In *Albert v. Carovano* (1988), for example, the court stated that inferences of racial discrimination could not be drawn from allegations concerning a private college's failure to discipline students in "other circumstances" because none of the allegations of nonenforcement involved circumstances reasonably comparable to those surrounding the suspension of students who conducted a "sit-in."

Discrimination against students because of gender or race flies in the face of the equal protection clause of the 14th Amendment, which states that the state should not " . . . deny to any person within its jurisdiction the equal protection of the laws." Additional measures preventing discrimination based on gender include Title IX of the Education Amendments Act of 1972, which provides that no " . . . person in the United States shall, on the basis of sex, be excluded from participation in, be denied the benefits of, or be subjected to discrimination under any education program or activity receiving Federal financial assistance."

An interesting case illustrating fairness of treatment concerning sexual discrimination is *Hall v. Lee College* (1996). This case involved the rejection of a sexual discrimination claim under Title IX brought by a male nursing student. Despite allegations, the student had not presented any real evidence that his evaluations were false or biased or the standards applied were inappropriate. The analysis of nursing faculty seemed reasonable. Thus there was ample evidence to demonstrate that his exclusion from further study was due to clinical shortcomings, not his male gender.

Additional protections regarding racial discrimination can be found under Title VII of the Civil Rights Act of 1964, concerning equal rights under the law. Hence

> all persons within the jurisdiction of the United States shall have the same right in every State and Territory to make and enforce contracts, to sue, be parties, give evidence, and to the full and equal benefit of all laws and proceedings for the security of persons and property as is enjoyed by white citizens. . . .

Educational Malpractice

This type of action is unlikely to cause nursing faculty major concern. The courts are reluctant to oversee the quality of academic or clinical guidance for public policy reasons in higher educational institutions. See for example, the case of *Swidryk v. Saint Michael's Medical Center* (1985), which involved an educational malpractice claim arising out of an alleged failure to train a physician adequately during his medical school residency. The main issue was whether a physician may assert a claim for educational malpractice. The superior court held that recognition of the claim would result in unwarranted judicial intervention in everyday academic decisions. See also the case of *Tolman v. CenCor Career Colleges* (1992), wherein an appeals court dismissed a case raised, in part, on the grounds of educational malpractice concerning medical and dental education. The cause of action was dismissed on the facts, since it is very difficult (though not impossible) to prove that a student was not deficient or that an array of many other external factors was not responsible for the failure.

■ External Forum

Copyright

It is common to see copyright notices, even in nursing textbooks, which state that no one may copy any portion of the book without the prior written consent of the publisher (usually the copyright holder). Yet, according to the provisions of section 107 of Title 17 of the Copyright Act (1976), the law states that " . . . the fair use of a copyrighted work, including such use by reproduction in copies . . . is not an infringement of copyright." This point is further clarified in the section where " . . . teaching (including multiple copies for classroom use), scholarship, or research . . . " are considered to be specific examples of fair use. Section 107 goes on to mention four factors to be considered when assessing fair use: (a) the purpose and character of the use (commercial or not for profit); (b) the nature of the copyrighted work (fact versus creative); (c) the amount and substantiality of the portion used (proportionality); and (d) the effect of use on the potential market for, or value of, the copyrighted work.

What is a member of the nursing faculty to make of this? On the one hand, publishers issue seemingly blanket prohibitions. On the other hand, "fair use" provisions seem quite vague concerning questions of scope. We sympathize with the predicament of trying to be on the right side of the law but can only offer a few summary remarks for guidance here. Further assistance can be gained by reading a set of nonstatutory guidelines considered by a Committee of the House of Representatives when examining the fair use provisions of the 1976 Copyright Act (Ad Hoc Committee, 1976). See also the articles by Spalding (1993) and Patterson (1997) on copyright use in the educational setting.

A clear case of unfair use would be for a faculty member to make multiple copies of an entire course text available to a class, considering it too expensive for students to buy. Here the faculty member would be breaching both the proportionality requirement and the effect on potential market requirement of the copyrighted work.

The *spontaneous* reproduction of multiple copies of a copyrighted article from a journal, to be distributed to a class, for use on a one-time-only basis, would probably fall within the scope of fair use. This one-time-only use would also apply to multiple copies of excerpts from a copyrighted book for class distribution (providing, of course, that the excerpts did not represent a substantial portion of the work). When considering the question of proportionality, proper regard must be given to whether or not the proportion of the work being copied is, so to speak, of the "heart of the work." Thus proportionality is not simply a *quantitative* criteria but also a *qualitative* one. For example, to copy all the chapters in the Nursing Theory section of this textbook would breach copyright, since this section is central to the nature of the work. An appeal to the spontaneous nature of one-time-only copying does not bring with it license to undermine the property interest an owner has in the work. When in doubt, it is better to err on the side of protecting the copyright and obtain permission from the publisher for copying.

The spontaneous, one-time-only compilation of an internal "course pack" created and manufactured by and distributed solely for use within the nursing school— and only on a cost recovery basis—would also likely fall within the scope of fair use, providing that each entry in the course pack can stand or fall on its own terms and that, collectively, individual entries *would not* constitute a substantial aggregate from a single source.

When making *subsequent use* of an item previously reproduced and distributed in class, a faculty member should seek the appropriate permissions from the copyright holder. Spontaneity is no longer an appeal that can be made. There can be no reasonable excuse for neglecting this requirement when there is time to request and obtain permission. Nursing faculty should not form the habit of *falling into a pattern* of repeated multiple copying for class distribution.

The reproduction and display of copyright materials via the Internet is a new and uncertain area of the law (Colyer, 1997). However, it seems reasonable to assume (by analogy to printed sources) that the electronic display of copyrighted materials similar to an article, course pack, or excerpts from a book, as previously described, would be governed by the same considerations. Of particular importance with reference to the education-only use of materials, is the need to restrict access to the posted material. Restriction of access to students enrolled in a course is usually handled by creation and use of appropriate security and password control.

As a concluding caveat on the topic of copyright, nursing faculty ought to be aware that when they write and publish under contract they will often have to relinquish the copyright of their work to the publisher. If they have relinquished the copyright, they need to seek permission for reprints of that material in their other works. They are no longer free to make use of the work as they see fit. The moral of the tale here is for nursing faculty to read and understand the terms of a contract before signing it.

Public Safety

General Duty

Clearly, there is an expectation that accredited schools of nursing must comply with and meet the standards of accrediting bodies as well as state and federal law. Some of those standards and laws are general with regard to the educational institution and some are specific to the education of people who will become registered nurses. Nursing faculty must recognize that they have a responsibility not only to their students but also to protection of the public. This obligation to public safety is important and should be transmitted to students by nursing faculty throughout the educational process. Every nursing course should rely on this underlying theme. Moreover, safety information should be clearly written and provided to students in school bulletins and orientation materials. This information serves as a foundation for the evaluation of students as they progress toward graduation and for the students' careers following graduation.

Clinical Contracts and Agency Agreements

Several legal issues affecting nursing programs center on questions pertaining to clinical contracts or agency agreements. With these contracts and agreements come questions of a school's role in public safety and the protection of patients. At this juncture, it is important to point out that a school of nursing, while cooperating with outside clinical bodies for its students to provide needed services, cannot sacrifice important student interests simply for the expeditious renewal of a contract or continuance of an agency agreement. Further, nursing programs should be careful to minimize the creation of additional burdens on students beyond the requirements of the university itself. An example would be for an agency to attempt to require the physical examination of students by a physician before allowing them to participate in patient care in a facility.

School administration should educate nursing faculty both about the need for contracts before arranging clinical experience with an agency and the implications for the school of contract terms to which parties agreed. One example of a contract term would be the distinction between a "medical malpractice" claim and a "property" claim. If a student discards a multiple dose vial of medication that belongs to a patient and results in the financial harm to the patient, that is a "property" issue not a "medical malpractice" issue. Thus the contract should specify whether or not the university has a responsibility for the loss of patient property by a student during clinical practice.

External Clinical Activities Under Own Auspices

Another consideration for the school and faculty is the carrying out of clinical activities that are not conducted by, or do not take place on, the premises of any clinical agency. An example is a depression screening offered by undergraduate students (related to a class project) at a local shopping mall. This activity, while it should *not* be prohibited, carries with it heightened liability for the university due to a lack of any responsible clinical agency to vouch for the care of patients. Therefore an analysis of the specific activity, proposed benefit, and the amount of faculty supervision available are important questions to assess. Nursing faculty, of course, in such screening activities bear liability for patient care, being licensed professionals directing others. Further, the university, being the employer of nursing faculty, will likely be held liable for any action that may ensue. Possible safeguards would be to have an agreement with providers who are willing to have clients referred to them (and to see them) without regard to insurance status or ability to pay. Also, the treatment of minors should be prohibited due to questions of parental consent. The wise course of action is to seek out the advice of legal counsel prior to carrying out an activity. *Students should be well instructed in the technique to be performed or the nature of the health advice being given at least to the minimum standard of professional care.*

Another issue to be considered before setting up shop in a public area, municipal area, or a private business is that of property insurance. Issues not related to the specific activity but related to general safety, building maintenance, and people "just falling down," are not normally within the scope of the university's potential for liability. However, nursing faculty should discuss the issue of liability with the appropriate authority responsible for the area. A written reply to a request, granting permission to use the space, will probably be adequate.

Affiliates for Student Education

Relationships with clinical affiliates for student education are important and can make or break clinical placements. Individual faculty must develop a relationship with staff, unit manager, and nursing administrator. Both the nursing faculty and the school administration have a responsibility to foster those relationships and involve affiliates in the educational process. The creation of a community and agency advisory board is one way to foster such relationships. The board should be representative of the affiliates, nursing faculty, and administration. It can be further enhanced by representation from the state nurses association and, perhaps, the state board of nursing. Keeping the advisory board "in the loop" on curriculum changes and seeking their input on strategic direction help to keep those relationships effective.

Faculty Practice and Grants

The school of nursing enters into relationships with outside agencies as a representative of the university. The trend within many universities is toward responsibility centered management, and in these cases the financial risk is ultimately the responsibility of the school (McBride, 1999). Financial awards governed by contracts need to be reviewed by the appropriate internal offices prior to signing. Faculty are often responsible for the monitoring and management of risk. For example, if something changes and the award of a grant from an affiliate is reduced from what was budgeted, quick action must be taken to try and reduce the loss incurred. In general, the sooner action is taken to minimize loss, the better.

Particularly in the case of patient services, the school has an obligation to the people using the service and cannot abruptly end it. Likewise, people who are employed must be given appropriate notice of termination and be paid the appropriate level of benefits due them. It is the grant recipient's responsibility to monitor grant activity and identify problems as they arise. Grants that bind school and university should not be sought or accepted by nursing faculty without involving, at a minimum, the department chairperson and associate dean or dean. A school may well need the assistance of university attorneys or contract and grant officers to negotiate and enforce the terms of a grant contract.

Professional Malpractice Liability

One example of financial risk that a nursing school must concern itself with is the possibility of a medical malpractice lawsuit. The university can either self-insure or purchase medical malpractice insurance to cover professional licensed health care providers and health profession students. It is a necessary cost of educating students for the health professions.

Nursing faculty and administration must continually weigh and measure the ability of the student against the potential for risk to a patient. Thus the level of mastery a student must achieve in a laboratory setting before entering a patient setting and reasonable expectations to be placed on students within the patient setting must be determined. Close collaboration with professional colleagues is vital to create a sensible balance between laxity on the one hand and undue rigor on the other hand.

When students are admitted to schools of nursing, from the outset they are held accountable for professional nursing standards. The expectation of nursing education is to educate people to function as nurses and prepare them to demonstrate that ability by taking a licensure examination. Commitment to professional standards must be made patently clear to students. Nursing faculty must understand that it is their responsibility to assess competency and cultivate a commitment toward it in a variety of formal and informal settings. They must teach professional standards and implement steps, in appropriate cases, to dismiss students who are in violation. It is a clear faculty and school responsibility to hold fast to existing professional standards, not least for the sake of protecting the public, without being unjust to the legitimate interests of students.

■ Concluding Statement

Clearly, our account of the legal issues relevant to nursing education today is partial and incomplete. We have made no pretense of comprehensiveness in the scope of our coverage. That would require a whole book, not a chapter. Also, some of the issues covered may seem somewhat abstract. However, we believe that our analysis and commentary does tackle a significant number of issues in sufficient depth to offer nursing faculty a reasonable overview of the legal duties and responsibilities incumbent upon them. In doing so, we also hope to have conveyed something of the "spirit of the law" to nursing faculty, which may serve them in good stead as they consider issues that we have been unable to cover here.

■ References

Ad Hoc Committee on Copyright Law Revision. (1976). Agreement on Guidelines for Classroom Copying in Not-For-Profit Educational Institutions With Respect to Books and Periodicals. *House of Representatives Report* No. 94-1476.

Albert v. Carovano, 851 F.2d 561 (C.A.2 N.Y. 1988).

Americans with Disabilities Act of 1990, 42, U.S.C.S. §12101 et seq. (Lexus, Academic Universe 2000).

Antrobus, S., & Kitson, A. (1999). Nursing leadership: Influencing and shaping health policy and nursing practice. *Journal of Advanced Nursing, 29*(3), 746–753.

Betts v. Rector & Visitors of Univ. of Va., 191 F.3d 447 (4th Cir. Va. 1999).

Billings, D. M., & Halstead, J. A. (1998). *Teaching in nursing: A guide for faculty.* Philadelphia: W. B. Saunders.

Brent, N. J. (1997). *Nurses and the law: A guide to principles and applications.* Philadelphia: W. B. Saunders.

Civil Rights Act of 1964, 42, U.S.C.S. §1981 et seq. (Lexus, Academic Universe 2000).

Clements v. The County of Nassau, 835 F. 2d 1000 (2nd Cir. 1987).

Colyer, A. (1997). Copyright law, the Internet, and distance education. *American Journal of Distance Education, 11*(3), 41–57.

Constitution of the United States of America Amendments, U.S.C.S. Const. Amend. 14, §1 (Lexus, Academic Universe 2000).

Copyright Act of 1976, 17, U.S.C.S. §107 et seq. (Lexus, Academic Universe 2000).

Dixon v. Alabama State Board of Education, 294 F. 2d 150 (5th Cir. 1961).

Dorsett v. Board of Trustees for State Colleges and Universities, 940 F.2d 121, 124 (5th Cir. 1991).

Education Amendments Act of 1972, 20, U.S.C.S. §1681 et seq. (Lexus, Academic Universe 2000).

Gaspar v. Bruton 513 F.2d 843 (10th Cir. 1975).

Hall v. Lee College, 932 F. Supp. 1027 (E.D. Tenn. 1996).

Indiana University School of Nursing. (1999). *Annual report.* Indianapolis: Indiana University.

Leon, L., & Zareski, S. (1998). Changes in nursing education: Implications for faculty stress. *Nurse Educator, 23*(2), 7–8.

Massy, W. (1996). New thinking on academic restructuring. *AGB Priorities, 6,* 1–14.

McBride, A. B. (1999). Breakthroughs in nursing education: Looking back, looking forward . . . papers from the 25th anniversary of the American Academy of Nursing. *Nursing Outlook, 47*(3), 114–119.

Patterson, L. R. (1997). Regents guide to understanding copyright and fair use. *Journal of Intellectual Property Law, 5,* 243–305.

Reed, L., Blegen, M. A., & Goode, C.S. (1998). Adverse patient occurrences as a measure of nursing care quality. *Journal of Nursing Administration, 28*(5), 62–9.

Rehabilitation Act of 1973, 29, U.S.C.S. §701 et seq. (Lexus, Academic Universe 2000).

Rendell-Baker v. Kohn, 457 U.S. 830 (1982).

Rhodes, R. S., Davis, D. C., & Odom, B. C. (1999). Challenges and rewards of educating a profoundly deaf student. *Nurse Educator, 24*(3), 48–51.

Rossomando v. Board of Regents of the University of Nebraska, 2 F. Supp. 2d 1223 (D. Neb. 1998).

Southwell v. University of the Incarnate Word, 974 S.W.2d 351 (Tex. App. 1998).

Spalding, A. D. (1993). Fair use of research and course packets in the classroom. *American Business Law Journal, 31,* 447–481.

Swidryk v. Saint Michael's Medical Center, 493 A.2d 641 (N.J. Super.Ct.Law.Div. 1985).

Tolman v. CenCor Career Colleges, 851 P.2d 203 (Colo. App., 1992).

■ *Editor's Questions for Discussion*

Discuss the legal rights and responsibilities of nursing education programs in terms of faculty and students. What are the obligations, expectations, and responsibilities of faculty and students? How may qualifications and competencies of faculty be determined for teaching courses and providing supervision in a clinical setting? What suggestions may be offered for faculty to ensure fair and adequate *evaluation* and *documentation* regarding students' performance?

Discuss fair evaluation of students' clinical competencies. What constitutes fairness? How much "practice" must be provided for a particular skill before students are given a failing grade for a clinical experience? What remedial efforts are essential? To what degree is English language proficiency essential to success in a nursing program? How might and to what extent should programs provide remediation for "weaker" students?

What are the aspects of risk management that pertain to nursing programs? What policies and procedures are essential to minimize risk to faculty and students? What constitutes "reasonable accommodation" for students who may have disabilities? What nursing practices might make reasonable accommodation difficult?

8

Federal Health Policy

Issues for the Nursing Profession in the 21st Century

Janet Heinrich, DrPH, RN, FAAN
Mary Wakefield, PhD, RN, FAAN

As a nation, we have been concerned about cost and distribution of medical care since the beginning of the 20th century. The Committee on Costs of Medical Care (CCMC) reported medical services as maldistributed and badly organized, with no coordination beyond the walls of any particular hospital and clinic (Starr, 1982). The U.S. health care system continues to be diverse and pluralistic as we enter the 21st century, but with deepening concerns about cost, access, and quality. Costs continue to escalate in spite of efforts to use market forces to control them through competition. Although growth of expenditures has slowed for hospital and physician services, the rate of growth has increased in other sectors, such as outpatient services and

pharmaceuticals (Levit et al., 1998). Growing numbers of people are uninsured or underinsured, thus having limited access to basic primary and preventive care (Kuttner, 1999). Consumer groups and many providers voice fears of decreasing safety and quality as we try to decrease unit costs and increase productivity in ever changing health care systems (President's Advisory Commission on Consumer Protection and Quality in the Health Care Industry, 1998).

Policy makers and elected officials at federal and state levels are concerned about numerous health care issues. These are articulated in proposed legislation, appropriation bills, and regulations promulgated through federal and state agencies of the executive branch of government.

Nurses must understand the process by which health care issues receive attention at national and state levels, how issues are analyzed and by whom, and how legislation is implemented. Nursing as a profession needs to be thoughtful and strategic about where to focus its efforts. In this chapter we identify "hot" issues important to nurses, describe the process for federal health policy decision-making, and suggest strategies for nurses to affect health policies about which they are concerned.

■ Nursing Issues for the 21st Century

Many issues confronting the U.S. Congress each session are brought to the attention of legislators by constituencies from their home districts or states. With the current demographic trends in the United States, health issues regarding our aging population are likely to be central concerns for many years to come. The long-term financial future of Medicare and Social Security will continue to be discussed, as will issues related to quality and costs of long-term care in nursing homes, assisted living, and home care services. Access to new technology and new pharmaceuticals will continue to be debated as well as who will pay for these "state of the science" breakthroughs.

Consumer Participation

Recognition of the need for involvement of consumers in health care policy and decision-making is growing. Protection of consumers in legislation such as the "Patients' Bill of Rights Act" (56/HR 358, January 1999) that focuses on choice of health care providers—providing recourse for individuals and families when care is denied or they have objections to other managed care policies and practices—is an example of empowering individuals in making health care decisions. Pertinent legislation introduced

at the national level and in all 50 state legislative bodies is supported by a broad coalition of health care providers, consumer groups, and labor organizations. Additional legislation can be expected, which will encourage consumers to assume even more responsibility for their own health care and require that valid information be provided to individuals and families so that they can make informed choices. Protection of individual health information, especially as related to privacy issues, will continue to be an important area of concern with the advent of new computerized health information systems. Patient privacy and confidentiality legislation has been proposed in the past but not acted upon. Yet to be identified is the best approach for safeguarding patients' rights to privacy. Legislative proposals should balance privacy issues with the need for information that documents appropriateness, necessity, and quality of care required for quality assurance, payment of third-party payers, and for other research designed to improve care (Goldman, 1998).

Health Professions Education

Federal support for education in the health professions—nursing, medicine, public health, and other disciplines—will continue to be controversial. The increase in supply of physicians and nurses has been dramatic in the United States, to the point that some argue there is now a surplus. However, workforce studies have been inconclusive regarding supply and demand for physicians and nurses (Lohr, Vanselow, & Detmer, 1996; Wunderlich, Sloan, & Davis, 1996). Some conservative groups advocate a free and unregulated market approach, with no government involvement in workforce planning. Others argue for a highly centralized approach to match workforce supply with demand. Government funding, with minimal regulation of the number of people prepared for the health professions, has been provided since the early 1960s.

The Health Professions Education Partnerships Act of 1998 authorized federal support to (a) strengthen nursing education and practice, (b) support advanced nursing education programs, (c) sustain minority and disadvantaged education programs, and (d) provide traineeships and nursing student loan funds. The Medicare program has paid a major portion of costs of medical training through Graduate Medical Education (GME) expenditures. This subsidy amounted to approximately 38% of hospital costs for residency training programs in 1992 (Kovner, 1998). In 1994, Medicare provided approximately $248 million to hospitals in support of nursing education costs through GME (American Nurses Association [ANA], 1998).

Policy makers at state and national levels are developing proposals to support funding for education that align policies with needs for health professionals in (a) specific specialty areas such as primary care and (b) in rural and federally designated Health Professional Shortage Areas (HPSA). Policies important to monitor in relation to workforce issues include the National Health Service Corps (NHSC) and entry of foreign educated nurses and physicians through temporary visas. Continued development of global trade agreements—North American Free Trade Agreement (NAFTA) and General Agreement on Tariffs and Trade (GATT)—that encourage free trade of health services among participating countries need surveillance.

Devolution of Decision-Making

In the last several years, policy makers at state and national levels have engaged in major debates over authority for major social programs, such as Medicaid and welfare. At issue is the extent to which control of programs should be shifted from the federal government to the states. This migration, or devolution, often is known as the "New Federalism." States

have gained increased freedom to run Medicaid and other health programs that are responsive to local needs. The federal Balanced Budget Act (BBA) of 1997 repealed many federal requirements governing state reimbursement of nursing homes, hospitals, and community health centers. It also eliminated the need for states to obtain waivers to enroll most Medicaid beneficiaries in managed care organizations. At the same time that states have gained increased flexibility, major increases in the number of uninsured in most regions of the country have put additional burdens on state efforts to provide essential health care services to low-income populations (Kondratas, Weil, & Goldstein, 1998). Many contend that states are in the forefront of redesigning U.S. health and social policy. Opponents of devolution argue that many states will not adequately meet needs of low-income populations and that lack of uniform national standards could result in a "race to the bottom," with increasing economic competition among the states. Nurses need to stay involved at the local level while the "New Federalism" plays out and local decisions are made about services to uninsured and low-income populations.

Access to Health Care for Everyone

A major concern for the nursing profession will continue to be creation of a health care system that assures access to quality services at affordable costs to everyone. In 1992, major nursing organizations worked together to develop, publish, and disseminate *Nursing's Agenda for Health Care Reform* (ANA, 1992). It called for a basic "core" set of essential services to be available to everyone and located in convenient sites, focusing on health and prevention and away from illness and cure. A similar process to develop a policy agenda for the 21st century needs to be considered. To that end several health care foundations are funding efforts to convene forums for public discussions of the health care system and current problems in insurance coverage.

Public interests in health care reforms need to converge to address (a) access to cost-effective services for special populations such as older people, children, vulnerable groups, and the working poor; (b) the general population now covered through plans offered by employers; and (c) interests of health care providers who seek freedom from intrusive policies that curtail professional decision-making. As of 1999, the ranks of uninsured had grown to 43 million, up by more than 10 million from a decade earlier (Holahan, Wiener, & Wallin, 1998). The United States is the only industrialized nation in the world that does not assure health care for all its people. Yet the United States spends more money on its health care system than any other country.

■ An Overview of the Federal Legislative Process

Nursing Role in Identifying Needs

Knowledge and understanding of the legislative process represents power for nurses to effect change and participate effectively in the democratic process. Ideas expressed by constituents and organizations often are the genesis for new legislation. For example, nurses may identify a need for expanded child health services in rural and inner city areas. This idea might then be shared with one or more members of the nurses' congressional delegation through correspondence or face-to-face meetings. Concerns for child health might also be shared with the congressional member's legislative assistant responsible for health issues. Professional nursing organizations might approach congressional members and their staffs, asking them to consider drafting bills designed to address particular concerns. Nursing organizations can then focus on members who have a particular interest in the issue and who serve on the committee that will ultimately have jurisdiction over the bill.

Once a senator or representative has drafted a bill, incorporating the ideas expressed, the bill is introduced into the respective chamber and subsequently referred to committee(s) that has (have) jurisdiction over content of the bill. Although nurses may wish to ask their congressional delegation to vote for an introduced bill, support should be requested even earlier. It is useful to ask legislative members to cosponsor a bill that will be or has been introduced but has not yet come to the floor for a vote. Cosponsorship indicates commitment and large numbers of cosponsors enhance the likelihood that the bill will move through Congress.

Authorizing Committees

Two general categories of committees in both the House and Senate are responsible for considering bills. One type of committee is responsible for authorizing government programs. Generally, a program is first authorized and then, in separate legislation, money to support the program is appropriated. It is possible to have an authorized program, yet not have appropriations to support it—making it impotent.

Authorizing committees for most health legislation include the Senate Health, Education, Labor and Pensions (HELP) Committee, the House Commerce Committee, and the House Ways and Means Committee. Although many authorizing committees have jurisdiction over various programs, such as agriculture, defense, and health, there is only one appropriating committee in each chamber. Each appropriations committee, however, has 13 subcommittees with responsibility for different programs. Appropriations for most federally funded discretionary health programs are initiated by the Senate and House Appropriations Subcommittees for Labor, Health, and Human Services and Education. To illustrate the authorization and appropriation process, when the National Institute of Nursing Research was authorized in 1993, nurses needed to focus efforts each year on obtaining adequate funding for nursing research through the appropriations committees.

Characteristic of most federal programs is reauthorization that occurs at various intervals, often from 3 to 5 years. For example, the Nursing Education Act that includes all the programs carried out through the Division of Nursing was reauthorized in 1998. When authorization is allowed to lapse, arguing for appropriations to fund programs is more difficult. Considerable attention is given to evaluating program success and making programmatic changes based on information and comments from interested individuals and organizations.

Because of the role that various committees and subcommittees play in reviewing and shaping legislation, knowing who committee members are and committee assignments of your elected representatives is essential. Committee assignments often determine the issues with which House and Senate members will be most involved and can be most influential. Members with health care committee assignments are in a strategic position to influence the content and viability of the bills being considered to change federal health programs. If a bill is not moving out of committee, nurses can request assistance in obtaining action from members of their delegation serving on that committee (deVries & Vanderbilt, 1992).

Prior to a committee sending an authorization or appropriation bill to the full House or Senate, committee hearings ordinarily are held to allow input into provisions of the proposed legislation. Usually arranged by their professional organizations, nurses are asked to testify at relevant congressional hearings. This opportunity is important because testimony becomes part of the public record and nurses who testify have an opportunity to speak directly to committee members.

After hearings, the committee meets to consider and recommend changes in the bill—a process referred to as "mark up." If there are provisions that nurses believe should be added or deleted prior to a bill going to the full House or Senate for a vote, recommendations should be presented to committee members prior to mark up. Changes usually are much easier to accomplish in a relatively small committee than through amendments introduced on the Senate or House floor.

Senate and House Considerations

Once a bill has been forwarded to the full House or Senate, it is typically up to the Majority Leader in the Senate or the Rules Committee in the House to determine if and when it will be considered on the floor. After one chamber votes on the bill as forwarded by the committee, it is then sent to the other chamber. The other chamber may (a) ignore the bill and work on similar legislation that it is developing, (b) pass the bill in its original form as sent from the initiating chamber, or (c) after having been received, send the bill to the appropriate committee for evaluation and eventually return to the full chamber for a vote.

After similar bills are passed by each chamber, a conference committee consisting of members from both chambers is formed. The conference committee is composed primarily of members from committees of jurisdiction, and the purpose of their work is to eliminate differences in the bills. The two chambers frequently pass different versions of a bill, obliging members of conference committees to negotiate differences. Members of conference committees are not supposed to insert new provisions, but such activities are not uncommon. Whether any member of a nurse's congressional delegation is serving on the conference committee is important for the nurse to know because significant changes can still be made in the final version of the bill. Once the majority of committee members have signed the conference report, the report is sent back to both the House and Senate for a final vote. Upon passage, the bill is forwarded to the White House for action by the president.

White House Signature and Federal Agency Jurisdiction

After legislation has been signed by the president, it is forwarded to the federal agency that has jurisdiction over that legislation. The agency is charged with writing regulations to implement the new law that reflect accurately its intent. These regulations are subject to public comment before they become final. For example, when legislation was enacted that provided reimbursement for advanced practice nurses under Medicare, regulations to implement the bill came from the Health Care Financing Administration, Department of Health and Human Services—the agency with responsibility for Medicare policies.

Thus individuals and organizations can attempt to influence legislative outcomes at various points in the process. Often nursing and health care organizations employ health policy analysts and lobbyists to draft, track, and evaluate legislative proposals. Considering the magnitude of federal health care issues, nurses can influence the health care of individuals, families, and communities on a vastly greater scale by means of health policy than through virtually any other means. Involvement in policy formation not only is desirable, it is imperative.

■ Strategies for Influencing Policy

Channels for Nursing Legislative Input

Nurses can make their views effectively known to Congress through three different vehicles. First, individual nurses can cultivate ongoing working relationships with congressional offices. Second, nurses can work through membership in professional associations and interest groups to establish legislative agendas and priorities. Third, nurses can participate in national advisory groups mandated to advise Congress and the administration on specific issues such as Medicare policies or nursing education.

Individual Contact

In making contact with congressional members, working relationships also should be established with legislative assistants who handle the congressional members' health issues. These aides exercise considerable influence in shaping congressional attitudes and opinions. When communicating with members and staff, either through writing or personal meetings, nurses should indicate their educational background and expertise relevant to the positions they are advocating. Additionally, holding an office in a statewide or national nursing or other organization is advantageous if the individual's views are representative of organizational members' views. Financial implications of a proposal should be delineated, and the extent to which constituents would be affected should be identified. Facts should be offered and actions being requested specifically identified. In addition, if a proponent is asked about opposition, arguments of those who oppose the proposal should be articulated fairly.

Although appointments can be arranged in Washington, D.C., effective meetings with legislators and their staffs can occur in their home states, often over weekends or during congressional recesses. In addition, staff in the congressional member's state offices also can be contacted. Local staff are often underutilized for communicating information to congressional members.

To help a legislator or staff person to focus on issues of concern to nurses, arranging visits to schools or health care settings, allowing the legislator or assistant to observe a situation first hand and also to meet with other interested individuals. Lobbying by a coalition is effective, and indicating that views presented are shared by other groups is important. In general, personal interactions often make stronger impressions on the legislator and staff than limiting them to reading concerns expressed in a letter, mass postcard mailings, or e-mail messages.

Communication needs to be well organized and brief. In addition to expressing concerns about an issue or recommending a position on a particular bill, correspondence conveying appreciation for votes on particular issues is effective. Knowing that a particular vote or stand on an issue was well received by constituents is beneficial to legislative members. Communication should be made with knowledge of the legislative timetable (deVries & Vanderbilt, 1992). If, for example, support is being solicited for funding for nursing research, early interaction in the appropriations process via mail, telephone, and e-mail is important. Giving examples of promising studies and relevance of research findings to patient outcomes can be useful.

Working Through Nursing Organizations

In addition to individual nurses' interactions with a congressional delegation, significant strides in influencing policy are made when representatives of national nursing organizations develop ongoing relationships with congressional offices. The American Nurses Association, the American Association of Colleges of Nursing, and specialty nursing organizations such as the Oncology Nursing Society have developed effective working relationships with many offices on Capitol Hill. Policy analysts from nursing organizations spend considerable time educating legislative

assistants, congressional members, administrative officials, and representatives of other organizations on nursing and health care issues. Through professional organizations, nurses can be involved in drafting legislation, providing statistical and other factual information requested by congressional offices, testifying at hearings, and evaluating proposed legislation.

Nursing organizations that have committed time and resources to shape health policy provide immeasurable service to their members, other nurses, and health care consumers. Without the investment of time and expertise made by professional nursing associations to influence policy, both nursing and consumer health care would be affected adversely. The extent to which this investment can be made is contingent on continued and expanding support of nursing organization membership. Views shared by groups of people are typically more motivating to congressional members than single voices (Ornstein & Elder, 1978). When a nursing organization representative states that the position presented is supported by thousands of nurses, or 1 in 44 registered women voters, it is often difficult for congressional members to ignore the position.

National Advisory Committee Membership

Many opportunities are available for nurses to serve on national advisory committees that issue reports and advice to Congress. All agencies at the National Institutes of Health, the Bureau of Health Professions, Centers for Disease Control and Prevention, and the Agency for Health Care Policy and Research, to name just a few, have advisory councils that provide recommendations to the administration and issue reports to Congress. The Institute of Medicine (IOM) of the National Academy of Sciences is constantly putting together panels of experts for studies on a variety of topics mandated by Congress. Examples of past studies include quality issues in long term care, primary care, nurse staffing in hospitals and nursing homes, environmental issues, and child health.

The president may establish special advisory groups with a specified time frame for a report, such as the Advisory Commission on Consumer Protection and Quality in the Health Care Industry. Or, for ongoing advice Congress may create an entity such as the Medicare Payment Advisory Commission (MedPAC) that focuses on new payment methodologies for health care providers, access to care, adjusted community rates under Medicare, and disproportionate share payments to hospitals, among other controversial issues.

Getting appointed to an advisory committee often requires support from a broad network of congressional members, agency staff, and both nursing and nonnursing organizations. A nurse who wants to be so involved should develop a list of potential supporters with the help of colleagues. In considering these people it is important for the nurse to have determined where decision-making will occur and whose opinion will matter the most to the identified decision makers.

Then, to facilitate attaining support for committee appointment the nurse should

1. send a résumé with a request for support;

2. draft key points for inclusion in a letter of support;

3. articulate why it is critical that the specific nurse's perspective is represented "at the table";

4. emphasize the nurse's ability to work in interdisciplinary work groups, effectively express

views, and demonstrate concerns that extend beyond nursing specific issues; and

5. request that telephone calls be made in support of the individual nurse's request for committee appointment.

To be an effective member of an advisory group, nurses must do their homework and understand the issues being discussed. That usually requires reading volumes of material—some of which will be incomprehensible—ahead of meetings. The member should seek advice from outside experts and to ask colleagues for information and views. It is also desirable to obtain perspectives from professional organizations and consumer groups that may have concerns or recommendations on specific issues. Nurses bring useful clinical perspective on patient and family needs as well as knowledge of how health care systems work. Nurses also should have a healthy understanding of the group process and how and when to intervene and when to negotiate.

■ Concluding Statement

Health issues with which Congress is grappling are complex and far-reaching. That the nursing profession and individual nurses use their expertise to assist Congress in developing health policy is imperative. To accomplish that objective, nurses must make their views known on health issues and understand the process and the players, both at state and national levels. Nurses also need to capitalize on and support both broadly based professional and narrower specialty nursing organizations that are available to them.

■ References

American Nurses Association. (1992). *Nursing's agenda for health care reform.* Washington, DC: American Nurses Publishing.

American Nurses Association. (1998). *Legislative and regulatory initiatives for the 105th Congress.* Washington, DC: American Nurses Publishing.

Balanced Budget Act of 1997. (P.L. 105–33), August 1997, HR 3426-Medicare and Medicaid Health Insurance Act, *U.S. Statutes at Large* (Volume VII, pp. 251–788). Washington, DC: U.S. Government Printing Office.

deVries, C., & Vanderbilt, M. (1992). *The grassroots lobbying handbook: Empowering nurses through legislative and political action.* Washington, DC: American Nurses Association.

Goldman, J. (1998). Protecting privacy to improve health care. *Health Affairs, 17*(6), 47.

Health Professions Education Partnerships Act of 1998. (P. L. 105–392), November 13, 1998. Amendment to Title 7 and 8 of the Public Health Service Act.

Holahan, J., Wiener, J., & Wallin, S. (1998). *Health policy for the low-income population: Major findings from assessing the new federalism case studies.* Washington, DC: Urban Institute.

Kondratas, A., Weil, A., & Goldstein, N. (1998). Assessing the new federalism: An introduction. *Health Affairs, 17*(3), 17.

Kovner, A. R. (1998). *Jonas's health care delivery in the United States.* New York: Springer.

Kuttner, R. (1999). The American health care system: Employer-sponsored health coverage. *New England Journal of Medicine, 340*(3), 248–252.

Levit, K., Cowan, C., Braden, B., Stiller, J., Sensenig, A., & Lazenby, H. (1998). National health expenditures in 1997: More slow growth. *Health Affairs, 17*(6), 99.

Lohr, K., Vanselow, N., & Detmer, D. (Eds.) (1996). *The nation's physician workforce: Options for balancing supply and requirements.* Washington, DC: National Academy Press.

Ornstein, N., & Elder, S. (1978). *Interest groups, lobbying and policymaking.* Washington, DC: Congressional Quarterly Press.

Patients' Bill of Rights Act (56/HR 358, January 1999). (According to the library it appears that the final bill has not yet been passed!)

President's Advisory Commission on Consumer Protection and Quality in the Health Care Industry. (1998). *Quality first: Better health care for all Americans.* Washington, DC: U.S. Government Printing Office.

Starr, P. (1982). *The social transformation of American medicine.* New York: Basic Books.

Wunderlich, G., Sloan, F., & Davis, C. (1996). *Nursing staff in hospitals and nursing homes: Is it adequate?* Washington, DC: National Academy Press.

■ Editor's Questions for Discussion

How does Buerhaus' discussion (Chapter 10) support assessment and comments by Heinrich and Wakefield? Debate who should pay for the financial future of medicine and Social Security. To what extent should control of programs be shifted from the federal government to the states? What role should nurses and professional associations play in resolving the debate? How may the Thompson and Lavandero (Chapter 9) discussion about associations contribute to your response? What impact may free trade of health services among countries have on the profession of nursing, nursing education programs, and practice?

By what means and through what organizational groups or associations should nursing as a profession be involved in health care policy? How can nursing as a profession provide national leadership for converging public interests in health care reform? What interventions may nursing organizations provide in the legislative process of policy development? How can professional nurses best use their expertise in developing health policy?

How should nursing students be introduced to, learn about, and participate in legislative processes for health policy-making? What role modeling should faculty offer and how? Define one critical issue in health care. Propose a plan, strategy, and implementation for addressing the issue via legislation. Who, why, when, where, and at what level would you involve others in implementing your plan?

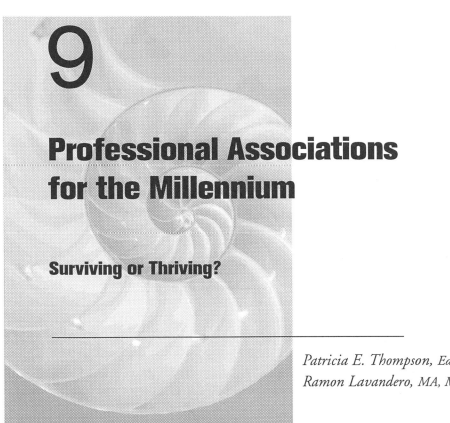

9

Professional Associations for the Millennium

Surviving or Thriving?

Patricia E. Thompson, EdD, RN
Ramon Lavandero, MA, MSN, RN

Associations spring to life when a group of people want to accomplish something that its members cannot do as individuals. Alexis de Tocqueville (1945) stated:

> Associations are formed by people who share a common interest in [a profession] and who are able to identify others with the same interests. In many cases, individuals are not aware of others who share their interest or concern until the association's founders articulate it and make it known. (p. 117)

Nursing associations support members by speaking for them in legislative and regulatory forums, improving working conditions, fostering practice standards, and promoting profes-

sional development (Bower, 1999). Such has been the case since American nursing associations began in the late 19th century. With an ultimate aim of promoting health and curing disease, nursing associations have organized to fulfill one or more of the following purposes: strengthening the profession, educating nurses to practice in particular situations or roles, credentialing practitioners, and recognizing professional accomplishment.

By representing critical masses of nurses, associations can be a mighty force to achieve professional unity. However, when they focus myopically on narrow special interests, associations are equally powerful in fostering fragmentation. Co-author Ramon Lavandero has observed the evolution of numerous nursing organizations, making him a frontline witness to many of the historical developments described in this chapter.

■ Development of American Nursing Associations

Established in 1897, the American Nurses Association (ANA) is the organization most often associated with strengthening the profession because of its commitment to improving education, working conditions, and public policy decisions affecting nurses and patients. Its subsidiary, the American Nurses Credentialing Center (ANCC), also makes ANA a hub of professional credentialing through voluntary certification and continuing education.

Other credentialing groups accredit either academic programs or individual practitioners. Until 1996, the National League for Nursing was sole provider of voluntary accreditation for all professional nursing education programs in the United States. That year, the American Association of Colleges of Nursing (AACN) established the Commission on Collegiate Nursing Education (CCNE), an autonomous voluntary accrediting agency for baccalaureate and graduate education. In addition to ANCC, dozens of certification boards accredit individual nurses for specific roles and practice areas. These include the American Association of Nurse Anesthetists, Certification Board Perioperative Nursing, and Oncology Nursing Certification Corporation.

Since the early 20th century, practice- and role-focused associations have played an important part in nursing's development. The public health nursing section of the American Public Health Association, founded in 1923, and the American Association of Nurse-Midwives (renamed the American College of Nurse Midwives–ACNM), founded in 1929, are among the oldest. More recent entries in these categories include the Association of Perioperative Registered Nurses (AORN) and the American Organization of Nurse Executives (AONE), an affiliate of the American Hospital Association.

As American health care became more complex and technologically sophisticated in the fourth quarter of the 20th century, the number of specialty associations exploded. As of 1999, ANA's Nursing Organization Liaison Forum counted more than 80 members. In 1973, the American Nurses Association established the American Academy of Nursing, a self-governing affiliate, to fulfill a vision of transforming health care so as to optimize the well-being of Americans and people in the world generally (Kelly & Joel, 1995). In recognition of their professional achievement and excellence, nurses may be nominated to become Academy fellows, joining a cadre of nationally prominent colleagues who bring their best thinking to address critical issues facing the profession.

Most nursing associations have been autonomous from the beginning, although some started as affiliates of their medical counterparts. For example, the Association of Women's Health, Obstetrics and Neonatal Nursing (AWHONN) began as the Nurses' Association of the American College of Obstetrics and Gynecology (NAACOG).

Occasionally, medical societies have evolved to become interdisciplinary organizations. Members of the Society of Critical Care Medicine (SCCM) include physicians, nurses, respiratory therapists, pharmacists, and other professionals who care for the critically ill. Other organizations, such as the American Burn Association (ABA), have been interdisciplinary from the outset.

Geographic Divisions

To become more accessible to members and carry out their missions more effectively, associations organize in a variety of geographic configurations. Most associations charter local chapters wherever there is a critical mass of interested members. Many specialty organizations also have regional or state councils. Regional or local units always are bound by their members' shared professional interests, although their legal relationships with the parent organization may differ.

Some associations, such as the ANA, are federations of affiliating state associations. The International Council of Nurses also is a federation. Its constituents are national nursing associations like the ANA. But there are also nonfederated international nursing associations, such as the International Society of Nurses in Cancer Care.

As the 20th century drew to a close, nursing associations were responding to demands of an increasingly global society. Sigma Theta Tau International, the honor society of nursing, has framed a strategic plan that will propel the organization onto the world scene through leadership provided by its members' commitment to improving the health of their communities. Interestingly, this interest in transnational linkages renews the seminal work of Lavinia Dock at the start of the century. Dock maintained lively and frequent correspondence with her European colleagues, even without the fax or Internet (M. S. Kennedy, personal communication, 1999).

■ The Work of Associations

Five Activities

How do nursing associations carry out their missions? Like other professional associations, nursing associations focus on five general kinds of activities: standards setting, professional development and education, credentialing, recognition, and group benefits.

Professional associations set the standards by which professionals practice and are evaluated. The goal is for health professionals to develop standards in concert with regulatory agencies, payors, and those they serve. In the United States, they often lobby for their standards to be included in health care legislation.

Logically, associations have become major providers of learning programs for their professions. Initially, they were the main continuing education source for American health professionals. However, since the 1980s, associations have faced heavy competition from for-profit education providers. Many times these companies are operated by the professional associations' own members. Competition has given consumers a wider variety of learning programs and, aided by new technology, propelled growth in distance learning. But competition also has jeopardized associations' main revenue stream, leading them to set up for-profit education, publishing, and consulting subsidiaries of their own.

Often associations assume responsibility for specialty credentialing in their profession. They typically do so through a separate credentialing corporation that is either independent from the association or its wholly owned subsidiary. For example, the American Board of Neuroscience Nursing operates independently from the neuroscience nursing association but maintains a liaison relationship with it. In critical care, the AACN Certification Corporation is a wholly owned subsidiary of the American Association of Critical-Care Nurses, which appoints its board of directors. Credentialing programs usually are voluntary, although some, like those in anesthesia and midwifery, are required for state licensure in the specialty.

Associations also support professional standards by giving awards to exceptional individuals and groups and by supporting funding research and demonstration projects. In 1936, Sigma Theta Tau awarded the first grant for nursing research. Today, grants are made increasingly in alliance with other professional groups. For example, Sigma Theta Tau International awards joint research grants with the

Emergency Nurses Foundation and the American Association of Diabetes Educators, among others.

As a service to members and a source of operating revenue, many associations offer a variety of discounted group benefits to their members. Typical benefits include health and liability insurance, credit cards, and discounted rates for books and software, educational programs, legal services, and car rentals.

Delivery of Services

How do nursing associations deliver their services? Traditionally, associations were born as a result of face-to-face contact among the founders. Postal and telephone communication were added, and many new groups now use electronic mail and synchronous online chat from the start. When today's nursing associations recognize that face-to-face contact, print materials, and electronic media are all tools in a kit and select the best tool for the job, they will reach their constituencies more effectively, efficiently, and economically.

Face-to-face communication is so embedded in the fabric of nursing that it is still the standard for communication. When resources allow, association leaders and working committees are likely to meet face-to-face. Conventions and education programs also tend to be face-to-face events. As technology improves, telephone meetings and synchronous online chat are being used to reach distant members and contain expenses, especially for transnational organizations such as Sigma Theta Tau International and the International Council of Nurses.

When an association cannot communicate with its members in person, it sends them print materials. Its print pieces serve several purposes—communicating professional news, announcing and providing professional education, disseminating scientific and clinical knowledge, helping members network, and

generating revenue. There may be separate pieces for each purpose; for example, newsletters, magazines, journals, and brochures, or a combined publication can be produced.

As computer technology becomes more widely available, associations are recognizing its value as a communication tool. Venturing into the online world, associations are beginning to use computers and the Internet to summarize face-to-face contacts and disseminate print materials. In the late 1990s, association magazines became available online in either abstracted or full-text format. And several online-only journals for nurses are published, such as Sigma Theta Tau's *Online Journal for Knowledge Synthesis in Nursing*. Online services are becoming an important way to reach members who are geographically inaccessible or who cannot attend face-to-face events for other reasons.

■ Life Stages of an Association

Associations develop in stages that mirror those of human beings, undoubtedly because they are created by people. Arthur D. Little, Inc., has described five stages in the maturation of industries—embryonic, growth, staff operation, maturity, and aging (Dunlop, 1989). Development of an association usually matches these stages.

Five Stages

An association's identity and purpose are molded during the embryonic stage when a group of professionals with shared interests decides to make its informal networking formal. This stage is characterized by high energy and excitement. The founders define the new association's purpose and gather human and financial resources to do its work. But embryonic energy often fuels crises that will punctuate every phase of the association's life. This first crisis is one in which conflicting visions and strategies must be reconciled. Crises frequently lead either to new found strength or to fragmentation and retrenchment. At times these crises propel the organization to a new stage.

The growth stage emerges when founders start paying for work. The founders recognize that, to prosper and grow, the organization needs more than random help from volunteers. They hire clerical help, perhaps by paying someone for work previously done as a volunteer or buying support time from an association management company. Either way, paying for work marks a significant developmental change. It also may incubate a new source of tension if staff members and volunteers have conflicting priorities or lack clarity about each other's roles.

An association moves into the staff operation stage as it grows in size and complexity in response to membership growth, expanded programs, and need for more resources. During this stage, its fundamental culture solidifies. The basic choreography of the volunteer–staff dance is also written at this time, although this happens accidentally more often than intentionally (Dunlop, 1989). Initially during the staff operation stage, volunteers and staff vigorously negotiate the boundaries of each other's authority. This action may become a source of great tension for nursing associations because the law invests governance authority in an association's members. The tension builds when key staff members who are nurses believe that they know more than their volunteer colleagues because of their dual identity as nurses and full-time association executives. Or tension may build when key staff members who are not nurses but are trained as association executives must prove repeatedly to volunteers that they understand the nuances of the nursing profession.

Driven by effective leadership or in response to a crisis, an association adopts a typ-ical way of operation and moves into maturity. Nursing associations exist to support the work of nurses, so associations mature as the profession matures. This maturity is marked by membership growth, subspecialization, and turf encroachment. Membership grows as more nurses choose the type of work supported by a particular association, but it begins to segment or diminish when members specialize.

Professional associations age when a profession declines—when the association responds ineffectively to changes in its profession or when it is confronted with a combination of related factors. Aging associations usually follow one of two paths. Many wither on the vine, dying along with their profession or with founders who did not identify viable successors. For others, aging becomes a catalyst for rebirth. Nursing associations can seize this unique opportunity to fend off the aging process and self-renew if they are guided by visionary leaders. Need for nurses will always exist, despite peaks and valleys of market demand. But, as a community's health care needs continue to evolve, nurses will need to keep their knowledge and skills current. When a nursing association recognizes or, ideally, anticipates and responds effectively to new demands, it can acquire a new lease on life. In the new millennium these associations will either just manage to survive, or they will truly thrive.

■ Quality Indicators for Thriving Associations

Several indicators mark a thriving association. The first indicator focuses on meeting needs of both the professional group and its members. A clearly focused mission statement effectively implemented is key to accomplishing this task. With overlap and duplication of goals by many organizations, identifying and marketing a unique function is critical for success of an association. Current and potential members need to know what the association and the profession can offer them that is not available elsewhere. With a large number of professional associations from which to choose, nurses are going to select carefully where they spend their time and money based on perceived returned value.

Meeting the needs of the membership centers on understanding who the members are. According to Kennedy (1997), effective associations in the future are going to have to focus on meeting member needs across generations. Historically, the majority of nurses are from the baby boom generation (1946–1959), and this group currently holds most leadership positions in associations. Boomers like to lead, care about what others think, and enjoy communicating on a personal level. The cuspers (1960–1965), busters (1965–1975), and post-TV (1975–1981) generations have a different work ethic, lifestyle, and methods of communicating, which results in a variety of different needs and expectations from an association. Cuspers can lead but are comfortable as followers. They enjoy working with people and are not computer literate. The busters and post-TV generation, however, understand technology and prefer to work alone. They are not interested in holding leadership positions. Associations must recognize these differences and market services accordingly. One approach is to have a basic membership fee for everyone and then self-selected add-on fees for services that members pick from available options. Twenty-four hour access to association services also will be desired. Associations that do not address these differences in generational needs will find themselves without members (Kennedy, 1997).

Relevance is another requisite for an association to thrive. Number of active members, goal-related work accomplished, and the association's reputation for pursuing its stated mission are measures of relevance. Maintaining active members who volunteer time and support is challenging. The association's respon-

siveness to its members and their needs is key in retaining and keeping members involved. Accomplishing the association's work is an important expectation. Members, as well as other constituents, expect the time and money they donate to result in definite outcomes. Relevance also is measured by an association's recognition, based on its reputation and the actions and competence of its individual members in terms of achieving its mission.

Thriving associations in the future will have visionary leaders who can scan the environment and project not only where the organization needs to be positioned for success, but also can move the group in that direction. Doing so requires both flexibility and risk taking on the part of the association. It also requires ongoing strategic planning with input from both internal and external constituents.

The structure of association governance will differ in the future from current models. With change becoming the norm, governance models need to be developed for rapid response to critical issues and member needs. Expanded use of technology is one way to accomplish this goal. Technology also will provide tools for boards to communicate and make decisions quickly (Blanken & Liff, 1998).

■ Resources Needed for the Future

Adequate resources are essential for associations to thrive. These resources include personnel, technology, and revenue. Personnel for an association involves leadership, membership, and staff. Each group provides infrastructure for the organization's survival. Leaders of the association must be visionaries as they position the group for the future. They must also be viewed as credible and having the expertise to make decisions for the association in a complex, ever changing environment. Leadership styles will change as members who are not boomers move into these positions.

The membership is a valuable asset for any association; the challenge is how to recruit and retain that asset. To stay involved, members must value the goals of the association and believe that their commitment of time and money is accomplishing worthwhile purposes. Competition for members will increase, so associations that are collaborative will thrive. One collaborative strategy could be discounted dues for members belonging to partnered associations. With baby boomers at or nearing retirement age, associations will recognize the potential pool of talent and expertise that this segment of the membership has to offer. Strategies should be developed to target recruitment of retirees into volunteer positions within the association.

Staff is a critical group in any association. To sustain the smooth operation of the association, staff members must be experts in their fields. The key staff position is Chief Executive Officer (CEO), who can either facilitate growth or evoke disaster for the association. Ability of the other officers and the CEO to work together and foster a true commitment to the organization from the staff is important for thriving associations.

Staying on the "cutting edge" of technology and its many uses will move an association into the new millennium successfully. The level of technology use in associations varies, but full use of this resource in meeting association and member needs has not yet occurred. Technology can connect people and groups to facilitate achievement of an association's mission. Interactive Web pages already are in use, but few associations with similar purposes have linked their Web pages. Holding meetings of the board or committees or both with people around the world no longer has to occur by telephone conference. Other options include real-time video and Internet meetings.

Associations will need to review revenue sources and carefully analyze use of available revenue. Potentially cost-effective strategies such as partnering with other organizations for activities like programming can prevent duplication of resources. After careful analysis many associations will outsource some services. Associations that thrive will move from a majority dues-financed operation to a multisource revenue base. Associations increasingly will focus on what they can market in services and sales. Another approach will be to emphasize philanthropic giving by members and supporters of the association.

■ Concluding Statement

Historically, associations have been an important part of professional nursing. The work they accomplish makes a difference for the profession, its members, and the health of the public. In the new millennium associations must adjust to constant change as the norm. To thrive and not just survive will require leadership to balance a variety of issues for an intergenerational membership. Not all associations will survive, but those that do will have implemented strategies to meet successfully the needs of both its members and the profession in a changing world.

■ References

Blanken, R. L., & Liff, A. (1998). *Facing the future: Preparing your association to thrive.* Washington, DC: The Foundation of the American Society of Association Executives.

Bower, F. L. (1999). The role of professional organizations. In E. J. Sullivan (Ed.), *Creating nursing's future: Issues, opportunities and challenges* (pp. 345–354). St. Louis: Mosby.

deTocqueville, A. (1945). *Democracy in America* (Vol. 2, p. 117). New York: Random House. (Original work published: Volume 1, 1835 and Volume 2, 1840, London: Saunders and Otley.)

Dunlop, J. J. (1989). *Leading the association.* Washington, DC: The Foundation of the American Society of Association Executives.

Kelly, L. Y., & Joel, L. A. (1995). *Dimensions of professional nursing.* New York: McGraw-Hill.

Kennedy, M. M. (1997). Can you communicate cross-generationally? *Career Strategies Inc.* (Manager's Intelligence Report). Wilmette, IL: Ragan Communications.

■ Editor's Questions for Discussion

What motivates nurses to join one or more professional organizations or associations? Should competition between nursing organizations be encouraged or minimized? Provide specific examples of issues or concerns addressed by each organization or association described by Thompson and Lavandero. Discuss the pros and cons of an umbrella organization for all nursing organizations. Which organization might you propose to be the umbrella organization and why? How might your choice be achieved?

How may nursing students become knowledgeable about the roles and functions of nursing organizations? What role should faculty fulfill in professional associations? Describe stages of members' involvement in professional organizations. What professional development process do members go through?

Identify the critical challenges that nursing organizations must meet. Provide criteria and measures for evaluating professional nursing organizations and association effectiveness. What additional measures of relevance may be used to evaluate the largest professional nursing organization? How does Heinrich and Wakefield's discussion (Chapter 8) apply to professional associations?

How can organizations deal with competing functions and interest groups within one organization? What results may be anticipated if ANA members vote to divide into two groups? How do collective bargaining issues get resolved in professional nursing organizations? How likely are other professions to develop subgroups within one association?

What distinctive leadership skills and requirements are more critical for professional organizations than may be required for leadership roles in health care service settings and academia? How does a leader strategically position a professional organization? What information must the leader have to position it effectively? What functions should organizations provide to thrive? Are associations and organizations in nursing to serve only needs of members or needs of the profession at large and the profession's impact on health care? What critical role should professional associations and organizations have in resolving health care issues such as access to care, types of services, and ethical dilemmas? How should leadership be provided to resolve international health care dilemmas related to cultural and ethical differences?

10

Future of Medicare

Implications for Nursing Practice, Education, and Research

Peter I. Buerhaus, PhD, MS, RN, FAAN

S ince its initiation in 1965, the Medicare program has been one of the federal government's most popular and important social programs. Medicare offers health insurance to nearly 38 million Americans, mostly older, for services provided by hospitals, doctors, nursing homes, and home health care agencies. For more than three decades the Medicare program has ensured access to needed health care to a large and growing segment of the U.S. population. Paying providers to deliver health care services to Medicare beneficiaries also has made the program an important source of revenue for mil-

lions of organizations that, in turn, employ millions of health care professionals and other workers. In 1996, the amount Medicare paid to providers exceeded the income that flowed into the program, thus requiring the program to use some of its financial reserves. Confronted with this problem, members of both political parties in Congress overcame partisan differences among themselves and, working with the Clinton administration, quickly enacted the 1997 Balanced Budget Act (P.L. 105-33, the BBA). The BBA immediately affected the Medicare program in two ways. First, it set forth the largest set of changes to

This chapter was written while Dr. Buerhaus was employed at the Harvard Nursing Research Institute. The opinions expressed do not necessarily reflect the views of the Institute.

the program since Medicare began, including over $100 billion in savings between 1998 and 2002. Second, it established the National Bipartisan Commission on the Future of Medicare to identify options and make recommendations on long-term restructuring of Medicare.

Eighteen months before the BBA was enacted, the nation's economy had begun to grow at an impressive pace. In 1998, rising employment and personal earnings resulted in record income tax collections, which meant that the federal government was suddenly awash in revenues. The ensuing budget surplus, together with effects of vigorous belt tightening by providers in response to growing market competition and anticipation of negative effects of the BBA, resulted in an equally sudden and dramatic easing of the financial pressure on the Medicare program. The BBA originally was expected to prevent the financial insolvency of Medicare to 2005, but in light of those economic changes the projections were pushed back several years. Easing of financial pressures on Medicare also had an impact on the work of the National Bipartisan Commission on the Future of Medicare (the Commission), which was only halfway through its deliberations. With urgency to develop recommendations removed, disagreements over various proposals took on greater importance—so much so that the Commission was unable to obtain the votes required to make any recommendations. Hence in March 1999, the Commission ended without voting on a package of proposals or even issuing a report (Vladeck, 1999).

Despite the Commission's failure to formulate recommendations aimed at ensuring the long-term survival of Medicare, the need to reform the program will remain a major domestic public policy concern during the next 10 years. In 2010, the first of 78 million baby boomers will reach 65 years of age. Thus, the number of Medicare beneficiaries will begin to expand rapidly, placing extreme stress on every aspect of the program (Wilensky & Newhouse, 1999). Leading up to this time, however, politicians probably will be reluctant to tamper with Medicare, given extension of the program's near-term financial stability and the fact that senior citizens—Medicare beneficiaries—vote at higher rates than any other segment of the population. Nevertheless, while the nation's political leadership looks the other way, forces already underway eventually will alter the Medicare program profoundly and, as they do, reverberate throughout the nation's health care financing, organization, and delivery systems. The purpose of this chapter is to identify and discuss the forces and problems facing Medicare, review options to restructure the program and assess prospects for their adoption, and discuss implications for the nursing profession.

■ Background on Medicare Financing, Benefits, Demographics, and Public Support

The Medicare program was modeled after traditional indemnity insurance plans offered by Blue Cross and Blue Shield policies that were dominant in the 1960s. Thus the Medicare program was developed with two major components. Part A, which is analogous to service benefit policies offered by Blue Cross (Wilensky & Newhouse, 1999), pays for inpatient hospital care, the first 100 days of home health care, 100 days of a skilled nursing facility following a hospital stay, and hospice care. Part B, which is analogous to the Blue Shield policy, pays for physician, outpatient hospital, and other services for the aged and disabled. Additional information regarding specific coverage and dollar benefits can be obtained through the Internet site: www.medicare.gov (2000).

Medicare Part A

According to the Board of Trustees of the Federal Hospital Insurance Trust Fund (1997a), when expenditures exceeded income in 1996 and precipitated the 1997 passage of the BBA, Medicare Part A covered 33 million aged and 5 million disabled beneficiaries. The total number of beneficiaries had increased 22.4% over the preceding 10 years, but only about one fifth of these individuals received medical services covered by Part A. Nevertheless, total benefits accrued by these beneficiaries in 1996 amounted to $128.6 billion and average expenditures per beneficiary were $3,400. Payments for costs of fee-for-service inpatient hospital care represented 67% of Part A benefits, skilled nursing and home health care accounted for 22%, managed care plans represented 9%, and hospice benefits accounted for 2%. Administrative costs were 1% of program expenditures.

Part A, also referred to as the Hospital Insurance (HI) program, is financed primarily by payroll taxes paid by workers and employers —FICA, the Social Security tax on earnings. Payroll taxes, which are paid by 147 million workers and account for 89% of total Part A income, are used mainly to pay benefits for *current* beneficiaries. Income not currently needed to pay benefits and related expenses is held in the HI trust fund and invested in U.S. Treasury securities. Interest represents about 8% and revenue from the income taxation of Social Security benefits contributes 3% of total Part A income (Board of Trustees of the Federal Hospital Insurance Trust Fund, 1997a).

Medicare Part B

The other major component of the Medicare program, Part B, provides protection against the costs of physician and other medical services to about 32 million aged and 4 million disabled persons. According to the Board of Trustees of the Federal Supplementary Medical Insurance Trust Fund (1997b), approximately 84% of these individuals receive medical services annually and total benefits on their behalf amounted to $68.6 billion in 1996. The number of Part B enrollees increased by nearly 20% between 1985 and 1996, and average benefits per enrollee amounted to $1,902.

Part B benefits have been growing rapidly and are expected to continue increasing faster than the economy as a whole. Total payments to providers increased by 45% over the past 5 years, and despite substantial government efforts to control Part B costs, payments grew about 14% faster than the economy as a whole. Payment for costs of physician and other professional services represent approximately 63% of Part B benefits, payments to facilities 24%, and managed care plans 13%. Administrative costs run about $1.8 billion, or less than 3% of program expenditures.

Part B also is referred to as the Supplementary Medical Insurance (SMI) program and is financed primarily by transfers from the general fund (i.e., tax revenues) of the U.S. Treasury (76%) and monthly premiums paid by beneficiaries (22%). Interest and other miscellaneous income account for the remainder, or about 2%, of income. In the future, premiums paid by beneficiaries are expected to cover a declining share of program costs—falling to 16% in 2006 and comprising a progressively lower share thereafter. Income not currently needed to pay benefits and related expenses is held in the SMI trust fund and invested in U.S. Treasury securities. The SMI trust fund is expected to remain adequately financed into the indefinite future because current law provides for establishment of program financing each year based on an updated calculation of expected cost per beneficiary (Board of Trustees of the Federal Supplementary Medical Insurance Trust Fund, 1997b).

■ Outdated Program Benefits

Wilensky and Newhouse (1999) assert that the present package of Medicare benefits largely reflects the thinking of the 1960s and therefore needs to be modified to reflect the way health care is organized and delivered at present. Medicare currently pays hospitals and physicians lower amounts than the private sector and does not cover outpatient pharmaceuticals or protect against large medical bills. Further, the program offers beneficiaries unlimited choice of providers, a feature that has stymied development of price competition among providers. The constrained nature of health plan choices and limited benefit package has resulted in most beneficiaries having to supplement their Medicare coverage with Medigap insurance policies—only 10% of senior citizens have no supplementary insurance (Wilensky & Newhouse, 1999). However, using Medigap policies to cover the mostly acute care services not included by Medicare has resulted in beneficiaries' paying supplemental premiums ranging from $1,000 to $3,000 annually, imposing additional economic burdens on the majority of the nation's elderly population.

The current Medicare benefit package, which emphasizes coverage for mostly acute care services provided primarily by traditional providers (hospitals and physicians), fails to provide adequate coverage for chronic and pharmaceutical health care services needed by millions of older Americans. In fact, Medicare now pays barely half the total costs of health care for an average beneficiary, and out-of-pocket costs for premiums, supplemental insurance, and noncovered services are growing faster than overall health care costs (Vladeck, 1999). The aging of the U.S. population and consequent increase in the prevalence of acute and chronic illness (Hoffman, Rice, & Sung, 1996) means that financial and access problems caused by current defects in Medicare benefits will grow for millions of

Americans in the years ahead, as will the political consequences for elected leaders.

■ Demographic and Financing Challenges Awaiting Medicare

Demographic changes in the United States will bring about important if not overwhelming challenges to the financing and overall structure of the Medicare program. Impact of these challenges is only a decade away: In just 10 years—by 2010—the first wave of the baby boom generation born between 1945 and 1965 will turn 65 years of age (see Figure 10.1) and begin to enroll in Medicare. By 2030, when the last of the baby boom generation reaches 65, the number of Medicare beneficiaries is expected to increase to 75 million Americans.

Fuchs (1999) estimates that if trends of the past two decades continue until 2020, the elderly's health care consumption in that year will be approximately $25,000 per person (in 1995 dollars) compared with $9,200 per person in 1995. Bruce Vladeck (1999), former administrator of the Health Care Financing Administration—the federal agency that oversees the Medicare and Medicaid programs—asserts that costs of benefits for the expanding number of beneficiaries almost certainly will exceed the capacity of Medicare's current sources of financing. In addition, he warns that Medicare will consume an ever-expanding share (currently about 12%) of the federal budget, thus reducing funds available for other worthy social programs.

Demographic problems confronting Medicare stem from the fact that not only will so many people be enrolling in the program, but also that many beneficiaries will live well into their 90s and beyond. At the same time that enrollment is expanding and life expectancy is increasing, the number of workers paying taxes who largely finance the program will decrease

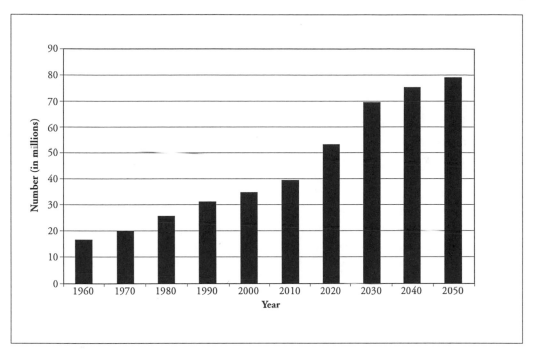

Figure 10.1 U.S. Population Over 65 Years of Age.

sharply through the first decade of the 21st century, falling to 3.6 workers per beneficiary by 2010 (McKusick, 1999). Thereafter the ratio of workers to beneficiaries is expected to decline rapidly to 2.3 by 2030. Thus not enough taxpaying workers will be available to offset increasing program expenditures associated with a growing number of beneficiaries and increased medical costs. As Dr. Katherine Swartz observes, "This means we will have more people drawing on Medicare and fewer people contributing to Medicare during their working years to make it a pay-as-you-go system, which is how Medicare has operated financially thus far" (Buerhaus, 1998a, p. 117).

■ Public Support for Medicare

Despite shortfalls in benefits covered by Medicare, numerous public opinion polls reveal strong intergenerational support for the pro-gram, and a desire to ensure the long-term financial well-being of Medicare (Bernstein & Stevens, 1999). The public has maintained a favorable opinion about Medicare despite increasingly negative views over the past three decades about the role of government, value received for tax payments, size of government, and trust in the government to do the right thing (Blendon et al., 1999). For example, a 1994 national poll found that three fourths of Americans considered the Medicare program important to their own families (Blendon et al., 1995), and a 1996 national survey reported overwhelming support for Medicare. More than 80% of respondents agreed that the pro-gram enables retirees to remain independent, and only 22% believed that persons aged 65 and older can afford private health insurance on their own (Bernstein & Stevens, 1999).

With respect to the public's view of government's role in health care, Americans repeatedly have expressed strong support for health care as a basic right for everyone, not just for the elderly or disabled (Jacobs & Shapiro, 1994), and polls have found support for the government's involvement in health care (International Communications Group, 1997). At the same time, Blendon and colleagues' (1995) review of poll data from 1994 and 1995 found that the public was not well informed about Medicare benefits, and many Americans were unclear about what services were covered by the program. In addition, the majority of Americans were unaware that Medicare does not pay for outpatient prescription drugs or for long-term nursing home care. Similarly, most people did not understand how Medicare is financed—fewer than one third knew that different funding sources, including separate trust funds and general revenues, pay for Medicare (Blendon et al., 1997). Finally, public opinion surveys done in the mid 1990s showed that 80% of Americans thought that Medicare was in financial trouble, and 60% believed that these problems were serious (Blendon et al., 1995). Further, most Americans under 65 years of age have doubts about whether Medicare will be there for them when they become eligible to enroll (Kaiser–Harvard Program, 1997).

In sum, current methods of financing Medicare Part A will be untenable as the ratio of workers to beneficiaries declines in the years ahead. The benefits covered are outdated and out of step with current and future health care practices and delivery systems. The soon to be retiring baby boomers will expand the number of beneficiaries rapidly, and increasing longevity of beneficiaries will raise demand for services and program costs substantially. Yet despite lack of knowledge about the program's benefits structure and financing problems, public support for Medicare remains strong. And, because the BBA has extended the time until the Part A Hospital Insurance Trust Fund will require replenishing, it will be difficult for politicians to legislate needed modifications

before another crisis in Medicare financing develops.

■ Options for Restructuring Medicare

To date, those concerned with preserving the future of Medicare have been unable to identify either a large number or a particularly satisfying set of options to restructure the program. Each option has certain benefits and drawbacks and therefore has provoked controversy and debate among policy makers, particularly over questions involving effectiveness and fairness. Thus, throughout this decade, we can expect more discussion and analysis of options that previously have been advanced to strengthen and preserve the Medicare program.

Raise the Eligibility Age

One way to offset some of Medicare's burdens would be to increase the age to 66, 67, 68, or beyond before an individual could enroll in the program. This option raises several questions. How much savings would result from each of these age adjustments? Would this option decrease access to needed care and, if so, for how many citizens? What would the political risk be to members of Congress and the administration?

Increase Taxes

Alternatively, taxes could be raised to ensure financial solvency of Medicare. But how much should taxes rise? When should the tax increase begin? Which groups should be taxed? Which should be excluded? And, again, what would the political risk be to members of Congress and the occupant of the White House? Swartz argues that the sooner taxes are raised, the lower the amount of tax that would be required, and the sooner Medicare's financial stability can be achieved (Buerhaus, 1998a).

The rationale for this view is that the number of working people upon which the tax could be spread over is decreasing over time. Further, Swartz observes that postponing a tax increase will mean that fewer and fewer workers whose earnings could be taxed will be in the workforce and that a tax hike would have to be higher than otherwise required. Conversely, Dr. Joseph Newhouse does not believe that a tax increase is needed in the near term because the BBA has forestalled the financial insolvency of the Hospital Trust Fund (Buerhaus, 1998a).

Raise Beneficiary Premiums and Copayments

Medicare could require beneficiaries to pay higher insurance premiums and raise copayments for services they receive, thereby increasing income for the program and perhaps reducing demand for some covered services. But how much should premiums and copayments increase? Would this option apply to all beneficiaries or only to higher income beneficiaries? How would such increases be adjusted over time? What would happen to beneficiaries who are the most severely sick or least able to afford the increase? And how much would this option reduce program costs and increase income received by Medicare? Overshadowing these questions is political concern that older citizens are likely to express in the voting booth their dissatisfaction over having to pay higher premiums and copayments.

Reduce the Level or Eliminate Certain Benefits

Medicare could decrease the number of benefits it now provides. But what benefits should be reduced? By how much? At whom should the reductions be targeted? By eliminating benefits, does this mean that Medicare would not have to reduce payments to providers, raise taxes, or increase premiums or copayments? However, because beneficiaries would directly bear the brunt of a loss in benefits, they would be expected to react negatively and express their dissatisfaction in the voting booth. Thus this option would be unattractive to bureaucrats and elected political leaders.

Increase Beneficiaries' Enrollment in Health Maintenance Organizations (HMOs) and Managed Care Plans

Having beneficiaries enroll in managed care health plans offers the possibility of increasing provider competition for enrollees and, conceivably, lowering total costs per Medicare beneficiary. In addition, managed care health plans can be expected to try to attract beneficiaries to their plans by competing in terms of the package of benefits offered, which could expand benefits substantially over what is currently available to beneficiaries (e.g., provide coverage for prescription drugs). Despite rhetoric critical of managed care emanating from the administration and Congress over the past several years, the proposal to enroll more beneficiaries into managed care plans was, in fact, included in the BBA as the Medicare+Choice program. Under this program, the BBA allowed for several new types of plans, including (a) Medicare preferred provider organization (PPO); (b) private fee-for-service plan, which can pay physicians more than the Medicare fee schedule and can charge beneficiaries an extra premium for the standard Medicare package of benefits; (c) provider-sponsored organization (PSO) in which physicians and hospitals may develop their own risk plan and compete directly with HMOs; and (d) demonstration project involving a medical savings account (MSA). Although the number of Medicare beneficiaries enrolled in HMOs grew during the 1990s, we currently do not know whether and to what extent the Medicare+Choice program has affected beneficiaries' movement into the new health plans offered by Medicare.

Pay Providers Less

The 1997 BBA produced more changes in Medicare than had occurred since the program began in 1965. In addition to creation of the Medicare+Choice program, other changes targeted providers, namely (a) requiring prospective pricing systems to be implemented for hospital outpatient visits, home health care, and skilled nursing facilities; (b) modifying the calculation of capitation rates to reduce variation in payments across various counties; (c) modifying and delaying portions of the physician fee schedule reform; and (d) shifting funding for a substantial share of home care visits from Part A to Part B. These proposals were expected to reduce payments to providers by $115 billion or more between 1998 and 2002. Further, lowered Medicare spending was anticipated for the 5-year budget cycle following enactment of the BBA to a nominal growth rate of less than 6% per year compared to 8.8% previously projected. But there is growing concern that after 2002 the financial status of hospitals, home health agencies, and long-term facilities will have deteriorated to such an extent that they will be unable to absorb further payment reductions without seriously jeopardizing beneficiaries' access to care.

■ Future of Medicare and Implications for Nursing

Because most nurses, including many involved in health policy, do not deal with the financing, demographic, and political intricacies of the Medicare program on a daily basis, the nursing profession could find itself participating at the periphery rather than at the center of activities aimed at influencing policies that will shape the future of Medicare. Such an outcome would be unfortunate because nurses not only have the trust of the public, but have great understanding and experience providing care to the elderly and disabled. Few professions are as well suited as nursing to offer information and perspective that would aid the development of sound Medicare health policy. But to fulfill this potential, nurses need to expand their understanding of the problems facing Medicare, and policy leaders must develop a commitment to participate in both the re-design of Medicare and help the profession prepare to serve the health needs of an increasingly older population of Americans. (Buerhaus, 2000, p. 117)

The demographic, financing, and benefits problems facing Medicare are not the only problems about which nurses should be concerned when contemplating the program's future and implications for nurses. Unfortunately, the professional nurse workforce is aging rapidly (Buerhaus, 1998b), with the average age of registered nurses (RNs) at 44.3 years in 1996 (Moses, 1996). Approximately three fifths of RNs in the workforce are between the ages of 35 and 50, one fifth of working RNs are between 50 and 65, and approximately one fifth are under 35 years of age (Buerhaus, Staiger, & Auerbach, 2000). The author's analysis of the impact of an aging RN workforce suggests that the number of full-time equivalent RNs will grow slowly through the first decade of the new century and begin contracting in about 2010, just when enrollment in the Medicare program is expected to increase substantially. The projected shortage of RNs will result in a reduction of full-time equivalent (FTE) supply, due both to the large number of RNs retiring and to increased demand for health care by aging nonnurse baby boomers. Thus, just when society (namely, Medicare beneficiaries) will need the nursing profession the most, it is unlikely that enough RNs will be available. Although this situation can be anticipated 10 years before it develops, what should the nursing profession do now both to strengthen the future of the Medicare program and ensure that enough RNs will be available to provide access and high quality care to the growing number of beneficiaries?

Nursing Policy

Nurses involved in policy-making should work closely with those in government and private organizations who are developing options for reforming Medicare. These individuals must be educated about the implications of a contracting RN labor force and become motivated to rectify the situation; it would be a pity if problems involving Medicare's financing and benefits structure were resolved during the next 10 years only to find that not enough RNs were available to make the restructured program work. In addition, policy makers in nursing should ensure that members of Congress realize the political implications of future RN shortages and how these shortages are likely to be viewed politically by both Medicare beneficiaries and health care providers.

Policy makers also need to focus on obtaining educational subsidies and influencing federal agencies to develop programs and funding aimed at increasing the future supply of RNs. And, because nurses rate highly in public opinion polls measuring Americans' view of how well health professionals and delivery organizations act to protect consumers, policy makers should involve nurses in shaping policies to redesign Medicare benefits. Nurses could also become involved in communicating reasons for these changes directly to the public. Further, clinical and organizational interventions and other programs judged to be effective from nursing's perspective need to be identified and then included in conversations involving the redesign of Medicare benefits.

Nursing Education

Educators could work more closely with employers to develop new programs to increase enrollment in nursing education programs (perhaps subsidized by grants from federal and state governments). Such programs could include fresh image and media campaigns, as well as new approaches to increase enrollment of men and minorities in nursing (Buerhaus & Auerbach, 1999). If educators embrace the goal of increasing the number of RNs during the next 10 years, then it would make sense for these new enrollees to be provided with considerable education and experience in geriatrics, managing chronic disease, and improving the mental health of seniors. Demand for nurse practitioners, particularly geriatric nurse practitioners, is likely to increase in the future as costs associated with relying on traditional hospital and physician dominance of Medicare make use of nonphysician clinicians more attractive to policy makers and the public.

Nursing Research

In addition to changes in the Medicare program, the 1997 BBA granted direct reimbursement to beneficiaries for care provided by nurse practitioners (NPs) and clinical nurse specialists (CNSs) in all geographic settings. This important, long sought after policy change (Wong, 1999) is likely to provide nurses in advanced practice with many new opportunities to improve the health of a large number of beneficiaries. However, with expansion in the role and influence of nursing comes responsibility to evaluate effects of this policy change. Topics needing to be addressed by nurse researchers include assessing (a) effects of NPs and CNSs on beneficiaries' access to primary and long-term care in all types of delivery settings—whether beneficiaries and their families experience improved health and how satisfied they were with outcomes obtained and nursing care provided; (b) effects on total Medicare spending—whether any innovations in clinical interventions and organization of care resulted; and (c) the financial and clinical effects on physicians, hospitals, insurers, and HMOs (Buerhaus, 1998c).

Nursing Practice

Not only will health care providers have to adjust to an older nursing workforce, but a larger portion of the people for whom they care will be Medicare beneficiaries suffering simultaneously with acute and chronic conditions. Contemplating challenges of managing clinical care of an aging population, using a rapidly aging nurse workforce, is sobering. To be sure, organizations will need to find better ways to restructure care delivery and utilizing increasing numbers of older and more experienced RNs so that these RNs will want to remain in the workforce. The work environment will have to change to respond better to the ergonomic needs of older RNs whose backs, feet, hearing, and eyesight are no longer those of 30-year-olds.

• If projected shortages of RNs materialize in 10 years at the same time Medicare enrollment accelerates, how will practicing RNs ensure that beneficiaries receive quality patient care and that appropriate clinical outcomes are achieved? This question suggests that new measures of quality need to be established that better reflect the perspectives of older patients and that also maintain the high standards of nursing practice. New models of nursing care delivery need to be developed that recognize RNs increasingly will manage nonnurse clinicians who likely will be giving more direct care in the face of RN shortages. These and many more challenges await nurses as the health care delivery system confronts effects of the nation's aging population.

■ Concluding Statement

Whatever happens to (a) restructure the highly popular Medicare program, (b) ensure long-term financing, and (c) modify benefits provided to a rapidly growing number of beneficiaries will exert highly visible social and political ramifications during the next several decades. Changes to the Medicare program will strongly influence evolution of the nation's health care delivery system and bring about many important opportunities and challenges for politicians, health care organizations, taxpayers, beneficiaries, and health professionals—particularly nurses.

Contemplating what may soon develop can be daunting and even frightening because the nursing profession may be on the verge of confronting the greatest challenge in its history in the United States. Thus, the sooner nurses in policy, research, education, and practice come to terms with the problems and implications discussed in this chapter, the better will be the chances for overcoming them. Only by dealing with these challenges swiftly and effectively can nurses hope to retain the high trust and confidence the American people have bestowed on the nursing profession.

■ References

Balanced Budget Act of 1997 (P.L. 105–33), August 1997, HR 3426–Medicare and Medicaid Health Insurance Act. *U.S. Statutes at Large* (Volume III, pp. 251–788). Washington, DC: U.S. Government Printing Office.

Bernstein, J., & Stevens, R. (1999). Public opinion, knowledge, and Medicare reform. *Health Affairs, 18*(1), 180–193.

Blendon, R., Altman, D., Benson, J., Matt, J., Roland, D., Neiman, P., Leitman, R., & Hyams, T. (1995). The public's view of the future of Medicare. *Journal of the American Medical Association, 274,* 1645–1648.

Blendon, R., Benson, J., Brodie, M., Brossard, M., Altman, D., & Morin, R. (1997). Trends: What do Americans know about entitlements? *Health Affairs, 16*(5), 111–116.

Blendon, R., Benson, J., Brodie, M., Altman, D., Morin, R., Deane, C., & Kjellson, N. (1999). The 60s and the 90s: Americans' political, moral, and religious values then and now. *Brookings Review, 17*(2), 14–17.

Board of Trustees, Federal Hospital Insurance Trust Fund. (1997a). *1997 Annual report of the board of trustees of the federal hospital insurance trust fund.* Washington, DC: Health Care Financing Administration.

Board of Trustees, Federal Supplementary Medical Insurance Trust. (1997b). *1997 Annual report of the board of trustees of the federal supplementary medical insurance trust fund.* Washington, DC: Health Care Financing Administration.

Buerhaus, P. (1998a). Financing, demographic, and political problems confronting Medicare in the United States. *IMAGE: Journal of Nursing Scholarship, 30*(2), 117–123.

Buerhaus, P. (1998b). Is another RN shortage looming? *Nursing Outlook, 46*(3), 103-108.

Buerhaus, P. (1998c). Medicare payment for advanced practice nurses. What are the research questions? *Nursing Outlook, 46,* 151–153.

Buerhaus, P., & Auerbach, D. (1999). Slow growth in the number of minority RNs in the United States. *IMAGE: Journal of Nursing Scholarship, 31*(2), 179–183.

Buerhaus, P., Staiger, D., & Auerbach, D. (2000). Implications of an aging registered nurse workforce. *Journal of the American Medical Association, 283*(22), 2948–2954.

Fuchs, V. (1999). Health care for the elderly: How much? Who will pay for it? *Health Affairs, 18*(1) 11–21.

Hoffman, C., Rice, D., & Sung, H. (1996). Persons with chronic conditions: Their prevalence and costs. *Journal of the American Medical Association, 276,* 1473–1479.

International Communications Group. (1997). *How Americans perceive the health care system: Report on a national survey.* Washington, DC: National Coalition on Health Care.

Jacobs, L., & Shapiro, R. (1994). Public opinions tilt against private enterprise. *Health Affairs, 15,* 285–298.

Kaiser–Harvard Program on the Public Health/Social Policy. (1997). *Post-election survey of voters 1997 health care agenda.* Cambridge, MA: Harvard School of Public Health.

McKusick, D. (1999). Demographic issues in Medicare reform. *Health Affairs, 18*(1), 194–207.

Moses, E. (1996). *National sample survey of the population of registered nurses.* Bethesda, MD: U.S. Department of Health and Human Services, Public Health Service, Health Resources and Services Administration, Bureau of Nursing, Division of Nursing.

U.S. Government. (2000). The Official U.S. Government Site for Medicare Information [On-line]. Available: http://www.medicare.gov/

Vladeck, B. (1999). Plenty of nothing—A report from the Medicare Commission. *New England Journal of Medicine, 340,* 1503–1506.

Wilensky, G., & Newhouse, J. (1999). Medicare: What's right? What's wrong? What's next? *Health Affairs, 18*(1), 92–106.

Wong, S. (1999). Reimbursement to advanced practice nurses (APNs) through Medicare. *IMAGE: Journal of Nursing Scholarship, 31*(2), 167–173.

■ Editor's Questions for Discussion

What implications exist for nursing education programs and program content with increasing numbers of Medicare beneficiaries? How should preventive and health maintenance care content change with increasing longevity of the elderly? What service needs and demands will increase with longevity? How can nursing prepare to meet increased demands for health services and care by an elderly population? How can nursing programs encourage students to be more interested in caring for the elderly? What attitudes regarding aging, quality of life, and life expectancy affect students' approaches to and experiences in elder care?

Address the questions posed by Buerhaus concerning options for restructuring Medicare. What role should professional nurses play in resolving issues raised in restructuring Medicare? What resocialization process needs to occur for professional nurses to be involved in health planning and policy-making?

How can nursing students learn about and respond to Medicare issues? How can nursing students become informed and inform the elderly regarding options for care, such as HMOs and managed care plans? What content should be taught concerning health policy issues? How does Buerhaus' policy for influencing health policy relate to Heinrich and Wakefield's discussion about health policy (Chapter 8)?

What can the nursing profession do to strengthen the future of Medicare? How can nursing prepare to ensure that sufficient RNs will be available to provide care? How can nursing students best learn policy-making and develop specific roles as policy makers? Discuss Buerhaus' predictions and suggestions for nursing's involvement in policy-making. Identify specific strategies for implementing Buerhaus' suggestions. Does Buerhaus' discussion about reimbursement apply to the content presented by Robinson, Griffith, and Sullivan-Marx (Chapter 41)? How do Porter-O'Grady's (Chapter 55) and Pinkerton's (Chapter 56) discussions address Buerhaus' plea for restructuring delivery of care and services?

11

The Future Registered Nurse Workforce in Health Care Delivery

Economic Considerations

Cheryl B. Jones, PhD, RN, CNAA

Few would argue that market forces in the United States, most notably managed care, have fundamentally changed the ways in which health care services are offered by providers, accessed by clients, and acquired by payors. Between 1988 and 1998, the proportion of persons insured in the United States enrolled in managed care—including health maintenance organizations (HMOs), point of service (POS) plans, and preferred provider organizations (PPOs)—increased from approximately 29% to 86% (Goldstein, 1999). Changes in the organization and financing of health care have shifted delivery from the hospital to the home and community. This shift essentially has changed the roles, functions, and expectations of various disciplines within the health care workforce.

Nursing, the largest of the health care disciplines, is faced with both opportunities and challenges. There are opportunities to (a) deliver care to those who are truly in need of services and who might not otherwise receive care; (b) reconceptualize health care delivery; (c) design new models of care; and (d) make

This chapter was written while Dr. Jones was employed as Senior Health Services Researcher at the Center for Primary Care Research, Agency for Health Care Policy and Research and Quality, Department of Health and Human Services, Public Health Service.

contributions to social change. There are challenges, however, because organizations that employ nurses are under great pressure to (a) control costs, (b) minimize treatment time, (c) minimize health care professional time with patients, (d) limit care to the growing population of uninsured, and (e) focus on those patients, treatments, and procedures that maximize income. Thus nursing moves toward the future facing potential conflicts between its professional view and the view of organizations for which nurses work, that is, between the provision of high-quality, cost-effective health care and an environment that seeks to limit that care.

In this chapter I discuss (a) the nursing workforce, (b) nursing's role in health care delivery, and (c) the effects of economics and market forces on nursing. I also make predictions about the evolution of the nursing workforce, based on historical patterns and anticipated market trends.

■ Economics and the Nursing Labor Market

Industry and market forces influence the discipline of nursing in a variety of ways, ranging from the education of nurses to practice differentiation across educational levels to types of nursing services offered to roles that nurses play in the health care sector. These forces and others either have roots in or intersect with economics (see, e.g., Aiken, 1982; Buerhaus, 1991a; Cleland, 1990; Coffman & Spetz, 1999; Feldstein, 1998; Griffith, 1984). Thus a brief discussion of economics is warranted to gain an understanding of current and future directions for the nursing workforce.

Nursing Shortages

Concern expressed in the nursing and popular literature about nursing shortages serves as a reminder that the nursing labor market cycled through periods of shortage and surplus throughout the 20th century (Aiken, 1982; Aiken & Mullinix, 1987; Buerhaus, 1991b; McCloskey, 1995; Yett, 1975). The American Association of Colleges of Nursing (AACN) (1999) reported that baccalaureate nursing school enrollments were down for the fourth consecutive year and that recent reports suggested occurrence of another shortage. Hospitals were closing beds, having difficulty recruiting and retaining nurses, and having problems acquiring competent temporary nurses to fill short-term staffing needs (Kilborn, 1999; National Journal Group, Inc., 1999a; Russell, 1999). Current anecdotal reports note increasing demand for nurses to work overtime, increasing nurse turnover, and increasing job dissatisfaction. Consequently, hospitals are reporting bed shortages (National Journal Group, Inc., 1999b) and the popular press is reporting incidents of unsafe care (Snyderman, 1999)—attributed, in part, to a shortage of nurses.

The confusion around shortages in the nursing labor market raises the questions: What is behind these recurring shortages? What can be done to mitigate effects of shortages? And what can be done to prevent future shortages? The word *shortage* often is used to refer to the quantity or supply of a good or service available in the marketplace relative to the need or demand for the good or service. From an economic perspective, discussions of supply and demand are predicated on the price of a given service or product—that is, supply and demand for a particular good or service are moderated by price. This price in labor market discussions refers to the wage offered in the market for a particular labor sector. The hallmark of a labor shortage is a wage rate that rises faster than average (Ehrenberg & Smith, 1991), an often overlooked point in nursing shortage discussions. Thus, to understand fully the dynamics of nursing shortages and their impact on the future workforce, three aspects of the phenomenon must be examined: supply, wages, and demand.

Supply of Nurses[1]

The supply of nurses in the United States has grown steadily over the past two decades. Table 11.1 provides detailed information on the supply of nurses. The Division of Nursing[2] reports that the number of licensed registered nurses (RNs) has grown at an average annual rate of 2.7%, from approximately 1.6 million in 1980 to more than 2.5 million in 1996 (Moses, 1982, 1986, 1990, 1994, 1998). The RN population experienced its greatest annual growth rate of 3.4% between 1992 and 1996, ironically at a time when the health care industry was downsizing, laying off employees, and implementing cost containment strategies.

The proportion of nurses employed in nursing—the labor participation rate—has increased steadily, from approximately 77% of licensed nurses working in 1980 to approximately 83% in 1996. The proportion of nurses employed full time also reached a high of 76% in 1996. *Thus, in 1996, the most recent year of nationally available statistics, there were more nurses, more nurses employed in nursing, and more nurses working full-time than ever before.*

Settings of Employment

Hospitals have been and continue to be the single largest employer of RNs, despite the fact that between 1980 and 1996 the proportion of nurses employed in hospitals declined from a high of 68% in both 1984 and 1988 to a low of 60% in 1996 (Moses, 1982, 1986, 1990, 1994, 1998). This shift was accompanied by increasing proportions of nurses working in community and public health (6.5% in 1980 and 13% in 1996) and ambulatory care (5.7% in 1980 and 8.5% in 1996).

Positions Held by Nurses

National Sample Surveys between 1980 and 1992 show that approximately two thirds of all employed nurses worked in staff-level positions—ranging between 65% and 67%. In 1996, the percentage of nurses employed in staff-level positions declined to 62%, although the actual number of staff nurses had increased. *This drop in the percentage of nurses employed as staff can be explained partially by an increase in the percentage of certain types of advanced practice nurses (APNs)[3] and other opportunities available to nurses between 1992 and 1996.* During this period, the percentage of nurses employed as nurse practitioners (NPs) and midwives increased from 1.4% to 2.1%, and the percentage of nurses holding a position labeled as "other" (e.g., case manager, discharge planner, outcomes manager, and patient care coordinator) increased from 6.5% to 10%. The proportion of clinical nurse specialists declined slightly from 1.9% of the nursing population in 1992 to 1.7% in 1996, despite the slight increase in the number of CNSs. These changes reflect the focus in nursing education on preparing NPs during the period.

Educational Preparation of Nurses

Figure 11.1 shows that the composition of the RN workforce by highest educational degree has changed over time. *The most remarkable changes were (a) decline in the numbers of nurses with the diploma, (b) increase in the number of associate and baccalaureate degree nurses, and (c) increase in the proportion of nurses with graduate degrees.* Nurses with an associate degree as their highest educational credential almost tripled during the 16-year period, with an annual growth rate of approximately 6.5%. RNs with a baccalaureate degree more than doubled over the same period, with an annual growth rate of approximately 5.2%. The 1.6% average annual decline in the proportion of

TABLE 11.1   Number of Registered Nurses, by Employment, Setting, Education, and Position (in thousands)

	1980	1984	1988	1992	1996
Total	**1,660**	**1,888**	**2,033**	**2,239**	**2,559**
Employed	1,273	1,486	1.627	1,853	2,116
Not employed	389	402	406	387	443
Settings					
Hospital	836	1,012	1,105	1,233	1,271
Long-term care	101	115	108	129	171
Nursing education	47	40	30	37	49
Community/public	83	101	111	180	278
Student health	45	43	48	51	64
Occupational health	29	23	22	19	22
Ambulatory care	72	97	126	144	179
Other	53	53	77	56	83
Education					
Diploma	903	855	821	755	697
Associate degree	295	430	512	633	812
Baccalaureate, nursing	326	430	510	612	736
Baccalaureate, related field	42	51	47	59	64
Masters/doctorate, nursing or related field	86	111	130	179	249
Positions					
Staff	825	993	1,088	1,234	1,310
Administration	61	77	98	115	112
CRNA	15	19	17	19	22
CNS	19	24	29	36	36
Consultant	8	11	18	17	27
HN/AHN	90	95	86	85	123
Instructor	60	66	63	64	73
Nurse clinician	8	15	18	25	30
NP/midwife	17	19	24	27	45
Private duty	23	23	20	12	16
Researcher	3	3	5	8	13
Supervisor/assistant	76	90	92	92	95
Other	61	53	65	120	212

1. All data used in this table were extracted from the National Sample Survey of Registered Nurses (Moses, 1982, 1986, 1990, 1994, 1998).

2. Many percentages cited in text were calculated by dividing the number of nurses for a particular year, and setting, education, or position by the number of employed nurses for that same year.

nurses with a diploma as their highest educational credential during this time is concomitant with a decline in the number of nursing diploma programs (Aiken & Gwyther, 1995).[4]

The proportion of nurses with master's or doctoral degrees in nursing or a related field almost tripled during the 16-year period, growing at a rate of 6.8% annually.

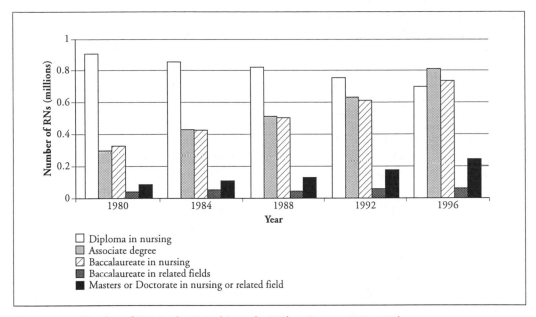

Figure 11.1   Number of RNs in the United States by Highest Degree, 1980–1996.
Note: Data used to create this figure were extracted from Moses, 1982, 1986, 1990, 1994, and 1998.

*Other Characteristics That
Influence the Supply of Nurses*

Beyond system changes, the demographics of the nursing labor market—age, race, and gender—also have an impact on the number and types of nurses available for the future nursing workforce. The aging of the nursing workforce has received a great deal of recent attention (Buerhaus & Staiger, 1999; Moses, 1998), with emphasis on the numbers of nurses expected to retire from the workforce in the near future and the need to recruit younger nurses. In 1996, the average age of the nursing workforce was 44.3 years, compared to an average age of 40.3 years in 1980. In 1996, less than 10% of the RN population was under the age of 30, compared to 25% in 1980.

Racial diversity in the nursing workforce is important as the health care system changes to meet needs of an increasingly diverse society. In 1980, 6.3% of the nursing population was represented by a race other than white, and this proportion increased to 9.7% of the population in 1996 (Buerhaus & Auerbach, 1999; Moses, 1998). In spite of these gains, the racial composition of the nursing workforce still does not reflect the diversity of the U.S. population as a whole (Buerhaus & Auerbach, 1999). *An increasingly diverse workforce will enable nursing to serve a diverse population better but will necessitate creation of a working environment that fosters and rewards cultural competency and sensitivity.*

Nursing remains predominantly a female profession, but significant gains have been made to increase the percentage of males. Males represented approximately 5.0% of the nursing population in 1996, compared to 2.7% of the population in 1980. However, the number of males in nursing almost tripled between 1980 and 1996. The annual growth rate for males in the RN population (6.6% annually) outpaced the annual growth rate overall (2.7% annually) during all time periods between 1980 and 1996. *Greater gender diversity in the nursing workforce has the potential to bring about an increase in wages and opportunities for all nurses.*

Nursing Wages[5]

Nursing wages are not the sole component of professional recognition, yet wages are an important component of professional recognition within an industry or labor market (Ehrenberg & Smith, 1991). Wages are set in the marketplace to reflect the "value" of a particular profession and they indicate opportunities within that market. Labor market wages also are a critical factor in an organization's hiring decisions, including the number of nurses to hire, their employment arrangements, and the roles they will fulfill. Beyond economics, wages are linked to employee loyalty, commitment, turnover, retention, and a host of organizational and individual factors that ultimately affect type and quality of the services provided, and the competency, productivity, and efficiency of the nursing workforce.

Nurses' earnings have increased steadily since 1980. On average, nurses' reported annual earnings of $17,394 in 1980 (Moses, 1982), $23,505 in 1984 (Moses, 1986), $28,383 in 1988 (Moses, 1990), $37,738 in 1992 (Moses, 1994), and $42,071 in 1996 (Moses, 1998). These figures represent an increase of approximately 142% during the 16-year period, or roughly 5.7% per year. The period with the lowest annual average salary increase of 2.8% occurred between 1992 and 1996; the period with the greatest annual average salary increase of 7.8% occurred between 1980 and 1984.

These numbers can be misleading, however, unless inflation during this period is also considered. In "real," or inflation-adjusted dollars, nurses' earnings increased 84%, or 3.9% per year, during the 16-year period. Real earnings increased an average of 6.1% between 1980 and 1984, 3.1% between 1984 and 1988, 3.9% between 1988 and 1992, and 2.5% between 1992 and 1996. Note that inflation-adjusted nursing salaries increased at or above the 16-year average rate during only two time periods—in the early 1980s and late 1980s when nursing shortages were widely reported. Salary increases during other periods outpaced inflation but were less than the 16-year average rate. The year 2000 and future National Sample Surveys will provide key information on nurses' earnings and the existence of a true nursing shortage at the turn of the century.

Demand for Nurses

Demand for nursing is difficult to determine, even though the supply of nurses in the United States and nurses' salaries are reasonably well known. *The demand for nurses is determined largely by the organizations that employ them—hospitals, long-term care facilities, public and private clinics, and so forth.* The largest employer of nurses, hospitals, tends to dictate demand for nurses, although other employment settings have some impact on the demand for nurses. Hospitals report nursing vacancies, which often are interpreted by the market as demand. These reported vacancies can be derived from actual data or based on perceived need. Additionally, estimated demand for nurses may be based on demographic trends and nurse-to-population ratios.

Unfortunately, both of these estimation methods are problematic. First, use of demographic trends and nurse-to-patient ratios do not necessarily capture the willingness of employers or payors to hire or reimburse nurses to serve those populations. Second, use of hospital vacancy rates reflects vacancies in only one setting within the health care industry. Moreover, hospitals may inflate reported nurse vacancy rates because of inherent economic incentives to do so.[6] These "inflated" vacancies exist at a current and prevailing wage rate, not necessarily at an increased wage—an amount hospitals may be unwilling to pay to attract employees to fill those vacancies. Hospitals obviously want to hire as many nurses as possible without raising wages. Moreover, hospitals would get more for their money: "more" in terms of numbers and "more" in the sense that nurses function across a broad range of skills and abilities. *If a shortage of nurses is reported, one way to determine if, in fact, a shortage exists is to document that wages are rising faster than the average increase for some historical period. Such a situation existed twice during the past two decades.*

Substitution Effect

Increasing use of unlicensed personnel in hospitals and nurse practitioners and other advanced practice nurses (APNs) in primary care over the past 10 years has caused much discussion about substitution in the health care workforce. In economics, substitution means that, as the price of one good or service rises, the demand for that good or service will stall or decline and that consumers[7] of the good or service will begin using another good or service for which the same level of satisfaction is derived. This is not to say that both alternatives are the same, but rather, that the same outcome is achieved at a lower cost (Folland, Goodman, & Stano, 1993).

Organizations combine inputs—namely labor, capital, technology, and other resources—to achieve a certain level and quality of outcome relative to their available budgets (Folland, Goodman, & Stano, 1993). In health care, when nursing salaries increase to the point that employers cannot or will not bear the costs of the increased wages, employers often change labor inputs in an attempt to achieve the same level of outcome at a lower cost. The question relevant to this discussion is whether the same level of outcome—quality of care—is actually achieved when substitution occurs. In other

words, can unlicensed assistive personnel be equal substitutes for licensed nurses and can APNs be equal substitutes for primary care physicians? Nursing has embraced the idea of assuming a greater role in primary care, but the profession generally has resisted the notion of unlicensed personnel taking on a greater role in hospitals and other settings. Nursing's reaction is predicated on the belief that substituting NPs for primary care physicians is an equal substitution in some cases but that substitution of unlicensed personnel for licensed nurses is not an equal substitution in situations involving direct patient care.

Discussion of demand and substitution highlights the complexities and intricacies of the health care labor market. We cannot consider supply and demand within one sector of the health care labor market without considering the labor market in general, and the effects of changes in one sector of the market on other sectors. Thus it is short-sighted to examine the nursing labor market in isolation or without consideration of the health care and public policy systems.

■ Policy Influences on the Nursing Workforce

The nursing workforce is influenced by policies established at the levels of practice, health systems, and public policy. These policies can influence the number of nurses, where they work, the positions they hold, their roles and functions, how they are educated, their nursing salaries, and even the racial and gender mix of the nursing workforce.

Clinical Practice Policies

Policies at the level of *clinical practice* are aimed at facilitating decision-making for delivering care to patients (Eisenberg, 1998). Clinical practice–level policies relevant to the nursing workforce include those related to staffing: when and who should provide care, when to take certain actions, when to use specific procedures for taking action, and which protocols to use for treatment. These policies may be based on recommendations from professional groups or experts. Examples of such policies are ANA's standards of practice, clinical guidelines developed by the Agency for Healthcare Research and Quality (AHRQ), and unit-level standards of care. Theoretically, clinical practice–level policies are translated into practice through continuing education, quality improvement programs, and other means. In turn, these policies should guide decisions about methods of health care delivery, interface of disciplinary and interdisciplinary practice, and interactions at the point of delivery.

Health Systems Decisions

Health systems "have the resources to base their decisions on careful analysis and review of the evidence" (Eisenberg, 1998, p. 102). Decisions within health systems may be at the organizational level (e.g., hospital, network, or plan) or at the operative unit level (e.g., a division of nursing and patient care services, a clinic, or a center). Other organizational and professional systems, such as the Joint Commission for the Accreditation of Healthcare Organizations (JCAHO) and the American Nurses Credentialing Center (ANCC), also influence health system and practice policy by setting requirements for organizational accreditation and professional credentialing.

Public Policies

Policies made at the *public or societal level*—whether aimed at ensuring quality, protecting privacy, or paying for health care—have an impact on health care systems, professional practice, and individuals. For example, passage of Medicare and Medicaid legislation in the 1960s affected the services provided to (a) aging, disabled, and poor individuals in our society; (b) the hospital, home health care, long-term care, and other delivery programs and services offered by organizations, state, and local governments; and (c) the preparation and education of health professionals. Moreover, this legislation affected the conditions under which health services would be paid for, financial responsibilities of program participants, and funding processes for educating health care professionals.

One important influence on the number and types of nurses prepared in the workforce, in fact, is the mechanism of paying for nursing education. Paying for nursing education usually occurs in one of three ways: self-pay, scholarships, or federal reimbursement to health care organizations. Self-pay and scholarships are fairly straightforward and generally understood, but the mechanism of federal funding for nursing education—part of which is in the form of Medicare pass-through reimbursements and part of which is designated through Title VIII Public Health Service funding—is quite complex (see Aiken & Gwyther, 1995, for a detailed discussion of this process).

Medicare pass-through reimbursements designate hospitals with affiliated nursing programs (i.e., diploma nursing programs) as the recipients of nursing educational funding. Unfortunately, this funding mechanism designates the majority of Medicare funding (66% in 1991) for diploma, hospital-based programs, the type of nursing education program that is producing a dwindling proportion (10% in 1991) of nursing graduates (Aiken & Gwyther, 1995). In contrast, Title VIII funds are directed to nursing educational institutions and represented approximately 19% of all federal funding for nursing education in 1994 (Aiken & Gwyther, 1995). Thus the important distinctions between these two sources of federal funding is that Title VIII funds go directly to nursing education; whereas, Medicare pass-

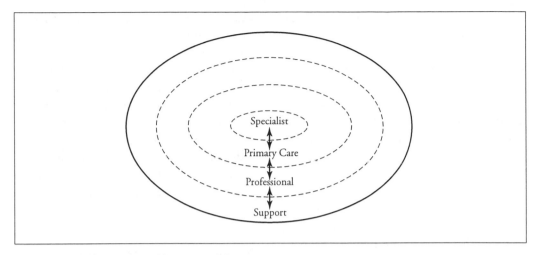

Figure 11.2 The Future Health Care Workforce.

through funds (a) go to hospitals' general revenues, (b) support a declining proportion of nursing programs and graduates, and (c) are not necessarily set aside for nursing education per se (Aiken & Gwyther, 1995).

■ Outlook for the Nursing Workforce

Over the past two decades, nurses have become more highly educated; the number and percentage of nurses with a diploma as the highest educational credential have decreased, whereas the number and proportion of nurses in all other educational groups have increased. This growth, coupled with changes in types of positions nurses hold (i.e., increases in the proportion of nurses employed as APNs, researchers, outcomes managers, and in other nontraditional positions) point to the success of nursing's efforts in knowledge development. This development is consistent with knowledge growth and technological capability-building in our society in general, which Drucker (1994) calls a shift from an industrial society to a knowledge society.

Economists refer to knowledge, skills, and abilities possessed by individuals as *human cap-*

ital. Theoretically, as knowledge, skills, and abilities increase, so too do productivity and wages. Nursing has increased its stock of human capital, as nurses' education and salaries have increased since 1980. What is not clear, however, is whether nurses' human capital—in terms of productivity, output, competencies, and "quality"—has increased sufficiently to meet market demands.

The health care marketplace is changing faster than any of the health care disciplines can respond, and advances in technology will foster even faster change in the future. One thing is certain, however: The health care purse strings are not likely to be loosened in the future; costs of care will continue to be a concern as technological advances make the best possible care increasingly expensive. Consequently, health care payors and organizations likely will place less emphasis on disciplines, per se, and more emphasis on ensuring quality through qualifications, capabilities, and competencies across disciplines.

Figure 11.2 illustrates that the health care workforce of the future can be conceptualized as a large professional group (RNs, CNSs, and multidisciplinary health professionals), working in concert with primary care providers (physicians, NPs, midwives, and physician assistants) and health care specialists (physicians and doctorally prepared nurses), and supported by a group of licensed and unlicensed personnel (licensed practical nurses [LPNs] and unlicensed assistive health care personnel). These categories are not mutually exclusive; for example, some ANPs (NPs and CNSs) may be in the professional segment of the workforce, whereas others may be in the primary care or specialist segments. The important point is not how individuals are categorized in the future, but rather the fact that individuals in all segments of the health care workforce must possess a specialized set of knowledge, skills, and abilities to function within any of its segments. Advancing from the support segment of the workforce to the professional segment, from the professional segment to the primary care segment, or from the primary care segment to the specialist segment necessitates increasing levels of knowledge, skills, and abilities. Thus, the more education possessed by individuals in the future, the greater will be the potential for advancement in the health care workforce; the less education possessed by individuals relative to others, the more difficult it will be to remain or advance in the workforce. As technology continues to develop and proliferate, there will be increasing pressure on individuals to expand competencies to remain in a particular segment or to advance in the workforce.

Now more than ever health care professionals have greater access—through the media, the Internet, and other sources—to information about jobs and career opportunities in the health care sector. Data are readily and widely available regarding health care downsizing and layoffs, pressure on remaining staff to carry heavy workloads, low nurse staffing levels, stress and burnout, job dissatisfaction, concerns about quality of care, and generally bad working conditions for nurses. Widespread availability of this information makes the concern about recruitment into nursing and declining nursing school enrollments even more critical. Changes in the health care system and subsequent impacts on health care professionals and the work environment have the potential to make nursing an unattractive option for those who are at the point of making a career decision. The current competitive labor market calls for long-term investments in recruiting and retaining individuals in the nursing profession—especially those under the age of 25—that focus on making it attractive, lucrative, and rewarding.

■ *Nursing Workforce Needs*

Innovations

The health care market functions predominantly according to economic expectations; thus it behooves nurses to understand the economics of the nursing labor market. As McCloskey (1995) suggests, improving working conditions within which nurses practice requires concurrent consideration of not only health care costs, but also the quality and cost–quality trade-offs that influence decision-making in health care. Efforts to attract and retain nurses also should emphasize values and beliefs of the profession, which are immune to the ups and downs of the health care marketplace, as well as continued advances in the way nursing care is provided. Focusing on aspects of nursing that do not change is impossible because, after all, nursing does not exist in a vacuum and the health care field is constantly changing. Yet, although it must be prepared for constant change, nursing also should focus on the contributions that it can make to health care and ultimately society's health that will withstand the winds of change: serving as patients' advocates; advancing the provision of safe, high-quality, and cost-effective care; researching and developing ways of improving care; and enhancing health care and health for all.

Profession or Commodity

Historical and current practice suggests that nursing is a commodity, in the sense that its product—nursing care—is bought and sold in the marketplace at the price established by purchasers. For example, during times of shortage, purchasers are willing to pay the increasing price of nurses' wages; at other times, purchasers are unwilling to increase the amount paid to nurses and they have no incentive to do so. The challenge to nursing is that it views itself as a profession, yet purchasers view it as a commodity.

A case in point is that there is, effectively, a one for one substitution by employers of nurses prepared at the baccalaureate, associate degree, and diploma levels (Botelho, Jones, & Kiker, 1998). The curricula for these three levels of nursing preparation differ to some degree, yet there is conflict within the profession whether nurses prepared at these three levels of education are, in fact, interchangeable. Thus it is not surprising that purchasers of nursing services see little distinction between entry-level nurses. Until the marketplace appreciates the differences of entry-level nursing preparation, the profession will be plagued by outside perceptions of its status as a commodity. Purchasers will change their view of nursing *only* if there are benefits to do so and if nursing offers something that other disciplines cannot provide. Nursing therefore must aggressively (a) seek out and creatively identify ways to differentiate services across levels of the workforce, (b) document its value, and (c) widely disseminate information about its many contributions to health care.

Segments of the Health Care Workforce

In the future nurses can expect to participate in three segments of the workforce—professional, primary care, and specialist— and interact with individuals at all levels of the workforce. The majority of the nursing workforce currently practices in the professional segment of the workforce. Tension is felt at the margins of workforce segments, that is, at the points of economic substitution. Because nursing currently experiences tension from downward substitution to assistive personnel and upward substitution as primary care providers, the tension that nurses experience is not likely to lessen. To alleviate tension, open discussion across all levels of the workforce is needed to clarify existing and potential ambiguity between roles and to recognize and emphasize the importance of all roles within the health care workforce of tomorrow.

Nurses in the future workforce must recognize the importance of management and research at all levels of practice. This requirement reflects the changing role of nurses at all levels, such as (a) the staff RN who is required to supervise increasing numbers of unlicensed and licensed staff and (b) the APN who must track patient and organizational outcomes to document effectiveness of care. Nurses of the future must possess more knowledge, skills, and abilities (i.e., human capital) to maintain the same relative present position or advance in the health care workforce. To meet these needs, nurses of the future will need (a) basic skills to function across levels of the health care workforce; (b) advanced skills in delegation, collaboration, and interdisciplinary practice to work effectively with individuals and groups at various levels of the health care workforce; (c) advanced skills in leadership, management, and research to envision, implement, coordinate, integrate, and evaluate care delivery; (d) ability to think conceptually, critically, and analytically; (e) a mind-set of lifelong learning and continuous adaptation to change; and (f) aspirations to capitalize on advancement opportunities in practice, education, and research.

Workforce Research

The lag time to (a) identify changes and needs in the workforce, (b) prepare a response, and (c) educate students to meet these needs can span several years, presenting challenges for nursing, the educational system, and health care generally. Although long-run solutions ultimately are needed to address nursing workforce needs—particularly cyclic nursing shortages and working conditions—short-run efforts are necessary to overcome this time lag, alleviate cyclic nursing shortages when they occur, and meet immediate needs in the provision of health care. One solution implemented in the late 1980s and reintroduced at the turn of the century is federal legislation to allow foreign nurses to work in underserved and shortage areas (National Journal Group, Inc., 1999c). Other short-run efforts to meet nursing workforce needs include (a) use of temporary agencies to fill nursing vacancies and outsource the provision of nursing care, (b) encouraging or mandating existing nursing staff to work overtime, and (c) closing of hospital beds due to short staffing.

These care delivery decisions may be needed to meet care demands, yet unfortunately, the ultimate impact of such decisions on care and care delivery are largely unknown. Nursing and the entire health care system must build an evidence base for the work environment and workforce planning to improve decision-making about health care delivery and nursing services, similar to evidence-based research efforts that have occurred in clinical practice. Several data needs exist that call for development of such an evidence base: (a) more complete and accurate data on the nursing workforce; (b) more complete and accurate structure, process, and outcomes data at the public, systems, unit, and patient care levels; (c) identifiers to link workforce and outcomes data; (d) data on other health professions that can be used to model the interdisciplinary effects of care delivery; (e) faster means of data development, collection, and analysis; and (f) secure data depositories.

Availability of such data will facilitate forecasting nursing demand and enable the linking of nursing supply and demand data. Other labor market analyses to examine issues such as wage disparities between certain groups in nursing and the impact of mandating staffing ratios, employing foreign-trained, and utilizing temporary nurses on care delivery also are needed. An in-depth examination of these issues will provide insight into (a) responses of the nursing labor market to clinical practice and systems-level changes, (b) turnover, (c) mobility, and (d) other behaviors of the nursing workforce that result from market-level and public policy decisions.

■ Concluding Statement

The supply of and demand for nurses has fluctuated greatly over time, as manifested in cyclic shortages of nurses. Whether a true nursing shortage exists at the beginning of the 21st century remains to be seen. Both nursing and the health care system generally must actively take steps to (a) improve working conditions in health care, (b) make nursing a more attractive and lucrative career option, and (c) address cyclic nursing shortages by implementing long-term strategies to invest in the future of the nursing workforce. Short-run strategies may help organizations cope with staffing and cost containment issues, but they do not address long-term needs of nurses, health care organizations, other health care employees, or patients. Investments aimed at increasing nurses' human capital and making nursing a viable and attractive career option for future generations has the potential to mitigate future shortages, improve the quality of patient care, and increase organizations' return on investment. Investments made in the workforce of today influence the quality of the outcome achieved, that is, the caliber of the nursing workforce of tomorrow and its ability to meet future societal needs.

As the health care system struggles to balance the costs of providing care and the quality of care provided, conflicts will increase between organizations and employees and between groups of health care professionals. Resolution of these conflicts will depend upon acceptance of a new model for the health care workforce—one that recognizes the importance of human capital in the delivery of high-quality care and one that reduces tension at the margins between support personnel, professionals, primary care providers, and specialists. Nursing must use its unique capabilities, and its role as patient and family advocate to help meet challenges and seize opportunities associated with the implementation of a new workforce model. The future of the nursing workforce and the health of society depend on it.

■ Notes

1. All data reported in this section were extracted from reports of the National Sample Survey of Registered Nurses, 1980 (Moses, 1982), 1984 (Moses, 1986), 1988 (Moses, 1990), 1992 (Moses, 1994), and 1996 (Moses, 1998).
2. The Division of Nursing (DON), Bureau of Health Professionals, Health Resources and Services Administration [HRSA], Department of Health and Human Services), routinely conducts the National Sample Survey of Registered Nurses to gather descriptive data on educational preparation, employment status, and general demographic characteristics of the registered nurse population. The first of these studies was conducted in 1977, and beginning with the 1980 survey, the DON initiated a 4-year cycle for survey distribution and data collection.
3. Advanced practice nurse is defined here as RNs prepared at the graduate degree level to practice as a Clinical Nurse Specialist (CNS), Nurse Anesthetist, Nurse-Midwife, or Nurse Practitioner (NP) (AACN, 1999).
4. In 1996, the proportions of newly licensed RNs by type of educational preparation were 7% diploma, 59% associate degree, and 34% baccalaureate (National Council of State Boards of Nursing, 1999).
5. Unless otherwise noted, all data reported in this section were extracted from reports of the National Sample Survey of Registered Nurses, 1980 (Moses, 1982), 1984 (Moses, 1986), 1988 (Moses, 1990), 1992 (Moses, 1994), and 1996 (Moses, 1998).
6. Hospitals have the ability to influence nursing wage rates through monopsony power. Hurd (1973) studied vacancies and monopsony and the nursing labor market and concluded, " . . . monopsony power is exerted in the labor market for nurses in order to hold wages down" (p. 239). A few employers that have the ability to influence wages or collude in setting wages within a particular market are called an *oligopony;* a single employer that has this ability is called a *monopsony* (Ehrenberg & Smith, 1991). The word *monopoly* is often used to refer to the case of a single employer or a few employers who have the ability to control wages within a labor market. The profit-maximizing monopsony model may be more relevant in health care today than when Hurd reported the phenomenon, given recent increases in the number of for-profit health care organizations.

7. As used here, *consumer* means either the entity that pays for services or the entity that actually receives the service, which may be different. Although *consumer* also implies the notion of choice, that inference should not be made here.

■ References

Aiken, L. H. (1982). The nurse labor market. *Health Affairs, 1*(4), 30–40.

Aiken L. H., & Gwyther, M. E. (1995). Medicare funding of nurse education, the case for policy change. *Journal of the American Medical Association, 273*(19), 528–532.

Aiken, L. H., & Mullinix, C. F. (1987). The nurse shortage. Myth or reality? *New England Journal of Medicine, 317*(10), 641–646.

American Association of Colleges of Nursing. (1998, January 28). *AACN position statement: Certification and regulation of advanced practice nurses.* Washington, DC: Author. AACN [On-line]. Available: http://www.AACN.nche.edu. March 25, 1999.

American Association of Colleges of Nursing. (1999, January 25). *AACN news release: Nursing school enrollments lag behind rising demand for RNs, AACN survey shows.* Washington, DC: Author. (Retrieved March 25, 1999).

Botelho, A., Jones, C. B., & Kiker, B. F. (1998). Nursing wages and educational credentials: The role of work experience and selectivity bias. *Economics of Education Review, 17*(3), 297–306.

Buerhaus, P. I. (1991a). Economic determinants of annual hours worked by registered nurses. *Medical Care, 29*(12), 1181–1195.

Buerhaus, P. I. (1991b). Dynamic shortages of registered nurses. *Nursing Economics, 9*(5), 317–328.

Buerhaus, P. I., & Auerbach, D. (1999). Slow growth in the United States of the number of minorities in the RN workforce. *IMAGE: Journal of Nursing Scholarship, 31*(2), 179–183.

Buerhaus, P. I., & Staiger, D. O. (1999). Trouble in the nurse labor market? Recent trends and future outlook. *Health Affairs, 18*(1), 214–222.

Cleland, V. S. (1990) *The economics of nursing.* Norwalk, CT: Appleton & Lange.

Coffman, J., & Spetz, J. (1999). Maintaining an adequate supply of RNs in California. *IMAGE: Journal of Nursing Scholarship, 31*(4), 389–393.

Drucker, P. F. (1994). The age of social transformation. *The Atlantic Monthly, 274*(5), 53–80.

Ehrenberg, R. G., & Smith, R. S. (1991). *Modern labor economics: Theory and public policy* (4th ed.). New York: HarperCollins.

Eisenberg, J. M. (1998). Health services research in a market-oriented health care system. *Health Affairs, 17*(1), 98–108.

Feldstein, P. J. (1998). *Health care economics* (5th ed.). Albany, NY: Delmar.

Folland, S., Goodman, A. C., & Stano, M. (1993). *The economics of health and health care.* New York: Macmillan.

Goldstein, A. (1999, October 10). How HMOs became the enemy; from nonprofit ideals to corporate horror stories. *Washington Post,* pp. A1, A8, A9.

Griffith, H. (1984). Nursing practice: Substitute or complement according to economic theory. *Nursing Economics, 2*(2), 105–112.

Hurd, R. W. (1973). Equilibrium vacancies in a labor market dominated by non-profit firms: The "shortage" of nurses. *The Review of Economics and Statistics, 55*(2), 234–240.

Kilborn, P. T. (1999, March 23). Registered Nurses in short supply at hospitals nation-wide. *New York Times,* p. A-14.

McCloskey, J. C. (1995). Breaking the cycle. *Journal of Professional Nursing, 11*(2), 67.

Moses, E. (1982). *1980: The registered nurse population, findings from the national sample survey of registered nurses.* Rockville, MD: Division of Nursing, Bureau of Health Professions, Health Resources and Services Administration.

Moses, E. (1986). *1984: The registered nurse population, findings from the national sample survey of registered nurses.* Rockville, MD: Division of Nursing, Bureau of Health Professions, Health Resources and Services Administration.

Moses, E. (1990). *1988: The registered nurse population, findings from the national sample survey of registered nurses.* Rockville, MD: Division of Nursing, Bureau of Health Professions, Health Resources and Services Administration.

Moses, E. (1994). *1992: The registered nurse population, findings from the national sample survey of registered nurses.* Rockville, MD: Division of Nursing, Bureau of Health Professions, Health Resources and Services Administration.

Moses, E. (1998). *1996: The registered nurse population, findings from the national sample survey of registered nurses.* Rockville, MD: Division of Nursing, Bureau of Health Professions, Health Resources and Services Administration.

National Council of State Boards of Nursing. (1999). *Research and statistical data: demographic data, newly registered nurses and licensed practical nurses, 1996 and 1997.* [On-line]. Available: http://www.ncsbn.org/research/statistical/. (Retrieved December 13, 1999).

National Journal Group Inc. *Bed shortage: MA hospitals surprised by reverse trend.* (1999, March 31). American Health Line [On-line serial]. Available: American Health Line 03/31/99, http://www.cloakroom.com.

National Journal Group Inc. *Nursing shortage: Relief bill reaches president.* (1999, November 4). American Health Line [On-line serial]. Available: American Health Line 11/4/99, http://www.cloakroom.com. (Retrieved November 5, 1999).

National Journal Group Inc. *Nursing shortage: Shortfall may be long term.* (1999a, March 23). American Health Line [On-line serial]. Available: American Health Line 3/23/99, http://www.cloakroom.com. (Retrieved March 24, 1999).

Russell, S. (1999, December 10). Severe nursing shortage ahead in California, report says. *San Francisco Chronicle,* p. A7.

Snyderman, N. (Medical Correspondent). (1999, November 26). "Disappearing nurses." *20/20* [Television series]. New York: American Broadcasting Company (ABC).

Yett, D. (1975). *An economic analysis of the nurse shortage.* Lexington, MA: D.C. Heath.

■ *Editor's Questions for Discussion*

Discuss the relationships among supply, wages, and demand concerning the future nursing workforce. What impact has increasing numbers of APNs had on the nursing workforce? What factors may contribute to changes in settings for the largest employers of RNs? How may racial and gender diversity increase the workforce? What difference may such diversity make in the available RN workforce in terms of type of nursing education programs from which RNs graduate? What data are needed regarding wages and type of nursing education programs from which RNs graduate?

How should the profession demonstrate differences in practice, quality of care, outcomes of care, and cost? Is it possible to attribute cost to value and quality of care? How might unlicensed personnel be a legitimate "substitution" in the health care workforce? Debate whether the same level of outcome at a lower cost can be achieved in substituting unlicensed assistive personnel for RNs. How might nursing programs be affected if such personnel can be substituted for RNs and if APNs are substituted for physicians?

What strategies could the profession use to increase Title VIII funds for nursing education programs? Should Medicare funds be decreased for diploma programs? How might evidence be obtained regarding RN productivity, competence, and quality of care pertaining to graduates of each type of nursing program? How do the discussions by D. Jones (Chapter 31), Deets and Choi (Chapter 34), and Titler (Chapter 35) suggest ways of addressing concerns pertaining to outcomes and the nursing workforce? What impact should additional education have on advancement in the workforce?

Which suggestions by Jones for increasing the nursing workforce are also evident in discussions by Felton (Chapter 1) and Koerner (Chapter 2)? How might professional nurses in practice "sell" nursing when recruiting potential students? Indicate strategies that nursing can use to increase positive views of itself as a profession rather than as a commodity. What differences exist between a profession and commodity? Discuss the implications for nursing education programs and entry into practice if nursing is viewed as a profession or as a commodity. How does Jones reinforce points made in other chapters in this volume for Parts on Nursing Education, Nursing Practice, and the Future of Nursing? What health care delivery decisions may have an impact on future nursing programs? How should nursing as a profession prepare for future needs and changes in the health care workforce? What additional variables may be included in projecting a future workforce model?

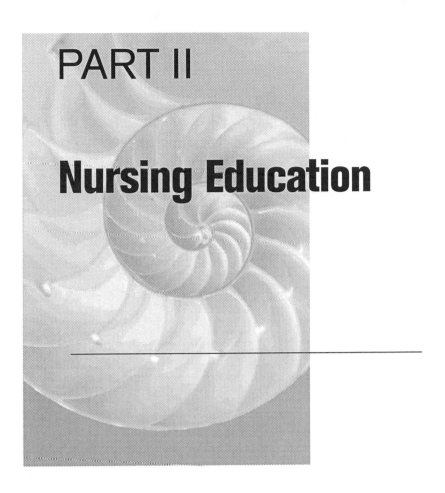

PART II

Nursing Education

"Two roads diverged in a yellow wood,
And sorry I could not travel both . . .
. . . And took the other, just as fair,
And having perhaps the better claim . . . "

These lines by Robert Frost may well describe the educational adventure of developing nursing programs, instructing students, and acquiring resources. Although multiple directions and options now exist in education, the beginning for nursing education lies in its basic programs. Thus, in introducing Part II, it is appropriate to provide an example of the content of such programs, as addressed by the authors of the various chapters.

Proposals reflecting "two roads" for basic practice in education have long been fraught with controversy. Frost's reference to a "yellow wood" lends itself to an embellished interpretation. All involved in the education enterprise may well take heed. "Yellow" may imply lack of courage (as the Thesaurus describes the word). Frost acknowledges regret that he could not travel both roads, perhaps similar to those in nursing who would "travel" (retain) all the avenues for basic nursing education and not make a clear choice.

Frost's next two lines exemplify avoidance in making clear distinctions between paths available. In choosing the path of "indecision" about entry education programs, that choice appears to be "the better claim." Such avoidance and perception of entry paths as being equal ("just as fair") has resulted in increasingly numerous obstacles on the road to nursing's effectiveness.

Writings in this Nursing Education Part provide evidence of that interpretation of Frost's lines. Indeed, his entire poem could be applied not just to the basic nursing program and outcome dilemma but to all aspects of nursing education. An entire revolution in education is occurring. Massive change is related to technology, advocacy for integrated and collaborative systems, increase of graduate programs, and global education. Educators, students, and administrators are urged to apply Frost's poem in its entirety in considering these authors' writings. The "paths" are abundant in the future of nursing education. Given the multiple perspectives available, Frost's poem provides an avenue for objectivity and choice on the road of education.

12

From Revolution to Transformation

Curriculum Development in a New Millennium

Barbara C. Gaines, EdD, RN

From the time of the first Nightingale schools in the United States (1873), program standardization has been a major criterion for quality control in nursing education (Anderson, 1981). Program standardization was useful to early hospital school educators and to faculties involved in nursing's struggle to gain disciplinary status in the mainstream of higher education. Unfortunately, as the 20th century progressed, program standardization came to mean that all nurses needed the same knowledge and skills. As a result, all nursing curricula were essentially the same. Single models of curriculum development predominated. As we enter a new millennium in which change appears to be the only constant, program standardization as a major criterion for curriculum development has lost much of its utility.

■ *The Curriculum Revolution: The Chink in the Armor*

The idea that transformational change was needed in nursing curriculum was introduced in 1987 at the National League for Nursing's Fourth Conference on Nursing Education, "Curriculum Development Revolution" (National League for Nursing [NLN], 1988). The purpose of the conference was to scrutinize current curriculum practices, using the principles of alternative curriculum development models. Much of the work presented was influenced by reconceptualist thinking, associated with the inquiry methods of "ethnography, hermeneutics, phenomenology, politics and economics" (Harris, 1991, p. 3). Substantive arguments were presented against (a) a single definition of what nursing accepted as knowledge, (b) continuing emphasis on technical skills rather than emphasis on skills associated with professional clinical judgment, (c) teacher-driven curriculum, and (d) the hegemony of Tylerian rationale—the predominant curriculum development model in use (NLN, 1988). Considered marginal by many in 1987, the reconceptualist approach has become, in less than 15 years, mainstream in some baccalaureate and higher degree program options. In others this approach continues to add a rich new dimension to our understanding of the "lived experience" of students and faculty, in what is known as the "hidden curriculum."

The pioneering work of these reconceptualist thinkers provided other nurse educators with the impetus to engage in curriculum development in the deliberative curriculum inquiry paradigm—characterized by curricula developed in professional schools to foster reflective practice (Harris, 1991; Schon, 1983, 1987). Still other nurse educators, working in the traditional empirical or analytic paradigm, were encouraged to raise new questions about both the substance and process of curriculum development. Research and inquiry in different curriculum models is now the norm. Hence these variances suggest that the most significant contribution of the reconceptualist revolutionaries was in forcing nurse educators to realize that no single model of curriculum (what we know, how we know it, and how we transmit it to students) would ever be sufficient again. The ability to appreciate alternative world views is integral to success in curriculum development in an uncertain future.

■ Transformational Change

Higher education has not proven immune to the reinvention phenomenon sweeping the nation. Systematic, overarching change is occurring in most institutions. The language of restructuring, accountability, continuous quality improvement and the learning organization permeate mission statements, position papers, and even the routine interoffice memoranda circulating in our schools and colleges. Incremental organizational change in academia is no longer as highly valued by administrators as it once was, nor is it viewed as innocuous (i.e., having an effect only on the unit initiating the change). The purpose of transformational change is to refocus the lens from preoccupation with process to emphasis on achievement of desired outcomes (Guskin, 1996; Marchese, 1998b). This intent has been acknowledged in nursing accreditation standards and in various organizational position papers. New models are guiding change from the traditional institution to the learning organization (Senge, 1990). Fitzpatrick (1998) reminds nurse educators of the benefits of using models in organizational change efforts. Nurse educators contemplating substantial curriculum revision focused on outcomes—and understanding the increasing complexities of practice—will find that a deliberative change framework provides overall direction and cohesion for their work.

■ Issues for Curriculum Development in the 21st Century

Faculty Role

Curriculum development in nursing education, at least for a while, will appear similar to that which is ongoing in schools and colleges today. That is, faculty will continue to select content, organize its presentation, and evaluate student performance. Under conditions of transformational change, however, familiar processes must yield new understandings about "what" it is critical to know and "how" we know it. Faculty synthesize and translate findings of research and inquiry and expert panels—and the realities of the health care environment—into sets of learning experiences for nursing students in a variety of programs. In so doing, faculty must identify the knowledge and skills critical to students at that program level. Because all nurses and practice are not the same, thoughtful consideration about differing roles is required. In organizing the appropriate learning experiences for a program, faculty will be expected to use an organizing framework that encourages attainment of identified, critical outcomes. And finally, along with evaluating student performance in authentic ways, faculty will be reevaluating program administration policies and practices to ensure that program flexibility is facilitated.

Preparation for Practice Entry

New student groups, new providers, and the availability of electronic education modalities are making it possible for schools to offer a wide variety of program options. The first question that must be answered about programs (other than community college programs) is the level—baccalaureate, postbaccalaureate, master's, or professional doctorate—at which they will prepare students for entry into practice. A second question is whether they will prepare a generalist, in nursing's traditional usage of the term, or a specialist who has enough generalist knowledge to pass the licensure exam. Answers to both of these questions are critical in that they define what faculty will agree is the substance of the discipline and hence the central knowledge for the curriculum. A final question—how faculty will facilitate student progress through the selected options—adds unwanted but necessary complexity to the decision-making process. Nursing programs are not only very expensive to operate, they must also compete with each other for students in a time of decreasing resources.

Program Delivery

Solutions that have been successful to date in dealing with the conceptual and economic dilemmas that programs face include (a) modularizing courses, (b) delivering courses as distance learning and on-line; (c) initiating certificate programs; (d) establishing individually focused and population focused tracks within single-level programs; and (e) conducting associate degree to master's degree (ADN–MS) "fast track," generic master's degree, and clinical doctorate programs. How many of these options will continue to provide viable alternatives beyond the next decade is unclear. Viability depends not only on wise decisions with regard to which programs to offer, but it also depends on external forces and economic vagaries.

■ Selecting What to Teach

Faculty will continue to use several sources of nursing knowledge to ensure that the developed curriculum meets programmatic aims. Texts such as this one will influence content decisions, as will (a) acknowledged guidance provided by expert panel reports (e.g., pain management as a fifth vital sign; Fitzpatrick, 1999), (b) accreditation standards, (c) surveys of local need, (d) faculty and student interests, and (e) college and university resources. Research findings on quality outcomes and evidence-based practice will become major sources of influence as well. The potential sources of content will increase, and there will always be too much to learn! What will be different, however, is that we will be not be able to prepare nurses with the necessary sets of knowledge and skills in the usual way. We cannot continue to see curriculum development as simply adding content to what we already teach or as a simple reorganization of what we have always done. We must give credence to using the principles of transformational change as we develop programs and curricula compatible with educational reform. If we do not begin to frame curriculum decisions as a process of critical selection, we will find ourselves squarely in the middle of the dilemma posed by Tanner (1998): Are we developing a "curriculum for the 21st century—or is it the 21 year curriculum?" The question will not be answered easily.

Knowledge for Practice

Along with our reluctance to forgo what we know, several different scenarios about practice are developing within the profession. One point of consensus has emerged (AACN, 1998; AACN, 1999; O'Neil, 1999; Stevens & Valiga, 1999; Tagliareni, Pollock, Horns & LeDane, 1999). Nursing, like all health care, needs a knowledge worker for the information-age. A knowledge worker nurse is one whose practice is grounded in skills associated with (a) critical thinking and clinical judgment; (b) teamwork and communication; (c) new technologies; and (d) leadership, management, and delegation. Which of the many knowledge bases useful to nurses should provide the context for skill acquisition is once again moot, especially in entry-level programs. The following example provides one explanation.

Over the past decade, knowledge in the areas of systems, negotiation, collaboration and conflict resolution, health promotion, cultural competence, and case management have provided the framework for changes in curricula. Once the preserve of public and community health nursing and leadership and management courses in baccalaureate programs, this content has been used to reorganize programs at all nursing education levels. Substantial effort has gone into these revisions because community-based practice is believed by many to be the future of nursing practice (Cahill et al., 1998; Irons, 1998; Jamieson, 1998; Mitty & Mezey, 1998).

However, we find ourselves in the midst of yet another nursing shortage in hospitals and long-term care settings, the traditional practice sites for nursing. In these practice settings, the knowledge and skills associated with individual care of the seriously ill have primacy. And as should be expected, student interest and faculty expertise in the practice of individual care remains high. The dilemma of what content to choose as context for the newly agreed upon skill sets is complicated. The uncertain health care environment in which students will practice makes planning difficult. That knowledge is the crux of disciplinary status and faculty reward systems also affects choice of content. Therefore that knowledge viewed as central to the discipline of nursing will remain a significant question for faculty.

Consensus for Content

At all program levels, conventional wisdom dictates that curriculum developers start their selection process with areas in which there is agreement. Currently, it suggests that successful programs, regardless of level, will (a) embrace program flexibility and new ideas as a way to accommodate complex knowledge needed for practice in a variety of settings (O'Neil, 1999; Tagliareni et al., 1999; Bellack, 1999); (b) emphasize cognitive skill development rather than technical skill proficiency (Rapson & Rice, 1999); and (c) foster a preventive, systems, and population focus for care without losing the ability to help students gain the clinical judgment that will allow them to apply knowledge wisely in individual patient care situations (Eisenhauer, 1998).

To make sense of choices for specific program curricula, faculty are seeking help from colleagues outside academia. Many schools and colleges are reporting on community conferences (vision conferences) at which mission statements and necessary curriculum revisions supporting refined missions have been formulated through a joint process, outlining alternative futures for nursing in the community. Faculty at these schools and colleges find that practitioners provide a sensitive lens that genuinely reflects core values of nursing and the realities of multiple competing demands of various practice settings.

■ Partnerships

School–community partnerships also may be the best example of an increasingly viable mechanism in the implementation of outcome-oriented nursing curriculum. These partnerships, descriptions of which fill the pages of current journals, have developed primarily in baccalaureate and higher degree programs. Available descriptions suggest their evolvement far beyond the first faculty practice models and traditional preceptor programs. Focused on real practice considerations and defined in terms of vulnerable populations or specific social and health concerns, these partnerships have strong potential for increasing student understanding of disease prevention and health promotion. Partnerships may also help them develop new skills in communication, leadership, and delegation. Partnerships also provide an opportunity to reinforce nursing values of service and social responsibility (Faulk & Mancuso, 1998; Mitty & Mezey, 1998).

Partnerships between schools and colleges and their communities have taken on an additional dimension. Regional and national site-based initiatives have begun to disseminate findings from their respective projects with reports that provide direction for national policy and curriculum development at the school or college level (Rapson & Rice, 1999; Shoultz, Kooker, & Sloat, 1998; Simoni & McKinney, 1998).

The common theme in all the partnership literature is recognition that the nursing curriculum at every level must recognize the centrality of practice and plan learning experiences for students that reinforce this concept (Bellack, 1998). Selecting critical content for this new world view, in the face of the continuing knowledge explosion and increasing accessibility of information, remains one of faculty's biggest challenges. One avenue of promise is the learner-centered curriculum. In a learner-centered curriculum faculty see their discipline through a student's eyes, choosing content and learning experiences that support the student's growth toward identified outcomes.

■ Organizing for Learning

For much of the 20th century, we assumed that students learned best in higher education if they were educated in a paradigm focused on transmitting the structure of the discipline. In most disciplines structure is equated with the essential questions and methods that create knowledge amassed through research. In nursing, the structure of the discipline—at least in the organization of curriculum in entry-level programs—has been framed in terms of (a) historical practice skills, the so-called "fundamentals"; (b) assumptions about simple versus complex nursing; and (c) demands of providing safe care in real patient environments. Many nurse educators believe firmly that this way of organizing learning is student-centered. Literature coming out of the reconceptualist, curriculum revolution paradigm and deliberative, problem or inquiry-based programs persuasively contradict this long-held assumption of student-centered learning. Additionally, serious national concern about how well we are preparing graduates reinforces the available research. Successful student outcomes with regard to critical thinking, clinical judgment, and teamwork require that we reorganize curricula to emphasize how students learn the discipline. But what does it mean to "organize for learning"?

Elements

Probably the most comprehensive and understandable answer to this question (how to organize for learning) is found in a synthesis of papers presented at a recent American Association of Higher Education meeting. Ewell (1997) sorts the research on learning into three categories: "What we know about learning," "What we know about promoting learning," and "What we know about institutional change" (pp. 4–6). Principles outlined in the section on what we know about promoting learning provide a strong framework for thinking more deeply about learning per se. Ewell suggests we start thinking about "remaking instruction" using approaches that

- emphasize application and experience;
- constructively model the learning process;
- emphasize linking established concepts to new situations;
- emphasize interpersonal collaboration;
- emphasize rich and frequent feedback on performance; and
- consistently develop a limited set of clearly identified, cross-disciplinary skills, publicly held to be important.

Nursing education has a rich history of using many elements addressed in clinical learning situations. Yet the disconnect remains between our perceived need to cover even more content so that our students will perform well on licensure and certification examinations and the need to organize for learning so that

students will be successful practitioners. Increasing evidence from research in the cognitive sciences makes it apparent that allowing the disconnect to persist is a real disservice to students.

Requirements

Organizing for learning requires that students be actively engaged with real problems from which they will, in unique ways, create, reflect on, and modify what they learn. Learning in this manner fosters the deeper understanding necessary for the student to become the knowledge worker desired by society. Deep learning, interdisciplinary education experiences, and curriculum models (e.g., problem-based, case-based, and inquiry-based) that foster student engagement highlight ways that nurse educators can further enhance the critical thinking and clinical judgment necessary in a culture where expertise is valued. Strategies such as active learning, cooperative learning, and authentic assessment are essential to success in these programs. The importance of these strategies to development of teamwork and cognitive skills is gaining recognition in the literature.

Strategic Goals

Simply put, active learning strategies provide

. . . opportunities for students *to talk and listen, read, write, and reflect* as they approach course content through problem-solving exercises, informal small groups, simulations, case studies, role playing, and other activities—all of which require students to *apply* what they are learning. (Meyers & Jones, 1993, p. xi)

Many of these activities occur regularly in nursing programs, and it is tempting to argue therefore that our curricula are "organized for learning." However, several problems exist with the argument. First, using active learning strategies is a choice of individual faculty members, but students may progress through a program with little or no experience in active learning. Second, early evidence indicates that use of a strategy, without clearly defining its purpose and methods to students, means that it is unlikely to succeed. For support of this conclusion, consider the following nonnursing example from Grinnell College (Trosset, 1998).

Open discussion is believed to encourage critical thinking about sensitive issues. Yet when Trosset asked approximately 200 students at varying levels in the college curriculum about its value, she found that students overwhelmingly believed that the purpose of discussion was to advocate their own views and, in some cases, to be protected from the views of others. For them, the objective was comfort in the discussion situation. In contrast, faculty believed that the purpose of discussion was to encourage critical thinking as students (a) learned from others, (b) used evidence, and (c) were persuaded to new views when the quality of the evidence warranted a change in position. Many of us have had similar experiences in clinical conferences, in ethics courses, or in dialogues with students about pathophysiology. We often assume that students share our understanding of the purpose of an activity when that may not be the case. So, although we are engaged in discussion with our students, if differing assumptions persist, critical thinking necessary to the development of clinical judgment may well not occur

Cooperative Learning

And finally, new research on cooperative learning (Johnson, Johnson, & Smith, 1998) outlines five conditions that must exist in the learning experience if the desired goal of teamwork is to occur, in addition to cognitive gains. Learning experiences promoting teamwork require that all students in the group perceive that, even though they are individually ac-

countable for their own performance, no student can succeed unless every one does. The authors of the study state further that faculty must teach students the "needed social skills [for teamwork] and ensure that they are used appropriately" (p. 30). O'Banion (1997) argues that associate degree programs in nursing are using principles of collaborative and cooperative learning successfully:

> Nursing programs in community colleges have some of the highest success rates in all of education, at least in part because a cohort is guided together through a rigorous competency-based curriculum. Nursing students study together and support each other, and there is no disincentive for all to succeed at high levels because students are not graded relative to each other (as on a Bell curve) but relative to a performance standard. (p. 55)

Organizing for learning provides a useful approach to resolving the content overload dilemma at all levels of nursing curricula. Undertaken thoughtfully, it also will help remove unnecessary program administration variables.

■ Credits, Competencies, Certification, and Articulation

Degrees and certificates in higher education are awarded on the basis of successful completion of credits. Credits serve as a proxy measure of knowledge and competence associated with successful completion of the curriculum. What would be called "seat time" in elementary school translates into the generic 3 credit, 3 meetings a week course that spans a term of 10 to 15 weeks. Course credits are multiplied until the requisite number of hours for the degree have been amassed.

Credit hours, as a method of program standardization, are integral to determining tuition and very important in determining transferability of student courses between programs

(Schneider & Schoenberg, 1999). But as nursing curriculum experiments in the 1960s and 1970s (e.g., integrated curricula and modular curricula) revealed and as RN completion and certificate programs today show, credit hours and levels of competence are not always easily equated. Nowhere is this phenomenon more apparent to faculty than in the attempt to award credit for prior learning, especially learning that occurred outside the traditional college setting. As Schneider and Schoenberg (1999) put it, the credit hour is a "persistent feature of college life" (p. 30) and is increasingly problematic.

The current emphasis on (a) outcomes and accountability, (b) need for continuing education for workers changing positions within agencies or in need of developing new competencies, (c) availability of online and distance education programs, and (d) the plethora of new providers entering the higher education and health care marketplace add yet another dimension to challenges encountered by traditional credit-based programs (Marchese, 1998a). If school and college-based nursing education programs are to emphasize the quality of learning offered and compete with new providers, these programs will need mecha-

nisms for within-program assessment that recognizes competence, not seat time (Luttrell, Lenburg, Scherubel, Jacob, & Koch, 1999). Additional cross-program strategies, such as the few noncredit-based articulation agreements between community college and baccalaureate programs also are needed. Fortunately, administrative practices, such as the credit-degree formula, that were once considered immutable are now being questioned.

■ Concluding Statement

Transformational change in nursing programs is not only necessary, it is possible. Curriculum research and inquiry in multiple paradigms and enhanced communication with practitioners provide the foundation for new understandings of what nurses practicing in different roles need to know. Adopting a learner-centered framework for curriculum decisions provides the mechanism to cope with the abundance of information and changing health care environment. The process of reinvention occurring in our parent institutions allows for innovation and change in administrative policies and procedures.

■ References

American Association of Colleges of Nursing. (1998). *The essentials of baccalaureate education for professional nursing practice.* Washington, DC: Author.

American Association of Colleges of Nursing. (1999). Position statement: A vision of baccalaureate and graduate education: The next decade. *Journal of Professional Nursing, 15,* 59–65.

Andersen, N. E. (1981). The historical development of American nursing education. *Journal of Nursing Education, 20,* 18–36.

Bellack, J. P. (1998). Community-based nursing practice: Necessary but not sufficient. *Journal of Nursing Education, 37,* 99–100.

Bellack, J. P. (1999). Emotional intelligence: A missing ingredient? *Journal of Nursing Education, 38,* 3–4.

Cahill, M., Devlin, M., LeBlanc, P., Lowe, B., Norton, B., Tassin, K., & Vallette, E. (1998). Reexamining the associate degree curriculum: Assessing the need for community concepts. *Nursing and Health Care Perspectives, 19,* 158–161.

Eisenhauer, L. A. (1998). The reconstruction of professional knowledge. *Journal of Nursing Education, 37,* 51–52.

Ewell, P. T. (1997). Organizing for learning: A new imperative. *American Association of Higher Education Bulletin, 50,* 3–6.

Faulk, D., & Mancuso, F. (1998). A collaborative effort for sex education in rural school settings. *Nursing and Health Care Perspectives, 19,* 271–273.

Fitzpatrick, J. J. (1998). Learning organizations . . . and other benefits of the Senge culture. *Nursing and Health Care Perspectives, 19,* 259.

Fitzpatrick, J. J. (1999). The fifth vital sign: An agenda for nurse educators. *Nursing and Health Care Perspectives, 20,* 67.

Guskin, A. E. (1996). Facing the future: The change process in restructuring universities. *Change, 28,* 27–37.

Harris, I. B. (1991). Contributions to professional education from the field of curriculum studies: Research and practice with new traditions of investigation. *PERQ, 13,* 3–16.

Irons, P. D. (1998). A community college responds to changes in health care delivery. *Nursing and Health Care Perspectives, 19,* 162–165.

Jamieson, M. K. (1998). Expanding the associate degree curriculum without adding time. *Nursing and Health Care Perspectives, 19,* 161–162.

Johnson, D. W., Johnson, R. T., & Smith, K. A. (1998). Cooperative learning returns to college: What evidence is there that it works? *Change, 30,* 26–35.

Luttrell, M. F., Lenburg, C. B., Scherubel, J. C., Jacob, S. R., & Koch, R. B. (1999). Competency outcomes for learning and performance assessment. *Nursing and Health Care Perspectives, 20,* 134–141.

Marchese, T. (1998a). Not-so-distant competitors: How new providers are remaking the postsecondary marketplace. *American Association of Higher Education Bulletin, 51,* 3–7.

Marchese, T. (1998b). Restructure?! You bet! An interview with change expert Alan E. Guskin. *American Association of Higher Education Bulletin, 51,* 3–6.

Meyers, C., & Jones, T. B. (1993). *Promoting active learning: Strategies for the college classroom.* San Francisco: Jossey-Bass.

Mitty, E., & Mezey, M. (1998). Integrating advanced practice nurses in home care: Recommendations for teaching home care program. *Nursing and Health Care Perspectives, 19,* 264–270.

National League for Nursing. (1988). *Curriculum revolution: Mandate for change.* New York: Author.

O'Banion, T. (1997). *A learning college for the 21st century.* Phoenix: Oryx Press.

O'Neil, E. (1999). Refocusing the lens: The opportunity that is nursing. *Nursing and Health Care Perspectives, 20*(1), 10–14.

Rapson, M. F., & Rice, R. B. (1999). Colleagues in caring: Regional collaboratives for nursing workforce development—educational policy implications. *Journal of Nursing Education, 38,* 197–202.

Schneider, C. G., & Shoenberg, R. (1999). Habits hard to break: How persistent features of campus life frustrate curricular reform. *Change, 31,* 30–35.

Schon, D. A. (1983). *The reflective practitioner.* New York: Basic Books.

Schon, D. A. (1987). *Educating the reflective practitioner.* San Francisco: Jossey-Bass.

Senge, P. M. (1990). *The fifth discipline: The art and practice of a learning organization.* New York: Doubleday.

Shoultz, J., Kooker, B.M., & Sloat, A.R. (1998). Community-based nursing education research study from the NLN vision for nursing education: Hawaii/phase II. *Nursing and Health Care Perspectives, 19,* 278–282.

Simoni, P. S., & McKinney, J. A. (1998). Evaluation of service learning in a school of nursing: Primary care in a community setting. *Journal of Nursing Education, 37,* 122–128.

Stevens, K., & Valiga, T. M. (1999). Formulating priorities for research in nursing education: A consensus-building approach. *Nursing and Health Care Perspectives, 20,* 167–169.

Tagliareni, M. E., Pollock, C. P., Horns, P. N., & LeDane, S. (1999). The councils respond. *Nursing and Health Care Perspectives, 20*(1), 15–17.

Tanner, C. A. (1998). Curriculum for the 21st century—or is it the 21 year curriculum? *Journal of Nursing Education, 37,* 383–384.

Trosset, C. (1998). Obstacles to open discussion and critical thinking: The Grinnell College study. *Change, 30,* 44–49.

■ Editor's Questions for Discussion

What factors contribute to content change in curricula? Discuss implications for the Gaines chapter (12) of the discussion by Dooling and Gaines as shown in Chapter 13. Given perpetual curricula change, should accreditation of programs be required? What other variables may be more important for high-quality nursing programs? Should nursing faculty undergo a certification or accreditation process?

What impact will changes in faculty roles have on future curriculum development? Apply implications from the discussions by Lindeman (Chapter 63), Hoffman (Chapter 64), Keating and Perry (Chapter 65), Flood (Chapter 66), Biordi and McFarlane (Chapter 67), Lindell (Chapter 69), and Shaver (Chapter 76). How will options available to programs affect the future role of faculty?

What data and processes are essential for deciding program level to prepare students for entry into practice? What principles of transformational change should be used in developing programs and curricula? To what extent should practice settings and health care delivery systems influence curriculum content? Which should be the most significant determinant for content: beliefs of the profession and faculty, health care delivery systems, or health care status and needs of the population?

How is a learner-centered curriculum similar or different from problem-based learning? What parts of the discussion by Nichols and Renwanz-Boyle (Chapter 16), M. Fisher (Chapter 17), Yeaworth et al. (Chapter 14), Billings (Chapter 15), Fitzpatrick (Chapter 18), and Boland (Chapter 71) are applicable to curriculum development? What does it mean to "organize for learning"? Identify specific approaches for each element suggested by Ewell.

How can the need to address essential content for licensure and the need to organize for learning be connected? How can understanding and consensus about purposes of active learning strategies occur? Discuss the pros and cons of various methods for organizing learning. What variables influence the effectiveness of one method compared to the others?

What factors should be considered in planning and developing partnerships in implementing curriculum? How should partnerships be evaluated?

What other options should be considered instead of credit-degree formulas as evidence for knowledge competence? What implications exist in Jones-Dickson's (Chapter 4) presentation about measurement of competence for curriculum and programs?

13

Program Evaluation in Nursing Education

Shirley L. Dooling, EdD, RN
Barbara C. Gaines, EdD, RN

*How are you going to know you've arrived if you
don't know where you are going!*

(*Alice in Wonderland,* by Lewis Carroll, 1898/1940)

The purpose of program evaluation is to determine whether a nursing program has met its mission and goals. It is easier to determine whether goals have been met if they are stated specifically, with nouns well defined by indicator behaviors. Because goals must be achievable, most people select those that are measurable by direct indicator behaviors, and better yet, by the degree of those behaviors. However, more complex program goals (e.g., developing lifelong learners or preparing culturally competent practitioners) may need to be stated broadly, with proxy measures identified to allow progress toward the broad aim to be ascertained. For decision-making, trends evident from aggregate data that are valid and reliable are essential.

This chapter is not intended to provide information on "how to" conduct programmatic evaluations. Rather it provides (a) definitions of various types of evaluation undertaken by faculty teaching in nursing programs,

(b) historical perspective on trends in programmatic evaluation, and (c) brief discussion of some of the issues that academic nursing faculties face when engaging in programmatic evaluation. Because the majority of program evaluation efforts have occurred, at least in the past, in response to regulatory and accreditation requirements, examples from these arenas are featured.

■ Types of Evaluation

Program evaluation in nursing education generally consists of three types: (a) *in-house,* (b) *approval,* and (c) *accreditation.* Though often regarded as mutually exclusive activities because the purpose of each is somewhat different, similar processes are employed and thus can be undertaken simultaneously.

In-house

In-house evaluation is conducted for purposes of measuring outcomes of a curriculum, a course, a specific teaching–learning strategy, or perhaps a new or changed admission or progression policy. The motivation for in-house evaluation is to find out whether X has made a difference. In other words, what difference in outcome, if any, resulted when X was instituted?

Approval

Approval evaluation is a periodic process conducted by state boards of nursing for the purpose of determining whether minimum educational standards have been met to ensure adequate preparation of program graduates for safety in nursing practice. In most states, approval is mandatory. It is required of any program before graduates are eligible to take the examination for licensure as a registered nurse. Nursing programs cannot be considered for voluntary or specialty accreditation until state approval has been granted. In fact, most states will not even allow a program to recruit prospective students until approval, at least in the first stage, has been granted.

Accreditation

Accreditation is another periodic (which may be as long as 10 years) form of evaluation. Its purpose is to determine whether standards of quality in education have been achieved. During the accreditation process, what a school does is compared to a standard from which specific criteria have been derived. These criteria deal with key elements determined by members of the accrediting body to be important to education in all institutions or programs within the scope of the accrediting agency. Accreditation fosters a continuous process of self-evaluation that results in aggregate data, by which trends or patterns related to processes and outcomes can be identified. These results then are used as the rationale for decisions about development, maintenance, or revision of program activities.

Accreditation in nursing is a voluntary process based on the concepts of self-assessment and peer-review. It is directed by the U.S. Department of Education (DOE) so as to be free from influence by any professional organization.

Forms of Accreditation

Regional accreditation is a voluntary form of evaluation for any institution of higher education, be it a community college, 4-year college or university, or single-purpose institution. Although regional accreditation does involve making judgments about the quality of individual programs within an institution, such as a School of Nursing, it does not provide accreditation for individual programs. Accreditation is granted to the institution as a whole.

The six regional accreditation associations are the Northwest States Association of Colleges and Schools, Middle States Association of Colleges and Schools, New England Association of Schools and Colleges, North Central States Association of Colleges and Schools, Southern Association of Colleges and Schools, and Western Association of Colleges and Schools.

Specialty accreditation is offered to programs within an institution of higher education, usually only after that institution has attained regional accreditation. Although specialty accreditation also is a voluntary process, attaining specialty accreditation provides certain benefits to students. Students who complete an accredited nursing program generally are able to enter government employment (e.g., Veterans Administration Hospitals) and hold a higher rank in the military than students completing nonaccredited nursing programs. Similarly, the likelihood of graduates from an accredited nursing program being admitted to a master's or higher degree program is greater than for graduates from nonaccredited nursing programs.

Accreditation Organizations

Baccalaureate and higher degree nursing programs may be accredited by two organizations: (a) the National League for Nursing Accrediting Commission (NLNAC) and (b) the Commission on Collegiate Nursing Education (CCNE). Although neither organization currently accredits doctoral programs in nursing, both groups are studying this issue. Only NLNAC provides accreditation for practical nurse, associate degree, and diploma nursing programs. The CCNE (1998) has stated five purposes of specialty accreditation in nursing:

1. To hold nursing education programs accountable to the community of interest—the nursing profession, consumers, employers, higher education, students and their families—and to one another by ensuring that

these programs have mission statements, goals and outcomes that are appropriate for programs preparing individuals to enter the field of nursing.

2. To evaluate the success of a nursing education program in achieving its mission, goals and outcomes.

3. To assess the extent to which a nursing education program meets accreditation standards.

4. To inform the public of the purposes and values of accreditation and to identify nursing education programs that meet accreditation standards.

5. To foster continued improvement in nursing education programs and thereby in professional practice. (p. 3)

The American Nurses Credentialing Center Commission on Accreditation (ANCC-COA) accredits providers of continuing education in nursing. The value of this specialty accreditation is twofold. Some states require a specific number of continuing education hours for relicensure or certification as an advanced practice nurse. ANCC-COA accreditation is reciprocal in all states and is recognized by the majority of nursing specialty organizations.

■ History of and Trends in Programmatic Evaluation

Early nursing programs, like early medical schools, generally were proprietary organizations. Evaluation against agreed upon standards were almost nonexistent. The Flexner Report (1910–1972), an evaluative program report, had a major impact on medicine as a profession, on medical education, and subsequently on nursing education. During this period, some students in medical schools and many students in nursing programs had not even completed high school. As a result of Flexner's findings and because of new discoveries in the biological and psychosocial sciences, medicine was moved into institutions of higher education, ushering in the era of scientific medicine. Additionally, the affluence of a rising middle class, fueled by the influx of immigrants seeking opportunities for sons to become professionals, resulted in increased demands by the public for well-prepared and well-educated physicians (Bledstein, 1976).

By 1920, there were an estimated 2,000 diploma nursing schools (Notter & Spalding, 1976). Programs varied in length from 6 months to 2 years. Most of the lectures for nursing students at these schools were delivered by physicians, who also owned the hospitals. Apprenticeship experience occurred at the patient's bedside. Shortly after entering a nursing program, students were put in charge of an entire patient unit at night, and during the day they supervised probationary students who were just beginning the program. In most instances the driving force behind opening a hospital school was the inexpensive labor that "student nurses" provided. In fact, when needed, they provided additional hands in the operating room suite. If a student was viewed as especially competent in an area of patient care such as labor and delivery, the student was given responsibility for patients in that area. Lectures were viewed as less important than experience in the education of the student. Hence training and service were the key elements to the preparation of nurses, not education or a standardized program of study.

Florence Nightingale is well known among nurse educators for her stance that nurses needed an education that included a standardized curriculum in both theory and practice. She further believed that nurses should be prepared in educational institutions supported by public funds. She believed that nursing schools should be associated with a medical school and affiliated with a teaching hospital. However, it was important to Nightingale that the nursing school be independent of both. She further

maintained that professional nurses should be responsible for the administration of the school and the instruction of students and that they should be paid specifically for these services; that students should be required to attend lectures, write papers, and keep diaries. Additionally, Nightingale believed that records should be maintained on the students; each student should have her own bed; and students should be carefully selected and should reside in nurses' homes where discipline and character formation were also a part of the educational process (Ashley, 1976; Notter & Spalding, 1976).

Many superintendents of training schools were aware of how far short of the Nightingale standards the proliferating U.S. diploma program fell. In 1893, several years before the Flexner Report, the American Society of Superintendents of Training Schools for Nurses was created (National League for Nursing Accrediting Commission [NLNAC], 1999b). Its goal was the establishment and maintenance of a universal standard for the training of nurses. In 1912, this society was renamed the National League for Nursing Education (NLNE) (NLNAC, 1999b). In 1917, the NLNE published the first *Standard Curriculum for School of Nursing* (NLNE, 1917). In 1923, *Nursing and Nursing Education in the United States,* known also as the Goldmark Report, found that teachers in nursing programs were poorly prepared for their role and recommended that nursing education be moved into colleges and universities in order to raise the standards of nursing education (Goldmark, 1923). Several other evaluative studies followed; many produced similar findings and recommendations (Kalisch & Kalisch, 1995). While the profession appeared slow to follow the recurrent recommendations in these studies, some of the slowness to change occurred because of the powerful resistance of physicians and hospitals to increasing the content and length of the education of nurses.

In 1952, NLNE, the National Organization for Public Health Nursing (NOPHN), and the American Association of Colleges of Nursing (AACN) joined together to establish the National League for Nursing (NLN) (NLNAC, 1999b). The NLN assumed responsibility for the specialty accreditation of nursing education programs, from practical nursing to baccalaureate and higher degree programs. In 1992, new U.S. Department of Education (DOE) regulations required that accrediting programs demonstrate independence from influence, direct or indirect, of the NLN on its accreditation process (NLN, personal communication, 1992). The apparent conflict of interest was attributed to several circumstances involving the structure of the organization. Among the reasons given were that (a) school membership in NLN resulted in a lower fee for the site visit, (b) site visitors to programs being accredited or reaccredited were expected to be NLN members, and (c) councils for the various types of nursing programs were an organizational unit of the NLN. The DOE requirements resulted in the creation of the National League for Nursing Accrediting Commission (NLNAC) in June 1997 (NLNAC, 1999b).

In 1996, the membership of the American Association of Colleges of Nursing (AACN) decided to establish an independent arm of its organization, the Commission on Collegiate Nursing Education (CCNE), to accredit baccalaureate and higher degree programs in nursing (AACN, 1996). One major concern with the existing NLNAC, which might have fewer members from baccalaureate and higher degree programs, was that the accreditation process could not truly be a peer-review. Further, nursing faculties and heads of nursing programs contended that the existing processes for writing the self-study and the subsequent visit for accreditation or reaccreditation were tedious, too detailed, costly, and prescriptive. Many others argued that existing criteria did not allow for experimentation and thus did not yield information of value to help identify the quality or weaknesses of a baccalaureate and higher degree program. Concerns were also expressed about the preparation of visitors, including the fact that often they did not come from nursing programs with characteristics similar to the program being visited. Some members of the AACN questioned whether all the criteria being used were relevant measures of nursing program quality. Additionally, they expressed frustration in dealing with NLNAC.

The advent of CCNE provides baccalaureate and higher degree programs in nursing with a choice of accreditation agencies. Strong similarities exist in the criteria and accreditation procedures used by NLNAC and CCNE. In their reconfiguration as independent of the parent organization, both agencies have been responsive to criticisms from nursing schools and external reviewers. It is too early to tell whether both agencies will be successful in a market economy, but it is clear that market factors will be important. In a recent study, Bellack, Gelmon, O'Neil, and Thomsen (1999) declared:

> What are the services nursing education programs need and should demand for accreditation to be relevant and add value? This study's findings show the greatest perceived values added by specialized accreditation are not federal fund entitlement, response to accountability demands of external groups, or leverage for institutional resources. Instead the greatest perceived benefits are program excellence (and recognition for such), marketability and mobility of the school's graduates in the market, and continuous improvement of an educational program's services and products. The study findings also suggest the nursing education community, as reflected by the response of its academic leaders, is ready for accreditation to offer more than it does presently. Time will tell if nursing education's accreditors are able to respond with new and expanded services to meet the needs and demands of current nursing education programs and their faculty and students. (p. 60)

While it is clear that program evaluation currently is closely linked to accreditation standards, it seems clear from the study cited that both accrediting organizations must continue, insofar as possible, to evolve in response to user demand. Sometimes academic leaders' lack of knowledge of DOE regulations has resulted in unrealistic expectations regarding what accrediting organizations can and cannot do. Accreditation could be eroded if it is not responsive to changing educational norms or if it can be demonstrated that individual, rather than program, credentialing should be the new norm (Lindeman, 1999).

■ Program Evaluation Models and Associated Issues

A major decision for faculties designing and conducting program evaluations is the selection of a framework that will provide effective direction for the multiple purposes that program evaluation serves. Whether evaluation of a course, curriculum, or teaching–learning strategy, evaluation of a grant or contract, or evaluation of a regional or specialty program, an efficient design and implementation strategy is paramount. External factors—especially those associated with approval, accreditation, or grant and contract regulations—weigh heavily in design and data collection priorities. At least three approaches to framework design are popular with nursing faculties: evaluation models, process-oriented designs, and outcome-oriented designs. In comprehensive evaluations, it is common to find combinations and components of two or three of the approaches.

Evaluative Models

The *evaluative model* is generally based on an accepted or emerging theory of evaluation. Classic models in education include judgmental strategies, exemplified in Cronbach's work,

and decision-management strategies such as Stuffelbeam's model (Cronbach et al., 1980; Stufflebeam, 1983). Newer designs include an existing nursing theory or information processing models (Ingersoll & Sauter, 1998; Rossi & Freeman, 1993; Worthen & Sanders, 1973). The comprehensive educational evaluation models have been most popular in colleges and universities that have institutional research units to support various disciplinary units' evaluative needs. One nursing program reflecting successful application of concepts from several educational evaluation models to its program evaluation efforts is that of Thomas Jefferson University (Bevil, 1991). Nursing programs without strong institutional research support generally rely on program evaluation designs that directly address accreditation or grant and contract requirements.

Process-Oriented Strategies

The *process-oriented model* begins with a strong assumption: The design of a specific measurable plan of action leads to a predictable expected outcome. This model has been used extensively in nursing accreditation evaluations. Three examples of NLNAC's process-oriented strategies are found in its Criterion 3, Criterion 5, and Criterion 14. Criterion 3 reads: "Nursing unit is administered by a nurse who is academically and experientially qualified and who has authority and responsibility for development and administration of the nursing program" (NLNAC, 1999a, p. 5). One of five forms of documentation acceptable as evidence that this criterion has been met is that the nurse administrator holds a master's degree in nursing and an earned doctorate from a regionally accredited institution. If that is not the case, a strong rationale for acceptance of other credentials is required. The assumption is that the quality of the nursing leadership will be greater if the condition defined in the criterion exists.

Criterion 5 reads: "Faculty members (full- and part-time) are academically and experientially qualified and maintain expertise appropriate to teaching, service, and scholarly responsibilities" (NLNAC, 1999a, p. 7). This criterion is based on the assumption that the degree and experience of faculty is related to the quality of teaching, service, and scholarly activities.

Criterion 14 is another example of a process-oriented criterion: "Practice learning environments are selected and monitored by faculty and provide opportunities for a variety of learning options appropriate for contemporary nursing" (NLNAC, 1999a, p. 11). Documentation that this criterion has been met includes a statement of faculty judgment as to adequacy of clinical facilities and existence of agreements and contracts, with expectations and responsibilities of all parties identified. This criterion is based on the assumption that, if clinical facilities are adequate and agreements exist, the practice learning environment meets curricular objectives for each and every student.

The impact that process-oriented criteria have had on the quality of nursing education in the past must not be overlooked. It is now commonplace for the nursing education unit to be administered by a master's degree prepared nurse who also holds a doctoral degree. Criterion 5 also has been responsible for the increase in nurse faculty holding at least a master's degree in nursing, or returning to school to earn a master's degree in nursing, even though already holding a master's degree in another field. Once Criterion 5 became associated with accreditation by NLNAC, state boards of nursing also supported this minimal education requirement, at least for faculty teaching in baccalaureate and higher degree programs. Today few nursing programs will hire as faculty individuals who do not hold at least a master's degree in nursing. Thus Criterion 5 represents a belief by most to have had widespread benefit in nursing education.

Many other process-oriented criteria also have had a direct, or at least an indirect, positive impact on the quality of nursing education. However, many believe that use of Criterion 14, on the other hand, represents a position many have found less than satisfactory in ensuring the intended result. Patient and client availability for all students cannot be ensured, and the mere presence of an agreement does not ensure that a learning environment exists. Criterion 14 therefore illustrates a potential inadequacy associated with the use of process-oriented criteria.

Outcome-Oriented Strategies

The *outcome-oriented model* begins with the premise that there are many different ways to achieve the same result. Emphasis is not on how an outcome is achieved, but rather on the outcome desired and how it can be demonstrated that the outcome did or did not occur (or to what degree it occurred). The question then that must be asked is: What data and data collection procedures or processes will best demonstrate achievement of the outcome? Care must be taken to ensure that, if the outcome is found, the data collection method was valid and reliable, that the data did not yield spurious results.

Supporters of the outcome-oriented evaluation approach appreciate that not every school must use the same data collection methods or tools, or even define outcomes in the same way as another nursing program at the same level. In this way outcome-oriented evaluation promotes innovation and experimentation. Likewise, outcome-oriented evaluation provides greater motivation to faculty to undertake evaluation because they truly desire the data for programmatic information and action: maintenance, development, or revision of the program. Faculty can define outcomes according to their curriculum, their program's mission and goals, and the characteristics of their students.

Two troublesome aspects that exist in use of outcome-oriented evaluative models, especially in relationship to accreditation, include the following questions. First, what is the rationale for determining required versus elective outcomes and how prescriptive should the evidence be for the required outcome? Second, how can there be assurance that outcome data are not spurious (i.e., the outcome is not manipulated by supportive data that would not be considered the same by two independent evaluators). These issues continue to be significant in the accreditation debate because in recent years some outcomes in higher education have been mandated either by regional accrediting agencies or by the DOE. Three outcomes receiving considerable attention in colleges and universities as a whole, as well as in nursing programs, include demonstration of (a) critical thinking skills, (b) communication skills, and (c) patterns of employment (i.e., type of work and setting for the work role). The ability to think critically and the ability to communicate always have been important skills to faculty, but they often view the addition of patterns of employment as a response to a political concern. Despite their support for the outcomes of critical thinking and communication, nursing faculty have found measurement of these complex constructs difficult and in many cases beyond their expertise.

One example of difficulty is determining which indicators differentiate the expected level of critical thinking or communication in graduates from different program levels. Use of the same definition suggests that no difference in outcome stems from advanced education. The few existing instruments available to measure a construct such as critical thinking are often of questionable value for nursing students. A body of research suggests that nursing students may utilize different skills or employ critical thinking skills in a different way (Tanner, 1996).

A second difficulty occurs when narratives, such as case studies and papers, are used as measures of critical thinking and communication. Many faculty lack a firm understanding of the issues of reliability and validity when applied to narrative data; many faculty are even more uncomfortable with the concept of the student-driven portfolio as an outcome measure, although a few examples are beginning to appear in the literature (Wenzel, Briggs, & Puryear, 1998). Narrative measures hold promise, especially if sufficient faculty development occurs to enable faculty to authenticate narrative assessment as reliable and valid outcome measures.

A third difficulty centers on issues of practicality and economics. A faculty risks wasting both time and money collecting copious amounts of data, only to be overwhelmed in trying to collate and analyze it. Careful thought invested in (a) determining definitions of outcomes appropriate to the program, (b) identifying the type of data needed to show that the outcome has been achieved, and (c) agreeing upon benchmarks for the outcome goes far in avoiding this problem.

■ Concluding Statement

Because this chapter provides only an overview of program evaluation, specifics on how to conduct a program evaluation were not included. However, general guidelines that can assist faculty approach the conceptualization and design of a program evaluation were presented.

Although to date the spirited dialogue among the DOE, regional accrediting agencies, boards of nursing, and specialty and regional accrediting agencies has been uncomfortable for many, this discourse has highlighted the need for a more flexible program evaluation environment. Continuing change in identifying the really important indicators of safety and quality in nursing programs in a rapidly changing health care system is to be expected.

One area of consensus arising from this dialogue is that, at least for the near future, outcomes will remain important. Outcome orientations allow programs the flexibility to innovate and be responsive to changing student needs. Trends in aggregate program evaluation data provide a useful means of measuring progress toward outcome-oriented program goals.

A second area of consensus is that cost-effective and efficient instruments or processes, which allow regular and systematic collection of reliable and valid program evaluation data,

are necessary as the use of aggregate trend data increases in reporting outcomes. Of continuing interest and increasing discussion, though not yet an area of consensus, is the use of "authentic assessment," portfolios, case studies, and other qualitative measures as faculty search for ways to describe their programs meaningfully to new markets and other external groups. Fortunately for nursing faculty, access to information useful in program evaluation is readily available. Most regulatory and accrediting agencies have web sites with the latest information, and burgeoning general and professional education literature is available in the areas of evaluation and assessment.

■ References

American Association of Colleges of Nursing. (1996). *AACN moves to establish alliance to accredit nursing higher education.* (News release, November 5). Washington, DC: Author. AACN [On-line, 2000]. Available: http://www.aacn.org.

Ashley, J. (1976). *Hospitals, paternalism, and the role of the nurse.* New York: Teachers College Press.

Bellack, J. P., Gelmon, S. B., O'Neil, E. H., & Thomsen, C. L. (1999). Responses of baccalaureate and graduate programs to the emergence of choice in nursing accreditation. *Journal of Nursing Education, 38*(2), 53–61.

Bevil, C. A. (1991). Program evaluation in nursing education: Creating a meaningful plan. In M. Garbin (Ed.), *Assessing educational outcomes: Third national conference on measurement and evaluation in nursing* (pp. 53–67). New York: National League for Nursing Press.

Bledstein, B. (1976). *The culture of professionalism.* New York: W. W. Norton.

Carroll, L. (1940). *Alice in Wonderland.* Mount Vernon, NY: Peter Pauper Press. (Originally published 1898)

Commission on Collegiate Nursing Education. (1998). *Standards for accreditation of baccalaureate and graduate nursing education programs.* Washington, DC: Author. [On-line, 2000]. Available: http://www.aacn.nche.edu.

Cronbach, L. L., Ambron, S. R., Dornbusch, S. M., Hess, R. D., Hornik, R. C., Phillips, D. C., Walker, D. F., & Weiner, S. S. (1980). *Toward reform of program evaluation.* San Francisco: Jossey-Bass.

Flexner, A. (1910–1972). *Medical education in the United States and Canada: A report to the Carnegie Foundation for the advancement of teaching.* (Series title: Sourcebook series, Vol. 3, xvii, 346 p. 24 cm). Washington, DC: Science & Health Publications.

Goldmark, J. (1923). *Nursing and nursing education in the United States.* New York: Macmillan.

Ingersoll, G. L., & Sauter, M. (1998). Integrating accreditation criteria into educational program evaluation. *Nursing and Health Care Perspectives, 19*(5), 224–229.

Kalisch, P. A., & Kalisch, B. J. (1995). *The advance of American nursing* (2nd ed.). Boston: Little, Brown.

Lindeman, C. A. (1999, August). *The future of nursing education.* Keynote address at the Northwest Nursing Education Institute, Portland, Oregon.

National League for Nursing Accrediting Commission. (1999a). *Interpretative guidelines for standards and criteria.* New York: Author. [On-line, 2000]. Available: http://www.accrediting-comm-nlnac.org.

National League for Nursing Accrediting Commission. (1999b). *Orientation to NLNAC.* New York: Author.

National League for Nursing Education (NLNE). (1917). *A curriculum guide for schools of nursing.* New York: Author.

Notter, L. E., & Spalding, E. K. (1976). *Professional nursing: Foundations, perspectives, and relationships.* Philadelphia: Lippincott.

Rossi, P. H., & Freeman, H. E. (1993). *Evaluation: A systematic approach.* Newbury Park, CA: Sage.

Stuffelbeam, D. L. (1983). *Evaluation models: Viewpoints on educational and human services evaluation.* Boston: Kluwer-Nijhoff.

Tanner, C. A. (1996). Critical thinking revisited: Paradoxes and emerging perspectives. *Journal of Nursing Education, 35*(1), 3–4.

Wenzel, L. S., Briggs, K. L., & Puryear, B. L. (1998). Portfolio: Authentic assessment in the age of the curriculum revolution. *Journal of Nursing Education, 37*(5), 208–212.

Worthen, B. R., & Sanders, J. R. (1973). *Educational evaluation: Theory and practice.* Worthington, OH: Charles A. Jones.

■ Editor's Questions for Discussion

What should be the role of faculty and students in the evaluation process of a nursing program? What relationship may exist between various accreditation bodies that would be beneficial for nursing programs? How might such relationships be fostered and developed?

Discuss evaluation models for nursing programs. How may NLNAC Criterion 14 cited by Dooling and Gaines be rephrased or developed to be addressed more effectively? What outcome-oriented evaluation data should be available as valid and reliable evidence for such models? How may such valid and reliable data be developed and made available on an ongoing basis in nursing programs.

Discuss the future of evaluation and accreditation for nursing programs. Debate the pros and cons of discontinuing national nursing accreditation versus accreditation of programs jointly with regional processes and accreditation or certification of faculty for nursing programs. What changes nationally, regionally, and at the state level would need to occur for alteration in accreditation requirements, process, and criteria for acceptance by universities, programs, and faculty?

How will market factors determine whether both accrediting agencies (NLNAC and CCNE) will be successful, or which one will be more successful? Should individual accreditation rather than program credentialing be the new norm? If individual credentialing for faculty becomes the norm, what role(s) might the American Nurses Credentialing Center, state board regulatory bodies, regional accrediting bodies for higher education programs, or universities have in the evaluation of faculty?

14

Distributed Learning Strategies

Improving Educational Access in Nursing

Rosalee C. Yeaworth, PhD, RN, FAAN
Carol H. Pullen, EdD, RN
Lani Zimmerman, PhD, RN
Bevely J. Hays, PhD, RN

For more than 20 years, distance education has been regarded as a tactic for reaching primarily rural areas where there are no nursing education programs. A more recent educational approach, distributed learning, seeks to improve access to all levels of nursing education in both urban and rural settings. When educational programs are offered outside the traditional campus, employed nurses can obtain advanced degrees or complete certificate programs and continuing education requirements without leaving the communities where they work. Likewise, they are able to avoid having to arrange special schedules to accommodate their studies, incur expenses in time and money, and face risks of travel.

Is distributed learning really different from distance education, or is it merely the latest jargon for schools' efforts to package programs and improve marketing? In this chapter we use the term *distributed learning,* as it was defined by Saltzberg and Polyson (1995): "Distributed learning is an instructional model that allows instructor, student, and content to be located in different, non-centralized locations so that instruction and learning occur independent of time and place" (p. 10). Providing education in new areas has great appeal, but schools and their administrators, faculty, and students need to be fully informed about the choices and costs and the positives and negatives of using distributed learning strategies.

■ Brief History

Distance learning occurred to some degree, but at much slower pace, when it took the form of correspondence courses delivered via U.S. mail. Initially these courses consisted of printed syllabi and reading material, with tests to validate learning. Advancing technology led to inclusion of audiotapes and videotapes in the packets. The correspondence courses qualified as distributed learning because they were noncentralized and learning could occur independent of time and place.

This independence of time makes possible what is known as *asynchronous learning*. It has been greatly advanced by development of the World Wide Web (or, simply, the Web), which has led to Web-based courses, discussion groups, e-mail, and streaming video that provide audio and video of lectures and other activities. In contrast, synchronous learning takes place when all the students and faculty participate in the learning experience at the same time, even though the participants may be widely dispersed geographically. Synchronous learning over distance evolved as telephones and television became common in homes, leading to telephone conferences and a variety of options in television. A model for synchronous learning through television was established by schools of agriculture, engineering, and business who formed consortia and offered degrees through such TV networks as Ag*Sat and CorpNet (Yeaworth, 1996). Currently, the use of desktop video conferencing over the Internet is providing synchronous learning among widely dispersed sites. Nursing schools have used both synchronous and asynchronous learning to provide degrees to stu-

dents separated by distance (Yeaworth, Benschoter, Meter, & Benson, 1995).

■ World Wide Web Options

In addition to the Internet tools already mentioned, the Web offers options such as Web-based courses, chat rooms, and desktop video conferencing. Web-based courses can be conducted with completely asynchronous discussion groups or with a combination of asynchronous and synchronous learning. Syllabi, assignments, and some discussion questions on the Web (asynchronous) and desktop video conferencing allow faculty and students to see and talk with each other (synchronous). Desktop video conferencing uses small cameras, speakers, and software such as CUSeeMe and NetMeeting to link computers located at many widely separated sites (Yeaworth & Schmidt, 1998).

The ever-increasing number of Internet tools offer exciting possibilities for expanding and enriching student learning experiences. For example, students in a health policy course can gain real-life experience in exerting political influence by going to the Web pages of their state legislature or Congress to check on a bill, perhaps watching a legislative session in progress, and sending an e-mail message about their concerns to legislators. The Web pages of agencies—such as the Health Care Financing Administration, the Agency for Health Care Policy and Research, and the Robert Wood Johnson Foundation—can also be checked for information on policies, grants, professional meetings, and other interests. Students can interact directly with families or patients with particular illnesses by selecting e-mail addresses from a Web-based support group or chat group. Through telemedicine and telehealth, an advanced practice nursing student or a faculty member can interact with specialists, participate in simulated cases, or consult with a rural nursing home. As sophistication in technology increases and the bandwidth for accessing the Internet continues to expand, the potential for dynamic multimedia technology increases (Saltzberg & Polyson, 1995).

■ *Shift to a Student-Centered Learning Paradigm*

Along with enriching learning through the Web, distributed learning requires shifting from an instruction paradigm prevalent in much of today's education to a student-centered learning paradigm (Van Dusen, 1997). Many nursing educators in the past decade have urged just such a refocusing of the approach to educating new nurse professionals (Bevis & Murray, 1990; Chally, 1992; Quinn, 1989). The primary message within that curriculum revolution movement (Tanner, 1990) is the importance of creating critical thinkers, of moving away from imparting knowledge to more actively engaging the student in the learning process. In the instruction paradigm model, faculty impart knowledge mainly through live lecture and discussion, and the student plays a passive role. In the learning paradigm model, the focus is shifted from instruction to learning.

To implement fully a learning paradigm model, the roles of faculty and students must change. Faculty act as coaches and mentors to facilitate access to information (Forsyth, 1996), and the student becomes a more active participant in the teaching–learning process. Three principles, based on student feedback, have emerged for establishing and maintaining a student-centered learning community (Shotsberger, 1997). Faculty should (a) be responsive to students, (b) be competent with technology, and (c) organize interaction regardless of the technology employed for the course. Faculty help define questions rather than just handing out facts (Alley, 1996). Faculty help students discover and structure problems and questions

and then coach them in how to seek answers. According to Alley (1996),

> if a sage on a stage is the metaphor for traditional passive learning environments, then learner on-stage, and support staff as stage hands, with professor directing it all is a metaphor for the student-centered learning we want to achieve. (p. 51)

■ *Issues in Using Today's Technology*

As with most change, distributed learning can represent both exciting opportunities and disturbing problems for institutions, faculty, and students. It raises issues with regard to state licensing of professionals and evaluation of students and faculty. Institutions are confronted by costs of hardware, software, and installation; of motivating and training faculty; and of maintaining adequate support services. These facilities and services are not one-time expenses but require funding for ongoing maintenance and upgrading.

Issues for Educational Institutions

Faculty or administrators with interests and skills in technology may be the initiators and impetus for distributed learning, but it should not be undertaken haphazardly. Before starting a serious program in distributed learning, each educational institution or unit will need to consider carefully its own vision, role, mission, and goals. The institution or unit should have an overall plan that has been reviewed by faculty, students, and other major players in the system. Expressed and unexpressed goals may include (a) increasing their market share of students and income, (b) broadening the territory served, (c) promoting ability to attract more part-time faculty who desire to teach from their homes or businesses, (d) preparing students for practice in rural and underserved areas, (e) preparing students to use the technology that will increasingly be a part of health care delivery, or (f) providing opportunities for students to have greater access to educational programs and courses. To be successful and accomplish worthwhile goals, a plan must identify sufficient resources to allow development of an adequate infrastructure for delivery of courses, such as the library, bookstore, and student services. Accessing institutional resources from a distance is especially important for the rural student. The implementation time line should be realistic, taking into consideration the length of time necessary to develop both infrastructure and courses.

A critical element of implementation is strong faculty development and student orientation programs. The learning curve with regard to technologies is steep for both faculty and students, particularly for those who are technology novices (Berge & Collins, 1995; Hill, 1997). Because technology is constantly changing, ongoing technological support for faculty and student development is essential. Intimidation and fear of equipment compound learning and user problems. Technological difficulties add frustrations, whether they be inability to connect to a network, time for downloading materials, or problems with a personal computer (Hill, 1997). Faculty and students may have difficulty determining whether a problem involves the system (based in the institution or local Internet provider), the personal computer, or the user. Troubleshooting mechanisms should be in place prior to the start of the course. Some methods currently used include phone, fax, e-mail, and even a handout or Web site answering frequently asked questions (FAQs). Information should be provided as to how soon students or faculty can expect feedback (Rasmussen, Northrup, & Lee, 1997).

In the rush to use new technologies, particularly the Internet, some institutions and faculty unfortunately have tended to adapt the curriculum to the technology. In many cases, the result has been poorly designed courses that do not meet student or faculty needs. Much of the rush to use technology has resulted from the sense of competition, as virtual universities offer video and Internet-based courses, or full degree and certificate programs in what established universities have long considered their turf. Individual states generally have laws or agreements about mission and turf, but competition is no longer limited to institutions within a state or neighboring states. For example, the Western Governors University (W.G.U.) and Britain's Open University are forming a distance consortium known as the Governors Open University System to offer video and Internet-based courses and assessment of knowledge to students around the world. Existing institutions may view this effort as an invasion of their turf and competition for their students or as relief from the responsibilities of offering so many course and specialty options and thus as a good use of resources. They may also recognize the potential for participating in consortia, which provide faculty with a global source of colleagues and consultants and allow students to take courses from recognized experts in various fields of endeavor.

Issues for Faculty

In distributed learning, faculty role changes are necessitated by changes in the way courses are designed and implemented and the new skills that are needed. The teaching role does not diminish; in fact, demands on faculty may increase (Forsyth, 1996). Willis and Dickinson (1997) acknowledge that the challenges are imposing because distributed learning necessitates looking at courses in terms of adapting them to the unique environment of distributed learning. As faculty shift from content provider to content facilitator, they must consider not only mastery of content but also ability to draw on the varied backgrounds and talents of students. Faculty must be comfortable and proficient in using technology, and, in many instances, must learn to teach effectively without visual cues provided by direct eye contact with students. An understanding of and appreciation for distant students' lifestyle require sensitivity and flexibility in designing learning experiences (Rasmussen, Northrup, & Lee, 1997).

A critical issue in the implementation of distributed learning courses is preparation and organization of course materials well in advance of the actual delivery of the course (Pande & Hart, 1998). Students who are taking courses at a distance must have course materials before the start of the course. For programs that use synchronous methods such as desktop videoconferencing or interactive television, a back-up plan must be in place in case of problems with technology at scheduled course times. Waiting until the day of class to fax handouts may mean that distant sites do not receive the materials.

In developing distributed learning courses, faculty have the primary responsibility, but a team approach is essential (Saba, 1998). Faculty members are content experts; other team members may include an instructional designer, graphic artist, evaluator, technician, and programmer. The "ideal" team may not be available in the institution, but community resources, such as technology experts or consultants, may be engaged. One approach is to train and support strong lead faculty and staff who will then provide leadership to others in the institution. Saba advocates initially selecting faculty for new course development who are "technology ready," that is, who have basic skills and are willing to develop additional skills. Further, faculty who already have a strong commitment to distributed learning are essential to the success of the course.

Faculty development will need to be based on the institution's overall plan for distributed education. Robbins (1997) recommends that a faculty development program include the knowledge that faculty members need to develop distance learning courses while providing sufficient resources (release time, overload pay, and travel funds for professional development) for course development. Course development should address (a) pedagogical methods appropriate for various distributive learning environments, (b) application of various instructional technologies as appropriate to course content, (c) specific training on hardware and software, and (d) a mentoring system. Faculty will need initial and ongoing instruction and follow-up support. In many cases, learning has to be "just in time," or, in other words, when it becomes most relevant to the person. In addition, learning must accommodate busy schedules with their competing demands (e.g., research, professional service, and practice).

Issues for Students

Distributed learning requires a student-centered learning model that promotes self-discipline and requires students to take more responsibility for their learning. In changing to the new model, both faculty and students have to develop different expectations for themselves, for each other, and for interactions between faculty and students. New skills must be acquired to achieve expectations. Transition time may be necessary to help students move toward and adopt a new way of learning (Berge & Collins, 1995).

Student motivation is a key issue in student self-responsibility. Three factors have been identified that are indicative of student success in a distance education course: (a) intention to complete the course, (b) early submission of work, and (c) completion of previous distance education courses (Cornell & Martin, 1997). Other components are course design, degree of interaction between students and faculty, and interaction among students. For students who need more structure, short self-contained segments in courses with specific questions to answer and assignments to complete are helpful. For many students, especially adult learners, linking course content to real-life work is effective.

Just as faculty development for technology is important in distributed education programs, student development of skills also is necessary. Some institutions have taken the approach that students must have certain competencies and skills when they enter the program; other institutions teach students the skills they need when they enter and as they progress. Another model is a combined approach, in which certain skills are required in advance and other skills are acquired during the program. Disadvantaged students, such as minority group members, rural residents, or the poor, may not have had the technological advantages of other students. Consequently, such students may require more support to ensure that they have the same opportunities as other students.

The cost of technology to students cannot be overlooked. Even though they may save money and time on travel, students often later discover costs that they had not anticipated. They may find that their computers have inadequate memory or their modems inadequate speed. In rural areas, the problem may lie not with individual hardware and software but with limitations of the local telephone company or an Internet or TV provider.

Students often complain of feeling isolated and unconnected when they use distributed learning technologies (Berge & Collins, 1995; Hill, 1997). Strategies that encourage both cooperative and independent work, as well as interaction, will help overcome this barrier to learning. Adequate and frequent feedback by faculty is essential. With student-centered and active learning, students also can provide feedback to other learners, which enhances interac-

tivity (Saba, 1998). Concerns remain, however, about just how increased use of distance teaching and learning will influence socialization and mentoring of students.

Issues for Clinical Teaching and Learning

Delivery of the clinical component in nursing curriculum and health science education has always been more complex, expensive, and challenging than the classroom portion. Examples of didactic courses delivered via the Web using distributed learning strategies are becoming commonplace, but how can students stay in their home communities to do clinical work? Among the more traditional methods is use of clinical preceptors in the community, combined with having faculty going out to sites or students coming into the educational setting. Written care plans and logs give faculty an opportunity to evaluate students' thinking processes. A more recent tactic involves having students send faculty videotapes of themselves completing an exam or interacting with a patient.

Some of these methods have proven very useful in delivering the clinical component of the curriculum to the distant student, but such methods also can be very costly to the student and to the educational institution. Faculty or student travel could involve a 4-hour or 5-hour (or longer) drive and the costs of transportation and overnight lodging. Such a trip could occur two or three times a semester. Many students living in rural, underserved areas may not be able to leave their families and jobs to come to a campus site for their clinical rotations. So what are some alternatives? With explosion of the use of technology in delivery of health care, it seems only reasonable that a strategy such as desktop video conferencing also could be used to deliver much of the clinical portion of a course.

Goals for Practice

Distributed learning that uses advanced technology can meet the dual goals of providing high-quality, student-centered courses and incorporating in curriculum design the kinds of information technology needed for current and future practice. Technologies such as video conferencing, video streaming, and transmitting clinical assessments and evaluations over the Internet will continue to transform the way health care is delivered. Innovations such as (a) computer-based records, (b) hospital information systems, (c) computer-based decision support tools, (d) community health information networks, (e) telemedicine, and (f) new ways of distributing health information to consumers are beginning to affect the cost, quality, and accessibility of health care.

Home health care delivery by nurses via computer-assisted video conferencing affords an efficient solution for clients discharged early from hospitals by providing support, education, and monitoring—all of which have an impact on health and quality of life for clients. Video conferencing by nurses would be especially useful in providing follow-up care in rural and underserved areas. When clinical educators use technology to monitor and supervise the clinical portion of a curriculum, their students gain experience in using that technology, which can then be applied to direct care for clients.

Portable Computer Stations

Use of portable computer stations with home monitoring equipment is a distributed learning strategy that will revamp traditional ways of monitoring and evaluating the clinical component of home and community health courses. Some systems available today include a laptop computer with video camera, sound card, speakers, microphone, and modem with attached electronic stethoscope, pulse oxime-

ter, and other equipment to measure physiologic parameters such as blood pressure, heart rate, temperature, blood oxygen, and weight. The monitoring system is connected by modem and phone line (or cellular phone if the client does not have a phone) to a permanent campus computer station. Images and data can be transferred immediately to the campus, and faculty can give students advice and feedback as necessary. Faculty (from the campus station) can evaluate student performance during client evaluation and provide consultation in care management decisions, if needed. All interaction between client and student and the vital signs can be recorded and stored in the computer for self-learning and evaluation. This process provides a backup that faculty can later review. Computer-assisted video conferencing technology also can be used to hold meetings involving student, preceptor, and faculty. This method is feasible because all computer-assisted video conferencing equipment can be connected through regular telephone lines. Soon to become available throughout the country—to add transmission speed—are a new digital transmission technology cable modem, Digital Subscriber Line (DSL), and Integrated Service Digital Network (ISDN). These innovations will be adapted to educational technology whenever their use becomes economically feasible.

Issues in Licensure

Individual state licensing laws can become an issue in delivering education, consultation, and care across state lines. Presently, states require that health care professionals be licensed in the states in which they practice. Faculty who cross state borders to teach classes and supervise clinical experiences may be expected to be licensed in all the states in which they serve in the faculty role. In addition, some state boards of nursing have interpreted teaching by distance technology to be the practice of nursing and have required licensure of faculty in any state to which technology may carry their teaching, even though they may never be physically present in any state but the one where they are employed. As more people travel to transplant centers or other specialty centers for care, the need to call their nurses or physicians for advice and consultation after returning home can become a legal issue. The National Council of State Boards of Nursing is trail-blazing for nursing and other health care professions by promoting mutual recognition of licenses, comparable to the way drivers' licenses are recognized. Nurses would be licensed in their state of residence and could practice in other states as long as they know and practice under the laws of that state. This policy will require changes in licensing laws of individual states (National Council of State Boards of Nursing [NCSBN], 1998).

Issues for Evaluation

Evaluation of student learning and satisfaction is crucial and always difficult. The idea of evaluating students whom faculty have never met face-to-face can be especially intimidating, although some might argue that such evaluation eliminates the possibility of bias on the basis of a student's physical features and appearance. A body of literature shows that there is no significant difference in learning based on the media used and that there is even some evidence that students do better on-line (McCollum, 1998). Although not yet well documented, many faculty using distributed learning believe that it is contributing to improving the critical thinking and writing abilities of students. Learning of facts has always been straightforward to evaluate, and application of knowledge has been tapped through case studies, care plans, and situational questions. But in nursing, as in all health care, evaluation of outcomes is what is really needed. Faculty need to (a) establish desired

outcomes, (b) decide what data are required for measurement, and (c) determine what should be used as benchmarks. These outcomes and benchmarks require continual refinement. Faculty also may be concerned that failures in or frustrations with technology may influence students' evaluations of them as teachers. In fact, emphasis on "customer satisfaction" by educational institutions, coupled with requirement that students evaluate faculty performance, has no doubt contributed to the grade inflation problem.

■ Future Directions

Technology associated with personal computers and the Internet is moving so rapidly that it is difficult to imagine what will be happening in distributed learning in even the near future. But it seems certain that use of technology is not going to decrease. In "A Vision of Baccalaureate and Graduate Education: The Next Decade," the American Association of Colleges of Nursing (1999) states:

> Technology has dramatically altered the practice, teaching and learning environments in nursing as well as the way in which nurses, educators, and students communicate. Although easier to access, information is often harder to control because of the speed at which it is generated and communicated. (p. 61)

The idea of how technology contributes to lack of control of information and speed of generation and communication ties to O'Neil's (1999) warning:

> While we argue over who rightly owns this or that domain of care or who should educate the entry-level nurse, someone is spending time digitizing our precious knowledge base and making it available to other health care workers and, increasingly, directly to the patient. . . . [Nursing must] transform education with the best of organization, pedagogy, and technology. (p. 14)

As a part of their practice, nurses have always made their knowledge available to patients and families. However, nurses now must face the dilemma of keeping abreast of technology and pedagogy, while recognizing that their interpersonal relationships have been defining elements of their practice and teaching. For, as Fitzpatrick (1999) notes,

> there is a value in face-to-face interactions with colleagues that will never be replaced by technology, no matter how sophisticated our tools. As nurses we thrive on personal connections with others, those we care for and those nurses who are our colleagues in caring. (p. 3)

Although nursing faculty and students may desire and thrive on personal connections, the economics of higher education and ease of accessing information require that some of those personal connections in teaching, learning, and practice be accomplished through technology. Experience shows that it is possible to do so.

■ Concluding Statement

Distributed learning not only improves access to all levels of nursing education in both urban and rural areas, but, according to some evidence, also improves learning. Educational institutions, faculty, and students should set goals and develop a plan for the use of distributed learning strategies. Development of the plan will raise issues for institutions, faculty, students, and licensing that should be resolved insofar as possible. Improved technology, educational economics, and increasing use of and comfort with personal computers are likely to lead to even more distributed learning in the future.

■ References

Alley, L. R. (1996, March/April). An instructional epiphany. *Change, 49,* 50–54.

American Association of Colleges of Nursing. (1999). A vision of baccalaureate and graduate nursing education: The next decade. *Journal of Professional Nursing, 1*(1), 59–65.

Berge, Z. L., & Collins, M. P. (1995). *Computer mediated communication and the online classroom.* Cresskill, NJ: Hampton Press.

Bevis, E. O., & Murray, J. P. (1990). The essence of the curriculum revolution: Emancipatory teaching. *Journal of Nursing Education, 29,* 326–331.

Chally, P. S. (1992). Empowerment through teaching. *Journal of Nursing Education, 31,* 117–120.

Cornell, R., & Martin, B. L. (1997). The role of motivation in Web-based instruction. In B. H. Khan (Ed.), *Web-based instruction* (pp. 93–100). Englewood Cliffs, NJ: Educational Technology Publications.

Fitzpatrick, J. J. (1999). Global nursing education, visited and revisited, today and in the future. *Nursing and Health Care Perspectives, 20*(1), 3.

Forsyth, I. (1996). *Teaching and learning materials and the Internet.* London: Kogan Page.

Hill, J. R. (1997). Distance learning environments via the World Wide Web. In B. H. Khan (Ed.), *Web-based instruction* (pp. 75–80). Englewood Cliffs, NJ: Educational Technology Publications.

McCollum, K. (1998). Is distance learning any good? [On-line]. Available: http://teleeducation.nb.ca/anygood/betteronline.shtm.

National Council of State Boards of Nursing. (1998). Mutual recognition of nursing licenses benefits both nurses and health care consumers. *Issues, 19(4)*, 3.

O'Neil, E. (1999). The opportunity that is nursing. *Nursing and Health Care Perspectives, 20*(1), 10–14.

Pande, J. S., & Hart, A. L. (1998). An online course in health policy: Pearls and perils of cyberspace teaching. *Distance Education Report, 2*(10), 4–5.

Quinn, J. (1989). *Empowering the teacher–student relationship.* Presented at the National League for Nursing's 6th National Conference of Nurse Educators, Philadelphia.

Rasmussen, K., Northrup, P., & Lee, R. (1997). Implementing Web-based instruction. In B. H. Khan (Ed.), *Web-based instruction* (pp. 341–346). Englewood Cliffs, NJ: Educational Technology Publications.

Robbins, C. (1997). Training faculty to teach at a distance. *Distance Education Report, 1*(8), 1, 3.

Saba, F. (1998, August). What faculty need to put their courses on the Web. *Distance Education Report. Special Report: World Wide Web,* 3–4.

Saltzberg, S., & Polyson, S. (1995). Distributed learning on the World Wide Web. *Syllabus, 9*(1), 10–12 [On-line]. Available: http:/www.syllabus.com/.

Shotsberger, P. G. (1997). Emerging roles for instructors and learners in the Web-based instruction classroom. In B. H. Khan (Ed.), *Web-based instruction* (pp. 101–106). Englewood Cliffs, NJ: Educational Technology Publications.

Tanner, C. A. (1990). Reflections on the curriculum revolution. *Journal of Nursing Education, 29,* 295–299.

Van Dusen, G. C. (1997). *The virtual campus: Technology and reform in higher education.* ASHE-ERIC Higher Education Report Volume 25, No. 5. Washington, DC: George Washington University, Graduate School of Education and Human Development.

Willis, B., & Dickinson, J. (1997). Distance education and the World Wide Web. In B. H. Khan (Ed.), *Web-based instruction* (pp. 81–84). Englewood Cliffs, NJ: Educational Technology Publications.

Yeaworth, R. C. (1996). Consortia arrangements and educational telecommunication. *Journal of Professional Nursing, 12*(3), 147–153.

Yeaworth, R. C., Benschoter, R. A., Meter, R., & Benson, S. (1995). Telecommunications and nursing education. *Journal of Professional Nursing, 11*(4), 227–232.

Yeaworth, R. C., & Schmidt, S. (1998). What you need to know about distance learning in nursing education. *Peterson's guide to nursing programs* (4th ed.). Princeton, NJ: Peterson's, 21–23.

■ Editor's Questions for Discussion

What is the difference between asynchronous and synchronous learning? How does distributed learning differ from distance education? What planning and development are essential prior to implementation of a distance learning program? What resources and infrastructure are essential for a distance learning program? Propose strategies for ensuring high-quality learning material and library resources being available in a timely fashion. How should these programs be evaluated? What suggestions by Deets and Choi (Chapter 34) should be taken into account in designing measurement of outcomes?

What changes are critical for faculty in providing distance education? Discuss the instruction paradigm versus learning paradigm model and implications for faculty and students. How can changes in thinking be promoted among traditionally prepared faculty? Propose specific content for faculty development in distributed learning. To what extent may promotion and tenure requirements be altered when distance education is in place? Should all faculty be technologically prepared for distance education? What issues regarding workload distribution may be more crucial for distance education than traditional programs? How may workload equity and balance in expectations be achieved?

How will Yocom and Thomas' "mutual recognition" (Chapter 3) resolve licensure issues raised by Yeaworth, Pullen, Zimmerman, and Hays? Are there any regulation concerns that "mutual recognition" cannot resolve? If so, what are they?

How may clinical teaching and learning be provided in distance education? What ethical issues may arise in the clinical component of distance education? How may they be anticipated and resolved? What cost-effective measures may be utilized for clinical evaluation of students in distance education?

What similarities, differences, and applications are there between Yeaworth et al. and Billings (Chapter 15), Schroeder and Long (Chapter 47), and Boland (Chapter 71)? What nursing courses may be more or less appropriate for distance and distributed learning? How amenable are curricula in master's degree and doctoral programs for distance education in contrast to undergraduate curricula?

15

Teaching and Learning in On-Line Communities of Professional Practice in Nursing

Diane M. Billings, EdD, RN, FAAN

The dawn of the knowledge age brings new opportunities for teaching and learning in nursing. Who is learning, what is being learned, when it is being learned—the present-day state of each of these matters is changing the face of nursing education. Students entering nursing schools directly from high school are already sophisticated computer users, active knowledge seekers, and savvy consumers. Those pursuing higher education later in life place high value on their time and require convenience and easy access to education that meets their needs. Nurses who are already employed find themselves continuously assessing their competencies and updating personal and professional skills that fit increasing demands for nurses with advanced degrees and certificates.

To meet the educational needs of these learners, nursing degree and continuing education programs are using information technologies such as the Internet to make courses accessible and convenient in on-line communities. As these associations mature, they become "communities of professional practice" (Norris & Olsen, 1997)—virtual places where the best practices in the profession are developed and disseminated. These communities are reshaping the way faculty and students interact to acquire and use professional knowledge and skills.

Teaching and learning in on-line nursing communities require new technical and pedagogical skills and also new approaches to inquiry and learning in the discipline. The purposes of this chapter are to (a) introduce the vision of an on-line community of professional practice in nursing, (b) describe how the community is established and sustained, (c) discuss new ways of teaching and learning, and (d) propose an approach to assessing success in these communities.

■ On-Line Communities of Professional Practice

Nursing has a long history of using print, video, and audio technologies to connect learners and faculty who are separated by time and space (Billings & Bachmeier, 1994). These technologies met access needs for nurses and nursing students who were unable to participate easily in courses at the locations where they were offered. However, with the advent of the Internet, barriers of time and space are minimized and abundant opportunities exist for learning any time, any place, and with any number of experts and colleagues. Learning communities are referred to variously as learning networks, electronic learning communities, authentic communities, advanced learning networks, and asynchronous learning networks. These groups use networked communication and collaborative learning tools to establish dynamic interaction among members who work together to explore, critique, reflect, teach, learn, develop, and disseminate the knowledge of the profession (Brown & Duguid, 1996; Harasim, Hiltz, Teles, & Turoff, 1996; Norris & Malloch, 1997; Norris & Olson, 1997). The communities are characterized by access and convenience, common purpose, and shared use of resources. Members of the communities are connected through social relationships formed to accomplish mutual

tasks and goals (Brown & Duguid, 1996). Although many such communities are informal and self-emergent, most exist within formal institutions and professional organizations (Norris & Malloch, 1997).

■ On-Line Communities of Professional Practice in Nursing

On-line communities of professional practice in nursing (OLCPPs) are forming to meet the educational needs of their members. For example, schools of nursing are offering Internet courses designed to provide basic and advanced education. Other communities are forming to (a) offer continuing education, (b) meet needs of special interest groups, (c) provide staff development, (d) develop and disseminate knowledge, (e) recruit and socialize nurses to the profession, or (f) promote international access and cross-cultural sharing. These communities are flexible and fluid; nurses and students may be members of one or more communities at any given time.

Basic and Advanced Education in Distributed Learning Communities

In response to the need for access and convenience or to recruit and retain students, schools of nursing are using the Internet to offer courses and even full degree programs. And, as students' need for connection and community increase, schools of nursing are enhancing traditional and on-campus programs, using community building tools of e-mail, electronic distribution lists, course home pages, and on-line testing and assessment. Learning is increasingly interactive, modularized, and individualized. Emphasized are (a) course-specific and program-specific outcomes, (b) mastery of content, (c) application of learning to real-life problems, (d) collaboratorybased research, and (e) socialization to the profession through mentoring and apprenticeship (Bonk & Cunningham, 1998; Norris & Malloch, 1997). Resources of the academic community can be extended by partnerships and strategic alliances with health care agencies, consortia, and other affinity groups, whose own members have mutual interests and needs that are supported by alignments with the academic institution.

Lifelong Learning, Perpetual Learning, and Continuing Nursing Education

In the knowledge age, focus is no longer on education and training, but on learning. Lifelong learning in the 20th century required "time out" for learning, with nurses attending "stand-alone" courses and conferences. In the knowledge age, learning is pervasive and learners are linked with experts in interactive networks (Norris & Malloch, 1997). Learning is fused with work, as rapid change in knowledge and practice require all nurses to become "perpetual" learners (Norris & Malloch, 1997).

With fusion of learning and work, OLCPPs are forming to support personal and professional development. These communities are developing rapidly as nurses seek accessible and convenient opportunities, either for certification and career development or to meet requirements for renewal of nursing licenses and prescriptive privileges for advanced practice. Nurses use career planning services of the OLCPPs and prepare portfolios that demonstrate competence for professional advancement or entry into degree granting or certificate programs. Networked communities link learning with practice, and provide access to human and material learning resources— the ultimate fusion of work and education. Earning continuing education credits is only one way of learning and documenting learning outcomes.

Workplace Communities

With continuous changes in health care and ease of dissemination of best practices, health care agencies are looking to networked communities to provide staff development and professional education. Intranets—networks internal to an agency—deploy just-in-time learning modules and competency assessments and link new employees with preceptors and mentors. Workplace communities and academic communities are natural partners for strategic alliances.

Special-Interest Communities

Special-interest communities arise from existing membership groups (within professional organizations and specialty groups) and use network communication tools such as listservs, newsgroups, Usenets, and discussion boards to keep members informed about (a) activities of the organization, (b) new products, (c) educational opportunities, and (d) changing practice standards. Members of these communities have immediate access to information and resources of peer experts; likewise, an organization has immediate access to its members to provide services or calls for action.

Knowledge Development and Dissemination

OLCPPs also form to develop and disseminate knowledge. Nurse researchers have access to databases, patients, and interdisciplinary colleagues who join them in discovery. Students and research assistants easily become members of the community and learn discovery strategies, with expert researchers serving as role models for using research methods. As instruments and surveys are posted on-line, patients and other participants in the research become integral team members and can benefit from the knowledge as soon as findings yield recommendations for tailored interventions. This type of community is enhanced by access to electronic resources such as literature databases, search engines, full-text articles, and links to best practice standards.

Apprenticeship and Socialization

Nursing is inherently an "apprenticeship profession," a profession in which novices learn the knowledge and skills by observing experts and are socialized to norms and practices by working with mentors and preceptors. The cognitive apprentice model is a socially interactive relationship similar to the one used in skilled trades wherein newcomers observe expert practice and gradually assume greater responsibility for role acquisition (Bonk & Cunningham, 1998). In apprenticeship relationships, experts and peers (a) pose questions, (b) provide information, (c) guide use of resources, (d) demonstrate skills and techniques, (e) provide consultation, (f) solve real-life clinical problems, and (g) model knowledge development, critical thinking, and decision-making processes. Because learning occurs best when it is anchored in the real world, the OLCPP is well suited for supporting socialization to the profession.

The OLCPP also lends itself to serving as a forum for networking with colleagues and experts and thus provides a valuable professional support system (Bachman & Panzarine, 1998; Halstead, Hayes, Reising, & Billings, 1995). Through such dialogues, values and traditions of the profession are transmitted and new roles are acquired.

Global Communities

Use of the Internet removes barriers of time and communication worldwide. Access to information, shared course development and implementation, real-time collaboration using on-line video networks are possible in communities drawn from geographically or culturally diverse or both types of populations. These communities are ideal for increasing global awareness, broadening learner perspectives, and developing cultural competence. In these communities, members have an opportunity to respect diversity and participate in learning experiences that would be otherwise unavailable (Anderson, 1995; Kirkpatrick, Brown, & Atkins, 1998).

■ Creating and Sustaining the Community of Professional Practice

Creating and sustaining communities of professional practice involve establishing networked environments, developing and supporting members, and modifying educational practices. A resource team of content experts, instructional designers, Web programmers, Web masters, librarians, database managers, and software specialists provides consultation and support services.

Establishing Networked Environments

OLCPPs depend on an organizing infrastructure and sufficient resources to meet the purposes and goals of their members. Two ingredients are key: (a) well-developed and supported network infrastructure and (b) abundant learning (physical, virtual, and human) resources.

Network Infrastructure

A reliable and easy-to-use infrastructure is required to support the OLCPP. Although membership in the community is composed of individuals with computers connected to the Internet, communities of professional practice depend on communication tools such as electronic mail, listservs, and discussion groups and collaborative work tools such as course management software, computer conferencing, and testing. Discipline-specific tools also are shared, including those that guide clinical decision-making and expert decision support or those that aid and model knowledge-building processes of the profession or develop critical thinking skills (Ribbons, 1998; Todd, 1998). The infrastructure must also support easy entry and exit from the community. For example, student advisement, registration, and on-line payment services must be available. Additional services include learning assessment, portfolio procedures, competency assessment, and cumulative recording of participation (diplomas, certificates, and continuing education credits).

Learning Resources

Access to learning resources is the value-added benefit of membership in the community. Resources may include those traditionally found in physical libraries and learning resource centers (e.g., textbooks, references, mannequins, models, and videotapes). Assets comprise those that are also available electronically (e.g., full-text services and multimedia, electronic text, drug interaction references, and clinical databases). Virtual laboratories, virtual patient simulations, and other learning resources that can be delivered on demand through the networked community are essential.

Although traditional models of learning depended on physical resources, the OLCPP depends on human resources—peers, mentors, experts, clinical practitioners, patients, students, faculty, and interdisciplinary colleagues—and access to authentic professional activities. Access to these resources will distinguish the OLCPP and determine its success.

Developing and Supporting Community Members

Teaching and learning in an OLCPP changes the focus from emphasis on teaching to emphasis on learning (Barr & Tagg, 1995; Dolence & Norris, 1995; Skiba, 1997). Orientation and development of both educators and learners for new roles and responsibilities is critical to ensuring success of the community.

Faculty

The role of faculty in the OLCPP is to create active learning environments in which students can explore and solve real-life problems. Faculty are content experts and become instructional planners as they work with a team of pedagogical and technical experts to develop the module, course, or curriculum (Bachman & Panzarine, 1998; Carlton, Ryan, & Siktberg, 1998; Clark, 1998).

Faculty facilitate learning through coaching, guiding and supporting students. Faculty and capable peers provide learning scaffolds—supports that help learners complete a task or solve a problem that they could not otherwise accomplish without expert assistance (Bonk & Cunningham, 1998). Faculty establish clear expectations, provide feedback, and assess progress toward learning outcomes. Finally, faculty select appropriate strategies for assessing learning outcomes and certifying competency.

Development opportunities must be available to orient faculty both to new pedagogy of Web-based teaching and learning and to technology and use of course management software and collaborative work tools. These activities must be available to faculty during course development and also on an ongoing basis as they make transitions to new roles.

Further reward systems must be in place to sustain faculty membership in the community.

Intrinsic rewards, such as challenge and self-satisfaction, or teaching awards from student and peer review sustain many faculty; support in terms of recognition from colleagues and administrators also is critical. Other rewards include workload credit; financial compensation; and favorable promotion, tenure and merit reviews.

Learners

Roles and rewards in the community change for learners as well. Learning in the community is active and self-directed. Learners assume responsibility for identifying their own learning needs and make learning plans and contracts to attain learning goals.

As with faculty, learners need orientation to membership in the community. Such orientation involves use of the technology infrastructure and course management and collaborative work tools. Learners also must be oriented and enculturated to the norms of professional practice in the OLCPP. In learning communities all members share responsibility for outcomes. The community thrives on respect for diversity, active participation, collaboration, and ethical use of information.

Changing Educational Practices

Because learning nursing occurs through social interaction with professionals, learner-centered, constructivist, and sociocultural models of education provide theoretical grounding for teaching and learning in on-line learning communities (Bonk & Cunningham, 1998; Chickering & Gamson, 1987; Dolence & Norris, 1997; Graveley & Fullerton, 1998; Harasim, Hiltz, Teles, & Turoff, 1996; McGonigle & Mastrain, 1998; Norton, 1998). These models emphasize human interaction, engagement in authentic and real-world learning, and shared and collaborative learning experiences. Emphasis is on high expectations, active learn-

ing, respect for diversity, rich and rapid feedback, and interaction with faculty and peers to meet learning outcomes and competency standards. Table 15.1 summarizes benchmarks for educational practices that guide teaching and learning in OLCPP.

■ Assessing Practices and Outcomes in On-Line Communities of Professional Practice

As on-line communities of professional practice (OLCPPs) in nursing become integral to nursing education, it is essential to (a) understand what contributes to formation of these communities, (b) know what constitutes best practices in teaching and learning in them, and (c) identify the extent to which intended outcomes have been attained. That includes accrediting agencies, commissions of higher education, schools of nursing, health care agencies, and members of the communities themselves.

Teaching and learning in OLCPP involves dynamic interaction among use of the technology and collaborative work tools, educational practices, and development and support that are available to create and sustain a community (Barr & Tagg, 1995; Billings, 1997; Chickering & Gamson, 1987; Chickering & Ehrmann, 1997; Cobb, 1998; Harrison et al., 1991). Each component of the teaching, technology, and support triad and its contribution to overall outcomes must be assessed.

Assessment is a process that provides information about outcomes, teaching–learning practices, faculty, students, and related costs (Stark & Thomas, 1994). Assessment also involves understanding changes that occur during and after participation in an educational event (Angelo & Cross, 1993). Findings from assessment activities are used to improve teaching and learning practices, processes,

TABLE 15.1   Benchmarks for Best Practices in Teaching and Learning in Web-Based Nursing Courses

Outcomes

Learning	Learners attain learning outcomes (as specified in module, course, curricula).
Access	Learners are able to participate in the educational offering because it is available in the on-line community.
Convenience	Courses are offered at a convenient time, place, and pace, allowing learners to manage multiple responsibilities.
Recruitment, retention, completion, and graduation	Learners enter and complete (and graduate) from the course or program.
Preparation for real-world work	Course activities prepare learners for clinical practice.
Productive use of time	Study and learning time contributes to learning outcomes; availability of resources facilitates use of time; course management software and collaborative work tools facilitate effective use of learning time.
Proficiency in technology use	Members become proficient in using technology, collaborative work tools, and knowledge work tools of the profession (databases, spreadsheets, clinical decision-making models, and expert systems).
Socialization to the profession	Course activities contribute to the development of professional roles and responsibilities.
Satisfaction	Members are satisfied with and enjoy the experience of teaching and learning in the on-line community; members would choose this experience again.

Educational Practices

High expectations	Members establish high expectations and standards for achievement; progress is monitored continuously by students, faculty, peers, and experts.
Active learning	Members are actively engaged in learning and take responsibility for their own learning; members complete assignments on time, share responsibilities for collaboration; construct own knowledge and meaning.
Prompt feedback	Members seek, provide, and use feedback to improve performance.
Time on task	Members spend sufficient time on course-related activities to achieve course goals.
Respect for diverse talents, ideas, and ways of learning	Members respect varying abilities; options are provided for learning and demonstrating learning; members demonstrate respect for multiple views and diverse cultures; members reinforce and observe the norms of the community.
Collaboration and interaction among peers	Members pose problems, ask questions, discuss, and share information and resources to elicit greater understanding for all members; members assume responsibility for completing collaborative work assignments
Student–faculty interaction	Faculty create learning environments and communities; faculty provide cognitive structures and use learning scaffolds to help learners solve problems; faculty provide access to authentic contexts and opportunities to explore and solve real-life problems; faculty are accessible both inside and outside class to discuss students' personal and professional goals; faculty and learners assume responsibility for overcoming isolation or other barriers to meaningful student–faculty interaction.

continued

TABLE 15.1   *continued*

Development, Orientation, Rewards, Resources, and Services

Development for teaching and learning in the OLCPP	Programs are available for developing faculty and learners for teaching and learning in the OLCPP; instructional support (e.g., instructional designer, Web programmer, librarian, database manager) is available for helping faculty design courses.
Orientation to use of technology	Established orientation programs can be used to help learners and faculty use course technology and course management software and tools.
Faculty workload, recognition, and rewards	Formal plans and policies exist to compensate and recognize faculty (workload, merit, promotion, tenure).
Learning resources and services	Learning resources (library, multimedia, patients, experts, real-world learning experiences) and services (learning assessment, career assessment, advising, testing, registration, bursar, financial aid, transcripts, portfolios) are available on-line to members.

Technology Use

Technology	Hardware and software are appropriate to support teaching and learning goals; technology is used appropriately; access to hardware and software is available and reliable.
User support	Twenty-four-hour technical support is available for course development and maintenance.

---

courses, and programs. Assessment works best when programs have clear purposes and makes a difference when issues of concern to stakeholders are examined. Assessment is ongoing and ensures accountability to stakeholders and the public (AAHE Assessment Forum, 1994).

Benchmarking is one specific assessment method that can be used to assess outcomes, practices, and services of a program or organization. Benchmarking is a discovery process that reveals best practices—that is, activities and strategies that contribute to improved performance by focusing on the customer (learners), emphasizing outcomes, and using resources and support systems effectively (Czarnecki, 1996; Ellis & Morris, 1997). Use of benchmarking procedures can create a shared vision of ideal practices among stakeholders (learners, faculty, institutions, and

organizations) and focus attention on performance shortcomings that can be addressed immediately.

Several national groups are spearheading efforts in higher education to develop assessment models, methods, and instruments to guide assessment of technology outcomes (Ehrmann & Zuniga, 1997; Johnstone & Krauth, 1996) and in nursing (Cobb, 1998; Cobb & Billings, 2000). One such project is the Nursing Benchmarking Project—part of a larger assessment effort by the Flashlight Program of the TLT Group, the Teaching Learning and Technology Affiliate of the American Association of Higher Education. Participants have developed a model and benchmarks for use in understanding the best practices in teaching and learning in on-line communities of professional practice in nursing (see Table

15.1). The model focuses on (a) outcomes of concern to nursing education, (b) educational (teaching–learning) practices that enable outcomes, (c) development, orientation, rewards, resources, and services that sustain the community, and (d) accessibility and reliability of technology, infrastructure, and user support services. Variables contained in the model are not exhaustive; educators may add or select variables of concern to particular faculty, school, or program assessment activities.

Also being developed is a benchmarking process and survey instruments for students, faculty, and administrators, adapted from survey items in the Flashlight Evaluation Handbook (Ehrmann & Zuniga, 1997). This survey can provide data for benchmarking best practices in OLCPPs to improve course or program-specific processes and outcomes for local (internal) use or to compare results to the best practices of peers. The survey is administered on-line from the Flashlight Project database and provides national norms and benchmarks from peer institutions. By undertaking such assessment activities, on-line communities of professional practice can continue to improve to meet needs of their members.

■ Concluding Statement

In the knowledge age, many, if not most, nurses will become members of on-line communities of professional practice. These communities will meet members' needs for knowledge generation and dissemination to support basic, advanced, and continuing nursing education and professional affiliation. Through membership in these communities, nurses will use resources and services for professional development; learners will have access to authentic professional activities and use collaborative work tools to build and maintain professional competence. Sophisticated network infrastructure and new professional alliances will enable and sustain the communities of teachers and learners—the nurses whose professional practice is tomorrow's vision.

■ References

AAHE Assessment Forum. (1994). Principles of good practice for assessing student learning. In J. S. Stark & A. Thomas (Eds.), *Assessment and program evaluation* (pp. 769–771). Needham Heights, MA: Simon & Schuster.

Anderson, D. G. (1995). Electronic education: E-mail links students and faculty. *Nurse Educator, 20*(4), 8–11.

Angelo, T. A., & Cross, K. P. (1993). *Classroom assessment techniques: A handbook for college teachers.* San Francisco: Jossey-Bass.

Bachman, J. A., & Panzarine, S. (1998). Enabling student nurses to use the information superhighway. *Journal of Nursing Education, 37*(4), 155–161.

Barr, R., & Tagg, J. (1995). From teaching to learning—a new paradigm for undergraduate education. *Change, 27*(6), 13–25.

Billings, D. M. (1997, January 23). *Current status and future directions of distance education in nursing.* Paper presented to Division of Nursing, U.S. Department of Health and Human Services, Alexandria, Virginia.

Billings, D. M., & Bachmeier, B. (1994). Teaching and learning at a distance: A review of the literature. In L. R. Allen (Ed.), *Review of research in nursing education* (pp. 1–32). New York: National League for Nursing.

Bonk, C. J., & Cunningham, D. J. (1998). Searching for learner-centered, constructivist, and sociocultural components of collaborative educational learning tools. In C. J. Bonk and K. S. King (Eds.), *Electronic collaborators* (pp. 25–50). Mahwah, NJ: Lawrence Erlbaum Associates.

Brown, J. S., & Duguid, P. (1996). Universities in the digital age. *Change, 28*(9), 11–19.

Carlton, K. H., Ryan, M. E., & Siktberg, L. L. (1998). Designing courses for the Internet: A conceptual approach. *Nurse Educator, 23*(3), 45–50.

Chickering, A. W., & Ehrmann, S. (1997). Implementing the seven principles: Technology as lever. *American Association of Higher Education* [On-line]. Available: http://www.tltgroup.org/ehrmann.htm.

Chickering, A. W., & Gamson, Z. F. (1987, March). Seven principles for good practice in undergraduate education. *American Association of Higher Education Bulletin,* March, 306.

Clark, D. J. (1998). Incorporating an Internet Web site into an existing nursing class. *Computers in Nursing, 16*(4), 219–222.

Cobb, K. (1998, June). *Evaluation by students enrolled in nursing courses offered via the World Wide Web: Using the flashlight in the dark.* Paper presented at Distributed Education Conference, Indianapolis, Indiana.

Cobb, K., & Billings, D. (2000). Assessing distance education programs in nursing. In J. Novotny (Ed.), *Distance learning in nursing* (pp. 85–112). New York: Springer.

Czarnecki, M. T. (1996). Benchmarking: A data-oriented look at improving health care performance. *Journal of Nursing Care Quality, 10*(3) 1–6.

Dolence, M. G., & Norris, D. M. (1995). *Transforming higher education.* Ann Arbor, MI: Society for College and University Planning.

Ehrmann, S. C., & Zuniga, R. E. (1997). *The flashlight evaluation handbook.* Washington, DC.: Corporation for Public Broadcasting.

Ellis, J. M., & Morris, A. (1997). Pediatric benchmarking: A review of its development. *Nursing Standard, 12*(2), 43–46.

Graveley, E., & Fullerton, J. T. (1998). Incorporating electronic-based and computer-based strategies: Graduate nursing courses in administration. *Journal of Nursing Education, 37*(4) 186–188.

Halstead, J., Hayes, R., Reising, D., & Billings, D. (1995). Nursing student information network: Fostering collegial communications using a computer conference. *Computers in Nursing, 13*(2), 55–59.

Harasim, L., Hiltz, S. R., Teles, L., & Turoff, M. (1996). *Learning networks, a field guide to teaching and learning on-line.* Cambridge, MA: MIT Press.

Harrison, P. J., Seeman, B. J., Behm, R., Saba, F., Molise, G., & Williams, M. (1991). Development of a distance education assessment instrument. *Educational Technology Research & Development, 39*(4), 65–77.

Johnstone, S. M., & Krauth, B. (1996). Some principles of good practice for the virtual university. *Change, 28*(2), 38–41.

Kirkpatrick, M. K., Brown, S., & Atkins, T. (1998). Electronic education: Using the Internet to integrate cultural diversity and global awareness. *Nurse Educator, 23*(2) 15–17.

McGonigle, D., & Mastrain, K. (1998). Learning along the way: Cyberspacial quests. *Nursing Outlook, 46*(2), 81–86.

Norris, D. M., & Malloch, T. R. (1997). *Unleashing the power of perpetual learning.* Ann Arbor, MI: Society for College and University Planning.

Norris, D. M., & Olson, M. A. (1997). Preparing for virtual commerce in higher learning. *Cause/Effect, 20*(1), 40–44.

Norton, B. (1998). From teaching to learning: Theoretical foundations. In D. M. Billings & J. A. Halstead (Eds.), *Teaching in nursing, a guide for faculty* (pp. 211–245). Philadelphia: W. B. Saunders.

Ribbons, R. M. (1998, July/August). The use of computers as cognitive tools to facilitate higher order thinking skills in nurse education. *Computers in Nursing,* 223–227.

Skiba, D. (1997). Transforming nursing education to celebrate learning. *Nursing and Healthcare Perspectives, 18*(3), 124–129.

Solence, M. G., & Norris, D. M. (1997). *Transforming higher education.* Ann Arbor, MI. Society for College and University Planning.

Stark, J. S., & Thomas, A. (Eds.). (1994). *Assessment and program evaluation.* Needham Heights, MA: Simon & Schuster.

Todd, N. A. (1998). Using e-mail in an undergraduate nursing course to increase critical thinking skills. *Computers in Nursing, 16*(2), 118.

■ Editor's Questions for Discussion

Discuss the purposes of on-line communities for professional practice (OLCPP). Who benefits from on-line communities and how? How can they be developed? Describe a plan and process for implementing and establishing an OLCPP. How are OLCPPs used to provide distance education courses? How might individual practitioners tap into on-line community courses and professional education for personal and professional development?

What professional accountability exists for on-line communities and to whom? How are accountability and quality control addressed for information, courses, and programs offered through on-line communities? How may OLCPPs be addressed in accreditation and regulation standards?

How might nursing centers, rural areas, and other underserved areas benefit from OLCPPs? Address issues raised by Yeaworth et al. (Chapter 14), Purnell (Chapter 37), Todero (Chapter 51), Barger (Chapter 52), and Duffy (Chapter 53) that could be resolved through OLCPPs. How can geographic areas, persons, or programs that have limited infrastructure networks begin to plan and use OLCPPs? What faculty role change, relearning, and reorientation are essential for establishing OLCPPs for nursing programs? How does Lindeman's (Chapter 63) predictions regarding faculty roles affect development of OLCPPs? Provide strategies to motivate faculty for change. What additional concerns may be related to OLCPPs? How might they be prevented or resolved?

16

Strategies for Successfully Educating Nursing Students in the 21st Century

Amy A. Nichols, EdD, RN
Andrea Renwanz-Boyle, DNSc, RN

Education of students in the 21st century will focus increasingly on development of clinicians prepared to work in rapidly changing, multicultural environments strongly influenced by technological advances and fiscal constraints. Technological changes also will significantly alter traditional educational structures, forcing educators to rethink how physical classrooms, teaching resources, and discrete discipline-specific content are used (Tanner, 1997; Office of Educational Research & Improvement, 1999).

These changes present challenges to nursing educators throughout the world. In commenting on the World Health Organization's identification of the current explosion of scientific information, Frost (1996) noted that this explosion makes traditional educational approaches increasingly irrelevant. Traditional curricula are based on what is known today, to the exclusion of how to learn what will be known tomorrow. To meet these challenges, nurse educators will be required to redirect their teaching to areas that promote critical thinking and other requisite skills so necessary for future nursing practice.

In this chapter we initially identify major limitations of traditional educational methods in light of current and projected trends. We then present and discuss strategies to enhance education, including service learning, portfolios, and problem-based learning.

■ Limitations of Traditional Educational Methods: Why Traditional Education Will Not Work in the 21st Century

Nurses preparing for practice in the 21st century will work within an environment in which less costly but high-quality health care is delivered to patients with complex health problems (Pickersgill, 1998). Clinicians must be prepared to be scholars as well as practitioners, with the intellectual capabilities to question, speculate, research, and synthesize information (Zorn, Clark, & Weimholt, 1997). Acquisition and development of skills that support self-directed inquiry are crucial for practitioners practicing in this reconfigured health care industry (Doddato, 1995). Additionally, many authors cite active and autonomous decision-making as important for all nurses (Biley & Smith, 1998; Glen, 1995; Heliker, 1994; Rideout, 1994). Conway-Welch (1996) commented that educators must remove the redundancy and repetition existing in current educational systems. Targeted were programs that prepare nurses who in part develop and analyze data for continuous care delivery improvement, use data to enhance clinical outcomes, and become highly skilled in information systems technology.

Traditional educational approaches have been structured around separate academic disciplines, fostering development of analytical skills, as opposed to skills required for problem-solving or synthesis of materials (Creedy, Horsfall, & Hand, 1992). Andrews (1996) noted that, as nursing education continues to move toward higher education, a conceptual shift will be required to integrate associated subjects with unique epistemological bases and methodological approaches.

Students educated traditionally have demonstrated less interest in continuing professional development, an essential element in an environment of technological changes and continual learning due to rapid growth in medical knowledge (Dowie & Elstein, 1993). Townsend (1990) commented that much learning occurring in traditional nursing education requires memorization of facts, considered to be mostly irrelevant by many students. Traditional approaches also have limited the use of teamwork, thus serving to promote a gap between theory and practice, as well as poor development of intellectual inquiry skills (Boud & Felitti, 1991). Thus the traditional educational approach will not prepare clinicians adequately for an environment characterized by evidence-based practice, technological advances, and ongoing information exchange.

Additionally, traditional educational approaches have been problematic for many nontraditional and adult learners, two rapidly increasing student groups within nursing. Knowles (1984) asserted that use of the traditional teacher-centered, subject-based educational strategies (that assume student experiences to be of lesser value than that of teachers) makes it difficult for adults to control their own learning. Rideout (1994) further noted that, when students are able to participate in their own learning, they develop those qualities of autonomy and independent decision-making sought after within the nursing profession.

■ Strategies to Educate Nurses in the 21st Century

Traditional educational methods do not prepare clinicians to work within a changing, technologically advanced and culturally diverse health system. However, certain educational strategies have the potential to prepare students for changes that they will encounter.

TABLE 16.1   Differences Between Clinical Practicum and Service-Learning

Clinical Practicum	*Service Learning*
"Doing for"	"Doing with"
Placing students	Selecting community partners
Linking activities with exams and care plans	Linking activities with journals and reflection assignments
Bridging clinical practice and theory	Bridging classroom and the street
Presenting abstract lessons	Strengthening abstract lessons with practical activity
Responding to curricular needs	Responding to community-identified and curricular needs

Three of these strategies are service-learning, use of portfolios, and problem-based learning.

Service-Learning

Service-learning is an established range of pedagogies and educational methodologies that provide opportunities for structured reflection and link academic theory to experience. Giles and Eyler (1993) describe service-learning as an instructional methodology built on a foundation of experiential learning, enhanced by critical, reflective thinking. The Health Professions School in the Service to the Nation (HPSISN) defines service-learning as a structured learning experience, combining community service-learning with preparation and reflection (Conners & Seifer, 1997). Students in service-learning must provide direct community service, learn about the context in which the service is provided, and understand the connection between service and academic course work. Through community service, students enhance civic and social responsibilities, develop critical thinking skills, and work on group problem-solving competencies.

As part of their mission and strategic planning, most nursing programs include commitment to community and service, but that alone is inadequate to prepare students to meet the needs of communities they will serve. Nationwide, students are encouraged to volunteer in their communities as a means of developing long-term civic responsibility. The concept of courses designed specifically for service-learning within nursing curricula are rare. Although many clinical courses take place within community or public health agencies serving disenfranchised populations, such courses are very different from service-learning experiences. In service-learning, content, reflection, and experience work interactively and reciprocally to enhance each other.

Confusion frequently occurs concerning differences between service-learning and clinical practica. Major differences are identified in Table 16.1.

Over the past 12 years, U.S. educators have made significant attempts to combine community service with academic, civic, and career development. Numerous educational associations, such as the American Association for Higher Education, the United Negro College Fund, the Council of Independent Colleges, and the American Association of Community Colleges, have placed service-learning on their agendas (Langseth & Troppe, 1997). Many college and university presidents have formed a coalition based on the belief that institutions of higher learning hold primary responsibility for fostering students' sense of civic responsibility and helping them contribute to the welfare of their communities.

Some faculty believe that service-learning will weaken the academic rigor of a course. Contrary to this opinion, service-learning programs can intensify the level of critical thinking and problem-based learning efforts by students. When students participate in service-learning in community settings and combine this learning with critical dialogue from classroom discussion, students are drawn closer to, not farther from, the center of relevant course content.

The strongest component of service-learning involves use of community partners. Student placements and assignments in agencies are in direct response to community needs. Service-learning involves the community as an active partner in course development, program design, and implementation of service-learning assignments. Linking service-learning and nursing courses connects theory with application and practice, promotes critical thinking, and creates a special learning environment that cannot be replicated in any classroom environment.

Implementation of Service-Learning

Implementation of service-learning requires many changes on the part of faculty, particularly in the areas of assignments and faculty role. Student assignments must maintain academic rigor. Journal writing and reflection papers are very different types of assignments than given in the past, and the quality of the assignment directly relates to meaningfulness of the community service-learning project and the student experience. Faculty must remember that assignments and learning experiences

must be balanced, students must be prepared to enter the community, and placements must be appropriately related to the course of study.

Faculty must also adjust to a new role in the classroom. Implementation of service-learning changes the focus of class learning from teacher to student. Many faculty, accustomed to traditional methods of instruction, fear loss of control in the classroom. Change to accommodate learning that comes from students instead of being driven by the instructor actually provides more control and stability in the classroom.

Faculty who want to integrate service-learning into a nursing course often have other challenges, typically from other faculty not familiar with the concept of service-learning or from faculty and institutional resistance to change generally. Faculty who are unsure about the concept of service-learning commonly do not understand the differences between service-learning and clinical training, state concerns over adding service-learning to already overloaded curricula, and express fears regarding potential loss of control and uncertainty of community resource availability.

One strategy to assist with overcoming obstacles is to propose pilot testing of service-learning in one course for one semester, to collect data and determine whether permanent integration into nursing courses is feasible. Unsure faculty often are willing to pilot test curricular changes because that is a safe method of trying something new without making any initial long-term commitment. Once data have been collected, evaluated, and presented to faculty, permanent integration may be easier to achieve than if pilot testing did not occur.

Use of Portfolios in Assessment of Nursing Students

The use of portfolios to assess professional development of nursing students has not been widely used. Nor has much been written about the use of portfolios to document nursing educational competencies and critical thinking. A portfolio is a focused, purposeful accumulation of work that documents evidence of both traditional and nontraditional sources of student learning over time (Wenzel, Briggs, & Puryear, 1998).

Portfolio use provides opportunities for both students and faculty to assess progress throughout a course or an entire program of study. Content of the portfolio will vary depending on (a) the course, (b) purpose of the portfolio, (c) level of the student, (d) extent of self-reflection, (e) integration of past experiences related to the course, and (f) inventiveness of the portfolio process. An additional advantage for educators in changing educational systems is that a portfolio can also be used for assessing students' employment potential.

Problem-Based Learning

Problem-based learning has been defined differently by many authors. In general, though, the term describes learning that is problem centered or focused (Boud, 1985; Maudsley, 1999), that results from a process of working to resolve or understand a problem (Barrows & Tamblyn, 1980), and that involves a hypothetical-deductive approach to inquiry (Barrows, 1996). As Barrows and Tamblyn (1980) have noted, the use of problem-solving in learning is not a new educational strategy. Traditional educational approaches provide students with problems after the students have received information, facts, or principles. Problem solving has served to reinforce information or apply knowledge. This approach contrasts to problem-based learning, where a problem is presented initially as a stimulus for active learning.

A model of problem-based learning has been proposed by Barrows (1996). The core components of this model stress that (a) learning is student centered; (b) learning occurs best in small student groups; (c) teachers are viewed as facilitators and guides rather than as experts; (d) problems serve as the organizing focus and stimulus for the development of clinical problem-solving skills; and (e) students acquire new information through self-directed learning. Martin (1996) asserted that a problem-based curriculum is designed to provide opportunities for (a) cumulative learning, where subject material is introduced repeatedly and at increasing levels of complexity during a course of study; (b) integrated learning where students are introduced to problems rather than specific content; (c) progressive learning that provides students with opportunities to acquire knowledge at levels consistent with their abilities; and (d) consistent learning with development of a learning environment that integrates all aspects of teaching and learning.

Several major assumptions underscore problem-based learning. Key among them is the premise that the student is at the center of the learning process and will be a participant in an active, rather than passive, learning process (Alavi, 1995).

Proponents of problem-based methods and curricula identify significant differences between this approach to education and more traditional approaches, including (a) reliance on the use of problems, (b) shift in emphasis from content acquisition to mastery of process, (c) changes in both student and faculty roles, and (d) focus on integration of knowledge across traditional course or subject boundaries.

Implementation

Use of problems within the context of problem-based learning is designed to serve as both an initial stimulus to engage students intellectually and to trigger acquisition of information relevant to the problems (Frost, 1996). According to David and Patel (1995), the nature of the problem is crucial: It must be stimulating, contextual, and designed to provide students with opportunities to meet identified or designated learning goals and objectives. Although traditional case studies, care vignettes, and computer simulations also require the development of stimulating, clinically relevant problems, the format of problems in a problem-based format must resemble closely problems as they would occur in the "real world" (Barrows, 1996). Problems presented in this way are incomplete, sometimes confusing, and open to a number of interpretations by students. This approach contrasts to problems presented in case studies, for example, where students are presented with discrete information and expected to arrive at one answer or a series of correct answers. Problems used in problem-based learning (a) are not easily resolved, (b) are not always resolved using the same approach, and (c) may serve to generate additional questions rather than answers or solutions. Barrows (1994) stated that students, in problem-based learning, are not being asked to solve problems so much as they are being required to analyze underlying concepts or dynamics inherent within the problem structure itself.

Focus

The term *problem-based learning* is, in fact, a misnomer because the focus is on addressing knowledge acquisition rather than problem resolution or mastery of discrete content. Problem-based learning may be viewed as "explanation-based learning," emphasizing integration of professional knowledge into a coherent whole (Andrews, 1996). The intellectual work required for problem identification, explanation, and understanding becomes the primary goal of problem-based learning rather than acquisition of specific facts. This approach is in direct contrast to traditional educational strategies that emphasize presentation (usually in lecture format) of specific facts to be memorized for future recall by students

(usually measured by tests). In many medical and nursing schools, problem-based learning is organized around actual patient problems, enmeshed with clinical reasoning processes necessary for knowledge recall and application in clinical settings (Barrows, 1994).

Many comparisons can be made between the roles of students and faculty in problem-based and standard nursing education programs. Traditionally, faculty have assumed the role of content expert, designated to providing knowledge and guidance to students or novice learners. In addition, faculty and student roles have been fairly well defined, with faculty assuming responsibility for structuring the learning environment—determining what and how content is to be provided and evaluated. Students traditionally have assumed the responsibility to learn what faculty require for each course.

Roles of faculty and students within a problem-based context contrast to those traditional roles. In the problem-based setting, students assume responsibility for identifying what they want to learn, structuring the format in which learning occurs, and evaluating their own learning. Faculty serve in facilitative rather than authoritative roles, serve as guides rather than experts, and avoid direct control of classroom proceedings (Barrows & Tamblyn, 1980). Students are active in what can be described as a student-centered learning process; faculty serve in a colearning capacity (Frost, 1996). Roles within the problem-based setting become more flexible and less well designed.

Problem-based curricula also can be compared to traditional nursing curricula. A problem-based curriculum, by design, integrates core knowledge from a variety of disciplines and areas. In contrast, a traditional curriculum divides content into discrete areas or courses. Traditional strategies for identifying specific content do not work well when applied to problem-based curricula.

A number of advantages for the use of problem-based learning in 21st century nursing education are apparent. Many authors argue that a problem-based approach to learning improves the integration of theoretical knowledge into the clinical or practice arena. This concept correlates with improved transfer of theoretical knowledge and experiences from the classroom into the clinical or practice setting. Additionally, many authors note that use of the active learning associated with problem-based learning promotes and improves the critical thinking capabilities of students and their problem-solving and clinical reasoning skills. Use of problem-based learning also is associated with improved long-term retention of knowledge (Barrows, 1994).

■ Concluding Statement

The 21st century promises to bring changes and challenges both for nurses and nurse educators. Increased attention to multiculturalism, increased use of technology in health care settings, changes in clinical roles, and increased emphasis on quality, cost-effective health care are forces that will shape future nursing practice. Educators using traditional educational models will have limited success in providing students with essential problem-solving, critical thinking, and practice skills.

Service-learning, student portfolios, and problem-based learning are educational strategies that have the potential to provide students with these critical skills. Service-learning can provide students with opportunities to work in multicultural community settings and thus work toward cultural awareness within professional nursing roles. Portfolios can provide educators with a comprehensive yet flexible strategy for evaluating not only individual students, but also for evaluating educational programs. Problem-based learning can provide students with critical thinking and problem-solving skills required for practice in a changing, technologically advanced health care system. The use of service-learning, student portfolios, and problem-based learning can be used to transform nursing education in the 21st century.

■ References

Alavi, C. (Ed.). (1995). *Problem-based learning in a health sciences curriculum.* London: Routledge.

Andrews, M. (1996). Problem-based learning in an undergraduate nursing programme: A case study. *Journal of Advanced Nursing, 23*(2), 357–365.

Barrows, H. S. (1994). *Practice-based learning: Problem-based learning applied to medical education.* Springfield, IL: Southern Illinois University School of Medicine.

Barrows, H. S. (1996). Problem-based learning in medicine and beyond: A brief overview. In L. Wilkerson & W. H. Gijselaers (Eds.), *Bringing problem-based learning to higher education: Theory and practice* (pp. 3–12). San Francisco: Jossey-Bass.

Barrows, H. S., & Tamblyn, R. M. (1980). *Problem-based learning: An approach to medical education.* New York: Springer.

Biley, F. C., & Smith, K. L. (1998). "The buck stops here": Accepting responsibility for learning and actions after graduation from a problem-based learning nursing education curriculum. *Journal of Advanced Nursing, 27*(5), 1021–1029.

Boud, D. J. (1985). Problem-based learning in perspective. In D. J. Boud (Ed.), *Problem-based learning in education for the professions* (pp. 12–20). Sydney: Higher Education Research and Development Society of Australia.

Boud, D., & Felitti, G. (1991). *The challenge of problem-based learning.* London: Kogan Page.

Conners, K., & Seifer, S. (1997). Service learning in health professions education: What is service learning, and why now? Community–campus partnerships for health. *A guide for developing community-responsive models in health professions education.* San Francisco: University of California, San Francisco Center for the Health Professions.

Conway-Welch, C. (1996). Who is tomorrow's nurse and where will tomorrow's nurse be educated? *Nursing & Health Care: Perspectives on Community, 17*(6), 286–290.

Creedy, D., Horsfall, J., & Hand, B. (1992). Problem-based learning in nurse education: An Australian view. *Journal of Advanced Nursing, 17,* 727–733.

David, T. J., & Patel, L. (1995). Adult learning theory, problem based learning, and paediatrics. *Archives of Disease in Childhood, 73*(4), 357–363.

Doddato, T. M. (1995). Advanced practice education for the twenty-first century. *Nursing & Health Care: Perspectives on Community, 16*(5), 266–269.

Dowie, J., & Elstein, A. (1993). Introduction. In J. Dowie, & A. Elstein (Eds.), *Professional judgement reader in clinical decision making.* Cambridge, U.K.: Cambridge University Press.

Frost, M. (1996). An analysis of the scope and value of problem-based learning in the education of health care professionals. *Journal of Advanced Nursing, 24*(5), 1047–1053.

Giles, D., & Eyler, J. (1993). *FIPSE service-learning proposal.* Nashville: Vanderbilt University.

Glen, S. (1995). Towards a new model of nursing education. *Nurse Education Today, 15,* 90–95.

Heliker, D. (1994). Meeting the challenge of the curriculum revolution: Problem-based learning in nursing education. *Journal of Nursing Education, 33*(1), 45–47.

Knowles, M. (1984). *Andragogy in action.* San Francisco: Jossey-Bass.

Langseth, M., & Troppe, M. (1997). *Expanding boundaries: Building civic responsibility within higher education* (Vol. II). Cincinnati: Cooperative Education Association.

Martin, K. (1996, June). University of Western Australia, Centre for Staff Development [On-line]. Available: http://www.udel.edu/pbl/.

Maudsley, G. (1999). Do we all mean the same thing by "problem-based learning"?—A review of the concepts and a formulation of the ground rules. *Academic Medicine, 74*(2), 178–185.

Office of Educational Research & Improvement, U.S. Department of Education. (1999). *Technology & educational reform research project.* Washington, DC: Author.

Pickersgill, F. (1998). Time to catch up. *Nursing Standard, 12*(37), 26–27.

Rideout, E. M. (1994). Letting go: Rationale and strategies for student-centered approaches to clinical teaching. *Nurse Education Today, 14*(2), 146–151.

Tanner, C. (1997). Innovations in nursing education. *Journal of Nursing Education, 36*(6), 243.

Townsend, J. (1990). Problem-based learning. *Nursing Times, 86*(14), 61–62.

Wenzel, L. S., Briggs, K. L., & Puryear, B. L. (1998). Portfolio: Authentic assessment in the age of the curriculum revolution. *Journal of Nursing Education, 37*(5), 208–212.

Zorn, C. R., Clark, W. J., & Weimholt, C. J. (1997). Educating the nurse scholar for the 21st century: How an interdisciplinary writing course can help. *Journal of Nursing Education, 36*(6), 244–249.

■ *Editor's Questions for Discussion*

What is the difference between service-learning and clinical practice? Does service-learning draw upon a theoretical base in application to the community? If so, how is the theoretical base for application in service-learning different from that applied in a clinical practicum? What is the difference between a community and a clinical practice setting? How does service-learning bridge the classroom and street?

How may portfolios be used for all nursing education programs? What are some advantages and disadvantages of portfolios? What criteria should be developed for portfolio assessment? Who should develop criteria for using portfolios? How may portfolios be used to evaluate student placement in a nursing program? How comparable are assessment of portfolios and NLN achievement tests in evaluating students? To what extent may portfolios be used in admission of students to levels in nursing programs for baccalaureate, advanced standing, master's, or doctoral studies? What content should be included in a portfolio? Who determines content and criteria for acceptance of portfolios? How may standardization occur in development, presentation, and review of portfolios?

How does M. Fisher (Chapter 17) demonstrate problem-based learning as described by Nichols and Renwanz-Boyle? Should all undergraduate curricula be developed as problem-based learning? Provide specific examples of problem-based learning at each level for undergraduate curricula. Who initially defines the problem in problem-based learning? How applicable is problem-based learning for master's program curricula?

17

Preparing Tomorrow's Nursing Leaders

Changing the Paradigm

Mary L. Fisher, PhD, RN, CNAA

The past five years have been difficult for nursing administration (NA) programs throughout the United States. In addition to the normal cycles that the nursing staffs have undergone historically—ebbs and flows of shortages and oversupplies—the most recent retrenchment in health care in the early 1990s hit nursing leaders especially hard. Health care reform efforts, guided by external financial pressures, led to redesigned delivery systems with fewer leaders. The number of middle managers and opportunities for them in traditional settings declined as spans of control broadened (Beyers, 1995; Davidhizar, 1995; Doerge & Hagenow, 1995). Service line realignment accounted for additional loss of

leadership opportunities for nurses as less emphasis was placed on clinical (operational) expertise and more emphasis was placed on business skills—marketing, finance, and acquisition (Haynor & Wells, 1998).

What happens in practice quickly gets translated into reality for education. In a 1995 study of nursing administration programs, "14 of 48 responding schools (29%) had discontinued or were closing their administration programs. . . . of the remaining 34 (71%), 19 (56%) reported a decrease in enrollment, and 15 (44%) remained the same or had increased enrollment" (Haynor & Wells, 1998, p. 15). If nurses perceive lack of opportunity in administration, it is natural for them to flock to other programs viewed as having career potential. Most recently, the career trend has been nurse practitioner (NP) programs. Nursing administration graduates still are moving into exciting careers, but the word has not gotten out to mainstream nursing that the specialty is alive and well.

■ Need for a New Vision

By rethinking the definition of leadership opportunities, we can move administration careers into new venues for creative leadership. Nurse-managed centers are a growing segment of health care as communities seek cost-effective care options. In these centers, nursing leaders must excel in operations management, human resources, marketing, budgeting, information systems design, and program evaluation (Patronis Jones, 1994). Nursing administration graduates should be well positioned to move into entrepreneurial roles and be able to have a direct impact on consumer outcomes beyond those of traditional institutional settings. Innovative practicum experiences with nurse entrepreneurs may pave the way for such endeavors (Ludemann & Loveridge, 1992).

Opportunity also exists for nursing leaders who are willing to relocate to underserved areas. Lack of geographic mobility of many NA graduates due to family responsibilities continues to limit their career paths. Building concepts of career tracking and networking with executive recruiters into NA programs may help socialize students to expect career moves as a normal part of career development, as many male-dominated professions demonstrate.

Nursing leaders are being asked to expand their roles to promote a transdisciplinary vision. They are becoming vice presidents of patient care services with several missions: "To do more with less, to continually improve care, and to exceed customer expectations" (Haynor, 1996, p. 61). Nonnurses increasingly are reporting to these new-age leaders who must bring the many clinical disciplines together to improve care, often for the first time. The old solo model of disciplines marching to their own drummer no longer works. New-age leaders must bridge language and communication barriers to meld people from different disciplines into teams with a patient focus. Hence old communication and relationship patterns must change.

These factors come together to emphasize that a new vision is needed for NA programs if the specialty is to survive into the future. Business as usual clearly will not do the trick.

■ Where We Are Now

Examining the current picture of nursing administration education is helpful in understanding where we need to go. Our past can be clue to a preferred future.

Administrative Inbreeding Within Organizations

Many organizations prefer to promote from within. They often reward previous achievements with promotion, regardless of educational preparation for the role or the future potential of the candidate. The "known entity" who is seen as a team player is preferred to an expensive external search that may result in a candidate who brings external influences into the organization. Executives also may bring leaders from their previous organizations to build a team with whom they are familiar and comfortable. Men and women may prefer to hire executives of their own gender for the same reasons. All these possibilities may limit nurse administrator mobility.

Deep Cuts in
Middle Management Roles

Middle managers find themselves faced with burgeoning responsibilities. They now perform duties that were limited to executive positions in the past and do so in increasingly complex settings that may span the continuum of care in a service line setting or multiple operating units in a more traditional organizational structure. Consequently, many nurse middle managers seek additional education to cope with these new realities. Displaced leaders are often disillusioned with health care in general. Many leave not only administration but nursing altogether, using their considerable talents in other service sectors (e.g., real estate, insurance, or other public-oriented employment). Such moves represent a great loss of leadership from nursing.

Lack of Standard
Preparation

Many nursing executives currently in practice lack a graduate degree in any field. Scalzi and Wilson (1990) studied nursing executives in acute care, home care, and long-term care. They found that 12% working in long-term care, 42% in home care, 55% in occupational health, and 69% in acute care held graduate degrees in nursing, business, or public health administration (p. 523).

Nursing leaders are educated in various ways. In addition to the traditional nursing administration master of science in nursing (MSN) degree, dual degree programs combining NA with business, public health, health administration, or public administration are available. Institutions also try to develop their own leaders through continuing education efforts. Certificates in administration can be obtained from both proprietary and academic institutions.

Even certification programs do not always guarantee standard preparation. Only certification in Nursing Administration, Advanced, from the American Nurses' Credentialing Cen-

ter recognizes a master's level of preparation, although the original degree does not have to be in nursing administration. Interdisciplinary certification as a health care executive has been available through the American College for Healthcare Executives (ACHE) since 1967.

Within NA programs, there also is great variability of curricula. Haynor and Wells (1998) reported wide variations in field experiences in nursing administration programs from 88 hours to 515 hours per program (mean = 214, SD = 119.73) (p. 16). Little leadership has been exercised nationally to correct these faults until recently.

Image of Weak MSN Curricula to
Prepare Nursing Leaders

The image of nursing administration programs in some circles is that of preparing leaders only for nursing leadership—in a sense, perpetuation of isolation from other clinical services that marks nursing's history (Malloch, 1998). Nursing executives report strong nursing identities (Scalzi & Wilson, 1990) that may isolate them from mainstream health care executives.

Instead of discipline-focused programs, Malloch (1998) argues for consumer-driven leadership that integrates multidisciplinary systems thinking, preferably through MBA programs rather than discipline-specific preparation. The proliferation of MBA-prepared health care executives may, in fact, be related to falling opportunities for MSN-prepared nursing leaders. Haynor and Wells (1998) postulated that executives prefer to hire leaders with degrees similar to their own, "thus limiting career advancement opportunities for those with nursing administration masters" (p. 18). Continuing growth of organizational structures in which managers lead multidisciplinary groups may further this discounting of the MSN-prepared administrator (Minnick, 1998).

Falling Numbers of Graduate Students in the Specialty

In their study of nursing administration programs, Haynor and Wells (1998) found an enrollment trend that supported closing or downsizing NA programs. This trend toward eliminating or weakening existing NA programs through neglect of faculty recruitment and attrition is evident in many schools. Long-term consequences of such decisions on the viability of the nursing profession must be addressed. If we relegate ourselves to a future of weaker nursing leaders, advocacy for the profession may be threatened. Without a strong nursing leadership voice and vision for the future, bean counters who value only dollars will increasingly advocate the use of less skilled and unskilled workers.

Renewed Nursing Shortage and Rising Turnover

Early signs of consequences from actions that effectively reduced the voice of nurses in reengineering decisions of the 1990s already are visible. Despite introduction of unlicensed assistive personnel (UAPs), we are again entering a time of nursing shortage. Pressures exerted on staff nurses brought on by broader patient responsibilities of larger teams of care givers for increasing numbers of patients have moved many nurses out of acute care and, in some cases, out of nursing altogether. Many hospitals now report acute registered nurse (RN) shortages, costly turnover approaching that of the peak seen in the 1980s shortage and mandatory overtime in order to keep units open. Those of us with a history in nursing administration see these signs as recurring themes, due in part to lack of a nursing leadership voice to maintain safe practice conditions, regardless of the "oversupply" during retrench-

ment. Nurses, indeed, have longer memories of injustices than business-only oriented executives who are dictating many clinical practice changes.

These current trends continue to place great pressure on nursing administration educators and practitioners to exercise a vision for the future. Only through such collaboration between practice and education can we hope to reverse the downward spiral that could be our fate.

■ Future Vision

Unification of clinical skills and business proficiency is vital for the future of nursing leadership education. The unique perspective that nursing leaders bring to the table is a patient focus and holistic view of the care process. We understand the fundamental business of health care—the services rendered.

Nursing Administration as Advanced Practice

Shortly after the American Association of Colleges of Nursing (AACN) and the American Organization of Nurse Executives (AONE) crafted their joint statement, *The Essentials of Master's Education for Advanced Practice Nursing* (1996), they issued their *Joint Position Statement on Education for Nurses in Administrative Roles* (1997). It covers core abilities, content, and practicum experiences to overcome the current lack of standard preparation for nursing leaders (AACN & AONE, 1998). Overall intent of the document is to achieve a parallel in the advanced education of nursing administrators with that of advanced practice nurses (APNs, which include clinical nurse specialists, nurse practitioners, nurse midwives, and nurse anesthetists). Both groups must share common grounding in theory, research, roles, legal and ethical considerations, and health policy. Nursing administrators, who need to value and hire APNs, must speak the language of advanced practice. The main difference is the focus of practice—the nursing administrators' clinical and field experiences are focused on the system, whereas the advanced practice nurses' clinical and field experiences are focused on the individual patient, family, or both.

Emphasizing Administrative Practice Experience

Nursing Administration majors must be prepared in such a way that they are "fully operational" upon graduation (Haynor & Wells, 1998). Programs that emphasize administrative experience, contextual learning, analytic skills, and mentoring relationships will put their graduates ahead of the competition. Practicum mentors representing a broad cross section of the health care community must be drawn into the program as resources for student learning.

Students should accumulate management portfolios during their programs of study. Evidence of community projects—group learning such as concept maps, writing samples, organizational assessments, practicum, and research projects—can serve as an exit evaluation tool to measure attainment of program outcomes. Students should face a panel for formal presentation of their portfolios, which should serve as graded components of capstone experiences.

Using Systems Focus to Assess the Changing Scope of Practice

Nursing leaders are in a unique position, possessing both the clinical background and leadership skills needed to influence decisions

about the future role of nurses. Nursing roles are evolving as UAPs are introduced through redesign of practice models. "Staff nurses are floundering . . . often reinforcing the very behaviors they find so problematic—inefficient use of time and overlap of responsibilities" (Ingersoll, 1998, p. 13). Questions such as What are the unique skills the RN brings to health care that must be preserved for quality care? and How can RNs best utilize UAPs to maximize patient outcomes and efficiency of care? must be addressed.

The nursing leader must be "clinically centered" with passion for excellent patient care (Fralic, 1993). Such a philosophy of practice must be fostered in the graduate program to produce leaders who are "grounded" and who can consistently act from a larger context. That larger context includes ethical considerations. Examination of personal philosophy, ethical principles inherent in the leadership role, and ethics of resource allocation decisions are minimum requirements for the role (Ludemann & Loveridge, 1992).

Fostering Critical Thinking and Leaders Who Are Team Players

Graduate education that does more than impart concepts is needed. Students must work in teams during their education to appreciate team responsibilities in real life. Group problem-solving models, used in context of a case study approach, help NA students gain consensus-building skills. Ability to view situations from a variety of perspectives fosters leaders who can suspend judgment long enough to seek solutions that will work for the larger good.

Rather than NA faculty serving as the "sage on the stage," new learning models encourage students to seek their own truths through more active learning. Such learners gain vital lifelong learning skills to become self-motivated learners.

Emphasizing Nontraditional Leadership Roles

To maximize student placement, the NA program of the future must expose students to cases that address issues across practice settings, across leadership levels and structural models, and across disciplinary lines. Practical experience in developing business plans for new ventures gives students opportunities to work in uncharted territory. Crafting a project plan for a new venture builds entrepreneurial skills.

Encouraging NA students to maintain their clinical background and skills, while perfecting leadership and business skills, can maximize their opportunities to have an impact on quality care. Case management positions allow for maximum use of both sets of skills. Accountability for patient outcomes and ways to measure them should be added to such curricula.

Educating Across the Continuum of Practice Settings

Future nursing leaders will need expertise that spans practice settings. Programs can no longer focus on hospital-based practice issues, as more care occurs in other settings. Knowledge of a broad range of regulatory bodies, political acumen, contract negotiation, new practice models, insurance savvy, and team building will be prominent skills for nursing leaders in the new millennium. Leaders who can assist nurses in identifying unique contributions in these new settings will help mold the basis for practice of the profession and the future. The nursing leader of the future will need vision and political skill to unify care across practice settings and to fight for models of care that maintain quality outcomes while being cost-effective.

Practicing Consultation Process

Consultation is a vital role of nursing administrators. Whether the consultation is internal to the organization or external for other agencies, NA students need experiences that build consultation skills. Because many nursing leaders engage consultants for projects within their organizations, fully understanding the consultation relationship and process will also help them become better consumers of consultation services.

Leading Change Successfully

If any skill is likely to be highlighted in the future, it will be the ability to lead change positively and effectively. Fundamental skills in building the kind of organizational culture that can respond to demands in a timely manner is needed (Feldman, 1995). The incessant change expected in the future demands leaders who can deal with the ambiguity and uncertainty that restructuring brings, both on a personal and leadership level. Constant readjustments needed during change (which should be an evolving process) can engender distrust and anxiety in employees (Ingersoll, 1998). Tomorrow's nursing leaders must demonstrate proficiency in both minimizing unnecessary changes through clear vision and leadership and positively leading associates through the change process with egos and professional role identities intact.

Maximizing use of APNs as change agents, fostering development of their influence for improved practice, and ensuring their involvement in establishing consistent nursing standards all will serve the nursing leader well (Nichols, 1992). Having such respected and highly skilled nurses on the change team will help ensure project success and clinical relevancy. APNs can also help measure change outcomes and "fine tune" changes to maximize their benefits.

Sitting at the Policy Table

Future nursing administrators must sit at important policy tables. The skills needed for such involvement in decision-making can be developed or enhanced in NA graduate programs. Exercises that engage groups of NA students in policy projects help them to learn the players in and the process of policy formulation. When their efforts have an impact on policy, students get a dose of real power. Power is often a maligned concept for nurses. Learning to accept power and channel it for good is a valuable skill that will enhance their administrative careers.

■ Evidence-Based Practice in Nursing Administration

Many changes that are initiated in healthcare fall under the "bandwagon" category; that is, if competitors redesign, then our institution must follow. As a result, administrators often mimic a redesign process without understanding what worked or did not work. Industry leaders often blindly initiate change without regard to possible consequences, with change often evolving through expensive and time-consuming trial and error. Future NA programs must develop nursing leaders who are resistant to such knee-jerk responses. As a discipline, nursing administrators must model evidence-based practice insofar as possible in all major projects they undertake. They need to know in advance whether changes will make things better or worse, not just for consumers, but also for staff.

Focusing on Outcomes Research

Tomorrow's nursing executives must initiate generation of data and analyses that document nursing's contributions to quality care. Additionally, each nursing leader has a duty to further a broader research agenda, such as that promoted by the American Organization of Nurse Executives (AONE, 1999). How can that be best accomplished? Through research consortia of nursing administrators monitoring practice using a minimum standard data set, we can monitor effects of change and systematically begin to address AONE's research agenda.

Evaluating Change

Nothing is more disruptive to an institution than change. Inherent to committing to change is an obligation to do it well and to understand its outcomes. Unfortunately, many in practice do not have the skills necessary to evaluate change. This area presents an opportunity for NA faculty. They can initiate links with service for the purpose of helping service evaluate change. Such relationships can provide a laboratory for graduate students to participate in outcomes research. Identifying outcomes to measure, determining how to monitor them within existing data systems, and sharpening data collecting skills all will be valuable tools for NA students to master.

Research Utilization Models

Established research utilization models can be used in NA programs to help students plan an evidence-based implementation project. Laschinger, Foran, Jones, Perkin, and Bovan

(1993) provided a template for such a graduate project. They proposed that students identify an area of administrative interest, research the literature, and develop a protocol to adopt in practice, using an existing model such as the Conduct and Utilization of Research in Nursing (CURN) model (Horsley, Crane, & Bingle, 1978) or the Steler-Marram (Goode, Lovett, Hayes, & Butcher, 1987) model. Skill in using such models serves the graduate of NA programs well as they transition to service.

■ Problem-Based Learning as a Model for Change

The learning environment must mimic workplace realities. If real-life nursing leaders must work in teams, then team-building and team-maintenance skills must be built into the learning model. If no one feeds the real-life nursing leader "content" for critical decision-making, then self-directed learning must be part of the learning model. Problem-based learning (PBL) is a pedagogical model that supports such real-life learning. Realistic problems are simulated in cases designed to accomplish the curriculum's major goals (Gordon & Puglia, 1998). Concepts such as multicultural needs of both employees and clients can be explored at depth. Application of concepts to multiple levels of workers and to clients in different settings and from various backgrounds (Ingersoll, 1998) are also fostered in PBL.

Borrowing from Successes in Medicine and Dentistry

Medicine and dentistry are two academic disciplines immersed in PBL. Accrediting bodies for both disciplines have encouraged conversion of programs to PBL in an effort to produce professionals for whom lifelong learning is ingrained. McMaster University Medical School in Hamilton, Ontario, Canada, is generally considered to be the focal point for the revolution in PBL.

Case-Based Curriculum Designed to Foster a Disciplined, Lifelong Learner

Contextual learning through a case-based curriculum allows students to explore content within the framework of a situation. Problem-based learning is learner centered. A group of students are responsible for determining their own learning needs and ways to solve problems presented by the cases (Gordon & Puglia, 1998). The ability to think critically is learned in the process. Typical components of the process include data identification, analysis, hypothesis generation, research on areas of knowledge deficit, and so on. This looping process helps students narrow possibilities through logical processes in an attempt to resolve problems presented by the case. Refinement of a concept map that explains intricacies of relating issues in the case is an example of mental work done in the case-solving process. To sustain inquiry to this level, the case must generate a compelling need to know (Gordon & Puglia, 1998).

Using the Cohort Group Model to Foster Teamwork in Case Solving

Teamwork is hard work. Nurses have a history of avoiding conflict, which often is associated with teams. If a nurse knows that she or he will not have to work with a partner again for a period of time, it is easy to forgo the stress of dealing directly with conflicts and failed expectations. Bringing a cohort group of students together for PBL forces resolution of natural group conflict issues. The NA faculty takes on the roles of facilitator, coach, and mentor, but the students are forced to do the hard work of group process (Woods, 1994).

Evaluating individual and group performance is built into the PBL model at the end of every session. Students learn to hold one another accountable for assignments because the entire group is dependent on all members pulling their weight. Nursing students hate this dependency, whether it be of the PBL group or of their team members in their clinical leader roles. However, it is a vital workplace lesson that needs to be learned. How to resolve effectively and move through such inherent conflicts is a valuable lesson.

Involving Community Nursing Leaders as Experts

Partnering with community nursing leaders to write relevant cases and to serve as resident expert consultants to the student PBL group can help increase both the depth and breadth of an NA program. Having these nursing leaders available as external consultants to the PBL group fosters mentoring relationships that can last a lifetime.

Such connections with reality can be further strengthened by faculty who have practice obligations in addition to their teaching responsibilities. Faculty projects can involve students in real-life learning opportunities. Seeing faculty interact with nursing leaders as peer role models for students cannot be simulated in a case.

Building Real-Life Consultation Cases into the Curriculum at Intervals

Engagement of community nursing leaders in the education of future nursing leaders can serve both parties. Students can come into the community facility and collectively serve as

consultants, with faculty support, which provides a consultation role and process learning experience for students. Similarly, consultation cases provide valuable service to the institution receiving the consultation. New ideas and perspectives are infused into the organization—a plan can be devised and perhaps even implementation can be overseen. Such service-learning also teaches students the service ethic. Everyone wins by reaching out to a new model of relationship between academia and service. Town and gown distances can be bridged by such efforts.

Tomorrow's nursing leaders must know how to access and interpret data from real life scenarios. They must understand their data needs and be able to use spreadsheets for choosing from "what-if" options. Moreover, the future will demand skilled leaders who are linked to national databases such as that of the American Hospital Association and the nursing minimum data set that is in progress (Ludemann & Loveridge, 1992).

Integration of Outcome Research for Evidence-based Practice of Nursing Administration

An outcomes research model can be integrated into each case study. Students would identify research protocols and select outcome measures and data collection tools for each case. Under this model, accountability for measuring outcomes would be part of the NA role from the beginning.

Changing the Role of Faculty

Problem-based learning requires a fundamental change in the role of faculty. New skills must be learned if NA faculty are to facilitate student-centered learning. Faculty are not a source of content in PBL. Instead, faculty facilitate the small-group process, serve as one resource for student self-directed learning, provide one level of evaluation, generate learning objectives and context for learning (cases and the problems they represent) (Gordon & Puglia, 1998).

■ Concluding Statement

In this new millennium, only by changing our paradigm of nursing administration education can we hope to prepare leaders who will survive future challenges. Many of those challenges are unknown, but a leader who is flexible, is committed to lifelong learning, is a team player, and is a visionary can flourish in the midst of this uncertainty.

Such leaders can be developed only if we, as nursing administration faculties, are ready for change. We cannot continue in our traditional roles, isolated from action. We have to gain the very skills that have been outlined for NA students of the future. Problem-based learning is one learning environment that allows students and faculty to develop fully these survival skills.

■ References

American Association of Colleges of Nursing & American Organization of Nurse Executives. (1996). *The essentials of master's education for advanced practice nursing* [On-line]. Available: http://www.aacn.nche.edu/specproj/mastessn.htm.

American Association of Colleges of Nursing & American Organization of Nurse Executives. (1997). *Joint position statement on education for nurses in administrative roles* [On-line]. Available: http://www.aacn.nche.edu.

American Association of Colleges of Nursing & American Organization of Nurse Executives. (1998). Position statement: Education for nurses in administrative roles. *Journal of Professional Nursing, 14*(2), 127–129.

American Organization of Nurse Executives. (1999). AONE research priorities. [On-line]. Available: http://www.aone.org/priorities.htm.

Beyers, M. (1995). Is there a future for management? *Nursing Management, 26*(1), 24–25.

Davidhizar, R. (1995). Nurse administrator vulnerability. *Nursing Leadership Forum, 1*(4), 132–136.

Doerge, J., & Hagenow, N. (1995). Management restructuring: Toward a leaner organization. *Nursing Management, 26*(12), 32–37.

Feldman, H. R. (1995). Preparing the nurse executive of the future. *Nursing Leadership Forum, 1*(1), 18–22.

Fralic, M. F. (1993). The new era nurse executive: Centerpiece characteristics. *Journal of Nursing Administration, 23*(1), 7–8.

Goode, C., Lovett, M., Hayes, J. E., & Butcher, L. (1987). Use of research based knowledge in clinical practice. *Journal of Nursing Administration, 17*(12), 11–18.

Gordon, P. R., & Puglia, C. D. (1998). *An introduction to problem-based learning fundamentals for facilitators.* Philadelphia: Allegheny University of the Health Sciences.

Haynor, P. A. (1996). Revisioning graduate education in nursing administration: Preparation for a new paradigm. *Nursing Administration Quarterly, 20*(4), 59–70.

Haynor, P. A., & Wells, R. W. (1998). Will nursing administration programs survive in the 21st century? *Journal of Nursing Administration, 28*(1), 15–24.

Horsley, J. A., Crane, J., & Bingle, J. (1978). Research utilization as an organizational process. *Journal of Nursing Administration, 8*(7), 4–6.

Ingersoll, G. L. (1998). Organizational redesign: Changing educational needs of midlevel nurse administrators. *Journal of Nursing Administration, 28*(4), 13–16.

Laschinger, H. K., Foran, S., Jones, B., Perkin, K., & Bovan, P. (1993) Research utilization in nursing administration: A graduate learning experience. *Journal of Nursing Administration, 23*(2), 32–35.

Ludemann, R. S., & Loveridge, C. E. (1992). Trends in nursing administration graduate education. *Journal of Nursing Administration, 22*(11), 9–10.

Malloch, K. (1998). The demise of nursing administration graduate programs. *Journal of Nursing Administration, 28*(7/8), 14–15.

Minnick, A. (1998). Education in administration: Trends in MSN/MBA and MSN in nursing administration. *Journal of Nursing Administration, 28*(4), 57–62.

Nichols, L. M. (1992). Estimating the costs of underusing advanced practice nurses. *Nursing Economic$, 10*(5), 343–351.

Patronis Jones, R. A. (1994). Graduate education in nursing administration: Necessity or nicety for nurse-managed centers? *Journal of Nursing Administration, 24*(9), 13–14.

Scalzi, C. C., & Wilson, D. L. (1990). Empirically based recommendations for content of graduate nursing administration programs. *Nursing and Health Care, 11*(10), 522–525.

Woods, D. R. (1994). *Problem-based learning: How to gain the most from PBL.* Hamilton, Ontario, Canada: McMaster University.

■ Editor's Questions for Discussion

Discuss types of practical experiences that best prepare nursing administration students for entrepreneurial roles. How will the role of nursing administrators change at entry and middle management levels in the future? What factors will contribute to that change?

Debate the pros and cons of discipline-specific preparation for administration. Why have the profession, generally, and nursing education, specifically, been insufficiently supportive of NA programs? Why have organizational structures discounted MSN-prepared administrators? Why has it been difficult to sell the value of NA preparation and programs? Suggest some strategies for changing past beliefs to obtain positive results in nursing administration and practice.

How may clinical skills and business proficiency best be combined and emphasized in graduate programs? Should management content, such as financial management and personnel administration, be required for graduate students in clinical nursing programs? How should leadership content appropriate for undergraduates be differentiated from that required for graduate students? Can hospital administrators or nursing administrators or both expect nursing professionals to supervise and be responsible for unlicensed assistive personnel if the nursing professional has no or limited management preparation? How and to what extent are nursing administrators in various types of care institutions and educators collaborating for future preparation of nursing administrators?

Discuss the pros and cons of problem-based learning (PBL) models. Propose strategies to resolve potential problematic issues. Address the strengths and limitations of the PBL examples provided by M. Fisher. What criteria are essential for faculty, preceptors, and mentors in NA programs? How can faculty best be prepared as instructors for NA programs?

How do administrative program experiences and content advocated by M. Fisher differ from those of the past? What outcomes may result and what outcome measures should exist in administration programs? To what extent and how should NA students maintain their clinical background and skills while perfecting leadership and business skills?

How do M. Fisher's suggestions for program content pertain to those addressed by McClure (Chapter 62), Gerber (Chapter 57), and Conger (Chapter 58)? How does Kerfoot's vision (Chapter 75) match M. Fisher's predictions? What relationship exists between evidence-based practice in NA and the discussions by Deets and Choi (Chapter 34) and Titler (Chapter 35)? Identify how Porter-O'Grady's (Chapter 55) discussion about structures applies to M. Fisher's plea for evaluation and collaboration between service and education.

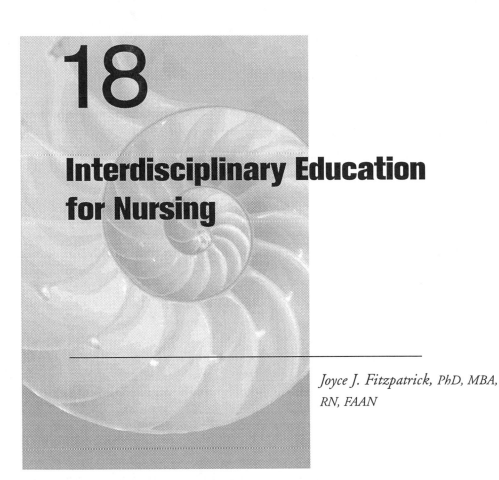

18

Interdisciplinary Education for Nursing

Joyce J. Fitzpatrick, PhD, MBA, RN, FAAN

Within the past decade, health care delivery has focused increasingly on managed care. Because this model of health care delivery is more likely to include a team approach, there has been a renewed call to interdisciplinary education within the health professions. This emphasis is strongly embedded in the several reports of the Pew Health Professions Commission published in the 1990s (Pew Health Professions Commission, 1991, 1993, 1995).

■ Definitions

Prior to a discussion of the key components of interdisciplinary education and practice, it is important to define the term. The literature lacks a clear definition of the term, and, in fact, the terms interdisciplinary, multidisciplinary, transdisciplinary, and interprofessional are often used interchangeably. In this chapter, my focus is on interdisciplinary education, and I use the following definitions.

- **Interdisciplinary:** The integration of contributions from members of two or more disciplines; often the disciplines have shared decision-making and shared goals. The collaboration among members of the disciplines may be in education, practice, or research.

- **Multidisciplinary:** Collaboration among members of two or more disciplines working toward parallel goals; the work, however, can be on the same project or issue or with the same patient or client.

• **Interprofessional:** Collaboration among members of two or more disciplines; the term is used to refer to collaboration in clinical practice.

• **Transdisciplinary:** Collaboration that goes beyond interdisciplinary or multidisciplinary collaboration in that the boundaries among the disciplines are blurred.

■ Levels in Interdisciplinary Practice

Levels in interdisciplinary practice have been elaborated in a model described by Huff and Garrola (1995). The ranges include "taking turns" in which nursing and medical students, faculty, or clinicians alternate in assuming responsibility for activities. Unfortunately, much of what currently occurs in interdisciplinary education is a process by which nursing and medical faculty members "take turns" and lecture to classes. Parallel learning may occur, and it is likely that the members will learn something about the other disciplines. The second level is one of collaboration and coordination of activities. There may be mutual shared goals for patient care or for student learning, but there is no depth of understanding of the other discipline's perspective. The third level is that of interdisciplinary or transdisciplinary education and practice, in which there are shared and mutual goals and in which the learning that occurs transforms that which could not have been possible without members of another discipline. Transdisciplinary work requires a merging of the disciplines and a blurring of disciplinary boundaries. Because of the lack of research, it is not clear what outcomes are expected, either in student learning or patient care.

■ History of Interdisciplinary Education and Interprofessional Team Practice

Baldwin (1996) summarized the long history of interprofessional team care, with particular emphasis on care delivered collaboratively by nurses and physicians. He traced the roots of collaborative care to that of the missionaries in India in the early 1900s. Later, following World War II, considerable efforts were made in Boston to deliver care to the chronically ill through teamwork among health professionals. However, the surge of interprofessional education and practice occurred in the 1960s through the 1980s when the federal government made funds available for collaboration. During the 1990s, with an increased emphasis on managed care as the preferred delivery model, there has been an increased emphasis on the need for interprofessional care and interdisciplinary education.

Specific benefits of team care have been documented: enhanced patient compliance and greater patient satisfaction (Bellin & Geiger, 1970); increased efficiency, less hospitalization, and reduced costs (Garfield et al., 1976); and a lower rate of broken appointments (Beloff & Korper, 1972). There is consensus in the literature that team practice is obtained through interdisciplinary education (Baldwin, 1996).

In the early 1990s, the American Association of Colleges of Nursing (AACN) appointed a task force to explore issues in interdisciplinary education. The position statement prepared by this group was adopted formally by the organization and made available to all member schools (American Association of Colleges of Nursing [AACN], 1996). The specific recommendations made for schools of nursing were broad and inclusive: (a) develop mechanisms for undergraduate and graduate students in all nursing programs to interact with students from a range of disciplines in the provision of health care; (b) establish mechanisms with other disciplines for joint planning and decision-making to identify shared content and clinical experiences; (c) collaborate with other health care disciplines to develop, implement, and evaluate models of interdisciplinary education; (d) seek opportunities to provide clinical experiences for interdisciplinary practice; and (e) conduct research to evaluate outcomes of interdisciplinary models of education and practice (AACN, 1996, pp. 121–122).

■ Recent Contributions

National League for Nursing Panel

Based on recommendations from a report delivered to the Institute of Medicine (IOM) as part of the IOM/American Academy of Nursing/American Nurses Foundation Scholars Program (Fitzpatrick, 1997), the National League for Nursing (NLN) commissioned a Panel on Interdisciplinary and Transdisciplinary Education. Members of the panel represented nursing, medicine, and allied health professions. A synopsis of its work was published as a report in key professional journals, but the primary report was published in the NLN journal, *Nursing and Health Care Perspectives* in 1997 (National League for Nursing [NLN], 1998). Significant aspects of the report included the delineation of underlying assumptions for interdisciplinary education and interprofessional practice and the core content that should be taught across disciplinary boundaries.

The following assumptions were outlined.

1. Interdisciplinary education is better served by a health, rather than a medical, model.

2. Learning together will lead to working together.

3. Learning together will enhance understanding of the problems and solutions.

4. Learning necessarily involves self-awareness and self-disclosure; a person must develop integrity that is both personal and professional.

5. Professionals have a responsibility for lifelong learning.

6. Professionals must accept responsibility and accountability for their own actions.

7. Professionals can learn to respect and trust people from other disciplines.

8. Models of authority do not foster relationship-centered practice.

9. Professional identity (collegiality) is strengthened by sharing and diversity.

10. Solutions should be need-based (demand-side rather than supply-side oriented).

11. Community building is a basic human need.

12. Professional service and stewardship is rooted in the principle of social justice. (NLN, 1998, pp. 2–3)

The panel identified core content to be taught across disciplinary boundaries. Further, its members asserted that, in teaching core content, values and process components (e.g., aspects of professional socialization) should be integrated. The panel recommended that the following skills and knowledge areas be included in interdisciplinary education: (a) behavioral sciences; (b) change and the change process; (c) common terminology; (e) community health; (f) death and dying; (g) ethics and values; (h) growth and development; (i) health assessment, health care systems, and health promotion and disease prevention; (j) interpersonal and communication skills; (k) relationship-centered care; (l) role theory, and (m) skills for community building (NLN, 1998).

■ Barriers to Interdisciplinary Education

The barriers to interdisciplinary education are many. They have been addressed repeatedly in the literature but most often have not been successfully overcome in attempts to sustain interdisciplinary education programs beyond the initial start-up funding stages. The disparities in educational background between physicians and nurses and unevenness in the power held by physicians in contrast to nurses in all aspects of health care delivery make it extremely difficult to build successful programs. This situation is further complicated by the considerable overlap among professional roles in care delivery, particularly between some subsets of physicians and advanced practice nurses. Given the historic tensions between nursing and medicine, current power balance, and perceived concerns about the future of health care, interdisciplinary education is difficult for academic administrators and faculty to support.

Faculty who engage in interdisciplinary education programs have not been rewarded. In fact, educational systems support disciplinary boundaries. In a study of health science programs that featured both nursing and medicine, only 5 of 35 respondents offered even one interdisciplinary course throughout the programs (Larson, 1995). Further, many faculty did not perceive any benefits to interdisciplinary teaching.

The summary of barriers to interdisciplinary education provided by the American Association of Colleges of Nursing (AACN) in its 1996 position statement is most helpful in grasping the extent of related issues. According to the AACN (1996), challenges may be philosophical and include (a) differences in commitment to interdisciplinary education; (b) lack of congruence in disciplinary goals and focus; (c) and lack of knowledge and valuing of other professions. These differences in philosophy provide the greatest challenges and barriers to interdisciplinary education. Barriers may also be sociological, including differences in gender and class between professions. Organizational barriers cited were (a) political factors within the schools and universities and differences in the sources of financing; (b) structural barriers identified included difficulties in scheduling and geographical separations; and (c) academic or professional problems, including issues of converging roles among members of different professional groups, need for faculty development, and lack of awareness of overall benefits of interdisciplinary education.

As with many other innovations in health professions education, there have not been many sustained programs in which innovations have been mainstreamed. Rather, often when the special outside funding is no longer available, programs revert to a preinnovative stage. Also, there are no clear rewards for participation in interdisciplinary education. And, importantly, there is little research of this approach that demonstrates overall positive outcomes for either student learning or patient care.

■ Benefits of Interdisciplinary Education

The core component of interdisciplinary learning is to bring the best understandings from more than one discipline to a more comprehensive and holistic perspective of the issue or problem being addressed. Learners are encouraged to share their perspectives and gain insights from the perspectives of their colleagues from other disciplines. The trust required in the teaching–learning process is extremely important; there is no room for political turf battles. Nursing education has been focused on defining the disciplinary boundaries in education, research, and practice. This intense inward focus—so necessary in positioning the nursing discipline for key roles in society—interferes with opportunities to implement interdisciplinary education.

Interdisciplinary education between nurses and physicians most often has been implemented in community-based settings. During the past two decades the W. K. Kellogg Foundation has supported a number of educational programs focused on interprofessional practice, with community involvement at all levels of teaching and learning. Projects involving both medical students and students from other professions have been supported for undergraduate and graduate education in nursing. Zungolo (1994) described the challenges in implementing such programs, despite the strong funding and support offered through foundation support. Among the barriers Zungolo identified are (a) attention to the comprehensive differences between nursing and medical education in philosophy and structure, (b) the respective place of nursing and medicine in higher education, and (c) differences between the learners.

■ *Future Opportunities and Challenges*

Several opportunities exist for demonstrating the benefits of interdisciplinary education. As health care delivery continues its transformation to more efficient and effective care, with higher quality and lower costs, leaders in the health professions will increase the search for new ways of teaching and learning.

Also, the fundamental shift of priorities from acute care institutions to community-based settings and managed care models of service delivery, will exert additional pressure on clinicians to function as members of interprofessional teams. Service priorities may then shift the focus in both medical and nursing education toward more collaborative and interdisciplinary programs, courses, and clinical experiences.

An example of an educational innovation that enhances interdisciplinary education is the recent "service-learning" models of education for health professionals. In these projects, students from nursing, medicine, or any of the other health professions commit to an extended learning project within a community targeted to achieve community-defined health goals. The educational focus is on helping students develop critical thinking skills and learning values focused on sensitivity to the needs of others different from themselves.

■ *Concluding Statement*

Health professionals must be responsive to the needs of patients and society and must be open to interprofessional models of care to achieve enhanced patient and community health outcomes. We must be prepared to set aside traditional disciplinary concerns and engage in creative dialogue with members of other professional groups. In this chapter the primary emphasis in the discussion of interdisciplinary education has been on collaboration between nurses and physicians, as these two professional groups are viewed as the core of health care delivery. There are many opportunities to extend principles of interdisciplinary education beyond the two core groups. Yet, leaders in nursing education cannot accomplish the goals of interdisciplinary education alone. There must be a commitment and willing collaboration among all partners.

■ *References*

American Association of Colleges of Nursing. (1996). Position statement on interdisciplinary education and practice. *Journal of Professional Nursing, 12,* 119–123.

Baldwin, D. C. (1996). Some historical notes on interdisciplinary and interprofessional education and practice in health care in the USA. *Journal of Interprofessional Care, 10,* 173–187.

Bellin, S. S., & Geiger, H. J. (1970). Actual public acceptance of the neighborhood health center by the urban poor. *Journal of the American Medical Association, 214,* 2147–2153.

Beloff, J. S., & Korper, M. (1972). The health team model and medical care utilization. *Journal of the American Medical Association, 219,* 359–366.

Fitzpatrick, J. J. (1997). Interdisciplinary education for primary health care: Report on the American Academy of Nursing/Institute of Medicine/American Nurses Foundation Scholars Program. Unpublished paper.

Garfield, S. R., Collen, M. F., Feldman, R., Soghikian, K., Richart, R., & Duncan, J. (1976). Evaluation of an ambulatory medical care delivery system. *New England Journal of Medicine, 294,* 426–431.

Huff, F., & Garrola, G. (1995). Potential patterns. *Journal of Allied Health, 25,* 359–397.

Larson, E. (1995). New rules for the game: Interdisciplinary education for health professionals. *Nursing Outlook, 43,* 180–183.

National League for Nursing. (1998). *Building community: Developing skills for interprofessional health professions education and relationship-centered care.* New York: Author.

Pew Health Professions Commission. (1991). *Healthy America: Practitioners for 2005.* San Francisco: Center for Health Professions.

Pew Health Professions Commission. (1993). *Health professions education for the future: Schools in service to the nation.* San Francisco: Center for Health Professions.

Pew Health Professions Commission. (1995). *Critical challenges: Revitalizing the health professions for the 21st century.* San Francisco: Center for Health Professions.

Zungolo, E. (1994). Interdisciplinary education: The challenge. *Nursing and Health Care, 15,* 288–292.

■ *Editor's Questions for Discussion*

To what extent has the third level of interdisciplinary education and practice been attained between nursing and medicine? What strategies may be employed, particularly in academic health centers, to increase interdisciplinary practice? What effect has managed care had on interdisciplinary practice? Provide specific examples.

How might interdisciplinary education be increased? How do nursing accreditation requirements affect implementing interdisciplinary education policies and practices?

What specific core content is beneficial across disciplinary boundaries? What qualifications are essential for teaching such core content?

Provide examples of overlap in professional roles in care delivery. How might such overlap be diminished via interdisciplinary education? What specific strategies might be implemented to reduce interdisciplinary education barriers? How might innovations in health professions education be sustained?

How does nursing's focus on positioning the discipline for key roles interfere with opportunities to facilitate interdisciplinary education? How might balance, compromise, and negotiation be encouraged between nursing and medicine for interdisciplinary education? What specific strategies may result in valuing interdisciplinary practice?

19

Global Perspectives on Graduate Nursing Education

Opportunities and Challenges

Shake Ketefian, EdD, RN, FAAN
Richard W. Redman, PhD, RN

Graduate education in nursing has been the subject of much attention in recent years. This attention has been due to transformations occurring in health care and the need for nursing to ensure that personnel are prepared appropriately to respond to societal needs. The purpose of this chapter is to take a global view of graduate nursing education, both at the master's and doctoral levels, determine emerging trends in the preparation of nurses at the graduate level, and identify issues and directions for the future.

■ Background

In discussions of graduate education we must contend with the basic education provided for nursing practice, on which graduate education ostensibly builds. However, it is clear that great variation in the educational systems exists across countries of the world. In some countries, basic nursing education is obtained at the university level; in others, at regional colleges, college preparatory programs, vocational schools, upper or lower years of secondary schools, or possibly, at the primary school level.

The authors would like to express appreciation to many international colleagues who provided information and insight on graduate education in their respective countries.

219

As space does not permit delineation of this issue, we simply recognize that a common foundation of basic nursing education cannot be assumed. It does appear, however, that various countries have systems and requirements in place on which graduate education for advanced practice or other roles can be built. Therefore in this chapter we are concerned with graduate level preparation only (in some countries referred to as postgraduate education).

■ The Framework and Conceptions of Graduate Education

We have taken a descriptive approach in this chapter. We present information gleaned from various regions of the world on the aims of graduate education, components and structure of the curriculum, and roles for which graduates are prepared. Due to the paucity of international literature related to conceptions of graduate education, we use approaches described in the U.S. literature as the starting point in delineating frameworks. It is not our intention to use these approaches as yardsticks for evaluating graduate education in other countries. Rather, we present them as starting points to provide a context for discussion. Variations can then be noted and unique features identified in different parts of the world.

Master's Degree Education

Concerns with regard to nursing education at the graduate level involve societal needs, competencies, outcomes to be achieved—both intellectual and clinical—and quality. The American Association of Colleges of Nursing (AACN) (1996) undertook a study of master's education with the aim of developing "a more coherent and consistent set of curricular standards" (p. 2). We utilize the report by AACN and its supplement as the basis for a framework for master's degree education.

The central thesis originally advanced is that "the primary focus of the master's education program should be the clinical role" (AACN, 1996, p. 3). This assertion was later amended to address the advanced content needed to prepare nurses for administrative responsibilities (AACN, 1997). The curricular model proposed to achieve this advanced practice focus includes three components.

1. *Nursing core, general:* This content is the foundation for all master's students regardless of specialty chosen. It includes research; policy, organization, and financing of health care; health policy; organization of health care delivery; financing; ethics; role development; theoretical foundations; human diversity and social issues; health promotion and illness prevention.

2. *Advanced nursing core:* This content is intended to provide direct advanced clinical services (advanced health assessment; advanced physiology, and pathophysiology; and advanced pharmacology) or administration of nursing services (leadership, continuous quality improvement, strategic management, and financial management).

3. *Specialty curriculum:* This content comprises learning experiences defined by specialty nursing organizations. (AACN, 1996, pp. 4–5; AACN, 1997)

Doctoral Education

The AACN has spearheaded development of quality indicators for nursing doctoral programs, which we utilize as the framework for doctoral education in this chapter. The document addresses six areas (AACN, 1993).

1. *Faculty:* Qualifications, scholarly activities of faculty, their ability to provide mentorship, intellectual diversity of views.

2. *Programs of study:* Philosophy of science, substantive nursing knowledge, analytic and leadership skills, research methods, guided independent study and research experiences; nature of core content; cognate studies in

related fields; role development to support career goals.

3. *Resources:* Availability of human, financial, library, equipment, clinical, technical and other resources and supports.

4. *Students:* Admission criteria; congruence between student goals and faculty research; involvement in active scholarship.

5. *Research:* A component of institutional mission; sufficient support for faculty and student research; development of programs of research; critical mass of research to support doctoral student experiences.

6. *Evaluation:* Comprehensive evaluation plan, both in terms of educational process and outcomes (AACN, 1993, pp. 1–4).

■ International Graduate Education: Locating Data

As there is no comprehensive, current directory of international nursing graduate programs, alternative approaches were utilized in making contacts and seeking information relevant to this chapter. For several years one of the authors, S. Ketefian, has been maintaining and updating a list of international doctoral programs. Key individuals from this list were contacted for information. This "invisible college" approach was augmented by contacts made during several international conferences where presentations were made on specific graduate programs. In addition, a manual search of recent issues of international journals was conducted for topic-relevant writings and authors were contacted via mail or electronic mail. What we present in this chapter reflects the results of these efforts. Unfortunately, the information yield is uneven. For some regions or countries we obtained sufficient material while for other regions the information is scant. We believe that this disparity reflects in part the state of nursing literature across countries, and in part indicates the number of individuals in a country who are working scholars that are writing and reporting their work in internationally circulated publications.

In the next section, we describe graduate education by regions of the world and focus on countries from which information was available.

■ Graduate Education in Regions of the World

Africa

Egypt

Egypt has a number of master's degree programs preparing individuals in specialized areas of nursing, administration, or education. Typically, 2 years of study are required, with the first year devoted to coursework and the second year to research. The majority of graduates enter teaching careers, as the advanced practice role has not yet been developed there. Some graduates seek administrative or management positions. The curriculum includes core, specialty, and related courses. Egypt has seven doctoral programs; these lead to careers in the nursing specialties, teaching, or administration of education or nursing service programs. Coursework is not specified; students conduct research. A number of these institutions collaborate with universities in other countries and appoint a faculty member from overseas to participate in supervising doctoral students; in some cases, students are able to travel to the country of the international mentor for short-term research experiences. Students prepare dissertations as a requirement for graduation.

South Africa

Fourteen schools in South Africa are thought to offer nursing preparation at the master's degree level, with nine offering doctoral degrees in nursing (Beukes, 1995). Doctoral programs are highly individualized, are intended to meet the needs of the country and those of nurse leaders who are expected to make original contributions to knowledge. The format for study varies; for example, at the University of South Africa, distance education is the mode, whereby students reside in their home country and obtain supervision long-distance, with a cosupervisor appointed closer to the student's location. In other institutions supervision is obtained from the university faculty. Beukes (1995) maintains that master's and doctoral prepared nurses make major contributions in generating relevant research and in contributing to health care innovations.

The Americas

Brazil

Brazil offers 13 master's degree programs in clinical areas. The advanced practice role is implemented in major hospitals in large health centers; some of these individuals also function in health policy roles. The typical curriculum involves 1 year of coursework concerned with nursing research, theories, and clinical concepts, and 1 year devoted to thesis work. Eight doctoral programs are offered and are intended to prepare individuals for leadership positions in research and teaching, although some function in clinical roles as well. The program involves approximately 2 years of coursework and an equal amount of time for dissertation work. Both master's and doctoral candidates have one major professor supervising their research.

Canada

Master's programs in Canada focus on advanced nursing practice—preparing individuals for clinical roles—although some programs focus on research—preparing individuals for investigative work—and view this level

of study as laying the foundation for doctoral study. Students may elect a thesis or a nonthesis option. The elements of the program are nursing core, advanced practice core, specialty core, and elective. Doctoral programs are intended to prepare individuals for knowledge development. Those programs are flexible as to number and type of courses required; students write a dissertation. There are six programs, two of which are collaboratively developed and taught.

United States

Master's degree education in the United States began at the turn of the 20th century and was intended to prepare educators and managers. Master's degree programs have gone through many phases since then, as a result of changes in educational systems and health care needs. Currently, the overwhelming trend is to prepare individuals for advanced nursing practice, as clinical specialists or as nurse practitioners. Some institutions have consolidated these roles into a single advanced practice role; more and more individuals are moving into community health settings, though others continue working in acute or chronic care facilities. The curriculum typically comprises the elements proposed by AACN, described previously (AACN, 1996). Some institutions require a master's thesis; others offer options.

Seventy-two institutions are offering 74 doctoral programs in nursing. Over 75% of these programs grant the Doctor of Philosophy (PhD) degree; the remaining are professional degrees, such as Doctor of Nursing Science (DNS, DNSc) and Doctor of Education (EdD). The curricular components are research and theory in substantive nursing subjects, research methods and design, theory building and philosophy of science, cognate studies in related fields, supervised research practicums, one or more research projects, and a dissertation. The graduates of doctoral programs are expected to be leaders in their respective areas; graduates teach, conduct research, lead or direct health-related enterprises, and function in a variety of settings, including the policy arena, private businesses, and the like.

Asia

China

Currently, there are 10 State Education Committee approved master's degree programs in nursing. The focus of these programs is education or administration, with some clinical practice. Advanced practice roles have not yet been developed in China; specialized and general nursing care are provided by registered nurses prepared at the basic level. Graduates of master's degree programs are hired as teachers of nursing. Courses required at the graduate level include English and politics, with other requirements or electives varying across institutions.

Republic of China (Taiwan)

Several master's degree programs are offered. Advanced practice roles have not yet been developed; thus graduates go into education, teaching, research, or management. Those desiring to remain in practice hold regular staff nurse positions, similar to nurses without graduate degrees. Taiwan has one doctoral program (PhD), which is in its first year of operation; the program follows the pattern of education in the United States, which includes advanced nursing theory and research, cognate studies in other fields, and a supervised dissertation. Achieving integration of clinical practice, education, and research is a special focus of the program, as this particular institution has a system whereby faculty hold joint appointments within the university hospital.

Japan

A number of master's degree programs are offered in Japan, focusing on research, theory development, and, increasingly, specialization with a thesis requirement. Three doctoral programs are offered, with minimal coursework focused on individually supervised research.

Korea

Twenty-three universities offer master's degree programs, nine of which also offer doctoral programs. Master's degree study involves extensive work in theory development in nursing, research, statistics, study in a specialization (usually without a clinical component), and a thesis. The advanced practice role is not fully developed, although some institutions require the master's degree for mid-level managerial positions. Nurse specialists are certified in kidney transplantation and in psychiatric nursing. Graduates assume teaching positions within universities.

Philippines

There are several master's degree programs with a thesis requirement; graduates assume teaching roles, as advanced practice has not yet been developed. One institution offers the PhD degree in nursing, which is similar in design to those in the United States.

Thailand

Five master's degree programs and five doctoral programs are offered. These programs prepare individuals in a variety of clinical specialties and to function in roles as educator, administrator, or clinical specialist (which is a newly emerging role). Some institutions prepare nurses for public health nursing—in some cases within faculties of public health. In addition, some universities offer special international master's degree programs to assist other countries in meeting their needs. The curriculum comprises core, specialty, and related studies and allows a thesis or nonthesis option. Nearly a decade ago doctoral education (DNS) was offered through a collaborative program involving four institutions with governmental funding. Freestanding doctoral programs now are being developed. Collaborative relationships are being established with institutions within the United States, to have American faculty on some student committees or to enable students to spend short periods of time on other campuses for enrichment and exposure to research-intensive environments.

Doctoral programs prepare scholars and scientists to provide leadership in various areas of nursing and health care. In some settings students may choose between a thesis-only approach, whereby they conduct research during the course of the program, or an option that combines coursework and thesis.

Australia

Master's degree programs offer a number of choices to students. These choices include master's by coursework, master's mainly by coursework with a "minor" thesis in the final year, and a master's with a dissertation that is literature-based but not research-based. Students select a strand, with a management, education, or clinical focus. Graduates hold clinical consultant roles whereby they carry a patient load, consult with nurses, serve as preceptor for students, or might carry out clinical research. Distance education is widely available to serve rural areas of the country or international students who continue residing in their countries.

Australia has 36 universities, all of which may admit and award PhD degrees; however, only 12 of these institutions currently seem to provide this level of training. Similar to tradition in the United Kingdom, there is no coursework; rather, a student works independently, under supervision of a mentor and writes a thesis. In the past several years, a view emerged that focusing on a single piece of research and a single method is too narrow and not responsive to the broad range of responsibilities doctoral graduates are expected to fulfill. Thus several institutions have developed the Doctor of Nursing degree, wherein students are expected to develop a broad range of preparation in both subject matter and methodology through the portfolio approach. This method requires students to contribute to knowledge more broadly and assemble evidence of their learning, reflection, and advanced practice activities in multiple ways (Borbasi, Pearson, & Gott, 1998). The degree requires 3 years of full-time study or 5 years of part-time study; students come to campus twice a year for a week of intensive coursework with faculty and visiting scholars, enabling interaction with international faculty and peers.

Europe

Hamrin (1997) indicated that there are now 51 countries in Europe, but in the majority of them, nursing is not an academic discipline. Hamrin reported on the status of doctoral education in 10 of those countries. Some require doctoral level coursework, but others do not. In many cases, work was interdisciplinary (course and supervision), and nursing was embedded in medical, social science, or other departments. In other cases, nursing studies occurred within a department of nursing or caring sciences. Public defense of the dissertation or publication of a thesis in book form were expectations of the programs.

European Network for Doctoral Nursing Programs

Eleven European nursing programs have developed a "taught" component, whereby participating doctoral students study together in intensive workshops that address a European perspective to research. The workshops are of 2 weeks duration the first year and 1 week during years two and three (Crow, 1998).

Belgium

A number of nursing master's degree and doctoral programs are offered. Master's degree study requires 3 years full-time, with a focus in one of several clinical areas. Students carry out small-scale clinical projects. Doctoral study in Belgium historically has consisted of independent, individually supervised study; more recently, coursework elements have been added. Some institutions have developed strategies that link master's theses to doctoral dissertations (Evers, 1995).

The Netherlands

The master's degree was first initiated through international collaboration; subsequently, the country established master's and doctoral degree offerings at several universities. An interesting feature in this case is that development of graduate studies occurred in tandem with concerted efforts to develop nursing research (Diepeveen-Speekenbrink, 1992).

Nordic Countries

Historically, graduate-level preparation in the Nordic countries has focused on educator and administrator roles; more recently, programs focused on nursing science have been receiving emphasis. Three universities in Norway provide master's degree and doctoral education in nursing; six universities in Finland offer graduate education, including master's-level clinical specialties. In Denmark and Sweden nurses may obtain doctoral preparation in several colleges and schools ("faculties") within universities. In Iceland a master's degree in nursing science is offered. Clinical specializa-

tion in Nordic countries is obtained within hospitals, following basic nursing studies. However, these courses are not counted toward graduate degrees for those pursuing that level of education; nurse clinicians prepared at the graduate level are expected to promote research and assist in developing the expertise of other nurses (Lorensen, Jones, & Hamilton, 1998).

In Norway, master's degree study in nursing science, education, and administration is offered over a 3-year period; an additional 3 years of work is required for a doctoral degree in nursing science. One avenue of doctoral study requires 200 hours of work and an advisor. A second avenue allows the student to study alone, with or without an advisor, prepare a thesis, and present it to the faculty of choice (Lorensen, Jones, & Hamilton, 1998).

United Kingdom (U.K.)

Within the United Kingdom, primary care (general) practitioners are educated at the diploma level, whereas specialist practitioners (e.g., psychiatric nurses) are educated at the degree level (baccalaureate); all are recognized by the regulatory body. There are now calls for advanced practice roles for which individuals are to be prepared at the master's degree or doctoral level; graduates would possess a complex set of competencies and fulfil multiple roles (e.g., expert practitioner, educator, researcher, or consultant) (Manley, 1997).

Nurses desiring to prepare for educational roles obtain a master's degree in education, and those preparing for management roles obtain a degree in management, such as an MBA. Within nursing, there are several avenues to attain a master's degree. One such is a research master's degree (MRes), which has coursework elements; another degree titled master's of philosophy (MPhil) does not have coursework but the student is examined on a 20,000 word thesis. The last option requires one year of full-time study (or two years of part-time study).

Graduates with these degrees seek academic positions teaching and conducting research. It is possible to obtain a master of science (MSc) in advanced practice; graduates seek careers in practice settings as managers or clinical leaders.

More than 30 universities in the United Kingdom may award the PhD degree to nurses, although how many of these institutions have enrolled students is unknown. As the PhD is a "research" degree, institutions need not have in place a formally approved doctoral program. Students spend 3 years full-time or 5 years part-time conducting their research under faculty supervision; faculty may be drawn from the social sciences, nursing, or medicine. No courses or examinations are required, although students attend some research seminars. The student writes a 100,000 word thesis, which is expected to make a contribution to the subject under consideration.

Recently, concern has been expressed that the PhD degree does not deal with practice issues and the substantive concerns of nursing. Thus the doctor of nursing science degree (DNSc) has emerged; it is a "taught" degree involving coursework. The degree focuses on nursing practice, theory, and research. Some institutions offer both the DNSc and the PhD degrees (McKenna, 1997).

■ Issues and Trends

A number of issues and trends are apparent in the development and evolution of international nursing graduate education. They present both challenges and opportunities, examples of which are presented in the following section.

Diversity of Approaches

The picture of international graduate education that has emerged is clear. There is much variation in the way different countries provide this level of preparation and in how graduates

of such programs are utilized. Both preparation and utilization are a function of a country's health needs and the state of nursing development in that country. We have wondered previously about the desirability or feasibility of standardizing graduate education (Redman & Ketefian, 1997) in view of the global community that is emerging. Yet, it has become clear that standardization, though desirable at some level, is neither feasible nor realistic at this time. Nursing education is an integral part of educational systems; in view of existing differences in educational patterns, standardizing graduate education would be well nigh impossible to achieve. Yet, with the movement of nurses across national boundaries for practice, modalities need to be found for identifying common ground and for better interpreting educational systems across countries. This task might require flexibility in thinking on everyone's part and recognition that knowledge and expertise can be gained through different means and methods.

Some of the variations noted in graduate education can be accounted for by the degree to which organizational, scientific, and related infrastructures in various settings are sufficient to support science development and scientifically oriented graduate education. In some countries, technological resources may be rich, whereas scientific, labor force, and nursing infrastructure may still be under development.

Diversity in Roles of Graduates

At the master's degree level, many countries are utilizing graduates as educators, and thus the type of education these individuals receive would need to reflect the educator role they fulfil upon graduation. Countries need to be aware of other roles that graduates may accept and develop curricula preparing persons to meet those needs. Advanced practice roles, such as clinical specialist and nurse practitioner, are newly emerging in many countries, and their utilization in health facilities is just beginning. In countries where there is no shortage of physicians, the nurse practitioner role has not developed. Further, the clinical specialist role and preparation for it has emerged in ways that are most responsive to the needs of a particular country.

At the doctoral level, there also are major variations in the conduct and delivery of education, program content, and the functions and roles that graduates serve. Two basic patterns could be noted: (a) the "European model" of doctoral education, which is obtained mainly through individually supervised research; and (b) the "North American model," which combines coursework with research and a dissertation. Variations of these models are emerging in many countries, tailored to meet local needs. In some countries, the PhD degree is sufficiently flexible to meet various goals, as in PhD study in the United States, where investigation of clinically relevant nursing problems and generation of knowledge for patient care is a clear direction. In other countries, the PhD degree is viewed as nonresponsive to patient problems, with the result that alternative doctoral degrees are being developed to address this unmet need. In many countries PhD-prepared individuals are pursuing academic careers; in some countries, such as the United States, PhD-prepared faculty are expected to contribute directly to nursing science. In other regions of the world this role may not be an expectation, with the result that these individuals either are not conducting research or may be engaged in research with no relevance to nursing practice. Therefore it would be fair to say that the AACN quality indicators do not provide guidance that is universally relevant. It behooves each country and institution offering doctoral degrees to have expressly stated criteria for evaluating the success of its programs in a manner that has validity for the setting of concern.

Continuing development of doctoral graduates into mature scientists is an issue in some countries; this concern has led to development of postdoctoral training. However, that level of training may neither be feasible nor realistic in other settings. Some countries are establishing collaborative relationships with others to provide postdoctoral training in their areas of need. This type of collaboration is clearly the order of the day, and this trend is noted both within and between countries and institutions. Significantly, much informal networking and interaction is taking place among individuals; networking opportunities are being made available through groups such as the Global Network of World Health Organization (WHO) Collaborating Centers for Nursing and Midwifery Development and the International Network for Doctoral Education in Nursing, among others. International research by scientists in different nations is another potential area for collaboration. Some projects of this kind exist, and the benefits of increasing these opportunities can be both rich and mutual.

Faculty Preparation

In many countries individuals prepared at the graduate level tend to be recruited to teach; yet severe shortages of faculties continue. Faculty responsibilities in some instances are so onerous that conducting nursing research to enlarge the body of knowledge and to address needs of patient populations is not feasible. Questions that could not be addressed in this chapter are: To what extent do international graduate programs focus on the education of the student? and To what extent is there systematic effort to have graduate student research address socially relevant and beneficial health concerns? Answers to these questions can lead to desirable goals, and the deliberate merging of these goals can meet important societal needs for research while training individuals at the graduate level.

Historically, many countries have hosted international students who travel to obtain graduate education. Funding constraints are making this option more difficult. At the same time, a growing number of institutions are offering courses and degrees through distance learning technologies, which can be accessed from any location; however, the extent to which systematic use is being made of such opportunities is not known at this time.

Collaborative Partnerships

Complexities of societal problems today often require collaborative solutions that bring institutions together as equal partners. In the United States, many partnerships have developed between communities and educational institutions to build on assets, strengths, and capacities of each to address health professions education, health care delivery, research, communitywide health improvement, and economic development in communities. This model of equal partners also has begun to develop between schools of nursing in the United States and international nursing education programs. These partnerships have provided opportunities such as student and faculty exchanges, curriculum development and implementation, and collaborative research programs.

International collaborative efforts in nursing are essential to knowledge development and the examination of issues related to provision of culturally competent care (Ketefian & Redman, 1997; Meleis & Regev, 1995). The development of partnerships among schools of nursing around the world are an important step in addressing issues specific to nursing. These partnerships face many challenges, however, including economic constraints, institutional barriers, and political obstacles. In addition, faculty perspectives and values that foster local versus international frameworks and priorities also present challenges to the development of collaborative efforts (Meleis & Regev, 1995).

Technology Infrastructure

Advances in technology open collaborative opportunities between nursing educational programs in the United States and their counterparts in other countries. Yet, the technology infrastructure varies considerably. Use of interactive video technologies is dependent on the fiber-optic infrastructure available in a given location. For many parts of the world, this technology simply is not available for routine instructional purposes. Where it is available, cost and scheduling challenges often make it a less than reliable medium for routine use.

Although the Internet is available globally, this medium also presents many challenges. The university-based educational community throughout the world is one of the sectors more likely to have access to the Internet. However, this access is both variable and somewhat unreliable. Using electronic mail as a communication device is probably the most feasible application of the technology at present.

Comprehensive Listings of Educational Programs

An on-line source of potential information is Healthweb (http://healthweb.org), which provides access to health care information on the World Wide Web. This collaborative project collects and organizes on-line resources in 77 allied health care and medical specialties, one of which is nursing. Within that section, current lists of nursing education programs are provided, some of which are international nursing education programs. Another directory within the nursing section provides a list of nursing education programs with on-line offerings. Healthweb is also developing a directory of international doctoral programs in nursing.

International Nursing Literature

A variety of resources are available for accessing the international nursing literature.

This literature is varied, but it provides an index to the level of organization of the nursing community, both academic and clinical, within a country. The International Nursing Index (2000), available through the National Library of Medicine's Medline (2000), provides routine indexing of an extensive array of international nursing journals. In 1999, 109 nursing journals from countries other than the United States were listed in the International Nursing Index. Another source of international nursing literature is the African Index Medicus (AIM) project, maintained by the World Health Organization's library (2000). This initiative was begun by WHO because few African health and biomedical information sources are included in the world's leading bibliographic databases.

■ Concluding Statement

Different factors have influenced both the development and direction of international graduate education in nursing. The impetus for health care reform appears to be present in many regions of the world. Systemic planning for health needs of a population is linked inextricably to consideration of type, quality, and credentials of health care personnel, including nurses. In addition, the AIDS epidemic has altered the social fabric fundamentally in many countries and has influenced the way nursing is taught and practiced.

Interest and involvement of several major foundations have contributed significantly to the development of graduate nursing education internationally. Foundation support has been provided in the form of fellowships for personnel training overseas, initiation of graduate programs, ongoing faculty development, consultations, and the like.

The Fulbright program is being utilized increasingly by nurses; although the program is not yet widely used, the impact of individual visiting scholars through it and other arrangements and exchanges is being felt both by host schools and individual visitors.

Exchanges of nurse scholars, institutional partnerships, individuals providing consultations are occurring to an unprecedented degree across national boundaries. Opportunities are being created thereby for mutual learning and sharing. Nurses who provide consultation and advice to international colleagues and institutions are challenged in their task by multiple imponderables inherent in settings which are unfamiliar; the need for the exercise of cultural sensitivity and competence has never been greater.

Progress in graduate nursing education in the past decade has been unprecedented. Much remains to be done, however because the health and nursing personnel needs of many countries are great. The types of collaboration whereby individuals and institutions take initiatives and begin in small steps with limited resources are significant and clearly are having impact. We hope that such collaborative activities will continue and expand in the future.

■ *References*

American Association of Colleges of Nursing. (1993). *Indicators of quality in doctoral programs in nursing.* Washington, DC: Author.

American Association of Colleges of Nursing. (1996). *The essentials of master's education for advanced practice nursing.* Washington, DC: Author.

American Association of Colleges of Nursing. (1997). *Joint position statement on nursing administration education: Supplement to the essentials of master's education for advanced practice nursing.* Washington, DC: Author.

Association for Health Information and Libraries in Africa (AHILA) & World Health Organization. (2000). *African Index Medicus.* [On-line]. Available: http://www.who.int/hlt/countrysup/aim/english/aime.htm

Beukes, M. (1995, June). Doctoral programs in South Africa: Issues and challenges. In S. Ketefian (Ed.), *Generating nursing science in the global community. Proceedings of the 1995 annual forum on doctoral education in nursing* (pp. 37–52). Ann Arbor: University of Michigan, School of Nursing.

Borbasi, S., Pearson, A., & Gott, M. (1998). Rethinking the single topic, single method approach to the PhD thesis: Moving towards research training that accommodates and values the innovation in the world of practice. In T. W. Maxwell & P. J. Shanahan (Eds.), *Professional doctorates: Innovations in teaching and research* (pp. 67–74). University of New England, New South Wales, Australia.

Crow, R. (1998, November). *European network for doctoral nursing programmes.* Paper presented at the Second International Conference on Expanding Boundaries of Nursing Education Globally, Pattaya, Thailand.

Diepeveen-Speekenbrink, J. C. M. H. (1992). Nursing science in the Netherlands: The Utrecht contribution. *Journal of Advanced Nursing, 17,* 1361–1368.

Evers, G. C. M. (1995). Graduate education at Catholic University of Leuven, Belgium: Scientific organizing framework. Issues and challenges. In S. Ketefian (Ed.), *Generating nursing science in the global community. Proceedings of the 1995 annual forum on doctoral education in nursing* (pp. 53–58). Ann Arbor: University of Michigan, School of Nursing.

Hamrin, E. (1997, June). *Models of doctoral education in Europe.* Paper presented at the First Meeting of the International Network of Doctoral Education in Nursing, Vancouver, BC, Canada. [On-line]. Available: http://www.umich.edu/~inden.

Ketefian, S., & Redman, R. W. (1997). Nursing science in the global community. *IMAGE: Journal of Nursing Scholarship, 29*(1), 11–15.

Lorensen, M., Jones, D. E., & Hamilton, G. A. (1998). Advanced practice nursing in Nordic countries. *Journal of Clinical Nursing, 7,* 257–264.

Manley, K. (1997). A conceptual framework for advanced practice: An action research project operationalizing an advanced practitioner/consultant nurse role. *Journal of Clinical Nursing, 6,* 179–190.

McKenna, H. (1997, June). *The mission and substance of doctoral education in nursing.* Paper presented at the First Meeting of the International Network of Doctoral Education in Nursing, Vancouver, BC, Canada. [On-line]. Available: http://www.umich.edu/~inden.

Meleis, A., & Regev, H. (1995, June). Strategies for international collaboration: A challenge to doctoral nursing education. In S. Ketefian (Ed.), *Generating nursing science in the global community. Proceedings of the 1995 annual forum on doctoral education in nursing* (pp. 91–100). Ann Arbor: University of Michigan, School of Nursing.

National Institute of Health. (2000). National Library of Medicine Medline [On-line]. Available: http://www.nlm.nih.gov/databases/freemedl.html.

Redman, R.W., & Ketefian, S. (1997). The changing face of graduate education. In J. C. McCloskey & H. K. Grace (Eds.), *Current issues in nursing* (pp. 160–168). St. Louis: Mosby-Year Book.

U.S. National Library of Medicine. (2000). *International Nursing Index* [On-line]. Available: http://www.aker.uio.no/Biblioteket/tidsskrift/tb332.htm.

U.S. National Library of Medicine. (2000). *MEDLINE (Medical Literature, Analysis, and Retrieval System Online)* [On-line]. Available: http://www.nlm.nih.gov/databases/freemedl.html.

■ Editor's Questions for Discussion

How are quality indicators operationalized for doctoral programs? What additional or other criteria indicate high-quality doctoral programs in nursing? To what extent are there collaborative graduate programs with other universities or disciplines internationally and in the United States? What criteria should be used in developing collaborative models?

How are faculty recruited for graduate programs internationally? What types of research are conducted in international programs? How does that research compare in quality and subject matter to research conducted in U.S. programs? How applicable are internal nursing research findings applicable to nursing practice globally?

How appropriate are distance learning technologies for master's degree and doctoral programs? What course(s) may or may not be particularly amenable to distance learning technology? What suggestions are made by Yeaworth et al. (Chapter 14)? What concerns and suggestions by Davis (Chapter 6) and Purnell (Chapter 37) should be considered in global education? How may Billings' discussion (Chapter 15) about OLCPPs apply to international graduate programs? What differences appear between international doctoral education as discussed by Ketefian and Redman and that presented by Lenz and Hardin (Chapter 20)?

Should more standardization exist in programs in the United States than in international programs? If so, why? What positive and negative lessons have been learned in developing doctoral education in the United States that should be shared with international programs? How is quality information best shared for doctoral programs?

20

Doctoral Nursing Education

Approaches to Achieving Quality When Resources Are Limited

Elizabeth R. Lenz, PhD, RN, FAAN
Sally Brosz Hardin, PhD, RN, FAAN

D octoral programs, with their faculty and students, define the science, sculpt knowledge boundaries, and become the idea brokers of a discipline. Doctoral programs are desired highly by schools because they establish a cultural milieu of inquiry, are regarded as prestigious, and enhance an institution's reputation. However, doctoral programs also present unique challenges, which include rigorous scholarly productivity for faculty, high economic costs for administration, and high demand on resources.

The resource needs of doctoral programs are great. Generally, these programs include small numbers of students; thus they lack economies of scale that are present at other curricular levels. Learning experiences, such as conducting research under guidance of a faculty mentor, are intensive and prolonged, with much of the learning taking place outside formal classroom settings in expensive one-to-one interactions with faculty. Economic costs are high not only because faculty-to-student ratios are low, but also because only the most experienced and productive faculty are selected to teach doctoral students. Financial support of full-time students and an excellent faculty are virtually mandatory if a school is to compete favorably for the best-qualified doctoral applicants.

Despite high costs, the consensus seems to be that doctoral programs are "worth it." More than helping to bring prestige to a school, doctoral programs are essential for recruiting highly qualified faculty who desire the challenges and rewards associated with teaching and directing dissertation research (American Association of Colleges of Nursing [AACN], 1996). Importantly, the presence of doctoral students tends to have a catalytic effect on research and scholarship within a school, often changing the milieu to one that values these elements highly (Lenz, 1989). The presence of a doctoral program also can result in improvement in a school's other course offerings because it places them in the context of the terminal degree. Benefits such as these have encouraged the proliferation of doctoral programs in schools of nursing in the United States and abroad. Presently, there are 74 nursing doctoral programs in U.S. institutions (at least 17 more are being planned), and a growing number of programs are being offered abroad (Anonymous, 1996; Berlin, Bednash, & Hosier, 1999). Although some of these newly evolving programs are strong, a longstanding and recurrent concern has been that, in the rush to join the ranks of schools of nursing offering doctorates, those with insufficient resources may generate programs, and hence graduates, of questionable quality.

■ Quality in Doctoral Nursing Education

What do we mean by quality in doctoral education and where does the discipline of nursing currently stand when compared with other fields? When we speak of quality in doctoral education, standards vary somewhat among disciplines; however, some general characteristics of successful programs and approaches to evaluating program quality have been set forth by the Council of Graduate Schools (1990a, 1990b).

AACN Quality Indicators

The document most frequently cited regarding quality in doctoral education in nursing is the American Association of Colleges of Nursing's (AACN) position statement on quality indicators of doctoral programs in nursing (AACN, 1997). The process of identifying indicators began at an invitational conference in 1984 that was sponsored jointly by AACN and the Division of Nursing, U.S. Public Health Service (USPHS); included were deans and program directors from most of the doctoral programs in nursing existing at that time (Jamann, 1985). Some decisions made at that conference had implications for future directions in the discipline. For example, a decision was made not to differentiate criteria for quality in academic Doctor of Philosophy (PhD) versus professional Doctor of Nursing Science (DNS, DSN, and DNSc) programs, but rather to focus attention on elements common to both types. The result was a document that neither clarified nor facilitated program differentiation. After a task force drafted a document from the conference proceedings and circulated it to member schools, the final AACN position statement was approved in October 1986.

Characteristics of Quality Indicators

Some characteristics of the AACN quality indicators need to be pointed out. First, AACN indicators are normative statements, that is, stated as recommendations about what should be present or done to achieve high quality. AACN "quality indicators" therefore are different from indicators commonly used in measurement or social policy literature. Authors writing in policy and the social sciences tend to describe indicators as "value free" variables that provide proxy evidence for the existence, strength, or characteristics of a given phenomenon. For example, the indicators commonly used to measure social class are education, income, and occupation. AACN indicators are not stated as variables, although they could be easily reconfigured to reflect program characteristics that could vary. Rather, AACN indicators are criteria or standards that should be met if a program is to be designated as high quality. Taken together, these criteria represent an "ideal type" that presents a standard for comparison but probably exists nowhere in reality.

Second, like most consensus statements and almost by definition, AACN indicators of quality are generic and noncontroversial. Rather than being cutting-edge, AACN indicators reflect the traditional academic model, summarizing and highlighting elements that all doctoral programs can agree are desirable. Thus these statements are written to accommodate diversity in academic and professional doctoral programs and foci.

Third, AACN quality indicators place more emphasis on the structure and process of doctoral education than on the outcomes of this process. Process is emphasized even in the sections dealing with the program of study. For example in this respect, AACN indicators speak not to specific disciplinary content, but to distribution between nursing and cognate courses, identifiability of core content, opportunities for role development, and sequencing of requirements. Thus AACN indicators emphasize syntax more than substance. That is, the content areas that are specified for inclusion deal more with the process of how knowledge building is done (philosophy of science, processes of theory and knowledge development, research methods, data analysis techniques) than with content of the discipline of nursing.

Continuing Evolution

The AACN quality indicators reflect a state of continuing evolution. They were updated with relatively minor changes in October 1993, following discussion at an AACN-sponsored conference. Nevertheless, "quality" remains a topic of ongoing discussion and debate. One reason why it is difficult to achieve consensus on what constitutes quality

in doctoral nursing education is that the desired outcomes for different types of programs may differ. Another factor is that within schools of nursing, faculty have earned doctorates in various disciplines, each of which may differ in definition of high quality in doctoral education. Basic science doctorates, for example, prioritize intensive involvement in the faculty advisor's research, whereas doctorates in education may place more emphasis on coursework. These very different world views likewise project very different implications for standards of quality. As currently formulated, AACN indicators have some limitations, not the least being their failure to differentiate quality in academic and professional degree programs and their relative neglect of both substance and desired outcomes. Another major revision is now being carried out by an AACN task force (G. L. Bednash, personal communication, May 1999).

In this chapter, we examine the current state of doctoral nursing education, using as a backdrop AACN's existing indicators of quality. In cases where quality is judged to be problematic or when quality may be threatened by financial cutbacks, we suggest strategies for maintaining and improving conditions. Suggested strategies are based on likely assumptions that most institutions have limited resources to allocate to any given program and that nursing doctoral programs are taxing universities' already stretched academic, faculty, and economic resources.

■ Students

Indicators of Student Quality

According to Anderson (1999), serious discrepancies exist between other disciplines' recognized standards, regarding characteristics of high-quality doctoral students, and those of nursing doctoral students. Generally accepted in doctoral education are the ideas that quality students are . . . intellectually gifted, chosen from a large pool of applicants, students who commit to full-time study, immersing themselves fully in the program. Intellectually gifted students are eager to learn, capable of intense discussion and debate, students who have an insatiable appetite for new information, who are inquisitive, energetic, and possess keen problem-solving abilities. (Anderson, 1999)

Anderson claimed that according to these and other academic standards frequently applied to judging the quality of doctoral applicants (e.g., grade point averages, Graduate Record Examination (GRE), or other standardized test scores), nursing doctoral students do not compare favorably to those in other fields. In particular, nursing doctoral students' standardized test scores tend to be mediocre. Low test scores may reflect a combination of limited exposure to mathematics beyond high school or a possibility that nursing may have suffered a "brain drain." That is, the most able of high school graduates are entering more prestigious and lucrative fields, whereas nursing increasingly attracts those who want jobs rather than careers. If that is the case, the implications for the discipline's future and its doctoral programs are frightening. An additional issue is whether standardized test scores reliably predict successful outcomes for nursing doctoral students or graduates.

Unlike the high-quality doctoral student that Anderson described, a majority of nursing doctoral students enroll part-time, rather than making a full-time commitment. In part, this difference is related to nursing doctoral students being older than doctoral students in other fields. Nursing doctoral students typically remain employed in relatively responsible and high-paying positions while simultaneously engaging in doctoral study. They often are balancing responsibilities of full-time employment, part-time study, and family, so have limited time to immerse themselves in studies or to be the "inquisitive,

energetic" quality student that Anderson (1999) described.

Currently, the total number of students enrolled in doctoral nursing programs is stable and relatively small. In 1998, the average number of full-time and part-time students per program was 16 and 26, respectively. Correspondingly, the number of doctoral graduates produced is small, averaging 5.8 in 1998, a 5% decrease from the number of graduations the previous year (Berlin, Bednash, & Hosier, 1999). In 1997–1998, 81% of nursing doctoral programs graduated 10 or fewer students (Anderson, 1999). In part, this low number is because many programs are relatively new and have not yet reached their full complement of students or graduates. However, because of limited faculty resources, many nursing doctoral programs have imposed limits on enrollment, with the intent of remaining small. Although small size is not inherently negative or positive, programs with few students may not provide ample opportunity for challenging interactions with peers and may lack economy of scale.

Increasing Student Quality

Strategies that might be considered for attracting higher quality students at the doctoral level include (a) setting high standards for admission and matriculated students and having the courage to reject mediocre applicants or students; (b) encouraging full-time, or close to full-time enrollment; (c) advocating postbaccalaureate entry into nursing doctoral education; and (d) placing less emphasis on clinical experience requirements and more on academic achievements in evaluating applicants. High admission and student standards often are difficult to enforce because of administrative pressures to admit and retain a sufficiently large cohort of students to justify the high expenditure for doctoral programs. At admission, it often is difficult to differentiate between the student who should be rejected because she or he is mediocre academically and will not perform well at the doctoral level and the student who is borderline on admission criteria—particularly standardized tests—because of a disadvantaged background or lack of recent exposure to the content examined. In making this decision, it is important to consider multiple indicators of potential success. For example, grades in research and statistics courses and a publication history may be more indicative of success in research than the quantitative score on the Graduate Record Exam, which may be heavily dependent on geometry and algebra concepts that a mature applicant may not have studied for decades. Indicators of "drive," scholarly performance, and perseverance may be particularly meaningful predictors of success at the doctoral level.

Full-Time Enrollment

Encouraging full-time enrollment in doctoral programs requires a combination of strategies. First, it is necessary to provide financial incentives to those who are willing to enroll full-time. A financial investment by the institution in the form of tuition and stipend support is generally required. Although providing the salary that an experienced nurse can earn in the clinical setting is not possible, full-time study often can be encouraged by providing tangible benefits of tuition remission and a stipend, together with intangible benefits of an experiential basis for future career choices, and publication and networking opportunities. The institution benefits by receiving skilled teaching and research assistance at a slightly reduced cost. Strategies that encourage doctoral enrollment of younger students can result in a higher percentage of full-time students. Approaches such as encouraging postbaccalaureate entry similar to the basic sciences and humanities and eliminating the requirement of extensive clinical experience prior to admission

may facilitate enrollment. Younger students tend to have fewer financial obligations and family commitments than their older counterparts. Further, such students are less likely to have lucrative or highly responsible positions that they are reluctant to give up in order to return to school. Enrolling younger students also would have the advantage of generating scholars with a longer career trajectory in which to fully develop and carry out their programs of research.

Streamlined Progression

Postbaccalaureate entry options are being developed increasingly by doctoral nursing programs, to encourage potential students who clearly want to earn the doctorate in a streamlined fashion (AACN, 1998). This motivation is especially true for more mature students who want a baccalaureate degree or have a second degree. Such students are either registered nurses who received their education in diploma schools or technical colleges but do not have a bachelor's degree, or those who are not registered nurses but have earned a baccalaureate or higher degree in another discipline. Typically, these optional curricular models allow the student to earn a master's degree "along the way." However, a recent trend has been to make the master's degree truly optional and to structure a postbaccalaureate doctoral program that is not based on prerequisite master's-level clinical skills. Such programs are offered as being appropriate for individuals who envision a research or administrative career that would not require in-depth clinical preparation and who do not desire to be credentialed as a nurse practitioner or clinical nurse specialist. Postbaccalaureate entry programs may be controversial because they do not include clinical content, and graduates may not be as fully attuned to complex clinical issues as their master's-prepared counterparts. Such postbaccalaureate programs do, however, begin to call into question the validity of the assumption that extensive clinical experience is needed prior to nursing doctoral study or that such experience be given priority in evaluating doctoral applicants. Students who are academically outstanding, but who have only limited clinical experience prior to entry, are, in fact, performing very satisfactorily in doctoral coursework and research and may acquire clinical experience concurrently.

Policy and Curricular Strategies

Additional strategies, at a more macroscopic level, will need to be employed ultimately if the number of full-time nursing doctoral students is to increase substantially. For example, to have sufficient funding to attract able full-time students, efforts to increase the amount of federal funding allocated to doctoral education and doctoral students will be necessary. Currently, a maximum of 10% of federal Advanced Nurse Traineeship funding can be allocated to doctoral students (Department of Health and Human Services [DHHS], 1998). This policy needs to be reexamined in the light of the projected oversupply of nurse practitioners and undersupply of nursing faculty (AACN, 1999; Anderson, 1998a). The National Institute for Nursing Research (NINR) and other federal agencies currently award funds for predoctoral research training. These funds traditionally have been limited and are often awarded late in the student's program of study. Funding needs to be increased and criteria reexamined to take into account those entering doctoral study without master's degree preparation. Moreover, incoming students should be encouraged to submit grant proposals prior to completing their first semester of doctoral study. Because of the amount of time required for review, even very highly rated proposals submitted just prior to the student's matriculation are not likely to be funded before the end of the first year of doctoral study.

Another broad strategy that would help encourage academically able students to pursue nursing doctoral study is to make curricula at all levels of the nursing education program more interesting and challenging, so that strong students would be attracted and retained. Ideally, faculty and courses at all levels would encourage and reward creative thinking and demand rigorous and scholarly approaches.

Mentoring of Students

Finally, a key to attracting and retaining high-quality nursing doctoral students may be in the quality and quantity of professional support and mentoring provided to students by their faculty, dissertation chair, committee members, and research sponsors. Faculty mentors must be role models who perform, as well as write about, research. Faculty must be available to students. An often-cited complaint of nursing doctoral students, even those in large prestigious institutions, is the unavailability of faculty advisors or lack of true research mentors or both. This unavailability may be a factor related to students' being "ABD" (i.e., completing all doctoral requirements except for the dissertation).

■ Faculty

Indicators of Faculty Quality

Generally recognized indicators of faculty quality in nursing doctoral programs include characteristics of both individual faculty members and the program as a whole. Individual indicators of faculty quality include (a) an earned doctorate in nursing or a related discipline, preferably from a prestigious institution and program; (b) an active program of research for which at least some external funding has been received; (c) a history of scholarly productivity in the form of multiple publications in peer-reviewed journals; and (d) for faculty who earned their doctorates relatively recently, post-doctoral research training. For the program as a whole, indicators of quality include (a) a sufficient number of doctorally prepared faculty, generally a faculty-to-student ratio of no more than 1:6; (b) sufficient faculty expertise to address both core program requirements and substantive offerings; (c) a good match between the program's goals and specialty areas and faculty research; (d) a very low percentage of faculty who are graduates from the home institution and, conversely, a high percentage of faculty who represent a number of diverse institutions; and (e) sufficient faculty experienced in teaching at the doctoral level and guiding doctoral student research.

Currently, doctoral nursing programs vary markedly in the degree to which their faculty reflect these indicators of quality. Approximately half the faculty members in schools and colleges of nursing have earned doctorates, so within academia nursing is, in effect, marginal with respect to faculty preparation in general (AACN, 1996; Anderson, 1999). A school may have a sufficient number of doctorally prepared faculty to sustain adequate faculty-to-student ratios and to cover core curricular elements, such as philosophy of science, nursing theory, theory development and evaluation, research methodology, and statistics; however, often there are not enough faculty with requisite research expertise and external funding to serve as role models and advisors for doctoral student research. The requirement that faculty be externally funded can be difficult to meet, particularly if this requirement is interpreted to mean federal funding. Federal research funding is concentrated in but a few schools. In fiscal year (FY) 1997 (October 1997 through September 1998), 26 schools with nursing doctoral programs had no NINR funding and 13 others had only one project funded (Anderson, 1999). Even if funded early in their research

careers, *relatively few nursing faculty sustain funded research programs over time.* Additionally, even nursing faculty who are actively conducting research may not enjoy a good fit between their teaching and their research. Faculty may be trying to balance multiple demands or be expected to teach content with which they have only limited familiarity.

A current pattern in many schools is to require all faculty to teach across multiple curricular levels. Often, this dictum comes from higher administrative levels within the university who confront complaints that undergraduate students have no exposure to senior faculty. Although such a policy may be appropriate in more senior or research-productive departments, to assign nursing's most senior faculty to undergraduate students may be an insupportable luxury at this point in the development of nursing doctoral programs. At the doctoral level, it is essential that courses be taught only by faculty having depth of expertise in the content.

Within a given program there also may be a lack of fit between the expertise and active research programs of faculty and the program's identified specialty research areas and current student interests. Ideally, the specialty research areas identified for a doctoral program reflect the research strengths of clusters of faculty. However, faculty turnover can lead to changes that produce a less than optimal fit.

Programs differ in philosophical stances regarding the degree of fit required between student and faculty research. In some programs, a student cannot be admitted unless a faculty member agrees to mentor him or her in a particular research topic. In other programs, more of a team approach is used to provide the expertise needed to guide a student. In such programs, content-based limitations on admissions are less stringent and students are permitted more latitude in selecting a research topic. Both approaches have some limitations. A very close faculty–student match works well unless the faculty member leaves or the student's interests change. Too loose a connection between the student's research topic and faculty expertise may result in inadequate guidance. Therefore the most reasonable stance is to identify specialty areas that are sufficiently broad to encompass the research of several faculty members and to encourage students to pursue research topics that fall within these identified areas.

Faculty Recruitment and Retention

Faculty are the most expensive, yet most important, resources of any doctoral program; they are also the major determinants of its quality. Possible strategies for maximizing a program's doctoral faculty resources and ensuring adequate support for a strong nursing doctoral program include (a) increasing scholarly productivity of faculty already on board, (b) attracting additional qualified faculty, and (c) expanding the faculty resource base by involving faculty from outside the school, college, or university. Doctorally prepared individuals already on the faculty may need assistance to increase scholarly productivity and research funding and to strike a reasonable balance among their various roles. Possible strategies include (a) allocating workload carefully to allow time for research and grant writing, (b) ensuring consistency between faculty research focus and teaching responsibilities, (c) providing incentives and assistance in preparing research grant proposals, and (d) providing support for travel to research conferences and continuing education programs that help develop valuable networks and state-of-the-science knowledge and research skills (Lash, 1992; Lenz, 1989; Norbeck, 1998). Supportive resources such as research assistants also have the dual benefit of providing funding and experience for nursing doctoral students.

Well-qualified, highly productive doctorally prepared faculty—particularly those whose research programs are federally funded—are highly in demand, and schools often compete with one another for them. Successful recruitment efforts generally include generous salaries and benefits, including workloads that are compatible with research productivity, and "start-up packages" that include research assistants and generous equipment allowances. An alternative to recruiting already funded faculty is to recruit new faculty with a high probability of securing funding in the future. Those who have had 1 or 2 years of postdoctoral research training often are poised to move ahead quickly and already may have submitted proposals for funding.

Collaborative Strategies to Enhance Faculty Quality

Intra-institutional Collaboration

For many nursing doctoral programs with marginal numbers of high-quality doctoral faculty, strategies to collaborate with other departments and institutions may be helpful. For example, few doctoral nursing programs provide all the instruction to their students. Most require that students take cognate courses in related disciplines or arrange for students to take some of their core courses—most often philosophy of science and statistics—in other university departments. Some dual-degree programs exist in which students earn degrees both in nursing (PhD or DNSc) and another school or department, such as business, public health, or law. Virtually all institutions require that nursing dissertation committees contain at least one member from another department. Ideally, such intra-institutional arrangements are reciprocal, with nursing's courses open to being selected by doctoral students from other departments who offer courses to doctoral nursing students. To date, however, this option has been sought infrequently. Nursing doctoral courses are selected relatively infrequently by students outside the health sciences. Doctoral nursing students' access to courses in other departments may need to be negotiated administratively, particularly with departments that have heavy graduate enrollments of their own and whose courses fill rapidly. An effective "bargaining chip" in such negotiations may be to offer courses that are sufficiently generic and interesting to appeal to students from other departments. Examples might feature courses concerning health promotion and disease prevention strategies, vulnerable populations, health policy, or clinical research study coordination. In some nursing doctoral programs, faculty have considerable methodological expertise and offer courses in statistics, research design, and measurement that are taken by students in other departments.

It is generally preferable for doctoral nursing students to sit in courses with students from other disciplines, rather than to have "special sections" designed for them alone. However, in certain instances in which required content is needed from another department and appropriate courses are not available, special arrangements may be necessary. A frequent example is the requirement that doctoral nursing students take a graduate-level course in the philosophy of science. Such courses are advanced, assuming much greater prerequisite familiarity with basic concepts and works of philosophy and physics than most nursing students possess. Strategies that have been used successfully are to have a philosopher of science team-teach a course with a nursing faculty member or offer a philosophy module within a doctoral nursing course that addresses nursing theory or intellectual development of the nursing discipline.

The choice of dissertation committee members is an important one. Frequently, nursing doctoral students have a difficult time accessing faculty from other departments with relevant expertise and compatible world views to serve on their committees. Cognate courses provide a vital link to potential committee members. Equally important, if not more so, are linkages provided by doctoral nursing faculty to colleagues and collaborators from other fields. Doctoral nursing programs are well advised to maintain lists of potential dissertation committee members from other departments of their universities.

Inter-institutional Collaboration

A number of collaborative relationships have been established between and among schools of nursing in order to share, and thereby expand, doctoral faculty resources. One approach is to provide joint course offerings in which courses are developed and offered jointly by faculty from more than one nursing doctoral program. Another strategy is to allow students to take another institution's courses to satisfy specific core or elective requirements. This approach is most likely to be used when institutions have formalized consortium agreements regarding tuition. Shared courses are particularly beneficial when a renowned faculty member or one with unique expertise is offering a course, or when esoteric or highly specialized content is being provided. Frequently faculty members in one institution agree to guide independent study experiences or supervise research residencies for students in other schools. A growing number of doctoral courses are being made available via the Internet. Institutional policies dictate whether the student's home school or the other institution awards credit for the experience.

A common practice in nursing is for doctoral faculty from one institution to serve as members of dissertation committees in another institution. In such cases, either the student or his or her school pays for the individual's travel, if any; a small honorarium also may be provided. Because of the relative scarcity of doctorally prepared nursing faculty with expertise in any particular research topic, it may be advisable to establish regional, national, or even international pools of research mentors or advisors. Such groups might include productive faculty and faculty experienced in research who would be willing to serve as members of dissertation committees or sponsors for predoctoral National Research Service Awards (NRSAs). An organization with national scholarly membership and sustained interest in doctoral nursing education and research, such as AACN or Sigma Theta Tau International (STTI), would be the logical choice to establish such a resource. Alternatively, it may be possible to establish regional or national "dissertation research or mentoring groups," similar to research interest groups established by the regional nursing research societies (e.g., the Western Interstate Council on Higher Education in Nursing and the Southern Regional Education Board) in the 1970s and 1980s. These regional organizations or AACN and STTI at the national and international levels, respectively, would seem to be appropriate coordinating and organizing bodies.

Joint Programs

Currently, there are seven formally constituted joint doctoral nursing programs that were developed as a shared undertaking between two institutions. Motivating factors for these arrangements have tended to be mandates from state-level organizations that approve doctoral programs contingent on inter-institutional collaboration. Models for these joint programs differ. The University of Massachusetts houses one collaborative program wherein schools of nursing on the Amherst and Worcester campuses admit students to either campus, but the two faculties jointly develop program policies and curriculum. Class sessions for a given course alternate between the two campuses and are taught by faculty from both (Hardin, Fain, & Lenz, 1998). Other joint programs involve shared program administration resources and divided responsibility between two institutions.

A major benefit of joint programs is the provision of a richer array of faculty resources than would be available at only one school of nursing. Such programs, however, can be cumbersome to administer and costly. The complex communications involved and the seemingly continual need to work out compromises require considerable skill on the part of all involved, but particularly those in charge. Seemingly minor issues, such as inconsistency between the calendars of the two schools, can be very troublesome to students and faculty alike. More major issues, such as determining which institution will grant the doctoral degree, also can be problematic unless criteria are clearly identified at outset. Success is highly dependent on clear lines of communication and authority and on a spirit of cooperation and good will between the institutions.

■ Program Administration and Resources

No single administrative structure characterizes doctoral nursing programs; rather, several different configurations exist. Examples include (a) administration by a program director whose responsibility is either limited solely to the doctoral program or combined with other levels of the curriculum; (b) administration by a committee or small group; (c) decentralization of the program to departments, with department chairpersons administering them; and (d) extreme decentralization to the individual faculty sponsor level (i.e., virtually no program administration per se). The first example describes the most common model in the United States. No model is inherently superior. Rather, the fit of model to the overall philosophy and structure of the university and school of nursing is an important consideration. The developmental stage of the nursing doctoral program, the program's success in achieving AACN quality indicators, and its success in meeting both outcome and process indicators should provide basis for the decision regarding administrative structure.

The goals of nursing doctoral program administration are to ensure that (a) all applicants and students are treated fairly; (b) standards exist and are applied equally to all students; (c) program processes such as recruitment, admission, progression, advisement, and research guidance occur smoothly; (d) communication about and within the program is clear, accurate, and effective; (e) sufficient resources are procured and allocated; and (f) all aspects of the program are evaluated regularly. Quality-related issues to consider in evaluating adequacy of an administrative structure include (a) adequacy of oversight and guidance to students and faculty; (b) consistency of standards and policy implementation; (c) evaluation of student experiences and progression (e.g., coursework, comprehensive examinations, dissertation and graduation completion, student research funding, and faculty and student publication); and (d) advocacy for the program and its students in university, professional, and scientific communities.

A key responsibility of nursing doctoral program administrators is to secure adequate resources with which to operate the program. Nursing doctoral program faculty and student financial aid—both vital resources—were discussed previously. Additional resource needs identified in AACN (1997) quality indicators include (a) laboratory, office, classroom, and study space; (b) computers and related technological equipment, software, support services, and expertise; (c) library and database materials and related support services; (d) support for small-scale, pilot research projects; (e) up-to-date instructional technology; and (f) centralized processing of admissions, progressions, student services, and program finances. Library and computer support are particularly important in doctoral education and need to be updated and supplemented regularly because of the rapid changes in technology.

■ Curriculum

Indicators of Curriculum Quality

The AACN (1997) quality indicators regarding nursing doctoral curricula acknowledge that program content should be based on faculty expertise. These indicators also list general areas of core content recommended for inclusion in all programs: (a) history and philosophy of science, (b) development of nursing knowledge, (c) approaches to theory and knowledge development, (d) analytical and leadership strategies for dealing with professional and research issues, (d) research methods, and (f) data analysis techniques. In addition, programs are expected to include substantive nursing knowledge, but the nature of that substantive knowledge is not specified. Guided and independent research experiences also are considered an important part of doctoral curricula. No differentiation is made between curricula of programs offering the academic doctorate (PhD) from those offering the professional doctorate (DNSc). Although curricular quality indicators have been used by nursing doctoral programs as standards for evaluating completeness of curricula, a number of issues continue to be raised. These issues concern (a) homogeneity of program design and content, (b) focus on process rather than the substance of nursing science, (c) lack of clarity about the product being produced, and (d) potential emphasis on formal courses versus out-of-classroom experiences.

Differentiation by Type of Degree

Historically, in doctoral nursing education there has been little differentiation of content by type of degree offered (Lenz, 1990; Ziemer et al., 1992). Although reasons for this homogeneity are not entirely clear, a contributing factor was the decision in many early programs to offer the professional doctorate (DNS, DNSc, or DSN)—dictated more by institutional policy than by the desired competencies of graduates. Curricula for professional doctoral degree programs tend to be research focused and closely resemble those of PhD programs designed to produce researchers.

During the past decade, the trend in nursing is toward offering the PhD; several schools that originally offered the professional doctorate have changed to the PhD. However, faculty in a small, but growing number of nursing schools, have made deliberate decisions to offer the professional doctorate in order to provide scholarly clinical leadership and innovations in practice; such a trend is advocated by some nursing leaders (Henry, 1997). These professional doctoral nursing programs are designed to be very different from PhD programs in that there is more emphasis on clinical practice and applied research and less emphasis on theory testing and development or on basic research.

The program at the University of Texas at Houston, for example, includes three semesters of clinical practica and emphasis on practice prevails throughout (Starck, Duffy, & Vogler, 1993). Similarly, the DNSc program at the Columbia University School of Nursing comprises both a research practicum and a practicum in either health policy or clinical leadership. The DNSc program at the University of Tennessee, Memphis (Veeser, Stegbauer, & Russell, 1999) contains core courses that provide the background for analyzing and evaluating clinical practice outcomes in "epidemiology, health policy, health economics, philosophy of practice, research utilization, health care quality improvement, health information systems, and leadership" (p. 40), and an individualized advanced clinical practica series. Of interest, the AACN quality indicators for cur-

riculum do not differ by program type, despite the Council of Graduate School's (CGS) assertion that products of programs offering academic and professional doctorates are expected to have different competencies.

Emphasis on Substance and Outcomes

To date in doctoral curricula, emphasis has been more on syntax or the process of doing science and the tools required to develop and apply knowledge (e.g., philosophy of science, history and development of the discipline, theory development, qualitative and quantitative research designs, and statistics) than on substantive content of the discipline, including middle-range theories that guide nursing research and practice (see Lenz, 1998a, 1998b; Liehr & Smith, 1999). Although the importance of syntax cannot be denied in curricula for preparing scientists (DiBartolo, 1998), nursing leaders have recommended that more emphasis be given to substantive content in nursing science (Ketefian, 1993). However, only limited agreement exists as to the specifics of that nursing content. It may not be useful, or even possible, to identify essential content for the nursing discipline as a whole. Instead, it may be more desirable to focus at the level of (a) particular clinical populations such as oncology patients or adolescents, (b) settings or types of practice such as primary care, (c) nursing phenomena such as pain or fatigue, or (d) middle-range theories that cross clinical populations (Liehr & Smith, 1999). Considerable forward movement is being made, particularly at the subspecialty level, in developing substantive nursing content and establishing research-based knowledge on which evidence-based nursing practice can be based.

Perhaps because of the emphasis on process, rather than outcomes, relatively little attention has been paid to describing the desired products of nursing's doctoral programs and the specific competencies that graduates should possess. Some have argued that insufficient attention has been paid to the "real-world" that nursing doctoral students will confront upon graduation. A similar criticism has been leveled regarding doctoral education in general (LaPidus, 1997). Specifically, the critics argue that doctoral nursing education has focused too much on developing theoretical and research skills and has not done an adequate job of preparing graduates for roles and responsibilities that they will be expected to assume after graduation, such as teaching (Anderson, 1998b, 1999; Ketefian, 1991), clinical research facilitation (Dennis, 1991), and practice leadership (Henry, 1997; Starck, Duffy, & Vogler, 1993). Questions also have been raised about the adequacy of preparation for a lifetime of scholarship and research productivity (Meleis, Hall, & Stevens, 1994; Schmitt, 1998). Some programs devote specific courses, required assistantships, or practicum experiences to preparing graduates for specific roles, such as teachers. The AACN's 1999 annual conference on doctoral education in nursing gave explicit consideration of the kinds of experiences that would be needed to provide adequate preparation of doctoral graduates for clinical leadership and scholarly practice, research and knowledge development, scholarly teaching, and preparation for the academy.

Emerging Trends

Several patterns—changes from the past—can be predicted to emerge as quality indicators of nursing doctoral programs. One of the most important will be increased emphasis on differentiating professional and academic program curricula. Another will be explicit attention to competencies expected of graduates, kinds of learning experiences and program requirements that will help students attain them—and some consideration of competencies needed for the kinds of roles anticipated.

Regarding the nature of core and specialized content, increased emphasis will be placed on substantive nursing content, including the generic concepts and middle-range theories that are of interest across the nursing discipline and specialty-specific concepts, theories, and research. A trend toward permitting postbaccalaureate entry into nursing doctoral programs will emerge. The question of whether a master's degree should be earned "along the way" to the doctorate, or at least a substantial amount of master's-level content be required, will continue to be debated; the decision ultimately may lead to more flexibility in requirements for roles, such as faculty positions that currently require master's degrees. Three areas that can be predicted to grow in importance in nursing doctoral programs will be information technology: (a) its uses in and impact on practice, (b) measurement and assessment of clinical processes and outcomes, and (c) accrual of empirical evidence on which to base nursing practice patterns and decisions. Finally, international perspectives are anticipated to gain increasing import in nursing doctoral education, spurred by the increase in international collaboration among nurse scholars and educators (see Ketefian and Redman's Chapter 19).

Criticism can be raised that nursing doctoral curricula have changed little since the late 1970s. The time is at hand for both institutions and the discipline as a whole to take on the challenge of reviewing and updating curricula that may be outmoded. Many hard-held assumptions about presumably "vital" content need to be reexamined in the light of current literature and practice patterns. For example, a debate is under way in many nursing schools about the desirability of including philosophy of science and the grand nursing theories in doctoral curricula. A critical examination of each institution's curriculum based on the kind of products desired should lead to more differences among programs than currently exist. Such examination should base substantive nursing foci of the program on its strengths, strengths of other departments within the university, and unique aspects of the institutional environment. For example, a school that has a strong clinically competent faculty—many of whom are engaged in advanced nursing practice and applied research, would be in a better position to consider offering the professional doctorate than a school whose faculty are more heavily engaged in basic research.

■ Concluding Statement

Ensuring quality in doctoral nursing programs remains a challenge. Continuing debates about what a high-quality program should be like and how quality can best be achieved and maintained encourage new opinions to be aired, new approaches tried, and "tried-and-true" traditions scrutinized. Intense activity by AACN to revisit its quality indicators and to generate a new document early in the new century, should provide a wonderful opportunity to debate the issues that we have identified, to question feasibility and desirability of perpetuating traditional patterns, and to determine standards for the next decade. The high cost of nursing doctoral education, both to the student and the institution, require ongoing attention to quality as a necessary investment of time and energy.

■ References

American Association of Colleges of Nursing. (1996, July). Nursing schools seek balance of teaching and research skills in effort to boost the PhD supply. *AACN Issue Bulletin,* pp. 1–5.

American Association of Colleges of Nursing. (1997). Position statement: Indicators of quality in doctoral programs in nursing. *Journal of Professional Nursing, 13,* 200–202.

American Association of Colleges of Nursing. (1998, June). As RNs age, nursing schools seek to expand the pool of younger faculty. *AACN Issue Bulletin,* pp. 1–4.

American Association of Colleges of Nursing. (1999, April). Faculty shortages intensify nation's nursing deficit. *AACN Issue Bulletin,* pp. 1–4.

Anderson, C. A. (1998a). Academic nursing: A desirable career? *Nursing Outlook, 46*(1), 5–6.

Anderson, C. A. (1998b). PhD graduates and the demands of faculty roles. *Nursing Outlook, 46*(2), 53–54.

Anderson, C. A. (1999, January). *Current strengths and limitations of doctoral education in nursing: Are we prepared for the future?* Presented at the AACN 1999 Annual Conference on Doctoral Education in Nursing, Sanibel, Florida.

Anonymous. (1996). Doctoral nursing schools outside the U.S. *Reflections, 22*(3), 36.

Berlin, L. E., Bednash, G. D., & Hosier, K. L. (1999). *1998–1999 enrollment and graduations in baccalaureate and graduate programs in nursing.* Washington, DC: American Association of Colleges of Nursing.

Council of Graduate Schools. (1990a). *Academic review of graduate programs.* Washington, DC: Author.

Council of Graduate Schools. (1990b). *The doctor of philosophy degree: A policy statement.* Washington, DC: Author.

Dennis, K. E. (1991). Components of the doctoral curriculum that build success in the clinical nurse researcher role. *Journal of Professional Nursing, 7*(3), 160–165.

Department of Health and Human Services, Health Resources and Services Administration, Division of Nursing. (1998). *Federal guidelines for advanced nursing training grants.* (Grant Application. Form PHS-6025-1, p. 27).

DiBartolo, M. C. (1998). Philosophy of science in doctoral nursing education revisited. *Journal of Professional Nursing, 14,* 350–360.

Hardin, S. B., Fain, J., & Lenz, E. R. (1998, January). *The University of Massachusetts-Amherst-Worcester PhD Program.* Presented at AACN 1998 Annual Conference on Doctoral Education in Nursing, Sanibel, Florida.

Henry, B. (1997). Professional doctorates for professional practice. *IMAGE: Journal of Nursing Scholarship, 29*(2), 102.

Jamann, J. S. (1985). Proceedings of doctoral programs in nursing: Consensus for quality. American Association of Colleges of Nursing. *Journal of Professional Nursing, 1*(2), 90–121.

Ketefian, S. (1991). Doctoral preparation for faculty roles: Expectations and realities. *Journal of Professional Nursing, 7*(2), 105–111.

Ketefian, S. (1993). Essentials of doctoral education: Organization of program around knowledge areas. *Journal of Professional Nursing, 9*(5), 255–261.

LaPidus, J. B. (1997). Doctoral education: Preparing for the future. *Council of Graduate Schools Communicator, 30*(10), 1–10.

Lash, A. A. (1992). Determinants of career attainments of doctorates in nursing. *Nursing Research, 41*(4), 216–222.

Lenz, E.R. (1998a). The role of middle-range theory in nursing research and practice. Part I. Nursing research. *Nursing Leadership Forum, 3*(1), 24–33.

Lenz, E. R. (1998b). The role of middle-range theory in nursing research and practice. Part II. Nursing practice. *Nursing Leadership Forum, 3*(2), 2–6.

Lenz, E. R. (1989). *Doctoral faculty as a community of scholars: Positive environments for doctoral programs.* In S. Hart (Ed.), *Doctoral education in nursing: History, process and outcomes* (Pub. No. 15-2238) (pp. 75–93). New York: National League for Nursing.

Lenz, E. R. (1990). Doctoral nursing education: Present views, future trends. In N. L. Chaska (Ed.), *The nursing profession: Turning points* (pp. 114–120). St. Louis: C. V. Mosby.

Liehr, P., & Smith, M. J. (1999). Middle range theory: Spinning research and practice to create knowledge for the new millennium. *Advances in Nursing Science, 21*(4), 81–91.

Meleis, A. I., Hall, J. M., & Stevens, P. E. (1994). Scholarly caring in doctoral nursing education: Promoting diversity and collaborative mentorship. *IMAGE: Journal of Nursing Scholarship, 26*(3), 177–180.

Norbeck, J. S. (1998). Teaching, research, and service: Striking the balance in doctoral education. *Journal of Professional Nursing, 14*(4), 197–205.

Schmitt, M. H. (1998). Assuring the production of scholars who will continue to build nursing knowledge into the next millennium. *Research in Nursing and Health, 21*(3), 187–188.

Starck, P. L., Duffy, M. E., & Vogler, R. (1993). Developing a nursing doctorate for the 21st century. *Journal of Professional Nursing, 9*(4), 212–219.

Veeser, P. I., Stegbauer, C. C., & Russell, C. K. (1999). Developing a clinical doctorate to prepare nurses for advanced practice at the University of Tennessee, Memphis. *IMAGE: Journal of Nursing Scholarship, 31*(1), 39–41.

Ziemer, M. M., Brown, J., Fitzpatrick, M. L., Manfredi, C., O'Leary J., & Valiga, T. M. (1992). Doctoral programs in nursing: Philosophy, curricula, and program requirements. *Journal of Professional Nursing, 8*(1), 56–62.

■ *Editor's Questions for Discussion*

What forces have contributed to delay in addressing deficiencies regarding criteria for quality of doctoral programs? How should faculty teaching in doctoral programs provide leadership in developing quality indicators? What role should doctoral faculty play in the administration of doctoral programs? What criteria should differentiate quality between academic and professional programs? What differences might be expected in revision of quality indicators anticipated in the year 2000? What process should occur for consensus about quality indicators and implementation of doctoral programs? What minimum doctoral faculty (number and type) should be in place prior to starting a doctoral program?

What evidence is available regarding relationships between standardized test scores such as the GRE and students' success in doctoral programs? What are the most reliable predictors of such success? Debate the pros and cons of encouraging postbaccalaureate entry into doctoral programs. How much clinical experience should a person have prior to doctoral study? What assumptions are involved in marketing postbaccalaureate doctoral programs for individuals who do not have master's-level clinical skills? What impact may postbaccalaureate entry programs have on the ability to attract persons for research or administrative careers? How may doctoral students be utilized in teaching undergraduate students? What criteria are essential for doctoral students for teaching in undergraduate programs?

Discuss strategies for balancing doctoral teaching faculty workload with other requirements of the faculty role. What negotiations are essential with doctoral faculty prior to hiring? What suggestions are offered by A. Fisher and Habermann (Chapter 21) about doctoral faculty development? How can new doctoral prepared faculty be oriented or prepared for teaching and advising doctoral students? How important is the degree of "fit" between present doctoral faculty and potential doctoral students prior to admission of students? How can a nursing school's administration reconcile conflicts between the need to hire doctoral faculty for master's degree and doctoral programs, having doctoral faculty teach in undergraduate and graduate programs, and the preferred choice of some doctoral faculty *not* to teach undergraduate students?

Describe a process for planning and implementation of inter-institutional and intra-institutional collaboration for a doctoral program. Debate the pros and cons of joint programs. What are the most critical administrative issues pertaining to doctoral programs? How might they be resolved?

How likely is it that curricula will be differentiated between PhD and DNSc programs? What structure and process are essential for quality and distinctions in outcomes to occur? Based on the discussions by Donnelly (Chapter 28), Miller (Chapter 36), and other authors in the Theory and Research Parts of this volume, what substantive content of the discipline should be taught in both or differentiated between PhD and DNSc programs? Should nursing educators focus more on specific competencies and outcomes or process? What evidence supports Lenz and Hardin's predictions regarding substantive areas for future doctoral programs? What are the implications of Shaver's (Chapter 76) and Ketefian and Redman's (Chapter 19) discussions for Lenz and Hardin's suggestions to increase quality and collaboration? How does Miller's (Chapter 36) discussion about preparing researchers apply to curricula changes and development advocated by Lenz and Hardin?

21

Transitions

From Doctoral Preparation to Academic Career

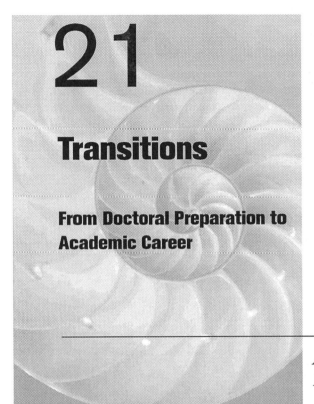

Anastasia Fisher, DNSc, RN
Barbara Habermann, PhD, RN

I n this chapter we examine transition from doctoral education to academic career. For those who choose to pursue an academic career, completion of the doctoral degree marks transition from role of student to that of faculty member. This transition, though critical to development of a successful academic career, is complex (Ketefian, 1991). Having obtained the Doctor of Philosophy degree (PhD), or another research-based doctorate, the recipient is assumed to have received necessary training to establish an academic career that includes building a program of research. In this chapter we question for several reasons the assumption that completion of a doctoral program adequately prepares individuals for a career in academia.

First, we challenge the position that all doctoral programs in nursing are of equal caliber and able to prepare students adequately as scientists. Second, because of role complexity and variability in institutional environments, we question whether any doctoral program adequately prepares potential scholars for successful transition to an academic career. Among the issues discussed in this chapter are (a) discrepancies between doctoral preparation and the demands of academia, (b) different academic

During the preparation of this chapter Dr. Fisher received support from NIH/NIDA 5T32 DA 07257-08 and Dr. Habermann from NIH/NINR 2T32 NR 07039-11.

contexts, and (c) individual and institutional responsibilities and strategies for career development. We conclude with a discussion of the future trends and career options in nursing academia.

■ Doctoral Education

The first doctoral programs in nursing were established in 1933 and 1934 at Teachers College, Columbia University, and New York University, respectively. These programs offered the degree of Doctor of Education in Nursing (Ketefian & Redman, 1994). In 1970, there were 16 doctoral programs (Murphy, 1981) in nursing. By 1991, the number had increased to 54 (Sigma Theta Tau International [STTI], 1991) and by 1999 to 74 programs (STTI, 1999). Today, 75% of all doctoral programs in nursing offer the PhD degree (Ketefian & Redman, 1997).

Although acknowledging increased geographic accessibility and capacity to prepare the number of nurse scientists needed, numerous authors have reemphasized need for evaluation of doctoral education (Germain, Deatrick, Hagopian, & Whitney, 1994; Meleis, Hall, & Stevens, 1994). The issue of quality in doctoral programs has always been pivotal in the discipline because of the critical nature of knowledge development. To better understand this issue, we offer a brief review.

Quality and Evaluation

The goals of doctoral education are twofold: (a) to develop the scientific knowledge base for the discipline through research and scholarly activities, and (b) to meet the increasing demand for doctorally prepared educators in university-based schools of nursing (Downs, 1978; Ketefian, 1991). Although these goals are as valid today as they were several decades ago, how to evaluate whether doctoral programs are meeting them has received limited attention.

Research evaluating doctoral programs was conducted in the 1980s when there were fewer programs (Holzemer & Chambers, 1986). Because evaluation of doctoral education, unlike undergraduate and other graduate education, is not subject to review by external accreditation agencies (Germain, Deatrick, Hagopian, & Whitney, 1994), the issue of quality has been difficult to resolve. Although the American Association of Colleges of Nursing (AACN) (1997) identified indicators of quality in doctoral programs, evaluation of programs is left to individual institutions. How extensively AACN indicators or other quality indicators are used or whether external accreditation would ensure program quality is not clear.

Due to rapid program expansion, multiple demands of an academic role, and social responsibility of an academic nursing career, evaluation of doctoral programs has become more critical (Meleis, 1998; Sullivan, 1997). Rapid program expansion burdens the profession in ensuring that resources are available for developing scholars who possess knowledge and characteristics necessary for an academic career. Meleis, Hall, and Stevens (1994) identified the presence of "communities of scholars working in concert, collaboration, and competition" (p. 179) within university settings as critical to developing scholars. Presence of this community creates an environment in which scholarship thrives and can be instilled in students (Meleis, Hall, & Stevens, 1994). Embracing values and characteristics of scholarship lays the foundation necessary for an academic career. Ability of academic settings to sustain a community of mentors and scientists may be compromised in light of the exponential program growth.

Individuals with academic appointments are required to balance research, teaching, and service demands (Hodges & Poteet, 1992; Stevenson, 1988). Academic context (e.g., research institutions versus liberal arts colleges) influences the priority given each of these roles within the setting, but competency in all of them is required for tenure. Doctoral programs have focused traditionally on preparing scientists with necessary skills to be competent novice researchers (Downs, 1978; Meleis, Hall, & Stevens, 1994), and skills required for other roles often were acquired on the job. Academic roles always have been multifaceted, but recent changes in society and health care have increased the complexity of academic nursing careers and make reforms in higher education crucial.

The social responsibility of an academic nursing career requires responsiveness to changes in both society and health care (e.g., technological innovation, emphasis on cost-effective outcomes, and demographic trends). The higher education environment, of which nursing is a part, has a responsibility to demonstrate to students, funding sources, employers, and the public that it is producing both graduates and scientific accomplishments that have value to society (Sullivan, 1997). Nurse scholars have the additional responsibility to conduct socially relevant research that makes a difference in the lives of people and has an impact on health care policy decisions (Meleis, 1998).

In summary, doctoral-level nursing education is committed to preparation of nursing scientists. Extensive efforts by the discipline to meet the needs for faculty in academic settings have resulted in increasing the number of doctoral programs. Less attention has been paid the transition from novice researcher to success in an academic career, including individual and institutional responsibilities for facilitating the transition.

■ Academic Contexts—
Finding the "Best Fit"

There is no one model for a successful transition to an academic career. However, a number of different types of academic contexts, with each institution having its own mission and priorities, directly affect faculty work life and productivity. Before making the transition to an academic environment, potential faculty members would benefit from defining their professional goals and abilities and matching them with the mission and priorities of the institution (Gropper, 1998). Potential for successful transition is increased when an individual's goals match those of the institution. Potential faculty members also will benefit from assessing productivity within the institutional setting, as their own productivity will be enhanced by working in a highly productive institution (Holzemer & Chambers, 1988).

Table 21.1 outlines the 1987 Carnegie classification system that categorizes institutions on the basis of degrees offered and comprehensiveness of mission (Boyer, 1990). This classification provides the general focus of the institution relative to teaching and research. While central aspects of a faculty role remain—teaching, research, and service—goals and missions inherent in various institutional types establish different priorities for faculty performance.

Individuals considering positions within one of these types of settings will want additional information—particularly promotion and tenure criteria—that more specifically delineate role expectations. Individuals have a responsibility to assess their abilities and gauge whether they are likely to be successful in a given system, and institutions have a responsibility to hire those who have potential for success in their settings. When institutions both (a) hire faculty members who have potential to attain tenure and (b) provide workloads and needed resources that permit them to teach,

TABLE 21.1   Carnegie Higher Institution Classification

Type	Description
Research university I and II	Offer a full range programs—baccalaureate through doctorate. Give high priority to research, receive federal support, and award at least 50 PhD degrees yearly.
Doctorate granting universities I and II	Offer a full range programs—baccalaureate through doctorate. The distinction between I and II is the number of PhD degrees awarded yearly and the number of disciplines in which they are awarded.
Comprehensive colleges I and II	Offer baccalaureate programs with most offering graduate education through the Master's degree
Liberal arts college I and II	Primarily undergraduate colleges.

Adapted from Boyer, E. L. (1990). *Scholarship reconsidered: Priorities of the professoriate.* Princeton, NJ: Carnegie Foundation for the Advancement of Teaching.

conduct research, and publish appropriately, those hired are more likely to succeed in their quests for promotion and tenure (Gropper, 1998).

Tenure

Tenure as a condition of continued employment in colleges and universities is a long-standing tradition. Each institution has written criteria for appointment, promotion, and tenure based on the American Association of University Professors (1984) guidelines. These criteria, although general, are designed to assess faculty competence and effectiveness in areas of research, teaching, and professional and/or community service (University of Washington, 1999). Traditionally, research universities place higher value on research effectiveness, and liberal arts colleges value teaching and service more (Hodges & Poteet, 1992).

Increasingly, these criteria are coming under scrutiny. Several recent publications have suggested that these expectations are now even more unrealistic than in the past (Anderson, 1998; Boyer, 1990; Henry, 1998; Sneed et al., 1995) and have called for broader definitions of scholarship (Boyer, 1990). This reevaluation is being driven by (a) the general trend in academia to have faculty back in the classroom teaching both undergraduate and graduate students and (b) the more specific trend in schools of nursing to have faculty engaged in revenue-generating community-based practice. In response to these added demands, some schools of nursing have adopted new models for tenure, which we discuss later in this chapter. What is important here is that these issues are far from resolved, making transition to an academic career more risky than ever.

■ Perils in Early Transition to an Academic Career

Transition from doctoral education to an academic position is complex. Several authors have discussed perils inherent in the first years of an academic career (Fox, 1985a; Hodges & Poteet, 1992). These perils may be workload or work-environment related.

Workload

One of the most significant workload perils is excessive or inappropriate teaching and service commitment. Although teaching and service demands are integral parts of a faculty role, a problem arises when these responsibilities take precedence over furthering scholarship. This problem is particularly challenging for nurses who often begin their academic careers after having held responsible positions in nursing or health care and also have previous teaching experience. These individuals are especially vulnerable to using their time in teaching and service activities, as opposed to developing their novice skills in research and publication. Rather than spending time immersed in curricular revisions, undergraduate teaching, or work of task forces or committees, Fox (1985a) recommends that faculty time during this transition be spent in research-related activities. These activities include acquiring grants, directing seminar groups, or advising graduate students in the faculty member's substantive area. Others too have found that the percentage of time spent teaching and advising students, at an individual and program level, was significantly and negatively associated with faculty productivity (Holzemer & Chambers, 1988). We suggest that, during this critical transition, newly prepared doctoral faculty be protected from activities that interfere with a focus on research. Once these faculty have established their programs of research, their committed time and activities in service and teaching can be renegotiated.

Work-Environment Issues

Equally important to workload considerations is the issue of the setting of an individual's first academic position. Most PhD recipients are products of large research universities that have considerable resources and facilities to support scholarship. Thus they have received mentoring in highly productive environments. With the increased number of doctorally prepared nurses, graduates may find themselves in settings where (a) a community of scholars has not been established, (b) resources to support research are scarce, and (c) there is heavy emphasis on undergraduate or master's degree or both types of education and few or no doctoral students. Such environmental factors take their toll on the intellectual, creative, and research productivity of faculty (Barhyte & Redman, 1993) and result in an inability to demonstrate a pattern of achievement in being published and obtaining grant funds. This inability to document success in these areas has an impact on a scholarly career well beyond the initial transition period.

These issues are particularly salient for nurse scholars, as data show women in general are less productive in scholarly activities than their male counterparts (Astin & Davis, 1985; Cole & Zuckerman, 1984; Fox, 1985b). This situation is further compounded by findings that, among women academics, nurses are involved in more administrative activities than their nonnurse colleagues who spend significantly more time in research and publishing (Lia-Hoagberg, 1985). Patterns of professional activities may be established early and maintained throughout a career. Not establishing a pattern of scholarly activities and publication can well result in failure to achieve promotion and tenure.

■ Building a Career— Individual Strategies, Institutional Resources and Responsibilities

After accepting that first academic appointment, a person's success in the position is enhanced if the individual and institution remain committed to furthering the development of the novice researcher to become a seasoned scientist. This commitment involves both individual strategies and institutional resources. Individual strategies include pursuing a postdoctoral fellowship, entering into a partnership with a senior scientist, and establishing a 5-year plan to facilitate successful transition.

Postdoctoral Education

Postdoctoral education is widely accepted as a necessary component of a research career in other disciplines and is increasingly recognized as an important stage in the maturation of nurse scientists (Hinshaw & Lucas, 1993). National Institute of Nursing Research statistics indicate that, between 1986 and 1993, 257 individual and institutional postdoctoral fellowships were awarded (Waters, 1996). Although postdoctoral training will not address all the challenges inherent in the transition from doctoral education to an academic career, a well-designed fellowship provides additional focused research work at a vulnerable point in a person's career. A fellowship can enable an individual to enter into the faculty role with additional mentorship in research, some ongoing research activity, and a viable proposal that can be submitted for funding (Williams, 1988).

To accomplish these goals postdoctoral programs aim to provide developing scientists with opportunities to refine skills learned in the doctoral program, including reflecting, writing, and conducting research on a targeted topic (Albrecht & Greiner, 1992). Objectives for the scholars are to develop new skills and methods (Chenitz & Swanson, 1981) and prepare for employment as beginning independent researchers (Albrecht & Greiner, 1992). Different models of postdoctoral education provide fellows with a combination of educational opportunities including participating in formal coursework, seminars, and independent study, as well as obtaining mentoring with a senior scientist in the area of study. Fellows are encouraged to work closely with nurse scholars and other professionals across disciplines.

People undertake postdoctoral education for a variety of reasons, including commitment to a research career or a desire to expand their substantive area of concentration. Whether an individual decides to pursue further education immediately after the doctorate or wait until later in his or her career, the time spent in postdoctoral education gives fellows an opportunity to work free from the distractions of teaching, administration, clinical practice, and service commitments that characterize positions in academia. Using postdoctoral experience to develop skills in grant writing, expand methodological skills, and publish research—all in an environment of intense scientific activity modeled by a successful mentor—can further develop the foundation acquired during doctoral education and aid transition to an academic career.

At the time this chapter was written both authors were postdoctoral fellows with different institutional training grants in the School of Nursing at the University of Washington. Although at different stages in their academic careers, both came to these fellowships with some academic experience but with the goals of gaining additional research and methodological expertise and expanding their substantive areas of interest. The fellowships allow them to devote their time to research, a factor not encountered in their previous academic positions and an opportunity to accomplish their identified goals.

Partnerships with Senior Scientists

The most productive scientists have a network of colleagues for consultation, critique, advisement, and research (Hood, 1985). These networks can be fostered within the same or different institutions and may be interdisciplinary. Examples include faculty research teams, writing and research support groups. Faculty research teams can provide novice scientists the opportunity to be mentored by senior faculty members who have similar research interests. It is essential therefore that new faculty members make their interests known to lead researchers in their institutions (Magnussen, 1997) and that these senior faculty create opportunities to mentor beginning scientists.

In addition to welcoming new academicians as members of research teams, faculty can provide guidance in support of their publication and research efforts through other forums. For example, in voluntary writing and research support groups, faculty work together—formally and informally—to critique articles, help develop research proposals, or review grant applications. These groups work best when kept small and when members share similar interests. They can be established either informally by individual faculty members or more formally with the assistance of a department chair (Magnussen, 1997). Perhaps more important than the forum chosen is recognition that the most successful academicians have an established network of colleagues with whom they work. Developing and nurturing these relationships early in a person's career therefore is important—in a doctoral program, as a postdoctoral fellow, or in the initial phase of a 5-year development plan.

The 5-Year Plan

As noted earlier, establishing a consistent pattern of scholarly activities within a substantive area early is crucial to building a career. According to Hodges and Poteet (1992), establishing a pattern requires careful planning, self-discipline, and perseverance. They also identified the conduct of research, publication and presentation of scholarly work, and receipt of funding for support of research as elements of successful scholarship that an individual needs to achieve within the first 5 years. Having a plan for achieving these basic requirements of tenure and the tenacity to maintain focus on these activities is essential. A well-constructed plan is precise and includes measurable, time-specific outcomes. It forms a basis for faculty development and periodic assessment of progress (Magnussen, 1997; Hodges & Poteet, 1992). Without steadfast focus, multiple demands of a faculty role will invade on time and energy required for scholarly activities. Equally important to success is need to negotiate the plan and pertinent resources in collaboration with mentors, colleagues, and academic administrators. Even the most well-developed plan constructed by an individual with demonstrated potential will fail without the necessary supporting institutional resources.

Institutional Resources and Responsibilities

Ultimately, individual faculty members are the most committed to ensuring academic success. The institution has an investment in persons and thus a large stake in their productivity, which reflects on the institution. Just as there are individual strategies for success, institutions have resources they must use to ensure that persons are successful. These resources must be tangible, as opposed to informal support mechanisms. Examples of such resources are protected workloads, an intramural grant program, and a research support program—including research design and statistical consultation, data processing services, grant preparation, and research assistants. Other basic services include poster and slide preparation, editorial services, and travel support for faculty development. Other than material resources, tangible mentoring and partnering with senior faculty is important.

Developing healthy relationships between new and senior faculty is critical because new academicians are extremely vulnerable. Senior faculty have the right and responsibility to recommend faculty appointment, promotion, and tenure (deTournyay, 1985). Because of this vulnerability, senior faculty must act in the best interest of novice scientists, insulating them from the complexity of the full faculty role by assuming additional leadership. Examples of such leadership include assuming responsibility for course development and class instruction, volunteering for additional committee work, introducing the individual to resources and relevant persons on campus, and facilitating the individual's career development. Not every senior faculty is capable of assuming this role, but each institution requires a certain number to perform this function if new faculty are to survive the transition and be successful.

So far, we have discussed relevant institutional responsibilities and individual strategies to increase the likelihood of successful transition to an academic career. We have focused on the transition to a traditional academic system (i.e., the tenure track). Historically, it has been the prevalent model, but new trends are emerging in academia. They involve a shift from tenure as the predominant model toward a more eclectic paradigm that includes research tracks, clinical tracks, and adjunct and joint appointments (Leatherman, 1999; Messmer, 1989; Norbeck, 1998; Sherwen, 1998; Sneed et al., 1995).

■ Future Directions

Although controversial, the practice of hiring full-time faculty members in non-tenure track positions is now a permanent fixture of academia (Leatherman, 1999). This trend began partially in response to decreased federal and state monies for higher education and increased public scrutiny of higher education (Norbeck, 1998; Sneed et al., 1995). The most frequently cited argument in favor of this trend is that it provides greater flexibility and potential financial savings for institutions (Leatherman, 1999). Although there are advantages, there also are some other consequences of a two-tiered system. A recent study confirms growth in non-tenure track positions across institutional types (cited in Leatherman, 1999). This study's preliminary report identified significant differences between tenure and non-tenure track faculty when comparing involvement in governance, salary and benefits, status, and written policies covering recognition of performance. Generally, for non-tenure track faculty, institutions grant fewer sabbatical leaves, provide less financial support for professional development activities, and offer less opportunity for participation in faculty governance. The researchers concluded that academia needs to address the status of non-tenure track faculty by creating an equitable system that recognizes good performance and long-term service (cited in Leatherman, 1999).

■ Concluding Statement

Increase in non-tenure track positions is evident in nursing by a multiplicity of alternative models including research tracks, clinical tracks, and adjunct and joint appointments. At this time there appears to be no consensus among nursing academicians as to which of these models is most effective for addressing needs of the discipline, nor have these alternative tracks been developed and implemented consistently. Thus, for example, a research track appointment in one setting may have different responsibilities and criteria for appointment than in another. Issues previously discussed, such as equity, have yet to be addressed fully in nursing academe. Although it is not likely that the tenure system will end in the near future, the increasing numbers of non-tenure track positions is expected to continue. Therefore novice scientists have more choices to consider when making the transition to an academic career. The challenge that remains is to find the "best fit" between an individual's talents, abilities, and career goals and the type and setting of academic position that will best promote that person's success.

References

Albrecht, M., & Greiner, P. A. (1992). Postdoctoral study: The importance for nursing. *Journal of Nursing Education, 31*(8), 373–374.

American Association of Colleges of Nursing. (1997). Indicators of quality in doctoral programs in nursing. *Journal of Professional Nursing, 13*(3), 200–202.

American Association of University Professors. (1984). *Policy documents and reports.* Washington, DC: Author.

Anderson, C. A. (1998). Academic nursing: A desirable career? *Nursing Outlook, 46*(1), 5–6.

Astin, H. S., & Davis, D. E. (1985). Research productivity across the life and career cycles: Facilitators and barriers for women. In M. F. Fox (Ed.), *Scholarly writing & publishing: Issues, problems, and solutions* (pp. 147–160). Boulder, CO: Westview Press.

Barhyte, D. Y., & Redman, B. K. (1993). Factors related to graduate nursing faculty scholarly productivity. *Nursing Research, 42*(3), 179–183.

Boyer, E. L. (1990). *Scholarship reconsidered: Priorities of the professoriate.* Princeton, NJ: Carnegie Foundation for the Advancement of Teaching.

Chenitz, W. C., & Swanson, J. M. (1981). The postdoctoral research fellow in nursing: In between the cracks in the academic wall. *Nursing Outlook, 29*(7), 417–420.

Cole, J. R., & Zuckerman, H. (1984). The productivity puzzle: Persistence and change in patterns of publication of men and women scientists. In M. W. Steinkamp & M. Maehr (Eds.), *Advances in motivation and achievement* (Vol. 2, pp. 217–258). Beverly Hills, CA: JAI Press.

deTournyay, R. (1985). Dealing with tenured faculty. *Journal of Professional Nursing, 1*(1), 9–13.

Downs, F. S. (1978). Doctoral education in nursing: Future directions. *Nursing Outlook, 26,* 56–61.

Fox, M. F. (1985a). The transition from dissertation student to publishing scholar and professional. In M. F. Fox (Ed.), *Scholarly writing & publishing: Issues, problems, and solutions* (pp. 6–16). Boulder, CO: Westview Press.

Fox, M. F. (1985b). Publication, performance, and reward in science and scholarship. In J. C. Smart (Ed.), *Higher education: Handbook of theory and research* (Vol. 1, pp. 255–282). New York: Agathon.

Germain, C. P., Deatrick, J. A., Hagopian, G. A., & Whitney, F. W. (1994). Evaluation of a PhD program: Paving the way. *Nursing Outlook, 42*(3), 117–122.

Gropper, R. G. (1998). Tenure in nursing education: How are we doing? *Nursing Outlook, 46*(5), 202–205.

Henry, B. (1998). Practice, teach and research too. *IMAGE: Journal of Nursing Scholarship, 32,* 102–103.

Hinshaw, A. S., & Lucas, M. D. (1993). Postdoctoral education—A new tradition for nursing research. *Journal of Professional Nursing, 9*(6), 309.

Hodges, L. C., & Poteet, G. W. (1992). The first 5 years after the dissertation. *Journal of Professional Nursing, 8*(3), 143–147.

Holzemer, W. L., & Chambers, D. B. (1986). Healthy nursing doctoral programs: Relationship between perceptions of the academic environment and productivity of faculty and alumni. *Research in Nursing and Health, 9*, 299–307.

Holzemer, W. L., & Chambers, D. B. (1988). A contextual analysis of faculty productivity. *Journal of Nursing Education, 27*(1), 10–18.

Hood, J. C. (1985). The lone scholar myth. In M. F. Fox (Ed.), *Scholarly writing & publishing: Issues, problems, and solutions* (pp. 111–125). Boulder, CO: Westview Press.

Ketefian, S. (1991). Doctoral preparation for faculty roles: Expectations and realities. *Journal of Professional Nursing, 7*(3), 105–111.

Ketefian, S., & Redman, R. W. (1994). The changing face of graduate education. In J. McCloskey & H. K. Grace (Eds.), *Current issues in nursing* (4th ed.) (pp. 188–195). St. Louis: Mosby-Year Book.

Ketefian, S., & Redman, R. W. (1997). Nursing science in the global community. *IMAGE: Journal of Nursing Scholarship, 29*(1), 11–15.

Leatherman, C. (1999, April 9). Growth in positions off the tenure track is a trend that's here to stay, study finds. *The Chronicle of Higher Education,* A14.

Lia-Hoagberg, B. (1985). Comparison of professional activities of nurse doctorates and other women academics. *Nursing Research, 34*(3), 155–159.

Magnussen, L. (1997). Ensuring success: The faculty development plan. *Nurse Educator, 22*(6), 30–33.

Meleis, A. I. (1998). A passion for making a difference: Revisions for empowerment. *Scholarly Inquiry for Nursing Practice: An International Journal, 12*(1), 87–95.

Meleis, A. I., Hall, J. M., & Stevens, P. E. (1994). Scholarly caring in doctoral nursing education: Promoting diversity and collaborative mentorship. *IMAGE: Journal of Nursing Scholarship, 26*(3), 177–180.

Messmer, P. R. (1989). Academic tenure in schools of nursing. *Journal of Professional Nursing, 5*(1), 39–48.

Murphy, J. F. (1981). Doctoral education in, of, and for nursing: An historical analysis. *Nursing Outlook, 29*(11), 645–649.

Norbeck, J. S. (1998). Teaching, research and service: Striking the balance in doctoral education. *Journal of Professional Nursing, 14*(4), 197–205.

Sherwen, L. N. (1998). When the mission is teaching: Does nursing faculty practice fit? *Journal of Professional Nursing, 14*(3), 137–143.

Sigma Theta Tau International. (1991). Nursing doctoral programs in the United States. *Reflections, 17,* 23.

Sigma Theta Tau International. (1999). STTI Library [On-line]. Available: www.sttiiupui.edu/library.

Sneed, N. V., Edlund, B. J., Allred, C. A., Hickey, M., Heriot, C. S., Haight, B., & Hoffman, S. (1995). Appointment, promotion, and tenure criteria to meet changing perspectives in health care. *Nurse Educator, 20*(2), 23–28.

Stevenson, J. S. (1988). Nursing knowledge development: Into era II. *Journal of Professional Nursing, 4*(3), 152–162.

Sullivan, E. J. (1997). A changing higher education environment. *Journal of Professional Nursing, 13*(3), 143–148.

University of Washington, School of Nursing (1999, February 9). *Criteria and examples for appointment, reappointment, promotion and tenure*. Unpublished draft.

Waters, C. M. (1996). Professional development in nursing research—A culturally diverse postdoctoral experience. *IMAGE: Journal of Nursing Scholarship, 28*(1), 47–50.

Williams, C. A. (1988). Career development of the nurse-scientist: The new doctorate faces a postdoctoral. *Journal of Professional Nursing, 4*(2), 73.

■ Editor's Questions for Discussion

Discuss the purpose and goals of doctoral education in nursing. To what extent have these goals been changed or reinforced to meet the demands of multiple types of doctoral degree programs? How are A. Fisher and B. Habermann's views regarding quality programs reinforced or challenged by Lenz and Hardin (Chapter 20), Ketefian and Redman (Chapter 19), and Miller (Chapter 36)?

What disparate beliefs exist about how to develop a scientific knowledge base for nursing education? What role should nursing practice play in knowledge development? Should nursing scientists have expertise in nursing practice?

Discuss the multifaceted academic role. How can people balance academic role requirements? What implications for future academic roles are presented by Fleming (Chapter 22) and Lindeman (Chapter 63)? What queries should potential faculty make in determining a match between themselves and institutions? Concerning information offered, how might perceptions be validated? What data would be helpful for prospective faculty? What obligations do institutions have in the recruitment of prospective faculty?

How may workload misunderstandings and problems be prevented? What administrative and management variables affect workloads? Present negotiation strategies that may be used to resolve workload concerns. What negotiations are needed regarding non-tenure track faculty if scholarship expectations are to occur?

Should postdoctoral programs be developed in accordance with different purposes of multiple types of doctoral programs in nursing? What should be qualifications for mentors in postdoctoral programs focused predominantly on developing a scientific knowledge base for nursing? What networks in practice settings should be established for postdoctoral fellows? How might such networks be developed through mentors in postdoctoral programs? Propose quality indicators for evaluation of postdoctoral programs. What developmental process needs to occur for faculty to become mentors?

22

Tenure

A Continuing Issue for Academic Nursing

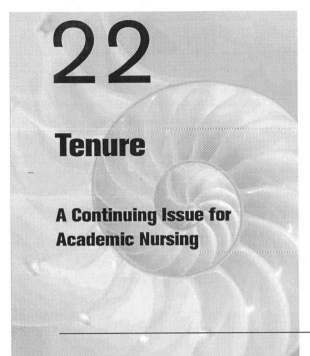

Juanita W. Fleming, PhD, RN, FAAN

A s we enter the 21st century, tenured faculty are expected to remain in the vanguard of academic nursing. These leaders are responsible for the continued high quality of nurse preparation in the face of rapid advances in knowledge, science, and technology. Economic factors and anticipated radical changes in the health care delivery system present further challenges. In this chapter, I present an overall view of academic staffing in institutions of higher learning and ultimately focus on the niche of tenured faculty as it exists now.

■ Academic Staffing in Institutions

Types of Institutions

The system of higher education in the United States is diverse and complex. Institutions include community colleges, liberal arts colleges, comprehensive colleges and universities, land grant universities, and major research universities. Some of these institutions are public—and receive assistance from state or local government or both. Some are private and have large endowments. Some are supported by religious organizations or other groups such as the military. All taken together are significant in terms of reputation and services provided to the nation.

Types of Academic Ranks

Academic ranks for appointments, listed in increasing order of importance, include instructor, assistant professor, associate professor, and professor. Specific criteria for each rank in the series are provided by each institution of higher learning. Additionally, lecturers may be employed; these faculty are basically qualified teachers hired for a fixed term.

Types of Appointments

Institutions of higher education have two types of appointments—tenured and non-tenured. *Tenured* appointments are those in which a faculty member is on full-time continuous assignment in an academic rank. Non-tenured appointments are those in which either (a) the faculty member is not eligible for tenure because of the nature of the position or (b) an arrangement whereby faculty may be considered for tenure in the future. We briefly describe non-tenured appointments first and then focus on tenured appointments.

Non-Tenured Appointments

Non-tenured appointments include temporary, voluntary, adjunct, shared, and (at some institutions) clinical and research appointments. *Temporary faculty* are those assigned duties and responsibilities for a specified period, usually for a year or less. *Voluntary faculty* are those with official appointment in a specific college or area who devote some of their time to an academic program for which no salary is received. *Adjunct faculty* are qualified professionals who contribute to teaching,

research, or other academic work in the university or an agency outside the university. *Shared faculty* meet needs of both the institution and appointees in a special way. Examples of such appointments are women or men who wish to work only part-time and are employed to share and perform responsibilities with another appointee but for one faculty position. *Clinical faculty* are clinically competent professional practitioners who provide care and counseling to clients in locations where students have clinical experiences. Such faculty expose students to professional expertise and direct students' work in these clinical settings. *Research faculty* operate under contracts, grants, or other designated funds. These faculty participate in university academic programs through research or other creative activity of specified duration.

■ Tenure in Academia

Academic tenure is defined as an arrangement under which a faculty appointment at an institution of higher education is continued until retirement for age or physical disability. Exceptions to this agreement are (a) dismissal for adequate cause or (b) unavoidable termination due to financial exigency or change of an institutional program. Tenure in academia, rightly understood and properly administered, is thought to provide the most reliable means of ensuring faculty quality and educational excellence, as well as the best guarantee of academic freedom.

Components and Criteria

Tenure is explicitly tied to the academic function of faculty in an institution of higher education. Faculty work is traditionally divided into three broad categories: teaching; research, creative productivity or both; and service. These three components comprise (a) effective teaching of students in undergraduate and graduate programs, which also involves advising and counseling students (pre-first-year students to postdoctoral students); (b) scholarly activity, which involves research or creative works or both, publications, presentations, or performances; (c) nondisciplinary activity, which involves serving on departmental, college, or institutional committees, assuming leadership roles in the institution, serving on external committees, task forces, and commissions; and (d) professional service, which involves applying expertise in the discipline to help the institution, governmental agencies, business, industry, and citizen groups or organizations.

Institutions of higher education have a great deal of autonomy and discretion in making appointments, reappointments, promotions, and tenure decisions. Accordingly, criteria for tenure are set by each institution, documentation of teaching, research, and service is measured. Diamond (1993, 1995) provides excellent guidance for documenting effectiveness of research faculty members, creative teaching, student learning, advising, scholarly professional, and creative work. Prior to obtaining tenure, a probationary period for the faculty member hired in a tenure track position is often required. This probationary period, often 7 years, is allowed for the faculty member to meet the institution's criteria for tenure.

Review for Tenure

For the most part, institutions grant tenure only after extensive review of an individual's performance. In this review, performance is judged by self, students, and committees of internal and external faculty, the department chair, and other administrators. Tenure is rarely automatically given, as it is viewed as a privilege, not as a right. Although obtaining tenure itself is not a right, once it has been granted, tenure confers certain rights—the primary one being continuous employment,

with the understanding that the individual and the institution continue to meet certain conditions.

Some faculty may be recommended for tenure early in their probationary period; others are considered for tenure only near end of the period. For example, if an individual has 7 years of probation, he or she may be considered for tenure at end of the fifth year or beginning of the sixth year. If tenure is not granted, a paid terminal period (often a year) is provided whereby the faculty member has a year to find other employment.

Tenure and Academic Freedom

For many years, tenure has been tied to academic freedom.

> In 1940, following a series of joint conferences begun in 1934, representatives of the American Association of University Professors and the Association of American Colleges agreed upon a restatement of the principles set forth in the 1925 conference statement on Academic Freedom and Tenure. (Kreiser, 1990, p. 3)

This restatement, known as the 1940 Statement of Principles on Academic Freedom and Tenure, was endorsed by a number of other organizations.

Institutions of higher education exist for the common good, not to further the interests of faculty or the institution as a whole. Consequently, the common good depends on the freedom to search for truth and its exposition. Academic freedom is essential to both teaching and research. Freedom in teaching is fundamental to the protection of the rights of the teacher in teaching and the student in learning.

Institutional Differences

Tenure appointments may vary by institution. The University of Kentucky, for example, has a Regular, Special, Library, and Extension Title Series in which an appointment for tenure may be made. The Regular Title Series is similar to that of other major research-oriented universities. Thus tenured faculty or faculty appointed to an academic rank position where tenure may be considered generally are expected to meet criteria that demonstrate excellence in the three basic areas—teaching and research or creative productivity, or both, and service. In the Special Title Series, faculty must meet the specific criteria delineated with excellent performance. However, in this series conduct of research is not required. The Library Series is designated especially for Librarians who hold academic appointments. The Extension Series is reserved for faculty whose primary assignment involves one of the University Extension programs serving citizens of the Commonwealth of Kentucky. Because the University of Kentucky is a land-grant institution, for all tenured positions the requirement for service involves meeting needs of communities in the commonwealth.

Other differences among institutions also affect expectations of faculty. In some private liberal arts colleges, Bukalski and Zirpola (1993) noted that

> a good teaching record and completion of modest committee assignments within the college may be considered sufficient for tenure or promotion. Faculty members are also expected to "keep up" with their fields through reading. Teaching is vigorously evaluated. Quality of education provided to the students is emphasized. (p. 7)

Liberal arts institutions are concerned with increasing human intellectual abilities and helping students gain appreciation for life experiences. Faculty in liberal arts colleges that exempt the research criteria for tenure likely will be judged on how well they help students develop through transmission of knowledge associated with a liberally educated person.

Comprehensive institutions may emphasize teaching, small land-grant institutions may emphasize service and teaching, and larger land-grant institutions may emphasize research and service. Both public and private institutions that are considered major universities have the broad mission of education, research, and service and expect faculty with tenure to be triple threats. Most expect tenured faculty in major research institutions at the associate professor level to have funded research with regional and national reputations and at the professor level to have national and international reputations.

Discipline Differences

Differences in the scholarship perspectives of disciplines may have ramifications affecting tenure. How a discipline perceives scholarship is very important. Organizations representing several disciplines have published statements proposing definitions of scholarly work in their fields. Institutions of higher learning may use these statements to develop criteria for evaluating scholarly, intellectual, and creative work at the institution. Diamond (1995) provides examples of scholarship proposed by the American Historical Association, the American Assembly of Collegiate Schools of Business, the National Office of Arts Accreditation in Higher Education, the American Chemical Society, the Joint Policy Board for Mathematics, and the American Academy of Religion. Perspectives of these disciplines vary considerably, with some being more traditional than others. For example, nursing is among the newer disciplines and may not be viewed in the same way as a traditional discipline.

Differences may be problematic in situations when colleagues from a different discipline assess scholarly achievement. What is effective or outstanding teaching in a discipline? One view of teaching is that it is a form of scholarship (Glassick, Huber, & Maecroff,

1997). How that is operationalized may vary among disciplines. Nursing educators must continue to help others in higher education understand how scholarship in nursing is demonstrated.

■ Unresolved Concerns Related to Tenure

Scholarship in Nursing

In nursing education, how investigative skills are developed, how research is transmitted to students, and how knowledge is used in practice need to be communicated effectively. As a result, evidence-based practice is emerging in nursing. As practices in nursing based on evidence are defined, they will need to be explained to colleagues in higher education so that nursing faculty seeking tenure can be judged objectively and fairly.

Scholarship in nursing like other disciplines is dependent on knowledge—the core business of institutions of higher education. Faculty who are successful in meeting criteria of an institution will demonstrate their scholarship by an activity (or a combination of activities) that discovers, creates, advances, integrates, applies, or transforms knowledge. Moreover, the need for lifelong learning is important.

Institutions of higher learning want engaged scholars. The University of Kentucky College of Arts and Sciences noted that engaged scholars are those who are wholeheartedly committed to the principles and aspirations of the academy and who vigorously participate in a full range of scholarly activities (J. Morreale, personal communication, March, 1999). During his or her career, an engaged scholar is a (a) dedicated and patient teacher, (b) learned resource, (c) mentor for students, (d) mental stimulant for colleagues, (e) public and active participant in the campus's intellectual culture, (f) contributor of scholarly publi-

cations, and (g) valued contributor to the larger success of the community of scholars and to the achievement of faculty responsibilities.

Workload Issues

Workload may be defined as all faculty activities related to essential professional activities and responsibilities. It includes interaction with students, colleagues, service to the university and the community, teaching, research or creative productivity, and professional development. Many institutions have specific workload policies. Faculty know how many courses they should teach for a full load and how to distribute their efforts in research or creativity, teaching, professional development, and service.

Issues related to workload for tenured faculty often center on productivity. Does productivity decrease when someone becomes tenured? Is teaching and advising as effective? Has research output declined? What is the interaction between research, teaching, and service? Should some faculty have research-only or service-only assignments? Should faculty teach only undergraduates or only graduates?

The need to have more tenured faculty in undergraduate classes has become an issue. Expectations of faculty and outcomes expected may need to be negotiated.

Post-tenure Review

Nursing educators in colleges and universities who have received tenure are subjected to post-tenure review. Demand for accountability, end of mandatory retirement, faculty demographics, need for flexibility, fiscal concerns, and debates about tenure are some of the reasons that post-tenure review has become an often popular topic among educators. Senior Scholar, Dr. Joseph C. Morreale, of the American Association of Higher Education, noted that in the public sector, 32 state systems have policies on post-tenure review, 8 states do the reviews on a case by case basis, and 6 states have a legislative mandate for post-tenure review (J. Morreale, personal communication, March 1999). He further pointed out that, in ongoing survey work in which he was involved, 46% of private institutions have post-tenure review in place and 28% have it under consideration.

Three basic models of post-tenure review have been identified (J. Morreale, personal communication, March 1999): (a) annual review, which is not viewed as a comprehensive review; (b) comprehensive periodic review; and (c) triggered consequential review, which occurs when performance is perceived as unsatisfactory. Arguments in favor of post-tenure review are that it (a) supports continuous faculty development, (b) helps the public recognize that institutions are accountable, (c) keeps tenure viable, (d) supports differentiated staffing models, and (e) forestalls further external interference. Arguments against post-tenure review are that (a) the process is unnecessary and duplicative, (b) an erosion of collegiality, (c) overadministration, (d) overtaxing resources, and (e) threatening tenure.

C. Licata (1998) summarizes the unifying principles of post-tenure review. Basically these principles include the notions that (a) post-tenure evaluation is not in opposition to the standard of tenure, (b) post-tenure review can strengthen rather than diminish the value of tenure, (c) tenured faculty represent an important intellectual resource, and (d) faculty have stake not only in their own contributions and accomplishments but in those of others. As higher education becomes more accountable and nursing practice based on evidence emerges, nursing faculty will, like other faculty, engage in helping resolve the issues associated with post-tenure review.

■ Concluding Statement

Tenured faculty in nursing likely will be expected to serve as leaders in the 21st century. They must help ensure that the educational enterprise provides programs that are effective and of excellent quality. Knowledge is the key, the core business of institutions of higher learning. Academic nursing is or should be about preparing its future professionals in discovery of new knowledge, its transmission, and its application to enhance health care. Faculty are obligated to help prepare individuals who can function globally and who are able to perform as excellent practitioners, educators, entrepreneurs, and administrators in nursing. Institutions of higher learning must demonstrate excellence through faculty. Questions about tenure remain. How should nursing education provide future leadership in helping to resolve tenure concerns?

■ References

Bukalski, P. J., & Zirpola, D. J. (1993). *Guide for nontenured faculty members: Annual evaluation, promotion, tenure.* [Monograph No. 6.] Atlanta: University Film and Video Association.

Diamond, R. M., & Adam, B. (1993). *Recognizing faculty work: Reward systems for the year 2000.* San Francisco: Jossey-Bass.

Diamond, R. M. (1995). *Preparing for promotion and tenure review: A faculty guide.* Boston: Anker.

Glassick, C. E., Huber, M. T., & Maecroff, G. I. (1997). *Scholarship assessed: Evaluation of the professorate.* San Francisco: Jossey-Bass.

Kreiser, B. R. (Ed.). (1990). *American Association of University Professors policy documents and reports* (7th ed.). Washington, DC: Author.

Licata, C. M. (1998). Post-tenure review: At the crossroads of accountability and opportunity. *American Association of Higher Education (AAHE) Bulletin, 50*(10), 3–6.

■ Editor's Questions for Discussion

Which of Fleming's suggestions have implications for faculty engaged in activities in managed care environments? Discuss the advantages and disadvantages of non-tenured university appointments. How typical are non-tenured clinical appointments in private and state universities?

Discuss the pros and cons of tenure track appointments. How are weights decided in assigning importance to the three standard criteria for tenure? What types of variation are related to different types of university? To what extent are differences in disciplines a factor in meeting tenure criteria? Should tenure criteria be the same for all disciplines? Do you agree with Fleming's statements about criteria and institutional differences for tenure? Provide examples in your response.

Debate the pros and cons of post-tenure review. What functions may or may not be served by post-tenure review? How may post-tenure criteria differ from tenure criteria? Address the workload issue and questions posed by Fleming. How realistically might these issues be resolved in the future?

What impact is Boyer's model (Keating & Perry, Chapter 65, and Boland, Chapter 71) likely to have on tenure and post-tenure review of nursing faculty? Should reviews by clinical agencies be evidence provided in tenure evaluation? How likely is tenure to be abolished by universities in the future? What factors may contribute to abolishing or maintaining tenure? Suggest means other than tenure or post-tenure review for assessing competency and maintaining highly qualified faculty.

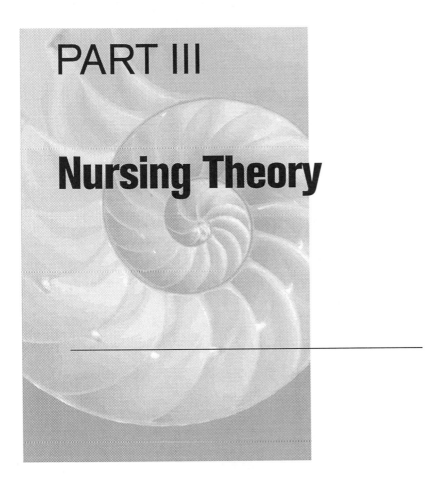

PART III

Nursing Theory

"... And both that morning equally lay
In leaves no step had trodden black ... "

Frost's lines can imply that numerous methodologies are available for developing nursing knowledge. Further, they may suggest that paths of theory construction are relatively fresh and untrodden, hinting that the state of theory development and application is virtually virgin territory.

The disparate views and approaches of the authors in this Part clearly show that diversity is healthy. In many respects the variation allows the professional to meditate on the value of developing an empirical base for knowledge and practice. Are all the approaches illustrated in these chapters of equal value? How important for nursing is it to engage in dialogue about advances and methodologies?

23

Directions for Theory Development in Nursing

For an Increased Coherence in the New Century

Hesook Suzie Kim, PhD, RN

Nursing's knowledge development during the past three decades has followed multiple paths, shaded by various commitments to different epistemologies and alternative linkages among philosophy, theory, and methods of inquiry. The resulting pluralism in the nursing knowledge system (i.e., pluralism in philosophies, ontology of human nature, theories and scientific explanations, scientific methodology, and conceptualization of nursing practice) raises critical concerns about issues pertaining to both nursing knowledge development and application of knowledge into practice. More than a decade ago, Stevenson and Woods (1986) suggested that nursing seems to have embraced a pluralism based on two philosophies of science—positivism and historicism—more readily than other disciplines. Diversity in approaches to nursing knowledge development is suggestive of intellectual vitality and seems to have provided much stimulation to seek alternative and sometimes competing explanations for nursing questions. This diversity has become more pluralistic during the current decade, going beyond just those two philosophies of science. However, it also has created disarray and unsystematic collection of knowledge bits in nursing, which has potential for causing confusion in practice applications. Kim (1993) addresses the problematic nature of this state of affairs for nursing practitioners who must contend with multiple claims of knowledge.

In moving into the new century, we need to seek a more systematic, coherent development of nursing knowledge. There is a need to embrace an epistemological perspective for nursing that can pull the various aspects of pluralism together and guide the future of theory development in nursing. To verify such a need, I present first the current picture of pluralism in nursing. I then present an epistemological perspective for nursing, which can transform nursing's individualistic and collective knowledge development into a coherent and unified whole.

■ Pluralism in Nursing Knowledge

Pluralism in science can be viewed within a levels framework from which different sets of scientific understandings and theories develop, as shown in Figure 23.1. Such a view is organized around pluralistic positions that can be used to pose questions about the philosophy of science, ontology, paradigm orientations, theoretical formulations, and methods. These levels seem to be interrelated and thus point to possible coherent linkages running through a set of knowledge being developed within a discipline.

Level One

The first level comprises the nature of scientific knowledge from the philosophy of science perspective. It encompasses two sets of positions regarding philosophy of science questions: (a) three positions of scientific realism, relativism, and pragmatism, which tend to specify fundamentally different ideas about the nature of scientific theories and scientific endeavor; and (b) three positions of scientific monism, dualism, and multiplism, which point to varying notions about differentiation in sciences. Debates regarding the ramifications of scientific realism, relativism, and pragmatism are ongoing and active on the current

postpositivistic scene; such arguments take place amid the waning of logical positivism both within the philosophy of science (see Laudan, 1990) and within different scientific fields, including nursing. Pluralism in sciences at various levels can be traced to these fundamental positions. In addition, philosophers of science have long argued for acceptance of scientific monism, scientific dualism, or scientific multiplism as a specific way of describing how the total scientific enterprise must deal with its work.

Scientific Monism

Scientific monism stemmed originally from the positivistic tradition, especially with regard to the social sciences, as enunciated by Auguste Comte (1865) in his discussion of economy, political science, and sociology in relation to the natural sciences. Specific monism adheres to the notion that one type of scientific explanation is thought to be viable logically and fundamentally, for all scientific disciplines; the basis of this concept is that all phenomena are believed either to be reducible to a certain common essential nature, to share fundamentally the same characteristics, or to belong to a unified explanatory structure.

This position, of course, advanced the notion of the science unity with "the thesis that the physical sciences afforded the paradigm of what was to be a science, *a fortiori,* a human science" (Margolis, 1990, p. 167). This proposal therefore is based on a commitment to both physicalism and extentionalism. Although the literature indicates demise of this sort of scientific monism in recent decades, scientific monism with orientations to materalism, naturalism, unitarianism, and holism is gaining a renewed favor. In nursing, advocates for holism and systems perspective can be considered holding the scientific monistic position. The major limitation of this position is in its adherence to reductionistic thinking in

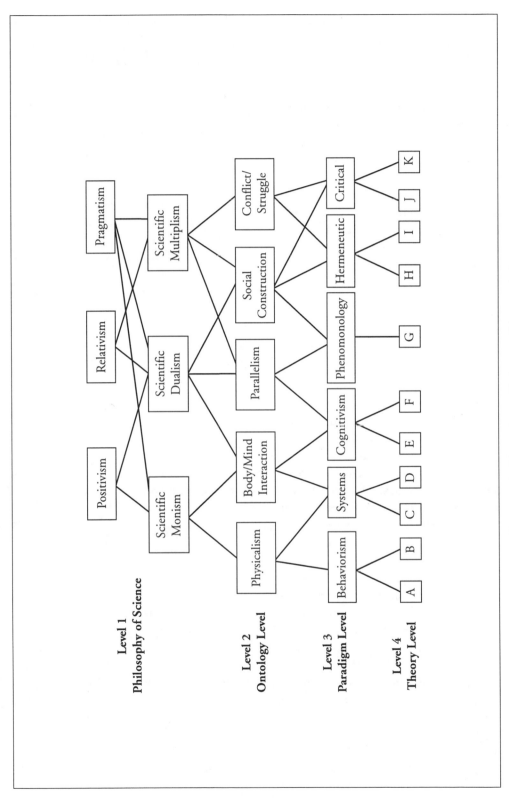

Figure 23.1 Depiction of Pluralism in Nursing at Different Levels. (Categories specified are possible examples.)

dealing with phenomena of concern specific to different disciplinary interests.

Scientific Dualism

Scientific dualism pits the human sciences against the physical and natural sciences in various respects. Margolis (1989, 1990) claims that three essential points (which are interrelated, however) separate the human sciences from the physical sciences because human sciences are entailed with (a) the inherent nature of human limitation in what we can know, (b) the characteristics of human phenomena that are basically tied to human intentionality, and (c) a human being's inseparable tie with its world through language and culture.

In a similar vein but with a different emphasis, Taylor (1985) suggests that it is not possible to understand "human life and action" with theories in the human sciences modeled on the natural sciences. He thus argues for a hermeneutic conception of the human sciences to be differentiated from major tenets of the natural sciences, in the same perspective argued by hermeneutic philosophers such as Dilthey (1988), Ricoeur (1981), and Bernstein (1983). In nursing, especially during the past decade, there has been a growing sentiment to align nursing science with the human sciences from the hermeneutic, interpretive perspective, and distancing it from medicine and the natural and physical sciences. This position, then, holds that nursing science is a branch of the human sciences, which are aimed at providing explanations and understanding of human phenomena from hermeneutic perspectives. The focus is on the historicity, culture-boundedness, language-embeddedness, and intentionality of human beings in terms of both the subjects of knowing and the knowers (i.e., scientists) themselves. The ramification of this position for nursing rests on the kinds of knowledge possible from this perspective only.

Scientific Multiplism

Scientific multiplism was most credibly articulated by Habermas (1971). He presented three types of human cognitive interests, arguing that human cognitive interests can be differentiated as technical, practical, and emancipatory interests. The technical cognitive interest focuses on technical control with emphasis on practical reasons in dealing with objects and thus points to the empirical-analytic sciences. The practical cognitive interest is oriented to understanding social life with an emphasis on reflective judgment and interpretive understanding and hence points to the historical-hermeneutic sciences. The emancipatory cognitive interest focuses on the freeing of individuals from constraints and domination with emphasis on critical reflection and self-reflection for mutual understanding and thus points to critical-oriented sciences.

From a different angle, Ford (1990) offered the concept of systematic pluralism, which

> asserts that, although the world may be one, there are plural routes to responsible knowledge, though the number of responsible approaches— or at least the number of classes into which they can be appropriately grouped—may be quite small, . . . that the foundational condition of systematic pluralism rests with the notion that each system must be logically prior to all the others, *in toto* and with respect to each of its basic constituent elements, its principles, methods, interpretations, etc. (p. 336)

Such pluralism begins at the level of pluralism in world views, which leads to pluralism at the level of the sciences. In addition, many scientists claim uniqueness of each discipline as the basis for differentiation of scientific knowledge—for example, differentiating biology from medicine, physics from engineering, and nursing from medicine.

From this position, then, nursing science is a distinct discipline with specific knowledge claims, for which unique sets of scientific methodology and epistemological positions need to be defined. Earlier, attempts were made to delineate nursing science from this position. Examples are the work of Carper (1978) in her articulation of fundamental patterns of knowing in nursing and the exposition by Donaldson and Crowley (1978) on the structure of nursing discipline. However, nursing as a scientific discipline has not yet developed a unifying position that sets it apart from other disciplines as a field of knowledge.

Nursing scholars have accepted pluralism at the philosophy of science level mainly at face value. On the one hand, Allen, Benner, and Diekelmann (1983) proposed that the viability of pluralism is based on three different philosophies of science—(i.e., analytical empiricism, Heideggerian phenomenology, and critical social theory) as "fruitful" in generating nursing research. On the other hand, Gortner (1993) suggested the need for convergence on "a nursing's developing syntax" through "scientific realism and explanatory power" to address both the natural and social aspects of nursing's subject matter; nonetheless, she accepted the necessity of multiple "world views" as the basis for substantive theory development in nursing (p. 486).

Level Two

The second level of pluralism is oriented to the ontology of sciences' subject matter. As nursing is concerned with human phenomena in terms of both patients as recipients of care and nurses as providers of care, the ontological focus has to be on human nature, on which specific models of human being are formulated. Ontologies of human nature vary according to positions taken on its different dimensions—for example, the dimension regarding body and mind interplay and structure of human being, the dimension regarding fundamental processes of human life, or the dimension regarding the nature of human existence.

Variation in Models

Among many models of human being espoused by scientists at present, few examples would be sufficient to suggest the variations in philosophies regarding human nature: physicalism, epiphenomenalism, parallelism, interactionism, rationalism, social or cultural determinism, intersubjective constructivism, and conflict philosophy (see Stevenson, 1987, and Rakover, 1989, for illustrations). Such ontological models view differently (a) the essential nature of biological (i.e., the body), metaphysical (i.e., the mind or spirit), and social aspects of human beings, (b) relationships, interrelationships, or integration among different aspects of the human entity, and (c) human beings' relations with the environment and universe. In nursing, the dominant ontological beliefs regarding human nature seem to be holism, bio-psycho-social integrationism, and social constructivism. Stevenson and Woods (1989) went so far as to suggest that "nursing's philosophical value of holism" could be the base from which scientific work in nursing may ensue. However, the ontology of holism is not the only perspective with which nursing theories have been developed in nursing.

Level Three

The third level of pluralism refers to paradigmatic pluralism. Contrary to Kuhn's suggestion that singular paradigm dominates a scientific discipline as in normal sciences (Kuhn, 1970), most sciences are developing with multiple paradigms. Staats (1989) talked of psychology as having developed into fields of study identified as separate entities holding oppositional positions as "nature versus nurture, situationism versus personality, scientific versus humanistic psychology" (p. 143), with little or no planning with respect to their relationships to the rest of psychology.

Good (1994) also identified four different approaches to the anthropological study of illness and health as "the rationalistic-empiricist" tradition, the cognitive tradition, the "meaning-centered" tradition, and the critical medical anthropology. Bhaskar (1986) suggested that it is inevitable that "on the new, integrative-pluralistic world-view that emerges, both nature and the sciences (and the sciences in the nature) appear as stratified and differentiated, interconnected and developing" (p. 101).

Nursing Paradigms

Similarly, nursing knowledge has been progressing with commitments to various paradigmatic orientations (a) based on holistic (unitary), adaptation, functional, and humanistic paradigms, which are evident in nursing's grand theories; (b) based on psychological and sociological paradigms, such as behaviorism, cognitivism, psychological humanism, interpretivism, structuralism, functionalism, symbolic interactionism, and critical philosophy; and (c) based on the natural sciences, such as biobehaviorism, biochemical determinism, and relativity. These so-called paradigms in nursing are scientific camps differentiated by a haphazard mixture of scientific philosophies and ontologies. No parallel features set apart the so-called paradigms in nursing.

Level Four

The fourth level of pluralism points to development of multiple theories from various paradigms. There are two aspects of theoretical pluralism: (a) multiple theories coming from partitioning of subject matters for theoretical focus and (b) multiple theories based on specific paradigm orientations. These two sources of differentiation produce multiple theories with different scopes, explanatory formulations, and scientific purposes, which often exist as fragmented, competitive, or rival in their explanations and scientific claims. Theoretical pluralism can be illustrated by an example of multiple theories providing explanations of behavioral change and prescriptions for compliance-gaining interventions identified by Wiseman and Schenck-Hamlin (1981). In nursing, for example, multiple theories exist regarding health behavior, pain and suffering, chronic illness experience, and caring, which are based on various ontological and paradigmatic orientations.

This illustration of pluralism in the sciences and nursing suggests a need for direction for the new century if nursing is to be systematic and coherent in its knowledge development. Different views exist regarding the way nursing must deal with pluralism. On the one hand, Reed (1995) suggests a "neo-modernist" world view, which she specifies as the "developmental-contextual" world view, to be the unifying perspective for nursing's knowledge development. On the other hand, several voices suggest the acceptance and necessity of multiparadigm epistemology for nursing that embraces multiplicity of theories, perspectives, and philosophies (Booth, Kenrick, & Woods, 1997; Engebretson, 1997; Geanellos, 1997; Schultz & Meleis, 1988). The framework presented in the following section was developed in the spirit of this second position; it is oriented to coalescing pluralism with an integrative epistemological framework. The purpose for this epistemological framework is to provide a guide for knowledge development in nursing and to specify directions for theory development.

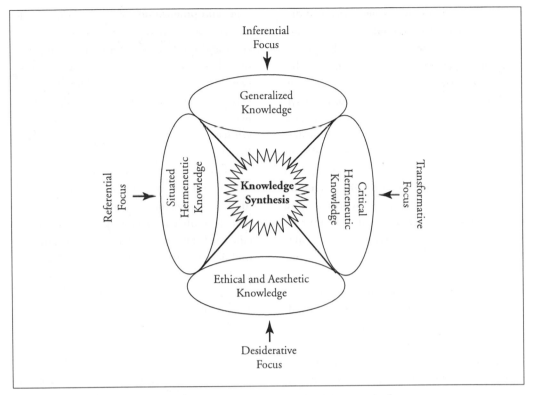

Figure 23.2   Epistemological Schema for Nursing Knowledge—Four Spheres.

■ *Applying a Unifying Epistemological Framework for Nursing Knowledge Development*

The position taken here is based on the belief that nursing science as a field of study must be considered a *practice science* that is oriented to developing knowledge not only of description and explanation, but also of practice and change. It must consist of knowledge of human phenomena that are of interest to nursing and how those phenomena must be understood and explained. In addition, nursing science must consider critical knowledge of how to transform, change, and correct human affairs of nursing concern and of what the desired states of those human condition are and should be. Nursing science hence must be concerned with what kinds of knowledge are needed for prac-

tice. Nursing practice is a form of social activity involving human agents who provide help in the context of other human beings' specific needs for that help. Nursing practice is an individual form of engagement, taking place in specific social contexts, with unique individuals, and for specified goals. Hence the knowledge needed for such practice must be developed as an organized system of science with multipronged orientations. From these premises, a unifying epistemological framework (Kim, 2000) has been developed to embrace cognitive needs for nursing practice, as depicted in Figure 23.2.

Nursing Science Orientations

Four specific orientations for nursing science are critical to this unifying epistemological framework:

- Inferential focus for generalized knowledge
- Referential focus for subjective hermeneutic knowledge
- Transformative focus for critical hermeneutic knowledge
- Desiderative[1] focus for ethical and aesthetic knowledge

Inferential Focus

Nursing knowledge with an inferential focus provides knowledge on which to base inferences about specific situations, drawing from various levels of generalized understanding, explanation, and prediction. Knowledge in this sphere *(generalized knowledge)* is developed under the assumption that certain sets of human phenomena must be understood, explained, and predicted because certain features, underlying processes, and mechanisms are relatively regular and patterned, allowing generalizable conclusions to be drawn and stated as theories. Generalized theories of description, explanation, prediction, and prescription are the key features of knowledge in this sphere. Generalization as used here does not necessarily mean universal generalizations; it also refers to context-specific and limited-scope generalizations.

Systematization of knowledge in this sphere must be oriented to refining ways to identify and delineate the nature of regularity and patterning in human phenomena of interest to nursing. Although the major form of explanation within this sphere can be based on causality, chaos theory and other forms of dynamic explanations have recently fostered new insights to thinking about patterning in human phenomena of interest to nursing. In addition, there must be further clarification regarding how context-specified and scope-limiting nursing theories can be advanced in the emerging scientific culture in which scientific realism, relativism, and pragmatism are paradoxically juxtaposed.

Referential Focus

Need for knowledge with a referential focus is most apparent because nursing practice involves individual engagements of clients and practitioners. This sphere of knowledge *(situated hermeneutic knowledge)* is critical for nursing under the premise that human beings are experiencing, subjective entities involved in creating and attaining meanings of their experiences. Although each individual experiences occasions of life through specific meanings that are created and attained uniquely in given situations, human beings share certain affinities that can be used for referential understanding. Hence knowledge with a referential focus provides points of reference for understanding any given situation through illumination, elaboration, depiction, and enlightenment gained from subjective experiences. The key method of knowledge development for this sphere is interpretation of meaning. Unlike generalized knowledge, the focus of referential knowledge is not regularity and patterning, but is singularity, variation, and situatedness. Knowledge in this sphere can provide nursing with an enrichment of understanding that is so necessary to individualize nursing practice. Major problems faced with knowledge development in this sphere have been the lack of models for accumulating knowledge of this type. In the new century, nursing must develop ways to systematize referential knowledge so as to accentuate variations and differences in human experiences.

Transformative Focus

Nursing knowledge with a transformative focus addresses knowledge regarding human life as a form of social praxis in which individuals engaged in coordinated living experience various forms of struggles, constraints, domination, and disharmony. This sphere of knowledge *(critical hermeneutic knowledge)* refers to the knowledge of interpretation, critique, and emancipation regarding human beings' inter-subjective and contextual coordination. It aligns with the critical scientific knowledge specified by Habermas (1971) and encompasses the postmodern critique of human life.

Knowledge with a transformative focus is necessary for nursing because (a) human living in the context of health and illness not only entails a person's specific experiences, but also entails experiences associated with living with other people in social contexts; and (b) nursing is a form of social practice that involves human to human engagements (i.e., between clients and nurses, nurses with other nurses, and nurses and clients with other health care practitioners). Transformative knowledge is about the nature of social praxis in the context of health and nursing with orientations in understanding, interpretation of meanings, identification of distortions and disharmony, and development of emancipatory projects.

Knowledge in this sphere is to be gained through description, interpretation, and critical and emancipatory analysis. Theories in this sphere may be developed that identify systematic distortions and disharmony in the social praxis of health and nursing; these theories also may specify forms of emancipatory projects oriented to increasing "autonomy and responsibility" and eliminating (or decreasing) distortions and domination. Transformative knowledge provides the base from which the coordinated work of practice, of getting well, and of living together can be formulated for nursing.

Desiderative Focus

Nursing knowledge with a desiderative focus is oriented to nursing's needs as a discipline to develop knowledge about how practice, as a profession, should be guided. Knowledge in this sphere *(ethical and aesthetic knowledge)* reflects normative ideas, ethical standards, value orientations, and aesthetic

expectations that need to be developed for the discipline to ensure that practice be quality oriented, ethically based, and aesthetic in its presentation. It provides grounding for orienting individual nursing practice to the professional values of ethics and aesthetics. Theories for this sphere of nursing knowledge need to be developed through philosophic analysis, dialectics, consensus building, and discourse analysis. Values and value standards not only are embedded in our practice, but also need to be formulated through the understanding of contextual requirements within which various forms of practice can be designed. Hence knowledge in this sphere not only addresses the nature of ethical and aesthetic frameworks for nursing practice, but also how frameworks become established, generated, or changed, and what the relationships are between such frameworks and the larger culture, society, and context.

Table 23.1 summarizes these four spheres of knowledge for nursing with respect to (a) their epistemological orientations, (b) the key underlying assumptions for knowledge development in nursing, (c) the main orientations of nursing theories, and (d) the forms of theories to be developed in nursing.

These four spheres of knowledge are viewed to be necessary for providing the foundation from which nursing practice must be shaped for the discipline and for individual practitioners. Although current nursing theories could be classified under these four spheres of nursing knowledge, their development has not been guided by the unifying epistemological position undergirding this framework. This schema of nursing epistemology moves nursing's discourse beyond debating about whether nursing knowledge system should be positivistic, humanistic, or hermeneutical to the critical issue of the sorts of knowledge required for nursing practice. This schema is a framework to view knowledge in terms of nursing's epistemological requirements of inference, reference,

TABLE 23.1 Epistomological Schema for Nursing Knowledge and Its Specification for Theory Development in Nursing

Epistemological Focus	Knowledge Sphere	Underlying Assumption	Focus of Theory Development	Forms of Theories in Nursing	Approaches to Theory Development
Inferential focus	Generalized knowledge	Presence of regularity and patterns in human phenomena (both universal and context-specific)	Understanding generalizable features and explaining how regularities and patterns occur or are produced	• Description • Explanation • Prediction • Prescription	• Induction and generalizations • Deduction and analytic models • Reconstruction • Prescriptive model-building
Referential focus	Situated hermeneutic knowledge	Situation-specific, subjective nature of human experiencing and meaning making	Gaining insights into singularity, individual-specific variations, and situatedness of human experience	• Elaborative, enlightening, and interpretive description	• Phenomenologic description • Existential analysis • Interpretive description
Transformative focus	Critical hermeneutic knowledge	Human life, as well as nursing practice, as social praxis entrenched with socially constructed meanings and processes	Discovering the existence of systematic distortions and disturbances in human beings' social life, and projecting toward mutual emancipation and transformation	• Interpretation • Critique • Emancipatory projects	• Hermeneutic analysis • Deconstruction • Critical methods of emancipation
Desiderative focus	Ethical and aesthetic knowledge	Nursing's commitment to optimal health, service ideals, and aesthetic authenticity	Advancing value priorities, ethical standards, and aesthetic ideals for various aspects of nursing practice	• Identification and specification of values, value-standards, and normative guidelines for nursing practice • Identification of aesthetic features of nursing practice	• Dialectics • Philosophical analysis • Consensus building • Case analysis • Model-case description

transformation, desirability, and normativity. Understanding these four epistemological orientations as the *necessary* requirement for nursing knowledge directs that pluralism be viewed in a complementary perspective. At the same time, through this schema, pluralism in nursing theories can be examined systematically for significance in terms of a heuristic and practice.

A cursory examination of existing nursing theories and research suggests that, although a rich array of nursing theories have been developed, tested, and reformulated in the *generalized sphere,* only a beginning has been made in developing knowledge in the other spheres (i.e., *the situated hermeneutic, the critical hermeneutic,* and *the ethical/aesthetic spheres).* Knowledge development in nursing must forge ahead with studies of and in-depth discourses regarding clients' and nurses' experiences in various contexts and problem areas for referential and transformative knowledge. There is also a need to address philosophical and ideological issues pertaining to ethical and aesthetic requirements, standards, values, and desiderata in nursing in the changing technical, social cultural arena.

■ Concluding Statement

Theories and knowledge must be developed in all four spheres of nursing knowledge to produce nursing practice that results from synthesis of inferential, referential, reformative, and desiderative knowledge. Knowledge synthesis also must be one of the priorities in nursing knowledge development in the new century as a way to deal with pluralism and to ground nursing practice in the knowledge being accumulated.

Theory development in nursing in the new century thus must be guided by these four-pronged cognitive orientations that provide delineation of different types of knowledge in nursing. Acknowledging that there are different forms of theory development in nursing, depending on the focus of epistemological attention, is important to acceptance of pluralism as a complementary and necessary framework. As knowledge in these spheres are perceived as complementary, this epistemological framework can be used as a unifying schema that identifies just how that complementary nature of knowledge in nursing must be developed and systematized.

■ Note

1. The term *desiderative* is used to indicate an idea of "desirability," that is, the aspect to be desired, expected, and held high in value. I coined the term *normative* for this focus with the same meaning; however, *normative* seems to connote control and regulation, which may not be appropriate in referring to knowledge oriented to determining what is valued and desired.

■ References

Allen, D., Benner, P., & Diekelmann, N. L. (1983). Three paradigms for nursing research: Methodological implications. In P. Chinn (Ed.), *Nursing research methodology* (pp. 23–38). Washington, DC: Aspen Systems.

Bernstein, R. J. (1983). *Beyond objectivism and relativism.* Philadelphia: University of Pennsylvania Press.

Bhaskar, R. (1986). *Scientific realism and human emancipation.* London: Verso.

Booth, K., Kenrick, M., & Woods, S. (1997). Nursing knowledge, theory and method revisited. *Journal of Advanced Nursing, 26,* 804–811.

Carper, B. (1978). Fundamental patterns of knowing in nursing. *Advances in Nursing Science, 1,* 13–23.

Comte, A. (1865). *The general view of positivism* (J. H. Bridges, Trans.). London: Trubner.

Dilthey, W. (1988). *Introduction to the human sciences* (R. J. Betanzos, Trans.). Detroit: Wayne State University Press.

Donaldson, S. K., & Crowley, D. M. (1978). The discipline of nursing. *Nursing Outlook, 26,* 113–120.

Engebretson, J. (1997). A multiparadigm approach to nursing. *Advances in Nursing Science, 20,* 21–33.

Ford, J. E. (1990). Systematic pluralism: Introduction to an issue. *The Monist, 73,* 335–349.

Geanellos, R. (1997). Nursing knowledge development: Where to from here? *Collegian, 4,* 13–21.

Good, B. J. (1994). *Medicine, rationality, and experience: An anthropological perspective.* Cambridge, U.K.: Cambridge University Press.

Gortner, S. R. (1993). Nursing's syntax revisited: A critique of philosophies said to influence nursing theories. *International Journal of Nursing Studies, 30,* 477–488.

Habermas, J. (1971). *Knowledge and human interests.* (J. J. Shapiro, Trans.). Boston: Beacon Press.

Kim, H. S. (1993). Putting theory into practice: Problems and prospects. *Journal of Advanced Nursing, 18,* 1632–1639.

Kim, H. S. (2000). *The nature of theoretical thinking in nursing* (rev. ed.). New York: Springer.

Kuhn, T. S. (1970). *The structure of scientific revolution* (enl. ed.). Chicago: University of Chicago Press.

Laudan, L. (1990). *Science and relativism: Some key controversies in the philosophy of science.* Chicago: University of Chicago Press.

Margolis, J. (1989). Monistic and dualistic canons for the natural and human sciences. In B. Glassner & J. D. Moreno (Eds.), *The qualitative-quantitative distinction in the social sciences* (pp. 155–178). New York: Kluwer Academic.

Margolis, J. (1990). The methodological and metaphysical peculiarities of the human sciences. *Midwest Studies in Philosophy, 15,* 167–182.

Rakover, S. S. (1989). Incommensurability: The scaling of mind–body theories as a counter example. *Behaviorism, 17,* 103–118.

Reed, P. G. (1995). A treatise on nursing knowledge development for the 21st century: Beyond postmodernism. *Advances in Nursing Science, 17,* 70–84.

Ricoeur, P. (1981). *Hermeneutics and the human sciences.* (J. B. Thompson, Trans. & Ed.). Cambridge, U.K.: Cambridge University Press.

Schultz, P. R., & Meleis, A. I. (1988). Nursing epistemology: Traditions, insights, questions. *IMAGE: Journal of Nursing Scholarship, 20,* 217–221.

Staats, A. W. (1989). Unificationism: Philosophy for the modern disunified science of psychology. *Philosophical Psychology, 2,* 143–164.

Stevenson, L. (1987). *Seven theories of human nature* (2nd ed.). New York: Oxford University Press.

Stevenson, J. S., & Woods, N. F. (1986). Nursing science and contemporary science: Emerging paradigms. In *Setting the agenda for the year 2000: Knowledge development in nursing* (pp. 6–20). Kansas City, MO: American Academy of Nursing.

Taylor, C. (1985). *Philosophy and the human sciences.* Cambridge, U.K.: Cambridge University Press.

Wiseman, R. L., & Schenck-Hamlin, W. (1981). A multidimensional scaling validation of an inductively-derived set of compliance-gaining strategies. *Communication Monographs, 48,* 251–270.

■ *Editor's Questions for Discussion*

What relationship exists between Kim's discussion of knowledge development and Donnelly's (Chapter 28)? Of what benefit is pluralism in nursing knowledge? How can an epistemological perspective for nursing guide future theory development in nursing? To what extent have nursing scholars accepted pluralism at the philosophy-of-science level? Provide examples of the four levels of pluralism in nursing for developing nursing knowledge. What evidence exists of theoretical pluralism in nursing? Because multiple theories may compete with each other, what benefit or function is served by holding multiple theories?

How can nursing systematize knowledge from inferential, referential, transformative, and desiderative foci? Propose a methodology for addressing specific nursing practice problems, using those four orientations. How do situation-specific theories, as described by Meleis and Im (Chapter 72), utilize the four spheres of nursing knowledge advocated by Kim? Examine systematically the nursing theories addressed by Chinn (Chapter 24), Watson (Chapter 25), Fawcett and Bourbonniere (Chapter 26), Neuman (Chapter 27), and Donnelly (Chapter 28) for their significance in a heuristic process and practice.

24

Toward a Theory of Nursing Art

Peggy L. Chinn, PhD, RN, FAAN

The purpose of this chapter is to present a philosophic theory of nursing art. The theory was developed to deepen understanding of that aspect of nursing that moves practice beyond purely technical or interpersonal skills into a realm that is a healing art form. The healing art form of nursing involves integrating all aspects of nursing into a coherent whole, and the theory describes, and explains philosophically, how this happens.

It is important to understand that I am not projecting empirical theory. Rather I am presenting a philosophic theory that offers a conceptual definition of the art of nursing—explanations as to how nursing art evolves as a distinct aspect of nursing practice and explanations of artistic validity in nursing. Unlike

empirical theory, what I propose is not intended to be subjected to empirical testing but rather to be considered from a logical, philosophic, and aesthetic perspective. In philosophy, aesthetics is the study of that which is artistically valid. Notions such as beauty, for example, enter into logical explorations, but cannot be subjected to empirical investigation. Likewise, in developing this theory, I considered the notion of a unitary, coherent whole within a complex action and interaction—the art and act of nursing. This idea is analogous to the idea of beauty in traditional aesthetics.

The following section explains the background from which this theory has been developed. The subsequent sections present assumptions on which the theory is based—a conceptual definition of nursing art as a pattern of knowing in nursing and as a distinct way of being in nursing and theoretical explanations as to how nursing art evolves as a distinct aspect of what nursing is.

■ Developmental Background

Ideas that have come together to form this theory are grounded in an investigation conducted in Denver, Colorado, from 1990 through 1996 (Chinn, 1994; Chinn & Kramer, 1999; Chinn, Maeve, & Bostick, 1997). In the course of this investigation, I worked with nurses in five different units of two hospitals. I also worked with two colleagues, M. Katherine Maeve and Cynthia Bostick, who were doctoral students during the course of the study. Kathy pursued work in the area of nursing narrative and story telling (Maeve, 1994). Cynthia, who is also a professional dancer, pursued her doctoral dissertation on movement and its relationship with creativity in practice (Bostick, 1997).

I observed 12 nurses in their practice for three to four 2-hour sessions. We each reflected on the observation period and journaled. About 2 to 3 days later, we discussed our experience and reflections on their practice. Because a main purpose of my inquiry was to develop a method for developing aesthetic knowledge in nursing, I used a discussion approach that integrated hermeneutic interpretation and aesthetic criticism (Chinn, 1994). In other words, I shared insights concerning (a) meanings that I perceived in their practice, (b) symbolic messages conveyed in what they did and how they did it, and (c) reflective details about aesthetic qualities such as rhythm, synchrony of movements and interactions, and overall coherence of their practice in relation to the whole scenario in which they acted. For example, in one observation, I noticed that the nurse, upon

entering a patient's room, moved around the space, briefly touching various things. The space that she touched became the space within which she maintained her practice for the duration of her stay in the room. In some instances she moved within a broad space that included others in the room; in other instances she moved within a relatively confined space that included only bed and patient. When we met for our discussion, I reflected on the symbolic meanings of "setting the stage" for her practice encounter in this time and space.

Groups of nurses who volunteered to participate in the inquiry met weekly to discuss ideas concerning the art of nursing and to share stories of practices. Charlene Eldridge volunteered to take black and white photographs of selected nurses as they practiced; these were spontaneous photographs that were not rehearsed in any way. We met in groups to discuss what the photographs revealed about the art of nursing.

Steps for Personal Grounding

Because staying focused on the art of nursing as aesthetics—and not as an empirical phenomenon—was so difficult, I took steps to keep myself grounded in art experiences and in healing as an art form. I completed a 1,000-hour massage therapy program at the Colorado School of Healing Arts in Denver. This program explicitly taught massage as a healing art, integrating motive, intention, action, and spirit into the skill of therapeutic massage. Although there were similarities in philosophy between what we learned in massage therapy and what I believed about nursing, never in my nursing education had I experienced the same kind of explicit acknowledgment of, and intentional focus on, nursing as a healing art. Needless to say, this discovery inspired for me a very different vision of what nursing can become and how it can be taught.

The study of music deepened my understanding of what it means to learn an art form and what it means to teach an art form effectively. I have had the good fortune of working with master teachers and continue to study and practice, playing a traditional folk harp. This experience provides grounding in aesthetics and brings to awareness some distinctions between empirical methods and aesthetic methods.

Exploratory Course Offering

At the University of Connecticut in the Spring of 1998, I proposed and taught a one-time exploratory course titled "An Introduction to the Art of Nursing" for freshmen and sophomore students. (See the Web site http://www.nursing.uconn.edu/ to find a link to the syllabus for this course.) I remain in touch via e-mail with these students to explore further ideas and insights that have emerged in developing a theory of nursing art. The course's content and processes were designed from the findings of my Denver study. After the first three weeks of focusing on the art form of nursing, the course integrated allopathic and holistic skills, practicing in class with a focused eye toward developing the skill as a nursing caring/healing art form. Skills included those that can be used by any lay person, such as taking vital signs, wound care, foot care and massage, use of hot and cold, and so forth. Each week we discussed an excerpt from Nightingale's "Notes on Nursing" (1969) pertinent to the topic of the week, focusing on the significance of what we were learning for developing nursing as a caring and healing art form. For example, the week that we worked with music and movement as a therapeutic modality, I read Nightingale's note on the healing properties of music and the type of music that is beneficial to the sick (Nightingale, 1969, p. 67). This reading prompted rich discussion of how nurses facilitate healing by mindful, intentional use of music and movement.

The 1998 course was based on a premise that directly challenges preconceived ideas that students need to master technical skills before beginning to integrate elements of interpersonal dynamics into their practice. Instead, I felt that introducing students to nursing as an art form first, using basic technical skills as the "carrier" of the art form can have a number of advantages. With that sequence, students will acquire skills more easily, they will view the worth of what they do as nurses differently, and they will perceive themselves to be actively engaging in a caring and healing process. From everything that I have observed to date, this indeed is the case.

■ Assumptions

Assumptions on which my theory of nursing art is based come from my beliefs about nursing and about the nature of art. First, nursing is a healing art. This concept is growing in significance as nurses turn increasingly to holistic healing modalities that enhance their participation in healing processes. Even though holistic modalities can greatly expand nursing's potential, I also believe that everything that traditionally has been a part of nursing practice can be viewed as a medium for the healing process.

Art requires two kinds of knowledge (Chinn & Kramer, 1999; Eisner, 1985). The first is knowledge of human experiences toward which our art form is directed—suffering, pain, birth, life transitions, stress, illness, and so forth. Art also requires knowledge of the art form itself, which is the focus of my own work and substance of this theory.

Art is present in all activity that involves forming elements into a whole. Most instances of art are not subjected to critical reflection nor valued as art. However, when we bring elements together to form a whole, we experience art.

Art expands perceptual abilities beyond what is, to what might be. Art moves us to another plane, another potential, another possibility. When someone reads a novel or views a painting or sees a performance, he or she is moved into the realm of experience represented by the art form. This "move" is an inner, emotional, mental, spirit-self move that is in a realm of perception that arises from aesthetics.

All art requires skill in technical aspects of the art. My experience in learning to play the harp certainly brought this into focus. However, I also learned during the first two weeks of lessons that, because of what my teacher imagined a simple song could sound like and her ability to convey that possibility to me, I could produce a beautiful, artistically valid song. The technical skill for the simple song was not difficult and so, as I mastered the relatively easy technical skill, I also could focus on artistic qualities that my teacher guided me to integrate as I played. At first, I could only play one song, but it sounded heavenly!

Art requires imagination and intuition to bring elements into a creative whole. When I play the harp, I do need skill to pluck the right strings, in a particular order and with rhythm to produce a recognizable tune. This technical skill needs to be developed "in my fingers" for each new tune I play, and technical challenges gradually progress as I gain expertise and skill. What makes a tune a beautiful song is the imagination of feeling that I want to bring into the sound and the intuitive following of various musical possibilities that emerge in the song. This creative imagination, when nurtured from the moment of beginning to learn the skill, multiplies the meaning of the skill a thousandfold and moves the skill into a place of the imagination so that the emerging and developing skill becomes a carrier for the art. Because of this dynamic, even as the skill is developing, artistic quality comes through, making learning a thing of joy and beauty.

Art seeks unique expressions. One of my first songs—the Quaker hymn "Simple Gifts"—speaks to deep satisfaction that comes from giving and taking, of living in company of friends and finding joy and delight in simple gifts we offer one another. This common human experience is conveyed both in words and in the music itself, which has a soothing tone, with movements of notes and rhythm that also suggest a deep longing for the kind of nurturing connections that are possible in community. Each time I play the song, it acquires unique expressions that emerge in the moment.

Finally, art is a bodymind experience and it elicits bodymind responses. This is the aspect of art that makes it difficult to understand as a component of nursing. We are accustomed to understanding nursing as a mind experience only. To move to the bodymind concept is a considerable challenge.

■ Conceptual Meanings of Nursing Art

Joy Johnson (1994) conducted a philosophic analysis of nursing literature that used the term "art of nursing." Johnson found five distinct meanings associated with idea of the art of nursing. I will discuss each of these briefly in terms of the assumption that nursing art requires knowledge of the experience toward which our art is directed, and knowledge of the art form itself.

Johnson (1994) found that the art of nursing meant the grasping of meaning in a situation. Grasping meaning is associated primarily with knowledge of the experience toward which our art form is directed. Nurses must know the nature of the experiences of illness, life transitions, grief, tension, stress, and so forth. Nurses must be able to sense the nature of a particular experience in any situation. It is within the contexts of these experiences that nursing art is practiced, and it is toward these experiences that nursing art is directed. But this reality does not address the art form itself.

Another meaning that Johnson found is the ability to establish a meaningful connection. This ability repeatedly appeared in my discussions with practicing nurses in the Denver study. Those nurses clearly identified meaningful connection as the reason for practicing artfully. The art, those practicing nurses said over and over, is what makes connection possible. Consistent with Jeanne LeVasseur's ongoing work (LeVasseur, 1999), this aspect of nursing art suggests something about outcome, or the object of nursing art. However, the connection that is established as nursing art is practiced still does not address the art form itself.

Johnson also found that the art of nursing has been associated with ability to perform nursing activities skillfully. This aspect of nursing art also appeared frequently in my discussions with nurses in the Denver study. Those nurses often said: "It is not what you do, but how you do it." Still, they were at a loss to speak to the form, to describe exactly what they meant by "how you do it."

Johnson (1994) further identified meanings associated with the ability to determine rationally a course of action and the ability to conduct practice morally. These two abilities are part of what enters into the picture when all elements of nursing practice come together to form a whole, but as distinct entities of practice these abilities do not address the art form.

■ *Conceptual Definition of the Form of Nursing Art*

The definition of nursing art that emerged from the Denver study remains the conceptual foundation for this theory of nursing art and focuses on the art form itself (Chinn & Kramer, 1999):

> The nurse's synchronous arrangement of narrative and movement into a form that transforms experiences into a realm that would not otherwise be possible. The arrangement is spontaneous, in-the-moment, and intuitive. The ability to make the moves that are transformative is grounded in a deep understanding of nursing, including relevant theory, facts, technical skill, personal knowing, and ethical understanding; and this ability requires rehearsal in deliberative application of these understandings. (p. 90)

This definition first identifies elements that nurses use to form a whole: narrative and movement. Using these elements in a synchronous fashion, the nurse transforms experiences into a realm that would not otherwise be possible. Although it is possible to focus on the nurse's movement or narrative, what emerges is a whole that is greater than the sum of the parts and includes the total picture of the situation, including others with whom the nurse interacts.

Arrangement of narrative and movement is spontaneous, in-the-moment, and intuitive. This component of our definition emerged from nurses in the art study, using improvisational theater as an analogy for what they experience as the art of nursing. However, consistent with improvisational arts, in order to interact spontaneously and intuitively in the situation, nursing art requires rehearsal. In the art study, nurses spoke of their years of practice as "rehearsal time," but also began to imagine what it might have been like if they had been able to work in a studio, with expert teachers, coaches, and directors to help them refine their artistic potential early in their practice.

The ability to form art in nursing practice is also grounded in deep understanding of nursing, including theory, technical skill, personal knowing, and ethical understanding. The studio

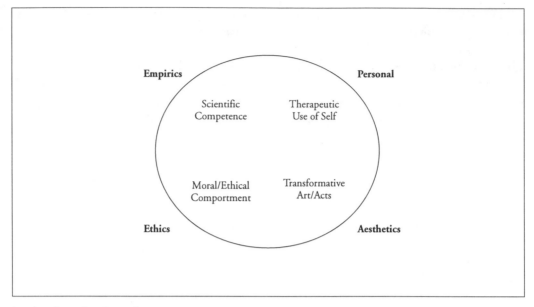

Figure 24.1   Ontology of nursing practice.

Excerpted from Chinn, P. L., & Kramer, M. K. (1999). *Theory & nursing: Integrated knowledge development* (5th ed.). St. Louis: Mosby.

can provide some practice that integrates this understanding, but clinical experience is truly the ground from which this integration arises.

In Barbara Carper's initial presentation of nursing's patterns of knowing, she spoke to the tension between elements of an art form and that which emerges as the whole (Carper, 1978). Carper said: "The design, if it is to be esthetic, must be controlled by perception of the balance, rhythm, proportion and unity of what is done in relation to the dynamic integration and articulation of the whole"(p. 18).

■ Ontology of Nursing Art

Art is a distinct aspect of nursing practice. Nursing art arises from aesthetic knowing. Empirical, personal and ethical knowing cannot give rise to nursing art. For example, an empirical theory of pain and comfort informs what a nurse does and contributes to making

judgments in alleviating pain, but such a theory does not, and cannot, provide insight as to *how* to carry out the nursing actions and interactions involved in alleviating pain. *How* the nurse *is* in this context comes from the nurse's aesthetic sensibilities and senses.

In our work with Carper's patterns of knowing, Maeona Kramer and I distinguished between knowledge, which is the epistemological dimension that focuses on what we know and how we come to know it, and the ontological dimension, which is what it means to be a nurse, to experience the practice of nursing (Chinn & Kramer, 1999). We conceptualized the core of nursing as practice as the ontological perspective of what nursing is.

Nursing is that which arises from each of the four fundamental patterns of knowing in nursing. Each pattern of knowing has a nondiscursive form of expression, which is what we can discern in nursing practice and what forms the ontological elements that form nursing practice, as depicted in Figure 24.1.

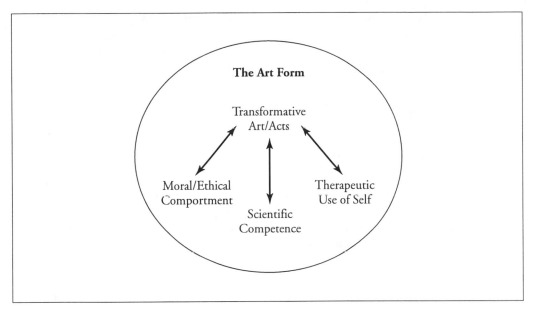

Figure 24.2   Art as an Integrating Pattern.

Scientific competence arises from empiricism. Moral and ethical comportment arises from ethics. Therapeutic use of self arises from personal knowing and transformative art and acts arise from aesthetics. When we witness nursing practice, we perceive the whole of what is happening and cannot perceive the elements of practice in isolation from the whole. At the same time, we can discern what we would characterize as scientific competence and differentiate it from moral and ethical comportment. As an example, consider what it takes to recognize a person. You know the sound of a person's voice, appearance of that person's face, and size and configuration of that person's body. You can distinguish each of these elements that make it possible to recognize the person, but all are required for a full and accurate perception of who the person is.

For purposes of developing a theory of the art of nursing, I am proposing a shift in focus for basic elements of nursing practice. From the perspective of nursing art, aesthetics is viewed as an integrating pattern, whereby the art form itself provides foundation for transformative art and acts, which in turn integrate moral and ethical comportment, scientific competence, and therapeutic use of self, as illustrated in Figure 24.2. That is, it is the art that brings all elements together to form a whole of nursing practice.

■ *How Nursing Art Evolves*

Nursing art evolves in four ways—the four "R's":

- refining synchronous narrative skills,

- refining synchronous movement skills,

- rehearsal and connoisseurship, and

- reflective practice in nursing, with a critic or connoisseur.

Each of these processes requires more than learning skills. They require developing a mindful way of bringing caring and healing intention into being, into experience.

Refining Synchronous Narrative Skills

Narrative skills involve both what is said or not said, as well as how it is said. In developing narrative skills, the major focus is on how a person speaks, sounds, and develops timing and rhythm to convey caring and healing intention. Voice tone is an important aspect of artistic narrative skill. In the "Introduction to the Art of Nursing" class, we used various exercises to explore possible voice tones and considered which tones conveyed caring and healing intention. The students then used different voices in narrative exchanges, giving and receiving feedback as to what voice tone and expression conveyed.

Effective story-telling is a skill that, until now, most nurses have taken for granted. In the Denver art study, we began to recognize the central role that story-telling played in the day-to-day practice of nursing. Nurses talked about stories they told their patients, stories they told one another at end of the day, and how they used story-telling to try to understand and improve their practice. Many nurses wrote down their stories for the group, which provided opportunities for recasting stories and rehearsing alternative story lines (Maeve, 1994). Recasting stories became a form of rehearsal, whereby nurses challenged one another to envision different possibilities for the story and to rehearse narratives that would move struggles of the story toward a different end. With each telling of a story, reflective insights deepened and possibilities for future encounters broadened. For example, one of the nurses told of being asked by a dying woman: "Will I know when I am dead?" The actual response to this question had been very unsatisfactory. In response to her account

of what happened, many different story lines emerged, with different ways of responding, different rhythms, timing, and synchrony in how various scenarios could unfold. This process deepened everyone's perception of what might be possible in a similar situation.

Artistic Validity of Narrative

Developing narrative skills requires an understanding of what constitutes artistic validity: What are the artistic qualities of narrative? Overall, artistic quality depends on the formation of a valid whole. From a narrative perspective, this means that the nurse's voice tone, expression, and substance of the narrative interaction are synchronous with intentions brought to the interaction. Within a nursing context, intention is consistent with caring and healing. Artistic quality depends on a "right relationship," which is also reflected in the idea of synchrony. A right relationship between what is expressed and how it is expressed must be evident, involving synchrony with movement of the self and the other and the nurses' timing and rhythm in bringing the experience together to form a valid whole that conveys caring and healing intention.

Refining Synchronous Movement Skills

Narrative skills have been given some attention in nursing, but movement has been reduced to a brief introduction to body mechanics. Movement skills involve much more than body mechanics, and indeed, when viewed from an artistic perspective, body mechanics take on new and significant meanings. Movement skills involve personal style in both large and fine motor movement, refined balance, finesse, timing, and synchrony. Skills include knowing how to deliberately form movements to convey a motive, intention, or feeling. Touch, which we often consider as a separate entity, from an artistic perspective is one phase in an entire movement sequence. It is the movement that brings touch to actuality that conveys meaning of the touch. We actually gained this insight by studying black and white photographs of nurses in the art study. The photographs prompted many different stories around what might have been happening when the pictures were taken. When a photograph showed a nurse touching a patient, the story could not emerge by focusing on the touch itself. The story and meanings symbolized in the situation came from imagining what moves had preceded and what moves followed the moment of touch.

Artistic Validity of Movement

Artistic qualities of movement, like those of narrative, focus on forming a valid whole, characterized by balance and finesse in both large and fine motor movements. Movement exhibits synchrony in timing and rhythm. Each nurse exhibits a personal style of movement that is refined over time but, like personality itself, has an enduring quality that conveys unique ways in which this particular nurse moves. In order to be artistically valid, movement in a nursing art context conveys caring and healing intentions. Movement of the nurse must be synchronous with both the narrative and with movement of others in the situation.

■ Rehearsal and Connoisseurship

The next element that explains how nursing art evolves is rehearsal and connoisseurship. Rehearsal can be done without a connoisseur (e.g., teacher, coach, director, or critic), but presence of a connoisseur enhances awareness

of what the art form is expressing and how well it is conveying the intended message.

Rehearsal brings movement and narrative together. Exercises that we used in the art course to refine narrative and movement skills focused largely on one or the other, but when we began rehearsal, one could not happen without the other. For example, at first we rehearsed what to say when first approaching a new patient, with particular attention on voice tone and words that convey caring and healing intention for interactions and relationships. Then we focused on how to move into a new situation, examining various body moves and stances that convey different intentions. These separate exercises constituted refining narrative and refining movement skills. When we began to work with particular nursing modalities, narrative and movement came together. We rehearsed entire sequences that included (a) the first approach, (b) introduction, (c) questions to become acquainted, (d) explanations as to what will happen in this encounter (e.g., taking a blood pressure reading), (e) movement of the body and hands to accomplish the task in a way that conveyed caring and healing intention, (f) explanations as to what happened or what was observed, and (g) words and movements to bring the encounter to a close.

Rehearsal Purpose

Each rehearsal included students who were "acting" the scenario and one or more student observers who were specifically noticing artistic qualities in the rehearsal (the connoisseurs). This kind of rehearsal nurtures reflective capacities that refine artistic capabilities. It gives the nurse artist an opportunity to notice differences between good timing and rhythm from poor timing and rhythm, for example. The observer or connoisseur provides feedback to students who are enacting the scenario, encouraging them to reach new dimensions— feeling what it is like to achieve coordinated movement, for example, when that has seemed particularly difficult. Learning to become a connoisseur and learning and rehearsing an art form at the same time are essential for reflective practice. Connoisseurship makes it possible to see the art form beneath what appears on the surface, to notice artistic qualities, and to reach toward the intended artistic expression.

Rehearsal reveals creative potential because the connoisseur encourages the artist to take risks. The connoisseur is able not only to "mirror" what actually has happened, but also to show, demonstrate, and inspire something else that might happen in the scenario—some new possibility for developing the art form. Even if the connoisseur is a student colleague, the connoisseur is an expert teacher, the best of coaches, the most inspiring of directors. The connoisseur provides a "mirror" for the artist's technical skill and artistic qualities. The best connoisseur gives accurate feedback as to how performance is executed. If it is not done well, the focus is on how to do it better. My harp teacher, for example, never says, "That sounds terrible." Instead, she says, "Try playing it like this (and she demonstrates) and listen to the difference. Now try it again."

Connoisseur Role

The connoisseur interprets perceived motive, intention, and feeling. My harp teacher says in an excited voice, for example, "That made me feel like I was running and now I am breathless." Now changing her voice to a slow pace, lower pitch, and lilting rhythm, she says, "This is a lullaby—slow it down and make me feel like going to sleep!" Then, when I play the piece like a lullaby (and not like a march), she says, "Oh, how sweet that sounds! I can just imagine holding this little baby until it sleeps."

The connoisseur presents imaginary situations and helps the student imagine new situations and project new creative possibilities. In "Introduction to the Art of Nursing Class" for

example, we imagined situations that were different from those we had rehearsed, changing story lines and playing out scenarios with new story lines that called forth new creative skills and possibilities.

Most important, the connoisseur interprets artistic validity, giving the artist a way to see the art from another perspective. Doing so involves

- explaining symbolic elements that hold promise for transforming experience,
- connecting specific elements of artistic quality with perceived meanings and intentions that are conveyed, and
- connecting what art inspires as new possibilities for the future.

Reflective Practice with a Connoisseur

Finally, what emerges—from refining narrative and movement and from rehearsal with a connoisseur—comes into play as reflective practice. Reflective practice is the ultimate rehearsal studio and makes possible refinement of practice itself. Reflective practice brings what is rehearsed into practice and brings skills of connoisseurship to bear on nursing practice for the nurse and for others. Practice presents infinite complexities that usually are not present in rehearsal and provides infinite possibilities for reflection. Practice reveals ethical, empirical, and personal insights that emerge in artistic practice and provides a ground from which to envision new possibilities for the nurse artist.

■ Concluding Statement

In this chapter, I presented a theory of nursing art that includes assumptions, conceptual meanings of nursing art, a definition of the form of nursing art, and explanations as to how nursing art evolves. This theory can inform the teaching and practice of nursing art and can lead to scholarly aesthetic inquiry in the form of artistic criticism that arises from connoisseurship.

The question remains: Why nurture the art of nursing? My response to this critical question lies within our definition of nursing art, which states that "nursing art transforms experience from what is, to what might be possible." This transformation is the heart of our caring and healing practice—the ability to participate in experiences in such a way as to inspire new possibilities and to facilitate a healing path.

■ References

Bostick, C. (1997). *Dance movement and its effects on rhythmic flow and nursing practice.* Unpublished PhD dissertation, University of Colorado, Denver.

Carper, B. A. (1978, October). Fundamental patterns of knowing in nursing. *Advances in Nursing Science, 1*(1), 13–23.

Chinn, P. L. (1994). Developing a method for aesthetic knowing in nursing. In P. L. Chinn & J. Watson (Eds.), *Art & aesthetics in nursing* (pp. 19–40). New York: National League for Nursing Press.

Chinn, P. L., & Kramer, M. K. (1999). *Theory & nursing: Integrated knowledge development* (5th ed.). St. Louis: Mosby.

Chinn, P. L., Maeve, M. K., & Bostick, C. (1997). Aesthetic inquiry and the art of nursing. *Scholarly Inquiry for Nursing Practice, 11*(2), 83–96.

Eisner, E. (1985). *Learning and teaching the ways of knowing: Part II*. Chicago: University of Chicago Press.

Johnson, J. L. (1994). A dialectical examination of nursing art. *Advances in Nursing Science, 17*(1), 1–14.

LeVasseur, J. J. (1999). Toward an understanding of art in nursing. *Advances in Nursing Science, 21*(4), 48–63.

Maeve, M. K. (1994). Coming to moral consciousness through the art of nursing narratives. In P. L. Chinn & J. Watson (Eds.), *Art and aesthetics in nursing* (pp. 67–89). New York: National League for Nursing.

Nightingale, Florence (1969). *Notes on nursing: What it is and what it is not.* New York: Dover. (Original work published 1860)

■ Editor's Questions for Discussion

What is the difference between an empirical and philosophic theory? How may philosophic theory be most appreciated? Define the art form of nursing. How might the art of nursing be taught in nursing programs? How is movement and narrative essential to nursing art? How are interpersonal dynamics inherent to nursing's art form? What learning from Chinn's exploratory course has implications for placement and sequencing of communication skills and interpersonal dynamics in curriculum? To what extent is creative imagination nurtured in teaching nursing skills? How do nursing students obtain "knowledge of experience" toward which nursing art is directed? What application may be made from Watson's discussion (Chapter 25) to teaching nursing art? How is skill defined in nursing? What relationship may exist between nursing competence, nursing art, and nursing skill? What is the nature or being of nursing art?

Propose additional strategies to refine synchronous narrative and movement skills. How is personal style in nursing relevant to nursing practice? What types of nursing scenarios may be rehearsed in learning nursing art? How may faculty fulfill the role of "connoisseur" in teaching nursing art?

What requirements are essential for aesthetic inquiry? How may aesthetic inquiry provide meaning for nursing practice? What relationships may exist between aesthetic inquiry and development of situation-specific theory as presented by Meleis and Im (Chapter 72)?

How might Watson's journal (Chapter 25) facilitate learning the art of nursing as described by Chinn? Describe how journaling may be a method for aesthetic inquiry of nursing as an art. How are meanings of every day experience signifiers for the art of nursing? How does Watson's journal reflect transpersonal caring?

25

Postmodern Nursing and Beyond

Jean M. Watson, PhD, RN, HNC, FAAN

■ *Background–Postmodern Developments*

The term *postmodern* has become code for the crisis of confidence in the nursing profession, whereby the "modern" models of nursing and society are being critiqued and deconstructed (Lather, 1991; Watson, 1995b). Postmodern thinking has challenged the modern idea of a single view of reality, of one way to know or develop knowledge.

Origins of Postmodernism in Architecture

The term *postmodern* originated in the field of architecture. Straight lines of structures were critiqued and challenged by new ways of thinking—thinking that moved beyond straight lines, square or rectangular buildings, and block structures to free forms and new experiments in shape, color, and integration of design. This postmodern approach juxtaposed previous shapes into current and futuristic styles, leading to a liberation and creative freedom in architecture and designs worldwide. Toulmin (1990) stated that an American architect, Robert Venturi, argued that the age of "modern" is past and must yield to a new postmodern style. Medical facilities, in particular during the modern era, were designed and built with the clean sterile look of progressive modernity—an efficient functional block appearance of sameness and anonymity. The design of hospitals is just beginning to shake off the modern burden, with architects now creating hospitable, friendly, and even healing spaces that accommodate souls as well as physical bodies. Postmodern hospitals are reintroducing elements of beauty, historical reference, and even mythological archetypal designs, including aesthetics, integration of nature, local landscape, and space. In the most sophisticated versions of this thinking we can see evidence of "sacred architecture," intentionally designed to potentiate comfort, calmness, healing, and wholeness (Watson, 1995, 1999).

Origins of Postmodernism in Literature

The second major field to embrace postmodernism came from literature early in the 20th century (Derrida, 1976; Foucault, 1972; Sarup, 1988). The rise of postmodern thinking—in the sense of literary critique of the modern mindset and its one model of reality—emerged dramatically throughout the century, especially in Europe. Early efforts in this direction became evident through the angst of existential philosophical movements and then led to phenomenological attempts to grasp the human experience. From there it moved to hermeneutics, feminism, language critique, and deconstruction of dominant models of Western reality (Sarup, 1988; Skinner, 1990).

The result has been a deconstruction of a one view of the world, one view of truth, one view of science, and one view of reality itself. Such critiques have promoted an uprising against all theory (any one "master narrative"), rationality, objectivity, and hard science as a basis for what is real. Nursing itself now has become part of this shifting world view and critique of reality and taken-for-granted assumptions.

Postmodern Meanings

Just what does *postmodern* mean? It has come to mean almost anything that anyone says it is. In this chapter, I use the term *postmodern* in contrast to the modern, industrial world view of Western civilization and medical science, including modern nursing. In that sense, postmodern is both a period concept (i.e., time bound, referring to an era in human history that is beyond what we have known as "modern") and a time in human history in which the world no longer conforms to our former objective reality. At another level, postmodern represents a thought system that points toward a new way of perceiving reality and life itself (Watson, 1999a).

In the postmodern view, reality, science, and problems alike are not to be "solved," rather, they are "deconstructed" (Reed, 1995) through analysis of language, text, knowledge, and power structures. For example, what is missing from a text is as important as what is included. What is hidden in the silent or not so silent margin of a text or discourse is as crucial to meaning as what is made explicit. As a result of postmodern critique and deconstruction efforts across diverse fields, new questions and dilemmas have been generated. Alternative views to established assumptions about reality itself have emerged.

Literature and discourse (Watson, 1995a, 1995b) reflect debates and critiques of world views, knowledge, science, and methods in the following contrasting dialectics:

Natural Science–Human Science

Received Views of Science–Perceived Views of Science

Old Paradigm Research–New Paradigm Research

Separateness Science–Wholeness Science

Paradigm I, II, III Contrasts and Evolutions

In other circles modern–postmodern tensions have been reflected in debates during the past two decades. Examples include hard science versus soft science and quantitative versus qualitative. This movement toward constructivist, critical, and interpretative frames of complexity has led to disownment of theory or dominating systems that restrict human liberation and evolution.

Nursing's Internal Dialogue

Postmodern tensions have engaged nursing in its own internal dialogue. At this point in the modern–postmodern debate, prominent questions include the following:

"Why do we need continuously to deconstruct medicine, science, nursing, and the human condition?"

"Why do we need an alternative to modern Western science and modern medicine's influence on nursing science and practice?"

"How can we reconcile the paradox between continuously rejecting dominant discourse, disowning any master narrative (e.g., grand theories), and remaining in a critical, postmodern future on the one hand, while on the other hand still adhering to a professional, ethical ground for nursing science and practice?"

Answers to these postmodern questions involve dimensions that embrace nursing's search for wholeness for self and others. Examples reflect experiences and meanings associated with integrative caring and transpersonal dimensions of nursing's work that tap into inner healing processes. These multifaceted, transdimensional aspects of health and healing go far beyond modern models of science and medical diagnosis and treatment and cure approaches.

Converging Themes

A second reality in contemporary postmodern nursing science and practice is emerging, with themes about nursing's phenomena for inquiry and informed action converging. These themes include concepts such as energy fields, unity of being and becoming, subjectivity, intersubjectivity, transcendence, relation, context, meaning, spirit, consciousness, intentionality, and transcultural caring practices. Such practices and processes all reside in the paradoxes and patterns of inner healing, healing environments, and the healing arts—processes associated with unknowns of human self-caring and self-healing possibilities. These dimensions encompass the physical and the nonphysical alike. They enter the spiritual and sacred realms, inviting a fuller actualization of human growth and evolution of persons and humanity.

An ironic twist of the modern–postmodern debate within nursing is the fact that nursing can make a case for answers to the preceding questions—offering an alternative to modern thinking in medicine and Western views of science and reality that parallels other disciplines. Simultaneously, consistent with postmodern angst, like other disciplines, nursing can reject any "master narrative" whether it is medicine, science, patriarchal views, or nursing theory itself.

Inherent in the deconstruction of modernist thinking is suspicion of any overriding discourse, any one truth. Rather, a call for multiple voices and multiple truths found through experience is raised. Momentum for ongoing critique and deconstruction exists, with hope for a new discourse and an evolving consciousness of humanity itself.

Paradoxical Twists Between Modern and Postmodern Dialogues

As part of this evolving postmodern direction, suggestions to abandon nursing theories and reject any metanarrative for the profession have emerged (Whall, 1993). Such suggestions encompass middle-range theories or theories that are extracted only from practice—and silent with respect to a priori ways of viewing reality. However, some critique of deconstruction of the modern era has given rise to postmodern bleakness, whereby problems are deconstructed rather than rethought in an attempt to find creative solutions. Thus, at some point, postmodern deconstruction discourse places us as a profession and a people in an abyss.

At the same time, it is through awareness of the modern–postmodern dichotomy that the debate turns in on itself, and we are all helped ironically to awaken to the fact that body, mind, soul, and spirit—the human condition—cannot be reduced to Western material thinking alone. Confronting us is the reality that we no longer live in a temporally fixed universe of matter but are part of a dynamic universe that we help create.

This paradoxical twist of awareness within and between modern and postmodern dialogues takes nursing both backward and forward. In going through the problematic dissonance in nursing's past and present, we are invited to surrender and, at end of the process, to relocate nursing within its grand theories and metanarratives. Some of these dialogues and narratives even are premodern notions of timeless dimensions and calls for human service—acts of caring and love—caritas—that are eternal notions that sustain humanity and civilization. Otherwise, to reside in the deconstructive side of the postmodern debate without hope for reconsideration leaves us bereft, without ground beneath our feet.

Consequences of Postmodern Deconstruction Debate

If nursing (and for that matter, society) is stripped of all metanarratives and an ungrounded route to the postmodern critique, we are left personally and professionally abandoned without a raison d'etre. However, we are entering a new space in the postmodern that embraces critique, ambiguity, and paradox—a space in which questions of reasons for being and purpose have to be asked anew. As a result, nursing is being called on to critique its own world view and return to its core values, philosophies, and theoretical metanarrative (Reed, 1995). Thus part of postmodern deconstructive development is a counterreaction toward what might be called reflective reconstruction.

Reflective Reconstruction

In nursing, this reconstructivist movement is rooted in nursing's historic covenant with the public, which seeks to sustain an ethic, philosophy, and authenticity of caring practices—practices that are relational, integrative, and based on human science. This historic and, at the same time, most contemporary nursing covenant is likewise tied to Nightingale's (1992) assumptions about accessing the natural healer within. To address those assumptions means working to affect environmental health, critiquing policies and politics that interfere with human wholeness, health, and healing—the spirit-filled foundation of nursing's work.

Thus contemporary, postmodern direction in scholarship and action invites nursing and its caring–healing theories and practices to move from medicine's modern treatment practices to a new informed, visionary center. That is, reemergence of wholeness, healing, art, and even spirituality of practice—congruent with nursing's past—is what the public now seeks within this postmodern era.

The emerging center, evolving from deeply informed postmodern discourse, is consistent with nursing's ancient traditions and most contemporary theories, offering caring and inner healing directions for self and others. Contemporary nursing theory and ancient caring–healing knowledge across time now serve as a hopeful paradigm and metanarrative linking worlds and time. Such reconstructive thinking will help nursing find a way to bridge and integrate modern and postmodern debates. The result—a reflective, postmodern perspective on nursing's timeless values and knowledge that unifies the past, present, and future of nursing science and practice. Finally, nurses within this postmodern framework are invited as individuals to first deal with their own caring and healing needs (wounded healers are we). They can then participate fully as mature caring–healing practitioners, in partnership with the public and with other health professionals, in this new millennium.

Modern–Postmodern Shifts

Major critiques have led to dramatic shifts from modern to postmodern mindsets in nursing and in other fields of study. These shifts are manifest in ways of knowing, as well as ways of being and doing. They can be highlighted in the following ways.

- From an impersonal, strict rationalist curing and treating perspective to a personal holistic caring–healing perspective

- From objective, analytic facts to subjective, intersubjective meaning; critical inquiry; and coconstructed meaning in methods and practices

- From separatist, distancing professional roles to relationship-centered caring and being in "right-relation" (full use of self-in-relation) roles

- From a dominant, outer-directed, medical treatment emphasis, to inner healing with a personal-symbolic meaning emphasis

- From physical to nonphysical phenomena as the locus of concern

- From conventional, biological, hard science to human science and art

- From body physical medicine (era I) to mind–body medicine (era II) to mind–body–spirit medicine and transformative medicine/nursing (era III) (Dossey, 1991; Watson, 1995a, 1995b, 1999a)

- From nursing as "doing technology" (e.g., medical tasks, procedures, and skills) to nursing as "being ontology" (e.g., integrating doing, knowing, and being into one integrative artistry of practice)

- From numbers and factual data alone to text, story, and narrative—extracting meaning and theory laden with personal experiences, self-reports, and actions

- From high-tech nurse as technician to high-touch nurse as someone who holds caring–healing consciousness and intentionality for self and others and the health care system and as an informed knowledge worker and expert in caring–healing practices

- From disregard for spirit to return to sacred dimensions of nursing and the human caring–healing processes

- From the nursing qua medicine model for nursing science development to the nursing qua nursing model for disciplinary and professional practice focus (Watson, 1999a)

- From institutionally based nursing to personally based practices, grounded in overall expertise, experience, talents, gifts, skills, competencies, and full use of self.

Inside Out and Upside Down

Identifying and coming to terms with modern–postmodern shifts displaces everything toward which we thought we had been working. At some basic level of reality and thinking, postmodern critiques and deconstruction efforts have turned our usual ways of thinking inside out and upside down.

For purposes of this chapter, I want to demonstrate modern–postmodern contrasts, as upside down and inside out through my own personal experience. The use of a personal story or narrative is congruent with postmodern style and with emerging models of caring–healing.

In presenting ideas this way, I hope that you will be able to experience postmodern thinking. Further, I hope that, through these ideas, you can also gain new insights into the debates and discourse between modern and postmodern perspectives and changing mindsets that can, do, and must inform nursing's and nurse's personal and professional future.

■ Personal Story as Exemplar of Modern–Postmodern Thinking

Journal Entry: June 22, 1998

"BENDICION POR HORRIFICO Y SANTISIMO:
BENEDICTION FOR THE HORRIBLE AND THE HOLY"
I live in pain. Yet I dwell in a semblance of peace. I know fear. Yet I dwell in love.

I know terror and life's horrors, yet I glimpse joy. I live in darkness; yet I experience light. I know despair; yet I live in hope. I know doubt, I reside in faith.

I live with and witness suffering for myself, my two daughters, my grandchildren, my family, friends and loved ones. I learn about deep caring and healing. I am asked to learn how to bear the unbearable as one of my life journeys.

I live with a broken heart, which may never mend. Yet the blood of life still flows through my veins and my life;— reminding me of the Sacred flow.

I am blind in one eye. Yet I see. I move at the speed of sound. Yet I am still.

I weep; yet I rejoice still.

I am lonely and alone. Yet I am never alone. I am sad; yet I laugh and cry.

I lost my eye. Yet I am sighted. I lose my husband. Yet I am wedded.

I lose my home. Yet I am housed. I lose my balance. But I still dance.

I lose my identity, Yet I am finding myself. I lose my life, as I have known it—Now full of tears.

Yet I now seek and glimpse another, inner life of life's blessings through tragedies.

I lose my "I" as I have lived it for 57 years. I find a greater "I", an humble "i," and the Divine I AM!

I am fragile, vulnerable, and labile. Yet I am softened and purified and strengthened by my wounds and my wonder at life and death.

I will never be cured, I may be healed.

(Watson, 1998. Personal journal entry. Printed with permission of author.)

Published as "Private Psalms: Surrendering to the Sacred" (p. 50) in "Aesthetic Expression," *International Journal of Human Caring, 3*(2) p. 50. Reprinted with permission of author.

■ Outer Story from the Modern, Clinical–Logical Side

IN JUNE, 1997 I suffered a traumatic eye injury, being hit by a golf club in a freak golfing accident; my eye could not be saved after up to three months of treatments, multiple, extensive surgeries and attempts at repairing and fixing it. I did everything possible to "save the eye," but to no avail. I ended up having to have the eye surgically removed and replaced with the highest level of technology and scientific advancements of materials and surgical repairs, implants, and prostheses. It was a so-called successful operation and implantation.

NINE MONTHS* after my injury and after needing and receiving full time care, provided by my husband, I was "hit again" by my husband's sudden, onset of situational depression, which never could be reversed medically, with all treatment efforts. He ended up committing suicide to the shock and dismay of all who knew him as a life-loving peaceful, spiritual being.

(Watson, 1999b. Unpublished personal journal. Printed with permission of author.)

■ Personal Story Within the Postmodern and Beyond Frame

I can never reveal, nor explain my story through logic, academic format, or the framework of modern medical science. I may be able to reveal it as a form of postmodern context, coming into being from time past, present, and future contained in the emerging now of human experience.

My story has been and remains, an out-of-the-ordinary experience, of Greek mythic proportions. It approaches the Great Unknown, the Mystery, the Void, of which there is nothing greater. This is not just my story, only one story. It is a story of the human condition that we all know; it is a story we all have access to, as we learn to bow down and be present to that which goes beyond what we have previously known as medical treatment and enter into inner healing.

■ My Inner Story

Journal Entry: July 1997

I have been blinded in my left eye, from an uncanny, freak golf club accident with my innocent grandson. He and I now are both joined and maimed by this event. How could such a life-changing event occur, so completely out of the blue, in such a literal blink of the eye, I lost my eye?

This accident occurred June 7th, on the eve of my sabbatical, filled with international travels, plans, and expectations of life as usual, as unusual as my/our life is, has been, it was a life for me, being in the world. Traveling throughout abroad and US had become a life style.

My work was university, academic life of the mind; my work was and has been about nursing theory and philosophy and human caring knowledge and practices. For my sabbatical I was scheduled for two trips to Finland, one to United Kingdom, with several lecture engagements in Wales, London, Oxford.

I am still scheduled to be in Hawaii at the University, to be in Thailand, and other places not yet determined. I had plans for concentrated writing time in Mexico.

And now I am confined to home and head cradle, at least for two months. My travels have been mind and heart travels, limited to my monastic cell: my cradle has been my rocking and wailing site, rocked with pain, wailing with despair at such a shock and calamity, to interrupt such a busy, worldly life; to interrupt self as I know myself to be; to knock me cold with disbelief and reality—a reality yet to be comprehended.

While I have journaled for these past 3 months, this computer effort marks my attempt to make meaning of such despair and disorientation for others and myself.

I write to orient myself as I re-enter the public world. Yet, I am not ready to re-enter the public world, I still resort to falling into my cradle, so to speak. The cradle meaning the head cradle of the massage table, which I had to recline on in the prone, downward position, 45 minutes out of each hour—for 6 weeks, and then weaned from 45 minutes to 20 minutes each hour, for another two weeks.

August 12 marked the day of being able to be up, to look up, and to lie on my back. Oh, for such sweet pleasures, one cannot imagine. The sheer luxury of lying back in a hot tub and feeling the warm water and bubbles on my neck and shoulders. How quickly we must learn to enjoy the small pleasures as major life events.

How can it be that I still am falling into my cradle, not knowing where to go from here? I have no choice it seems but to resort to making my space a holy space and falling down before my blessings in the midst of despair, with both praise and humility and thanksgiving, honoring the sacred healing process, creating sacred space for healing at many levels. The eye (I) has to heal and needs quiet, uncontaminated space and lessons in love, patience, and learning to wait.

Wait, I say, wait upon the Lord.

My time out, has been time in; this change in time, has grounded me; My time out/in, has required me and my family to seek new meaning, new ways of seeing and being. I am calling my time out a Sacred Inter-mission, realizing the INTER aspect as critical to this unnaturally imposed penance/gift experience I am forced to face and admit and surrender to.

I have to go through it, and it is not going away. It is up to me and my God to understand and find the blessings from the other side of this tragedy. For now, it is still a tragedy, evoking terror and pity from others, including myself.

Fifteen Months Later: November 24, 1998
4:30pm; Sea of Cortez, Mexico; All Alone*

IT is now November, 1998 as I return to these computer notes here in Mexico, making my way from the underside, the other side of that accident, only to be reeling and healing from even more calamity after my eye accident; the other side now finds me here for some time out again; time in again to be still and quiet after actually losing my eye in October last year (1997)— this occurred in spite of all kinds of quiet and loving devoted care from Doug my husband of almost 37 years; the eye could not be saved; the trauma was too great, the pressure never really returned, so I surrendered my eye, as I have/am continuing to learn, to surrender my life.

For you see, even more profound than the loss of my eye, soon was followed by loss of Doug, first from stark acute depression— that manifested on the day of my eye removal surgery and accelerated, unabated with only small moments of relief, such as walks in the mountain trails nearby our home; simple meals with candlelight and flowers, and being together; just being together. In spite of treatment and multiple medication regimes, nothing ever worked. He lost 30 pounds, he complained of constant ringing in his ears; he described a block in his head, he was not able to think straight. He became agitated, guilt ridden, and as I look back on it now, I admit he became irrationally paranoid. We were both so distorted in our view of reality for this time, so it was hard to sort out what was real and what was irrational. He had a CAT scan; it was normal. In spite of psychiatric treatment, all medication regimes and schemes, there was never any true improvement; he never established an alliance with his therapist. He absolutely refused to consider any type of hospitalization. He became

more and more a ghost of himself; the Doug I knew, spirit was gone. It disappeared somewhere between my accident and my supposed recovery. After my injury or after learning that my eye could not be saved, life was never available to him again it seems, for whatever reason. His soul seemed to be gone since the day of my surgery. None of it made any "rational sense". He seemed tormented.

And then the morning/afternoon of March 2, 1998, when I was hopeful he was improving; (we made plans to go to Mexico for recovery and were anticipating positive options for the future)— he ended his despair and sought his eternal peace by going out, buying a gun, going to the mountains we loved, on the trail we took almost daily, and shooting himself— by a quiet stream in Chautauqua, McClintock Trail, parallel to Enchanted Mesa Trail, our special place for over 30 years. I feel compelled to tell this story as part of my healing.

So, here I am some 15 months later, in profound shock, but somehow learning to be still to all the pain, misery, and mystery; I am here appreciating life and all its blessings in the midst of unimaginable wounds of suffering, despair, loss and changes that have taken me from my previously, supposedly balanced life.

So, I write, walk, meditate, pray, and journal here almost continuously to find new meaning, to discover the sacred and the holy amidst the horrific and unimaginable turns in my life's Earth plane journey; I do so now with an openness to finding and experiencing the Divine in all; the sacred in the midst of the profane; the Holy in the midst of the Horrible.

How can that be? What are my lessons? What are the meanings and where have I found my refuge from such tragedy? This story is one version of my experience and learnings from my cradle and from my close encounter with the death and loss of my husband, my lover, my closest friend, soul mate, and companion— through suicide— supposedly triggered by my accident and overwhelming despair over the loss of my eye.

I know, we all have to know that his death was not just my accident; there was something much deeper, longer standing, even past life, early life, soul, issues, mysteries than can never be comprehended from this side. It is soul business from another time and space, manifest here in all its harsh reality for us to cope with, sort out, and move beyond. Impossible task that is, but must occur.

The tragedy is compounded by the fact that his death came after devoted care and healing attempts that depleted his life energy and spirit; whereby he seemingly could seek peace only from the spirit realm, from his God; I pray that he is in peace as I make my way without him.

So, I come before you now to share this personal story as a postmodern view of a medical–health crisis and a journey toward inner healing, not just an impersonal case of medical–nursing science. It is this contrast between the impersonal, exterior view of "the problem", and the inner experience and search for meaning, wholeness, caring and healing in the midst of a medical crisis.

(Watson, 1999b. Unpublished personal journal entries: June 1997–November 1998. Printed with permission of author.)

■ Transition: Modern to Postmodern Healing

Confining my story to the modern perspective alone, I could say that I had the finest of medical–surgical interventions and the most contemporary, technological care during hospitalization and surgical procedures. I had the finest doctors and surgeons that money could obtain. I had the most advanced "modern care and cure" model available. But it was the caring, the caring modalities, and relationship-centered caring (the metanarrative of nursing's stance across time) that allowed for the shared search for meaning, the being-with-me along the way that became my inner healing journey and, as the famous Robert Frost line goes, "It made all the difference" (1964, p. 131). One of the blessings during that time was that I had the privilege of "experiencing my own theory from the inside out" as a recipient of loving, caring practice offered to me by my husband as a sacred gift. It is this personal, inside out story

which has contributed to my healing. My healing could not be confined to modern, medical–surgical treatment alone. That was only one small part of my journey toward wholeness, which is lifelong.

■ Postmodern Nursing and Beyond

Despite evolving insights gained through postmodern discourse and critiques of the Modern taken to the extreme, nursing is left void of a professional and disciplinary stance. For it is through its conceptual, philosophical, ethical, and theoretical systems that nursing contains a coherent disciplinary framework and most salient philosophical assumptions (Smith, 1994). In light of an abyss of values represented by the deconstructionist movement, nursing models provide a unifying framework of ethical and moral values that cannot be obtained from free-floating critique that attempts to strip the overriding moral structure from the profession.

Values of Metanarratives

Reed (1995) refers to these roots found in grand theories, not as *artifacts* to be discarded within postmodernist tradition, but rather as *archetypes* that depict, inspire, and represent philosophical and ethical frameworks for both the profession and discipline. Thus metanarratives provide ethical and intellectual grounding for moral universals that make a difference in patient care and in society alike.

Rather than "totalizing the discourse," these metanarratives now can be seen as external correctives to the movement to reject values. As such, these models now can serve as open metanarratives for further theoretical development and scientific inquiry. The models provide for further liberation of the human spirit and movements toward wholeness and emancipation while allowing us to still stand with ground beneath our feet.

In reconsidering the modern and postmodern turn in nursing and society, we can choose both to embrace and reject postmodern critique by continuing to deconstruct the mechanical, industrial, and matter-based model of humanity and the evolving human condition. Likewise, we can continue to question where critique ends and nihilism begins to avoid going into the abyss that rejects values and ethical stances. In so doing, nursing can participate in a process of "reflective and informed reconstruction"—a reconstruction that is based on critical postmodern discourse about nursing's extant theories, values, and philosophies. Reflection and reconstruction engages us in the postmodern while taking us beyond into new space.

■ Concluding Statement

Risky it is, but we need to blend the personal with the professional if we are going to learn and teach about the human condition with which we deal. As a result of reflection and reconstruction, a new space opens and liberates by integrating and embracing that which has come before. This new space converges and transcends dualities and holds diverse views. This new space for postmodern nursing is capable of dwelling in the present, eternal now, while embracing paradox and personal experiences. This new space offers sacred space for healing. Finally, this new space is an emerging paradigm that attends to processes and practices of caring, healing, and health at all levels. In this new free-floating postmodern space, we are enabled and liberated as professionals, as persons, as collective beings—growing into and becoming our already present, spirit-filled existence.

■ References

Derrida, J. (1976). *On grammatology.* Baltimore: Johns Hopkins University Press.

Dossey, L. (1991). *Meaning and medicine.* New York: Bantam Books.

Foucault, M. (1972). *The archaeology of knowledge and the discourse on language.* (A. M. Smith, Trans.). New York: Pantheon Books.

Frost, R. (1964). *Complete poems.* New York: Holt, Rinehart and Winston. (Original work published 1916)

Lather, P. (1991). *Getting smart: Feminist research and pedagogy within the postmodern.* New York: Routledge.

Nightingale, F. (1992). *Notes on nursing* (1992–The Commemorative Edition). Philadelphia: J. P. Lippincott. (Original work published 1859)

Reed, P. G. (1995). A treatise on nursing knowledge development for the 21st century: Beyond postmodernism. *Advances in Nursing Science, 17*(3), 70–84.

Sarup, M. (1988). *Post-structuralism and postmodernism.* New York: Harvester Wheatsheaf.

Skinner, Q. (1990). *The return of grand theory in the human sciences.* Cambridge, U.K.: Cambridge University Press.

Smith, M. C. (1994). Arriving at a philosophy of nursing: Discovering? Constructing? In J. F. Kikuchi & H. Simmons (Eds.), *Developing a philosophy of nursing* (pp. 43–61). Thousand Oaks, CA: Sage.

Toulmin, S. (1990). *Cosmopolis. The hidden agenda of modernity.* New York: Macmillan.

Watson, J. (1995a). Nursing's caring–healing paradigm as exemplar for alternative medicine? *Alternative Therapies, 1*(3), 64–69.

Watson, J. (1995b). Postmodernism and knowledge development in nursing. *Nursing Science Quarterly, 8*(2), 64–69.

Watson, J. (1998/1999). Closing refrain. In J. Watson, Private psalms. Cited in *International Journal of Human Caring (1999), 3*(2), 50. (Original work unpublished 1998 journal entry)

Watson, J. (1999a). *Postmodern nursing and beyond.* (Edinburgh, Scotland) U.K./ New York: Churchill-Livingstone/Harcourt Brace.

Watson, J. (1999b). Unpublished personal journal.

Whall, A. L. (1993). Let's get rid of all that theory. *Nursing Science Quarterly, 6,* 64–165

■ Editor's Questions for Discussion

Identify alternative views to modern assumptions about nursing knowledge developments and practice that have emerged from deconstruction efforts and critique. Identify postmodern tensions in nursing knowledge development and methods that may be reflected in the discussions by Kim (Chapter 23), Chinn (Chapter 24), Fawcett and Bourbonniere (Chapter 26), Neuman (Chapter 27), Donnelly (Chapter 28), and Meleis and Im (Chapter 72). To what extent do these authors address the prominent questions posed by Watson? What findings exist to answer the questions Watson raises? How are the themes addressed by those authors useful in guiding nursing's inquiry?

To what extent does Donnelly's assessment of nursing theories (Chapter 28) support Watson's description of postmodern direction and discourse regarding nursing theory? What service to the profession does Donnelly provide in her explication of nursing theory? Does Watson agree with Donnelly as to "where are we at"? How do either Donnelly or Watson or both address the question, "Where do we go from here?" in the postmodern debate? How does Watson's postmodern perspective apply to Pesut's plea (Chapter 70) for "inner work" by the profession?

Discuss Watson's personal story as an exemplar of modern–postmodern thinking. How are shifts from modern to postmodern mindset in nursing reflected in Watson's narrative and ways of knowing? Reflect on examples of "personal, inside-out" experiences that have contributed to healing within yourself. Identify "personal, inside-out" examples that could facilitate healing within the profession. How might those experiences personally and professionally be valuable and accomplish healing? How does healing within oneself affect healing within the profession? Describe how Watson's use of a journal might be an example for aesthetic inquiry of nursing as an art as discussed by Chinn (Chapter 24). As nurses, how can the personal be blended with the professional to learn and teach human conditions?

26

Utilization of Nursing Knowledge and the Future of the Discipline

Jacqueline Fawcett, PhD, RN, FAAN
Mary G. Bourbonniere, MSN, RN

In this chapter, we discuss contemporary utilization of nursing knowledge and its implications for the future of the nursing discipline. The discussion is in "one voice" reflecting more than a year of dialogue between a 20th century metatheorist (J. F.) and a nurse scholar for the 21st century (M. B.).

■ Four Fundamental Premises

Premise One

The discipline of nursing can survive and advance only if we celebrate our own heritage and utilize nursing knowledge.

This premise is predicated on the recognition of nursing as a distinct discipline with a distinctive body of knowledge. Modern nursing is and always has been a distinct discipline. Nightingale (1859/1946) captured its essence. She recognized that members of the disciplines of medicine and nursing collaborate in patient care, each contributing important perspectives and ways of caring that relate to cure and prevention, respectively. Furthermore, Nightingale recognized that nursing knowledge comes from recording and analyzing clinical observations. Donaldson and Crowley (1978) maintained that nursing is a professional discipline. They explained that the mission ascribed to nursing by society requires that knowledge not only be generated and disseminated but also be used for social good. Consequently, nursing is considered a professional discipline rather than an academic discipline. In a contemporary update, Watson (1996) characterized nursing as "a human science discipline as well as an academic-clinical profession" (p. 142). A discipline or profession, as Anderson (1995) noted, is distinguished from a trade by the existence of a "well-developed body of knowledge . . . a solid scholarly and scientific foundation upon which to base practice" (p. 247).

Premise Two

Nursing knowledge is formalized in explicit conceptual models of nursing and nursing theories.

The second premise asserts that nursing discipline knowledge is formalized in several conceptual models, grand theories, and middle-range theories. A conceptual model is a set of relatively abstract and general concepts and the propositions that describe and link those concepts. A conceptual model provides a distinctive frame of reference, a different lens or intellectual perspective, a "horizon of expectations" (Popper, 1965, p. 47) for viewing phenomena of particular interest to a discipline. Nursing's disciplinary phenomena are the person, the environment, health, and nursing (Fawcett, 2000). The most widely recognized nursing conceptual models are Johnson's Behavioral Systems Model, King's General Systems Framework, Levine's Conservation Model, Neuman's Systems Model, Orem's Self-Care Framework, Rogers' Science of Unitary Human Beings, and Roy's Adaptation Model.

Grand theories are rather broad in scope; they are made up of concepts and propositions that are less abstract and general than the concepts and propositions of a conceptual model but are not as concrete and specific as the concepts and propositions of a middle-range theory. The most widely recognized nursing grand theories are Leininger's Theory of Culture Care Diversity and Universality, Newman's Theory of Health as Expanding Consciousness, and Parse's Theory of Human Becoming.

Middle-range theories are narrower in scope than grand theories. They are made up of a limited number of concepts and propositions that are written at a relatively concrete and specific level. The most widely recognized nursing middle-range theories are Orlando's Theory of the Deliberative Nursing Process, Peplau's Theory of Interpersonal Relations, and Watson's Theory of Human Caring.

The importance of a distinctive body of nursing knowledge was underscored by Rogers (1994), who stated, "If we do not think in terms of real knowledge, we have no place in higher education. Our knowledge must be nursing knowledge" (p. 8). The importance of discipline-specific nursing knowledge as formalized in explicit nursing conceptual models and theories is underscored by postmodern writers, who "remind us that, without one's own language, 'You do not exist'" (Watson, 1996, p. 155). "Throughout history," Watson went on to explain, "nursing has adopted or adapted other's languages for nursing phenomena. Thus nursing, as the largest health care profession, ironically is not often seen as distinct in its own right. Instead, nursing is seen as an extension of modern medicine" (p. 155).

Nursing conceptual models and theories are unequivocally written in languages that are distinctively nursing. Consequently, nurses whose work is guided by nursing conceptual models and theories can securely follow in Nightingale's footsteps and articulate what nursing is and what it is not.

Premise Three

Advances in nursing knowledge can occur only by development of nursing research methodologies and nursing practice methodologies.

The third premise means that distinctive nursing methodologies are needed to advance nursing knowledge. Nursing research methodologies are used to generate and test nursing middle-range theories. Mitchell (1994) and Thorne, Kirkham, and MacDonald-Emes (1997) pointed to the need for research methodologies that adhere to the systematic reasoning of the nursing discipline.

Nursing practice methodologies are used to apply nursing conceptual models and theories in clinical situations. For many years, the nursing process has been regarded as the way to conduct nursing practice. A shift to the notion of practice *methodologies* extends the discussion of the reciprocal relationship between nursing knowledge and nursing practice (Fawcett, 1992) by focusing more explicitly on the contributions of practical activities to the advancement of nursing knowledge. Jacobs and Huether (1978) expressed concern that nursing cannot exist without the nursing knowledge–nursing practice link, reminding us that as we develop our science, we take control of practice. Donaldson (1995) and Christman (1995) echo that concern in ways that urge nursing to continue to move forward in developing the science and to critically appraise the way advanced practice nurses are prepared.

Premise Four

Nursing research methodologies and nursing practice methodologies are derived from the focus and content of conceptual models of nursing and nursing theories.

The fourth premise means that methodologies for development of new *nursing* knowledge must be associated with existing formal *nursing* knowledge. Considerable progress has been made on this front. Distinctive nursing research methodologies have been directly derived from Rogers' conceptual model; Leininger's, Newman's, and Parse's grand theories; and Watson's middle-range theory (Fawcett, 2000). Distinctive nursing practice methodologies have been derived from all the nursing conceptual models, grand theories, and middle-range theories cited earlier (Fawcett, 2000). Especially noteworthy are Newman's research as praxis methodology and Peplau's clinical methodology, both of which do double duty as a research methodology and a practice methodology.

■ Two Major Challenges to the Four Premises

Challenge One

Conceptual and theoretical frameworks for research and practice are largely implicit, private images of nursing that are grounded in the knowledge of other disciplines.

Despite dissemination of formal nursing knowledge through publications and presentations by authors of the nursing conceptual models and theories and nurses who are using those models and theories to guide their research and practice, little has changed since Reilly (1975) and Johnson (1987) pointed out that most nurses use private images or implicit, mental frameworks of nursing to guide research and practice. Johnson (1987) elaborated, noting that

> unfortunately, the mental images used by nurses in their practice, images developed through edu-

cation and experience and continuously governed by the multitude of factors in the practice setting, have tended to be disconnected, diffused, incomplete and frequently heavily weighted by concepts drawn from conceptual schema used by medicine to achieve its own social mission. (p. 195)

Even a limited review of nursing literature reveals that far more attention is given to developing knowledge of other disciplines than nursing knowledge. An examination of the 90 research reports published in two clinically oriented nursing journals *(Geriatric Nursing* and *Nurse Practitioner)* and two nursing research journals *(Nursing Research* and *Research in Nursing and Health)* during 1998 is enlightening. The clinical journals were chosen because they represent nursing areas that were created to deliver nursing to traditionally vulnerable, underserved persons. The research journals were selected because they are among the top-ranked, peer-reviewed nursing research journals. Of the 90 published studies, only 9 (10%) were guided by or based on explicit nursing conceptual models or theories. Of the remaining 81 (90%) studies, a few were guided by implicit frameworks, and the rest, by explicit conceptual models and theories from nonnursing disciplines or fields of study, including psychology, sociology, medicine, dentistry, physiology, biology, education, decision sciences, economics, ethics, epidemiology, management sciences, marketing, and communications.

Determination of the researcher's conceptual or theoretical viewpoint permits the study to be "measured against historical and intellectual loci" and enables an appropriate critique of the study within the context of "the extremely politicized world of health care today" (Gullifer, 1997, p. 157). The only conclusion that can be drawn from the review of the 90 research reports is that the editors of the four nursing journals sanction publication of research that contributes not to nursing but to

other disciplines, and that they are not paying sufficient attention to the politics of contemporary health care, which many nurses agree are focused on demeaning or eliminating nursing's role.

Is it any wonder, then, that nursing has been characterized as invisible (Gordon, 1997)? Moreover, the glaring absence of nursing conceptual models and theories in so many of the 90 research reports reviewed clearly reflects oppressed group behavior in nursing and contributes to the marginalization of nursing as a science with a unique theoretical basis (Roberts, 1983).

There is, of course, nothing wrong with nurse researchers' use of nonnursing conceptual models and theories, but their work contributes nothing to the discipline of nursing (Cody, 1998; Mitchell, 1994). As Rogers (1994) explained, such research contributes "nothing to nursing knowledge because [it is] not studying the same phenomenon. . . . Sociology [for example,] is a fine field of study, but theories derived from sociology, regardless of who derived them, are still sociological theories directed toward sociology" (p. 8).

Challenge Two

Rapid growth of advanced practice nurse practitioner programs has diverted attention away from development and utilization of nursing knowledge and toward medical knowledge.

Advanced practice nursing is increasingly interpreted as the nurse practitioner role. And nurse practitioners more and more resemble physician's assistants (Rogers, as cited in Huch, 1995), junior doctors (Meleis, 1993), pseudo doctors (Kendrick, 1997), or nursing qua medicine (Watson, 1996). Clearly, nurse practitioners are emulating physicians, perhaps because "the lure of following the medical model is sanctioned and well rewarded in some settings" (Hawkins & Thibodeau, 1993, p. 11).

An alarming example of society's interpretation of physician emulation is the appearance of employment advertisements indicating that *either* a nurse practitioner or a physician's assistant will meet job requirements. Additionally, the ongoing efforts to assimilate more of medical practice into advanced practice nursing certainly shifts the focus of the discipline from health and its restoration to illness and its diagnosis. Uncritically embracing and utilizing knowledge from other disciplines dilutes the pool of knowledge developed by and for nursing practice.

Watson (1996) warned that

> if [nursing] remains an extension of medicine, continuing to evolve within a Nursing-qua-Medicine [paradigm], it will not fulfill its mandate to the public, and its long effort to give society a mature caring-healing health profession will be vulnerable to termination. (p. 146)

Moreover, as Lubic (1995) noted, it would be

> folly to embrace [the medical model] and risk being seen as "more of the same" [at a time when medical practice] is being severely criticized as being self-serving and also because it has failed to serve all the people of the nation. (Presentation)

■ Two Strategies to Meet the Challenges

Strategy One

End nursing's intellectual and practical romance with the knowledge of other disciplines.

Ending the romance with the knowledge of other disciplines requires giving up behaviors associated with oppressed groups (Roberts, 1983). Nurses who work within the context of nonnursing knowledge certainly must regard themselves as oppressed or they would not embrace the nonnursing knowledge and ignore or denigrate extant nursing knowledge (Roberts, 1983). Furthermore, those nurses are making false claims when they maintain that they are contributing to the advancement of nursing knowledge. Thus all nurses must "have the courage to take a position about why people need nursing and about what nursing can and should be" (Orem, 1995, p. 414).

One solution to overcoming nurses' emulation of physicians is the provision in nurse practitioner education of "more substantive nursing content so that the distinctiveness of nursing is not lost in the wake of nurses' mimicking physicians" (Baumann, 1998, p. 90). An extension of that solution is an agreement that every nurse accepts the status of senior nurse (Meleis, 1993) and therefore practices nursing qua nursing (Watson, 1997). In addition, advanced practice nursing must not be regarded as a way to fill a medical practice gap. As Rogers (as cited in Huch, 1995) commented,

> I would wonder why in the world nurses want to extend into medicine. I will repeat again, Nightingale said medicine and nursing should never be mixed up. Nurses do not need medicine in order to practice nursing. And if we practiced nursing, we would know that. (p. 44)

In other words, true advanced practice *nursing* builds on the foundation of *nursing* conceptual models and theories to deliver safe and effective *nursing*.

Furthermore, state board of nursing laws must be changed. For how can nurses regard advanced practice *nursing* as that which, by a law regulating the practice of nursing, requires "practice for at least 24 months, under the supervision of a licensed physician or [employment] by a clinic or hospital that has a medical director who is a licensed physician" (Advanced Practice Issues, 1998, p. 4)?

Strategy Two

Fall in love with nursing knowledge and develop a passion for the destiny of the discipline of nursing.

Falling in love with nursing knowledge and developing a passion for the destiny of the discipline of nursing is greatly facilitated in nursing education by (a) introducing nursing models and theories in the very first nursing course, (b) using that knowledge as the base for all other nursing courses, and (c) using only those nursing textbooks focusing on the content and use of nursing conceptual models and theories. In nursing practice, this strategy is facilitated by using explicit nursing conceptual models and theories as the structure for delivery of nursing services in all clinical agencies. In nursing research, the strategy is facilitated by requiring nurse researchers to explicate the *nursing* conceptual model or theory that guides their studies and encouraging nurses who elect to continue to develop knowledge from other disciplines to publish in nonnursing journals.

■ *The Likelihood of Meeting the Challenges*

Nursing is unlikely to survive in the 21st century if nurses continue on the current path of conducting research within the context of conceptual models and theories from nonnursing disciplines and practicing nursing within the context of the medical model. Nursing is more likely to survive and advance as a discipline if the roles of nurse researcher and nurse practitioner are integrated into the single role of nurse scholar.

Nurse scholars use an explicit nursing conceptual model or theory to guide their activities, and they use the data from every encounter with a patient for nursing research purposes. In other words, nurse scholars use the clinical data

available to them in every patient situation to refine or reject existing nursing conceptual models and theories and to develop new models and theories and new research and practice methodologies. The use of an explicit nursing conceptual model or theory permits nurse scholars to articulate what nursing is and what distinctive contributions nurses make to collaborative practice and interdisciplinary research. Dodd (1997), for example, explained how use of Orem's Self-Care Framework helped her retain a *nursing* perspective in the interdisciplinary health care milieu. She stated,

> Orem's [framework] provides a nursing-based focus and systematic guidelines for examining the balance between a person's needs, capabilities, and limitations in exercising self-care actions to enhance personal health. . . . Orem's [framework] assisted us in maintaining a focus on issues salient to nursing practice. (p. 987)

Nurse scholars assume the role of "attending nurses" in practice situations. Watson (1996) described the attending nurse as one who works alongside other health team members while assuming responsibility for the "caring–healing focus of care" (p. 163). She envisions patients bringing "their own nurse to a hospital to assume responsibility for 'attending' to a full range of their individualized caring-healing needs, including mediating among multiple providers and systems, and ensuring continuity of their care needs" (p. 163).

Nurse administrators at the UCLA Neuropsychiatric Institute and Hospital already have developed and implemented a Johnson's Behavioral System Model–based version of the attending nurse (Dee & Poster, 1995). The major focus of their attending nurse is clinical case management. Role responsibilities include (a) direct patient care; (b) delegation and monitoring of selected aspects of nursing care; (c) provision of leadership, consultation, and guidance to nursing staff; and (d) collaboration with multidisciplinary team members. The attending nurse role has been well-received by members of the multidisciplinary team and by the nurses, who reported increased job satisfaction and retention, role clarity, and communication with patients' family members and decreased role conflict and role tension (Moreau, Poster, & Niemela, 1993; Niemela, Poster, & Moreau, 1992).

The attending nurse role can be realized most fully if nurses are self-employed, rather than serving as employees of ever larger and constantly merging clinical agencies. Thus we reissue Sills' (1983) call for the formation of nurse corporations.

"The conceptual key to the corporation proposal," Sills (1983) explained,

> . . . is that it changes the fundamental nature of the social contract. The professional nurse would no longer be an employee of the hospital or agency, but rather a member of a professional corporation which provides nursing services to patients and clients on a fee-for-service basis. . . . Such a change in the nature of the social contract is, it seems to me, fundamentally necessary for the survival of nursing as a profession rather than an occupational group of workers employed by other organizations. (p. 573)

Sills' proposal could be expanded so that nursing corporations, made up of nurse scholars in equal partnership with one another, would contract with individuals, families, communities, and clinical agencies (e.g., medical centers, community and specialty hospitals, and home care agencies) for the provision of distinctively nursing services guided by nursing conceptual models and theories.

■ Concluding Statement

Use of explicit, formal nursing conceptual models and theories as guides for nurse scholars' activities will advance the discipline of nursing. Moreover, if nursing practice "is the use of nursing knowledge" (Rogers, 1994, p. 5), why are Bruser and Whittaker (1998) concerned with the so-called "encroachment on traditional nursing practices" (p. 59) by other health professionals? Why, indeed, if the "incursions on nursing practice" (p. 59) are by pharmacists who want to administer medications and emergency medical services (EMS) personnel who want to do medical histories and physical examinations? We submit that nurses should rejoice that pharmacists want the opportunity to use the knowledge of pharmacology in practice and that EMS personnel want to use medical knowledge in practice. Such opportunities clearly would free nurse scholars from nonnursing practices and permit time for the use and further development of distinctive nursing knowledge.

Nursing must remember its social mission. The past and the present of the discipline have depended on the development and utilization of nursing knowledge. The future does, too.

■ References

Advanced Practice Issues. (1998, August). *Maine State Board of Nursing Bulletin, 4.*

Anderson, C. A. (1995). Scholarship: How important is it? *Nursing Outlook, 43,* 247–248.

Baumann, S. L. (1998). Nursing: The missing ingredient in nurse practitioner education. *Nursing Science Quarterly, 11,* 89–90.

Bruser, S., & Whittaker, S. (1998). Diluting nurses' scope of practice. *American Journal of Nursing, 98*(10), 59–60.

Christman, L. (1995). Science as the predictor of professional recognition and success. In A. Omery, C. E. Kasper, & G. G. Page (Eds.), *In search of nursing science* (pp. 291–294). Thousand Oaks, CA: Sage.

Cody, W. K. (1998). Critical theory and nursing science: Freedom in theory and practice. *Nursing Science Quarterly, 11,* 44–46.

Dee, V., & Poster, E. C. (1995). Applying Kanter's theory of innovative change: The transition from a primary to attending model of nursing care delivery. *Journal of the American Psychiatric Nurses Association, 1,* 112–119.

Dodd, M. J. (1997). Self-care: Ready or not! *Oncology Nursing Forum, 24,* 990.

Donaldson, S. K. (1995). Nursing science for nursing practice. In A. Omery, C. E. Kasper, & G. G. Page (Eds.), *In search of nursing science* (pp. 3–12). Thousand Oaks, CA: Sage.

Donaldson, S. K., & Crowley, D. M. (1978). The discipline of nursing. *Nursing Outlook, 26,* 113–120.

Fawcett, J. (1992). Conceptual models and nursing practice: The reciprocal relationship. *Journal of Advanced Nursing, 17,* 224–228.

Fawcett, J. (2000). *Analysis and evaluation of contemporary nursing knowledge: Nursing models and theories.* Philadelphia: F. A. Davis.

Gordon, S. (1997). *Life support: Three nurses on the front lines.* Boston: Little, Brown.

Gullifer, J. (1997). The acceptance of a philosophically based research culture? *International Journal of Nursing Practice, 3,* 153–158.

Hawkins, J. W., & Thibodeau, J. A. (1993). *The advanced practitioner: Current practice issues* (3rd ed.). New York: Tiresias Press.

Huch, M. H. (1995). Nursing and the next millennium. *Nursing Science Quarterly, 8,* 38–44.

Jacobs, M. K., & Huether, S. E. (1978). Nursing science: The theory–practice linkage. *Advances in Nursing Science, 1*(1), 63–73.

Johnson, D. E. (1987). Guest editorial: Evaluating conceptual models for use in critical care nursing practice. *Dimensions of Critical Care Nursing, 6,* 195–197.

Kendrick, K. (1997). What is advanced nursing? *Professional Nurse, 12*(10), 689.

Lubic, R. W. (1995, February). *Principles for a successful professional life.* Paper presented at the Annenberg Public Policy Center's Women in the Public Sphere 1994–1995 Lecture Series, "Women's Voices: Women's Choices—Nursing Responds." Philadelphia: University of Pennsylvania.

Meleis, A. I. (1993, April). *Nursing research and the Neuman model: Directions for the future.* Panel discussion at the Fourth Biennial International Neuman Systems Model Symposium (B. Neuman, A. I. Meleis, J. Fawcett, L. Lowry, M. C. Smith, A. Edgil, participants), Rochester, NY.

Mitchell, G. (1994). Discipline-specific inquiry: The hermeneutics of theory-guided nursing research. *Nursing Outlook, 42,* 224–228.

Moreau, D., Poster, E. C., & Niemela, K. (1993). Implementing and evaluating an attending nurse model. *Nursing Management, 24*(6), 56–58, 60, 64.

Niemela, K., Poster, E. C., & Moreau, D. (1992). The attending nurse: A new role for the advanced clinician—Adolescent inpatient unit. *Journal of Child and Adolescent Psychiatric and Mental Health Nursing, 5*(3), 5–12.

Nightingale, F. (1946). *Notes on nursing: What it is, and what it is not.* Philadelphia: Lippincott. (Original work published 1859; London: Harrison)

Orem, D. E. (1995). *Nursing: Concepts of practice* (5th ed.). St. Louis: Mosby.

Popper, K. R. (1965). *Conjectures and refutations: The growth of scientific knowledge.* New York: Harper & Row.

Reilly, D. E. (1975). Why a conceptual framework? *Nursing Outlook, 23,* 566–569.

Roberts, S. J. (1983). Oppressed group behavior: Implications for nursing. *Advances in Nursing Science, 5*(4), 21–30.

Rogers, M. E. (1994). Nursing science evolves. In M. Madrid & E. A. M. Barrett (Eds.), *Rogers' scientific art of nursing practice* (pp. 3–9). New York: National League for Nursing Press.

Sills, G. M. (1983). The role and function of the clinical nurse specialist. In N. L. Chaska (Ed.), *The nursing profession: A time to speak* (pp. 563–579). New York: McGraw-Hill.

Thorne, S., Kirkham, S. R., & MacDonald-Emes, J. (1997). Interpretive description: A noncategorical qualitative alternative for developing nursing knowledge. *Research in Nursing and Health, 20,* 169–177.

Watson, M. J. (1996). Watson's theory of transpersonal caring. In P. Hinton Walker & B. Neuman (Eds.), *Blueprint for use of nursing models: Education, research, practice, and administration* (pp. 141–184). New York: National League for Nursing Press.

Watson, J. (1997). The theory of human caring: Retrospective and prospective. *Nursing Science Quarterly, 10,* 49–52.

■ *Editor's Questions for Discussion*

How does Donnelly's assessment of nursing theories (Chapter 28) apply to the four premises presented by Fawcett and Bourbonniere? To what extent do Fawcett and Bourbonniere's challenges to the four premises reinforce Donnelly's evaluation? What explanations other than oppressed group behavior may account for absence of nursing conceptual models in research reports? Debate whether other disciplines may or may not contribute to the discipline of nursing. How relevant are debates such as whether advanced nurse practitioners are practicing nursing or medicine? How may such issues be resolved permanently?

What substantive nursing content should be taught in nurse practitioner programs that is not currently part of such programs? Provide examples of how advanced practice nursing specifically builds on a foundation of nursing conceptual models and theories. Why do nurses conduct research from nonnursing discipline conceptual models? Does not that practice reinforce Donnelly's assessment of nursing theories? Discuss potential effectiveness of strategies suggested by Fawcett and Bourbonniere to meet the challenges. What is the likelihood that—given varying views (Lenz and Hardin, Chapter 20; Miller, Chapter 36; A. Fisher and Habermann, Chapter 21; Deets and Choi, Chapter 34; and Titler, Chapter 35) regarding research, scholarship, and doctoral education—Fawcett and Bourbonniere's plea will be heard for an integrated role of nurse scholar? Would such a role result in situation-specific theories as espoused by Meleis and Im (Chapter 72)? Which Fawcett and Bourbonniere strategies and suggestions for future knowledge development are supported by Deets and Choi (Chapter 34)?

Is attaching the term "attending" to nurses in practice situations mimicking the traditional "attending physician" label used in medicine? Could such employment of attending be counterproductive for nursing distinctiveness? What relationship may exist between the attending nurse role and entrepreneurship as presented by Duffy (Chapter 53)?

27

The Neuman Systems Model

A Futuristic Care Perspective

Betty M. Neuman, PhD, RN, FAAN

This chapter focuses on the Neuman Systems Model (NSM), a widely recognized conceptual model of nursing. The chapter begins with an overview of the NSM and continues with discussion about the use of the NSM as a guide for 21st century international nursing research, education, administration, and practice. Additional discussion focuses on use of the NSM as a dynamic guide for interdisciplinary health care teams. The chapter concludes with a summary of the NSM contributions to the discipline of nursing.

■ Overview of the Neuman Systems Model

The NSM was developed as a way to organize nursing course content that addressed the breadth of nursing problems (Neuman & Young, 1972). Most recent refinements in the

I gratefully acknowledge my coauthors, Patricia Deal Aylward, Charlene Beynon, Diane M. Breckenridge, Jacqueline Fawcett, Anita Fields, Lois Lowry, Rae Jeanne Memmott, and Jane Toot, all of whom are true experts in the use of the Neuman Systems Model and all of whom contributed equally to the chapter.

NSM are presented in *The Neuman Systems Model* (Neuman, 1995).

Explication of the NSM

The NSM reflects nursing's interest in well and ill people as holistic systems and in environmental influences on health. Clients' and nurses' perceptions of stressors and resources are emphasized, and clients act in partnership with nurses to set goals and identify relevant prevention interventions. The individual, family or other group, community, or a social issue all are client systems, which are viewed as composites of interacting physiological, psychological, sociocultural, developmental, and spiritual variables.

The internal environment encompasses all forces within the boundaries of the client system and is the source of intrapersonal stressors. The external environment encompasses all forces outside the client system and is the source of interpersonal and extrapersonal stressors. The created environment is the client system's perceived safety net about situations and events; it supersedes and encompasses both internal and external environments.

The central core encompasses innate and genetic factors and strengths and weaknesses of the client system. It is surrounded by lines of defense and resistance. The flexible line of defense is the outermost protective buffer that prevents invasion of stressors. When the flexible line expands, it provides greater short-term protection against stressor invasion; when it contracts, it provides less protection. The normal line of defense is the second protective mechanism; it represents the client system's usual wellness state, which has developed over time. Expansion of the normal line of defense reflects an enhanced wellness state; contraction, a diminished state of wellness.

The normal line of defense is penetrated by one or more stressors when the flexible line of defense cannot withstand stressor impact. The result is reaction, in the form of client system instability or illness. The lines of resistance are closest to the central core. They are involuntarily activated when a stressor invades the normal line of defense and attempts to stabilize the client system. When they are effective, the client system can reconstitute; if they are ineffective, death may ensue. The amount of resistance to a stressor is determined by the interrelationship of the five variables of the client system.

Interventions

The goal of nursing is to facilitate optimal client system stability through primary, secondary, and tertiary prevention interventions. Primary prevention is action to retain client system stability and is selected when the risk of a stressor is known but a reaction has not yet occurred. Secondary prevention is action to attain system stability and is selected when a reaction to a stressor already has occurred. Tertiary prevention is action to maintain system stability and is selected when some degree of client system stability and reconstitution has occurred following secondary prevention interventions.

Utilization

Nurses who use the NSM develop skills in leadership and scholarship. Leadership is envisioning a course of action and carries with it the responsibility for scholarship. Scholarship is establishing the scientific adequacy of that course of action and carries with it the responsibility for leadership. The NSM provides steps or "markers" for the integration of leadership and scholarship (Neuman, 1997). The markers, which are a summary of the NSM nursing process, are the following.

1. Identifying the boundary of a particular client system. The boundary represents the

flexible line of defense, which meets the external environment.

2. Determining the usual wellness state of the client system. That state represents the normal line of defense.

3. Studying the interactions of the physiological, psychological, sociocultural, developmental, and spiritual variables of the client system. Those interactions represent the current wellness state of the client system.

4. Identifying the internal and external environmental stressors, their possible and actual effects on the stability of the client system, and validating those effects with the client system. Effects represent symptoms that reflect the degree of stressor reaction or client system variance from wellness.

5. Stating the condition of the client system and establishing and prioritizing goals that will promote optimal client system stability in conjunction with the client system.

6. Identifying and implementing primary, secondary, and tertiary prevention interventions that scientific research has shown to attain established goals.

7. Evaluating the degree of goal attainment reached by the client system.

The adoption and successful use of the NSM through application of the markers has increased steadily since its inception. In recent years, its utility has been documented in many different countries and cultures throughout the world.

■ The Neuman Systems Model and Nursing Research

The NSM has documented utility as a guide for nursing research. On the international front, faculty from Maalardaylens Hogskola, in Vasteras, Sweden, and from Göteborg University in Sweden are conducting NSM-based studies, as is a nurse researcher at Ewha University in Seoul, Korea.

Integrative Review

An integrative review of NSM-based studies from 1982 through 1997 yielded 200 publications, including 61 journal articles, 3 book chapters, 81 master's theses, and 55 doctoral dissertations. One-third of the studies focused on prevention interventions; another one-quarter, on perception of stressors; and almost 10%, on one or more of the five NSM variables. Thirty-seven percent of the studies were descriptive; 34%, experimental; 25%, correlational; and 4%, instrument development. Only 55% of the reports included an explanation of the linkage between NSM concepts and study variables, and 59% did not include conclusions regarding the utility or credibility of the NSM. Overall scientific merit was judged as adequate, although several reports did not include psychometric data.

Significance

Analysis of the 69 experimental studies revealed that just 13 (19%) had statistically significant findings for effects of prevention interventions, 17 (25%) had statistically nonsignificant findings, and 31 (45%) had some significant and some nonsignificant findings; statistical significance was not reported for the remaining 8 (11%) studies. The analysis indicated that programs of targeted NSM-based research are needed in the 21st century to better understand factors that contribute to efficacy of prevention interventions. The analysis also pointed to a need for workshops to help researchers explicate clear linkages between the NSM and study variables.

■ The Neuman Systems Model and Nursing Education

The NSM has documented utility as a guide for nursing education. The NSM is among the four conceptual models most frequently used by nurse educators in the United States and has been adopted as a curriculum guide by many nurse educators in other countries.

Curriculum Guide

An interdisciplinary team of faculty from Vanersborg University College have collaborated with a team from the University of South Florida to teach select topics in cultural sensitivity through satellite communication. Moreover, the Gereformeerde Hogeschool, a baccalaureate program in Zwolle, Holland, recently adopted the NSM; that school received national recognition in 1998 for the best nursing curriculum in the country.

International Liaisons

In addition, several nurse educators who are NSM experts are actively engaged in promoting international liaisons and encouraging use of the NSM in diverse cultures. A Brigham Young University faculty member accompanies baccalaureate nursing students to Guatemala each summer, where they practice in government-sponsored hospitals and clinics, and use the NSM to assess communities. A University of Portland faculty member serves as an external educational examiner for the Kuwait University School of Nursing.

An East Tennessee State University faculty member is working closely with faculty from Chiang Mai University in Thailand to write a book of NSM-based culturally sensitive case studies in the Thai language; this faculty member also is cooperating with nurses from the Veterans General Hospital in Taipei, Taiwan, to write a similar book in Chinese. Moreover, the NSM is used to guide curricula of the baccalaureate nursing programs at the University of Jordan, Yang Ming Medical College in Taiwan, the University of Guam, and Akureye University in Iceland. In addition, much of the content of the *Neuman Systems Model* (Neuman, 1995) has been translated for use by Japanese educators and students.

Interventions for Nursing Education Programs

The NSM guided analyses of stressors and lines of defense in contemporary nursing education that led to identification of proactive interventions will foster the stability of programs of nursing education far into the 21st century. These interventions are:

1. Develop unique partnerships, consortiums, or collaborations between nursing and other health care programs in state higher education systems to meet shared needs.

2. Promote a positive image of nursing education as a career choice.

3. Ensure that graduates are prepared for the current and projected marketplace.

4. Use state-of-the-art teaching and learning technologies.

5. Encourage interdisciplinary education in baccalaureate, master's, and doctoral programs.

6. Obtain creative funding.

7. Expand support services for students.

Model for Other Disciplines

Implementation of the interventions will lead to realization of a new nursing education model that can serve as a prototype for education in other disciplines. The model encompasses (a) dialogue among nurse educators in a spirit of community; (b) recognition of having to do more with less but not settling for less; (c) fewer faculty but faculty with enthusiasm for innovative, collaborative teaching and learning; (d) faculty gender and cultural composition reflecting student and community populations; (e) salaries that keep pace with the marketplace; and (f) time to attend educational forums, participate in clinical practice and research, publish results of practice and research projects, and network with nurses and other health care professionals in the community and faculty in other disciplines.

■ The Neuman Systems Model and Nursing Administration

The NSM has documented utility in nursing administration. Indeed, use of the NSM as a guide for nursing administration has been the subject of several published reports (e.g., Burke, Capers, O'Connell, Quinn, & Sinnott, 1989; Hinton-Walker, 1995; Kelley & Sanders, 1995; Kelley, Sanders, & Pierce, 1989).

Today's health care administrators are functioning in an especially turbulent work environment, an environment characterized by constant change and chaos. At the same time, administrators must address needs of today's employees, who want more control over their work and work environment, and want to work with management to shape the future work environment and have their contributions recognized. Consequently, traditional management models, in which the administrator retains power and control and assumes primary responsibility for planning, organizing, directing, and coordinating are no longer adequate. Clearly, new ways of thinking and behaving are required, as are new models that emphasize empowerment, teamwork, partnerships, risk taking, and experimentation (Block, 1993; Senge, 1990).

Guide for Administrators

The NSM offers clear direction and guidance for administrators of learning and "leaderful" organizations that are needed to advance delivery of nursing services into the 21st century. Learning organizations are those that are continually expanding their capacity to create their future (Senge, 1990). Learning organizations (a) engage in systematic problem solving, (b) experiment with new approaches, (c) learn from their own and others' experiences and best practices, and (d) disseminate knowledge quickly and efficiently throughout the organization (Garvin, 1993). "Leaderful" organizations are those in which leadership is encouraged at all levels and in which employees assume ownership and take responsibility for the future of the organization. Especially relevant to administrators of such organizations are the NSM's emphasis on seeking input of all who are involved in a particular situation, validating perceptions of stressors and resources, and mutually determining appropriate courses of action.

Application of NSM

Daily use of the NSM markers described earlier offers nurse administrators a concrete way to (a) seek input from others, (b) collaborate and engage others in dialogue, (c) foster strategic thinking, (d) promote the professional development and involvement of peers and subordinates, and (e) mutually identify actions based on available information. Assessing the degree of stressor reaction helps the administrator to determine priorities so that scarce resources can be used most efficiently and productively. Routine use of the markers yields data that can be used by the nurse administrator to make informed and rational decisions. The three types of prevention interventions provide direction away from a crisis management style, allow the administrator to look beyond the current situation, and lead to proactive strategic thinking. Organizational evaluation of prevention interventions then can focus on such criteria as strengthened viability (health) of the organization, increased productivity, and prevention or diminution of the impact of an impending crisis or current stressor.

■ The Neuman Systems Model and Nursing Practice

The NSM has documented utility as a guide for nursing practice in diverse settings, including clinics, hospitals, hospices, homes, and even the streets and sidewalks of a community. Given its applicability in so many contemporary health care settings, the NSM should be an effective guide for nursing practice in 21st century health care settings.

The markers described earlier represent a nursing process that is used by clinicians to (a) assess client systems, (b) set mutually agreed upon goals, and (c) implement and evaluate the effects of prevention interventions designed to assist clients to retain, attain, or maintain optimal client system stability. To date, the NSM has been used for nursing practice targeted to individuals, family, and community as the overall client system.

Client Systems

Specific client systems include children with acute clinical conditions requiring hospitalization and children with chronic conditions such as cancer, mental and physical impairments, psychiatric disorders, and hyperkinesis. Other client systems include (a) well adults and adults at risk for injury or illness who are in need of primary prevention interventions; (b) adults with acute clinical conditions such as cancer, multisystem failure, trauma, spinal cord injuries, cardiac disease, cerebral vascular accidents, and orthopedic problems; and (c) adults, including the elderly, with chronic clinical conditions such as substance abuse, cognitive impairment, diabetes, HIV disease, cancer, kidney disease, chronic obstructive pulmonary disease, multiple sclerosis, hypertension, and psychiatric illnesses.

Following from Neuman's (1983) explanation of how the Neuman Systems are used when the family is the client system, reports of nursing practice have focused on childbearing families and families with an acutely ill or chronically ill member. Nursing practice with communities as the client system also has been reported, as has nursing practice with the nurse as the client system.

Consultation Results

Consultation provided by NSM experts has led to adoption of the NSM to guide nursing practice in clinical agencies in such international locations as the Whitby Psychiatric Hospital in Whitby, Ontario, Canada; the Elizabeth Bruyere Health Center in Ottawa, Ontario, Canada; St. Joseph's Hospital Nursing Service in Reykjavik, Iceland; Rykov Hospital Nursing Service in Jonkoping, Sweden; the World Health Organization Collaborating Center for Primary Health Care in Maribor, Yugoslavia; and the Emergis Psychiatric Hospital in Zeeland, Holland. An especially innovative use of the NSM in international nursing practice is the "Hospital at Home" program being implemented in Bosnia, Slovenia, Austria, and Italy. A Dutch language book about use of the NSM with individuals, families, and populations has greatly facilitated adoption of the NSM in Holland, especially by social psychiatric nurses, who have a leadership role in interdisciplinary mental health centers throughout the country.

Health Promotion and Outcomes

Furthermore, with its emphasis on health promotion activities inherent in primary prevention interventions, the NSM is well suited as a framework for community health nursing practice. Canada is a recognized leader in use of the NSM in community health settings. For example, the NSM became the basis of community health standards for nursing in the province of Ontario in the early 1980s; other provinces followed by using the NSM in their community health district nursing units.

Implementation of NSM-based practice in many different countries has demonstrated cost-effective and high-quality client health care (Neuman, 1996). Moreover, clinicians describing use of the NSM in nursing practice generally have indicated their own satisfaction with resultant nursing practice in terms of comprehensiveness. Beynon (1995) reported that annual surveys of the staff of the Middlesex–London Health Unit Public Health Nursing Division in Ontario, Canada, revealed increasing acceptance and use of the model "when assessing individuals, families, and groups; when formulating nursing diagnoses, expected outcomes, and nursing interventions; in recording; and in case consultations with supervisors" (Beynon, 1995, p. 539).

■ The Neuman Systems Model and Interdisciplinary Teams

The holistic, comprehensive, and flexible nature of the NSM readily accommodates formation of interdisciplinary teams and interdisciplinary collaboration. Interdisciplinary teams maximize educational interchange while engaging in interdependent planning to provide patient services. Their primary concern is the quality and effectiveness of the outcome of the teamwork, not recognition of individual contributions (Stuart & Sundeen, 1991).

Interdisciplinary Health Care

Interdisciplinary teams are not new to health care organizations. Long-standing legal requirements, as in the case of special education, or clinical complexity, as in hospice care

and rehabilitation, mandate interdisciplinary teams. Although adherence to regulations is evident, varying degrees of "buy-in" are demonstrated by staff members and administrators when interdisciplinary teams are formed. Variations in interdisciplinary team "buy-in" are related to team members' and administrators' educational experiences and clinical experiences. Students frequently are informed about the idea of interdisciplinary teams and even may have clinical experiences with such teams. Too often, however, those experiences are what Bailey (1996) called a compartmentalized curriculum. There, the principles of interdisciplinary practice are evident in just one course or one module within a course, rather than a part of every course. Given the difficulties of arranging interdisciplinary educational experiences and the typical lack of institutional support, educators have little motivation to develop interdisciplinary-infused curricula (Bailey, 1996). In clinical settings, the dominant experience is discipline-specific practice. Administrators may assert expectations for interdisciplinary team practice but typically devote little thought or time to facilitating the development and ongoing operation of such teams.

Yet interdisciplinary teams offer opportunities for cooperative approaches that optimize the expertise of all team members. And, both health care professionals and clients speak positively of the interdisciplinary approaches' potential.

NSM for Interdisciplinary Settings

The NSM can be utilized as the "glue" to promote consistent interdisciplinary experiences in both educational and practice settings. If students enter the workforce with a solid background in use of the NSM as a guide for interdisciplinary practice, they will be less likely to see nursing as the only answer and will be more accustomed to listening to ideas and understanding the nomenclature of professionals in other fields.

The success of interdisciplinary teams has been documented at Grand Valley State University in Michigan where efforts have focused on a NSM-based infusion approach in physical therapy and occupational therapy. Future initiatives will focus on inclusion of physician assistant students in interdisciplinary teams and an NSM-based graduate program in gerontology that will encompass eight disciplines.

Additionally, clinical faculty at Brigham Young University discovered that use of the NSM overcomes barriers to development of interdisciplinary teams in the clinical setting. Potential problems are diminished by negating or facilitating resolution of issues related to the legal responsibilities of particular professions, leadership of the team, and primary responsibility for a particular client system. Using the NSM as the unifying framework for an interdisciplinary team facilitated the transformation of a collection of discipline-specific professional experts into a cohesive team by providing a common language for the team, a distinctive focus for the knowledge of each discipline, and a holistic perspective of the client system that brings to the forefront the importance of the collective expertise of team members.

■ Concluding Statement

The NSM is an exceptionally useful guide for nursing education, administration, and practice in many settings in several countries. The NSM is readily translatable to diverse cultures and therefore has the potential to facilitate important global sharing and resolution of universal nursing concerns.

The NSM fits well with the holistic concept of optimizing a dynamic yet stable interrelationship of spirit, mind, and body of the client system in a constantly changing environment and society. It joins the World Health Organization mandate for the year 2010, seeking unity in wellness states—wellness of spirit, mind, body, and environment. The NSM also is in accord with American Nursing Association initiatives, sharing concern about potential stressors and emphasis on primary prevention as well as world health care reform concern for preventing illness. Moreover, the NSM supports the Sigma Theta Tau Arista II proposals for preferred 21st century nursing activities in that the NSM provides a clear directive for cooperative programming, delineation of the nursing goals, and guidelines for delivery of nursing and other health services.

Use of the NSM markers helps all nurses to see the "big picture" of a client system and to identify empirically adequate strategies to retain, attain, and maintain optimal client system stability. Thus use of the markers closes any gaps between nursing research, education, administration, and practice. In closing that gap, nurses who act as scholarly leaders are able to direct their efforts toward (a) managing new and different roles for themselves and client systems, (b) establishing health team partnerships, (c) empowering other nurses and health team members, (d) coordinating health services, and (e) shaping health policies.

Evolution of the NSM in the 21st century was ensured through establishment of the NSM Trustees Group in 1988. Trustees and associate members from the United States and several other countries comprise an organization committed to supporting and promoting the NSM through scholarly work and professional forums, including biennial international symposia. Furthermore, the establishment of the NSM Archives at Neumann College in Aston, Pennsylvania, has facilitated access to important documents and thus should enhance NSM-based scholarly work for many years to come.

■ *References*

Bailey, D. B. (1996). Preparing early intervention professionals for the 21st century. In M. Bambring, H. Raub, & A. Beelman (Eds.), *Early childhood intervention: Theory, evaluation, and practice* (pp. 497–499). New York: de Gruyter.

Beynon, C. E. (1995). Neuman-based experiences of the Middlesex–London health unit. In B. Neuman, *The Neuman systems model* (3rd ed., pp. 537–547). Norwalk, CT: Appleton and Lange.

Block, P. (1993). *Stewardship: Choosing service over self-interest.* San Francisco: Berrett-Koehler.

Burke, M. E., Capers, C. F., O'Connell, R. K., Quinn, R. M., & Sinnott, M. (1989). Neuman-based nursing practice in a hospital setting. In B. Neuman, *The Neuman systems model* (2nd ed., pp. 423–443). Norwalk, CT: Appleton and Lange.

Garvin, D. A. (1993). Building a learning organization. *Harvard Business Review, 71*(4), 78–91.

Hinton-Walker, P. (1995). TQM and the Neuman Systems Model: Education for health care administration. In B. Neuman, *The Neuman systems model* (3rd ed., pp. 365–376). Norwalk, CT: Appleton and Lange.

Kelley, J. A., & Sanders, N. F. (1995). A systems approach to the health of nursing and health care organizations. In B. Neuman, *The Neuman systems model* (3rd ed., pp. 347–364). Norwalk, CT: Appleton and Lange.

Kelley, J. A., Sanders, N. F., & Pierce, J. D. (1989). A systems approach to the role of the nurse administrator in education and practice. In B. Neuman, *The Neuman systems model* (2nd ed., pp. 115–337). Norwalk, CT: Appleton and Lange.

Neuman B. (1983). Family intervention using the Betty Neuman health care systems model. In I. W. Clements & F. B. Roberts, *Family health: A theoretical approach to nursing care* (pp. 239–254). New York: John Wiley & Sons.

Neuman, B. (1995). *The Neuman systems model* (3rd ed.). Norwalk, CT: Appleton and Lange.

Neuman, B. (1996). The Neuman systems model in research and practice. *Nursing Science Quarterly, 9,* 67–70.

Neuman, B. (1997, November). *Leadership-scholarship integration: Using the Neuman systems model for 21st century professional nursing practice.* Keynote address presented at the University of Amman Third International Nursing Year 2000 Conference, Amman, Jordan.

Neuman, B., & Young, R. J. (1972). A model for teaching total person approach to patient problems. *Nursing Research, 21,* 264–269.

Senge, P. M. (1990). *The fifth discipline: The art and practice of the learning organization.* New York: Doubleday.

Stuart, G., & Sundeen, S. (1991). *Principles and practice of psychiatric nursing* (4th ed.). St Louis: Mosby.

■ *Editor's Questions for Discussion*

Apply concepts of the NSM to resolving a specific nursing practice problem, providing content for nursing curricula, addressing a nursing research question, or resolving an issue in nursing administration. How does the NSM provide steps for integration of leadership and scholarship? Specify strategies for evaluating NSM. How does NSM guide research? To what extent does integrative review of NSM-based studies presented by Neuman incorporate guides for reviews suggested by Androwich and Haas (Chapter 32)?

On what basis was NSM's scientific merit judged? How is NSM evaluated as a curriculum guide? Specifically apply NSM concepts to curriculum development. How might NSM be a prototype for education in other disciplines?

How is application of NSM in administration different from other current management and organization theories used by administrators? What types of administrative problems may be particularly amenable for resolution using NSM? How may NSM effectiveness specifically be evaluated?

To what extent is the NSM a normative framework for conceptualizing nursing practice rather than a scientific theory as discussed by Donnelly (Chapter 28)? How specifically does NSM accommodate formation of interdisciplinary teams? How can NSM be a unifying framework for various disciplines?

28

An Assessment of Nursing Theories as Guides to Scientific Inquiry

Eleanor Donnelly, PhD, RN

We have cast a spell upon ourselves and only we can break it. We are held in thrall by the idea that our nursing theories are the most discipline-relevant means by which we can generate a body of scientific knowledge for nursing. This is not to say that all of us are equally bound by this spell. Some of us actually manage to function productively in our professional lives as if neither the spell nor the nursing theories exist. Nevertheless, ample evidence for persistence of the spell abounds, along with indications of the continuing vitality of the nursing theories as foci for scholarly treatment. When I speak of the nursing theories, I am adopting common usage to refer to frameworks for conceptualizing the practice of nursing created by Leininger (1978),

Orem (1971), Peplau (1952), and Roy (1976), among others, and to Rogers' (1970) paradigm for a science of nursing. I think it is a fairly safe bet that there is not a graduate nursing program in the country that does not devote part of its curriculum to the study of these theories.[1]

■ Indicators of Unremitting Vitality

We have only to peruse *Books in Print 1998–99* (1998) to see that there is a thriving literature in nursing theory. Two sources in particular stand out as they have become the chief repositories of our knowledge about the theories. One is Marriner-Tomey and Alligood's (1998) *Nursing Theorists and Their Work,* now in its fourth edition. It is a collection of individually authored papers, the majority of which have as their focus one of the nursing theories. In addition to an in-depth description of a given theory, each theory paper provides biographical material on the theorist and an extensive bibliography of all recoverable primary and secondary sources on the theory.

The second notable repository is Meleis' (1997) *Theoretical Nursing: Development & Progress,* now in its third edition. Meleis not only explicates and analyzes all the usual nursing theories, but she also provides a history of theory development along with critiques and analyses of all the major theoretical writings in nursing. If someone is looking for sources on nursing theories and on theoretical writings in general in nursing, Meleis' book is the ultimate catalog. With these two volumes in hand, those curious about nursing theory are probably in possession of all the extant references to and about nursing theory that were of any scholarly significance as of the dates of the books' publication. The problem of lack of systematic retrieval strategies to locate materials on the nursing theories, pointed out by Silva (1986), has thus been partially resolved. Marriner-Tomey and Alligood (1998) and Meleis (1997) have done most of our homework for us.

As befits a contemporary vital force, nursing theories also have a presence on the Internet. Using the key words *nursing theory,* a search engine such as *Infoseek* will call up literally thousands of hits—not all of which, of course, pertain directly to our subject matter here. As in our print media, so in our electronic sources, a pair of sites stand out as repositories. The first is called *The Nursing Theory Link Page* (Eichelberger, March 1999). It is maintained by Lisa Wright Eichelberger, in the Department of Nursing at Clayton College and State University, who states that she is "trying to create a complete collection of Internet

resources of the various nursing theorists and their theories." The second site is called *The Nursing Theory Page* (Norris, 1999). It is maintained by Judy Norris at the University of Alberta, who states

> The Nursing Theory Page is a collaborative effort of an international group. We are interested in developing a collection of resources about nursing theories throughout the world. The project began on 21 May 1996 and will always be a work in progress (March 1999).

Both sites provide links to sites featuring nursing theorists and their theories and, as might be expected, there is considerable overlap in the links they identify. Both had been recently updated on the day I last accessed them, in March 1999.

■ *Origins*

Modern writings by nurses about how to conceptualize nursing began appearing in the 1950s. By the end of the 1960s, the nursing community had begun to identify as theories the work of, among others, Henderson (1966), Levine (1969), Orlando (1961), Peplau (1952), Travelbee (1966), and Wiedenbach (1964). Not that the so-called theorists themselves necessarily identified their work as theories. As Marriner-Tomey (1998) points out in her preface to *Nursing Theorists and Their Work,* "Many . . . do not consider themselves theorists and never intended to develop theory" (p. xiii). Identification of these works as theories took place in the context of collegiate-level nurse educators' heightening sensitivity to the discrepancy between the status they desired as peers among peers in academia and their actual status.

With the growing movement of basic nursing education into colleges and universities after World War II, nurse educators found themselves both needing to possess the kind of credentials their colleagues in other departments had and wanting to be able to point to a body of knowledge that was nursing's very own. Attainment of a critical mass of doctorally prepared faculty has come about gradually (Bullough & Bullough, 1984). Assembling of a body of knowledge seems to have happened in just slightly more time than the twinkling of an eye.

Meleis (1997) pointed to two events in particular that fueled identification of nursing theories as constituting nursing's body of knowledge. The first was the American Nurses Association's (ANA) (1965) position paper, *Educational Preparation for Nurse Practitioners and Assistants to Nurses,* in which theory development was distinguished as a priority professional goal. The second was a symposium, sponsored by Case Western Reserve University, "Symposium on Theory Development in Nursing," which was held in October 1967; the papers presented appeared a year later in *Nursing Research* (1968).

These publications supported what were previously considered simply perceptions and conceptions of theoretical nursing from an isolated number of theorists. Not only did a group of significant people in nursing get together to discuss theory in nursing, but the official scientific journal of the field also recognized the significance of these proceedings by publishing them (Meleis, 1997, pp. 38, 41).

At the Detroit symposium, two Yale philosophers, Dickoff and James (1968), presented what subsequently became one of the most highly influential papers in the nursing literature, "A theory of theories: A position paper". That paper and a subsequent one (Dickoff, James, & Wiedenbach, 1968), coauthored with Wiedenbach, a nurse theorist, were widely read and well received. The appeal of the ideas apparently lay with the authors' validation of the nursing community's theo-

retical aspirations—that theories were significant for practice, that practice was susceptible to theoretical development, and that nurses were capable of developing theories (Meleis, 1997).

■ Affect Laden Aspirations

It would seem that, almost from the start, nursing theory and its development were not principally reason-driven pursuits, but significantly affect laden ones, enmeshed as they were with concerns about status and legitimacy. Indeed, in the first edition of what became a nursing theory standard, *Theory and Nursing: A Systematic Approach,* Chinn and Jacobs (1983) made the argument that "professional autonomy and power will come from development of theoretical knowledge in nursing" (p. 6), an argument they have repeated in subsequent editions. For many nurses, the profession's most cherished hopes and dreams came to be associated with the fortunes of its nursing theories.

During the same period when we began to identify the nursing theories as theories, we took to referring to nursing as a science. And we established the practice of referring to knowledge relevant to nursing as nursing science. The theories were considered part of that knowledge. For many in the nursing community, the association between nursing science and nursing theories appeared obvious and fitting. From there it was but a short conceptual leap to think of the theories as scientific (i.e., to regard the nursing theories as scientific theories). That nursing theories have been thus regarded by main stream nurse scholars, or at least as precursors to scientific theories, seems to me indisputable on the basis of the extant literature. Open any text on the topic and the reader will find references to the philosophy of science and narrative sprinkled with the language of scientific inquiry—terms such as testing, assumptions, propositions, empirical indicators, and hypotheses (see, e.g., Fawcett, 1995; Marriner-Tomey, 1998; Meleis, 1997).

■ Parallel Discourses and the Making of a Muddle

The most significant initial contributions to nursing's literature on theory construction and testing from the perspective of philosophy of science (Hardy, 1974; Jacox, 1974) followed, rather than preceded, all the hullabaloo in the 1960s about nursing theories. It is one of the curiosities of nursing history that there apparently was little overlap in membership between nurse scholars invested in nursing theories and those invested in metatheoretical considerations (Silva & Rothbart, 1984). That seems to continue to be the case. Dialogs have proceeded separately, sometimes side-by-side, but have rarely merged. In *Nursing Theorists and Their Work* (Marriner-Tomey & Alligood, 1998), for example, the whole first section of the volume is devoted to a series of papers on metatheoretical matters based principally on literature in the philosophy of science. In none of the papers, however, are these understandings from the philosophy of science applied in an analysis of nursing theories as scientific theory candidates. One of the contributors, Bishop (1998), did concede that "the use of rigorous criteria for a scientific theory to critique nursing formulations will surely result in nursing theories being found deficient" (p. 51). She did not, however, offer a demonstration, but simply attributed this deficiency to construction of nursing theory being in its early stages.

In a paper titled, "Debunking myths in nursing theory and research," Chinn (1985) pointed out that scientific knowledge was not the only kind of knowledge of value to nursing and sought to debunk what she referred to as the "myths" about it. But, whereas the paper's title referred to nursing theory, Chinn's treatment of her topic omitted any consideration of nursing theories from the standpoint of their scientific significance. More recently, Schumacker and Gortner (1992) carefully analyzed and offered some sound correctives to what they had discerned to be misconceptions about science in the nursing literature. But neither did their paper take up the scientific status of the nursing theories. I view these additional examples of the separation of our metatheoretical dialog from our nursing theories dialog as also pointing to a slowly growing but nagging collective sense that, conceptually speaking, we are a bit muddled when it comes to matters scientific and theoretical.

Adam (1985) seemed to have experienced the muddle as being terminological in origin, as have apparently a good number of other nurse scholars. Nursing theory texts typically devote large portions to definitions and discussions of terminology (e.g., Barnum, 1998; Fawcett, 1995; Meleis, 1997). All this effort at clarification is for naught, however, when the *context of usage* is *neglected*. By neglecting to specify the context of usage, these authors never quite make clear what sort of enterprise is implied in their discussions. Are we talking about research, practice, education, or some combination thereof? If we are talking about research, is this research in the broad sense as scholarship or are we talking about empirical research and, if so, what kind of empirical research—scientific, evaluation, or historical?

Context of usage undeniably makes a difference in how we understand the significance of the concepts referenced. Though concepts such as theory, assumption, proposition, and hypothesis are not exclusive to scientific discourse, we can be forgiven for our tendency to associate them with that discourse. Whether purposeful or inadvertent on the part of authors, such decontextualized treatments of concepts such as theory, framework, and model have contributed to and have helped sustain the conceptual muddle in which we find ourselves. Coupled with absence of any critical examination of nursing theories as actual or possible scientific theories, a reader readily interprets the texts as being about the scientific enterprise and scientific theory. A close examination of those texts will reveal, however, that no such claim is ever directly made.

■ Testing

In a much-cited paper, Silva (1986) reported an analysis of 62 reports in the nursing empirical research literature in which investigators claimed to have used one of the nursing theories for their research. She assessed all the reports she could find that were based on five of the nursing theories: Johnson's (1980), Newman's (1979), Orem's (1971, 1980, 1985), Rogers' (1970, 1980, 1983), and Roy's (1970, 1976, 1984). Silva was interested in ascertaining to what extent nursing theories had undergone any testing. She stated that investigators used the theories in three ways.

The first was to identify a nursing theory or framework for research and then to do little more with it beyond describing it. This was the case in 24 of the 62 reports. The second way was to use a nursing theory in a descriptive rather than hypothesis-generating study, with the investigator making the implicit assumption that the theory's tenets were valid. Twenty-nine of the 62 reports fell into this category. Only 9 reports, examined according to Silva's evaluation criteria, were found to be examples of actual theory testing.

Although the criteria Silva enumerated would seem appropriate to analysis of reports of research carried out on scientific theories,

the question of nursing theories being scientific did not arise in her exposition. Instead, in the three detailed examples of theory testing that she supplied, it was the form of the studies' designs and the logic informing the relations between the design elements that were considered. A key criterion was the derivation of hypotheses from the theories' propositions. At the end of the section describing the examples, Silva (1986) concluded by stating:

> In summary, three research studies in which investigators have tested hypotheses derived from select propositions within Rogers', Orem's, and Newman's models have been presented. These studies were selected because they represent investigators' efforts to test nursing theory explicitly. (p. 8)

The scientifically naive reader could be forgiven, if at that point, she or he failed to recognize that hypotheses of various sorts can be derived or deduced from almost any kind of coherent set of ideas. Within the midst of this conceptual clutter, it is hard to remember that not all coherent sets of ideas are scientific theories or even possible descriptions of actual states of affairs, or to keep in mind that not all hypotheses or deductions pertain to matters potentially generalizable. In a subsequent paper on the testing of nursing theory, Silva and Sorrell (1992) criticized Silva's previous approach as " . . . primarily deductive and empirical, thus reflecting the philosophical position of logical positivism and the correspondence theory of truth . . . " (p. 14). Apparently, given this association of a perspective within a philosophy of science with Silva's notion of theory testing, Silva herself regarded the evaluation criteria for theory testing that she had used in the 1986 paper as applicable to scientific theory.

But matters became even more confused. Silva and Sorrell (1992) did something that Silva on her own did not do in her 1986 paper.

Together they provided a definition of nursing theory along with an expansion of the ways in which such a creation might be tested.

> We define nursing theory as a tentative body of diverse but purposeful, creative, and logically interrelated perspectives that help nurses to redefine nursing and to understand, explain, raise questions about, and seek clarification of nursing phenomena in their research and practice. (p. 14)

Note that nursing theory is not defined in scientific terms but in a way so broad as to encompass all the purposes to which the nursing theories have been put in research and practice. Compounding the confusion is the proposal that the notion of theory testing also embraces (a) verification through critical reasoning, (b) verification through description of personal experiences, and (c) verification through application to nursing practice. Testing thus becomes whatever anyone would like it to be.

■ Seeing the Theories for What They Actually Are

Earlier, I stated that separate dialogs about metatheory and nursing theories have rarely merged. Two especially important instances where they did merge were in the writings of Jan Beckstrand (1978a, 1978b, 1980, 1984) and Frederick Suppe (1996, 1997; Suppe & Jacox, 1984). Beckstrand was the first nurse scholar to examine nursing theories critically from the standpoint of the philosophy of science. When nursing theories became associated with the idea of practice theories, she took on the notion of practice theory, as characterized both by Dickoff, James, and Wiedenbach (1968) and by Jacox (1974). In a series of papers on the topic (1978a, 1978b, 1980, 1984), Beckstrand basically argued that a special category of theory designated as practice

theory was not needed because notions of a practice theory in nursing represented some combination of science, ethics, and logic. In other words, calling some combination of them a practice theory did not designate some unique form of knowledge. To do so simply obscured that fact.

In tandem with questioning the necessity for practice theory, Beckstrand challenged the idea that the nursing theories were scientific, contrasting their attributes with those of scientific theories. She described nursing theories as normative and pointed out that they were "legitimately alterable on the sole basis of personal or public discretion" (Beckstrand, 1980, p. 75). She also demonstrated that neither knowledge of the properties of nursing nor how nursing is constituted—the province of the nursing theories—would help nursing develop the kind of knowledge needed about patients' problems and how to deal with them (Beckstrand, 1980).

When I first came across Beckstrand's analysis, I was convinced that there would soon be a nursing theories funeral, and that she would be the chief pallbearer. It would be a quiet, dignified affair, marked by an initial flurry of papers of enlightenment followed by a gradual but steady disappearance of the subject matter in the nursing literature. Obviously that did not happen. Although the canons of scholarship dictated acknowledgment of some sort of four carefully argued papers in a peer-reviewed journal, much of the nursing community seemed not to have understood Beckstrand's work and its implications for the nursing theories. In part, this lack of understanding was probably due to there being few among us at that time with the requisite sophistication in the philosophy of science to appreciate both the points Beckstrand made and how she made them. Nevertheless, Beckstrand was and is regularly cited as contributing to the nursing theories dialog. Her papers also have been included in nursing theory anthologies. The nursing theories business itself went on as usual.

A short time later, I came to harbor similar funerary hopes with respect to Suppe's contributions to the literature. In a seminal paper jointly authored with Jacox (Suppe & Jacox, 1984), the relationship between the philosophy of science and the development of nursing theories was described and analyzed. Nursing theories were explicitly identified as teleological, and justification for this conclusion was provided. The authors clearly stated that, as teleological theories, evaluation of them should be conducted on the basis of "normative, not scientific, considerations" (p. 259). But once again the implications of this paper for the fortune of the nursing theories, were its claims to be judged valid, did not seem to have been fully appreciated by the nursing community. Like Beckstrand's papers, this one too is regularly cited.

In a more recent treatment of the nursing theories, Suppe made a presentation, at Indiana University School of Nursing's Annual Doctoral Forum entitled, "Nursing science as a mature discipline: Is there a place for nursing theory and philosophy of science?" (Suppe, 1996). He did not specifically advise interment, but he did relegate nursing theories to our history books. Comparing the early situation of sociology with that of nursing, Suppe argued that nursing theories had played a legitimating role for us in academia, much as grand theories in sociology had for sociology. In his opinion, nursing was now clearly established as a credible discipline, and we no longer needed nursing theories. Whatever usefulness they possessed was now spent. Nursing theories were not suitable guides for the conduct of inquiry, but they were part of our history, and as such, we might want to include content about them when addressing the historical development of scholarship in nursing curricula.

In a sizable audience comprised largely of nursing faculty and doctoral students, no one challenged Suppe's thesis. Indeed, the remarks and questions directed to him clearly suggested that he was preaching to the choir. I spoke to a number of my colleagues about Suppe's presentation, and I came away with the impression that his ideas had been very well received. I thought that, perhaps soon in our graduate curriculum committee, we would be addressing the issues he had raised. Thus far we have not. I would like to think it is because I regularly teach our introductory nursing theories course and that is sufficiently reassuring to my colleagues that our conceptual house is in order. But I really do not know.

Beckstrand's and Suppe's challenges to the significance of the nursing theories are notable because of their being launched from a philosophy of science perspective, but they are not the only scholars who have taken exception to the status that the community has accorded these theories. From across the Atlantic, in Sweden, came a particularly prescient paper by Lundh, Soder, and Waerness (1988) that critically questioned the use of nursing theories as a basis for research, principally on grounds of their being both normative and highly abstract in character. The authors argued that these theories, rather than facilitating research, actually made research development in nursing "more difficult" (p. 40). They described and illustrated the theories as "airy and consensus oriented."

Back in the United States, Florence Downs (1987), then editor of *Nursing Research* and Professor, Associate Dean, and Director of Graduate Studies at the University of Pennsylvania, minced no words with her assembled colleagues at the 1987 National Forum in Doctoral Education. In an invited paper, Downs declared that the nursing theories were "empty of content" (p. 66). She warned that insistence on use of these theories to inform research was "to deaden the critical abilities of students" (p. 65). More ominously, she counseled that affectation of a scientific posture was no substitute for the genuine article.

Kuhn (1970), in the book that revolutionized the philosophy of science, asserted that mature sciences were informed by what he called paradigms, or "universally recognized scientific achievements that for a time provide model problems and solutions to a community of practitioners" (p. viii). Deets (1990) pointed out that the nursing community had simply declared that its paradigm consisted of four major concepts: nursing, patient, health, and environment.

The famous four concepts first entered nursing's discourse via a paper by Yura and Torres (1975): "Today's conceptual frameworks with the baccalaureate nursing programs." Yura and Torres referred to nursing's focal concepts as person, society, health, and nursing. A number of writers picked up on this idea and promoted identification of a set of concepts that would serve as nursing's paradigm (Bush, 1979; Fawcett, 1978, 1983, 1984; Flaskerud & Halloran, 1980; Newman, 1983). Within a short space of time—less than 10 years—it became commonplace in the literature for authors to refer to nursing's paradigm and to identify person, nursing, health, and environment as the paradigm's four major concepts (Meleis, 1997). Many of the surviving nurse theorists amended their work to include reference to the four concepts, if they had not previously been addressed. Sometimes this was done for them (cf. Chinn & Jacobs, 1983; Kim, 1983).

Deets (1990) viewed nursing's declaration of a paradigm as an attempt at legitimization that ignored how a scientific paradigm actually came into being (i.e., that it emerged on the basis of activity of a scientific community and only became identifiable after the fact). Deets charged that "in its rush to mature, nursing has attempted to short circuit the process of developing a tradition, through the massing of research information by deciding on the paradigm's concepts and then conducting the research" (p. 150). In a review of 300 nursing research articles from 1986 through early 1988, Deets found only 6 that addressed concepts in their paradigmatic form. She concluded that there was little support for the viability of the concepts themselves, let alone as elements of a paradigm. More significantly, she disputed the very relevance of the famous four cornerstone concepts for development of nursing scholarship.

■ What Does a Real Scientific Theory Look Like?

So what does the genuine article look like? How would someone know that she or he was in the presence of a scientific theory? How would someone recognize a scientific investigation and differentiate it from other forms of inquiry? Although there is no single "official" set of definitions of scientific theory and inquiry to which all involved accede, there is some consensus among philosophers of science on certain key ideas (Gale, 1979). The first and most significant is that scientific inquiry entails posing a question about some set of phenomena in the realm of actual empirically observable events, whether natural or social. Though specific phenomena are what is observed, these are always regarded as representing larger classes of things. The goal is both to describe and to explain these specific events or objects as instances of more inclusive categories. The objective is knowledge that is neither time nor place bound. Indeed, development of a scientific theory is the outcome of a quest both to describe what has been observed and then to figure out what sort of principle must be operating behind those appearances. An example would be Darwin's theory of evolution. To oversimplify, Darwin's observations entailed descriptions of the morphological characteristics of living things in relation to their environments. He inferred the principle of natural selection to account for (i.e., explain) the variation and similarities he had observed (Darwin, 1859).

If we examine the historical record in science, stories of investigations and discoveries, we come to understand that the conduct of scientific inquiry is always driven by some question about the empirical world that scientists are doing their best to answer. Often the original impetus is practical in nature, as in the case of Pasteur, who was asked by the vintners of France to figure out some way of preventing the spoilage of wine and beer. Pasteur came to understand, in contrast to his contemporaries, that fermentation was not a chemical reaction but a consequence of the activity of living things, yeast. He supported this discovery with data collected and analyzed during the experiments he had conducted. He shared his ideas in papers and presentations and thus subjected his ideas to the scrutiny of his peers (Gale, 1979). The historical record makes clear that scientific inquiry and theory development take place within the context of a scientific community. Individual scientists' work is informed by that of their contemporaries and their predecessors. Indeed, part of the process of legitimizing a scientist's current efforts is to cite those of fellow investigators.

■ Breaking the Spell and Undoing the Muddle

Now back to the nursing theories. One clear give-away that the nursing theories reader is not in the presence of scientific theories is lack of reference to any systematic investigations having been carried out with respect to some question about how the world works. There is no material about how a given author arrived at her theory as a consequence of having pursued some burning empirical question. In addition, no references whatsoever are made to the investigative work of any contemporaries or predecessors informing or leading up to the theorist's ideas.

What are these things then that we call the nursing theories? With the exception of Rogers' theory, to which I shall shortly return, the nursing theories are all proposals about how the practice of nursing might best be conceptualized. They are descriptions of desirable ways for nurses to conceptualize practice—this is another key give-away. Scientific theories are about actual states of affairs in the world, not desirable ones. That is, the province of ethical inquiry. Suppose, however, that we treated the nursing theories as if they were possible descriptions about actual states of affairs. Would they then qualify as scientific theories? No. None of them include, as authentic scientific theories do, ideas that might serve as explanatory principles to account for what has been described (Hospers, 1980).

What is both curious and worthy of note about the nursing theories is that, with the exception of Rogers' (1970), they are all similarly structured. Practice is represented as actualized within the context of a relationship between nurse and patient. That relationship is dominated by a phenomenon that characterizes the patient as an object of nursing intervention and is, in turn, the focus of the nurse's interventions. The goal of nursing practice is to make a positive impact with respect to the phenomenon. In Roy's (1976) theory, for example, the phenomenon is adaptation. The patient is conceptualized from the standpoint of adaptation and the nurse should intervene so as to maximize the patient's positive adaptation. In Orem's (1971) theory, the phenomenon is self-care; in Leininger's (1978), culturally congruent care; in Nightingale's (1992), the reparative process; in Paterson and Zderad's (1976), becoming more; and so on.

Rogers' (1970) theory, in contrast to the others, is not about how nurses might best conceptualize their practice. It is, rather, a proposal to develop a body of knowledge that would be unique to nursing. To develop that unique body of knowledge, Rogers proposed that human beings be conceptualized as energy fields in interaction with the environment, which was also conceptualized as an energy field. She was suggesting that nurses carry out research on this relationship and that knowledge thereby gleaned would be knowledge of a uniquely nursing sort. With the stroke of a pen, Rogers brought into existence what she regarded as a science for nursing—the science of unitary human beings.

■ Concluding Statement

There is no doubt that the nursing theories inspired considerable scholarly activity, including the conduct of empirical investigations. They kept us busy and served as a significant focus for honing our collective intellectual acumen. But even though they kept us busy, they also distracted us from the examination and exploration of more fertile ideas to guide our research. One would expect that no would-be nurse scientist in her right mind would choose, as a theoretical framework to guide her investigations, a wholly untried set of ideas with no discernible connections to any previous work. And yet any number of us did that very thing.

It is past time to stop doing that. The nursing theories certainly deserve a place in our history, but not as scientific theories or even as embryonic ones. As so astutely described by Suppe (1996), they have been the innocent tools of a collective legitimizing process. It behooves us to recognize them as such and to abandon our misguided aspirations for them. It might also prove salutary to examine them for the brainchildren they are—normative frameworks for conceptualizing practice, or in the case of Rogers, a chimerical science of energy fields.

■ Note

1. I have, in general, limited myself to citing publications in which the nursing theories first appeared. I did so in the interest of space and efficiency of presentation, not from oversight. It is, of course, true that many of the nursing theories have been modified somewhat over time in terms of their content. However, I regard their basic structure as having been preserved, these modifications not withstanding. Readers who wish to pursue development of the nurse theorists' thoughts are encouraged to visit the extensive bibliographies in Marriner-Tomey and Alligood (1998) and in Meleis (1997).

■ References

Adam, E. (1985). Toward more clarity in terminology: Frameworks, theories, and models. *Journal of Nursing Education, 24*(4), 151–155.

American Nurses Association. (1965). *Educational preparation for nurse practitioners and assistants to nurses: A position paper.* New York: Author.

Barnum, B. S. (1998). *Nursing theory: Analysis, application, evaluation* (5th ed.). Philadelphia: Lippincott.

Beckstrand, J. (1978a). The need for a practice theory as indicated by the knowledge used in the conduct of practice. *Research in Nursing and Health, 1*(4), 175–179.

Beckstrand, J. (1978b). The notion of a practice theory and the relationship of scientific and ethical knowledge to practice. *Research in Nursing and Health, 1*(3), 131–136.

Beckstrand, J. (1980). A critique of several conceptions of practice theory in nursing. *Research in Nursing and Health, 3,* 69–79.

Beckstrand, J. (1984). A reply to Collins and Fielder: The concept of theory. *Research in Nursing and Health, 7,* 189–196.

Bishop, S. M. (1998). Theory development process. In A. Marriner-Tomey & M. R. Alligood (Eds.), *Nursing theorists and their work* (4th ed., pp. 43–54). St. Louis: Mosby.

Books in Print 1998–99. (1998). Volume 5: Subject guide N-R. New Providence, NJ: R. R. Bowker.

Bullough, V. L., & Bullough, B. (1984). *History, trends, and politics of nursing.* Norwalk, CT: Appleton-Century-Crofts.

Bush, H. A. (1979). Models for nursing. *Advances in Nursing Science, 1,* 13–21.

Chinn, P. L. (1985). Debunking myths in nursing theory and research. *IMAGE: Journal of Nursing Scholarship, 17*(2), 45–49.

Chinn, P. L., & Jacobs, M. K. (1983). *Theory and nursing: A systematic approach.* St. Louis: Mosby.

Darwin, C. (1859). *The origin of species.* (1999, March) [On-line]. Available: http://www.literature.org/authors/darwin-charles/the-origin-of-the-species/.

Deets, C. A. (1990). Nursing's paradigm and a search for its methodology. In N. L. Chaska (Ed.), *The nursing profession: Turning points* (pp. 149–154). St. Louis: Mosby.

Dickoff, J., & James, P. (1968). A theory of theories: A position paper. *Nursing Research, 17*(3), 197–203.

Dickoff, J., James, P., & Wiedenbach, E. (1968). Theory in a practice discipline, Part 1: Practice oriented theory. *Nursing Research, 17*(5), 415–435.

Downs, F. (1987). Toward the future. *Proceedings of the 1987 National Forum on Doctoral Education in Nursing* (pp. 62–66), June 25–26, 1987. Pittsburgh: University of Pennsylvania.

Eichelberger, L. W. (1999, March). *The nursing theory link page* [On-line]. Available: http://www.clayton.edu/eichelberger/nursing.htm.

Fawcett, J. (1978). The "what" of theory development. In Jacqueline Fawcett (Ed.), *Theory development: What, why, how?* (pp. 17–33). New York: National League for Nursing Press.

Fawcett, J. (1983). Hallmarks of success in theory development. In P. L. Chinn (Ed.), *Advances in nursing theory development* (pp. 3–15). Rockville, MD: Aspen.

Fawcett, J. (1984). *Analysis and evaluation of conceptual models of nursing.* Philadelphia: F. A. Davis.

Fawcett, J. (1995). *Analysis and evaluation of conceptual models of nursing* (3rd ed.). Philadelphia: F. A. Davis.

Flaskerud, J. H., & Halloran, E. J. (1980). Areas of agreement in nursing theory development. *Advances in Nursing Science, 3,* 1–7.

Gale, G. (1979). *Theory of science: An introduction to the history, logic, and philosophy of science.* New York: McGraw-Hill.

Hardy, M. E. (1974). Theories: Components, development, evaluation. *Nursing Research, 23*(2), 100–107.

Henderson, V. (1966). *The nature of nursing.* New York: Macmillan.

Hospers, J. (1980). What is explanation? In E. D. Klemke, R. Hollinger, & A. D. Kline (Eds.), *Introductory readings in the philosophy of science* (pp. 87–103). Buffalo: Prometheus Books.

Jacox, A. (1974). Theory construction in nursing: An overview. *Nursing Research, 23*(1), 4–13.

Johnson, D. E. (1980). The behavioral system model for nursing. In J. P. Riehl & C. Roy (Eds.), *Conceptual models for nursing practice* (2nd ed., pp. 207–216). New York: Appleton-Century-Crofts.

Kim, H. S. (1983). *The nature of theoretical thinking in nursing.* Norwalk, CT: Appleton-Century-Crofts.

Kuhn, T. S. (1970). *The structure of scientific revolutions* (2nd ed.). Chicago: University of Chicago Press.

Leininger, M. (1978). *Transcultural nursing: Concepts, theories, and practices.* New York: John Wiley & Sons.

Levine, M. E. (1969). *Introduction to clinical nursing.* Philadelphia: F. A. Davis.

Lundh, U., Soder, M., & Waerness, K. (1988). Nursing theories: A critical view. *IMAGE: Journal of Nursing Scholarship, 20*(1), 36–40.

Marriner-Tomey, A. (1998) Preface. In A. Marriner-Tomey & M. R. Alligood (Eds.), *Nursing theorists and their work* (4th ed., p. xiii). St. Louis: Mosby.

Marriner-Tomey, A., & Alligood, M. R. (Eds. 1998). *Nursing theorists and their work* (4th ed.). St. Louis: Mosby.

Meleis, A. I. (1997). *Theoretical nursing: Development and progress* (3rd ed.). Philadelphia: Lippincott.

Newman, M. A. (1979). *Theory development in nursing.* Philadelphia: F. A. Davis.

Newman, M. A. (1983). The continuing revolution: A history of nursing science. In N. L. Chaska (Ed.), *The nursing profession: A time to speak* (pp. 385–393). New York: McGraw-Hill.

Nightingale, F. (1992). *Notes on nursing.* Philadelphia: Lippincott. (Original work published 1859)

Norris, J. (1999, March). *The nursing theory page* [On-line]. Available: http://www.ualberta.ca:80/~jrnorris/nt/theory.html.

Orem, D. (1971). *Nursing: Concepts of practice.* New York: McGraw-Hill.

Orem, D. (1980). *Nursing: Concepts of practice* (2nd ed.). New York: McGraw-Hill.

Orem, D. (1985). *Nursing: Concepts of practice* (3rd ed.). New York: McGraw-Hill.

Orlando, I. (1961). *The dynamic nurse–patient relationship.* New York: G. P. Putnam's Sons.

Paterson, J. G., & Zderad, L. T. (1976). *Humanistic nursing.* New York: John Wiley & Sons.

Peplau, H. (1952). *Interpersonal relations in nursing.* New York: G. P. Putnam's Sons.

Rogers, M. E. (1970). *An introduction to the theoretical basis of nursing.* Philadelphia: F. A. Davis.

Rogers, M. E. (1980). A science of unitary man. In J. P. Riehl & C. Roy (Eds.), *Conceptual models for nursing practice* (2nd ed., pp. 329–337). New York: Appleton-Century-Crofts.

Rogers, M. E. (1983). Science of unitary human beings: A paradigm for nursing. In I. W. Clements & F. B. Roberts (Eds.), *Family health: A theoretical approach to nursing care* (pp. 219–228). New York: John Wiley & Sons.

Roy, C. (1970). Adaptation: A conceptual model for nursing. *Nursing Outlook, 18,* 42–45.

Roy, C. (1976). *Introduction to nursing: An adaptational model.* Englewood Cliffs, NJ: Prentice-Hall.

Roy, C. (1984). *Introduction to nursing: An adaptational model* (2nd ed.). Englewood Cliffs, NJ: Prentice-Hall.

Schumacher, K. L., & Gortner, S. R. (1992). (Mis)conceptions and reconceptions about traditional science. *Advances in Nursing Science, 14*(1), 1–11.

Silva, M. C. (1986). Research testing nursing theory: State of the art. *Advances in Nursing Science, 9*(1), 1–11.

Silva, M. C., & Rothbart, D. (1984). An analysis of changing trends in philosophies of science on nursing theory development and testing. *Advances in Nursing Science, 6*(2),1–13.

Silva, M. C., & Sorrell, J. M. (1992). Testing of nursing theory: Critique and philosophical expansion. *Advances in Nursing Science, 14*(4), 12–23.

Suppe, F. (1996, April 17). *Nursing science as a mature discipline: Is there a place for nursing theory and philosophy of science?* Invited lecture presented at the Indiana University School of Nursing Annual Doctoral Forum, Indianapolis, Indiana.

Suppe, F. (1997, March). *Middle-range theories: Historical and contemporary perspectives.* [On-line]. Available: http://www.comm.wayne.edu/nursing/suppe.html.

Suppe, F., & Jacox, A. J. (1984). Philosophy of science and the development of nursing theory. *Annual Review of Nursing Research, 3,* 241–267.

Symposium on nursing theory development. *Nursing Research, 17*(3), 196–227.

Travelbee, J. (1966). *Interpersonal aspects of nursing.* Philadelphia: F. A. Davis.

Wiedenbach, E. (1964). *Clinical nursing: A helping art.* New York: Springer-Verlag.

Yura, H., & Torres, G. (1975). *Today's conceptual frameworks with the baccalaureate nursing programs* (National League for Nursing Publication No. 15-1558, 17–75). New York: National League for Nursing Press.

■ Editor's Questions for Discussion

How relevant is Dickoff, James, and Wiedenbach's (1968) paper today? Discuss justifications for or against Donnelly's arguments. Have other authors expressed similar beliefs? What foundation exists for acceptance of Donnelly's polemic? What significant dialog might result from Donnelly's assertions? How important is it for the profession of nursing that valid and reliable nursing theories exist? What differences are there between developing nursing theory knowledge and developing conceptual knowledge for nursing practice? Explicate differences between nursing science and nursing practice. To what extent is any one or all the nursing theories scientific theories?

Why have understandings from the philosophy of science *not* been applied to an analysis of nursing theories? Is theory construction really in its "early stages in nursing" or are there other reasons why demonstrations have not occurred? Debate whether the "separation of our metatheoretical dialog from our nursing theories" may, can, or will ever become connected. What criteria are lacking for such linkages and clarification?

How can "context of usage" be defined to bridge the gap between nursing theories and scientific theory? Is it not possible to link the two? What criteria exist for legitimate theory testing? To what extent are such criteria evident in nursing?

How relevant are Beckstrand's (1978a, 1978b, 1980, 1984) arguments today and for the 21st century? Discuss Beckstrand's argument (referred to in Donnelly's Chapter 28) as to why knowledge of the properties of nursing would not help nursing develop knowledge about patients' problems. Why and to what extent has the nursing community not appreciated Beckstrand's work, the contribution by Suppe and Jacox, and the arguments presented by Deets? How likely (and why) is it that the "rebuttal" by Donnelly in this chapter might be ignored by the nursing community? What implications do Donnelly's conclusions have for content presented by other authors discussing theory in this volume (Kim, Chapter 23; Chinn, Chapter 24; Watson, Chapter 25; Fawcett and Bourbonniere, Chapter 26; Neuman, Chapter 27; and Meleis and Im, Chapter 72)? What might facilitate consideration and acceptance of Donnelly's beliefs?

If we accept that nursing theories have not been developed from systematic investigations, what has been the basis for their development? What should guide nursing research? Discuss Donnelly's statement that scientific theories are about actual states of affairs, not desired states of affairs. Do any of the present nursing theories serve as potential explanatory principles for nursing as a science? Why is nursing practice, "represented as actualized within the context of a relationship between the nurse and patient," an ill-founded base for a scientific theory? Is there a future for developing nursing theories as scientific theories? If so, what should be the basis? If the basis never has existed to date, how can nursing hope or attempt to develop nursing theories in the 21st century?

Have the efforts of nursing theorists to date been all for nothing other that to serve as a collective legitimizing process for nursing as a profession? How can past work serve as normative frameworks for conceptualizing nursing practice? Does not such conceptualization refute Beckstrand's arguments regarding "no need for a special category of theory designated as practice theory?" Should we "bury" our theory development aspirations as Donnelly suggests? What should guide us? Where do we go from here?

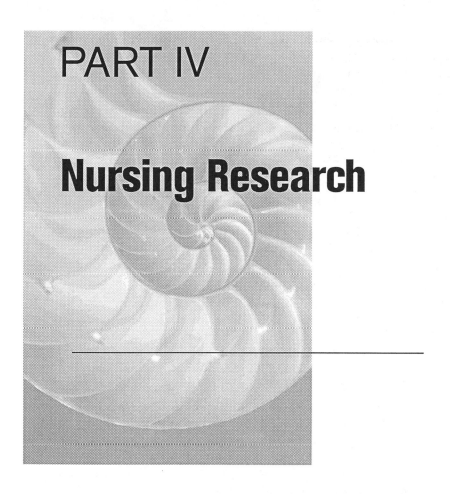

PART IV

Nursing Research

" . . . Oh, I kept the first for another day!
Yet knowing how way leads on to way,
I doubted if I should ever come back . . ."

Frost apparently understood that a search process is inherent in the road of life. Thorough examination of the paths is also part of the process. So, too, appraisal is necessary in nursing research.

Throughout scientific explorations nurse researchers may discard possible approaches and questions, realizing that they may never return to the original. Nurse researchers understand that one step leads to another for developing valid and reliable investigations. Careful thought and analysis in conducting research is demonstrated by the authors who address nursing research here. The paths for outcomes are clear, utilizing the various methodologies these authors suggest. Empirically conducted, theory-based, interdisciplinary and collaborative ventures, and, most important, evidence-based research are the means strongly advocated by these authors.

Assess carefully and consider the connections between these chapters concerning development of quality nursing research and the chapters in the other Parts of this volume. What is the best preparation for nurse researchers? Consider how standardization of nursing language can benefit interdisciplinary collaboration, nursing research, and the patient.

29

Interdisciplinary Efforts, Progress, and Promise

Cancer Nursing Research

Ada M. Lindsey, PhD, RN, FAAN

You are invited to go with me on a brief odyssey to see where we have been, where we are now, and where we need to go in cancer nursing research. This trajectory is not easy to distinguish clearly as its target continues to be a shifting panorama. Many of us are still beginning our research efforts, and some few of us have significant tracks. This odyssey reveals the promise for the next generation of cancer nursing research. What impressions do we want to make or need to make in the next 20 years? The answer shapes the direction for cancer nurse researchers.

As you think about this question, I hope that you will be inspired to (a) engage in interdisciplinary, collaborative research and to share findings more broadly, (b) develop and build on a program of focused research, and (c) engage in research to test effectiveness of interventions in improving patient outcomes or delivery of care or both.

This chapter was adapted from a keynote address given at the 5th National Conference on Cancer Nursing Research in Newport Beach, California, February, 1999. I wish to acknowledge consultation provided by Dr. Deborah McGuire and technical assistance provided by Ms. LaDonna Tworek in preparation of this chapter.

■ *The Past 20 Years*

This first section includes observations about where we have been in the past 20 years. Nursing research has been done, many projects have been delivered to faculty and to library shelves, but few of these studies have been published. We have kept our work relatively hidden from others, including nurse colleagues. In many cases, our research has not been of sufficient size or significance to attract attention or merit publication. Many of us have worked to make our research proposal and our resulting manuscript the best, in our perception, only to have reviewers be unimpressed. However, the critiquing process is essential. When initially rejected, some in our field have given up. But others, with better understanding of the process, seek the critique—valuing its input as helpful in striving for the ultimate goal of improving the research effort.

Past Deficiencies

Many factors have contributed to our lack of success in the past. One, our research projects often have been the easiest or most convenient to do. We need to move our research beyond those criteria. Some of us have been involved in projects for which we have not had the requisite expertise, most current information, or state-of-the-art scientific equipment. Maybe we did not know that we were in difficulty until the resulting proposal or manuscripts were not accepted. Most of our work has been done by junior investigators, but that is now gradually changing. Some of us were not well prepared as researchers. We completed our educational program but not with ideas about building a focused program of research—not knowing how to begin the next study or even what to study. Many of us completed programs in disciplines other than nursing. Consequently, many of the earlier research paths explored did not coalesce or develop; they remained scattered, sporadic attempts that did not lead to building a science base for nursing practice.

Lack of Mentoring

Some of us have not received mentoring, the opportunity of walking and working beside a more senior investigator. Senior or experienced investigators are still too few in number. In reality, many are still in the middle of their own maturational development with respect to a focused program of research. Thus much of nursing's early research was done by single investigators. The number of multiple-investigator studies has increased, but mostly the participants have been from a single discipline.

Lack of Resources

Many nurse researchers have had to choose between using modern state-of-the-art scientific equipment or using older methods to carry out research projects because of the lack of equipment or expertise available, or both. Additionally, many studies have been small due to funding limitations. It is difficult to conduct significant research without sufficient resources. Further, it is quite difficult for young investigators to obtain requisite funding if they do not become part of an experienced, funded research group.

National Support

During these past 20 years, the National Institute for Nursing Research (NINR) was created at NIH (it is now just over 10 years old). Even though the budget for NINR has increased during the organization's life, it has not kept pace with the increased demand for nursing research funding. In the recent past, the Oncology Nursing Foundation also has grown in its capacity to support cancer nursing research and has been able to increase some awards for targeted research areas. Work-

TABLE 29.1 Disciplines Represented by Research Article Authorship in *Oncology Nursing Forum* and *Cancer Nursing*, 1998

• Nursing	• Women's Studies
• Medicine	• Epidemiology
• Dentistry	• Psychology
• Public Health	• Statistics
• Pharmacology	• Anthropology
• Kinesiology	• Sociology
• Exercise Physiology	• Social Work
• Immunology	• Business

ing to enhance the funding for cancer nursing research is essential to its future.

Progress in Publications

Noteworthy is the increase in the number of research articles published in *Cancer Nursing* during the past 20 years. Only 2 were published in the journal's 1978 issues. The number increased to 10 in 1983, 16 in 1988, 20 in 1993, and in 39 in 1998 (Ash, 1998). Clearly, in the past 20 years, nurse researchers have been leaders in the field and they have made visible impressions for us to build upon.

■ Current Efforts

Our interdisciplinary research efforts are evident. I reviewed the published research in *Oncology Nursing Forum* (ONF) and *Cancer Nursing* (CN) journal issues for 1998. In ONF, 40 research articles were published in 1998—23 (58%) authored by nurses and 17 (42%) included authors from at least one additional discipline. Of the 23 authored by nurses, 7 (30%) were written by an individual author. Twenty-nine (73%) authors acknowledged receiving some funding, including traineeships, scholarships, and specific project funding.

A similar number (39) of research articles were published in 1998 in CN. More than half these articles (21) were authored by investigators from multiple disciplines; however, 4 of the 21 articles did not list a nurse as a coauthor. Considering the 17 articles that named nurses as coauthors, 44% of the research publications were multidisciplinary. These data suggest that nurses are leading or participating in multidisciplinary cancer nursing research projects with more than 40% of the research published in these two journals in 1998 demonstrating multidisciplinary authorship. Identifying the disciplines represented in the credits provided in these journals was not always easy; however, the list of disciplines in Table 29.1 represents those that were identifiable.

Cancer Nursing Research

Of concern is the paucity of cancer nursing research reported in the ONF and CN in which the effectiveness of nursing interventions was tested. Ten (25%) (Coward, 1998; de Moissac & Jensen, 1998; Ezzone, Baker, Rosselet, & Terepka, 1998; Griebel, Wewers, & Baker, 1998; Ippoliti & Neumann, 1998; Mock et al., 1998; Samarel, Fawcett, Davis, & Ryan, 1998; Sarna, 1998; Segar et al., 1998; Weinrich,

Weinrich, Boyd, & Atkinson, 1998) of the 40 research articles published in ONF reported testing an intervention. Only 3 (8%) (Benor, Delbar, & Krulik, 1998; McDaniel & Rhodes, 1998; Rustoen, Wiklund, Hanestad, & Moum, 1998) of the 39 research articles published in CN reported testing an intervention. Thus the large majority of research published in these two journals in 1998 was exploratory and descriptive.

Conceptual Frameworks

Only a few published research reports (5 or 6 annually in each of the two journals) referred explicitly to a conceptual or research framework or to basing the study on a middle-range theory. The conceptual frameworks referenced as underpinning the research included (a) Health Belief Model (Bakker, Lightfoot, Steggles, & Jackson, 1998; Choudhry, Srivastava, & Fitch, 1998; Tingen, Weinrich, Heydt, Boyd, & Weinrich, 1998); (b) Conservation Model (Mock et al., 1998); (c) PRECEDE (Weinrich, Weinrich, Boyd, & Atkinson, 1998); (d) Quality of Life (Ferrell, Grant, Funk, Otis-Green, & Garcia, 1998a, 1998b; Rustoen, Wiklund, Hanestad, & Moum, 1998; Yarbro & Ferrans, 1998;), (e) Integrated Fatigue Model (Woo, Dibble, Piper, Keating, & Weiss, 1998); (f) Science of Unitary Human Beings (Samarel et al., 1998); (g) Healthy Family Systems (Murtonen et al., 1998); (h) Decision-making (Kilpatrick, Kristjanson, Tataryn, & Fraser, 1998; Reaby, 1998); (i) Sense of Coherence (Andershed & Ternestedt, 1998); and (j) Symptom Management (Rutledge & Engelking, 1998). Investigator-developed frameworks also were reported by Porock, Kristjanson, Nikoletti, Cameron, & Pedler (1998).

Middle-Range Theories

The middle-range theories (MRT) referenced explicitly in the research articles were (a)

Uncertainty of Illness (Deane & Degner, 1998; Mast, 1998a, 1998b); (b) Self-regulation (Nail et al., 1998; Rhodes, McDaniel, & Matthews, 1998); (c) Grief (Chapman & Pepler, 1998); (d) Stress and Coping (Chapman & Pepler, 1998); (e) Transitions (Chapman & Pepler, 1998); (f) Self-transcendence (Chin-A-Loy & Fernsler, 1998; Coward, 1998); (g) Reasoned-action (Bakker, Lightfoot, Steggles, & Jackson, 1998); and, (h) Fulfillment (Kilpatrick, Kristjanson, & Tataryn, 1998). Nurse researchers have tended to use MRTs from other disciplines to guide nursing research (Moody et al., 1988). As the science base of the discipline develops, more MRTs will likely be developed from the nursing discipline's perspective, such as Mishel's theory of uncertainty of illness and Cox's interaction model of client health behavior (Cox, 1982; Lenz, Suppe, Gift, Pugh, & Milligan, 1995; Mishel, 1990). This development, however, may have implications for the direction of interdisciplinary research.

Phenomena of Interest in Cancer Nursing Research

To examine evidence of possible solid building, linking, and extending of research efforts in focused areas, I grouped these published studies by identified phenomena of interest. My impression is that we are still "becoming." In both ONF and in CN in 1998, most of the research articles could be categorized as shown in Table 29.2.

Some studies reported on disparate phenomena and thus were not categorized. Two examples were out of pocket expenditures (Moore, 1998) and alternative therapies (Montbriand, 1998). Thus, from the works published in the cancer nursing journals in 1998, some evidence of areas of focus exists— for example, screening, quality of life, side effects or symptoms (including fatigue), and varied psychosocial factors. Although catego-

TABLE 29.2   Categorization of Phenomena Identified from Research Published in *Oncology Nursing Forum* and *Cancer Nursing,* 1998

Category of Phenomena	Number of Articles	
	ONF	*CN*
Side effects/symptoms	9	4
Psychosocial factors	6	3
Fatigue	5	3
Screening	4	4
Family	3	5
Quality of life	3	4
Nurses: Experiences/perceptions	3	7
Information needs, knowledge	0	3

rization was possible, the actual phenomena grouped in these categories were still quite varied. For example, the nine side effects or symptoms or both appearing in the ONF research articles included (a) weight loss in nonsmall cell lung cancer (NSCLC) (Brown & Radke, 1998), (b) cancer-related pain (Burrows, Dibble, & Miaskowski, 1998), (c) diarrhea–drug management (Ippoliti & Neumann, 1998), (d) severity of radiation skin reaction (Porock et al., 1998), (e) symptom distress (DeKeyser, Wainstock, Rose, Converse, & Dooley, 1998; Sarna, 1998), (f) oral cavity status and high-dose antineoplastic therapy (Berger & Eilers, 1998), and (g) nausea and vomiting (Ezzone et al., 1998).

In the 1998 issues of *Oncology Nursing Forum* and *Cancer Nursing,* eight research articles included reports on the study of fatigue. Several investigations focused on determining psychometric properties of various measures of fatigue (Piper et al., 1998; Schneider, 1998; Schwartz, 1998b). In other studies, fatigue was measured in (a) patients receiving chemotherapy (Berger, 1998; Richardson, Ream, & Wilson-Barnett, 1998;), (b) in women receiving radia-

tion therapy (Irvine, Vincent, Graydon, & Bubela, 1998), and (c) in women undergoing different therapies (Woo et al., 1998). Correlates of fatigue (Mast, 1998a), and exercise and fatigue (Schwartz, 1998a), were studied. Thus, although fatigue was examined in several studies, different measures were used and the samples and clinical circumstances were varied. However, attention to measurement issues in the cluster of studies in which fatigue was examined demonstrated progress in understanding this complex phenomenon.

The varied psychosocial factors in the ONF research reports were (a) self-transcendence (Coward, 1998), (b) decision-making (O'Rourke & Germino, 1998), (c) illness uncertainty (Mast, 1998b), and (d) the emotional impact of breast cancer (Cohen, Kahn, & Steeves, 1998). The screening studies reported in CN examined an assortment of factors—for example, (a) benefits and predictors (Tingen et al., 1998), (b) barriers (Fitch, Greenberg, Cava, Spaner, & Taylor, 1998), (c) acculturation (Yi, 1998), and (d) follow-up for abnormal findings (Rajaram, 1998). Thus, although

TABLE 29.3   Categorization of Phenomena Identified from National Institute of Nursing Research Cancer-Related Grants, 1998

Category of Phenomena	Number of Grants
Side effects/symptom management	7
Psychosocial factors	5
Screening	4
Genetic testing	4
Family/children	3
Quality of life	3

categorization of phenomena studied is possible, continuing efforts are needed to extend the science base for practice. It is important, however, to acknowledge that some of these studies have examined the phenomena from a cultural perspective. This aspect of cancer nursing research is crucial and thus needs much more attention.

Cancer Related Funding by NINR

Because funding for cancer nursing research is critical to its development, I also examined cancer-related grants funded by the National Institute of Nursing Research (NINR) in fiscal year 1998 (NINR, 1998). Twenty-six cancer-related grants were funded (including R01, training, and center grants represented). Awards went to 21 institutions—3 institutions received two grants, and one institution had 3 grants—which are categorized in Table 29.3.

This review does not include information about funding that cancer nurse researchers received in 1998 from the National Cancer Institute, other institutes, and other funding agencies. It does, however, demonstrate the focus of the cancer nursing research funded by NINR in 1998.

Contributions to Cancer Research

Many nurse clinicians and researchers, both past and present, have made significant contributions to cancer research. They have been involved in clinical trials and have been a major resource in the progress of the research. An example of these contributions is reflected in a recent study (Freedman, 1998) and the Oncology Nursing Society (ONS) (1998) position statement about cancer research and cancer clinical trials. The following is an excerpt from that position statement:

> It is the position of ONS that . . . coordination of clinical trials (e.g., coordination of clinical sites, development of standardized treatment orders, symptom management, patient education and advocacy, facilitation of informed consent, and assistance with accrual and retention) is best accomplished by registered nurses who have been educated and certified in oncology nursing. (p. 973)

This statement clearly makes the point that cancer nurses have long been involved in interdisciplinary cancer research. Although this involvement has been and continues to be vitally important, it does not reflect nursing leadership of interdisciplinary research teams. It has, however, provided many opportunities for cancer nurses to be engaged in research. This on-the-job educational experience has motivated many nurses to pursue advanced degrees and to prepare themselves to lead research efforts.

Summary of Current Efforts

The evidence suggests that (a) only a small number of nurse researchers are prepared to lead interdisciplinary research teams, (b) only a few have stepped out to obtain postdoctoral research training or more research experience, and (c) too few are excited about the spirit of inquiry. Although nurse researchers increasingly have published research findings, especially within the past 5 years, the majority are still exploring, still seeking description. Little work is being done on testing effectiveness of interventions, and little cancer nursing research is being published on patient outcomes. We are beginning to see some clustering of work around selected phenomena but not yet much building on that work; as a result, efforts are still quite disparate. Fewer single investigator and single authored works are appearing. The difficulty of working in isolation without ready access to expertise, state-of-the-art scientific methods and equipment that are necessary to success is being recognized. We are beginning to see more nurse-led interdisciplinary research teams and more multisite studies. Happily, we are beginning to see a larger base of funding for support of cancer nursing research. However, competition for limited funding has increased, and it is likely to get worse even as nurse researchers continue to develop their research capacities. In cooperation with the ONS, the Oncology Nursing Foundation funded a Fatigue Initiative through Research and Education (FIRE) projects. This effort is a great example of progress being made in the increased funding of targeted cancer nursing research initiatives.

The foundation's Phase I Fatigue Initiative supported and promoted planning for multi-institutional studies to build the science base on commonly experienced phenomenon of cancer-related fatigue. In the *Oncology Nursing Forum* September 1998 issue, reports of the three FIRE-Phase I funded projects describe development of the research teams and their multisite projects (Grant et al., 1998; Mock et al., 1998; Nail et al., 1998). These research teams were led by nurse investigators but also included members from other disciplines to accomplish specific aims. Subsequently, the foundation supported a FIRE-Phase II project requesting proposals on instrumentation for measuring fatigue. These efforts also were funded. These two initiatives represent a major effort to move this field of study to what is required for the next generation of nursing research.

■ Transition to the Future

Passage of cancer nursing research into the next 20 years may seem formidable. We need to understand and celebrate its past and current achievements, but we also must have passion to move forward with comprehension of limitations of the past and imagination for the future. We must have the courage to move beyond where we have been, to build on where we are, and to develop the expertise needed to do what we need to do next. As a transition from where we are now to where we need to go, some comments about interdisciplinary, collaborative research are appropriate.

Need for Interdisciplinary Collaborative Research

About 20 years ago, Oberst (1980) wrote: "The nature of many clinical problems encountered in the acute care setting is such that an interdisciplinary study is likely to be the most effective approach" (p. 459). More recently, in a 1998 presentation to the National Advisory Council for NINR and in a subsequent article, McGuire (1999) noted that interdisciplinary research is more likely to yield science that is innovative, substantive, and applicable to the real world. The study of many clinical phenomena of interest to nurses requires integration of nursing science with other relevant sciences: (a) biobehavioral sciences, (b) socioeconomic sciences, (c) epidemiologic sciences, (d) genetics, and (e) others such as exercise physiology and nutritional sciences.

In addition to the multidisciplinary components of clinical phenomena and the expertise required to consider these components, interdisciplinary, collaborative research is attractive and necessary for several other reasons. They include (a) acquiring requisite expertise, (b) accessing subjects and other resources, (c) adding depth to the science, and (d) generating new ideas and innovation in the research. Beyond these reasons for engaging in interdisciplinary research, other incentives are increasing. They include pressures from within academic and clinical institutions, managed care groups, private foundation sponsored initiatives, and NIH (Lindeke & Block, 1998; McGuire, 1999).

Requirements for Collaboration

More than a decade ago, Williams (1987) noted the need for nurses to engage in interdisciplinary, collaborative research and described that collaboration:

- The entire collaborating group must have strong mutual interest in questions that are posed.
- The questions posed require resources beyond the capacity of one investigator or one discipline.

- The investigators must work together as colleagues.

Expanding on these ideas, Henneman, Lee, and Cohen (1995) stated that the defining characteristics of collaborative, interdisciplinary research are team members who (a) are committed to joint intellectual effort, (b) recognize that interdisciplinary efforts require investment of time and energy, (c) willingly participate from inception to conclusion of the project, (d) willingly share expertise and responsibility, and (e) honestly acknowledge contributions of the other collaborators. If the research team is successful as an interdisciplinary working group, evidence will show that (a) the efforts were truly a cooperative endeavor, (b) trust was developed among the professional colleagues, and (c) the investigators were peers with shared decision-making responsibilities (Lindeke & Block, 1998; Williams, 1987).

A successful interdisciplinary research team will not be a group with just one individual dictating its activities. McGuire (1999) and Lindeke and Block (1998) commented that, with interdisciplinary research teams, power is likely to be unequal—unequal by profession or discipline, unequal by position or title, unequal by educational background, unequal by socioeconomic class, and maybe unequal by gender. However, if a transition is made to a truly collaborative endeavor, power and authority are shared among group members to make the interdisciplinary group research effort successful (Henneman et al., 1995). These shared decision-making responsibilities include specifying project goals, setting priorities, distributing work based on expertise, and determining how results are disseminated (Williams, 1987). Values demonstrating an interdisciplinary spirit include working, trusting, supporting, sharing, respecting, and applauding (McClosky & Maas, 1998).

Challenges in Collaborative Efforts

If collaborative efforts enhance (a) importance of the work, (b) sophistication of the research, (c) mentorship of less experienced researchers, (d) opportunities for funding, and (e) potential for focus and building of research programs, why is interdisciplinary research not considerably more evident in cancer nursing research? A number of impediments to collaborative efforts have been identified (Lindeke & Block, 1998; McCloskey & Maas, 1998; McGuire, 1999). For example, some individuals simply do not want to participate in any group. Turf, loyalty, and ownership issues arise, as do workload concerns. Competing priorities and, in some cases, conflicting schedules may make follow-through on commitments problematic for the team. Some members may work in different physical or even geographic space. Insufficient funding or resource support, such as turnover of personnel, may impede collaboration. Differing values, viewpoints, opinions, and perceptions may also negatively influence collaborative group processes.

To be successful, interdisciplinary collaborative research requires competence, creativity, confidence, complementarity, commitment, communication, and cohesiveness at the very least. A team needs some members with a creative spark and others with a penchant for detail. Building an interdisciplinary research team takes time, effort, and energy and is likely to be an incremental process. The collaborative team must work in harmony with joint decision-making and collectively have the spirit of inquiry, adventure, and of going together on the research odyssey.

Nursing Perspective in Interdisciplinary Research

Tensions also exist with respect to doing interdisciplinary work (Lindeke & Block, 1998; McCloskey & Maas, 1998). How to develop and maintain a nursing discipline's perspective while engaged with individuals from other disciplines in interdisciplinary research is the issue. Nursing research should have considerable import for informing practice—that is acknowledged. Thus there is potential for conflict with that goal and with that of conducting interdisciplinary work. For example, as McCloskey and Maas (1998) stated, "An overemphasis on interdisciplinary research and practice could dilute nursing knowledge and further obfuscate the important role of the nurse in the planning and delivery of health care" (p. 160). This consideration is vitally important for nurse researchers, especially as nursing research and the discipline are still "becoming."

However, expertise from various perspectives may be essential in conducting significant research. Thus, a one-discipline perspective may not be sufficient to address many clinical or health-related phenomena (e.g., wound healing or healthy lifestyle change). One solution is to have more nurse-led interdisciplinary research teams and to maintain a disciplined focus for research questions being addressed.

In this next generation of research, nurse researchers must give increased attention to developing and testing more middle-range theories. Such theories form the basis for the theory–research–practice linkages that are needed for continued development of the discipline and professional practice—which ultimately should result in improving health care outcomes.

The Director of NINR, Dr. Patricia Grady, in a news column in the July/August 1998, issue of *Nursing Outlook,* reported on several nurse researchers who participated in an NIH sponsored conference titled "From Scientific Discovery to Practice—What Does It Take to Bring About Changes in Health Care" (Grady, 1998). Three notable characteristics of the efforts of these nurse researchers were that (a) they have worked with a diverse or interdisciplinary research team, (b) they have been building and extending their focused research over a considerable number of years, and (c) their research has tested and demonstrated the effectiveness of interventions or models of care delivery to improve the health outcomes of people and to influence health care costs. All are salient characteristics of leaders in nursing research.

Future Cancer Nursing Research

In thinking about the next 20 years of cancer nursing research, I concluded that three overarching questions need to be asked continuously to guide our research to make a difference:

1. Are the research questions being addressed truly significant? That is, do they have potential for making an impact on the delivery of care or on care outcomes?

2. Do we have confidence in the *quality* of our research? That is, do we believe that nursing's (a) research models or theoretical frameworks, (b) research designs, (c) instrumentations (equipment or other measures), (d) interventions (culturally sensitive and appropriate), (e) representativeness of samples, and (f) analyses measure up to the standards generally accepted for scientific research?

3. Is there evidence of focus, building, and extending the research, of adding depth to the science and particular phenomena or populations or both?

Resounding positive answers to these questions show us where we all must head in the next 20 years of cancer nursing research.

To achieve this vision in cancer nursing research—as well as for most nursing research efforts—we must assemble appropriately selected interdisciplinary research teams. We next must carefully design small feasibility studies (can it be done?) that can serve well as preliminary or pilot work, which are necessary to chart the way—and then not rest or stop with these small studies. We must have larger, significant studies that are sufficiently funded to obtain requisite personnel, sample sizes, and state-of-the-art scientific instrumentation—or we will not keep pace with other research efforts or even make progress in this next generation. We must have many more outstanding committed researchers who have a track record in making progress in a focused direction and who can lead the field. We also must make our work more visible to others, taking opportunities to tell others, enhance dissemination of findings, and publish more broadly.

■ Concluding Statement

Difficult or risk taking as it may seem at times, successfully establishing more interdisciplinary, truly collaborative, nurse investigator–led research teams is a direction that will make a difference. Doing so will affect our efforts positively in cancer research, in our science, and more importantly in health care for those with cancer and their families.

In concluding this brief odyssey, exploring the past and present of cancer nursing research and imagining the next 20 years, like Florence Downs, I declare "research is the news in the field" (Downs, 1998, p. 247). And, especially, the "news" is cancer nursing research—unless of course, prevention, treatment, genetic engineering, and antiaging research eradicate cancer. If that does not occur, what cutting edge, collaborative, and interdisciplinary work will you be undertaking? What impressions will you and your research team make on the next generation of cancer nursing research? The answer to that is the promise!

■ References

Andershed, B., & Ternestedt, B. M. (1998). Involvement of relatives in the care of the dying in different care cultures: Involvement in the dark or the light? *Cancer Nursing, 21*(2), 106–116.

Ash, C. R. (1998). Cancer nursing research: An international perspective. *Cancer Nursing, 21*(4), 225.

Bakker, D. A., Lightfoot, N. E., Steggles, S., & Jackson, C. (1998). The experience and satisfaction of women attending breast cancer screening. *Oncology Nursing Forum, 25*(1), 115–121.

Benor, D. E., Delbar, V., & Krulik, T. (1998). Measuring impact of nursing intervention on cancer patients' ability to control symptoms. *Cancer Nursing, 21*(5), 320–334.

Berger, A. M. (1998). Patterns of fatigue and activity and rest during adjuvant breast cancer chemotherapy. *Oncology Nursing Forum, 25*(1), 51–62.

Berger, A. M., & Eilers, J. (1998). Factors influencing oral cavity status during high-dose antineoplastic therapy: A secondary data analysis. *Oncology Nursing Forum, 25*(9), 1623–1626.

Brown, J. K., & Radke, K. J. (1998). Nutritional assessment, intervention, and evaluation of weight loss in patients with non-small cell lung cancer. *Oncology Nursing Forum, 25*(3), 547–553.

Burrows, M., Dibble, S. K., & Miaskowski, C. (1998). Differences in outcomes among patients experiencing different types of cancer-related pain. *Oncology Nursing Forum, 25*(4), 735–741.

Chapman, K. J., & Pepler, C. (1998). Coping, hope, anticipatory grief in family members in palliative home care. *Cancer Nursing, 21*(4), 226–234.

Chin-A-Loy, S. S., & Fernsler, J. I. (1998). Self-transcendence in older men attending a prostate cancer support group. *Cancer Nursing, 21*(5), 358–363.

Choudhry, U. K., Srivastava, R., & Fitch, M. I. (1998). Breast cancer detection practices of South Asian women: Knowledge, attitudes, and beliefs. *Oncology Nursing Forum, 25*(10), 1693–1701.

Cohen, M. Z., Kahn, D. L., & Steeves, R. H. (1998). Beyond body image: The experience of breast cancer. *Oncology Nursing Forum, 25*(5), 835–841.

Coward, D. D. (1998). Facilitation of self-transcendence in a breast cancer support group. *Oncology Nursing Forum, 25*(1), 75–84.

Cox, C. L. (1982). An interaction model of client health behavior: A theoretical prescription for nursing. *Advances in Nursing Science, 5*(1), 41–56.

de Moissac, D., & Jensen, L. (1998). Changing IV administration sets: Is 48 versus 24 hours safe for neutropenic patients with cancer? *Oncology Nursing Forum, 25*(5), 907–913.

Deane, K. A., & Degner, L. F. (1998). Information needs, uncertainty, and anxiety in women who had a breast biopsy with benign outcome. *Cancer Nursing, 21*(2), 117–126.

DeKeyser, F. G., Wainstock, J. M., Rose, L., Converse, P. J., & Dooley, W. (1998). Distress, symptom distress, and immune function in women with suspected breast cancer. *Oncology Nursing Forum, 25*(8), 1415–1422.

Downs, F. S. (1998). The rightful place of research in academia. *Nursing Outlook, 46*(5), 246–247.

Ezzone, S., Baker, C., Rosselet, R., & Terepka, E. (1998). Music as an adjunct to antiemetic therapy. *Oncology Nursing Forum, 25*(9), 1551–1556.

Ferrell, B. R., Grant, M. M., Funk, B., Otis-Green, S. A., & Garcia, N. J. (1998a). Quality of life in breast cancer Part II: Psychological and spiritual well-being. *Cancer Nursing, 21*(1), 1–9.

Ferrell, B. R., Grant, M. M., Funk, B., Otis-Green, S. A., & Garcia, N. J. (1998b). Quality of life in breast cancer survivors: Implications for developing support services. *Oncology Nursing Forum, 25*(5), 887–895.

Fitch, M. I., Greenberg, M., Cava, M., Spaner, D., & Taylor, K. (1998). Exploring the barriers to cervical screening in an urban Canadian setting. *Cancer Nursing, 21*(6), 441–449.

Freedman, T. G. (1998). The breast cancer prevention trial: Nurses' observations. *Cancer Nursing, 21*(3), 178–186.

Grady, P. A. (1998). News from NINR. *Nursing Outlook, 46*(4), 153.

Grant, M., Anderson, P., Ashley, M., Dean, G., Ferrell, B., Kagawa-Singer, M., Padilla, G., Robinson, S. B., & Sarna, L. (1998). Developing a team for multicultural, multi-institutional research on fatigue and quality of life. *Oncology Nursing Forum, 25*(8), 1404–1412.

Griebel, B., Wewers, M. E., & Baker, C. A. (1998). The effectiveness of a nurse-managed minimal smoking-cessation intervention among hospitalized patients with cancer. *Oncology Nursing Forum, 25*(5), 897–902.

Henneman, E., Lee, J., & Cohen, J. (1995). Collaboration: A concept analysis. *Journal of Advanced Nursing, 21,* 103–109.

Ippoliti, C., & Neumann, J. (1998). Octreotide in the management of diarrhea induced by graft versus host disease. *Oncology Nursing Forum, 25*(5), 873–878.

Irvine, D. M., Vincent, L., Graydon, J. E., & Bubela, N. (1998). Fatigue in women with breast cancer receiving radiation therapy. *Cancer Nursing, 21*(2), 127–135.

Kilpatrick, M. G., Kristjanson, L. J., & Tataryn, D. J. (1998). Measuring the information needs of husbands of women with breast cancer: Validity and reliability of the family inventory of needs—husbands. *Oncology Nursing Forum, 25*(8), 1347–1351.

Kilpatrick, M. G., Kristjanson, L. J., Tataryn, D. J., & Fraser, V. H. (1998). Informational needs of husbands of women with breast cancer. *Oncology Nursing Forum, 25*(9), 1595–1601.

Lenz, E., Suppe, F., Gift, A., Pugh, L., & Milligan, R. (1995). Collaborative development of middle-range nursing theories: Toward a theory of unpleasant symptoms. *Advances in Nursing Science, 17*(3), 1–13.

Lindeke, L. L., & Block, D. E. (1998). Maintaining professional integrity in the midst of interdisciplinary collaboration. *Nursing Outlook, 46*(5), 213–218.

Mast, M. E. (1998a). Correlates of fatigue in survivors of breast cancer. *Cancer Nursing, 21*(2), 136–142.

Mast, M. E. (1998b). Survivors of breast cancer: Illness uncertainty, positive reappraisal, and emotional distress. *Oncology Nursing Forum, 25*(3), 555–562.

McCloskey, J. C., & Maas, M. (1998). Interdisciplinary team: The nursing perspective is essential. *Nursing Outlook, 46*(4), 157–163.

McDaniel, R. W., & Rhodes, V. A. (1998). Development of a preparatory sensory information videotape for women receiving chemotherapy for breast cancer. *Cancer Nursing, 21*(2), 143–148.

McGuire, D. B. (1999). Building and maintaining an interdisciplinary research team. *Alzheimer Disease and Associated Disorders, 13*(suppl. 1), S17–S21.

Mishel, M. (1990). Reconceptualization of the uncertainty in illness theory. *IMAGE: Journal of Nursing Scholarship, 22,* 256–262.

Mock, V., Ropka, M. E., Rhodes, V. A., Pickett, M., Grimm, P. M., McDaniel, R., Lin, E. M., Allocca, P., Dienemann, J. A., Haisfield-Wolfe, M. E., Stewart, K. J., & McCorkle, R. (1998). Establishing mechanisms to conduct multi-institutional research—Fatigue in patients with cancer: An exercise intervention. *Oncology Nursing Forum, 25*(8), 1391–1397.

Montbriand, M. J. (1998). Abandoning biomedicine for alternate therapies: Oncology patients' stories. *Cancer Nursing, 21*(1), 36–45.

Moody, L. E., Wilson, M. E., Smyth, K., Schwartz, R., Tittle, M., & Van Cott, M. L. (1988). Analysis of a decade of nursing practice research: 1977–1986. *Nursing Research, 37,* 374–379.

Moore, K. (1998). Out-of-pocket expenditures of outpatients receiving chemotherapy. *Oncology Nursing Forum, 25*(9), 1615–1622.

Murtonen, I., Kuisma, M., Paunoness, M., Lehti, K., Koivula, M., & White, M. (1998). Family dynamics of families with cancer in Finland. *Cancer Nursing, 21*(4), 252–258.

Nail, L. M., Barsevick, A. M., Meek, P. M., Beck, S. L., Jones, L. S., Walker, B. L., Whitmer, K. R., Schwartz, A. L., Stephen, S., & King, M. E. (1998). Planning and conducting a multi-institutional project on fatigue. *Oncology Nursing Forum, 25*(8), 1398–1403.

National Institute of Nursing Research. (1998). [On-line]. Available: http://www.nih.gov/ninr/1998NINRgrants.html.

Oberst, M. T. (1980). Nursing research: New definitions, collegial approaches. *Cancer Nursing, 3*(6), 459.

Oncology Nursing Forum. (1998). *Oncology Nursing Society position cancer research and cancer clinical trials, 25*(6), 973–974.

O'Rourke, M. E., & Germino, B. B. (1998). Prostate cancer treatment decisions: A focus group exploration. *Oncology Nursing Forum, 25*(1), 97–104.

Piper, B. F., Dibble, S. L., Dodd, M. J., Weiss, M. C., Slaughter, R. E., & Paul, S. M. (1998). The revised Piper fatigue scale: Psychometric evaluation in women with breast cancer. *Oncology Nursing Forum, 25*(4), 677–684.

Porock, D., Kristjanson, L., Nikoletti, S., Cameron, F., & Pedler, P. (1998). Predicting the severity of radiation skin reactions in women with breast cancer. *Oncology Nursing Forum, 25*(6), 1019–1029.

Rajaram, S. S. (1998). Nonadherence to follow-up treatment of an abnormal pap smear: A case study. *Cancer Nursing, 21*(5), 342–348.

Reaby, L. L. (1998). Breast restoration decision-making: Enhancing the process. *Cancer Nursing, 21*(3), 196–204.

Rhodes, V. A., McDaniel, R. W., & Matthews, C. A. (1998). Hospice patients' and nurses' perceptions of self-care deficits based on symptom experience. *Cancer Nursing, 21*(5), 312–319.

Richardson, A., Ream, E., & Wilson-Barnett, J. (1998). Fatigue in patients receiving chemotherapy: Patterns of change. *Cancer Nursing, 21*(1), 17–30.

Rustoen, T., Wiklund, I., Hanestad, B. R., & Moum, T. (1998). Nursing intervention to increase hope and quality of life in newly diagnosed cancer patients. *Cancer Nursing, 21*(4), 235–245.

Rutledge, D. N., & Engelking, C. (1998). Cancer-related diarrhea: Selected findings of a national survey of oncology nurse experiences. *Oncology Nursing Forum, 25*(5), 861–872.

Samarel, N., Fawcett, J., Davis, M., & Ryan, F. M. (1998). Effects of dialogue and therapeutic touch on preoperative and postoperative experiences of breast cancer surgery:
An exploratory study. *Oncology Nursing Forum, 25*(8), 1369–1376.

Sarna, L. (1998). Effectiveness of structured nursing assessment of symptom distress in
advanced lung cancer. *Oncology Nursing Forum, 25*(6), 1041–1048.

Schneider, R. A. (1998). Reliability and validity of the multidimensional fatigue inventory
(MFI-20) and the Rhoten fatigue scale among rural cancer outpatients. *Cancer Nursing, 21*(5), 370–373.

Schwartz, A. L. (1998a). Patterns of exercise and fatigue in physically active cancer survivors. *Oncology Nursing Forum, 25*(3), 485–491.

Schwartz, A. L. (1998b). The Schwartz cancer fatigue scale: Testing reliability and validity.
Oncology Nursing Forum, 25(4), 711–717.

Segar, M. L., Katch, V. L., Roth, R. S., Garcia, A. W., Portner, T. I., Glickman, S. G.,
Haslanger, S., & Wilkins, E. G. (1998). The effect of aerobic exercise on self-esteem
and depressive and anxiety symptoms among breast cancer survivors. *Oncology Nursing
Forum, 25*(1), 107–113.

Tingen, M. S., Weinrich, S. P., Heydt, D. D., Boyd, M. D, & Weinrich, M. C. (1998).
Perceived benefits: A predictor of participation in prostate cancer screening. *Cancer
Nursing, 21*(5), 349–357.

Weinrich, S. P., Weinrich, M. C., Boyd, M. D., & Atkinson, C. (1998). The impact of
prostate cancer knowledge on cancer screening. *Oncology Nursing Forum, 25*(3), 527–534.

Williams, C. A. (1987). Collaborative research: A commentary. *Journal of Professional
Nursing, 3*(2), 82, 124–125.

Woo, B., Dibble, S. L., Piper, B. F., Keating, S. B., & Weiss, M. C. (1998). Differences in
fatigue by treatment methods in women with breast cancer. *Oncology Nursing Forum,
25*(5), 915–920.

Yarbro, C., & Ferrans, C. E. (1998). Quality of life of patients with prostate cancer
treated with surgery or radiation therapy. *Oncology Nursing Forum, 25*(4), 685–693.

Yi, J. K. (1998). Acculturation and pap smear screening practices among college-aged
Vietnamese women in the United States. *Cancer Nursing, 21*(5), 335–341.

■ Editor's Questions for Discussion

What factors have contributed to insufficient publication of nursing cancer research?
How might these contributing factors be reduced or eliminated? What patterns exist in
Lindsey's review regarding areas of focus, phenomena studied, utilization of tools and
measurement, and conceptual frameworks? How do Lindsey's findings concerning the
paucity of tested nursing intervention via cancer nursing research support Deets and
Choi's findings (Chapter 34)? How likely is it that middle-range theories will be developed as the science base for nursing research? What perspectives presented by Donnelly
(Chapter 28), Deets and Choi (Chapter 34), and Titler (Chapter 35) have implications
for interdisciplinary research? To what extent are Lindsey's findings regarding areas for
research supported or refuted by Deets and Choi (Chapter 34), Titler (Chapter 35), and
Androwich and Haas (Chapter 32)?

What appear to be the areas most focused upon in nursing research? Discuss the measurement issues raised by the studies about fatigue. What challenges exist in building on previous research? Provide evidence of nursing leadership on interdisciplinary research terms. Why is there little evidence on the testing effectiveness of interventions and patient outcomes? To what extent is this limitation true primarily for cancer interventions? What other patient conditions have limited research-based interventions? Given the cultural factors inherent in cancer research, what interventions from the writings of Froman and Owen (Chapter 33) may be applied?

What strategies will be most effective in fostering research collaboration? How may supportive and cooperative behaviors result? Because of the multidisciplinary components of many clinical phenomena, what implications does Jenkins' discussion (Chapter 54) have for collaborative research in genetics? How might impediments to collaborative efforts be resolved? How would increasing nurse-led interdisciplinary research teams ensure various perspectives in conducting research? How might overemphasis in interdisciplinary research dilute nursing knowledge? To what extent is such dilution realistic? To what extent does or should nursing research inform nursing practice? Based on the views expressed by Donnelly (Chapter 28), debate the roles of middle-range theories in research as a basis for professional practice linkages. What disparities in beliefs must be resolved within the profession for future cancer nursing research to occur, as envisioned by Lindsey? How might those differences and issues be resolved?

30

Emerging Research Issues in Mobility

Christine E. Kasper, PhD, RN,
FAAN, FACSM

The maintenance of mobility and skeletal muscle function are major goals in the care of individuals with impaired function. When the total daily amount of exercise in activities of daily living (ADLs) declines, skeletal muscle atrophy rapidly begins within 4–8 hours (Booth & Seider, 1979). Because the average daily level of activity serves as a set-point by which the body regulates the mass and strength of skeletal muscle, any decrease in activity from those set-points results in a rapid loss of muscle tissue, also known as atrophy (Kasper, 1990). Therefore progression of atrophy in skeletal muscle varies in accordance with the severity of immobilization of the patient.

Although skeletal muscle atrophy is often associated with debilitation and immobiliza-tion, the phenomenon also occurs during mechanical ventilation, certain drug therapies, bed rest during pregnancy, and injury to pelvic floor muscles resulting in urinary incontinence (Boyington, Dougherty, & Kasper, 1995; Jakobsson, Jorfeldt, & Brundin, 1990; Kelly & Goldspink, 1982; Khaleeli et al., 1983; Maloni & Kasper, 1991; Zeiderman, Welchew, & Clark, 1990). Unfortunately, the risk of skeletal muscle atrophy encompasses nearly all patient populations. More important, loss of functional mobility resulting from atrophy yields a decreased ability to perform self-care functions, such as shopping for food and standing for a period of time to cook (Kasper, 1990).

The goal of remobilization and physical rehabilitation is to restore the debilitated patient to the best possible level of mobility and function (Medicine, 1997). Each patient will vary in inherent functional capacity, degree of debilitation, and physiologic abilities in relation to rehabilitative outcomes. Emerging research issues in mobility flow from both the phenomenon of skeletal muscle atrophy and the rehabilitation required to recover from its effects. These issues also span the spectrum of the biologic basis of clinical nursing therapeutics and include (a) appropriate timing of rehabilitation following a period of disuse atrophy, (b) electrical stimulation of skeletal muscle, (c) determination of minimal level of strength needed to carry out normal ADLs, and (d) anticipatory measures for spinal cord repair.

■ Appropriate Timing of Rehabilitation Following a Period of Disuse Atrophy

The resumption of mobility after sustained bed rest following serious illness can be slow, requiring rehabilitative intervention. However, the appropriate timing of exercise during the rehabilitative process has not been clearly identified. Early vigorous exercise can lead to muscle weakness, soreness, and injury, which may delay or permanently inhibit recovery, especially in aged populations (Clarkson, Nosaka, Braun, 1992; Faulkner, Brooks, & Zerba, 1995; Fridén & Lieber, 1992; Lindle et al., 1997). Related studies have demonstrated that exercise damage induced by repeated injury can seriously affect the rate and magnitude of recovery (Kasper, White, & Maxwell, 1990).

In normal and regenerating muscle, physical conditioning of the appropriate intensity, duration, and frequency results in hypertrophy of muscle cells, increased strength, increased capacity for aerobic metabolism, and improved endurance. Although it seems reasonable to expect that an exercise program following prolonged inactivity might help to ameliorate the muscular atrophy and decrease fatigability of these muscles, previous studies (Kasper, 1995; Kasper, Maxwell, & White, 1996; Kasper et al., 1990) have shown that exercise may induce structural degeneration and damage in atrophied skeletal muscle. Usually the damage is widespread and can involve muscle cells, connective tissue, and associated nerves (Russell, Dix, Haller, & Jacobs-El, 1992).

Many of the cellular alterations that occur during prolonged inactivity, especially those that predispose atrophied mammalian skeletal muscle to injury during recovery from prolonged inactivity, have been described. These cellular alterations can be categorized broadly as either mechanical tearing due to high forces or rupture of the muscle fiber due to contraction against sarcomere nonuniformities. For example, the effects of reloading of atrophied skeletal muscle were studied to determine if weight-bearing alone would produce significant sarcolemmal membrane disruption or wounding prior to development of cell death. Wounding and damage of muscle fiber were found to be related to the muscle fiber cross-sectional area, and small fibers were more predisposed to wounding than larger fibers (Kasper, 1995). Damage to small atrophic cells, often Type I fibers, may be exacerbated by additional mechanisms. *The implications were that the extent of injury to skeletal muscle fibers from postatrophic reloading is far more extensive than previously predicted.* Further, conditions such as aging, concurrent systemic pathology, or drug therapy may inhibit resealing of membranes and may result in greater cell death than in control populations (Kasper, 1995).

Studies of changes in individual proteins during restricted mobility are ongoing (Thomason, Biggs, & Booth, 1989). Important to clinical nursing is the determination of physical readiness of the patient to resume weight-bearing, to increase the amount of daily activity, and to have sufficient muscle mass with appropriate fiber type composition to support self-care activities without fatigue or injury to the muscle.

Skeletal muscle can regenerate and eventually recover from exercise-induced damage in young animals; however, adult and aged animals may not be able to completely regenerate sufficient skeletal muscle tissue to produce contractile forces sufficient to resume activities of daily living. Although it is well known that normal skeletal muscle can be damaged by exercise and that atrophic skeletal muscle is more severely damaged by exercise, clinicians continue to prescribe exercise to debilitated patients without regard to potential risks. For example, the mechanical stress of reloading atrophic skeletal muscle occurs instantly upon removal of casts, initial weight-bearing after hip replacement, and standing for the first time following bed rest during pregnancy. Previous investigations have shown that damage to atrophic skeletal muscle decreases after 4 days of sedentary recovery (Kasper et al., 1996; Kasper & Xun, 1992; Thomason et al., 1989). However, the timing of rehabilitative exercise to minimize skeletal muscle cell injury has not been explored.

The investigation of appropriate exercise during recovery is an area unique to nursing research and of interest to investigators in physical therapy. Little has been done to determine other associated variables, such as the influence of concurrent pharmacologic therapies on effectiveness of exercised recovery. In addition, expansion of the concept of muscle atrophy and recovery is needed. Rather than focusing primarily on weight-bearing muscle, research of other applications to pelvic floor and respiratory muscle would be useful. Two examples are developing better strategies and methods for alleviating urinary incontinence and ameliorating the difficulty of weaning patients from mechanical ventilation.

■ Exercise-Based Interventions to Aid Recovery from Atrophy

Electrical Stimulation of Skeletal Muscle

Currently, electrical stimulation of skeletal muscle (EMS) is being increasingly employed in both research and clinical settings as a therapeutic method to increase skeletal muscle size and strength. However, electrical stimulation is being applied somewhat indiscriminately to the aged as well as to the athlete. Devices that produce EMS are advertised in popular magazines, but little is actually known about the effects of external EMS on skeletal muscle in human beings.

In human beings, EMS can contribute to improved fitness (Enoka, 1988), increase muscle strength in athletes, help in rehabilitation following spinal cord injury (Glaser, 1994), and aid in recovery from surgical procedures (e.g., anterior cruciate ligament repair). A large variety of stimulating protocols have been studied. The majority of this work involves short-term therapy (3 to 6 weeks) with higher frequency stimulation that causes about 20 individual maximal contractions over a period of 10 or more minutes. Strength increases of as much as 50% to 60% have been observed in healthy subjects using this type of protocol (Eriksson, Haggmark, Kiessling, & Karlsson, 1981; Hultman & Sjöholm, 1983; Kagaya, Sharma, Kobetic, & Marsolais, 1998; Söderlund & Hultman, 1991; Tarka, 1986; Valencic, Vodovnik, Stefancic, & Jelnikar, 1986).

EMS originally was used as a physiologic research tool to drive adaptation of skeletal muscle contractile proteins, biochemical content, and speed of contraction by invasive stimulation of specific muscles or motor units in animal models (Chi et al., 1986; Salmons, 1994). Electrodes implanted in rats are used to stimulate nerve and muscle directly and generally provide continuous stimulation for periods of up to 24 hours. Methods now used with human beings do not resemble those in animal studies, but data have been extrapolated to human beings and used as physiologic justification for application to the aged. To date, the currently used model of EMS for human beings, with external maximal stimulation of a limited number of contractions, has not been tested in an animal model. For EMS to be successful in recovering strength in human beings, the duration and frequency of stimulation must match that of the peripheral nerve in situ stimulating a specific muscle. These studies have yet to be done.

With progressive loss of muscle mass and strength in aging, resulting in loss of mobility, many practitioners have proposed and currently are using EMS in an attempt to recover these age-related losses of skeletal muscle strength, mass, and size. As strength is related directly to the cross-sectional area of a muscle, increasing contractile activity by EMS is assumed to increase the mass and cross-sectional area, yielding increased strength. Areas of emerging research interest include appropriate use of EMS in humans and selection of correct frequencies of stimulation.

Exercise of the Aged

With increasing age, skeletal muscle has been demonstrated to atrophy. This age-related atrophy is accompanied by a reduction in muscle strength and an altered speed and force of contraction (Alley & Thompson, 1997). Between the ages of 30 and 80, gradual loss of 40% in the lean body mass occurs, with an associated increase in the spread of fiber sizes (Borkan, Hults, & Gerzof, 1983). This loss of muscle mass is reflected in decreased cross-sectional area of the muscle and parallels a drop in muscular strength (Larson, Grimby, & Karlsson, 1979).

Isometric and dynamic maximal strength also functionally declines beyond age 50 (Kuta, Parizkova, & Dycka, 1970). Age-related atrophy is accompanied by reduction in muscle strength and altered speed and force of contraction (Alley & Thompson, 1997). Aging and inactivity exert similar deleterious effects on skeletal muscle function; however, the rate of atrophy due to inactivity is far more rapid than that of aging. When inactivity or immobilization is superimposed on aging muscle, the resulting atrophy may be more severe and require a longer period for recovery.

During growth, development, and remodeling, regulation of protein synthesis occurs through mechanisms that operate at the nuclear and cytoplasmic levels. Pluskal, Moreyra, Burini, and Young (1984) found that the decline in protein synthesis efficiency with aging appears to be due to a change in the level of mRNA (messenger ribonucleic acid) in cells, leading to a decrease in the polyribosomes. Therefore very old rats (30 months) would need to recruit increased numbers of myonuclei to maintain the "status quo" of contractile proteins, membranes, and associated structures. As the percentage of satellite cells depends on the total numbers of satellite cells and myonuclei, hindlimb unloading (HU)–induced atrophy may exhaust the satellite cell pool, as does denervation (Rodrigues & Schmalbruch, 1995). With the additional stressor of HU, these oldest rats appear to be unable to recruit additional satellite cells to aid in remodeling; this inability results in a greater magnitude of atrophy and a proportional decline in number of nuclei. In short, the aged are more likely not to recover from a period of disuse atrophy because they no longer possess the cells required for regeneration. Therefore careful study is needed to determine exercise response in different individuals in different states of mobility.

Central emerging issues for nursing research include: (a) is increasing strength in the aged sufficient, or do the aged also require endurance training to improve self-care; and (b) what is the minimal level of strength needed to carry out normal activities of daily living (ADLs) (Booth, Weeden, & Tseng, 1994; Buchner, 1997; Stockton, 1988; Strawbridge, Cohen, Shema, & Kaplan, 1996; Vita, Terry, Hubert, & Fries, 1998).

■ Anticipatory Measures for Spinal Cord Repair

During the past 10 years, new technologies were developed that may eventually prove successful in repairing spinal cord damage and reversing chronic paralysis. Studies conducted on mammalian animals have investigated various ways to induce healing in severed or damaged spinal cords (Schwab, 1996; Turbes, 1997a, 1997b). Other researchers have sought therapies utilizing remaining motor neuron and spinal reflexes to promote some level of walking and mobility (De Leon, Hodgson, Roy, & Edgerton, 1998, 1999; Edgerton et al., 1997; Roy et al., 1998a; Roy et al., 1998b).

Advances in this previously unimagined area of spinal cord repair are progressing rapidly. Within the next 10 years, methods likely will exist either to minimize or repair spinal damage due to trauma. An important nursing question lurks behind this future medical advance. Will a regenerated and repaired central nervous system (CNS) be able to reactivate severely atrophic and previously denervated skeletal muscle? And, at what level of function do we need to maintain the paralyzed patient for the patient to benefit from future repair and reinnervation of muscle?

■ Concluding Statement

Regeneration of skeletal muscle following peripheral nerve section has been previously demonstrated in classic studies (Arancio, Cangiano, Magherini, & Pasino, 1988; Carlson, 1981). That skeletal muscle can be transplanted and regenerated following relatively short-term denervation also has been shown (Baker & Poindexter, 1991; Bischoff, 1989; Carlson, 1976). Because skeletal muscle rapidly adapts to its new level of contraction or "exercise," the possibility exists that severely atrophic and denervated muscle may not be able to recover the necessary size, contractile proteins, and metabolic contents that are required to support coordinate activity. Research in this area is of the utmost importance.

■ References

Alley, K. A., & Thompson, L.V. (1997). Influence of simulated bed rest and intermittent weight bearing on single skeletal muscle fiber function in aged rats. *Archives of Physical Medicine & Rehabilitation, 78*(1), 19–25.

Arancio, O., Cangiano, A., Magherini, P. C., & Pasino, E. (1988). Effects of reinnervation with normal and tetrodotoxin-inactive nerves on resting membrane potential of rat skeletal muscle. *Neuroscience Letters, 88,* 179–183.

Baker, J. H., & Poindextor, C. E. (1991). Muscle regeneration following segmental necrosis in tenotomized muscle fibers. *Muscle & Nerve, 14*, 348–357.

Bischoff, R. (1989). Analysis of muscle regeneration using single myofibers in culture. *Medicine and Science in Sports & Exercise, 21*(5), S164–S172.

Booth, F. W., & Seider, M. J. (1979). Early change in skeletal muscle protein synthesis after limb immobilization of rats. *Journal of Applied Physiology: Respiratory Environmental & Exercise Physiology, 47*(5), 974–977.

Booth, F. W., Weeden, S. H., & Tseng, B. S. (1994). Effect of aging on human skeletal muscle and motor function. *Medicine & Science in Sports and Exercise, 26*(5), 556–560.

Borkan, G. A., Hults, D. E., & Gerzof, S. G. (1983). Age changes in body composition revealed by computed tomography. *Journal of Gerontology, 38*, 673–677.

Boyington, A. R., Dougherty, M. C., & Kasper, C. E. (1995). Pelvic muscle profile types in response to pelvic muscle exercise. *International Urogynecology Journal, 6*(2), 68–72.

Buchner, D. M. (1997). Preserving mobility in older adults. *Western Journal of Medicine, 167*(4), 258–264.

Carlson, B. M. (1976). A quantitative study of muscle fiber survival and regeneration in normal, predenervated, and marcaine-treated free muscle grafts in the rat. *Experimental Neurology, 52*, 421–432.

Carlson, B. M. (1981). Denervation, reinnervation, and regeneration of skeletal muscle. *Otolaryngol Head & Neck Surgery, 89*, 192–196.

Chi, M. M-Y., Hintz, C. S., Henriksson, J., Salmons, S., Hellendahl, R. P., Park, J. L., Nemeth, P. M., & Lowry, O. H. (1986). Chronic stimulation of mammalian muscle: Enzyme changes in individual fibers. *American Journal of Physiology, 251*(*Cell Physiology, 20*), C633–C642.

Clarkson, P. M., Nosaka, K., & Braun, B. (1992). Muscle function after exercise-induced muscle damage and rapid adaptation. *Medicine & Science in Sports & Exercise, 24*(5), 512–520.

De Leon, R. D., Hodgson, J. A., Roy, R. R., & Edgerton, V. R. (1998). Full weight-bearing hindlimb standing following stand training in the adult spinal cat. *Journal of Neurophysiology, 80*(1), 83–91.

De Leon, R. D., Hodgson, J. A., Roy, R. R., & Edgerton, V. R. (1999). Retention of hindlimb stepping ability in adult spinal cats after the cessation of step training. *Journal of Physiology, 81*(1), 85–94.

Edgerton, V. R., de Leon, R. D., Tillakaratne, N., Recktenwald, M. R., Hodgson, J. A., & Roy, R. R. (1997). Use-dependent plasticity in spinal stepping and standing. *Advances in Neurology, 72*, 233–247.

Enoka, R. M. (1988). Muscle strength and its development: New perspectives. *Sports Medicine, 6*, 146–168.

Eriksson, E., Haggmark, T., Kiessling, K. H., & Karlsson, J. (1981). Effect of electrical stimulation of human skeletal muscle. *The International Journal of Sports Medicine, 2*, 18–22.

Faulkner, J., Brooks, S., & Zerba, E. (1995). Muscle atrophy and weakness with aging: Contraction-induced injury as an underlying mechanism. *Journal of Gerontology, 50A*, 124–129.

Fridén, J., & Lieber, R. L. (1992). Structural and mechanical basis of exercise-induced muscle injury. *Medicine & Science in Sports & Exercise, 24*(5), 521–530.

Glaser, R. M. (1994). Functional neuromuscular stimulation. Exercise conditioning of spinal cord injured patients. *International Journal of Sports Medicine, 15*(3), 142–148.

Hultman, E., & Sjöholm, H. (1983). Energy metabolism and contraction force of human skeletal muscle in situ during electrical stimulation. *Journal of Physiology, 345,* 525–532.

Jakobsson, P., Jorfeldt, L., & Brundin, A. (1990). Skeletal muscle metabolites and fibre types in patients with advanced chronic obstructive pulmonary disease (COPD), with and without chronic respiratory failure. *European Respiratory Journal, 3,* 192–196.

Kagaya, H., Sharma, M., Kobetic, R., & Marsolais, E. B. (1998). Ankle, knee, and hip moments during standing with and without joint contractures: Simulation study for functional electrical stimulation. *American Journal of Physical Medicine & Rehabilitation, 77*(1), 49–54; quiz 65–66.

Kasper, C. E. (1990). Antecedent condition: Impaired physical mobility (disuse syndrome). In B. L. Metzger (Ed.), *Altered functioning: Impairment and disability, monograph series 90* (pp. 20–38). Indianapolis, IN: Nursing Center Press of Sigma Theta Tau International.

Kasper, C. E. (1995). Sarcolemmal disruption in reloaded atrophic skeletal muscle. *Journal of Applied Physiology, 79*(2), 607–614.

Kasper, C. E., & Xun, L. (1992). Adaptation of titin to short-term microgravity. *ASGSB Bulletin, 6*(1), 87.

Kasper, C. E., Maxwell, L. C., & White, T. P. (1996). Alterations in skeletal muscle related to short-term impaired physical mobility. *Research in Nursing & Health, 19*(2), 133–142.

Kasper, C. E., White, T. P., & Maxwell, L. C. (1990). Running during recovery from hindlimb suspension induces muscular injury. *Journal of Applied Physiology, 68*(2), 533–539.

Kelly, F. J., & Goldspink, D. F. (1982). The differing responses of four muscle types to dexamethasone treatment in the rat. *Biochemical Journal, 208,* 147–158.

Khaleeli, A. A., Edwards, R. H. T., Gohil, K., McPhail, G., Rennie, M. J., Round, J., & Ross, E. J. (1983). Corticosteroid myopathy: A clinical and pathological study. *Clinical Endocrinology, 18,* 155–161.

Kuta, I., Parizkova, J., & Dycka, J. (1970). Muscle strength and lean body mass in old men of different physical activity. *Journal of Applied Physiology, 29*(2), 168–171.

Larson, L., Grimby, G., & Karlsson, J. (1979). Muscle strength and speed of movement in relation to age and muscle morphology. *Journal of Applied Physiology, 46*(3), 451–456.

Lindle, R. S., Metter, E. J., Lynch, N. A., Fleg, J. L., Fozard, J. L., Tobin, J., Roy, T. A., & Hurley, B. F. (1997). Age and gender comparisons of muscle strength in 654 women and men aged 20–93 yr. *Journal of Applied Physiology, 85*(5), 1581–1587.

Maloni, J. A., & Kasper, C. E. (1991). Physical and psychosocial effects of antepartum hospital bedrest: A review of the literature. *IMAGE: Journal of Nursing Scholarship, 23*(3), 187–192.

Medicine I. (1997, chap. 1). Introduction. In E. N. Brandt, Jr., & A. M. Pope (Eds.), *Enabling America: Assessing the role of rehabilitation science and engineering* (pp. 24–39). Washington, DC: Committee on Assessing Rehabilitation Science and Engineering, Division of Health Science Policy, Institute of Medicine of the National Academy of Sciences.

Pluskal, M. G., Moreyra, M., Burini, R. C., & Young, V. R. (1984). Protein synthesis studies in skeletal muscle of rats. I. Alterations in nitrogen composition and protein synthesis using a crude polyribosome and pH 5 enzyme system. *Journal of Gerontology, 39*(4), 385–391.

Rodrigues, A., & Schmalbruch, H. (1995). Satellite cells and myonuclei in long-term denervated rat muscles. *Anatomical Record, 243,* 430–437.

Roy, R. R., Pierotti, D. J., Baldwin, K. M., Zhong, H., Hodgson, J. A., & Edgerton, V. R. (1998a). Cyclical passive stretch influences the mechanical properties of the inactive cat soleus. *Experimental Physiology, 83*(3), 377–385.

Roy, R. R., Talmadge, R. J., Hodgson, J. A., Zhong, H., Baldwin, K. M., & Edgerton, V. R. (1998b). Training effects on soleus of cats spinal cord transected (T12–13) as adults. *Muscle & Nerve, 21*(1), 63–71.

Russell, B., Dix, D. J., Haller, D. L., & Jacobs-El, J. (1992). Repair of injured skeletal muscle: A molecular approach. *Medicine & Science in Sports & Exercise, 24*(2), 189–196.

Salmons, S. (1994). Exercise, stimulation and type transformation of skeletal muscle. *International Journal of Sports Medicine, 15*(3), 136–141.

Schwab, M. E. (1996). Structural plasticity of the adult CNS. Negative control by neurite growth inhibitory signals. *International Journal of Developmental Neuroscience, 14*(4), 379–385.

Söderlund, K., & Hultman, E. (1991). ATP and phosphocreatine changes in single human muscle fibers after intense electrical stimulation. *American Journal of Physiology, 261 (Endocrinology, Metabolism, 24),* E737–E741.

Stockton, W. (1988, November 28). Can exercise alter the aging process? *New York Times,* p. B6.

Strawbridge, W. J., Cohen, R. D., Shema, S. J., & Kaplan, G. A. (1996). Successful aging: Predictors and associated activities. *American Journal of Epidemiology, 144*(2), 135–141.

Tarka, I. M. (1986). Changes in the probability of firing of motor units following electrical stimulation in human limb muscles. *Physiologica Scandinavica, 126,* 61–65.

Thomason, D. B., Biggs, R. B., & Booth, F. W. (1989). Protein metabolism and ß-myosin heavy-chain mRNA in unweighted soleus muscle. *American Journal of Physiology, 257 (Regulatory Integrative Comparative Physiology 26),* R300–R305.

Turbes, C. C. (1997a). Intercostal nerve neuroma (PNS) implantation in spinal cord anastomosis bridging spinal cord transection—Enhancement of central neurons (CNS) axonal regeneration. *Biomedical Sciences Instrumentation, 34,* 344–350.

Turbes, C. C. (1997b). Peripheral nerve (PNS) spinal cord anastomoses bridging spinal cord transection—Enhancement of central neurons (CNS) axonal regeneration. *Biomedical Sciences Instrumentation, 33,* 326–331.

Valencic, V., Vodovnik, L., Stefancic, M., & Jelnikar, T. (1986). Improved motor response due to chronic electrical stimulation of denervated tibialis anterior muscle in humans. *Muscle & Nerve, 9,* 612–617.

Vita, A. J., Terry, R. B., Hubert, H. B., & Fries, J. F. (1998). Aging, health risks, and cumulative disability. *The New England Journal of Medicine, 338*(15), 1035–1041.

Zeiderman, M. R., Welchew, E. A., & Clark, R. G. (1990). Changes in cardiorespiratory and muscle function associated with the development of postoperative fatigue. *British Journal of Surgery, 77,* 576–580.

■ Editor's Questions for Discussion

What maintenance of mobility role should nurses fulfill in caring for individuals with impaired function? Identify issues pertaining to clinical nursing therapeutics and immobile patients. How should nurses address those issues in clinical practice? How might nurses collaborate with researchers to address research issues pertaining to patients' remobilization and physical rehabilitation? What implications exist for nursing practice in the presentation by Kasper?

Identify implications of Kasper's discussion for further nursing research. What additional variables may be associated with effectiveness of exercise in recovery of mobility? How may appropriate exercise be determined? What factors might inhibit age-related muscle atrophy? How may exercise response in persons in different states of mobility be determined? How might Kasper's identification of specific nursing issues concerning strength and endurance training be addressed? Develop research questions and methodology in response to the questions Kasper raises related to spinal cord repair and reactivated muscle.

Do nursing programs have imbedded in them content related to the concepts of atrophy and exercise? At what program level and to what extent should such concepts be addressed? Although nurses often use EMS clinically, how might they better understand the science behind its application?

31

Linking Nursing Language and Knowledge Development

Dorothy A. Jones, EdD, RN, FAAN

As we begin the 21st century, changes in health care will continue to occur at a rapid pace. Advances in computer technology, improved management of illness, and the influence of holistic healing modalities will contribute to redefining health care practices, cost, and models of delivery. Professionals directly involved in patient care will continue to be challenged to describe their contributions to health care outcomes.

In recent years, attention paid to the language used to communicate patient care has increased significantly. Of importance is the inclusion of nursing language in development of a standardized, computer-based, patient medical record. Crucial to this effort is the clarity of the language used to describe the domain of nursing practice and elements of the care provided to individuals and groups. "The very survival of a profession may be at risk unless the discipline is defined" (Donaldson & Crowley, 1978, p. 4).

The purpose of this chapter is to explore nursing language and its link to knowledge development within the discipline. Current nursing vocabularies are discussed in terms of their potential for use within a standardized, computer-based patient record. Language developments within the discipline are explored to reflect nursing's perspective on health within an evolving system of information access and retrieval.

■ Focus of the Discipline

Nursing's disciplinary perspective values the whole person (individual, family, and community) within the context of a changing environment. Preserving the intrinsic worth and dignity of person dominates the focus of nursing practice. Nursing seeks to address the human experience in its totality, isolating individual and group responses and behaviors manifested in health and illness. The interaction between nurse and patient is unique, dynamic, and reciprocal. The connection created within the nurse–patient relationship fosters trust and discovery of the human experience. Nurses use knowledge to (a) promote growth, (b) facilitate decision-making and choice, and (c) address the physical, spiritual, emotional, and environmental responses that compromise and enhance healing and the human potential.

Nursing seeks to uncover meaning and comes to know the person through the use of dialogue (Radwin, 1996). The nurse is a patient's advocate, seeking to preserve human dignity and protect the person or group when rights are threatened or violated. The nursing experience manifests intentionality and presence within an environment that reflects the values and beliefs of nursing (Newman, 1986; Rogers, 1970; Roy & Andrews, 1991; Watson, 1999).

■ Phenomena of Concern

Nursing's contract with society is to "care and nurture both healthy and ill people," integrating the "science of caring . . . with the knowledge base for the diagnosis and responses to health and illness" (American Nurses Association [ANA], 1995, p. 6).

"Phenomena are those events and processes that form the core of nursing science and link it to the core nursing values and nursing outcomes" (Walker, 1997, p. 7). The fundamental nursing phenomena relate to "care and self processes, comfort, discomfort, pain, emotions related to experiences of birth, health, illness, and death . . . decision- and choice-making abilities . . . and social policies that affect health" (ANA, 1995, p. 8). This mandate reflects nursing's commitment to society. It guarantees that nurses will develop and use knowledge in the provision of nursing care to individuals, groups, and communities across the health care spectrum. As the scope of nursing practice expands and new knowledge is generated, language will be an essential vehicle used to communicate nursing's social mandate.

The naming of phenomena makes an experience real and gives scientists an opportunity to discuss it (Hayakowa & Hayakowa, 1990). "It is reasonable . . . for us to pursue inquiry to develop taxonomies such as those representing nursing diagnoses, nursing interventions . . . while at the same time pursuing phenomenological or critical inquiry to capture other aspects of these conditions" (Rogers, 1997, p. 37). Identification of phenomena of concern to nursing provides language to describe a scope of practice for which the nurse is accountable.

■ Problems Addressed By the Discipline

What are the problems for which nursing is accountable? In describing them, "we must remain cognizant of our own purposes, values and goals as we identify and define our problems" (Rogers, 1997, p. 38). On the one hand, Toulmin (1972) discussed problems as differences between the goals of a particular discipline and its current intellectual capacities. On the other hand, Lauden (1977) believed that, when a discipline identified a problem, it must view that problem as important to the discipline.

For nursing, multiple factors (e.g., social, cultural, environmental, and situational) influence and sometimes confound the identification of a problem. At times, the lack of a clearly identified scope of practice can add to the confusion. Exploring the human experience from a nursing perspective can help to direct knowledge development and contribute answers or raise new questions generated by emerging information to stimulate nursing inquiry (Lauden, 1977; Rogers, 1997).

■ Isolating a Disciplinary Focus

Multiple modes of inquiry are available to nursing as it seeks to isolate issues of disciplinary concern. Carper (1978) discusses four patterns of nursing knowledge: empiric, esthetic, personal, and ethical. Nurses use different strategies to access knowledge in practice. One familiar method is that of problem solving; another is process. Each approach attempts to link the philosophical values and beliefs of the discipline to strategies used to uncover the human experience.

Problem Solving

Problem solving relies on logical reasoning and critical thinking to isolate a problem, define goals, and seek a solution. *The Standards of Nursing Practice* (ANA, 1972) describes problem solving as assessment, diagnosis, goal setting, intervening, and evaluation of care. Through an organized approach, data are collected, analyzed, and synthesized. The result is the formulation and naming of a nursing judgment (nursing diagnosis), problem, or phenomenon of concern to nurses.

Problem identification, supported by data (e.g., defining characteristics), provides the evidence needed to name the phenomenon and describe the attributes needed to determine whether a problem actually exists, and, if so, the nursing diagnosis of it (Gordon, 1987).

Process

Process focuses on information as expressed by a person in response to questions used to uncover the human experience. Within the context of the dialogue, this approach moves away from the more linear, problem-solving mode to a process mode of inquiry. Uncovering a phenomenon of concern to the person or naming emerging themes is an evolving process requiring observation of a pattern over time and reflection on it (Newman, 1986, 1999).

The discovery of responses and behaviors manifests "an unbroken wholeness that captures expression and re-creates humanity itself (Gramling, 1999, p. 49). The use of dialogue reveals the need to represent and conceptualize an event as experienced by the individual(s). The process mode is reciprocal and centers on capturing reality as reflected through someone's experience over time and communicated through language.

■ Knowledge Development

Nursing knowledge development has been occurring over many years and is still evolving. Concept definition and nursing theory development are two structures that have helped to translate the ontology and teleology of the discipline into language that reveals and describes nursing practice. Both have given substance to the discipline and guided the generation, refinement, and advancement of nursing knowledge.

Concepts

"A concept is a mental image of a phenomenon, an idea or a construct" (Walker & Avant, 1995, p. 24). Concepts help persons cluster and organize experiences that can be discussed at various levels of abstraction. They reflect units of thought (Tuttle, 1999).

Concepts are developed through a process of analysis and synthesis and are refined through testing and evaluation. Naming a concept involves the use of language or application of a label to reflect adequately the definition (attributes) of the phenomenon or event being described. The label becomes the vehicle used to communicate our thoughts to others (Walker & Avant, 1995).

The testing and refinement of a concept enhances clarity, refines the definition, and helps differentiate one concept from another. Differentiation promotes accuracy and delineates unique manifestations and responses, attributable only to the concept being defined. Researching a concept decreases redundancy and aids in clarifying concept definition. Concepts that are measurable can be used in clinical research to expand the science.

Theory

When linked, concepts form statements. These statements can connect two or more concepts (*relational statements*), suggest *association* or *causality,* or present concepts that appear to be unrelated (*nonrelational statements*) (Meleis, 1985; Walker & Avant, 1995). Organization and pattern shape and characterize theory (Chinn & Jacobs, 1983). As a theory emerges, it presents a particular perspective about reality. "Theory development provides a way of identifying and expressing key ideas about the essence of practice" (Walker & Avant, 1995, p. 3). In general, theory builds on the values and beliefs of a discipline, expands knowledge, and is the hallmark of a profession (Bixler & Bixler, 1945).

Theory synthesis reflects knowledge gained through research and evaluation (Walker, 1998). When nursing develops a unique perspective (theory) about the dynamics of person, the environment, nursing, and health interaction (Fawcett, 1984), it provides a guide for nurses to use when exploring and describing events, behaviors, and responses from a particular point of view (Newman, 1986, 1999; Rogers, 1970; Roy & Andrews, 1991; Watson, 1999).

Theories have given nurses language to articulate a world view and reflect one perception of reality. *Grand theories* provide a global framework for describing, explaining, predicting, and controlling events and responses related to the human experience (Chinn & Jacobs, 1983; Meleis, 1985; Walker & Avant, 1995). These theories are abstract, highly synthesized conceptualizations of the lived experience that help give the nurse an approach to practice and discovery.

The evolution of *mid-range theory* provides a bridge between grand and practice theory and "shares some of the conceptual economy of grand theory" (Walker & Avant, 1995, p. 11). However, these concepts (mid-range theories) are less abstract (e.g., *caring:* Watson, 1999; *uncertainty:* Mishel, 1988) and provide a focus for research and practice that reflect responses to a phenomenon or experience. The language used in naming these concepts can be evaluated in a variety of clinical situations to reflect human behaviors and reactions.

Practice theory provides concrete representations of reality. It is focused on selected goals and the activities needed to accomplish the desired outcomes (Dickoff, James, & Weidenbach, 1968; Jacox, 1974). Practice theory directs care and offers the nurse a prescription for achieving selected outcomes. Use of nursing diagnosis (North American Nursing Diagnosis Association (NANDA), 1998–2000), interventions (McCloskey & Bulechek, 2000), and outcomes (Johnson, Maas, & Moorehead, 2000) are components of a practice theory.

Nursing theory can be used to (a) describe the focus of the discipline, (b) communicate areas of professional autonomy, and (c) create fields of study that lead to the generation, evaluation, and refinement of knowledge. The values and beliefs embedded in theory identify areas of accountability and link disciplinary knowledge and nursing expertise to patient care.

■ *Language Development*

Language is important to survival. It is a highly developed symbolic process, a vehicle for exchange, and a way to express thoughts (Hayakawa & Hayakawa, 1990). Language gives meaning, communicates a perspective, and provides information.

The development of nursing knowledge and the testing and refinement of knowledge across clinical settings has helped shape a disciplinary language. "What appears evident is that nursing knowledge has sharpened our ability to describe the content of practice and possibly extend the focus of the discipline" (Jones, 1998, p. 77). The naming of nursing phenomena offers nurse scientists an opportunity to discuss, accept, refute, or expand the experience being described (Hayakawa & Hayakawa, 1990).

Knowledge development and language appear to be iterative processes. Linking nursing knowledge with language development solidifies what is known and raises new questions that will help refine, validate, and expand the disciplinary perspective. Nursing knowledge provides the framework for understanding the patient experience in a unique way. Language offers nursing an opportunity to communicate that experience to others. As language evolves it can be grouped to communicate information about nursing care effectively and clearly.

Nursing Language: What It Doesn't Explain

The human experience is dynamic and continually changing. Some dimensions of this experience are easily described and others defy explanation. The art of nursing is an essential activity grounded by practice that is manifested by helping patients create coherence in lives that are threatened by multiple transitions (LeVasseur, 1998). The nurse uses knowledge and artistry to create the environment for the human experience to emerge (Watson, 1999).

"The complexity and density of the human interactive nature of nursing cannot be represented by traditional scientific scripts or objective queries. But nursing begs for language to describe the art" (Gramling, 1999, p. 2). Nursing art, language, and knowledge can be used effectively to describe elements of the nurse and patient encounter. There are times, however, when the essence of the experience may transcend language.

Nursing language can provide a changing, tangible description of reality. Artistry combined with science creates an opportunity for discovery and evolution from what is known. Current nursing vocabularies describe elements of the nurse–patient relationship, but they may never describe it all. Hayakawa and Hayakawa (1990) suggested that we experience only a small fraction of a phenomenon. As nurses expand their awareness of the human experience, language development can be informed by reality and knowledge can continue to expand.

Nursing Language and Standardized Vocabularies

Formal nursing vocabularies have been developing for more than 25 years. Standardized nursing vocabularies delineate the elements of nursing care (diagnoses, interventions, and outcomes) and provide a mechanism for capturing and describing the patient's experience from a nursing perspective. Because multiple nursing vocabularies exist, no one classification system can meet all the criteria for inclusion in a computer-based patient record (Henry, Warren, Lange, & Button, 1998).

TABLE 31.1 Nursing Classification Systems, Data Sets, and Nomenclatures
Officially Recognized by the American Nurses Association

Classifications[a]

The North American Nursing Diagnosis Association (NANDA) is a membership driven organization. Nurses from around the world have contributed to the development of more than 150 nursing diagnoses with definitions, risk factors, and defining characteristics (NANDA, 1998–2000). Each diagnosis is classified under nine patterns of human responses to illness and life transitions (Taxonomy I). Individuals submit a candidate researched diagnosis for evaluation by an expert review panel (Diagnostic Review Committee) and inclusion in the current taxonomy. NANDA has been classifying diagnoses since 1973. Taxonomy I is used in a variety of health care settings to document patient care, research studies, and in publications. Taxonomy II is currently under consideration by the NANDA members. If approved, it will be used as a framework for reclassifying nursing diagnoses under a new series of domains and classes. Access: http://www.nanda.org

The Nursing Intervention Classification (NIC) was developed by McCloskey and Bulechek (2000) at the University of Iowa Center for Nursing Classification. It is used by nurses to document nursing interventions. More than 433 nursing interventions have been generated by the research team. Each intervention is uniquely coded within a three-level taxonomy comprising 6 domains and 27 classes. The NIC is used in a variety of health care settings to document patient care, in research studies, and in various publications. Access: http://www.nursing.uiowa.edu

The Nursing Outcomes Classification (NOC) was developed by Johnson and Maas (1996) at the University of Iowa Center for Nursing Classification. It is used by nurses to document nursing outcomes. More than 190 nursing outcomes have been generated by the research team. Each intervention is uniquely defined with a set of indicators and measured on a five-point Likert scale to measure patient status. The NOC is used in a variety of health care settings to document patient care, in research studies, and in various publications. Access: http://www.nursing.uiowa.edu

The Home Health Care Classification (HHCC) was developed by Virginia Saba (1992, 1997) for more than 10,000 home health agencies. Nursing diagnoses and interventions were included in an effort to standardize vocabulary and code and to index, classify, document, and track home health care. Diagnoses (145) and interventions (160) are classified under 20 care components. Modifiers are used to evaluate outcomes. The HHCC is used in various sites to document care (e.g., HMOs and outpatient clinics) and in computer-based patient records, and it has been incorporated into critical paths.

Data Sets

The Patient Care Data Set was developed by Ozbolt (1997). It uses nursing diagnoses, patient care actions, and nursing outcomes to document nursing care, primarily in acute care settings. Data are organized under the 20 care components of Saba's HHCC and 2 components added to adapt the data set to acute care. The data set is used in several test sites, including the Patient Care Information System at Vanderbilt University.

The Omaha System was developed by Martin and Scheet (1992). It is used to document community and home health care. The system contains 42 nursing diagnoses and interventions and a problem rating scale to evaluate outcomes. It is used in many home health care agencies and promoted by the efforts of Martin through consultation, newsletters, presentations, and publications.

The Perioperative Nursing Data Set (PNDS) was developed by the Association of Operating Room Nurses to offer clinicians in a variety of perioperative settings with easy access to an automated, standardized nomenclature to describe specialty practice (Kleinbeck, 1996). Includes 68 selected NANDA-approved nursing diagnoses, 127 nursing interventions, and 29 nursing outcomes unique to perioperative nursing. Clinical testing and validation of PNDS is under consideration. Language approved by PNDS in 1999.

Nomenclatures

The Systematized Nomenclature of Medicine (SNOMED RT) was the first ANA-recognized nomenclature developed by the College of American Pathologists (CAP), a medical society serving more than

16,000 physician members (mostly pathologists) and laboratories globally. SNOMED was developed in 1976 to create a system for indexing, retrieving, aggregating, and analyzing patient medical record data. It originally contained 11 axes in the domain of medical language. In 1997, SNOMED committed $17 million to respond to a global direction that focuses on creating a way to capture, retrieve, analyze, and send data throughout the health care delivery system. The association is committed to having SNOMED content approved by the clinicians who develop and use the information in clinical practice.

Currently, a group called the SNOMED Authority makes the final decisions on content. They are informed by the SNOMED Editorial Board, which includes domain experts, terminology experts, and liaisons and collaborators. Nursing is a member of the editorial board and includes representatives from the American Nurses Association and current nursing vocabulary developers. SNOMED RT (a reference for terminology) has evolved from SNOMED and has several distinguishing characteristics. They include (a) hierarchies and relationships defined in a computer-readable format, (b) codes that are context-free, and (c) multiple parenting in coding, and (d) no reassignment of codes to different concepts or terms after they are retired (Kudla & Rallins, 1998). A group within SNOMED—called the SNOMED Convergent Terminology Group for Nursing (CTGFN)—is to become a work group of the SNOMED Editorial Board. The group was formed in January 1999 to ensure that content within the domain of nursing will be adequately represented in SNOMED (Kudla & Rallins, 1998).

[a]Work begun by NANDA, NIC, and NOC continues on identifying linkages among nursing diagnosis, intervention, and outcomes within each of the three classification systems.

Adapted from Warren, J., & Bickford, C. (1999, May 19). *ANA recognized nursing data sets, classification systems, and nomenclatures.* Washington DC: American Nurses Association Committee for Practice Information Infrastructure report.

The ANA's Steering Committee on Data Bases (now called the ANA Committee for Nursing Practice Information Infrastructure) was developed to "monitor and support the development and evolution of multiple vocabularies and classification schemes within the framework of the Nursing Minimum Data Set" (Henry, Warren, Lange, & Button, 1998, p. 321). Criteria have been developed to evaluate a classification system for use in a computer-based patient record. These criteria include (a) attention to clarity of concepts; (b) comprehensiveness in describing the clinical process; (c) definitions that are clear and concise; and (d) syntax, grammar, and defining attributes that distinguish and differentiate the concept under discussion. A list and description of ANA-approved classifications, data sets, and nomenclatures are discussed in Table 31.1.

Recently, the ANA also passed a resolution to create the Nursing Information and Data Set Evaluation Center (NIDSECsm) to evaluate information systems that are used to support the documentation of nursing practice. This group will continue to review terminologies in relation to the domain of nursing and the definition of specific criteria related to inclusion of a data set in an information system.

Language and Documentation: Future Directions

In recent years there has been a growing recognition of the contribution that nursing vocabularies can make in (a) documenting care, (b) linking nursing contributions to quality outcomes, and (c) costing out nursing care services based on patient acuity, age, gender, and so forth. Table 31.2 lists values associated with having a standardized nursing language.

Several additional forces continue to stimulate recognition of nursing language. They

TABLE 31.2   Value of a Standardized Nursing Language

- Creates a centralized database that represents important components of nursing practice.
- Identifies particular health problems and related health care of an individual or group based on nursing diagnoses, interventions, and outcomes.
- Establishes a database that describes patient (family, community) experiences and can differentiate responses by variables such as age, gender, health status, and the like.
- Provides researchers with a database that can be used to help direct new research initiatives.
- Facilitates a more accurate representation of patient phenomena, which can be used to guide the nurse–patient ratio by nursing problems.
- Helps nurses and administrators predict care costs more accurately.
- Improves communication across systems, states, countries, and continents.
- Fosters development of a standardized assessment model that can be used to describe responses and behaviors of populations based on events and to guide nursing judgments, interventions, and outcome evaluation.

include the (a) Health Insurance Portability and Accountability Act of 1996, (b) growth of information systems developers, (c) generation of reference terminology's, and (d) the *International Classification for Nursing Practice* (International Council of Nurses [ICN], 1996, 1999). Table 31.3 presents a description of these forces and the potential effects they will have on nursing language development.

Impact of Language Development

Nursing language and the development of a standardized, computer-based patient record will have an important impact on nursing knowledge development, education, practice, and research. The growth of electronic messaging development, refinement of nursing language, and inclusion of standardized languages in information systems will influence nursing in the years ahead.

Education

Developments in nursing language, informatics, and knowledge will shape courses taught in academic settings and promote inclusion of information on electronic messaging systems within curricula. Giving increased attention to articulating nursing knowledge (content and practice) within revised course structures (e.g., on-line computer-based courses) will enhance student learning. Documentation of care on information systems will be addressed in clinical practice sites, and role preparation will continue to respond to the complexities of practice and growth of the science.

Research

Nurse researchers will use a variety of methodologies to develop, test, and refine language. Qualitative researchers will continue to uncover the human experience through understanding meanings and responses associated with the lived experience. Quantitative approaches will isolate and analyze phenomena (concepts) in a more systematic way than before and test them across populations and health events.

Vocabulary research will continue to focus on (a) concept development, evaluation, and

TABLE 31.3 Forces Affecting Language Development

Health Insurance Portability and Accountability Act

In 1996, enactment of the Health Insurance Portability and Accountability Act (particularly, Section 263) stimulated increased interest in vocabulary development across all disciplines. The major thrust of this initiative was development of a computerized patient record. In response to this mandate the National Committee on Health and Vital Statistics (NCVHS) established the Sub Committee on Standards and Security (work group) to respond to the NCVHS request to develop the *Patient Medical Record Information (PMRI)* by August 2000.

In the spring of 1999, vocabulary developers across all disciplines responded to a series of questions from the perspective of the vocabularies that they were currently developing, using, and evaluating in clinical practice. The questions related to (a) the purpose of the vocabulary, (b) the scope of clinical practice covered by the vocabulary, (c) plans for expansion, (d) overall marketplace acceptance of the vocabulary, (e) translation of a particular vocabulary to other languages, (f) the current format used to communicate the vocabulary, and (g) the perceived long-term impact of the vocabulary on professional nursing.

Testimony will be reviewed and ultimately incorporated into a revised computer-based, patient electronic record. The emerging PMRI will be an official record used to document provider care and communicate patient information to insurers, administrators, and other groups, including information systems developers. It is essential that nursing continue to develop, test, and refine existing vocabularies and move toward a unified nursing language.

Information Systems Development—Health Level Seven (HL7)

Health Level Seven (HL7) was founded in 1987 by a consortium of health care providers and vendors "to develop and publish protocol specifications for application-level communication among diverse health care data acquisition, processing, and handling systems" (Beeler, 1999, p. 21). In 1994, HL7 began using an "open-consensus" process to develop standards for inputting, storing, and retrieving clinical data. The American National Standards Institute, (ANSI), accredits HL7. Each version of HL7 reflects improved technical capabilities and standards. The most recent version provides for a wide range of data to be incorporated into the information system, including drug prescriptions, discharge summaries, and clinical notes.

HL7's membership and organization is structured as multiple committees (e.g., Patient Care, Vocabulary and Data Warehousing) to work dimensions of the HL7 information system (Beeler, 1999). Nursing vocabulary developers are currently working with HL7 committees to ensure the inclusion of nursing information (language) within this system. Continued development and refinement of nursing vocabularies and related elements used to represent nursing language within HL7 will be essential to represent nursing adequately within this system.

Reference Terminology Model

The development of a *reference terminology* focuses on the inclusion of concepts that have formal definitions and are most effective when utilized within the framework of computer-based documentation system. A reference terminology model contains (a) terms or codes that are developed, tested, and validated; (b) generation of models that include clear attributes needed to reduce ambiguity of terms; (c) representational language within the science of informatics that is able to accommodate new terms as they emerge; and (d) software for processing, which includes rules, relationships, and attributes needed to accommodate the accessing of terms at various levels of abstraction (Bakken, 1999).

Current nursing vocabularies include terms for nursing diagnoses, interventions, and outcomes and contain language appropriate for inclusion in the development of a nursing reference terminology. The

(continued)

TABLE 31.3 *continued*

---

development of a reference terminology will (a) facilitate the move toward a unified nursing language, (b) create the semantic structure for those using different languages to talk to one another, and (c) generate an administrative model to evaluate cost and quality of outcomes. The current lack of a single unified language that contains the full range of concepts and terms used in nursing practice is viewed by some as limiting computer access for data analysis, costing out services, and reimbursing providers (Bakken, Cashen, Mendonca, O'Brien, & Zieniewicz, 2000). SNOMED is one example of a group seeking to develop a reference terminology (RT) of nursing languages.

International Classification for Nursing Practice (ICNP) Beta Version

For the past 10 years the International Council of Nurses (ICN) has worked to generate a common language that would increase nurses' visibility in describing and documenting care internationally. Support from the Kellogg Foundation and Kaiser Permanente has been used to develop and test an *International Classification for Nursing Practice, Unifying Language Framework* for nursing worldwide. Building on vocabulary developments in the United States (e.g., NANDA) the Alpha version (1996) of ICNP was published. After extensive feedback from nurses worldwide, the Beta version was published in 1999. This latest version contains a multiaxial structure that addresses nursing phenomena, nursing actions, and nursing outcomes. A series of axes are used to further amplify diagnosis and action. For example, the judgment axes include (a) the focus of nursing practice, (b) judgment, and (c) degree (severity). Language is used within each axis to further modify the axes (Coenen & Wake, 1999). Outcomes measure the status of nursing diagnoses after nursing interventions. The entire ICNP Beta version can be accessed at http://www.icn.ch/icnpupdate.htm. Currently, the Beta version of the ICNP continues to be validated through clinical testing internationally.

---

refinement of terms; (b) clarification of definitions used to describe the attributes of terms and avoid redundancy; and (c) improved translation of nursing vocabularies across languages (Chute, Cohen, Campbell, Oliver, & Campbell, 1996). A unified nursing terminology will emerge as an important component of vocabulary development as information systems evolve. As the reciprocal effect between language and knowledge development becomes more visible, nursing science will link nursing language to the continued expansion of nursing knowledge.

Practice

The development of a standardized, computer-based patient record will alter the way nurses document care. Data retrieved from new and improved information systems will (a) describe more accurately nursing's impact on patient outcomes, (b) provide a framework for costing out care and resource allocation, (c) identify patient problems within populations, and (d) link patient acuity and nurse provider mix more closely. Use of nursing language provides a clear way to articulate the patient's experience and the nurse's scope of practice. The refinement of language will reduce redundancy and increase the clarity used to communicate the message (Cimino, 1998).

■ Concluding Statement

The impact of nursing language and the growth of nursing science will enhance nursing's visibility in this millennium. To the degree that we are able to link the science with language and clearly articulate a disciplinary focus, nursing will continue to evolve as a central component of patient care. What is important to remember is that

1. Information systems that store, retrieve, analyze, aggregate, and compile all health care data will continue to become a reality;

2. The contribution of nursing language will continue to be recognized and valued as integral to patient care documentation internationally;

3. The patient medical record information (PMRI) will become an essential means of documenting and communicating care across providers;

4. Development of a standardized nursing assessment framework that complements nursing vocabularies will contribute new knowledge about the human experience; and

5. Research, development, utilization, and clinical testing of language will refine and expand nursing language and contribute to the evolution of disciplinary knowledge.

The knowledge and perspective that nurses bring to the patient experience will shape illness management and foster health promotion, personal transformation, and growth. The ability to communicate dimensions of patient experience through language will help make nursing's contributions to cost-effective, quality patient care more visible. Continued work on vocabulary development and standardization, such as the Nursing Vocabulary Summit held at Vanderbilt University in the spring of 1999 will bring together nursing scientists and information developers. The result will be an improved computer-based patient record that accurately represents the domain of nursing practice to patients, providers, and others worldwide.

■ References

American Nurses Association. (1972). *The standards of nursing practice.* Washington, DC: Author.

American Nurses Association. (1995). *Nursing: A social policy statement* (p. 8). Washington, DC: Author.

Baaken, S. (1999, October). *Toward a reference terminology in nursing.* Paper presented at Snomed Nursing Vocabulary Meeting, Snomed International, Chicago, Illinois.

Baaken, S., Cashen, M., Mendonca, E., O'Brien, A., & Zieniewicz, J. (2000). Representing nursing activities within a concept-oriented terminology system: Evaluation of a type definition. *Journal of the American Medical Informatics Association, 7*(1), 81–90.

Beeler, G. W. (1999). Taking HL7 to the next level. *MD Computing,* March/April 21–24.

Bixler, G., & Bixler, R. (1945). The professional status of nursing. *American Journal of Nursing, 45,* 730–735.

Carper, B. (1978). Fundamental patterns of knowing in nursing. *Advances in Nursing Science, 1*(1), 13–23.

Chinn, P., & Jacobs, M. (1983). *Theory and nursing: A systematic approach* (2nd ed.). St. Louis: Mosby.

Chute, C., Cohen, S., Campbell, K., Oliver, D., & Campbell, J. R. (1996). The content coverage of clinical classification. *Journal of the American Medical Informatics Association, 3,* 224–233.

Cimino, J. J. (1998). Diserata for controlled medical vocabularies in the 21st century. *Methods of Information in Medicine, 37*(4–5), 394–403.

Coenen, A., & Wake, M. (1999, June). *International classification for nursing practice: Beta version update.* Presented at the 100th Anniversary Conference of the International Council of Nurses, London, England.

Dickoff, J., James, P., & Wiedenbach, E. (1968). Theory in a practice discipline, Part II. *Nursing Research, 17,* 545–554.

Donaldson, S., & Crowley, D. (1978). The discipline of nursing. *American Journal of Nursing, 26,* 113–120.

Fawcett, J. (1984). The metaparadigm of nursing: Present status and future redefined. *IMAGE: Journal of Nursing Scholarship, 16,* 84–87.

Gordon, M. (1987). *Nursing diagnosis: Process and application* (2nd ed.). St. Louis: Mosby.

Gramling, K. (1999, April). *The art of nursing: Portraits from the critically ill.* University of Colorado, Dissertation (p. 49). University of Michigan: Dissertation Abstracts, (Microfilm).

Hayakawa, S. I., & Hayakawa, A. R. (1990). *Language in thought and action* (5th ed.). San Diego: Harvest Original, Harcourt & Brace.

Health Insurance Portability and Accountability Act of 1996, P.L. 104–191, August 21, 1996. *U.S. Statutes at Large* (Volume 110, pp. 1936–2104). Washington, DC: U.S. Government Printing Office.

Henry, S., Warren, J., Lange, L., & Button, P. (1998). A review of major nursing vocabularies and the extent to which they have the characteristics required for implementation in computer-based systems. *Journal of the American Medical Informatics Association, 5*(4), 321–328.

International Council of Nurses. (1996, 1999). *International classification for nursing practice, unifying language framework.* Geneva, Switzerland: Author

Jacox, A. J. (1974). Theory construction in nursing: An overview. *Nursing Research, 23,* 4–13.

Johnson, M., & Maas, M. (1996). Classifying nursing—sensitive patient outcomes. *IMAGE: Journal of Nursing Scholarship, 28*(4), 295–301.

Johnson, M., Maas, M., & Moorehead, S. M. (2000). *Nursing outcomes classification* (2nd ed.). St. Louis: Mosby.

Jones, D. A. (1998). Nursing knowledge and outcomes: An integrative perspective. In Sr. Callista Roy & D. A. Jones (Eds.), *Knowledge conference II: Linking knowledge with practice outcomes* (pp. 77–89). Chestnut Hill, MA: Boston College Press.

Kleinbeck, S. V. (1996). In search of perioperative nursing data elements. *Association of Operating Room Nursing (AORN), 63*(5), 926–931.

Kudla, K. M., & Rallins, M.C. (1998). SNOMED: A controlled vocabulary for computer-based patient record. *American Health Information Management Association, 69*(5), 40–44.

Lauden, L. (1977). *Progress and its problems: Toward a theory of scientific growth.* Berkeley: University of California Press.

LeVasseur, J. (1998). Plato, Nightingale and contemporary nursing. *IMAGE: Journal of Nursing Scholarship, 20*(3), 281–285.

Martin, K. S., & Scheet, N. I. (1992). *The Omaha system: Applications for community health nursing.* Philadelphia: W. B. Saunders.

McCloskey, J. C., & Bulechek, G. M. (Eds.). (2000). *Nursing interventions classification* (3rd ed.). St. Louis: Mosby.

Meleis, A. L. (1985). *Theoretical nursing.* Philadelphia: Lippincott.

Mishel, M. H. (1988). Uncertainty in illness. *IMAGE: Journal of Nursing Scholarship, 20,* 225–231.

Newman, M. (1986). *Health as expanding consciousness.* St. Louis: Mosby.

Newman, M. (1999). The rhythm of relating in a paradigm of wholeness. *IMAGE: Journal of Nursing Scholarship, 31*(3), 227–230.

North American Nursing Diagnosis Association. (1998–2000). *Nursing diagnosis: Definitions and classification 1998–2000.* Philadelphia: Author.

North American Nursing Diagnosis Association. (2000). [On-line]. Available: http://www.nanda.org

Nursing Intervention Classification. (2000). [On-line]. Available: http://www.nursing.uiowa.edu

Nursing Outcomes Classification. (2000). [On-line]. Available: http://www.nursing.uiowa.edu

Ozbolt, J. G. (1997). From minimum data to maximum impact. Using clinical data to strengthen patient care. *MD Computing, 14,* 195–301.

Radwin, L. (1996). Knowing the patient: A review of research on an emerging concept. *Journal of Advanced Nursing, 23,* 1142.

Rogers, B. (1997). Knowledge as problem solving. In D. A. Jones & Sr. Callista Roy (Eds.), *Developing knowledge for nursing practice: Three philosophical modes for linking theory and practice* (pp. 29–40). Chestnut Hill, MA: Boston College Press.

Rogers, M. (1970). *An introduction to the theoretical basis of nursing.* Philadelphia: Davis.

Roy, Sr. C., & Andrews, H. A. (1991). *The Roy adaptation model: The definitive statement.* Norwalk, CT: Appleton & Lange.

Saba, V. K. (1992). Home health care classification. *Caring Magazine, 11*(4), 58–60.

Saba, V. K. (1997). Why the home care classification is a recognized nomenclature. *Computers in Nursing, 15*(20), 567–573.

Toulmin, S. (1972). *Human understanding.* Princeton, NJ: Princeton University Press.

Tuttle, M. (1999, June). *"Problem lists" and other terminology: Lessons learned.* Paper presented at the Nursing Vocabulary Summit, Nashville, Tennessee. Lexical Technology, Inc.

Walker, L. O. (1997, November). Challenge of creating impact: Linking knowledge to practice outcomes. In Sr. Callista Roy & D. A. Jones (Eds.), *Knowledge impact conference II 1997: Linking nursing knowledge to practice outcomes* (pp. 5–16). Printed in 1998—not published—by Boston College Press, Chestnut Hill, MA.

Walker, L. O., & Avant, K. C. (1995). *Strategies for theory construction in nursing* (3rd ed.). Norwalk, CT: Appleton & Lange.

Warren, J., & Bickford, C. (1999, May 19). *ANA recognized nursing data sets, classification systems, and nomenclatures.* Washington, DC: American Nurses Association Committee for Practice Information Infrastructure report.

Watson, J. (1999). *Post modern nursing and beyond.* London, England, & New York: Churchill & Livingstone.

■ *Editor's Questions for Discussion*

Discuss factors that influence identification of a nursing problem. How does D. Jones' description of knowledge development relate to content in the Theory Part of this volume? What criteria exist for the use of vocabulary and classification schemes in a computer-based patient record? Why has language development seemingly been slower than development of classification systems for nursing diagnosis? What forces have contributed to language development? Propose methodologies for testing and refining nursing language. What relationships exist among the NANDA, NIC and NOC systems? Suggest directions for future development of classification systems.

How do Sills and Anderson (Chapter 77) address nursing language? What relationships exist between D. Jones' discussion and that of Stevens and Weiner (Chapter 38)?

32

Harvesting Knowledge

Conducting a Systematic, Integrated Literature Review

Ida M. Androwich, PhD, RNC, FAAN
Sheila A. Haas, PhD, RN

The abundance and availability of information in the literature is both a blessing and challenge. Today's clinical practitioners and researchers, far from suffering from a dearth of literature to synthesize, are surrounded by surfeit of published material that must be organized and managed. More than 2 million articles are published every year in more than 20,000 journals (Mulrow, Cook, & Davidoff, 1998). Harvesting this crop of knowledge and using it to inform and improve nursing practice presents an unprecedented opportunity for nurse researchers.

Most nurses are accustomed to narrative reviews, in which the relevant literature is abstracted, listed, described, and synthesized to some degree. On the one hand, a review that has been completed in a nonsystematic manner, although useful for gaining knowledge about a given topic, does not have the rigor to provide evidence that can be used for implementing practice changes. On the other hand, a precise and carefully completed systematic, integrated literature review can provide sufficient evidence for developing procedure protocols or clinical practice guidelines that will inform nursing practice.

Systematic literature reviews are defined as concise summations of the best available evidence. They require (a) use of rigorous, reproducible methods to formulate the question;

(b) exhaustive gathering of all pertinent evidence; (c) assessment of evidence for applicability to the specific question; (d) analysis and evaluation of available evidence; and, (e) presentation of findings in a clear and organized manner. Execution and presentation of a systematic, integrated review fully qualifies as research. Consequently, the methods used must be as rigorous, as reproducible, and as without bias as would be expected of any other study.

History of Systematic Reviews

Since the early 1940s when the first randomized, controlled, clinical trial (RCT) was published, more than 100,000 RCTs have been published (Mulrow et al., 1998). Many of the systematic, integrated reviews in medicine today include the review of RCTs that have been conducted and are amenable to quantitative methods such as meta-analytic techniques.

Nurses familiar with narrative reviews can differentiate them from systematic reviews by their focus and specificity. Narrative reviews tend to examine broad questions. Although evidence may be research-based, the methods used to garner, select, and appraise literature sources are not specified and thus may potentially introduce bias (Mulrow et al., 1998).

Many questions of interest to nurses are not best answered by "disease-oriented" or "organ-specific" evidence. Yet, these are the types of quantifiable outcomes that are the most prevalent in the health care literature. Evidence about the patient's well-being or choice by the nurse of alternative courses of action that would have an impact on quality of life are rarely found (Culpepper & Gilbert, 1999). Therefore attention must be paid to formulation of the question, including keywords used, so that the terms reflect a nursing practice focus.

Current Initiatives and Issues

Within nursing, there are several sources of reviews. The Cumulative Index to Nursing and Allied Health Literature (CINAHL) has a new journal, the *CINAHL Clinical Innovations Database* (CCID) (http://www.cinahl.com). In this quarterly online publication, comprehensive reviews are provided on the issue's topic, such as pain management or patient education. Another nursing journal, *The Evidence-Based Nursing Journal,* initiated in 1998, serves to "identify and appraise high-quality, clinically relevant research and publishes succinct, informative, and critical abstracts of each article" (http://www.evidencebasednursing.com, 1999).

Methods

Identification of a Well-Formulated Question or Problem

With thousands of potential answers available, the need to identify the question explicitly is central to a reliable and valid review. A well-formulated question is undoubtedly the sine qua non of a quality systematic review. The question serves as a guide for the entire review and provides rationale for subsequent decisions that will be made during the review. An unrefined topical area may yield a question that is too broad in scope to be useful (Shekelle, Woolf, Eccles, & Grimshaw, 1999).

A well-formulated question consists of a clinically, socially, or professionally important question, which addresses (a) a defined population; (b) a comparison; and (c) an outcome, on which basis a comparison is made. The content or topical area needs to be clearly circumscribed, but nontrivial. A number of considerations can drive question formulation.

What Types of People or Populations?

A good question explicitly identifies the type of population under review. For example, Is the topic of interest an older population? Which older population? The older adults who are living in long-term care (LTC)? The older adults living at home? How is the term "older" defined? Over 60? Over 80? Individuals may be further defined by gender, by age, or by disease condition.

Does the population of interest consist of individuals, families, communities, or aggregates sharing some identified risk factor? Is this population at home, coming to ambulatory facilities, in ICUs, or in LTC facilities? When a disease condition—say, diabetes mellitus—is being studied, certain factors that could possibly make a difference to results of the review need to be specified. Noting whether the focus is insulin-dependent diabetes or diet-controlled, adult-onset diabetes is important. In other conditions, for example, hypertension, a specific set of parameters (e.g., diastolic blood pressure of at least 90) must be noted. Conditions of measurement, such as sitting, standing, lying, or repeated measures also are relevant. As more is learned about DNA and the human genome project, questions for study may become as specific as limiting a population by DNA type.

What Types of Comparisons?

A comparison is merely the differentiating factor between the study group and the control group. Of interest are the conditions under which these comparisons will be made. For example, will there be comparison by a given intervention? If so, what specifically is the intervention? Are those using Drug A compared with those not using Drug A, or are they compared with those using Drug A and Drug B? How are Drug A users accepted or assigned—randomly, self-selected, self-reporting, or for convenience? A classic systematic, integrated review would typically require all assignments to be random. In nursing research, this requirement is not necessarily the case. Often, nurse researchers do not have the luxury of large numbers of randomized clinical trials (RCTs) in a particular content area; in such cases, casting a broader net than limiting the review to randomized clinical trials may be best. Further, in many cases the type of questions that are most important to nursing are not best answered by RCTs. Although RCTs traditionally have been used as the "gold standard" for research, some investigators have begun to criticize them. For example, Culpepper and Gilbert (1999) claim that RCTs are frequently not generalizable. The type of studies used for the review is an area of judgment by the reviewer.

What Types of Outcomes?

Being explicit about the types of outcomes to be compared is important. If the reviewer's interest is in looking at outcomes of patients' ability to tolerate Drug A or trying to assess a specific protocol for using Drug A, a study showing only mortality as an outcome would be of little use. Marek (1989) outlined classifications of outcome measures in nursing. The Iowa Nursing Outcomes Classification (NOC) (Johnson & Maas, 1997) provides a formalized classification of nursing-sensitive patient outcomes. Allowable criteria for establishing the presence of outcome achievement needs to be made explicit.

What Types of Study Designs?

At the outset, it is necessary to consider types of research designs that will be acceptable for inclusion in the review. Some questions

TABLE 32.1   Relationships Between Question and Design

Type of Question	Preferred Study Design
Therapy: Testing the efficacy of an intervention	Randomized controlled trial (RCT)
Diagnosis: Testing reliability and validity of a new diagnostic measure	Cross-sectional survey, using both new measure and "gold standard"
Screening: Testing value of test that can be applied to a population for early detection of disease	Cross-sectional survey
Prognosis: Determining likely course of disease	Longitudinal cohort study
Causation: Testing whether a putative harmful agent is related to development of an illness	Cohort, case-control study, or case report

lend themselves to a specific design and tend to exclude others. The important factor is a conceptual linking of the design to the problem or question. Greenhalgh (1997) suggested the relationships between question and design shown in Table 32.1.

Although the question often drives identification of the type of study designs that will be acceptable for review, the reviewer should not be too shortsighted early on and thus exclude studies that have the potential to contribute to evidence about the topic.

How strong is the evidence? There are a number of schemes for "grading the evidence." M. Chulay (personal communication, 1999) suggested the schema shown in Table 32.2.

■ Locating and Selecting Studies

The treasure hunt begins. Once boundaries have been set (year of publication, types of studies, and so forth), a good first step is to review completed systematic reviews, using available resources to determine whether other researchers are also working on similar review topics. At the beginning, a broad search strat-

egy is best for familiarizing a reviewer with available literature in the field and to assess its "maturity" (Brown, 1999). Major literature databases in health care include CINAHL (http://www.cinahl.com/) and MEDLINE (http://www.ncbi.nlm.nih.gov/PubMed/). The National Library of Medicine's (NLM) home page (http://www.nlm.nih.gov/) has links to many other useful sites and databases. Resources for evidence-based research include the Agency for Health Care Policy and Research (AHCPR) (http://www.ahcpr.gov/), the American College of Physicians (http://www.acponline.org/), and the Cochrane Collaboration (http://linux.chpt.es/cochrane/default/html). The Cochrane Controlled Trials Register, which is part of the Cochrane Library, contains references to more than 218,000 clinical trials.

In addition to automated searches, hand searches of journals in the field frequently yield studies that can be used. A technique, called "pearling," whereby references in an especially useful, pertinent study are screened for additional citations, is often useful. It is also important to check so-called fugitive literature, that is, material that has scientific merit but for one reason or another has never been published—

TABLE 32.2 Grading the Evidence

LEVEL VI	Clinical studies in a variety of institutions
LEVEL V	Clinical studies in two situations
LEVEL IV	Limited clinical studies to support
LEVEL III	Laboratory data, no clinical data to support
LEVEL II	Theory-based, expert consensus
LEVEL I	Common sense, manufacturer's guidelines

for example, research conference reports or well-designed studies not demonstrating significant findings.

Careful tracking and organization of references are essential. Several useful reference management software packages are available that are well worth the investment. Two examples are EndNote and ProCite.

■ Critical Appraisal of Studies for Inclusion in Review

Just as the skillful cook would not toss an egg of dubious quality in souffle or meringue, the skillful reviewer will not risk credibility of the entire review by including studies of doubtful value or relevance. Inclusion criteria should be based on the question and designed to ensure that findings will have relevance to the identified question or problem. For example, if the question were "What are the effects of exercise on weight gain in perimenopausal women with diabetes?," the criteria would include a definition of allowable "exercise," perhaps requiring that duration and intensity be specifically stated in the study. Criteria for "perimenopausal," for example, by age and history, would also indicate whether hormone replacement therapy (HRT) is allowable. Some metric (e.g., insulin dependence, glycosolated hemoglobin measures, and so forth) used for a subject to be labeled a diabetic would be desirable.

Once criteria have been established, it is useful to make a checklist with each criterion listed. This list then can be completed and attached to each study being considered for inclusion in the review. This paper trail allows the reviewer to ascertain quickly why a particular study was accepted or rejected for inclusion in the review. In the foregoing example, identified inclusion criteria were (a) age between 45 and 55, (b) exercise minimum of three times a week for at least 30 minutes, (c) target heart rate maintained for at least 20 minutes, (d) no history of hormone replacement therapy, (e) documented history of diabetes for at least 1 year, and (f) weight within normal limits at onset of the study. A sample checklist for the foregoing exercise study is shown in Table 32.3.

Use of such a checklist enables the reviewer to determine whether a given criterion was too stringent. When each study is rated and the rating checklist is attached, studies that previously were excluded because of that criterion can be readily reidentified. For example, if after a complete review, the reviewer found that most research reported participants as perimenopausal but did not give exact ages, the reviewer might reevaluate and opt to discontinue the greater than 45, less than 55 criterion for exclusion. Remember, the goal is to exclude studies that do not contribute to increased understanding of the research question but to include those that are well done and germane. Criteria serve the important purpose of having

---

TABLE 32.3   Sample Checklist for Exercise Study

STUDY #

Reviewer's Initials:

Criterion	Yes	No	Uncertain (include reason)
Age >45 and <55			
Target heart rate maintained during exercise for >20 min			
Exercise >30 min/3×/ wk			
No Hx HRT			
Hx of Diabetes documented for 1 yr			
Start weight WNL			

---

an objective metric for inclusion or exclusion, thus reducing bias as much as possible.

Having more than one reviewer allows for independence in selection, provides a check on the tools being used, and helps to prevent omission of good studies and inclusion of weak studies. This review process is used in graduate research classes. Even with seemingly explicit criteria, differences in interpretation arise and can benefit from discussion.

■ *The Funnel Effect*

The process of gathering evidence may be likened to a funneling process, with many studies gleaned during the broad search. A large number will be excluded after a brief glance at titles. Others will need a review of the abstract. During abstract review, more studies

will be excluded as the identified criteria are applied. Some few others only will be excluded after review of the entire study.

■ *Data Abstraction or Extraction*

Even if the reviewer is planning to be the only data abstractor, a form and code page will ensure that decisions made today will be recalled accurately tomorrow. This data abstraction, extraction, or summation form needs to be developed and tested. It should list, in a systematic manner, all the variables to be examined in each study and include an instruction page with necessary coding information.

Here again, it is necessary to test the data collection tool and directions to ensure that they display what is wanted, allow for exceptions, and are clear about how to deal with the vagaries, nuances, and exceptions that are bound to appear.

In the exercise example—effects of exercise on perimenopausal women with diabetes and weight gain—all the studies found will not define or report perimenopausal, diabetic, weight gain, and exercise exactly as the reviewer might wish. Nor will all studies conform perfectly to the tools used, no matter how well conceived the tools may be. Outcomes may be measured differently or defined differently. Judgment is used at every step.

Data Synthesis

Selecting Method of Analysis for Data Synthesis

A number of methods can be used for analysis. In the best of all worlds, studies would be conducted and reported in a manner that meta-analysis could be used and would allow a statistical measure of effect that would be reproducible. In the real world, other methods must be employed, along with efforts to ensure that results remain as reliable as possible. Quantitative methods, counts and weights, and qualitative methods all are acceptable.

In addition, complex statistical methods often are used to synthesize and interpret data in a systematic, integrated review. It is beyond the scope of this chapter to provide a detailed discussion of statistical analysis. However, an excellent overview and a discussion of this area were presented by Lau, Ioannidis, and Schmid (1998). Topics covered include (a) combining data, (b) evaluating the statistical heterogeneity of data, (c) exploring and explaining heterogeneity, (d) assessing the potential for bias, and (e) using meta-analytic techniques—including cumulative meta-analysis and meta-regression.

Interpreting and Presenting Results

Because of the pluralistic nature of nursing and the type and amount of research that has been conducted to date, strong *direct* evidence to answer a given research question is not always present. In the absence of research support for a direct causal link between specified variables, Cook and Campbell (1979) suggested building a "theoretical" model. The desire for causal links has given rise to development of evidence models. An example of a situation in which a researcher might want to build an evidence model is when there is no direct link between an institution using clinical ladders for nursing staff and increased patient satisfaction. Yet, evidence supports the use of clinical ladders for increased staff satisfaction, recognition, and productivity. Some evidence also supports linkage between increased staff satisfaction and increased patient satisfaction. Building an evidence model involves (a) identifying conceptual linkages to outcomes of interest, (b) collecting and analyzing the evidence related to each link, and (c) then combining the links (Mulrow, Langhorne, & Grimshaw, 1998). The outcome of a synthesized, integrated review is an evidence table that summarizes findings of the review and allows conclusions to be drawn about the strength and direction of the available evidence.

Final Report and Dissemination

The reviewer needs to report both what is known and what is not known because "proved" exclusions can be as significant as inclusions. In many cases, finding that there is not adequate evidence to support a practice change provides impetus for a clinical research study to provide evidence.

A systematic, integrated literature review is resource intensive and thus costly; the most scarce resource, the reviewer's time, is the prime resource required. Short cuts will always leave a mark in the form of a less robust review. Costs are associated with technology in copying for the paper trail. Unless the reviewer has significant expertise in searching the literature, many feel (with good reason) that a librarian's services in fine-tuning the search is apt to save time and thus money.

■ Concluding Statement

The value of systematic, integrated literature review is the confidence gained from having exhaustively and rigorously examined and synthesized all available evidence. From a risk-management perspective, asystematic, integrated literature review provides credible justification for practice innovation. In addition, deep familiarity with extant research in a given area allows not only the establishment of putative practice improvements but provides the ability to build protocol to evaluate practice changes. As richer literature databases are built and techniques in review methods are improved, nursing practice in the new millennium will become increasingly evidence-based.

■ References

Agency for Health Care Policy and Research (AHCPR). (1999). [On-line]. Available: http://www.nlm.nih.gov/.

American College of Physicians. (1999). [On-line]. Available: http://www.acponline.org/.

Brown, S. (1999). *Knowledge for health care practice.* Philadelphia: W. B. Saunders.

Cochrane Collaboration. (1999). [On-line]. Available: http://linux.chpt.es/cochrane/default/html.

Cook, T., & Campbell, D. (1979). *Quasi-experimentation: Design and analysis issues for field settings.* Boston: Houghton Mifflin.

Culpepper, L., & Gilbert, T. (1999). Evidence and ethics. *Lancet, 353,* 829–831.

The Cumulative Index for Nursing and Allied Health (CINAHL). (1999). CINAHL Clinical Innovations Database (CCID). (On-line). Available: http://www.cinahl.com/.

Evidence-Based Nursing Journal. (1999). (On-line). Available: http://www.evidencebasednursing.com/.

Greenhalgh, T. (1997). *How to read a paper: The basics of evidence-based medicine.* London: British Medical Journal Publishing Group.

Johnson, M., & Maas, M. (Eds). (1997). *Iowa outcomes project: Nursing outcomes classification (NOC).* St. Louis: Mosby.

Lau, J., Ioannidis, J., & Schmid, C. (1998). Quantitative synthesis in systematic reviews. In C. Mulrow & D. Cook (Eds.), *Systematic reviews: Synthesis of best evidence for health care decisions* (pp. 91–102). Philadelphia: American College of Physicians.

Marek, K. D. (1989). Developments in nursing classification: Classification of outcome measures in nursing care. In American Nurses Association (Ed.), *Classification systems for nursing practice* (pp. 37–42). (ANA Publication No. NP-74). Kansas City, MO: American Nurses Association.

Medline. (1999). [On-line]. Available: http:www.ncbi.nlm.nih.gov/PubMed/.

Mulrow, C., Cook, D., & Davidoff, F. (1998). Systematic reviews: Critical links in the great chain of evidence. In C. Mulrow & D. Cook (Eds.), *Systematic reviews: Synthesis of best evidence for health care decisions* (pp. 1–4). Philadelphia: American College of Physicians.

Mulrow, C., Langhorne, P., & Grimshaw, J. (1998). Integrating heterogeneous pieces of evidence in systematic reviews. In C. Mulrow & D. Cook (Eds.), *Systematic reviews: Synthesis of best evidence for health care decisions* (pp. 103–112). Philadelphia: American College of Physicians.

National of Library of Medicine's (NLM) home page. (1999). [On-line]. Available: http://www.hlm.nih.gov/.

Shekelle, P. G., Woolf, S. H., Eccles, M., & Grimshaw, J. (1999). Clinical guidelines: Developing guidelines. *British Medical Journal, 318,* 593–596.

■ Editor's Questions for Discussion

Discuss the research reviewed by Lindsey (Chapter 29) in terms of the qualifications for systematic review presented by Androwich and Haas. To what extent does Lindsey's review qualify as a systematic, integrated review? Pose further questions that might be addressed in the research reviewed by Lindsey.

Develop systematic review proposals suggested for the research advocated by Jenkins (Chapter 54), Kasper (Chapter 30), Froman and Owen (Chapter 33), Deets and Choi (Chapter 34), and Titler (Chapter 35). What elements are essential for valid and reliable systematic reviews? How explicit are criteria for outcome achievement in studies cited by these chapter authors? How strong is the evidence presented?

Suggest additional issues concerning criteria for variables included in systematic reviews. What other inclusion criterion may be relevant in the study example provided by Androwich and Haas? Identify limitations of systematic reviews. How may validity and reliability be established in building evidence models?

33

Instrumentation Concerns for Multicultural Research

Robin Dawn Froman, PhD, RN, FAAN

Steven V. Owen, PhD

Nurses profess to provide care to all individuals regardless of age, race, gender, or income. However, as our society becomes more multicultural, the provision of equitable care becomes more demanding. The problem is accentuated in our research efforts as we seek to study the scientific basis for our practices.

■ Challenges to Measurement

Although physiological data and measurements, such as temperature, blood pressure, cell count, ejection fraction, and glucose levels, may be assessed independently of biographic variables, the same cannot be said for many psychosocial variables of interest. Measures of attitude, affect, and perception often rely on self-report and are embedded in cultural and linguistic referents. These referents vary, sometimes dramatically, across ethnic groups, gender, and age.

Demographic Pluralistic Transformation

There is no question that the profile of demographic characteristics in the United States is changing rapidly. There is continuing pluralistic transformation in citizens and residents. In particular, Asian and Hispanic subgroups in the population are growing. The 1970s and 1980s brought an influx of Southeast Asian immigration. By 1992, 38% of immigrants to the United States were from Asia (U.S. Bureau of the Census, 1994). At the beginning of the 1990s, more than 22 million Hispanics lived in the United States (U.S. Bureau of the Census, 1991). Hispanics are expected to become the largest minority group in the United States, at a projected size of 53 million, and will represent more than 16% of the general population and 20% of children by 2020 (Sable & Stennett, 1998; U.S. Bureau of the Census, 1996).

These two large and growing ethnic groups share many characteristics that pose challenges to researchers. Unlike African Americans and Caucasians residing in the United States, Hispanics and Asians frequently have a primary language other than English. Many—particularly older adults or the elderly—are monolingual in their native language. Some 17 million Hispanic respondents to the 1990 census reported speaking Spanish in their homes, and more than 8 million stated that they could not speak English very well or at all (U.S. Bureau of the Census, 1996). Even among bilingual speakers, almost one quarter of Hispanics express preference for instruments written in Spanish (Marin & Marin, 1991). Additionally, educational levels in these ethnic subgroups tend to be lower than in the general population. Hispanics have the lowest high school graduation rate of any demographic group, only 50% nationally (Hayes-Bautista, Beazconde-Garbanaiti, Schink, & Hayes-Bautista, 1994), and approximately 45% of southeast Asian immigrants have only a primary grade or lower level of education from their native country or here (Devins, Beiser, Dion, Pelletier, & Edwards, 1997). Some researchers have recommended targeting a third-grade reading level when planning to collect self-report data from specific ethnic groups (Marin & Marin, 1991).

Health Problems of Ethnic Subgroups

Ethnic subgroups have significant acute and chronic health problems that are often managed by nurses. Diabetes and cardiovascular disease levels, asthma, and late stage breast cancer diagnosis are elevated in Hispanics (Bernal, Wooley, & Schensul, 1997; Sorlie, Backlund, Johnson, & Rogot, 1993). Southeast Asian immigrants and refugees are at particularly high risk for stress related disorders, depression, somatization, post-traumatic stress syndrome, and suicide (D'Avanzo, Frye, & Froman, 1994). Yet representation of these two ethnic groups in health care studies has been scanty, often impeded by shortage of adequately translated and validated research instruments. Limitations of using instruments developed and validated on the majority population are recognized, and caution should be exercised when interpreting findings from biographically different samples (Demi & Warren, 1995). But diverse subjects can at least be enrolled and represented in studies, as long as they are English-speaking. In the case of non-English-speaking individuals, such as many Asians and Hispanics, study subjects are not likely to be enrolled if instruments, regardless of adequacy or psychometric development, are not available. Thus the challenge currently facing researchers seeking to provide ethnic representation in samples is to develop, test, and validate instruments for use with subjects from alternative linguistic and cultural backgrounds.

■ Traditional Approach to Alternate Language Measurement Forms: Back-Translation

The need for alternate language forms of self-report instruments has been acknowledged for a while. Articles and texts have outlined traditional procedures for translations of English-language instruments. The most common and basic procedure is the use of translation and back-translation (Brislin, 1970; Brislin, Lonner, & Thorndike, 1973). Back-translation is sometimes referred to as double translation. In this procedure at least two bilingual speakers are needed. The first translator interprets the original language instrument into the desired second language, say, Spanish. This translation is the first, or forward, translation. The second translator subsequently translates the Spanish back into English. The back-translated items are compared to the original items for discrepancies in actual language or meaning. The translation and back-translation process continues until sets of items, original and back-translated, are deemed sufficiently close in both explicit and implicit language to be considered equivalent. Many examples in the nursing literature are cited whereby this process has been used as the initial step to generate alternative language scales for use with Hispanics or Asians (e.g., Bernal et al., 1997; Devins et al., 1997; Froman & Owen, 1999).

Limitations of the Back-Translation Approach

Back-translation is a good place to start, but it may lull researchers into a false sense of security in their use of translated scales if the process stops there. Unfortunately, back-translation often gives insufficient evidence about the equivalence of translated forms of instruments. Other, subtle measurement issues must be considered. For example, Hui and Triandis (1989) found evidence that, compared to Anglos, judgment styles of Hispanics create different patterns of responding in typical self-report surveys. Chen, Lee, and Stevenson (1995), and Si and Cullen (1998) found that Asians, more than Anglos, tend to drift toward the midpoint of self-report scales, particularly when there are an odd number of response options. Si and Cullen recommended omitting a midpoint

response option (i.e., giving preference to using an even-numbered response scale) when doing an Asian American cross-cultural study. Finally, in a cross-cultural study of adolescent depression, Iwata, Saito, and Roberts (1994) showed that, compared to Americans, Japanese youth responded quite differently to positively worded (but not negatively worded) items, invalidating the cultural comparison of scores. Failure to appreciate such subtleties may create bogus cross-cultural differences or similarities. The remainder of this chapter outlines other concerns, beyond merely moving items from English to a second language, which should be considered in creating alternative language scales. Methods of detecting differences between original and translated measures also are described.

Regional, Country, and Intracultural Dialectic Differences

Spanish and Asian-languages speakers are heterogeneous groups from a variety of homelands. Social and political differences both within and across countries are expressed in language. National and regional differences abound. Regional colloquialisms and idioms result in alternative interpretations of the same word or phrase. An English-language example may help to point this out. A sandwich may be called a "hero" in New York City, and at lunch it would not be uncommon to take orders for a hero or eat a hero for a meal. The same reference made in Utah might be either uninterpretable or perceived as cannibalistic intent on the part of the hungry person! Spanish-language expressions are notably different in Spain, Puerto Rico, Cuba, and Mexico. Similarly, Vietnamese, Cambodians, Laotians, Japanese, Chinese, and Koreans have different dialects, languages, and syllabaries.

If a translated instrument is intended for use with anything other than a geographically, socially, and politically homogeneous sample, the translation and back-translation process should include a range of bilingual speakers serving as both interpreters of items and evaluators of the sets of original and back-translated items. Whenever possible, the most standard form of the language, if one exists, should be used. The most basic form of the language selected for translation is preferred, with special attention to vocabulary, grammar, and syntax. This approach may be achieved with use of the committee method described by Guillemin, Bombardier, and Beaton (1993). This qualitative process requires two or more translators independently and simultaneously translating items into the second language. The translators come together after completing the translations and compare translated items for similarity. The goal is to produce consensus on translated items before back-translation. The consensual, agreed upon translated item is then back-translated by a third, independent translator.

Differences in Implicit and Explicit Meanings

Literal translations of words are relatively easy, with translation dictionaries, computer programs, and now, Internet translation sites. However, implicit or semantic meanings carried with translations may not be so apparent. In translating a measure of depression from English to Vietnamese, it may be possible to develop a literal equivalent for an item that asks respondents to indicate how frequently they have "the feeling I am going crazy." Flaskerud (1988) described just such a translation effort. She reported that most respondents queried in a study of 350 Vietnamese refugees in the Los Angeles area refused to answer the item. The problem was not in the wording of the item. The translation had legitimate semantic meaning and conveyed the intended notion of mental distress or illness. The high rate of refusal to answer was apparently the result of the Viet-

namese cultural norm to conceal or deny mental illness. Thus the explicit meaning of the item was clear, but authentic responses to the item were precluded by the implicit act of obscuring a culturally taboo condition.

■ Response Scale Considerations

The Likert-type response scale, whereby subjects respond to statements by indicating the degree to which they agree or disagree, is a commonplace format in measuring attitudes. The response format may be altered to have subjects respond by indicating their amount of confidence for performing specific tasks (Froman & Owen, 1999), or to indicate their frequency of engaging in particular behaviors (Gonzalez, Stewart, Ritter, & Lorig, 1995). These types of response scales and options are widely used because they spread respondents' scores out and often result in a normal distribution of scores across groups (Gable & Wolfe, 1993). Additionally, when response scales are used with more than a single item, as is typical with multiitem instruments, scores may be treated as equal-appearing interval data (Nunnally & Bernstein, 1994).

Few researchers look at item-level response patterns on scales after initial instrument development. In the case of translated scales, the inspection of such data may lead to some interesting discoveries. When translating an insulin management self-efficacy scale into Spanish, Bernal et al. (1997) found a number of difficulties with the self-report scale. The original English-language scale used a six-option format, with each option having a verbal and a numeric indicator. The original numeric indicators were "1," corresponding to the *strongest* agreement and "6" to the *least* agreement. Use of this numeric designation was troubling to Spanish-speaking respondents, as it was unclear how "1" could mean an indicator of strength and "6" could indicate weakness. Their cultural expectation was that the higher the number, the more there was of something. Thus the numeric rating needed to be reversed. Then, Bernal et al. (1997) found that the six response options, even with clearly stated verbal indicators, were too confusing. The clear majority of respondents could only meaningfully distinguish among four categories of response. This pattern of selecting only from four of the six possible response options was found upon visual inspection of item-level response patterns (H. Bernal, personal communication, April 15, 1997).

Flaskerud (1988) reported other difficulties in using the Likert-type format on translated scales. In the first example given, Spanish-speaking subjects were responding to a translated scale measuring alienation. Rather than producing item-level response distributions that resembled a bell curve, the format produced preferential responding at the extremes. Subjects did not distinguish between choices in the middle of the response format, and fully one third chose either *si* or *no* to respond to items rather than choosing midrange response options. These extreme responses were selected even after individual administration of questionnaires and encouragement to consider the entire range of response options. Flaskerud went on to report similar problems in use of the internal contrasts on scales translated into Vietnamese. When presented with a three-option response format (i.e., always, often, sometimes), about 50% of Vietnamese respondents answered merely *yes* or *no* to indicate the frequency of experiencing various affective states. These response patterns might have been masked if data analysis had been conducted on total scale scores. Inspection of individual item-level responses by subjects revealed that response formats commonly used on English-language instruments produced unanticipated response patterns in translated scales.

■ Empirical Assessment of Translated Instruments

Item-level analysis is not commonly used in translation efforts. Typically, item responses are combined to form one or more composite scores. For example, a 30-item self-report survey might have two subscores embedded in it. Thirteen of the items might comprise the first subscore and 17 items, the next. For many years, a typical method of developing and studying subscales has been to perform an exploratory factor analysis (EFA) on already collected data, to discover how many separate dimensions show up in the data. If, based on theory, the researcher expects a certain number of dimensions, the EFA may confirm that expectation or it may suggest how to alter the scale so that it produces the expected dimensions. The EFA may also suggest fewer or more dimensions than predicted. Focusing on an instrument's dimensions is essential because it is from this analysis that scoring rubrics are devised (DeVellis, 1991). But here, the instrument translation process can get short-circuited. Researchers interested in cross-cultural comparisons often assume that an instrument's dimensionality is the same for each compared group. To confirm that assumption, a researcher might do separate EFAs for subgroups. This step takes some courage, however, because many things can go wrong; for example:

- The original validation language group shows two dimensions on a scale, but the second, translated language group shows either three dimensions or one dimension on the translated scale.

- The analyst insists that the EFA program deliver the same number of dimensions for each subgroup, but doing so renders one or more dimensions uninterpretable for one of the groups.

- Both groups show the same number of dimensions, but different items and thus different interpretations comprise the dimensions.

Note that, when three or more groups are involved, say, with English, Spanish, and an Asian-language version of a scale, the likelihood of differences in subgroup dimensionality grows quickly. When evidence for common dimensionality across subgroups is not very supportive, there is little basis for cultural comparisons because such comparisons demand that the same constructs be used.

Using EFA to study an instrument's dimensions is artful work, and two researchers examining the same data might easily disagree about what they see. Today, there are more sophisticated tools to assess instrument dimensionality. Some statisticians have claimed that structural equation modeling (SEM) is the most significant analytic advance in the past 50 years (Stevens, 1996). That may or may not be true, but aspects of SEM certainly are invaluable in comparing translated scales. The SEM process of multigroup confirmatory factor analysis (CFA) is a form of strong inference about the equivalence of instruments. Whereas EFA is mostly a discovery process about instrument dimensionality, CFA is more "hard-headed." Now, the researcher must make an advance claim not just about how many dimensions are expected, but also must specify exactly which items belong on which dimension.

The CFA process will show how distant theory and data are, and when they are not congruent, it will suggest how to revise the instrument to conform to theory. When two (or more) groups are involved, CFA can test statistically whether the instrument dimensionality is the same for all groups. No matter how potent a multigroup CFA is, it cannot force the same dimensions to appear when the data resist it. In this case, the researcher may be left with a *descriptive* analysis of each culture in turn, stressing the apparent cultural differences in constructs.

■ *Balancing Art with Numbers*

Plainly, measurement can be the Achilles' heel of cross-cultural research. In converting an English-language instrument to another language, many opportunities exist for things to go wrong. When any single measurement episode is corrupt, the whole measurement process fails, and poor measurement virtually guarantees faulty research conclusions. When research is exploratory, the main harm of faulty measurement is probably that journal space is cluttered with irreproducible conclusions. In applied research, the measurement stakes are higher, because there results are often used to develop policy. Inept measurement will manifest itself as wrongheaded policy, a particularly troubling possibility with regard to cultural applications.

Some measurement specialists are so quantitatively biased that they imagine statistical programs will reveal and help to correct measurement flaws. That is only partly true. Statistical programmers did not have your research question in mind when they wrote the programs, and a particular program or analysis might be an unacceptable compromise for your data and objectives. Substituting mechanical calculation for substantive thinking is reckless. For example, in estimating a scale's internal consistency reliability, the "alpha-if-item-deleted" column of the printout is a favorite quantitative index (Ferketich, 1991). Using this column as the sole criterion to determine which items to toss out is badly shortsighted. It may be that perfectly credible items fail the threshold, *but still represent important data to collect*. The solution is to examine item content carefully. If you need such data to answer your research questions, keep the item(s); just do not insist that the item(s) be part of some subscale.

Remember that scale development and translation require as much art as statistical savvy. The following checklist can serve as a simplified guide to help you balance art with numbers.

√ Read a primer about instrument development. DeVellis (1991) authored a brief and readable introduction to scale development. Sage Publications (Fink, 1995) offers an excellent nine-volume paperback series called *The Survey Kit*. Volumes may be purchased separately or as a whole collection. If you need something more sophisticated, Nunnally and Bernstein (1994) is a classic work.

√ Before translating an instrument into target language, speak with someone knowledgeable about the culture. Show the person the English version of the survey items and response scale, and ask whether any cultural idiosyncrasies need to be considered in developing an equivalent version.

√ Recruit bilingual translators and back-translators who have a good working knowledge of the target culture. They should be familiar with idioms in both the U.S. and the target cultures.

√ Study existing research about how various response formats work (or do not work) with your target culture and use other researchers' experience in developing a sensitive response format. Beware of scoring the instrument, though, if the English version uses a five-point response scale and the translated version uses a four-point scale. Such a difference can render cross-cultural comparisons meaningless.

√ Enlist the help of a measurement specialist who can speak in plain language.

√ If you pursue factor analysis to study equivalence of dimensions on a translated scale, engage a statistician who can speak in plain language. This person might be the same as the measurement specialist. You should consider doing a little advance preparation. Statistics books are rarely fun reading, so try to locate understandable references, such as Bryant and Yarnold (1995), Kachigan (1991), or Tinsley and Tinsley (1987).

√ Try to get assistance from someone familiar with the target culture, who also knows about survey data. You will probably need clever suggestions about how to ensure a reasonable return rate. It will not be worth your—or your respondents'—time if you achieve only a 35% return on your surveys. An impoverished return rate will be almost assuredly biased and will probably lead to conclusions that are not representative of your target population.

■ Concluding Statement

Translation of scales is not a dauntingly difficult process, but doing it in a psychometrically sound way and preserving the intended meaning of instruments is a demanding task. It is clearly one that nurse researchers must address in the next century of research.

■ References

Bernal, H., Wooley, S., & Schensul, J. (1997). The challenge of using Likert-type scales with low-literate ethnic populations. *Nursing Research, 46,* 179–181.

Brislin, R. W. (1970). Back-translation for cross-cultural research. *Journal of Cross-Cultural Psychology, 1,* 185–216.

Brislin, R. W., Lonner, W. J., & Thorndike, R. M. (1973). *Cross-cultural research methods.* New York: Wiley Inter-Science Press.

Bryant, F. B., & Yarnold, P. R. (1995). Principal-components and exploratory and confirmatory factor analysis. In L. G. Grimm & P. R. Yarnold (Eds.), *Reading and understanding multivariate statistics* (pp. 99–136). Washington, DC: American Psychological Association.

Chen, C., Lee, S-y., & Stevenson, H. W. (1995). Response style and cross-cultural comparisons of rating scales among East Asian and North American students. *Psychological Science, 6,* 170–176.

D'Avanzo, C. E., Frye, B., & Froman, R. D. (1994). Stress in Cambodian refugee families. *IMAGE: Journal of Nursing Scholarship 26,* 101–105.

Demi, A. S., & Warren, N. A. (1995). Issues in conducting research with vulnerable families. *Western Journal of Nursing Research, 17,* 188–202.

DeVellis, R. F. (1991). *Scale development: Theory and applications.* Newbury Park, CA: Sage.

Devins, G. M., Beiser, M., Dion, R., Pelletier, L. G., & Edwards, R. G. (1997). Cross cultural measurements of psychological well-being: The psychometric equivalence of Cantonese, Vietnamese, and Laotian translations of the Affect Balance Scale. *American Journal of Public Health, 87,* 794–799.

Ferketich, S. (1991). Focus on psychometrics: Aspects of item analysis. *Research in Nursing & Health, 14,* 165–168.

Fink, A. (Series Ed.). (1995). *The survey kit.* Thousand Oaks, CA: Sage.

Flaskerud, J. H. (1988). Is the Likert scale format culturally biased? *Nursing Research, 37,* 185–186.

Froman, R. D., & Owen, S. V. (1999). American and Korean adolescents' physical and mental health self-efficacy. *Journal of Pediatric Nursing, 14,* 51–58.

Gable, R. K., & Wolfe, M. (1993). *Instrument development in the affective domain* (2nd ed.). Boston: Kluwer Academic.

Gonzalez, V. M., Stewart, A., Ritter, P. L., & Lorig, K. (1995). Translation and validation of arthritis outcome measures into Spanish. *Arthritis & Rheumatism, 38,* 1429–1446.

Guillemin, F., Bombardier, C., & Beaton, D. (1993). Cross-cultural adaptation of health-related quality of life measures: literature review and proposed guidelines. *Journal of Clinical Epidemiology, 56,* 1417–1432.

Hayes-Bautista, D. E., Beazconde-Garbanaiti, L., Schink, W., & Hayes-Bautista, M. (1994). Latino health in California, 1985–1990: Implications for family practice. *Family Medicine, 26,* 556–562.

Hui, C. H., & Triandis, H. C. (1989). Effects of culture and response format on extreme response style. *Journal of Cross-Cultural Psychology, 20,* 296–309.

Iwata, N., Saito, K., & Roberts, R. E. (1994). Responses to a self-administered depression scale among younger adolescents in Japan. *Psychiatry Research, 53,* 275–287.

Kachigan, S. K. (1991). *Multivariate statistical analysis* (2nd ed.). New York: Radius Press.

Marin, G., & Marin, B. V. (1991). *Research with Hispanic populations.* Newbury Park, CA: Sage.

Nunnally, J., & Bernstein, I. (1994). *Psychometric theory* (3rd ed.). New York: McGraw-Hill.

Sable, J., & Stennett, J. (1998). *The educational progress of Hispanic students. The condition of education 1998.* [On-line]. Available: http://nces.ed.gov/pubs98/condition98/c98004.html.

Si, S. X., & Cullen, J. B. (1998). Response categories and potential cultural bias: Effects of an explicit middle point in cross-cultural surveys. *The International Journal of Organizational Analysis, 6,* 218–230.

Sorlie, P., Backlund, E., Johnson, N., & Rogot, E. (1993). Mortality by Hispanic status in the United States. *Journal of the American Medical Association, 270,* 2464–2468.

Stevens. J. (1996). *Applied multivariate statistics for the social sciences* (3rd ed.). Mahwah, NJ: Lawrence Erlbaum.

Tinsley, H. E. A., & Tinsley, D. J. (1987). Uses of factor analysis in counseling psychology research. *Journal of Counseling Psychology, 34,* 414–424.

U.S. Bureau of the Census (1991). *The Hispanic population in the United States: March 1991.* Washington, DC: U.S. Government Printing Office.

U.S. Bureau of the Census (1994). *Statistical abstract of the United States, 114th ed.* Washington, DC: U.S. Government Printing Office.

U.S. Bureau of the Census (1996). *Statistical abstract of the United States, 116 ed.* Washington, DC: U.S. Government Printing Office. [On-line]. Available: http://www.census.gov/ population/projections/nation/nsrh/nprh1530.txt.

■ *Editor's Questions for Discussion*

Discuss the limitations of present instruments and methodologies in research, based on the diverse linguistic and cultural backgrounds of people in the United States. How may an investigator ensure the validity and reliability of translated scales? Provide examples of differing data interpretations due to differences between original and translated measures. What are implications of common nursing language as discussed by D. Jones (Chapter 31) and alternative language measurement concerns presented by Froman and Owen?

What research cited by Lindsey (Chapter 29) might be subject to challenges related to measurement issues? Why and to what extent may there be more measurement concerns in conducting interdisciplinary research than in conducting single-discipline research? How might investigators control for cultural variables that inhibit responses to items? What data analyses are essential to prevent masking of responses?

What implications does Froman and Owen's discussion about translated instruments based on theory have for the topics discussed by Deets and Choi (Chapter 34), Titler (Chapter 35), and Donnelly (Chapter 28)? Which of the areas of needed nursing research presented by Grady (Chapter 73) require expertise in scale development and translation? How might nurse researchers best gain that expertise? Apply the content presented by Froman and Owen to addressing ethical research questions raised by Davis (Chapter 6) and Kopala (Chapter 5). What distinctive translation and measurement problems arise in conducting ethics research?

34

Evaluating Theory-Based Interventions Using Evidence Tables

Carol Deets, EdD, RN
Euisoo Choi, MSN, MPH

T he original purpose for this chapter was to summarize a project with the aims of (a) identifying all systematically tested theory-based nursing interventions and (b) assessing the quality of intervention testing data using evidence tables. In the process of conducting the literature search to identify the theory-based interventions, it became clear that the project was not going to progress as planned. As is often the case in a well-planned study, one problem changes the project's parameters. The first of many changes was in the purpose of this chapter. The new purpose of this chapter is to relate the *process* followed in moving from evaluation of theory-based interventions to evaluation of a frequently tested intervention.

■ Overview

Clarity of communication is often difficult, but critical. That has been most true in construction of this chapter. The many changes necessitated by inability to meet the original purpose of the chapter resulted in a foundation of shifting sands rather than a foundation of hard rock for the research project. In an effort to improve communication of the process, changes, rationale for changes, and the results, several points of clarification are necessary.

Meaning of Theory

For purpose of this chapter, the term *theory* is used in a more restrictive sense than is usual in nursing. A theory is composed of a system of concepts and relationship statements (axioms, propositions, and so forth) that predict or explain a phenomenon. In order to predict or explain a phenomenon, there must be a body of evidence based on results of systematic testing of theoretical relationship statements. When developing this chapter, expectations were that advances in nursing science during the past 10 years would have resulted in research evidence supporting (a) development of theoretical relationship statements and (b) the use of interventions based on tested theories.

In nursing, the tendency is to limit theory by using modifiers such as "sociological" or "nursing." Use of theory in this chapter is not limited to a single discipline or profession. The concern was to identify theory-based interventions that have been studied in patient care situations, without regard to the discipline from which the theory originated. If a theory-based intervention is effective, will the client care which discipline developed and tested the theory?

Evidence-Based Tables

Other concepts that probably need amplification are evidence-based interventions and evidence tables. "Evidence-based" is the new "in" phrase in health care. The idea is not new to nursing; it just has a new label (Deets, 1998b). For evidence-based efforts, the process involves searching the literature for data related to a question, evaluating data from identified studies, and making decisions based on the evaluation (Jenicek, 1997). Use of evidence tables and meta-analysis are the two systematic techniques most frequently employed to summarize research data. Their use has produced positive and negative criticism. (See Crombie, 1998; Greco & Rudy, 1998; Linton, 1998a, 1998b; McGrath, 1998; and Williams, 1998, for examples of scholarly exchanges on the use

of evidence tables.) For this project the authors decided to use evidence-based tables because fewer assumptions are needed in constructing tables than with meta-analysis techniques *and* because it is the "in" thing to do.

An evidence table is nothing more than a summary of literature in tabular form. There may be an evidence table for each article or one that summarizes a series of related articles. In constructing evidence tables, the most important decisions concern the criteria to be used in evaluating the study and the data needed to evaluate the criteria. If too much is recorded, the table becomes cumbersome to use. If too little data are obtained, the table is useless. The best approach is first to decide on judgments that must be made as a result of evidence and then be sure that data needed to make these judgments are included in the table.

When using evidence tables, there are usually two judgments that result from data: quality of the study and quality of evidence supporting the intervention. The assumption has been that, if study quality is high, the quality of evidence supporting the hypotheses will be too. What if this relationship is not true? The U.S. Preventive Services Task Force (1993) recommended use of a six-category system to indicate quality of a study. The six categories ranged from systemic studies (highest) to published opinion (lowest). Others have employed less sophisticated category systems with as few as three categories. There is agreement that the highest quality studies include either random selection or assignment and employ an experimental design (clinical trial), whereas the lowest quality evidence is from opinion-based articles.

Another approach has been to determine whether research supported the intervention. The degree of support is categorized from good evidence to no evidence found. The number of categories used to represent the amount of evidence ranged from a high of eight to a low of three. This issue is not just one of significant differences or power of the study. On the one hand, if quality of the study was judged to be poor, the resulting evidence—even if significant and with considerable power (0.8)—would be questionable. On the other hand, if quality of the study was high but the power was low (0.2), the resulting evidence probably would be considered moderate if not poor. All such decisions are judgments and must be understood as such and not accepted as absolutes.

Assumptions

One assumption was that theory-based interventions existed. A theory-based intervention is developed from a theory's concepts and the relationship statements that connect them. The second assumption was that there were sufficient experimental studies with significant findings to justify use of interventions. The second assumption was a real concern in this project because Abraham, Chalifoux, Evers, and DeGeest (1995), in a review of six nursing research journals (two international journals and four North American journals), found that only 3.5% to 19.5% of the articles (N = 2,746) involved studies that included intervention. Their findings did not address whether reported interventions were based on theory. Many of the reported studies could have been, and probably were, designed to evaluate interventions currently employed in practice without regard to whether they had a theoretical basis.

■ Why Concern for Theory-Based Interventions?

If theories are the basis for understanding reality, then the most effective and efficient approach to advancing the nursing profession would be through generation of interventions derived from theories. The use of theory would result in an intervention that (a) would be usable in a wide range of parallel situations, (b) could be tested because the concepts were operationalized in prior research, and (c) would not be restricted to specific disease conditions. For instance, considerable research with diabetic patients concerns the approach that best results in patients' controlling their diabetes. Results from these research studies are not used with other populations, such as people with asthma and congestive heart failure because the intervention was tested with only diabetic patients. If the intervention had been theory-based, the disease status of clients would not have been a primary concern and the intervention could be used with other disease conditions.

Theory-based interventions need to be generated and tested because that is a more effective strategy than the trial-and-error approach used to develop and test most current interventions (if they are systematically tested at all). Why is it more effective? Because the theory's relationship statements allow the developer not only to determine what would most likely work, but also where it would work best, with what population of people, and in what kind of situations.

■ When Is an Intervention Theory-Based?

There are different answers to the question of when an intervention is theory-based, none of which are definitive. The most obvious answer is that a theory-based intervention is derived from the theory's concepts and relationship statements (a posteriori). But what happens more often in nursing is that an existing intervention is reconceptualized so that a theory's concepts and relationship statements explain how the intervention works (post hoc).

When an intervention is developed from a theory (a posteriori), the concepts and the relationship statements among the concepts lead to the intervention. The concepts with their relationship statements are not usually the basis for the intervention; rather, they indicate where an intervention should occur and what its outcome should be. For instance, Rosenstock's (1974) Health Belief Model was based on the relationship of four variables: perceived seriousness and susceptibility to the condition (could be, but does not have to be, a disease) and perceived barriers and benefits to taking a specific action (desired behavior) related to the condition. One theoretical statement is that the probability of an individual engaging in the desired behavior is low when perceived seriousness is low and the susceptibility, benefits, and barriers are moderate. Some research evidence indicates that the higher a person's perceived seriousness, the more likely it is that the person will engage in the desired behavior; thus the intervention should be designed to increase the person's perceptions of seriousness. The type of intervention is not addressed, and in this example it could be behaviorally or educationally oriented, as long as it is designed to change the person's perception of seriousness.

The post hoc approach is the one most often used in nursing. A time-honored intervention is reconceptualized and explained, or at least partially explained, by a theory. A nonnursing example of this post hoc approach is the current explanation that endorphins are the reason for effectiveness of acupuncture.

■ Why a Concern for Quality of the Research Results?

The main concern in evaluating the support for an intervention is whether obtained results are strong enough to recommend applying the intervention in the clinical setting. The answer is not an easy one. An effective intervention is one with demonstrated statistically significant

research evidence, replicated findings in several settings, and clinical importance. On the one hand, however clinically relevant they may be, interventions have not been studied enough to always yield statistically significant findings, nor have the studies always been replicated. On the other hand, because of its relative youth, nursing science cannot be expected to have amassed sufficient evidence to justify clinical use of all interventions. In the absence of research data, an intervention can be implemented as long as its effectiveness is systematically evaluated. Findings from carefully implemented interventions with built-in evaluation mechanisms for efficacy and cost-effectiveness can be shared with the community of scholars. Such findings are situation-specific and thus not generalizable. Because they are not generalizable, these findings must be consistent across multiple settings for there to be sufficient evidence of strength and efficacy of the intervention (Deets, 1998a).

All of these points are important, but they do not address the primary issue—judging the quality of the research and the quality of the evidence for intervention. A judgment must be made, and until the discrepancy between significant and clinically relevant results is more systematically addressed, the criterion of demonstrated significant results will remain primary for judging the quality of a research study.

■ The Process

The original plan for this project was to conduct a search of the current research literature (1989–1999) to identify studies that tested theory-based interventions. The most frequently studied interventions from this list were to be evaluated for quality of research. The expected end product was a list of interventions with sufficient data to justify use in patient care. Following is the process employed to fulfill this plan and rationale for deviations from the plan.

First Search

Both the Cumulative Index to Nursing and Allied Health Literature (CINAHL) and Medline were utilized in conducting the literature search. For CINAHL the search was guided by the following request: [Intervention or Clinical trial] AND [(Theory-based or Theory) or name of a specific theorist]. For Medline the search was guided by the following requests: Nursing AND [Intervention or Intervention study] AND [(Theory) or specific theorist]. These searches yielded only 24 studies that appeared to test theory-based interventions.

Of the 24 studies, four cited Orem's (1995) Self-care Model, seven cited Roy's (1991) Adaptation Model, six involved guided imagery with no specific theorist named, and seven involved therapeutic touch with references primarily to Rogers' (1990) theory. Studies involving Orem's Self-care Model and Roy's Adaptation Model were excluded because (a) different interventions were used for each study (e.g., diet and relaxation), and (b) the studies usually addressed multiple treatments (e.g., effect of an educational effort and use of imagery). A multiple treatment study results in confounded findings, thus limiting the quality of the results. Guided imagery studies were excluded because no one theorist was cited in relation to the identified studies.

In reality only one intervention—therapeutic touch (TT)—had been studied sufficiently to be included in this project. Unfortunately, this finding is consistent with that of Abraham, Chalifoux, Evers, and DeGeest (1995): that few intervention studies have been noted in the nursing literature. The majority of the articles that included TT as an intervention indicated that Rogers' (1990) theory was either the basis for the intervention or the authors implied that the theory explained why it was effective.

Since prior to 1989 there seemed to be only one intervention that had been studied employing some type of experimental design. Plans for the project were reassessed and reduced to conform to the reality of the data. Instead of summarizing the state of theory-based interventions, emphasis changed to summarize and illustrate steps taken when evaluating an intervention to determine (a) if it is theory-based and (b) if the quality of the research design and evidence for intervention are sufficient to recommend using the treatment in practice.

Second Search

Another search was conducted, seeking all TT studies between 1989 and 1999. Since there were only two studies that were seminal to TT research (Heidt, 1980; Quinn, 1984), these articles were evaluated to understand their impact on TT research. Other articles were reviewed, such as Daley's (1997) summary of TT research, but that summary was neither a meta-analysis nor evidence-based research, and thus the article was not evaluated as part of this project. Since the work of Straneva (1991) included communication in addition to TT in the intervention, it and other such articles were not included in the review. In the end, a total of 16 articles, representing 15 studies of TT intervention, were evaluated. The independent variables for one study were reported in separate articles (Peck, 1997, 1998). One study (Samarel, 1992) was descriptive in utilizing TT. But it did not address the effectiveness of TT, and thus was not included in the evidence tables that became the basis for the remainder of this chapter.

■ Decisions

Three decisions were required about each study in this project: Was the intervention used in the study based on a theory? Was there sufficient evidence to recommend use of the intervention in the practice setting? Did the quality of each study's design justify the evidence and support the intervention?

Theoretical Basis

First, a determination had to be made as to the relation between Rogers' (1990) theory and TT as an intervention. Earlier work cited Krieger (1979) almost exclusively. Later, Rogers' theory is mentioned as if the Krieger work evolved from it. Meehan (1993) conceptualized TT in terms of Rogers' theory and clearly explicated the post hoc nature of the relationship. She indicated how the energy fields in Rogers' theory and the energy transfer techniques of TT were compatible. Samarel, Fawcett, Davis, and Ryan (1998) combined TT with dialogue into one treatment in the belief that this compound intervention reflected Rogers' theory better than TT alone did. The compound intervention was developed a priori but the authors did not discuss the relationship between TT and Rogers' theory.

Clearly, TT as a treatment did not evolve from Rogers' (1990) theory (a priori). Although many authors cited Rogers' theory as a post hoc explanation for the intervention, they indicated a fit between TT and Rogers' theory because both TT and the theory dealt with energy fields. The authors did not discuss Rogers' theory as an explanation of how the treatment worked. The theory has not been extensively tested nor does it include explanations for how the concepts relate to one another. Once the theory has matured through rigorous testing, it may provide the explanatory power it currently lacks for TT.

Criteria Addressed in Evaluating the Quality of the Research

Next, the issue of research quality had to be decided. The authors of this chapter developed an evidence table from each of the articles they

reviewed. Those evidence tables, not shown in this chapter, made possible the evaluation and summarization of content as shown in Table 34.1. The first section of each evidence table included basic information, such as research questions, study design, sample, description of intervention, summary of results, and authors' conclusions. This information about each study had to be readily at hand for final analysis of the data collected in the remainder of that evidence table.

Remaining topics addressed in each evidence table included the usual criteria employed in evaluating a research study: (a) presence of inclusion and exclusion criteria, (b) appropriateness of data collection and analysis, (c) design threats to internal and external validity, (d) strength of the intervention (how often and for how long), and (e) time frame for the study. From these data two conclusions can be drawn: quality of the study and amount of support of an intervention for use in practice.

Evaluation of Quality

The quality of each study design was summarized on the basis of a simple three-category system:

A = experimental studies that employed random assignment or random selection of subjects and included a control group,

B = quasi-experimental studies (all research studies that did not qualify in category A), and

C = nonexperimental studies.

The amount of support for use of the intervention was described in a second three-category system:

A = significant differences that support the hypotheses (questions) and no major design issue,

B = significant differences that support the hypotheses (questions) but multiple design issues, and

C = no significant differences.

TABLE 34.1 Summary of Content Considered in Evaluating Quality of the Research

Content	Description
Research Questions	Report question(s) or hypotheses
Study Design	Indicate in random, blind, repeated measures
Population	Brief description
Sample	Details of sample characteristics
Inclusion/Exclusion Criteria	Indicate what author says about these criteria
Time Frame—study	How long was it conducted?
Time Frame—treatment	How long? How often? Other relevant data?
Intervention	Describe the total intervention and mock intervention
Data Collection	What was used for each dependent variable?
Analysis	Technique used and if inappropriate
Results	Reported in terms of research questions (hypotheses) if other findings are reported, they are included too.
Conclusions	Actual report of conclusions as stated in document
Threat to validity	
Randomization	What type was used?
Mortality	Describe subjects lost to follow-up
Blinding	Did person giving intervention know whether the subjects were in the experimental or control groups?
Homogeneity	Were groups equal at the beginning?
Groups treated equally?	Support for presence or absence of equality?
Comments	Major questions not answered in the study summarized
Remarks	Any interesting point not necessarily related to design or quality

■ Summary of Data from the Evidence Tables

The quality of studies has improved dramatically in the past 10 years, with 12 of the 15 studies rated "A." (See Table 34.2.) Of the 15 studies, only two received a "B" judgment and one a "C" judgment for quality of the study. The one "C" study was a qualitative study; thus it would have been inappropriate to include testing for significance. Even though the studies were evaluated positively, there were design issues, which may have been due to incomplete reporting. It was not possible to determine whether information was missing or whether there was a design flaw. For instance, subjects were lost to follow-up in many of the studies, but almost none of the authors stated reasons for their loss. When there appeared to be protocol variations, it was often impossible to determine why the variations occurred. Reporting variations allows others to anticipate the same problem in future studies and develop appropriate solutions. Equality of groups prior to intervention was an important issue not often addressed.

TABLE 34.2 Summary of Articles by Research Questions, Results, and Quality of the Study

Authors	Research Questions	Results	Quality of Study/Evidence
Gagne & Toye (1994)	Anxiety reduced for TT subjects (Ss) on state–trait anxiety inventory (STAI)	Sig reduction in STAI scores	A/B
	Anxiety reduction for both TT & RT groups would exceed MTT for STAI and physical movement	Sig reduction in STAI, but not physical movements for all groups. No real test for hypothesis	
Hughes et al. (1996)	Describe adolescent psychiatric patients' experience with TT	Two themes—therapeutic relationship and body/mind connection	C/C
Ireland (1998)	Decrease in posttest anxiety for TT than mock TT (MTT)	NS differences between TT and MTT	A/C
Kramer (1990)	Increase in relaxation scores for TT than MTT as measured by physical indicators	Insufficient information to determine direction of sig differences. TT is credited with decreased time needed to calm child	A/C
Meehan (1993)	Decrease in post pain scores for TT than MTT or Standard Intervention (SI)	Sig difference in TT and SI group with SI more effective. Nonsig between TT and MTT (p. 06)	A/C
Olson et al. (1992)	Stress decreases from pre to post TT	STAI scores significantly reduced for TT	B/B
	Decrease in stress will be greater for Ss who receive TT than sit still	Sig reduced STAI scores for TT than sitting still	
	Phy measurements will reflect relaxation response for TT Ss	NS	
	Amount of decreased stress related to length of treatment	Amount of decrease in stress is related to length related (0.48, 0.46)	B/B
Olson & Sneed (1995)	TT decreases anxiety (STAI, POMS, VASs) in episodic stress but not normal	NS T-tests even though means scores decreased for times 1 and 2	A/C
	TT does not decrease anxiety in healthy volunteers who are stressed in response to episodic stressor	NS	

Authors	Research Questions	Results	Quality of Study/Evidence
	TT more effective in decreasing anxiety in highly anxious Ss	NS but in the right direction	
	Greater decrease in anxiety in high and low anxious, non-TT Ss after occurrence of stressor	NS	
Olson et al. (1997)	Highly anxious Ss before exams who receive TT have less decrement in immunological indicators than control Ss	Sig difference for 2 of 7 tests	A/B
	Highly anxious Ss before exams who receive TT will have greater T-lymphocyte response	NS but in the correct direction	
	Highly anxious Ss before exams who receive TT will have a greater Haemophilus vaccine response	NS	
Peck (1997)	Post pain will be decreased from baseline following TT	Did not test this hypothesis	A/C
	TT Ss will have greater reduced pain than progressive muscle relaxation (PMR)	PMR was sig more effective	
Peck (1998)	Improved functional ability following TT compared to baseline	5 of 11 subscales were sig difference from baseline to post 6th treatment.	A/B or C
	TT Ss will have more functional ability than PMR Ss	TT sig. better for mobility and hand function (2 of 12 scales)	
Quinn (1989)	Decrease at post in anxiety, sys blood pressure (SBP), and heart rate (HR) for TT than MTT or control	NS findings	
	Decrease in anxiety, SBP and HR 1 hr post TT treatment than MTT or control	NS findings	
Quinn & Strelkauskas (1993)	Are there differences in immunologic profile post and follow-up TT?	No statistical testing— looked at % change in data	B/C
	Are patterns in profiles before, after, or delayed TT?		

TABLE 34.2 *continued*

Authors	Research Questions	Results	Quality of Study/Evidence
Quinn & Strelkauskas (1993)	Are there differences in psychological measures post and follow-up TT?		
	Are there patterns in psy measures before, post, and follow-up TT?		
	Are there patterns of effectiveness for TT and psychoimmunologic outcomes post TT?		
	Are there patterns in immunologic and psy measures post TT?		
	Are there patterns among time, effectiveness and psychoimmunologic outcomes?		
Samarel et al. (1998)	TT and dialogue Ss would have lower anxiety pre and post operatively, more positive mood pre and post operatively, and less postoperative pain intensity and distress than control Ss	NS	A/C
Sneed et al. (1997)	How do people describe first TT experience?	Qualitative study—description/themes	C/C
Simington & Laing (1993)	TT lower post anxiety score compared to back rub from RN not familiar with TT	Sig between Ss who received TT and back rub from RN not familiar with TT	A/B
	Sig lower anxiety for TT compared with RN familiar with TT	NS	
	No differences between RNs familiar with TT and RNs not familiar	NS	
Turner et al. (1998)	TT would reduce pain and anxiety over MTT	Sig for TT for 2 of 3 McGill (pain) scales, NS for VAS pain (2 scales), sig for VAS anxiety, NS for level of satisfaction, NS in medicine use and differences in phy measures were not tested due to small sample size.	A/B

The number of persons involved in administration of the intervention was another potential design flaw seldom addressed, even though evidence that the individual providing the treatment could affect the results is documented.

None of the 15 studies received an "A" judgment for quality of evidence supporting use of the intervention in the practice setting. In fact, only 5 of the studies were judged to have a "B" rating. In other words, 11 of the studies did not have evidence to support use of the TT intervention in practice. These findings are contrary to much of the current thought regarding TT. Three of the 5 studies rated "B" had one factor in common—use of Spielberger's State–Trait Anxiety Inventory (STAI) (Spielberger, Goruch, Luschene, Vagg, & Jacobs, 1983). Each of these articles included evidence on quality of the inventory's reliability and validity. One explanation for the finding of significant differences in these three studies is that the STAI is a sensitive instrument that captures subtle differences not measured by other instruments. Studies that improve their instrumentation probably would result in supportive evidence for the TT intervention.

■ Discussion

Two main issues are considered in this section. Because one of the purposes of this chapter was to illustrate the use of evidence tables, the value of the tables is discussed from several perspectives. As findings of this project are contrary to commonly held beliefs about research results in TT, possible reasons for these finding are considered.

Value of Evidence Tables

Daley (1997) and Mulloney and Wells-Federman (1996) have summarized much of the opinion and research-based literature on TT during the last 29 years. Comparing recommendations from their effort with results of this project is most instructive. Conclusions reached by the authors of this chapter concerning the value of TT and its use in practice and those reached by Mulloney and Wells-Federman (1996), as well as Daley (1997), differ sharply. Why do they?

Both the quality of the study's design and strength of the evidence for TT were assessed during this project. Most of the reviewed studies employed a randomized trial design with a control group. But identification and control of variables that could affect the results were questionable, allowing many competing hypotheses for the findings. Use of a more in-depth article evaluation led to the conclusion that, whereas the designs per se had improved, actual control of experimental situations with all their influencing variables needs to be enhanced.

The objective method of reporting results using the evidence-table criteria resulted in judgments that may not have been made using other techniques. Because the researchers evaluated each article individually, premature closure on any topic did not occur. As each topic was reviewed across tables, consistency in the topic was either obvious or questionable. When questionable, data were reexamined to identify reasons for inconsistencies. This strategy led to discovery of consistencies and inconsistencies that may not have been found if quality judgments alone had been used.

The articles were easy to abstract once content of the evidence tables had been determined. In reality, evidence tables are just a systematic method for recording information and are no more useful than their contents. The most important aspect of building tables is determining the pertinent contents to be recorded. Probably the next most important factor is creating a simple method within the tables to summarize the quality of the research design and the study's results. An unexpected observation was that the strategy for composing the evidence table related to TT research studies appears to be generalizable to most research articles. In other words, researchers could create a searchable database, using the evidence table criteria, which could be utilized with all the research literature in which they were interested. Searches of the database could result in a summary of (a) one article, (b) all articles using a specific method (or instrument), (c) articles dealing with a specific treatment, and (d) any other topic appropriate to the database. What a treasure this database would become over time!

A problem with the evidence-table system employed for this project was that the hypotheses (questions) section was separate from the result section. Combining these two sections into one would be advantageous. Presentation of results for hypothesis testing and findings without reference to the hypothesis (question) is problematic. To determine clearly whether there was support for the TT hypothesis, findings were reported for each hypothesis, as shown in Table 34.2. Results of other analyses were reported separately without reference to hypotheses (questions). Sometimes, reported significant differences in the reviewed studies were for data that did not address effectiveness of the intervention. Some study authors would include these significant findings in the article as if they were the main point of the study. For almost none of the articles the authors did not organize presentation of findings in terms of hypotheses (questions). Deciding which findings went with which hypothesis (question) was often difficult. No wonder there is so much confusion in this area!

Why the Nonsupportive Findings for TT?

Several reasons are suggested for the nonsupportive finding for TT intervention, including quality of instrumentation and different types of interventions under the TT label. Finally, inadequacy of reporting in some journals, specifically practice journals, influenced evaluation of some studies.

Instrumentation

The fact that the STAI instrument was used in three of five studies that reported significant support for use of TT is interesting. The STAI is a well-known instrument with considerable evidence for reliability and validity across multiple research settings. Sensitivity to change has been reported in many articles, so it is not surprising that STAI produced evidence of change due to TT intervention. In each of the studies the state version (how a person feels right then) of the instrument was used to measure change. A state-type instrument is more likely to measure change, but change is short-lived compared to traits. Selection of the instrument to measure expected change(s) in response to intervention is an important step in ensuring that the intervention has enough strength to produce desired changes.

Different Interventions

Examination of protocols for TT revealed different types of TT interventions. Not only were the TT techniques employed differently, but the duration of treatments and number of times TT was provided prior to measurement of the outcome variable also differed. If only one of these variables differed in a study, a case could be made that, for the most part, interventions were the same. This project demonstrated that several variables differed within each TT intervention.

A frequent criticism of early TT studies concerned a threat to design validity because of attention received by the treatment group. Two landmark studies by Heidt (1980) and

Quinn (1984) were instrumental in shaping quality of research studies in response to this criticism. Heidt designed a study that compared TT with casual touch (i.e., a control group). Use of the casual touch group addressed prior design criticism of internal validity by having as much time spent with subjects as in the real treatment. Quinn was the first to study how effects of TT were obtained. She contended that with an exchange of energy direct contact was not necessary. Her study involved two groups: Noncontact TT and a mock TT (MTT). The MTT procedure is the same for the TT procedure except that the nurse is counting backward to ensure that her or his energy is not being exchanged. Quinn contended that hers was the first study to use MTT as such. The noncontact TT group's anxiety scores were significantly lower than the control group's.

Since introduction of the MTT, almost all studies of TT as intervention included an MTT group, improving the quality of the research design. Even though almost all studies were judged to be in the "A" category, there were design problems. Major issues were (a) lack of a standard treatment duration, (b) variation in number of times a treatment was given, (c) impact (strength) of the intervention, and (d) amount of time between treatments when there were multiple applications.

Adequacy of Research Reports

Although some reports in research journals were not all that they could be, details found in most research journals are not reported in practice journals. Such inattention to detail left the reader wondering whether something had been omitted due to editing of the article or for some other reason. Decisions about internal and external validity of the study were extremely difficult to make, as few authors directly assessed their own studies. An excellent example is the internal validity criterion, mortality. As previously mentioned, even though several authors reported that subjects left the study, they provided no information as to why. This lack left reviewers with the task of trying to decide whether the reasons were within acceptable parameters or whether the design was flawed. Another good example was the issue of equality of the control and experimental groups prior to the intervention. Almost none of the authors addressed this critical issue.

■ Concluding Statement

Conclusions fell into several categories: theory related, use of evidence-based tables, content of the tables, and TT intervention. Because the basis for each conclusion is already noted in this chapter, the conclusions are simply listed here.

1. Theory-based nursing interventions have not been studied enough to produce sufficient findings to justify their use in the practice setting.

2. TT was not developed from a theory, even though many authors cited Rogers' theory.

3. Evidence tables allowed easy documentation of an article's content and summarization across articles.

4. Evidence tables as constructed in this project provided information on quality of the study's design and quality of research findings.

5. The value of evidence tables exceeds the cost of time needed to develop them.

6. Quality of research designs in TT studies has improved during the past 10 years, but problems still exist in meeting internal and external validity criteria for control of variables.

7. Little research evidence was found to support use of TT in the practice setting.

■ *References*

Abraham, I. L., Chalifoux, Z. L., Evers, G. C. M., & DeGeest, S. (1995). Conditions, interventions, and outcomes in nursing research: A comparative analysis of North American and European/international journals (1981–1990). *International Journal of Nursing Studies, 32*(2), 173–187.

Crombie, I. K. (1998). The limits of evidence-based medicine. *Pain Forum, 7*(1), 63–65.

Daley, B. (1997). Therapeutic touch, nursing practice and contemporary cutaneous wound healing research. *Journal of Advanced Nursing, 25,* 1123–1132.

Deets, C. (1998a). When is enough, enough? *Journal of Professional Nursing, 14*(4), 196.

Deets, C. (1998b). Evidence-based practice—Been there doing that. *Journal of Professional Nursing, 14*(6), 322.

Gagne, D., & Toye, R. C. (1994). The effects of therapeutic touch and relaxation therapy in reducing anxiety. *Archives of Psychiatric Nursing, 8*(3), 184–189.

Greco, C. M., & Rudy, T. E. (1998). In search of the superpractitioner. *Pain Forum, 7*(1), 60–62.

Heidt, P. (1980). Effects of therapeutic touch on anxiety level of hospitalized patients. *Nursing Research, 30*(1), 32–37.

Hughes, P. P., Meize-Grochowski, R., & Harris, C. N. D. (1996). Therapeutic touch with adolescent psychiatric patients. *Journal of Holistic Nursing, 14*(1), 6–23.

Ireland, M. (1998). Therapeutic touch with HIV infected children: A pilot study. *Journal of the Association of Nurses in Aides Care, 9*(4), 68–77.

Jenicek, M. (1997). Epidemiology, evidence-based medicine, and evidence-based public health. *Journal of Epidemiology, 7,* 187–197.

Kramer, N. A. (1990). Comparison of therapeutic touch and casual touch in stress reduction of hospitalized children. *Pediatric Nursing, 16*(5), 483–485.

Krieger, D. (1979). *The therapeutic touch: How to use your hands to help or to heal.* Englewood Cliffs, NJ: Prentice-Hall.

Linton, S. J. (1998a). In defense of reason: Meta-analysis and beyond in evidence-based practice. *Pain Forum, 7*(1), 46–54.

Linton, S. J. (1998b). The scientist-practitioner in the twenty-first century. *Pain Forum, 7*(1), 66–67.

McGrath, P. J. (1998). Best evidence meta-analysis is part of the solution, not part of the problem. *Pain Forum, 7*(1), 58–59.

Meehan, T. C. (1993). Therapeutic touch and postoperative pain: A Rogerian research study. *Nursing Science Quarterly, 6*(12), 69–78.

Mulloney, S. S., & Wells-Federman, C. L. (1996). Therapeutic touch: A healing modality. *The Journal of Cardiovascular Nursing, 10*(3) 27–49.

Olson, M., Sneed, N., Bonadonna, R., Ratliff, J., & Dias, J. (1992). Therapeutic touch and post-hurricane Hugo stress. *Journal of Holistic Nursing, 10*(2), 120–136.

Olson, M., & Sneed, N. (1995). Anxiety and therapeutic touch. *Issues in Mental Health Nursing, 16,* 97–108.

Olson, M., Sneed, N., LaVia, M., Virella, G., Bonadonna, R., & Michel, Y. (1997). Stress-induced immunosuppression and therapeutic touch. *Alternative Therapies, 3*(2), 68–74.

Orem, D. D. (1995). *Nursing: Concepts of practice* (5th ed.). St. Louis: Mosby.

Peck, S. D. (1997). The effectiveness of therapeutic touch for decreasing pain in elders with degenerative arthritis. *Journal of Holistic Nursing, 15*(2), 176–198.

Peck, S. D. (1998). The efficacy of therapeutic touch for improving functional ability in elders with degenerative arthritis. *Nursing Science Quarterly, 11*(3), 123–131.

Quinn, J. F. (1984). Therapeutic touch as energy exchange: Testing the theory. *Advances in Nursing Science, 6*(2), 42–49.

Quinn, J. F. (1989). Therapeutic touch as energy exchange: Replication and extension. *Nursing Science Quarterly, 2*(2), 79–87.

Quinn, J. F., & Strelkauskas, A. J. (1993). Psychoimmunology effects of therapeutic touch on practitioners and recently bereaved recipients: A pilot study. *Advances in Nursing Science, 15*(4), 13–26.

Rogers, M. E. (1990). Nursing: Science of unitary, irreducible, human beings: Update 1990. In E. A. M. Barrett (Ed.), *Visions of Rogers' science-based nursing* (pp. 5–12). New York: National League for Nursing Press.

Rosenstock, I. M. (1974). The health belief model and preventive health behavior. *Health Education Monograph, 2,* 354–386.

Roy, C., & Andrews, H. A. (1991). *The Roy adaptation model: The definitive statement.* Norwalk, CT: Appleton & Lange.

Samarel, N. (1992). The experience of receiving therapeutic touch. *Journal of Advanced Nursing, 17,* 651–657.

Samarel, N., Fawcett, J., Davis, M. M., & Ryan, F. M. (1998). Effects of dialogue and therapeutic touch on preoperative and postoperative experiences of breast cancer surgery: Exploratory study. *Oncology Nursing Forum, 25*(6), 1369–1376.

Simington, J. A., & Laing, G. P. (1993). Effects of therapeutic touch on anxiety in the institutionalized elderly. *Clinical Nursing Research, 24*(4), 438–450.

Sneed, N.V., Olson, M., & Bonadonna, R. (1997). The experience of therapeutic touch for novice recipients. *Journal of Holistic Nursing, 15*(3), 243–253.

Spielberger, C. D., Goruch, R. L., Luschene, R., Vagg, P. R., & Jacobs, G. A. (1983). *Manual for the state–trait anxiety inventory (Form Y).* Palo Alto, CA: Consulting Psychologists Press.

Straneva, J. E. (1991). Therapeutic touch: Placebo effect or energetic form of communication. *Journal of Holistic Nursing, 9*(2), 41–61.

Turner, J. G., Clark, A. J., Gauthier, D. K., & Williams, M. (1998). The effect of therapeutic touch on pain and anxiety in burn patients. *Journal of Advanced Nursing, 28*(1), 10–20.

U.S. Preventive Services Task Force. (1993). Screening for adolescent idiopathic scoliosis: Review article. *Journal of the American Medical Association, 269,* 2667–2672.

Williams, A. C. De C. (1998). Evidence-based health care: Applying fine words to one's fingertips. *Pain Forum, 7*(1), 55–57.

■ *Editor's Questions for Discussion*

Describe advances in nursing science that are fostering expectations to support theory relationships and theory-based interventions. Why were those expectations not met, according to Deets and Choi? Does it make a difference which discipline develops and tests a theory? If so, why?

How do evidence tables and meta-analysis differ from integrative research reviews? What similarities and differences exist between the issues identified by Lindsey (Chapter 29) and Androwich and Haas (Chapter 32), and those discussed by Deets and Choi? Could reviews by Lindsey, Androwich, and Haas also be presented as evidence-based tables? What criteria determine the quality of a research study and the quality of evidence supporting hypotheses? Because a small percentage of articles reviewed by Abraham et al. included an intervention, what value do those studies have? Discuss advantages and disadvantages of post hoc intervention explanations. Provide examples of "built-in mechanisms" for evaluation of implemented interventions in nursing clinical practice. How may findings of such interventions ever become generalizable? Discuss how influencing variables may be controlled in conducting and evaluating studies. What is a mock TT group?

Why have there been so few intervention-based research studies? Define steps for evaluating interventions. Why have nursing interventions not been based on theory? What agreement exists between Deets and Choi and Donnelly (Chapter 28)? Compare Deets and Choi's findings with Titler's (Chapter 35). How do the processes differ for determining whether intervention is theory-based and determining effectiveness for use in practice? What is necessary in nursing practice to systematically address discrepancy between significant and clinically relevant results?

Discuss reporting of findings in research publications. How can reporting be improved, particularly in practice journals? Discuss the validity and reliability basis for each conclusion presented by Deets and Choi. To what extent should each conclusion be further explored? If further exploration is advised, how might conclusions be further addressed? What are the advantages and disadvantages of evidence tables for reporting research results?

35

Research Utilization and Evidence-Based Practice

Marita G. Titler, PhD, RN, FAAN

R esearch utilization began with Florence Nightingale who used data to change practices that contributed to high mortality rates. The gap between the conduct of research and research utilization increased as the profession focused on transitioning education of nurses to colleges and universities, educating nurse researchers, and publishing research reports. In the 1970s, the need for greater use of research findings was identified as one of the 15 priorities in clinical nursing research. As nursing science became available to guide practice, the concept of research utilization emerged under the leadership of groups such as the Michigan Nurses Association, Western Interstate Commission for Higher Education in Nursing, Nursing Child Assessment Satellite Training Project, and the Moving New Knowledge into Practice Project (Titler, 1998).

As research utilization, evidence-based medicine, evidence-based practice, and translational research become more common in health care systems, several issues related to use

Special gratitude is expressed to Laura Cullen, Project Director of Research Utilization in the Department of Nursing Services and Patient Care at the University of Iowa Hospitals and Clinics for her thoughtful assistance and contributions to writing this manuscript. Kim Jordan is also acknowledged for her superb assistance in preparing this manuscript for publication.

of "best evidence" for clinical decision-making predominate in the nursing profession. These issues include

- definition of evidence-based practice and research utilization,

- typologies used to grade the evidence,

- format of EBP guidelines for use by practitioners, and

- science of applying evidence to use in practice (e.g., translational research).

In this chapter, I address these issues and suggest strategies for promoting evidence-based practice.

■ Evidence-Based Practice and Research Utilization

Cochrane, Sackett, and Haynes are credited as founders of evidence-based practice (EBP), which has gained increasing attention in the nursing literature during the past 5 years (Dickersin & Manheimer, 1998; Estabrooks, 1998; Geyman, 1998). Confusion exists, however, about the relationship between EBP and research utilization (RU) (Mitchell, 1997).

Evidence-based practice, as defined by some experts, is the synthesis and use of scientific information from randomized clinical trials (RCTs) (Long & Harrison, 1996; Mion, 1998; Rochon, Dikinson, & Gordon, 1997). RCTs are the "gold standard" for research evidence. Other forms of research, such as cohort designs and case studies, may be included in systematic reviews of research but are thought to be too weak to guide clinical practice. In contrast, some experts define EBP more broadly to include other types of scientific investigations and knowledge (e.g., case reports and expert opinion) as well as evidence from RCTs (Feinstein & Horwitz, 1997; Stetler et al., 1998; Titler, Mentes, Rakel, Abbott, & Baumler, 1999).

In nursing, evidence-based practice can be defined as conscientious and judicious use of the current best evidence to guide health care decisions (Sackett, Rosenberg, Gray, Haynes, & Richardson, 1996). Levels of evidence range from randomized clinical trials to case reports and expert opinions. Adopting this definition, research utilization is the subset of evidence-based practice that emphasizes the process of applying research findings from qualitative and quantitative studies for clinical decision-making. RU encompasses (a) disseminating scientific knowledge, (b) critiquing studies, (c) synthesizing findings, (d) determining applicability of findings to practice, (e) developing research-based practice guidelines, (f) instituting guidelines, and (g) evaluating the practice change.

■ Typologies for Grading the Evidence

As definitions of evidence-based practice emerge, typologies for grading the strength and level of evidence continue to proliferate (Lohr & Carey, 1999). For example, the American Association of Critical-Care Nurses (AACN) (1998) uses a six-level schema with level VI (the best evidence) being based on clinical studies in a variety of patient populations to level I (worst evidence) being manufacturers' recommendations only. In contrast, the Agency for Health Care Policy and Research (AHCPR) describes types of evidence ranging from I, which is a meta-analysis of multiple randomized clinical trials, to V, which is case reports and clinical examples. These types of research evidence then are used to grade evidence in making recommendations for practice. Grade A is some evidence of type I or consistent findings from multiple studies of types II, III, or IV; Grade B is evidence of types II, III, or IV with findings generally consistent; Grade C is evidence of types II, III, or IV, but findings are inconsistent; and Grade D is little or no evidence or there is type V evidence only (Jacox et al., 1994). Other experts suggest similar typologies for grading evidence, but there are inconsistencies in the methods used (Lohr & Carey, 1999). This inconsistency is confusing for practitioners.

The profession of nursing needs to provide leadership in adopting one method for grading evidence, which can be used consistently across the profession and among specialty organizations. Currently, no international consensus exists on the most appropriate way of classifying the strength of evidence on which guidelines and recommendations are based.

Evidence-Based Practice Guidelines

Evidence-based practice guidelines can be written as a protocol, policy, procedure, or CareMap; guidelines outline practice and designate components that are research-based and those that are consensus-based. Because evidence-based guidelines are general, patient care continues to require individualization based on patient needs and requests.

The process for development of an EBP guideline involves several essential steps, the first being identification of a clinical problem such as community acquired pneumonia or prevention of falls. After the clinical problem has been defined, a primary author or work group examines studies and other literature on the topic for purpose of assessing the research base. Relevant studies are critiqued using a two-stage process. During the first stage, type and quality of each study are examined using some schema such as that from AHCPR. During the second stage, applicability of study findings to clinical practice are assessed and practice recommendations or guidelines are formulated. Each recommendation usually is graded from A to D, based on quality and type of evidence from all studies that are critiqued.

Generally, EBP guidelines contain (a) a purpose statement describing the patient care problem; (b) operational definitions of major terms used in the protocol (e.g., fall or restraint); (c) a statement regarding the patient population(s) most likely to benefit from use of the protocol; (d) patient assessment criteria; (e) a step-by-step guideline on how to carry out the practice, with literature and research citations for each; (f) an evaluation guide to monitor process and outcome of implementing the protocol; (g) appendices with examples of tools for patient assessment and evaluation of protocol implementation; and (h) a reference list used in development of the research-based protocol (Titler, 1998).

Use of evidence to guide practice is difficult when (a) research results are conflicting, (b) research reports are difficult for staff to understand, (c) relevant studies are not compiled in one place, and (d) staff are isolated from colleagues knowledgeable about research (Atkins, Kamerow, & Eisenberg, 1998; Funk, Tornquist, & Champagne, 1995b).

The AHCPR has led national efforts that address barriers to use of evidence in practice. These include (a) developing evidence-based practice guidelines, (b) funding evidence-based practice centers, (c) formulating the National Guideline Clearinghouse, and (d) hosting an annual conference on Translating Research into Practice (Atkins et al., 1998; McCormick, Cummings, & Kovner, 1997). Emphasis on development and dissemination of evidence-based practice guidelines improves access to research evidence. Although much emphasis has been given to the process of grading evidence and developing evidence-based guidelines (Lohr & Carey, 1999), less attention has been given to testing strategies for effective implementation (Atkins et al., 1998; Geyman, 1998; Katz, 1999; Schneider & Eisenberg, 1998). When guidelines are implemented effectively, however, patient outcomes improve and resource use declines (Atkins et al., 1998;

McCormick et al., 1997; Schneider & Eisenberg, 1998).

Most guidelines are, by necessity, lengthy (e.g., more than 20 pages). This length is necessary for inclusion of essential research and for recommending practices that are evidence-based. A number of studies suggest that clinical systems, computerized decision-support systems, and prompts that support practice (e.g., decision-making, algorithms, and equianalgesic charts) have a significant positive effect on improving adherence to guidelines (Cook, Greengold, Ellrodt, & Weingarten, 1997; Hunt, Haynes, Hanna, & Smith, 1998; McCormick et al., 1997; Oxman, Thomson, Davis, & Haynes, 1995; Schmidt, Alpen, & Rakel, 1996). Computer-based decision-support systems can automate physician and nurse reminders and detail the evidence base of practice recommendations in settings that have automated medical records (Schneider & Eisenberg, 1998; Soumerai & Avorn, 1990). Other settings rely on written prompts such as bedside algorithms that visually map protocol strategy in an abbreviated manner. To move evidence from "book to bedside," information from evidence-based guidelines must be integrated into daily patient care processes, and information must be readily available and observable for practitioners.

■ The Science of Knowledge Transfer

Five federally funded projects have made major contributions to understanding the translation of research findings into practice: (a) the Western Interstate Commission for Higher Education (WICHE) regional project, (b) the Conduct and Utilization of Research in Nursing Project (CURN), (c) the Nursing Child Assessment Satellite Training (NCAST) project, (d) the Orange County Research Utilization in Nursing (OCURN) project, and (e) the Moving New Knowledge into Nursing Project (Funk et al., 1995a; Funk et al., 1995b; Horsley, Crane, Crabtree, & Wood, 1983; King, Barnard, & Hoehn, 1981; Krueger, Nelson, & Wolanin, 1978; Rutledge & Donaldson, 1995). In addition, the American Association of Women's Health, Obstetric, and Neonatal Nurses has implemented multisite research utilization projects on continence for women and nursing management of second stage labor (Niesen & Quirk, 1997; Sampselle et al., 1997). These projects have increased the awareness and use of research in practice, but much still needs to be done to move research findings from the scientific community to the bedside (Carroll et al., 1997; Funk et al., 1995b; Morin et al., 1999; Rutledge, Greene, Mooney, Nail, & Ropka, 1996).

The greatest challenge is persuading health care workers to adopt evidence-based guidelines as an integral part of practice (Bowers, 1998; Larsen & Thurston, 1997; Varcoe & Hilton, 1995). Influencing caregivers to let go of ritual-based practices is not an easy task. Diffusion of an innovation, such as an evidence-based guideline, is influenced by the guideline and the manner in which it is communicated (disseminated) to members (nurses) of a social system (organization, nursing profession) (Rogers, 1995). Characteristics of the organization; research knowledge, skills and attitudes of nurses; the manner in which research is communicated; and the quality of the research promotes use of research to inform and guide practice (Schnelle, Cruise, Rahman, & Ouslander, 1998; Wells & Baggs, 1994).

Characteristics of the Organization

A supportive organization that (a) values research, (b) provides time for staff to implement research-based practices, and (c) empowers staff to make changes in practice has a positive affect on use of research in practice (Carroll et al., 1997; Funk et al., 1995a; Titler, 1997; Varcoe & Hilton, 1995). Most RU projects and programs have been instituted in acute care settings with little knowledge or experience in implementation across health care systems, home health care, skilled care, and long term care (Goode & Titler, 1996; Shively et al., 1997; Titler, 1997). Chief nurse executives, nurse managers, and informal nursing leaders in an organization play pivotal roles in the success or demise of implementing research-based protocols (Stetler et al., 1998a; Titler, 1997).

Nurse Characteristics

Characteristics of the nurse who facilitates RU include (a) belief that research is valued by peers and administrators, (b) exposure to research reports, and (c) ability to understand and critique research (Carroll et al., 1997; Funk et al., 1995a; Titler, 1997; Varcoe & Hilton, 1995). Other facilitators of RU include willingness of nurses to change or try new ideas and perception of nurses that research-based practice will benefit both patients and staff (Funk et al., 1995b).

Communication Dissemination

Methods of communicating scientific knowledge to staff can facilitate or restrain adoption of the information. Barriers to RU include (a) research reports that are difficult for staff to understand, (b) relevant studies not being compiled in one place, and (c) isolation of staff nurses from colleagues knowledgeable about the research (Carroll et al., 1997; Funk et al., 1995b; Wells & Baggs, 1994). Facilitators of RU include (a) publication of research reports in practice journals, (b) inclusion of research columns in clinical journals, (c) publi-

cation of integrative research reviews, (d) development and dissemination of research-based and evidence-based practice guidelines, (e) national conferences that focus on research utilization, and (f) increase of nurses' access to research in the clinical setting via electronic media (Cronenwett, 1995; Titler, 1998). Emphasis on development and dissemination of evidence-based practice guidelines decreases the barrier of access to the most recent evidence.

Quality of the Research

Characteristics of the innovation or research itself also affects its adoption within a social system, such as a department of nursing or long-term care facility. Barriers that limit adoption of research in practice are methodological inadequacies of the research, conflicting research results, and limited availability of replicated studies on a specific topic (Funk et al., 1995b). Characteristics of the innovation, however, seem to be of less importance than the characteristics of the (a) adopter, (b) organization, and (c) dissemination and communication process (Carroll et al., 1997; Funk et al., 1995b).

Evidence-based practice centers funded by the AHCPR, Cochrane Collaboration, and Ontario Health Care Evaluation Network assemble, synthesize, and disseminate research evidence to practitioners (Brown, 1999; Guyatt et al., 1995; Jadad & Haynes, 1998; McCormick et al., 1997; Sibbald & Kossuth, 1998). Although access to research evidence by clinicians has improved during the past 10 years, little is known about the best methods for implementing, in practice, evidence discovered by the scientific community (Atkins et al., 1998; Carroll et al., 1997; Rutledge et al., 1996; Schneider & Eisenberg, 1998). Interventions that tend to be effective in promoting adherence to EBP guidelines are (a) system reminders (e.g., computer systems, stickers, and chart inserts), (b) outreach visits, (c) opinion leaders, (d) focus groups, (e) audits and feedback of performance measures, and (f) multifaceted interventions (Oxman et al., 1995; Schneider & Eisenberg, 1998; Shively et al., 1997; Soumerai & Avorn, 1990; Soumerai et al., 1998).

The Iowa Model of Research-Based Practice

The Iowa Model of Research-Based Practice to Promote Quality Care (see Figure 35.1) has been disseminated widely and adopted in academic and clinical settings.

Since the original publication (Titler et al., 1994a), we have received more than 50 written requests to reproduce the model for publications, presentations, graduate and undergraduate research courses, and clinical research programs. The publication has been cited 13 times in nursing journal articles (Social Science Citation Index, 1998). The University of Iowa Hospitals and Clinics, in collaboration with the College of Nursing, provides onsite educational opportunities for national and international constituents who wish to learn more about our highly successful RU program.

Knowledge and problem-focused triggers are the impetus for initiation of an EBP. Establishing a clinical issue as an organizational priority lends itself to administrative support, which is essential for successful completion. Team formation is followed by collection and critiquing of literature. The adequacy of the research base determines whether to pursue a pilot study, search for additional evidence, or conduct research. Implementation of a pilot study involves (a) selection of outcomes, (b) collection of baseline data, (c) guideline development, (d) pilot implementation, (e) evaluation of process and outcome data, and (f) modification of the guideline. When the pilot evaluation is completed, a decision is made regarding appropriateness of the EBP guideline for broader adop-

tion. Evaluative data include monitoring of structure, process, and outcome data from multiple sources (e.g., patient and family, environment, staff, and cost). The Iowa model offers a practical step-by-step approach for clinicians interested in evidence-based practice.

Use of this model is facilitated when it is incorporated into the work of existing committees, such as those dealing with quality management or research. This approach makes use of an established reporting channel within the existing organizational structure. Members of an existing committee or team have worked through group process, know the talents of each person, and thus can divide the workload to maximize the strengths of each member. Individuals with experience in quality management and research usually are experienced in data acquisition, data management, and transformation of data into information—all important components of evaluating the research-based changes in practice (Titler et al., in review).

Based on recent developments in the health care market and feedback from users, the original model was revised in 1998 to (a) incorporate new terminology and feedback loops, (b) reflect a more interdisciplinary focus, and (c) encourage use of other types of evidence (e.g., case reports and scientific principles) when research is unavailable to guide practice (Titler et al., in review).

■ Strategies for Promoting Research-Based Practice

Setting Priorities

Choosing a clinical issue is an essential first step in translating research findings into practice. Issues to consider when selecting a topic are summarized in Table 35.1.

A topic embraced by staff and aligned with strategic goals of the organization has a high

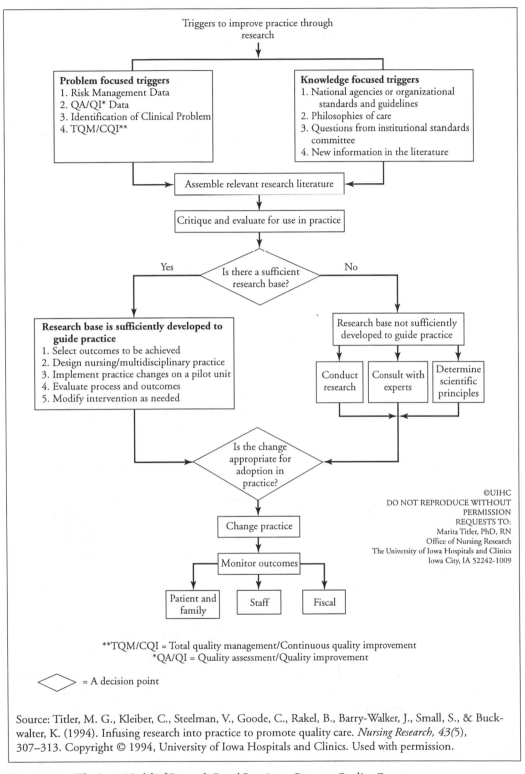

Figure 35.1 The Iowa Model of Research-Based Practice to Promote Quality Care.

TABLE 35.1   Issues to Consider When Selecting a Research Utilization Topic

Fit with the strategic goals (priorities) of the organization

Magnitude of the problem

Number of people and level of interest in the topic

Interdisciplinary support or opportunity for collaboration

Support of nurse leaders

Potential "landmines" associated with the topic/diffusion of the topic

Outcome and cost implications

Availability of baseline data from quality improvement or risk management sources

Probability of success:
- Potential barriers to change
- Sufficient facilitators

likelihood of being adopted by those providing care (Titler, 1998; Titler et al., in review). Selecting a topic that will be successful is especially important if the organizational (or unit) culture does not yet value or has little experience with evidence-based practice. If clinicians have a great deal of interest in a clinical issue but the topic is not considered an organizational priority, resolution may involve repackaging the proposal to include data that will secure administrative support by focusing on outcomes that are valued (e.g., patient satisfaction, potential cost savings, increased market share, and so forth).

Using Facilitators in Planning

Facilitators need to be considered before committing prematurely to a RU project. Facilitators include selecting a topic that is (a) aligned with the strategic plan, (b) has a sound scientific base, and (c) involves nurses who are enthusiastic (Cullen, in review). Increasing the number and amount of RU process facilitators is important.

Methods of Implementation

A number of studies have demonstrated that opinion leaders are effective in changing behaviors of health care practitioners (Bero et al., 1998; Elliott et al., 1997; Oxman et al., 1995; Soumerai et al., 1998). In fact, the combination of a trusted opinion leader with (a) outreach or (b) performance feedback has been shown to be quite potent in changing practice (Schneider & Eisenberg, 1998; Soumerai et al., 1998). Opinion leaders, by definition, are members of the local health care setting and are viewed as important and respected sources of influence among their peer group. The key characteristic of an opinion leader is that he or she is trusted to evaluate new information in the context of group norms. To do so, an opinion leader must be considered by associates as technically competent and a full and dedicated member of the local group (Oxman et al., 1995; Soumerai et al., 1998). Opinion leaders are evaluators who are trusted to judge the fit between a technology and the local situation. Change is accomplished by modeling, peer influence, and altering group norms.

Outreach Visits

Outreach visits, also known as academic detailing, involve a trained person who meets one-on-one with practitioners in their settings to provide information about an innovation. Information conveyed during outreach visits often include feedback on provider performance (Hendryx et al., 1998; Hulscher et al., 1997; Oxman et al., 1995). Studies have demonstrated that outreach visits alone or in combination with other strategies result in positive changes in practice behaviors of nurses and physicians (Hendryx et al., 1998; Jiang, Fieselmann, Hendryx, & Bock, 1997; Pippalla, Riley, & Chinburapa, 1995).

Change Champions

Use of change champions is another strategy for promoting use of evidence in practice (Backer, 1995; Rogers, 1995; Titler, 1998; Titler & Mentes, 1999). This strategy has been used more in organizational change than in converting behaviors of individual practitioners. Change champions are practitioners within the practice group who continually promote the new idea. Characteristics of successful change champions include (a) expert clinician, (b) informal leader from perspective of peers, (c) positive working relationship with other health professionals, (d) passionate about the topic of practice, and (e) commitment to improving the quality of care (Titler, 1998). The change champion believes in an idea, will not take no for an answer, is undaunted by insults and rebuffs, and above all persists. He or she circulates information, encourages peers to align their practice with the best evidence, convenes committees, arranges demonstrations, and orients new personnel to the idea. Observational studies suggest that champions of implementation of EBP guidelines are an important part of improving adherence to the guidelines (Hill, Fieselmann, & Nobiling,

1995; Schmidt et al., 1996; Shively et al., 1997; Titler et al., 1994b).

Core Groups

Adherence to EBP guidelines is facilitated by using a "core group" approach, in conjunction with change champions, for guideline implementation (Barnason, Merboth, Pozehl, & Tietjen, 1998; Pasero, Gordon, McCaffery, & Ferrell, 1999; Rischer & Childress, 1996; Schmidt et al., 1996). A core group includes practitioners with the mutual goal of disseminating information regarding a practice change and facilitating change in practice by other staff in their unit or peer group. Core group members are usually chosen by the change champion, in consultation with the nurse manager or medical director or both. Success of the core group approach requires that members represent those who work various shifts and days of the week. Responsibilities of core group members include (a) acting as ambassadors for change, (b) being knowledgeable of the evidence base for the guideline, (c) using the guideline in practice, (d) educating staff on use of the guideline, (e) providing regular feedback to staff regarding their use of the guideline, and (f) participating with the change champion and opinion leader in making decisions about adopting and implementing the guideline (Titler et al., 1994b). This approach results in a critical mass of practitioners championing the adoption of the guideline.

Trial Use

Users of an EBP usually try it for a period of time prior to adopting it in practice (Rogers, 1995). This trial can be a formal component of the implementation plan, or individual practitioners can try the EBP and subsequently decide whether to use it in practice. When "trying an evidence-based practice" is incorporated as part of the implementation process, users have an opportunity to try the innovation, provide feedback to those in charge of implementation, and modify the innovation if necessary (Goode, 1995; Shively et al., 1997; Titler et al., in review). If pilot evaluation demonstrates a problem with use of the research-based protocol and no further research or evidence exists to support an alternative approach to the method piloted, use of other types of evidence—such as expert opinion, scientific principles, or theory—can be used to determine the best practice (Titler et al., in review).

Leadership support, both at the upper management and middle-management levels, is a crucial to adoption of evidence-based guidelines (Katz, 1999; Schmidt et al., 1996; Stetler et al., 1998). The value of evidence-based practice is communicated to staff through the mission statement, philosophy, and strategic plan of an organization. Behaviors that support the use of research findings to guide practice must be built into job descriptions and performance evaluations of staff. Written and verbal feedback to staff who operationalize the research-based practice also is essential to the success of moving evidence into practice (Titler et al., 1999). The role of nurse managers and medical directors must include setting expectations for evidence-based practice, modeling use of evidence to guide practice, and overcoming system barriers (e.g., lack of availability of supplies and need for changes in documentation forms) that hamper evidence-based practice changes.

Such support is expressed not just verbally, but in commitment to provide (a) education of staff with regard to the knowledge and skills necessary to carry out the evidence-based practice, (b) financial support to purchase educational materials, (c) ownership of the new practice by nurses and all affected disciplines, (d) data showing that the change improves the quality of care, and (e) sufficient time to complete the process and carry out the EBP as intended (Titler et al., in review). And finally, if the guideline is to be an integral part of practice, education of new staff must occur to retain a critical mass of providers who practice according to the guideline (Barnason et al., 1998; Howell, Foster, Hester, Vojir, & Miller, 1996; Rischer & Childress, 1996; Titler et al., 1999).

Evaluation of the Practice Change

When changing practice based on research or other evidence, staff evaluation of the process and outcomes is critical (Goode, 1995; Titler, 1998). Evaluation allows modification of the practice as necessary. A desired outcome achieved in a controlled environment, when a researcher is implementing a study protocol to a homogenous group of patients as research clients, may not result in the same outcome as when the research-based practice is used by multiple caregivers in a natural clinical setting (Titler et al., 1999). Research-based changes in practice need an evaluative component, with findings from it incorporated into the quality and performance improvement program.

■ Concluding Statement

The need to use research findings in practice, as identified by nursing leaders almost three decades ago, in combination with a squeezed economic base for health care, has led to the emphasis on development, implementation, and evaluation of evidence-based practice. Although RU is a subset of EBP, the lessons learned from RU lend critical information for success with evidence-based practice. Aligning facilitators, limiting barriers, using an RU model to guide implementation, and planning use of diffusion strategies may lead to even greater successes for nurses, and even more important, for patients and families receiving nursing care.

■ References

American Association of Critical Care Nurses. (1998). *AACN protocols for practice: Creating a healing environment.* Aliso Viejo, CA: Author.

Atkins, D. M., Kamerow, D. M., & Eisenberg, J. M. M. (1998). Evidence-based medicine at the Agency for Health Care Policy and Research. *ACP Journal Club March–April, 128,* A1214.

Backer, T. E. (1995). Integrating behavioral and systems strategies to change clinical practice. *Joint Commission Journal on Quality Improvement, 21*(7), 351–353.

Barnason, S., Merboth, M., Pozehl, B., & Tietjen, M. J. (1998). Utilizing an outcomes approach to improve pain management by nurses: A pilot study. *Clinical Nurse Specialist, 12*(1), 28–36.

Bero, L. A., Grilli, R., Grimshaw, J. M., Harvey, E., Oxman, A. D., & Thomson, M. A. (1998). Closing the gap between research and practice: An overview of systematic reviews of interventions to promote the implementation of research findings. *British Medical Journal, 317,* 465–468.

Bowers, C. W. (1998). Development and implementation of evidence-based guidelines: A multisite demonstration project. *Journal of Wound, Ostomy, and Continence Nursing, 25*(4), 187–193.

Brown, S. J. (1999). *Knowledge for health care practice: A guide to using research evidence.* Philadelphia: W. B. Saunders.

Carroll, D. L., Greenwood, R., Lynch, K. E., Sullivan, J. K., Ready, C. H., & Fitzmaurice, J. B. (1997). Barriers and facilitators to the utilization of nursing research. *Clinical Nurse Specialist, 11*(5), 207–212.

Cook, D. J., Greengold, N. L., Ellrodt, A. G., & Weingarten, S. R. (1997). The relation between systematic reviews and practice guidelines. *Annals of Internal Medicine, 127*(3), 210–216.

Cronenwett, L. R. (1995). Effective methods for disseminating research findings to nurses in practice. In M. G. Titler & C. Goode (Eds.), *The nursing clinics of North America* (Vol. 30, pp. 429–438). Philadelphia: W. B. Saunders.

Cullen, L. (in review). Evidence-based practice: Strategies for success.

Dickersin, K., & Manheimer, E. (1998). The Cochrane Collaboration: Evaluation of health care and services using systematic reviews of the results of randomized controlled trials. *Clinical Obstetrics & Gynecology, 41*(2), 315–331.

Elliott, T. E., Murray, D. M., Oken, M. M., Johnson, K. M., Braun, B. L., Elliott, B. A., & Post-White, J. (1997). Improving cancer pain management in communities: Main results from a randomized controlled trial. *Journal of Pain and Symptom Management, 13*(4), 191–203.

Estabrooks, C. A. (1998). Will evidence-based nursing practice make practice perfect? *Canadian Journal of Nursing Research, 30*(1), 15–36.

Feinstein, A. R., & Horwitz, R. I. (1997). Problems in the "evidence" of "evidence-based medicine." *American Journal of Medicine, 103,* 529–535.

Funk, S. G., Champagne, M. T., Tornquist, E. M., & Wiese, R. A. (1995a). Administrators' views on barriers to research utilization. *Applied Nursing Research, 8*(1), 44–49.

Funk, S. G., Tornquist, E., M., & Champagne, M. T. (1995b). Barriers and facilitators of research utilization: An integrative Review. In M. Titler & C. Goode (Eds.), *The nursing clinics of North America* (Vol. 30, pp. 395–408). Philadelphia: W. B. Saunders.

Geyman, J. P. (1998). Evidence-based medicine in primary care: An overview. *Journal of the American Board of Family Practice, 11*(1), 46–56.

Goode, C. J. (1995). Evaluation of research-based nursing practice. In M. G. Titler & C. J. Goode (Eds.), *Nursing clinics of North America* (Vol. 30, pp. 421–428). Philadelphia: W. B. Saunders.

Goode, C. J., & Titler, M. G. (1996). Moving research-based practice throughout the health care system. *MEDSURG Nursing, 5*(5), 380–383.

Guyatt, G., Sackett, D., Sinclair, J., Hayward, R., Cook, D., & Cook, R. (1995). Users' guides to the medical literature. IX. A method for grading health care recommendations. *Journal of the American Medical Association, 274,* 1800–1804.

Hendryx, M. S., Fieselmann, J. F., Bock, M. J., Wakefield, D. S., Helms, C. M., & Bentler, S. E. (1998). Outreach education to improve quality of rural ICU care. Results of a randomized trial. *American Journal of Respiratory & Critical Care Medicine, 158*(2), 418–423.

Hill, M. G., Fieselmann, J. F., & Nobiling, H. E. (1995). Preventing cardiopulmonary arrest via enhanced vital signs monitoring. *MEDSURG Nursing, 4*(4), 289–295.

Horsley, J. A., Crane, J., Crabtree, M. K., & Wood, D. J. (1983). *Using research to improve nursing practice: A guide.* New York: Grune & Stratton.

Howell, S. L., Foster, R. L., Hester, N. O., Vojir, C. P., & Miller, K. L. (1996). Evaluating a pediatric pain management research utilization program. *Canadian Journal of Nursing Research, 28*(2), 37–57.

Hulscher, M. E., van Drenth, B. B., van der Wouden, J. C., Mokkink, H. G., van Weel, C., & Grol, R. P. (1997). Changing preventive practice: A controlled trial on the effects of outreach visits to organize prevention of cardiovascular disease. *Quality in Health Care, 6* (1), 19–24.

Hunt, D. L., Haynes, R. B., Hanna, S. E., & Smith, K. (1998). Effects of computer-based clinical decision support systems on physician performance and patient outcomes: A systematic review. *Journal of the American Medical Association, 280*(15), 1339–1346.

Jacox, A., Carr, D. B., Payne, R., Berde, C. B., Brietbart, W., Cain, J. M., Chapman, C. R., Cleeland, C. S., Ferrell, B. R., Finley, R. S., Hester, N. O., Hill Jr, C. S., Leak, W. D., Lipman, A. G., Logan, C. L., McGarvey, C. L., Miaskowski, C. A., Mulder, D. S., Paice, J. A., Shapiro, B. S., Silberstein, E. B., Smith, R. B., Stover, J., Tsou, C. V., Vecchiarelli, L., & Weissman, D. E. (1994). *Management of Cancer Pain. Clinical Practice Guideline* No. 9. Rockville, MD: Agency for Health Care Policy and Research, Public Health Service, U.S. Department of Health and Human Services, AHCPR Publication No. 94-0592.

Jadad, A. R., & Haynes, R. B. (1998). The Cochrane Collaboration: Advances and challenges in improving evidence-based decision making. *Medical Decision Making, 18,* 2–9.

Jiang, H. J., Fieselmann, J. F., Hendryx, M. S., & Bock, M. J. (1997). Assessing the impact of patient characteristics and process performance on rural intensive care unit hospital mortality rates. *Critical Care Medicine, 25*(5), 773–778.

Katz, D. A. (1999). Barriers between guidelines and improved patient care: An analysis of AHCPR's unstable angina clinical practice guideline. *Health Services Research, 34*(1), 337–389.

King, D., Barnard, K. E., & Hoehn, R. (1981). Disseminating the results of nursing research. *Nursing Outlook, 64,* 164–169.

Krueger, J., Nelson, A., & Wolanin, M. (1978). *Nursing research: Development, collaboration, and utilization.* Germantown, MD: Aspen Systems.

Larsen, L. L., & Thurston, N. E. (1997). Research utilization: Development of a central venous catheter procedure. *Applied Nursing Research, 10*(1), 44–51.

Lohr, K. N., & Carey, T. S. (1999). Assessing "Best evidence": Issues in grading the quality of studies for systematic reviews. *The Joint Commission Journal on Quality Improvement, 25*(9), 470–479.

Long, A., & Harrison, S. (1996). Evidence-based decision making. *Health Service Journal, 106* (5486 Health Manage Guide), 1–12.

McCormick, K. A., Cummings, M. A., & Kovner, C. (1997). The role of the Agency for Health Care Policy and Research in improving outcomes of care. *Nursing Clinics of North America, 32*(3), 521–542.

Mion, L. C. (1998). Evidence-based health care practice. *Journal of Gerontological Nursing, 24*(12), 5–6.

Mitchell, G. J. (1997). Questioning evidence-based practice for nursing. *Nursing Science Quarterly, 10*(4), 154–155.

Morin, K., Bucher, L., Plowfield, L., Hayes, E., Mahoney, P., & Armiger, L. (1999). Using research to establish protocols for practice: A statewide study of acute care agencies. *Clinical Nurse Specialist, 13*(2), 77–84.

Niesen, K. M., & Quirk, A. G. (1997). The process for initiating nursing practice changes in the intrapartum: Findings from a multisite research utilization project. *Journal of Obstetric, Gynecologic, & Neonatal Nursing, 26*(6), 709–717.

Oxman, A. D., Thomson, M. A., Davis, D. A., & Haynes, R. B. (1995). No magic bullets: A systematic review of 102 trials of interventions to improve professional practice. *Canadian Medical Association Journal, 153*(10), 1423–1431.

Pasero, C., Gordon, D. B., McCaffery, M., & Ferrell, B. R. (1999). Building institutional commitment to improving pain management. In M. McCaffery & C. Pasero (Eds.), *Pain: Clinical manual* (pp. 711–744). St. Louis, MO: Mosby.

Pippalla, R. S., Riley, D. A., & Chinburapa, V. (1995). Influencing the prescribing behavior of physicians: A metaevaluation. *Journal of Clinical Pharmacy and Therapeutics, 20,* 189–198.

Rischer, J. B., & Childress, S. B. (1996). Cancer pain management: pilot implementation of the AHCPR guideline in Utah. *Joint Commission Journal on Quality Improvement, 22*(10), 683–700.

Rochon, P. A., Dikinson, E., & Gordon, M. (1997). The Cochrane field in health care of older people: Geriatric medicine's role in the collaboration. *Journal of the American Geriatrics Society, 45*(2), 241–243.

Rogers, E. (1995). *Diffusion of innovations.* New York: Free Press.

Rutledge, D. N., & Donaldson, N. E. (1995). Building organizational capacity to engage in research utilization. *Journal of Nursing Administration, 25* (10), 12–16.

Rutledge, D. N., Greene, P., Mooney, K., Nail, L. M., & Ropka, M. (1996). Use of research-based practices by oncology staff nurses. *Oncology Nursing Forum, 23*(8), 1235–1244.

Sackett, D., Rosenberg, W., Gray, J., Haynes, R., & Richardson, W. (1996). Evidence based medicine: What it is and what it isn't. *British Medical Journal, 312,* 71–72.

Sampselle, C., Burns, P. A., Dougherty, M. C., Newman, D. K., Thomas, K. K., & Wyman, J. F. (1997). Continence for women: Evidence-based practice. *Journal of Obstetric, Gynecologic, & Neonatal Nursing, 26*(4), 375–385.

Schmidt, K. L., Alpen, M. A., & Rakel, B. A. (1996). Implementation of the Agency for Health Care Policy and Research Pain Guidelines. *American Association of Critical Care Nurses Clinical Issues, 7*(3), 425–435.

Schneider, E. C., & Eisenberg, J. M. (1998). Strategies and methods for aligning current and best medical practices: The role of information technologies. *Western Journal of Medicine, 168*(5), 311–318.

Schnelle, J. F., Cruise, P. A., Rahman, A., & Ouslander, J. G. (1998). Developing rehabilitative behavioral interventions for long-term care: Technology transfer, acceptance, and maintenance issues. *Journal of the American Geriatrics Society, 46*(6), 771–777.

Shively, M., Riegel, B., Waterhouse, D., Burns, D., Templin, K., & Thomason, T. (1997). Testing a community level research utilization intervention. *Applied Nursing Research, 10*(3), 121–127.

Sibbald, W. J., & Kossuth, J. D. (1998). The Ontario health care evaluation network and the critical care research network as vehicles for research transfer. *Medical Decision Making, 18*(1), 9–16.

Social sciences citation (1998). *Social sciences citation index.* Philadelphia: Institute for Scientific Information.

Soumerai, S., & Avorn, J. (1990). Principles of educational outreach ("academic detailing") to improve clinical decision making. *Journal of the American Medical Association, 263*(4), 549–556.

Soumerai, S. B., McLaughlin, T. J., Gurwitz, J. H., Guadagnoli, E., Hauptman, P. J., Borbas, C., Morris, N., McLaughlin, B., Gao, X., Willison, D. J., Asinger, R., & Gobel, F. (1998). Effect of local medical opinion leaders on quality of care for acute myocardial infarction: A randomized controlled trial. *Journal of the American Medical Association, 279*(17), 1358–1363.

Stetler, C. B., Brunell, M., Giuliano, K. K., Morsi, D., Prince, L., & Newell-Stokes, V. (1998). Evidence-based practice and the role of nursing leadership. *Journal of Nursing Administration, 28*(7–8), 45–53.

Titler, M. G. (1997). Research utilization: Necessity or luxury. In J. C. McCloskey & H. Grace (Eds.), *Current issues in nursing* (5th ed., pp. 104–117). St. Louis: Mosby.

Titler, M. G. (1998). Use of research in practice. In G. LoBiondo-Wood & J. Haber (Eds.), *Nursing research* (pp. 467–498). St. Louis: Mosby-Year Book.

Titler, M. G., Kleiber, C., Steelman, V., Goode, C., Rakel, B., Barry-Walker, J., Small, S., & Buckwalter, K. C. (1994a). Research-based practice to promote the quality of care. *Nursing Research, 43*(5), 307–313.

Titler, M. G., Kleiber, C., Steelman, V. J., Rakel, B. A., Budreau, G., Buckwalter, K. C., Tripp-Reimer, T., & Goode, C. J. (in review). Evidence-based practice and the Iowa model of research-based practice to promote quality care.

Titler, M. G., & Mentes, J. C. (1999). Research utilization in gerontological nursing practice. *Journal of Gerontological Nursing, 25*(6), 6–9.

Titler, M. G., Mentes, J. C., Rakel, B. A., Abbott, L., & Baumler, S. (1999). Putting evidence to use in the care of the elderly. *Joint Commission Journal on Quality Improvement, 25*(10), 545–556.

Titler, M. G., Moss, L., Greiner, J., Alpen, M., Jones, G., Olson, K., Hauer, M., Phillips, C., & Megivern, K. (1994b). Research utilization in critical care: An exemplar. *AACN Clinical Issues, 5*(2), 124–132.

Varcoe, C., & Hilton, A. (1995). Factors affecting acute-care nurses' use of research findings. *Canadian Journal of Nursing Research, 27*(4), 51–71.

Wells, N., & Baggs, J. G. (1994). A survey of practicing nurses' research interests and activities. *Clinical Nurse Specialist, 8,* 145–151.

■ *Editor's Questions for Discussion*

Discuss ways for classifying evidence in making recommendations for practice. What should be the primary criteria in developing such a system? How may consensus be developed for one method of grading evidence?

What is the difference between evidence-based practice and research utilization? How similar are typologies for grading evidence as Titler presents with methodology utilized by Deets and Choi (Chapter 34)? How do Deets and Choi's findings support Titler's conclusions regarding quality of research? What relationship exists between development of evidence-based tables and the methodology used by AHCPR to describe types of research evidence? Which method do you believe should be adopted for grading evidence? Provide a rationale for your recommendation.

How can nurses be motivated to use research findings in practice? How may informatics, as discussed by Stevens and Weiner (Chapter 38), facilitate evidence-based practice (EBP)? Discuss methods for implementing research evidence in practice. How may barriers be reduced in conducting and using research findings for EBP? Propose structure, process, and outcome for evaluating EBP for a specific clinical issue? How may someone determine the extent to which a clinical issue may be an organizational priority amenable for RU and EBP? To what extent may "opinion leaders" and "change champions" be valid and reliable resources for changing behaviors of health care practitioners? Propose additional strategies for increasing the use of RH and EBP.

36

Research Preparation in the 21st Century

Kenneth P. Miller, PhD, RN,
CFNP, FAAN

In this chapter, apparent research needs in nursing for the 21st century are discussed with the aim to delineate specific needs of nurse researchers and suggest possible areas for investigation. A brief review of the historical development of doctoral education for nurses, wherein research skills may be honed, also will be presented. Doctoral degrees include (a) EdD, doctorate in education; (b) DNS, DNSc, and DSN, doctor of nursing science with an emphasis on clinical practice; (c) PhD, doctor of philosophy and the Nurse Scientist program with an emphasis on basic science and social sciences; (d) PhD, doctor of philosophy in nursing, with program emphasis in clinical nursing research; and (e) ND, nursing doctorate, the newest program.

■ Historical Review of Nursing Doctorates

Nurse historians generally agree, with some variation in date, that doctoral education for nursing has spanned three distinct eras (Grace, 1978; Murphy, 1981; Stevenson & Woods, 1986). The first era (1924–1961) offered the doctorate in education (EdD) as the terminal degree. The second era began with initiation of the Nurse Scientist program in 1962 and ended with its demise in 1974. Finally, the current era began in 1974. Each of these eras had distinctive characteristics.

■ Doctor of Education in Nursing

The distinction of being the first university to offer a doctoral degree to nurses belongs to Teachers College at Columbia University, which established its program in 1924. The emphasis of this program was to prepare educators to teach or become administrators in schools of nursing. With this emphasis, it is not surprising that research in this era is often referred to as "nurses studying nurses." Curricular content, roles of administrators, and evaluation of teaching strategies were the common research trends.

Doctorates in Related Fields

The second era—the era of the nurse scientist—began in 1962 when the U.S. Department of Health and Human Services, Division of Nursing, funded Boston University to provide stipends for nurses to matriculate in the basic and social sciences doctoral programs with a minor in nursing. The purpose of the program was to develop a cadre of "research scientists" who could lead the nursing profession, through rigors of research, in developing its own scientific base for practice. According to Grace (1978), "the intent underlying the nurse scientist program was that of building a critical mass of faculty for the development of a doctoral program in nursing" (p. 21).

Ten universities participated in this program from 1962 through 1974, and each offered degrees in one or more of the following areas: Anatomy, anthropology, biology, communications and human relations, microbiol-

ogy, nursing, physiology, psychology, and sociology (Gortner, 1991). Upon completion of their training, these nurse scientists returned to their schools or colleges of nursing and began developing programs of research in their substantive areas.

Doctor of Nursing Science (DNS, DNSc, and DSN)

The first Doctor of Nursing Science program was established in 1960 at Boston University. The degree was established as a professional practice, or clinical, degree. The intent was for it to parallel the doctor of medicine (MD) degree and be an alternative to the doctor of philosophy (PhD) degree as a narrowly focused research degree. In essence, the doctor of nursing science became the clinical degree—at least in theory. The one aspect of the degree that has almost universal approbation is that the DNS has as its primary goal the preparation of advanced practitioners or applied researchers or both (Abdellah & Levine, 1994; Carpenter & Hudacek 1996; Forni 1989; Starck, Duffy, & Volger, 1993; Gortner, 1991).

Doctor of Philosophy in Nursing

Although the first PhD program in nursing can be traced back to New York University in 1934, followed by the University of Pittsburgh's in the 1950s, not until the 1970s did schools offering PhDs in nursing begin to flourish. During this time period, 5 schools developed new PhD programs, by 1982 there were 54, and in 2000 there are some 77 programs nationwide. The initial spurt of doctoral programs in nursing coincides with phasing out of the Nurse Scientist program in 1974. The PhD in nursing represents development of nursing knowledge through the process of nursing science.

The Nursing Doctorate (ND)

The Nursing Doctorate (ND) differs from other doctorates in nursing in that it is an initial rather than a terminal degree. My conceptualization of this degree is that it really is a "post masters, master's degree" that provides focused clinical experience without the depth or breadth of the other doctorates. As Forni (1989) noted, "Newman (1975, p. 705) advocated that the professional doctorate in nursing (the doctor of nursing degree) be offered as the first professional degree as a means of gaining recognition and authority for nursing" (p. 430). But it was Rozella Schlotfeldt (1978) who carried the banner for what initially was called "DN"—the first professional degree that would be equivalent to the MD degree. Later, it was referred to as the nursing doctorate (ND) and is currently offered at fewer than 10 schools. However, in attempts to entice candidates and shore up sagging enrollment figures, several schools are now pondering establishing ND programs.

■ Current Nursing Doctorates

The multitude of current doctorates in nursing represents both a "blessing and a curse" for the profession. The blessing derives from the fact that it offers a series of options for practitioners within the profession to find their niche and excel. It is a curse, in that it further complicates the public's perception and even the profession's perception, of what doctorally prepared nurses really do.

A Blessing

The spectrum of diversity in nursing is evident not only in its host of clinical specializations—including that for midwifes, nurse practitioners, clinical specialists, as well as for educators, administrators, and so forth—but also in its educational preparation. Nursing has been enculturated in diverse approaches from its earliest roots when paths for preparation allowed the diploma, associate, or baccalaureate degree to be the initial entrée to the profession. So, too, is it for the doctorally prepared nurse. Mandates of time and circumstance paved the way for doctoral education. As the profession began to grow it needed faculty who could educate young nurses in the professional role. What better preparation than a doctorate in education (EdD)?

As nursing matured professionally, it recognized the need for establishing a scientific basis for clinical interventions amid the need to be a member of the greater community of scientists. Initiated first was the Nurse Scientist program, resulting essentially as a PhD degree in another discipline and then the PhD in Nursing. Simultaneously with the latter, DNS, DNSc, DSN programs were developed for those who wanted to focus more on advanced professional practices rather than research.

By offering a multitude of venues in which to practice, nursing was able to recruit and educate the most motivated and goal-oriented individuals in specific content areas. For the past century these programs have served nursing well, even if nurses have not been able to reconcile program differences sufficiently for other academicians and for the public. And it is this latter point that defines "the curse" of having multiple degreed doctoral programs.

A Curse

The multiplicity of doctoral degree offerings for nursing has proven also to be a curse. The public perception is that "a nurse is a nurse is a nurse." It is difficult for the public to differentiate a technical nurse (associate degree) from a professional nurse (baccalaureate graduate), let alone a clinical doctorate

(DNS, DNSc, or DSN) from an academic doctorate (PhD)—the differences in the letters thereof, notwithstanding! But then add the Nursing Doctorate (ND), which represents an initial versus a terminal doctoral degree, and the morass is even more confusing. Newman (1975) argued that those who would subscribe to the former position that another degree would add to the confusion of those degrees already in existence, can be countered " . . . by pointing out that movement toward the professional doctorate will eliminate some of the confusion, rather than cause more, because there might be less question among nurses as to who is prepared to be the professional practitioner" (p. 705). However history has *not* borne out this assertion. Hudacek and Carpenter (1998) supported this viewpoint when they stated, "Leadership noted at the First National Conference on Doctoral Education [held in 1977] that the profession has not realistically addressed distinctions among degree types" (p. 14). Werley and Leske (1988) noted 11 years after this conference that

> one can read many articles about doctoral degrees in nursing and come away feeling that today's nurse leaders are no closer to taking a stand on the differences between the two [DNS & PhD] than were their predecessors during the days when university officials would not approve a PhD degree with study in nursing but would allow a nursing faculty to develop a DNS program. (p. 239)

Over the past two decades the operationalization of these distinctions in programs still has not been accomplished. Consensus has not occurred, in part because both PhD and DNS programs are striving to include the rigors of academic science. The degree of academic science rigor in programs remains an unresolved issue for some programs. So where does that leave nursing in terms of doctoral needs?

Doctoral Needs for the 21st Century

If the profession of nursing truly wants to be a leader in health care, consolidation needs to occur rather than diversification. As Grace (1978) noted, "Clinical practice and nursing research are proceeding on two separate and parallel paths that do not interact" (p. 26). What is needed is a hybridization of these roles into a "neopractitioner." She advocated

> development of a cadre of doctorally prepared nurses in clinical practice who are expert clinicians but also have a grounding in research enabling them to test out the effects of clinical interventions within the patient care setting be it hospital, home, or community. (p. 26)

Given the U.S.'s current socioeconomic situation and the trajectory of the current health care system, focus should be more on outpatient transitioning rather than inpatient care.

Patients are spending less time in the hospital and more recuperative time at home. Home health care services will be one of the greatest demands placed on the future nursing workforce. To meet this need, the "neopractitioner" will have to be grounded in critical thinking and become more process oriented, rather than content-based. Health care providers must understand better the healing process so as to provide appropriate interventions. Specialization will yield to generalization, and content will yield to process.

Changes in the U.S. health care system are occurring at an unparalleled pace. Developing practitioners who can respond to these changes will be nursing's greatest challenge. Research findings will have to be disseminated to clinicians who can apply them in community settings. It no longer will be sufficient for nurses to present findings at national and international conferences to the accolades of peers. Novel ways of sharing this information in easily understandable language must be developed so that the public can truly benefit from nursing science.

To this end nursing research scientists must "partner" with clinical colleagues to help disseminate findings to the clients to whom services are provided. This approach will involve breaching parochial boundaries and a willingness to think and act outside the traditional academic and clinical pathways in which nurses have been educated. What events have led to these conclusions? And, how best might nursing accomplish this task?

■ A Research Role for the 21st Century

Rapid developments in technology and science, as well as the sociopolitical milieu, are propelling nursing into the 21st century. Clients too will force nursing to be ever responsive to their needs for disease prevention and health data to enhance the quality of their lives. Because of their access to health information on the World Wide Web, they will be better educated and more willing to challenge "conventional wisdom" or treatments or both offered by their health care providers. Clients will want to be active partners in their care, wanting to know why a specific treatment or regime of drugs is appropriate to their care. They will want to know about newer treatments, drugs, and therapies that they have discovered at various Web sites on the Internet. They will no longer be content to "do what the health care provider says." Nursing's challenge then is to be responsive to these new demands of the clients.

Research Preparation

The "neopractitioner" of the 21st century will be charged with providing quality-based care (read as "scientifically based care") at remarkably reduced rates among a better educated clientele. This view suggests that researchers will have to be both academically and clinically competent. It means a blending of the heretofore ascribed PhD and DNS roles. To maintain nursing's ever-evolving status among peers in other disciplines, the PhD is suggested to remain the primary degree, with an enhanced clinical component (perhaps an internship). Horn (1999) noted that during the past 2 years several universities have prescribed for students in other disciplines mandatory internships to prepare them to (a) work in teams, (b) expose them to other cultural perspectives, and (c) develop their skills in problem identification and resolution. The model is there; nursing simply needs to adapt it to nursing's needs.

What better way is there to prepare researchers than to allow them to spend a year developing skills and acquiring knowledge that would serve them throughout their careers. Adding a year to the current doctoral program to participate in an internship would allow the doctoral student to (a) be exposed to interdisciplinary research; (b) participate in generation of researchable problems; (c) understand processes involved in initiating a project in a clinical setting; and (d) learn negotiation strategies for authorship of research papers, sharing of indirect costs, securing workspace for their projects, and the like. Having completed an internship, the doctoral student could return to the university and have much greater understanding and appreciation for the career on which she or he is about to embark. Sherwen, Bevil, Adler, and Watson (1993) suggested that "only by developing programs that can prepare scholars with research skills necessary to answer professionally mandated research questions can doctoral programs meet needs for nursing knowledge" (p. 197).

Shaffer (1999) foresees that

> the caretaker of the future is going to have to be a cross-trained generalist: a nurse who can draw upon a strong base of critical thinking to function efficiently and accurately across all health care settings, and a nurse who is prepared to see his or her practice as case management for populations along the continuum and not just episodic case management limited by institutions and boundaries. (p. 2)

Research will parallel this change in approach. More studies will be done across populations and outside the confines of inpatient facilities.

To affect this shift, resources are going to have to be increased. Hinshaw and Berlin (1997), in delineating the future of quality doctoral nursing programs, observed that one element of this formula involved not only doctorally prepared faculty but increased resources as well:

> The data suggest that the existence of doctorally prepared faculty is necessary but not sufficient, it is the scholarly productivity and research productivity which makes for quality doctoral programs. In addition the data suggest, the need for advanced research infrastructure and sharply increased resources for funding nursing research." (p. 12)

Nursing must not only identify mentors to guide fledgling researchers, but also must ensure that sufficient resources are made available to provide the infrastructure to carry out this research mandate. With the necessary resources and infrastructure, what might nursing's research agenda look like for the 21st century?

Potential Research Areas for the 21st Century

Nursing has a history of responding to fluctuating changes in the health care marketplace. O'Neil and Coffman (1998) noted that "this focus on immediate needs has yielded a capac-

ity for flexibility unequaled among health care providers, but it has also inhibited nursing's ability to institute long term changes" (p. 216). As examples of this phenomenon we need only consider issues such as entry into practice, doctoral degree differentiation, and the doctorate as an initial versus a terminal degree. Consensus has never been achieved on these issues despite the lengthy history of professional discourse. If nursing is to lead, rather than be overcome by the events of the new millennium, it is going to have to identify its sphere of influence along a health care continuum and chart a course. Part of this process will involve changing the way it has done business for the past century—not an easy task.

With health maintenance organizations (HMOs), diagnosis-related groups (DRGs), and federal guidelines being imposed on health care providers and practices, nursing will have to show that its contributions to the health care system add value. The profession must be able to provide substantive data to show that not only what it does makes a difference, but it must also identify where those differences occur. As interventions improve outcomes, nursing needs to be able to link those outcomes to specific variables. For example, if nurse researchers are able to show that nursing interventions have helped decrease the number of low birth–weight infants, the nursing profession will want to know whether it was due to prenatal care, presence of a case manager, or institution of critical pathways. Who, better than nurse researchers, can study this phenomenon and ferret out these variables?

Outcomes and evidence-based research will be the driving force that advances the body of nursing knowledge. O'Neil and Coffman (1998) believe that "the emerging system of care will value those inputs that can demonstrate a positive contribution to outcomes for both the individual and the population" (p. 221). White (1997) in her preface to Kane's

(1997) book, *Understanding Health Care Outcomes Research,* reinforces this viewpoint when she states:

> Outcomes research is providing the groundwork necessary to enable effective clinical decisions that relate to the context and quality of life. Moving the use of outcomes data into the course of clinical care increases the likelihood that medical care [read as "health care"] will improve the health functional status, and well being of patients. (p. vii)

Outcomes research should be the driving force behind nursing's research agenda.

A third fertile area for nurses to investigate will be new delivery of care models. In the past, most care has been provided on an inpatient basis. However, with economics driving the delivery of care, increasing amounts of care are being delivered on an outpatient basis in community settings. Consider, for example, the case of the new mother who, until last year, was being discharged within 24 hours of delivery. Prior to institution of this policy, there were little data to suggest that early discharge was feasible. Only after several deleterious events did insurance carriers begin to review the wisdom of such policy. And, even then, it took political intervention to mandate that new mothers could remain in the hospital a minimum of 72 hours and that insurance carriers had to provide reimbursement for these stays.

The proliferation of short stay units (<24-hour inpatient care) for procedures such as tonsillectomies, herniorrhophies, and so forth also mandated changes in nursing's schema of care delivery. Changes such as decreased hospital stays and increased outpatient care require baseline data to evaluate safety and effective-ness. Facilities that have in-house researchers, or who contract with researchers from local schools of nursing, will be able to provide data necessary for sound administrative and clinical decision-making.

Finally, nursing should explore ways of translating its research findings into health policy. For nursing to accomplish this feat, a shift is needed in how research is done. Historically, single studies from single institutions have been the modus operandi. If nursing is to have increased influence with legislators and health policy makers, the profession must broaden its horizons through establishment of multidisciplinary, multisite studies. Only when nursing is able to increase generalizability of results across large populations will its credibility with policy makers be enhanced. Some efforts have been made to achieve this goal through establishment of Centers of Nursing Excellence across the United States, but much work remains to be done.

■ Concluding Statement

In each of the endeavors mentioned, nursing can and should play a pivotal role. As the largest health care profession, with the most patient contact hours, nursing is well situated to identify researchable problems. However, to do so will involve commitment, collaboration, and willingness to change many of the practices enculturated during the past century. As Charles Darwin (1874/1999) noted, "It is not the strongest of the species that survive, nor the most intelligent, but the one most responsive to change." Can nursing meet the challenge?

■ *References*

Abdellah, F., & Levin, E. (1994). *Preparing nursing research for the 21st century.* New York: Springer.

Carpenter, D., & Hudacek, S. (1996). *On doctoral education in nursing: The voice of the student.* New York: National League for Nursing Press.

Darwin. C. (1874/1999). [On-line]. Available: http://www.cybernation.com/victory/ quotations/subjects/quotes change.html and http://www.aimmconsult.com/ quotes.html.

First National Conference on Doctoral Education [in Nursing]. (1977, June 23–24). *Proceedings of the 1977 forum on doctoral education in nursing.* Philadelphia: University of Pennsylvania.

Forni, P. F. (1989). Models for doctoral programs. *Nursing & Health Care, 8,* 430–434.

Gortner, S. (1991). Historical development of doctoral programs: Shaping our expectations. *Journal of Professional Nursing, 7*(1), 45–53.

Grace, H. K. (1978). The development of doctoral education in nursing: In Historical perspective. *Journal of Nursing Education, 17*(4), 17–27.

Hinshaw, S., & Berlin, L. (1997). The future for quality doctoral nursing programs—Are the resources there? *Proceedings of the AACN 1997 doctoral conference quality control: An evaluation of doctoral education,* Sanibel Island, Florida. January 31, 1997, 1–22.

Horn, M. (1999). Practical PhD's. (1999, March 21). [On-line]. Available: http://www.usnews.com/usnews/edu/beyond/grad/gbphd.htm.

Hudacek, S., & Carpenter, D. R. (1998). Student perceptions of nurse doctorates: Similarities and differences. *Journal of Professional Nursing, 14*(1), 14–21.

Kane, R. L. (1997). *Understanding health care outcomes research.* Gaithersburg, MD: Aspen.

Murphy, J. (1981). Doctoral education in, of, and for nursing: An historical analysis. *Nursing Outlook, 29,* 645–649.

Newman, M. A. (1975). The professional doctorate in nursing: A position paper. *Nursing Outlook, 23*(11), 704–706.

O'Neil, E., & Coffman, J. (1998). *Strategies for the future of nursing: Changing roles, responsibilities and employment patterns of registered nurses.* San Francisco: Jossey-Bass.

Schlotfeldt, R. (1978). The professional doctorate: Rationale and characteristics. *Nursing Outlook, 26*(5), 302–311.

Shaffer, F. (1999). Competencies: Preparing nurses for a new era. *Dean's Notes, 3,* 1–3.

Sherwen, L., Bevil, C., Adler, D., & Watson, P. (1993). Educating for the future: A national survey of nursing deans about need and demand for nurse researchers. *Journal of Professional Nursing, 9*(4), 195–203.

Starck, P., Duffy, M., & Vogler, R. (1993). Developing a doctorate for the 21st century. *Journal of Professional Nursing, 9*(4), 212–219.

Stevenson, J. S., & Woods, N. F. (1986). Nursing science and contemporary science: Emerging paradigms. In G. E. Sorenson (Ed.), *Setting the agenda for the year: Knowledge development in nursing* (pp. 6–20). Kansas City, MO: American Academy of Nursing.

Werley, H. H., & Leske, J. S. (1988). Pinning down the tracks to the doctoral degree. *Nursing and Health Care, 9*(5), 238–243.

White, E. B. (1997). Preface. In R. L. Kane (Ed.), *Understanding health care outcomes research* (p. viii). Gaithersburg, MD: Aspen.

■ *Editor's Questions for Discussion*

What factors have influenced the change in the focus on problems addressed by nursing research? To what extent does the PhD in Nursing degree represent today the development of nursing knowledge? What consensus exists regarding the PhD in Nursing according to Lenz and Hardin (Chapter 20), Donnelly (Chapter 28), Gray (Chapter 42), and Boland (Chapter 71)? Do you agree with Miller's conceptualization of the ND degree? Present arguments for your response.

Discuss the ND degree. To what extent is the content of that nursing program essentially undergraduate versus the content of graduate or postgraduate nursing programs? Provide specific examples and rationale for your response(s).

Discuss the advantages and disadvantage of multiple doctoral degree offerings for nursing. Provide specific examples of doctoral programs that do not grant a PhD in Nursing but prepare nurses for clinical research and promote development of nursing knowledge. What factors affect decisions about the types of doctoral programs offered in nursing? To what extent does nursing need to address variables influencing those decisions?

Present arguments for and against doctoral programs in nursing differing in name only. Given the lack of consensus regarding delineation between PhD and DNS programs in nursing, what difference does this lack make in the purpose, content, and outcomes of programs for nursing practice, research, and education?

Propose arguments for and against two-track doctoral programs in nursing: research and clinical practice. What difference does it make, if any, as to the type of doctoral degrees that are offered in nursing for the future? What impact might mandatory internships and interdisciplinary doctoral programs have on furthering the profession, practice, education of nurses, and research as advocated by Lindsey (Chapter 29)? What are some of the essential indicators for high-quality doctoral programs in the 21st century? How might nursing best prepare to provide high-quality programs?

What implications for research and case management cited by Miller are addressed by Gerber (Chapter 57)? How are Miller's statements about evidence-based research and outcomes supported or not supported by Deets and Choi (Chapter 34) and Titler (Chapter 35)? Provide examples of the health policy research cited by Miller that are also advocated by Heinrich and Wakefield (Chapter 8).

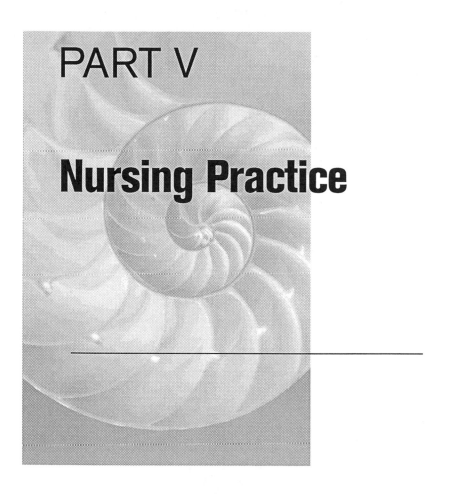

PART V

Nursing Practice

" . . . And be one traveler, long I stood
And looked down one as far as I could . . .
. . . Though as for that the passing there
Had worn them really about the same . . .
. . . Then took the other, as just as fair,
. . . Because it was grassy and wanted wear . . .
. . . I took the one less traveled by,
And that has made all the difference."

Perhaps at no time in the history of nursing have so many opportunities been available for practitioners and the profession both now and for tomorrow. The nurse "traveler" who plans a lifetime of professional service does need to look ahead. Long embedded ("worn") traditional nursing practice roles are changing dramatically.

Many factors have contributed to the expanding arena for professional practice. These elements include (a) increasing societal cultural diversity, (b) heightened consumer awareness in health care, (c) technology innovation and informatics, (d) emphasis on health and prevention of disease, (e) changes in health care delivery systems and settings for practice, (f) increasing collaboration in providing care, (g) focus on the community in health care, (h) alterations in funding and regulatory bodies, and (i) development of advanced practice nursing roles.

The paths for the future of nursing practice are varied, complex, and challenging. Fulfill-ment and goal attainment is there for the practitioner and the profession alike. The beginning practitioner may be inclined to choose a path that represents "greener grass." However, wisdom may lie in considering all the concerns, factors, and circumstances as portrayed in these contributing authors' chapters. So too, the profession will benefit from wise consideration of the content. Only then—may the practitioner and the profession realize the path or paths chosen "made all the difference."

37

Cultural Competence in a Changing Health Care Environment

Larry Purnell, PhD, RN, FAAN

As the United States becomes an increasing mosaic of cultures with globalization of the world economy and health care, nurses will care for clients from diverse cultures. Nurses also will work in new environments in other parts of the world. If they are to be successful in the future in a global health perspective, nurses must (a) understand their own culture, as well as those of their clients; (b) be aware of different perspectives on wellness and illness; (c) collaborate with nurses and other health care providers globally; (d) learn more about complementary and alternative therapies; and (e) understand the worldwide scope of travel and disease transmission. Additionally, nurses must study common problems on regional, national, and

international levels (Guevara et al., 1998), respect diverse beliefs and values, and incorporate their clients' world views and cultures into health care plans and interventions.

■ Cultural Competence

Important concepts for nurses to understand are the distinctions between cultural sensitivity, cultural awareness, and four levels of cultural competence—unconscious incompetence, conscious incompetence, conscious competence, and unconscious competence. Cultural sensitivity has more to do with using politically correct language and not saying things that may be offensive to another, such as WASP,

Negro, or illegal alien. Preferable terms would be European American or white, black or African American, and person with undocumented status. Cultural awareness has more to do with recognition and appreciation of diversity in arts, clothing, foods, and other external signs of diversity. Cultural competence means having knowledge and skills about an ethnoculturally diverse group that allows the health care provider to communicate in a manner congruent with the beliefs and practices of the group. An unconsciously incompetent person has no awareness that there are differences among clients. The consciously competent person is keenly aware that there are differences among their culturally diverse clients but does not know how to interact with them effectively. Conscious competence means the person has personal experiences with the group and is very deliberate in providing care to clients. The unconsciously competent person has multiple encounters and experiences with groups under care and has developed an intuitive grasp of how to be effective. For purpose of this chapter, culture is defined as

> the totality of socially transmitted behavior patterns, arts, beliefs, values, customs, lifeways, and all other products of human work and thought characteristics of a population that guides its worldview and decision making. These patterns may be explicit or implicit, are primarily learned and transmitted in the family, and are shared by the majority of the culture. (Purnell, 1998, p. 2)

Health care practices, beliefs, and values are inherent in this definition. Accordingly, culture affects how health and illness are perceived and defined. Culture has a powerful influence on what is acceptable and on the patient's interpretation of and response to health care. To be successful in the global village in the future, nurses must be prepared to (a) transfer knowledge from one culture to another, (b) share across disciplines by forming partnerships and integrating knowledge, and (c) then

distribute it globally. Otherwise, nurses' leadership is diminished and less effective (Dickerson-Hazard, 1998) in the future environment demanding a high level of wellness and cost containment.

Because they work with people in one-on-one, family, and community contexts, nurses are in unique positions to discover client's *emic* (viewed from within the culture) world view, which is a fundamental basis for providing culturally sensitive and competent care. Each person and culture has an outlook on life based on values and beliefs that are shared by the majority of the primary group to which the person belongs. Accordingly, nurses are in a position to provide high-quality care to diverse clients locally, nationally, and internationally. Additionally, many universities have initiated endeavors to promote an increase in multicultural understanding by adopting universities in other countries and engaging in international health care research.

In terms of the global workforce, it is essential to understand two opposing paradigms, individualism versus collectivism, that can affect working relationships. *Individualism* emphasizes individual outputs, rights, and rewards and values autonomy, competition, achievement, and self-sufficiency. Individualism is common among most English-speaking and European American cultures.

Collectivism emphasizes the need to maintain group harmony over the interests of individuals or subgroups. It values interpersonal harmony and group solidarity. Collectivism is common among the Asian, Amish (Andrews, 1998), and many Native American cultures (Still & Hodgins, 1998).

■ Globalization of Economics and Health Care

Globalization of economies and health care, with four of every five new jobs in the United

States being created by foreign trade, is helping drive need for cultural competence (Scarborough, 1998). Globalization is integration of one nation's economy and health care into the economy and health care of another nation, creating a global community. Within this global village, culture becomes an important element in economics and health care for both providers and consumers. Accordingly, businesses and the health care industry must recognize, respect, and integrate their clients' beliefs and practices into their own if they are to develop satisfactory working relationships. Creation of a good product is not enough if relationships between a business, in this case health care, and its clients are not managed in a culturally competent manner. Nursing programs must prepare nurses with a global perspective because they oversee the majority of health care in the world.

■ *Migration and Disease Risks*

Although immigration and population shifts occur worldwide, the United States with its growing economy and relatively low population density compared to countries from which people are emigrating, is receiving increased numbers of new immigrants with both legal and undocumented status. In the early part of the 20th century, immigrants to the United States came from the United Kingdom, Ireland, former United Soviet Socialists Republic, Latvia, Italy, Austria, and Hungary. By the late 20th century this pattern had changed and large numbers of immigrants were coming from China, Mexico, the Philippines, India, Brazil, Pakistan, Vietnam, Turkey, Egypt, and Thailand (Brunner, 1998).

Immigrants bring their own cultures and languages with them. Currently, some 32 million immigrants speak only their non-English native language—an increase of 34% during the past decade (Brunner, 1998). This potential language barrier has tremendous implications for the health care system. Health care organizations in all settings must procure interpreters and prepare educational materials in the language of choice, according to the client populations in their catchment areas. Today, nurses have increased opportunities for translation, with emergence of the AT&T translation services (AT&T, 1999) and other on-line resources (Diversity Rx, 1999) whereby many different languages can be accessed. The client can even be connected with someone who is bilingual in English and a native language.

Three blocs of countries are increasing the global perspective on trade and health care: the European Community (EC) formed by most of the countries in Western Europe; the North American Free Trade Association (NAFTA) among the United States, Mexico, and Canada; and the Japanese and Pacific Conglomerate. In addition, the Southern Hemisphere Coalition, with 34 Republics from Central America, South America, and the Caribbean, will further increase trade and health care globalization. These trade agreements and associations also are creating opportunities for joint research on problems that affect the delivery of health services worldwide.

As global trade, travel, migration, and immigration increase and economic development and health care become intertwined, so do internationalization of health risks and spread of infectious diseases, of which there is a high correlation (Lipson, 1996). Transmission can occur while people are on vacation or business travel. However, migrant and seasonal workers in the fruit, vegetable, and horticultural industries are at increased risk because they are exposed to pesticides and occupationally related injuries. Many times, migrant groups are at the low end of the educational system, are in low-pay positions, and are not familiar with the language of the host country, which makes it difficult for them to advocate for their rights and read labels on chemicals with which they work. Not only are workers themselves at increased risk, but the entire family, including children and pregnant women, is at risk because of inadequate housing, sanitation, and exposure to pesticides.

Exotic bacteria, viruses, and parasites along with reemergence of more virile old diseases, can traverse the globe in the time it takes for people and produce to move from one location to another, exposing people to diseases and illnesses to which they have no immunity. In less than a decade, there have been outbreaks of numerous powerful and deadly diseases. Since 1973, the World Health Organization (WHO) has added 28 pathogenic microbes to its list of human plagues. In addition to the human immunodeficiency virus, others are prevalent in North America (hantavirus and Legionnaires' disease), Central America (cholera, yellow fever, and dengue fever), South America (rabies, dengue fever, and cholera), Asia (avian flu, leptospirosis, and anthrax), Europe (shigella, E-coli, and typhoid), and Africa (Ebola virus, bubonic plague, and cholera) (World Health Organization [WHO], 1999). Some of these diseases have been introduced into countries through trade, such as cyclospora clusters from Guatemala into California, Texas, Nevada, Florida, and New York (Possehl, 1998). What new strains of tuberculosis and the human immunosuppressive virus are yet to occur? In poorer countries, infectious and parasitic diseases continue to be number one killers. Nurses must increase their skills and knowledge in epidemiology and public health surveillance worldwide.

■ *Paradigm Shifts
From Acute Care
to Wellness*

As society moves from a paradigm of acute care intervention to one of health promotion and wellness and of disease and illness prevention, nurses will increasingly encounter clashes between world cultures. In the wellness environment, nurses meet clients on their turf instead of the health system's turf, which dominates the acute care hospital environment. Furthermore, these clashes will occur more frequently, not only among clients and health care providers, but also among health care providers themselves. This new relationship will require new knowledge and skills if health prescriptions are to be effective and reduce costs to clients and society.

Wellness is a wholistic concept and a process that involves the biological, physical, sociological, cultural, psychological, and spiritual dimensions of a person's life. A high degree of wellness involves a person's ability to adapt to changes in health status. It allows the person to function at a high capacity. Additionally, it includes self-responsibility, self-knowledge, cultural self-awareness, self-expression, physical fitness, nutritional competence, and stress management. Wellness also is a process because it is constantly changing and moving a person toward greater awareness, even if the person has a terminal diagnosis, a chronic health problem, or developmental disabilities.

■ *Cultural Imperialism,
Relativism, and Cultural
Imposition*

As globalization of health care services increases, providers must deal with crucial issues such as cultural imperialism, cultural relativism, and cultural imposition. *Cultural imperialism* is the practice of extending policies and practices of one organization (usually the dominant one) to disenfranchised and minority groups. The U.S. government practiced imperialism in early 1800s. It forced Native American tribes to migrate, created reservations on which individual allotments of land were assigned to families instead of group ownership, and required Native American children to attend white people's boarding schools. Proponents of cultural imperialism appeal to universal human rights values and standards. Opponents of cultural imperialism posit that universal standards are a disguise for the dominant culture to destroy or eradicate traditional cultures through worldwide public policy (Amnesty International, 1999).

Cultural relativism is belief that behaviors and practices of people should be judged only in the context of their cultural system. Proponents of cultural relativism argue that issues such as abortion, euthanasia, female circumcision, and physical punishment in childrearing should be accepted as cultural values without judgment from the outside world. Opponents argue that cultural relativism may undermine condemnation of human rights violations and that family violence cannot be justified or excused on a cultural basis.

Cultural imposition intrusively applies the majority cultural view to individuals and families. Prescribing a special diet without regard to the client's culture and limiting visitors to immediate family—a practice in many acute care facilities—borders on cultural imposition. In this context, nurses must be careful in expressing their values too strongly, until cultural issues are more fully understood.

Genetic counseling is one area that has profound implications for cultural imperialism, cultural relativism, and cultural imposition, especially with racial and ethnic groups. Some ethnocultural groups have a high incidence of genetic and hereditary disorders, such as the Amish and Jewish. Additionally, Huntington's chorea and family planning with fertility drugs and birth control are areas that may involve all three of these cultural concepts. Should nurses encourage genetic testing? What does the nurse do with results after they have been obtained? What if the individual does not want to know the results? What if the results could have dele-terious outcome to an infant or mother or both? What if the results got into the hands of insurance companies that then denied payment or refused to provide coverage? Should public policy support genetic testing that may improve health and health care for the masses of society? Should multiple births from fertility drugs be restricted because of the burden of cost, education, and health imposed on the family? Should public policy encourage limiting family size in contexts of the mother's health, religious and personal preferences, and availability of potable water and food supply in the future? Given a nation with an aging population, decreasing family size, and decreasing numbers and percentages of younger people, what effect do these issues have on the ability of a country to provide health care to its citizens? Nurses must understand these three cultural factors and the ethical issues involved because they will be increasingly encountering situations in which they must balance the client's cultural practices and behaviors with health promotion and wellness and with illness and disease prevention activities for the good of client, family, and society. Other international issues that may be less argumentative include latex allergies, needle sticks, sustainable environments, pacification, and poverty.

■ Paradigm Shifts Toward Wellness and Alternative Medicine

Four Health Care Systems

There are four health care systems worldwide. The *biomedical allopathic health care system* combines Western biomedical beliefs with traditional U.S. values, such as self-reliance and individualism. It relies heavily on conquering disease and proving health care interventions, using the scientific method. Providers are specialized and licensed to practice. The *popular health care system,* which is most common worldwide, involves self-medication and treatment. When this first line of defense does not work, people then seek out other people for care, such as family, friends, or community leaders. The *folk traditional health care system* includes shamans or traditional healers who receive their gift from God or serve an apprenticeship. The *alternative health care system* includes homeopathic medicine, naturopathic medicine, chiropractic medicine, diet therapy, and pharmacological treatments (Luckmann, 1999). Most people move from one system to the other, depending on type and severity of illness. In some societies, allopathic care may not even be available; yet, people prosper and have high degrees of wellness because they practice health maintenance and illness prevention within their cultural contexts. Additionally, the concepts of preventive care and annual health evaluations by biomedical health care providers are unknown or not well accepted.

Traditional healing practices dominated health care from ancient times until the 1910 Flexner report (BeSaw, 1998). Today, allopathic medicine, with practice based on the scientific method, prevails in health care's practices and beliefs for illness and disease prevention, health maintenance, and health restoration in modern societies. Traditional medicine today, commonly referred to as complementary and alternative medicine (CAM), is making a resurgence in the United States because many people are dissatisfied with Western treatments and their negative side effects, unacceptable risks, and invasiveness.

Complementary and Alternative Medicine

The Office of Alternative Medicine (OAM) of the National Institutes of Health does not differentiate between the components of complementary and alternative medicine (CAM) and gives the following definition:

Complementary and Alternative Medicine is a broad domain of healing resources that comprises all health systems, modalities, and practices and their accompanying theories and beliefs, other than those intrinsic to the politically dominant health system of a particular society or culture in a given historical period. CAM involves all such practices and ideas self-defined by their users as preventing or treating illnesses or promoting health and wellbeing. Boundaries within CAM and between the CAM domain and the dominant system are not always sharp or defined. (CAM Panel, 1997, p. 50)

Additionally, the OAM is the collaborating center for the WHO. The Web site of the OAM can be accessed on-line at http://www.nih.gov/.

With demand for CAM well established, distinctions among curing, eradicating a disease, and healing are important concepts of wellness in arriving at a sense of wholeness and completeness. Because attempts to cure disease may have disastrous side effects on the client's quality of life for years, more and more people are seeking out more noninvasive techniques, such as those involved with complementary and alternative therapies. Kirby's (1992) survey of 1,165 households in Pennsylvania and Maryland reported that 33% of the households consulted chiropractors, 25% used massage therapists, and 16% used spiritual healers. Hufford's (1992) survey of cancer clients reported that 70% of them used folk treatments. In another study, of those who used CAM, 38% were between the ages of 25 and 59, and 44% had a college education with an income of more than $35,000 (Eisenberg et al., 1993). Visits to CAM providers were greater than visits to conventional providers, 425 million versus 388 million, mostly with an out-of-pocket expense rather than insurance reimbursement.

The Landmark Report (1998) showed that 42% of Americans had used some type of alternative therapy in the past 5 years, and 67% said that availability of an alternative health care component was an important consideration in choosing a health plan. The Agnes Reid Group (1998) showed that 42% of Canadians use alternative therapies and that the use of alternative therapies increases with age, with 40% of those aged 18 through 34 years using alternative therapies, compared with 57% of those aged 35 through 54 and 67% of those 55 and older. In 1997, CAM visits exceeded 455 million in the United States. Thus, to provide better care, health care providers need to know what CAMs clients are using. Many health care providers do not even ask clients whether they are using CAM therapies. When asked, clients do not respond honestly if the health care provider asks the question in a nonapproving manner. The majority of people in the United States who use complementary and alternative therapies seek them for prevention and chronic illnesses. Moreover, CAM remains the only medicine for 80% of the world's population (Dean, 1981; Hufford, 1992).

The U.S. Public Health Service, as part of its commitment to Healthy People 2000, offers postdoctoral training in complementary and alternative medicine. The OAM has funded 12 clinical research centers (2 of them nursing schools) in complementary and alternative medicine.

Complementary and Alternative Medicine Classifications

The components of CAM are categorized as (a) mind and body interventions; (b) alternative systems of medical practice; (c) manual healing; (d) bioelectromagnetic applications; (e) herbal medicine; (f) pharmacological and biological treatments; (g) diet, nutrition, and lifestyle changes; and (h) visual reality, which is this author's newest classification of CAM. In each of these categories, some of the therapies are widely accepted in the United States, but the efficacy of others is suspect or controversial. However, in other parts of the world these therapies are readily accepted.

Mind and body interventions, such as psychotherapy and hypnosis, meditation, guided imagery, biofeedback, dance therapy, art therapy, music therapy, and prayer, are readily accepted, in the United States and elsewhere in the world. Alternative systems of medical practice such as traditional Oriental medicine, acupuncture, Ayurvedic medicine, homeopathic medicine, naturopathic medicine, anthroposophically medicine, Native American Indian health care practices, and environmental medicine continue to get more acceptance in dominant cultures in the United States. Manual healing therapies comprise more than 20 different categories. Three prominent postural reeducation therapies (Alexander, Feldenkrais, & Trager) teach the client how to realign their body to improve function, coordination, and balance, which relieves structural and functional stress. These movement therapies are used in drama schools to improve performers' coordination. Successful medical applications include relief of back pain, whiplash, myalgia, hypertension, stress, and anxiety (Edelman, 1987; Ginsberg, 1986; Jackson, 1991; Kandel & Hawkins, 1992).

Virtual reality—a computer-generated therapy—combines visual display, audio input, and interactivity. It has been used successfully with clients who (a) fear flying, driving, spiders, heights, and public speaking; (b) have agoraphobia (Strickland, Hodges, North, & Weghorst, 1997); (c) are in rehabilitation (Greenleaf, 1997); (d) have attention and movement disorders (Wann, Rushton, Smyth, & Jones, 1997); and (e) are in special needs education (Kerr & Wilson, 1997). However, virtual therapy interventions may have deleterious health and safety issues, such as hearing disturbances, motion sickness, trauma related to falls, vertigo—both long range and short range physiological effects (Viire, 1997).

The public's desire for improved wellness through use of complementary or alternative therapies and medicine has had positive impacts on third party payors. Insurance companies, because of public demand, are beginning to reimburse for selected "unconventional therapies." Health centers and hospitals are beginning to incorporate these therapies into their allopathic practices. Additionally, 34 of the nation's 125 allopathic medical schools are now offering courses in alternative medicine (Neimark, 1997). A concern is: What are nursing schools doing to prepare their students for this "back to the future" paradigm shift?

■ Issues for Providers

As they encounter and even help create health care systems for culturally diverse clients worldwide, nurses must be sure that services are available, accessible, acceptable (Mokuau & Fong, 1994), and affordable. Health services that meet these criteria increase opportunities for early detection and management of health problems. *Available* means that services exist, there are adequate facilities, and health providers have requisite training and education and resource capacity to handle those in need of services. It can also mean availability of interpreters, bilingual personnel, and written educational materials in the preferred language of the clients.

Accessible health care means services are readily available in the community without barriers, such as transportation, geography, on-site baby sitting services, both walk-in and by appointment, and convenient hours of operation for people to access care and facilities.

Acceptable means that services are provided in a culturally adaptable manner and vary according to the values, beliefs, and traditions of the cultural groups served. Services may include having an on-site or referral source for indigenous and traditional healers, as well as a variety of complementary and alternative therapies.

Affordability means that the care is provided at a cost that does not take away the recipient's ability to provide the essentials of food, clothing, and shelter. When clients are not able to pay for all or part of their care, federal, state, and private funding should be available. Free preventive care, as in the case of pregnant women, may significantly reduce long-run costs to a society by reducing complications during pregnancy and postpartum for mother and newborn.

■ Concluding Statement

By definition, globalization requires people to interact with others in and from other nations—many times those with cultural world views, beliefs, values, and practices that may be similar to or different from those of the people delivering care. Quality of interactions and successful outcomes depend on quality of information, understanding and knowledge about the cultures with whom the person interacts, and a willingness to have an open mind and engage in cultural encounters. The only way to be successful and compete globally is to increase cultural knowledge and encounters and to collaborate with diverse cultures.

■ References

Agnes Reid Group. (1998). [On-line]. Available: http://www.agnesreid.com.
Amnesty International. (1999). [On-line]. Available: http://www.amnesty.org.
Andrews, M. (1998). Transcultural perspectives in nursing administration. *Journal of Nursing Administration, 28*(11), 30–45.

AT&T. (1999). [On-line]. Available: http://www.att/com/languageline.

BeSaw, L. (1998). Medical school make-over. *Texas Medicine, 94*(11), 67–69.

Brunner, B. (1998). *Information Please: Almanac.* Boston: Houghton Mifflin.

CAM Panel. (1997). Describing and defining complementary and alternative medicine. *Alternative Therapies in Health and Medicine, 3*(2), 49–57.

Dean, C. (1981). Self-care response to illness: A selected review. *Social Science Medicine, 15A,* 673–687.

Dickerson-Hazard, N. (1998). Nurses without borders. *Reflections,* 3rd quarter, 6.

Diversity Rx. (1999). [On-line]. Available: http://www.diversityRx.org/HTML/NEHOT. htm.

Edelman, G. (1987). *Neural Darwinism: The theory of neuronal group selection.* New York: Basic Books.

Eisenberg, D., Kessler, R., Foster, C., Norlock, F., Calkins, D., & Delblanco, T. (1993). Unconventional medicine in the United States. *New England Journal of Medicine, 328*(4), 246–253.

Ginsberg, C. (1986). The shake-a-leg body awareness training program: Dealing with spinal injury and recovery in a new setting. *Somatics,* spring/summer, 31–42.

Greenleaf, W. (1997). Applying VR to physical medicine and rehabilitation. *Communications of the American Academy of Medicine: New Technologies in Health Care, 40*(8), 43–46.

Guevara, E., Mendias, E., Goins, P., Drew, J., Heredia, A., Fellizzia, C., Ferraz, C., Mishima, S., de los Angeles Paz Morales, M., & Valdez Martinez, M. (1998). Values unlimited: Nurses say human needs come first. *Reflections,* 3rd quarter, 17–19.

Hufford, D. (1992). Folk medicine in contemporary medicine. In J. Kirtland, H. Andrews, C. Sullivan, & K. Baldwin (Eds.), *Herbal and magical medicine: Traditional healing today* (pp. 295–314). Durham, NC: Duke University Press.

Jackson, O. (1991). The Feldenkrais method: A personalized learning model. In M. Lister (Ed.), Contemporary management of motor control problems. *Proceedings of the II-Step Conference. Foundation for Physical Therapy* (pp. 131–135). Alberta, Canada: Acadia Physical Association.

Kandel, E., & Hawkins, R. (1992). The biological basis of learning and disability. *Scientific American, 267,* 78–88.

Kerr, D., & Wilson, J. (1997). *Communications of the American Academy of Medicine: New Technologies in Health Care, 40*(8), 72–75.

Kirby, J. (1992). *Moving toward a holistic lifestyle.* New York: Lightworks.

Landmark. (1998). *Landmark report on public perceptions of alternative care.* [On-line]. Available: http://www.landmarkhealthcare.com.

Lipson, J. (1996.) *Reflections,* 4th quarter, 10–11.

Luckmann, J. (1999). *Transcultural communication in nursing.* Albany, NY: Delmar.

Mokuau, N., & Fong, R. (1994). Assessing responsiveness of health services to ethnic minorities of color. *Social Work in Health Care, 20*(2), 23–34.

Neimark, J. (1997). On the front lines of alternative medicine. *Psychology Today, 30* (1), 52–68.

Office of Alternative Medicine, National Institutes of Health. (1999). [On-line]. Available: http://www.nih.gov/.

Possehl, S. (1998). Global hot spots. *Hospitals, and Health Networks, 72*(13), 28–31.

Purnell, L. (1998). Purnell's model for cultural competence. In L. Purnell & B. Paulanka (Eds.), *Transcultural health care: A culturally competent approach* (pp. 7–53). Philadelphia: F. A. Davis.

Scarborough, R. (1998). *Delaware foreign languages curriculum framework commission.* Dover: Delaware State University.

Still, O., & Hodgins, D. (1998). Navajo Indians. In L. Purnell & B. Paulanka (Eds.), *Transcultural health care: A culturally competent approach* (pp. 423–447). Philadelphia: F. A. Davis.

Strickland, D., Hodges, L., North, M., & Weghorst, S. (1997). Overcoming phobias. *Communications of the American Academy of Medicine: New Technologies in Health Care, 40*(8), 34–39.

Viire, E. (1997). Health and safety issues for VR. *Communications of the American Academy of Medicine: New Technologies in Health Care, 40*(8), 40–41.

Wann, J., Rushton, S., Smyth, M., & Jones, D. (1997). Rehabilitative environments for attention and movement disorders. *Communications of the American Academy of Medicine: New Technologies in Health Care, 40*(8), 49–52.

World Health Organization via the National Institutes of Medicine. (1999). [On-line]. Available: http://www.nih.gov/.

■ Editor's Questions for Discussion

Provide examples of how nursing programs can prepare nurses with a global perspective. To what extent is cultural competence emphasized in nursing curricula? What learning experiences will facilitate cultural competence? Discuss the impact of travel, migration, and immigration on nursing programs, nursing students, and health care services. What type of practice settings may be venues for increasing knowledge of and collaboration among diverse cultures? What views expressed by Ketefian and Redman (Chapter 19) will require knowledge of culture, as presented by Purnell?

What relationships exist between Purnell's discussion and points emphasized by Davis (Chapter 6) and Boland (Chapter 71) and those chapters presented in the Nursing Practice Part? Are culture clashes more likely to occur in wellness settings and broad health care environments than in acute care and hospital settings? Does cultural imperialism exist in nursing programs? To what extent is cultural relativism an issue for nursing students and faculty? How does cultural imposition by faculty affect counseling aspects of genetics, as presented by Jenkins (Chapter 54)? Indicate strategies and processes whereby nurses should balance their beliefs and values with clients' cultural practices and behaviors.

How does content offered by Snyder, Kreitzer, and Loen (Chapter 43) apply to Purnell's discussion about traditional healing practices? Identify nursing research conducted in complementary and alternative medicine. How are nursing programs preparing students for mind and body interventions and virtual reality therapy in nursing practice?

38

Informatics for Nursing Practice

Kathleen R. Stevens, EdD, RN, FAAN
Elizabeth E. Weiner, PhD, RN, FAAN

Envision nurses in the following practice environments: (a) communicating with patient support groups via electronic mail, chat rooms, or other electronic means; (b) serving as nurse experts to answer electronically posted health questions posed by anonymous clients from around the world; (c) using sophisticated data collection devices for purposes of documenting clinical patient outcomes; (d) analyzing research literature to determine knowledge strengths or gaps; or (e) inputting data into handheld data assistants for inclusion in larger patient databases. Nurses, today and in the future, are expanding their roles into practice arenas driven by nursing informatics.

■ *Informatics and Technology*

Nursing informatics became a popular term during the 1990s, but it is not well understood by either nurses or the general public. Perhaps in an effort to promote a contemporary image, speakers have often used these two words interchangeably with *technology*, which is really a tool that enables those working in the area of informatics to work more effectively and efficiently. The clinical setting offers the richest information environment that can most immediately be affected by the use of informatics. Understanding the possible uses and impact of informatics therefore becomes a professional imperative for practicing nurses in a variety of clinical settings. Nurses always have been in the business of processing information; only the methods have changed over time. Recently, the emphasis has shifted to further processing of information so that it becomes transformed into knowledge. Graves and Corcoran (1989) described informatics in their classic article as "the use of computers and information sciences to aid in the transition of data into information, and information into knowledge" (p. 227). Data are defined as discrete pieces of information that, when viewed alone, often have no meaning. When patterns or themes are discerned about data, they take on new meaning and become information. Further exploration of emerging information themes compared against some domain of knowledge results in the formation of knowledge. This knowledge then becomes the basis for nursing practice. A pragmatic description of nursing informatics is the "formalization and manipulation of information needed by nurses to practice and by patients to maintain self care" (Brennan, 1998).

The popularity, growth, and subsequent integration of technology into U.S. society have provided nurses with valuable tools that have become necessary for the data transformation process. Technology allows for data storage and graphical depiction of even the largest sets of data so that new meaning can be extracted from data that could not otherwise be readily understood. Patterns and themes can be identified and examined over time—yet another necessary skill that would be difficult without this tool. A wide range of possible uses of technology has emerged over the last decade making it inevitable that future nursing practice will become "informated."

Information Revolution

Toffler and Toffler (1995) describe three great waves of change affecting civilization. The agricultural revolution extended over thousands of years, but the industrial revolution took a mere 300 years. The authors suggest that the third wave, that of the information revolution, might take less than two decades to overtake cultures worldwide. As a result, educators, researchers, and practitioners in all disciplines are being called on to rethink the role of knowledge in order to grow from second-wave thinking into third-wave thinking. Integration of third-wave thinking will not only empower nurses for the future, but it will also enrich practice opportunities in ways never before thought feasible.

Effective third-wave thinking involves successful integration of technology into practice, an adaptation that has not come easy to some. Essential to successful integration is identification of ways to harness technologies to help achieve nursing's clinical goals (Brennan, 1999). A reengineering of practice then becomes possible and in some cases requires imagination and creativity. The ultimate reason for harnessing information technologies is to ensure quality patient care and promote growth of nursing knowledge.

Barriers to Integration

Change in itself is threatening, but incorporating new innovations into daily practice creates additional stress. The Diffusion of Innovation Theory provides a framework that helps explain how information is disseminated through a predictable social process (Rogers, 1995). Different types of adopters are described, such as the "innovators," who are the first to seek information about new ideas. "Early adopters" are respected members of an organization or social group who are followed by the "early majority," who adopt new ideas deliberately, just before the average member. The "late majority" usually learns of the change from peers rather than through formal channels. Those in the last group, the "laggards," are less responsive to new ideas, peer pressure, or other social influences.

Each practice setting must evaluate where members of the group are (or will be) classified along this spectrum. Implementation strategies can then be based on group characteristics and needs that capitalize on what the group needs, in order to fit the innovation with the needs of the organization. For example, integrating an automated information system in any setting should rely on innovators and early adopters both for input into the design of such a system and for their respected leadership. They, in turn, can assist with implementation strategies geared toward the early and late majority, along with the laggards.

Other barriers to successful integration include individuals who suffer from technophobia and information anxiety. One-on-one work with them will usually help decrease their fears and anxiety, but clear directions and well-designed user interfaces also are essential for success. Nurses in most settings are fast approaching the time when they will not be able to practice without simultaneously using technology.

■ The Merger of Technology with Nursing Practice

Why has technology become so important to nursing practice? The simplistic answer is "out of necessity." Weiner and Trangenstein (1999) describe in table format the crosscurrents of clinical nursing practice and technology. Examples from clinical practice are noted in conjunction with examples of simultaneous technology growth, and the synergy quickly becomes clear. For example, the earliest attempts to use technology centered on automation of the existing patient record. The major focus was on collecting data and information. Technology solutions centered on hospital information systems, which continue to be expanded today. As information management tools became available, nurses began to look at establishing relationships in data and organizing databases in a uniform fashion so that elements and connections could be determined. The database became the technological solution.

Storage of large amounts of data is readily enhanced with the use of technology. Document management has become an important topic for any organization seeking to rid itself of obsolete paper-based records. Benefits include (a) space savings, (b) simultaneous access to the same record, (c) immediate access to the record, (d) no lost records, (e) disaster recovery possibilities, and (f) no microfilm (Heinrich & Hinte, 1999). In addition, clinical data repositories and other data warehousing overcome any earlier data limitations. Administrators then have the basis for creating more effective administrative decision-support models.

Growth of the Internet and more advanced transmission techniques for audio, video, and still images has fostered a "virtual" practice arena. Emerging telehealth sites allow clinical consultation and diagnosis by health care providers from remote sites. New technology tools allow for better knowledge synthesis and expert clinical decision-making. The storage of data was an important prerequisite to data modeling. Data modeling is a process that allows the user to analyze data so that it becomes information, which then can be used to contribute to knowledge. The techniques of such modeling are outside the scope of this chapter, but you should be aware of the contribution of data modeling to the informatics process. In short, the conversion of current technology tools, with nursing's need to revise practice based on nursing knowledge, has pushed the profession into third-wave thinking.

Changing Nursing Practice

It should not be surprising that, as a result of this conversion, practice roles are changing. Not only has information technology changed the way nurses practice, but it is also changing the nature of practice. For example, information technology can greatly enhance the way nurses provide patient education. Information technology may also change the nature of practice, such as changing the role that the nurse assumes in an Internet cancer support group. Instead of meeting at a community center, the support group connects via an Internet chat room, changing the very nature of the nurse's interaction and practice with these patients. Likewise, readily available Internet health information may add new functions to patient education, such as evaluating Web sites for the quality of their content and interactivity so that these resources can be used confidently in patient intervention.

Using technology to communicate has expanded roles so that nurses now are being hired to answer health-related questions in call centers. "Call a Nurse" refrigerator magnets are common marketing practices of many health insurance companies and businesses selling certain health care products. However, the nature of interaction itself changes drastically when neither nurse nor patient has the benefit of nonverbal communication skills. Voice mail menus sometimes provide a frustrating experience for customers as they attempt to work through the maze of choices to get a question answered. Nurses employed in this type of environment may find that clients begin their initial exchange already feeling that additional frustration.

■ *Nursing Informatics*
   as a Specialty and a Role

Nursing informatics as a specialty emerged with the introduction of computers into health care. Computer applications expanded and merged with traditional central nursing functions, such as information management and nursing practice. Today, nursing informatics is recognized as a specialty, requiring knowledge and skills from a number of disciplines.

In 1992, nursing informatics was designated as a new nursing specialty by the American Nurses Association (ANA). This role was defined by the ANA (1994) as

> the specialty that integrates nursing science, computer science, and information science in identifying, collecting, processing, and managing data and information to support nursing practice, administration, education, and research; and the expansion of nursing knowledge. It supports the practice of nursing specialties in all sites and settings of care, whether at the basic or advanced practice level. (p. 3)

The ANA (1995) published practice standards for the informatics nurse, nursing informatics standards of professional performance, and domain standards for the informatics nurse.

Roles in nursing informatics vary widely in this new specialty. The work may be broadly described as ensuring that the information needed for nursing practice is available when practice is occurring and that the technology used to handle that information is specific, beneficial, and efficient in terms of nursing (Brennan, 1998).

Largely derived from a particular agency's organizational schema, position titles for nursing informatics specialists include clinical information systems coordinator, manager, or project director; clinical information analyst; clinical nurse specialist (CNS) for nursing informatics; and chief or director of nursing informatics (American Medical Informatics Association, 1999). One survey of position titles and role descriptions showed wide variation in title, scope, and functions of the nursing informatics specialist. As the nursing

---

TABLE 38.1   Examples of Educational Goals of Courses and Degrees in Nursing Informatics

- Analysis, design, implementation, and evaluation of clinical nursing information systems
- Research, model, and theory development in nursing informatics
- Clinical information systems and information handling
- Clinical and administrative decision making systems
- Processing, storage, and retrieval of nursing and patient care data
- Integrating evidence-based protocols into nursing information and patient care systems

---

informatics specialty stabilizes, standards of practice and preparation requirements will also stabilize.

Role Preparation

In response to the growing specialty knowledge in nursing informatics, a number of formal education and continuing education courses in the field are now available. Universities now offer courses and degrees in nursing informatics. These educational opportunities have been classified as (a) graduate programs (doctoral and master's) with a specialty nursing informatics focus; (b) graduate and undergraduate programs and courses in nursing informatics, including concentrations and minors; and (c) individual courses in nursing informatics in graduate and undergraduate programs. Educational goals specified across this range of courses and degree are listed in Table 38.1.

In addition to formal coursework in nursing informatics, numerous continuing education conferences also are available. These conferences include introductory short courses, networking opportunities, demonstration of new technologies, and discussions of current issues in nursing and health care informatics (e.g., confidentiality). Detailed information about these educational courses and conferences is available at two primary Web sites, as shown in Table 38.2.

Certification in Nursing Informatics

The American Nurses Credentialing Center (ANCC) administers the testing for Certification in Nursing Informatics. Requirements for this certification are that (a) the applicant hold a baccalaureate or higher degree in nursing; (b) have practiced as a licensed registered nurse (RN) for a minimum of 2 years; (c) have practiced at least 2,000 hours in the field of informatics nursing within the past 5 years or have completed at least 12 semester hours of credits in informatics in a graduate program in nursing and have practiced a minimum of 1,000 hours within the past 5 years; and (d) have 20 contact hours of continuing education in informatics specialty in the past 2 years. Further information is available from the ANCC, 600 Maryland Ave., SW, Suite 100 West, Washington, DC 20024-2571.

Nursing Knowledge in the Information Age

The tandem forces of information technology, health and nursing science, and public demand have resulted in a trend toward evidence-based practice. In evidence-based practice, nursing care is based on research evidence of the effectiveness of that care. The explosion of health knowledge presents particular challenges to

TABLE 38.2   Continuing Education for Nursing Informatics

Source	Web Address (URL)
Education Programs and Courses in Nursing Informatics American Medical Informatics Association (AMIA) Nursing Special Interest Group home page. This site includes a list of schools with classes and programs in Nursing Informatics.	http://amia-niwg.org/
Nursing Informatics Conferences University of Maryland School of Nursing, Susan K. Newbold's home page. The "Frequently Asked Questions" section lists a wide variety of upcoming conferences on health and nursing informatics.	http://nursing.umaryland.edu/

nurses, both now and increasingly in the near future. This knowledge explosion requires nursing information systems that enable nurses to access information and knowledge presented in synthesized form and evaluate the scientific evidence underlying nursing interventions (McCormick, 1997).

Information technology currently enables the nurse to access synthesized knowledge. Several sources highly relevant to nursing are the *Online Journal of Knowledge Synthesis for Nursing,* Agency for Health Care Policy and Research, and the Cochrane Collaboration (see Table 38.3). Each of these sources uses informatics-based approaches in addressing the combined challenge of the health knowledge explosion and the need for quality health care based on scientific evidence.

The *Online Journal of Knowledge Synthesis for Nursing* is an electronic journal, published by Sigma Theta Tau International, for nurses who base their practice on research. This journal is unique in that each of its articles is a synthesis of research on a given clinical topic. Acknowledging that extraction of clinical meaning from research articles is time intensive and difficult, the journal presents synthesis articles that review clinical research, extract clinical implications, and identify gaps in knowledge. It includes integrative reviews on such topics as agitation of persons with dementia, assessment of postpartum depression, maintaining patency of enteral feeding tubes, and external pinsite care.

A second major source for evidence-based practice is the Agency for Health Care Policy and Research (AHCPR). This federal agency produces syntheses of evidence on clinical topics and publishes them on its Web site. The AHCPR is charged with supporting research designed to improve quality of health care, reduce its cost, and broaden access to essential services. Its broad programs of research bring practical, science-based information to medical practitioners, consumers, and other health care purchasers.

The Cochrane Collaboration is an international organization that aims to help people make well-informed decisions about health care by providing systematic (meta-analytic) research reviews. The organization provides access to these reviews through its electronic publication, the Cochrane Library. The Library is designed to supply high-quality scientific evidence to inform people providing and receiving care and those responsible for research, teaching, funding, and administration at all levels.

TABLE 38.3   Resources for Evidence-Based Practice Knowledge

Source	Web Address (URL)
Online Journal of Knowledge Synthesis for Nursing	http://nursingsociety.org/
Agency for Health Care Policy and Research (AHCPR)	http://www.ahcpr.gov/about/overview.htm
Cochrane Collaboration and Library	http://www.cochrane.org/

■ Increased Access to Information

Recent growth of the World Wide Web, the Internet, and personal computers has opened the floodgates of information available to all health care consumers. Previous information may have been geared to health care professionals (e.g., grant opportunities, research databases, clinical trials, and so forth). But, currently, there is a shift to the provision of online information organized specifically for consumers of health care services.

Access and hardware previously were barriers to technology integration, but rapid advances in each of these areas have vastly expanded choices for the consumer and made the services irresistible. For example, America Online (July 29, 1999) describes itself as "the world's leader in interactive services, web and Internet technologies, and electronic commerce." Founded in 1985, the corporation now operates two worldwide Internet provider services, America Online (with more than 17 million subscribers) and Prodigy (with more than 2 million subscribers). The "virtual communities" in this case comprise at least 19 million subsets of the larger group.

People from varied ages and backgrounds think nothing of sharing their electronic mail (e-mail) addresses with one another. It has become standard practice to have e-mail or Web addresses printed on business cards. Even public buses and billboards carry catchy Web addresses designed to pull interested consumers toward use of their products.

Consumer Access

Consumer access is further being expanded by telephone and television companies venturing into new services that were not available even 5 years ago. For example, consumers continue to request faster and faster modems for transferring data across their telephone lines, but at some point the speed of the modem outstrips the capability for telephone wires to transmit data any faster. As a result, telephone companies such as Cincinnati Bell have expanded to include asynchronous digital subscriber line (ADSL) offerings for faster delivery of data. Packaged as a product line called Zoomtown (1999), this delivery uses the copper telephone wires already installed in private homes in such a way that the user can continue to talk on the telephone while enjoying data transmission rates that are as much as 50 times faster than the typical 28.8K modem. Television cable companies have been quick to follow suit with cable modem technology, which uses existing cable wiring for faster speeds that bypass the telephone system entirely.

Health Provider Access

Access for health professionals has been increasing with the addition of faster machines, vastly improved software, better security, and substantially lower costs being added to already stable networked practice environments. Many of these networks now interface with other systems housing needed client information. Increased speeds and collaboration possibilities also result from networks with increased bandwidth. More than 150 universities in the United States, working together with partners in industry and government, are leading efforts to expand bandwidth capabilities through the Internet2 (I2) initiative. The purpose of this collaborative effort is to develop advanced Internet technology and applications vital to the research and education missions of higher education. Internet2 is developing applications such as telemedicine, digital libraries, and virtual laboratories that are not possible with the technology underlying today's Internet. As a project of the University Corporation for Advanced Internet Development (UCAID), the Internet2 project is not a single separate network. Rather, it joins member network application and engineering development efforts to many advanced campus, regional, and national networks. Collaborative efforts with other countries, such as Canada, are just beginning to take place, and international networking possibilities are coming much closer to reality.

Impact of Access

Increased access to information has an impact both on the client and the health care provider. On one level, increased access expands possible nursing outreach and therefore changes traditional client characteristics. On another level, organization of data and information becomes critical as providers begin to rethink content, organization, and possible impacts on practice. One example of a client-focused Web site is Netwellness, http://www.netwellness.org/, an electronic consumer information service developed by the University of Cincinnati Medical Center and more than 35 community partners (Hern, Weitkamp, Haag, Trigg, & Guard, 1997). Nursing faculty have become involved in the "Ask an Expert" portion of the site. Other commercial providers are realizing the possible impact of providing health care information in this format and are designing sites with full-time experts involved.

These types of sites offer unique challenges to health care providers. How can the usefulness of a site be evaluated when the clients themselves may not be identifiable? How can publishers of databases of health care information better understand that these databases will no longer be used solely in medical center libraries but with an expanded user base extending well outside the usual boundaries of libraries? What sorts of licensing agreements are cost-effective, but reasonable, for those organizations delivering health care information? The "Web pioneers" are attempting to address all these questions, but it is clear that nursing has a role in the development, delivery, and evaluation of Web sites.

■ Health Information on the World Wide Web— The Issue of Quality

The Internet hosts a large number of high-quality health resources and offers grand opportunities to inform, teach, and connect health care professionals and patients. One concern, however, is that vast amounts of health information may be incomplete, misleading, or inaccurate. Although this new and exciting medium is highly attractive as a multimedia communication vehicle, the content remains the bedrock of health information and Internet resources must be evaluated for their substantive quality.

As Web health information and health services (e.g., support groups) are considered for use in patient care, health care providers will want to evaluate carefully their usefulness and validity. Various rating instruments are becoming available, but many are incompletely developed (Jadad & Gagliardi, 1998). Experts recommend a common sense approach and a review of web sites used in patient care. The core standards of a review include examination of (a) authors and their credentials and affiliations; (b) attribution of all content to references; (c) disclosure of Web site ownership, including advertising, sponsorship, and other arrangements; (d) currency disclosed in posted updates of the Web site (Silberg, Lundberg, & Musacchio, 1997); and (e) level of content validity, with evidence-based sources rated highest (Badgett & Lawrence, 1998).

■ *Standard Nursing Language for Health Information Systems*

Health care information has been the major focus of development in health and nursing informatics. The first step was computerization of patient care records. Computerized documentation systems are alternatively called clinical information systems, health information systems (HIS), or, in the case of nursing, nursing information systems. HIS provide great potential for information management. Informated patient and health care information potentially benefits quality of care, but cost-effectiveness is also a major incentive for development of such systems. Computer documentation provides information with which to control costs and streamline processes of care. This capability has given rise to development of evaluation of health care agency performance, as with the Health Plan Employer Data and Information Set (HEDIS). It provides a uniform reporting standard for health plans to specify, calculate, and report performance information in five categories: quality, en-

rollee's access and satisfaction, utilization, and financial data (Appleby, 1995).

Another significant advantage of HIS is the ability to mesh patient information, nursing care standards, research knowledge, effectiveness of care, and resource utilization information. The first step in the process of building health information systems is to describe accurately and reliably information to be entered into the system—in this case, nursing diagnoses, nursing interventions, and nursing outcomes. Standard languages or nomenclature allow for clear communication across disciplines, health care events, and health care settings.

Need for Common Language

The single most crucial phase in development of nursing informatics has been the creation of a standard vocabulary to describe what nurses do and the impact that it has. One of the foremost needs in a nursing-relevant health information system is to establish a stable model, or frame, of nursing data to allow better understanding and interpretation of patient care (Brennan, 1998).

The work to develop nursing data standards for computer-based systems has advanced on several fronts, using nursing process as the standard for documenting clinical nursing practice. In 1998, the ANA recognized the Nursing Minimum Data Set (NMDS) (Werley & Lang, 1988) as 16 elements necessary to document nursing care of patients and families across delivery settings. The four elements related to care—nursing diagnoses, nursing interventions, nursing outcomes, and intensity of nursing care—were proposed as minimal for computer systems, enabling comparison of nursing data across health care facilities, populations, and geographic areas (Werley & Lang, 1988).

A common language describing clinical nursing is crucial to development of automated health information systems. These standardized languages or vocabularies enable patient information to be integrated with health care information to provide seamless health care throughout a life span and across health care agencies. As nursing-focused elements are designed into computerized health information systems, these elements must be named and described with standardized classification systems and standardized languages. Only by using language systems that have been expertly and systematically developed and evaluated will essential information about nursing practice and its impact be documented and related to patient care and outcomes.

Standardized Systems

Standardized nursing information systems will evolve to be an integral part of the systematic inquiry process used in both quality assurance and research. Nursing information systems created with standardized language will allow examination of effectiveness and efficiency, either for monitoring quality of care or for producing new knowledge through research. With such systems in place, nursing research can more readily and inexpensively be accomplished on large databases and populations.

So important is the issue of standardized language use in health information systems that, in 1999, the American Nurses Association established the Nursing Information and Data Set Evaluation Center. The purpose of this center is to develop standards pertaining to information systems that support documentation of nursing practice and to evaluate voluntarily submitted information systems against these standards. The need for an evaluation center arose out of a long history of calls for standards pertaining to nursing data and information systems. The standards evaluate completeness, accuracy and appropriateness of four dimensions of nursing data sets and the systems that contain them: (a) nomenclature, (b) clinical content, (c) clinical data repository,

and (d) general system characteristics (Averill et al., 1998).

Currently, standardized clinical nursing information systems have been developed for nursing diagnoses, nursing interventions, and nursing outcomes. The ANA Nursing Information and Data Set Evaluation Center has recognized seven standardized language systems. A description of each of these standardized languages is presented in Table 38.4.

Linkage of Language Systems

Nursing informatics research continues to develop these and other language systems into reliable and valid ways of describing nursing care. In addition, the vision is for other information and knowledge resources to be linked to a well-developed nursing information system. To facilitate this goal, the Unified Medical Language System (UMLS) project was undertaken by the National Library of Medicine (1999). The UMLS project is intended to aid development of systems that help health professionals and researchers retrieve and integrate electronic biomedical information from a variety of sources. It also aims to help users easily link disparate information systems, clinical records, scientific literature, bibliographic databases, factual databases, knowledge-based systems, databanks, and directories of people and organizations (National Library of Medicine [NLM], 1999). Some of nursing's standardized language systems (NANDA, NIC, OMAHA, and HHCC) have been added to the UMLS to begin to link nomenclature through semantic networks and a metathesaurus. The UMLS Semantic Network provides consistent categorization of concepts represented in the metathesaurus and links terms across languages (Linberg, Humphreys, & McCray, 1993). Nursing also is moving forward with work on a Unified Nursing Language System. Extensive research is underway to enhance and refine the

TABLE 38.4 Standardized Language Systems Recognized by
the American Nurses Association (ANA)

Language System	Purpose	Description	Source
NANDA North American Nursing Diagnosis Association	Classifies nursing diagnoses	A classification system of nursing diagnoses developed by the North American Nursing Diagnosis Association. Nursing diagnosis is defined as a clinical judgment about individual, family, or community responses to actual and potential health problems and life processes. System includes a taxonomic structure for relating the groups within the system; 128 nursing diagnoses are included.	NANDA, 1996
NIC Nursing Interventions Classification	Standardizes the nomenclature of nursing treatment	A standardized language of treatments that nurses perform; NIC identifies both nurse-initiated and physician-initiated interventions performed to produce targeted patient outcomes and is comprehensive across setting and specialty; 433 direct and indirect care interventions are identified.	McCloskey & Bulechek, 1996
NOC Nursing Outcomes Classification	Provides a consistent nomenclature for describing patient and family caregiver status	A standardized taxonomy of nursing-sensitive client outcomes, useful across a continuum of care; 197 outcomes were published in 1997, and more have been added.	Iowa Outcomes Project, 1997
OMAHA Visiting Nursing Association Vocabulary	Provides a complete, structured approach to practice, documentation, and information management	A research-based vocabulary organized into Problem Classification Scheme, Intervention Scheme, and Problem Rating Scale for Outcomes. Originally developed in community health, it has been expanded to many settings.	Martin & Scheet, 1992 http://con.ufl.edu/omaha/
HHCC Home Health Care Classification	Provides standardized nomenclature to assess and document home health care	An empirically developed decision support system that categorizes home health care nursing services designed. It includes schema for coding and categorizing nursing diagnoses and interventions.	Saba, 1992; http://www.dl.georgetown.edu/research/hhcc/
Ozbolt's Patient Care Data Set	Provides a catalog of terms to name health issues or problems, orders for care, therapeutic goals, and goal evaluation status	A conceptual structure for statements with sets of atomic-level terms corresponding to each concept. By selecting terms and linked concepts, precise and complex descriptions of clinical realities can be composed that computers can understand and treat as data.	Ozbolt, 1999
Perioperative Nursing Diagnoses, Interventions and Outcomes	Provides perioperative nurses with a standardized language for documenting and thus evaluating the care they provide	An empirically validated standardized nursing language for perioperative and surgical settings. It includes schema for classifying nursing diagnosis, interventions, and patient outcomes.	Kleinbeck, 1996

languages and the system that connects them. Once the entire health record has become computerized, patient information will be linked directly to evidence-based knowledge that identifies effective interventions, anticipated outcomes, and related literature resources.

■ Empowering Nurses to Use Informatics Effectively

Undoubtedly, the specialty of nursing informatics will continue to develop, further defining standards of practice and the specialty role in nursing. Equally certain is that informatics will play an increasingly significant part in every nurse's role. The future will bring continued integration of informatics functions with all nursing roles, as nursing informatics becomes more and more integrated into the core processes of health care. This integration will occur as meaningful nursing information systems are folded into health information systems and as evidence-based practice knowledge becomes part of these health information systems.

The development and adoption phase of HIS provides a unique opportunity to integrate quality, utility, and unity into automated health information systems. Present needs must be assessed comprehensively and future needs anticipated clearly in order to design durable systems that communicate across present barriers.

Only an estimated 15% of health care agencies have comprehensive HIS. As the adoption rate increases, nursing informatics specialists will have an opportunity to determine HIS specifications—hardware, software, underlying language, and interface. This opportunity is unique because, once these costly systems have been adopted, major changes in HIS will not likely be supported by health care agencies. This situation is indeed a unique opportunity to evaluate technologies, platforms, and systems approaches during the adoption process. Such an opportunity will not likely present itself again until the next big shift from the Information Age to a future age. Nurses therefore are advised to use a broad approach, adopting a broad perspective in fashioning HIS. Individual health care agencies must overcome the temptation to develop specialized systems, using specialized languages and platforms that isolate the system from others. Without standardized nomenclature, such systems, lacking the necessary common language, will communicate ineffectively with others—or not at all—precluding the benefits of seamless health care.

■ Concluding Statement

Many nurses currently functioning in informatics roles have not received formal curricular training in this specialty. Some have expressed an interest in technology and were pulled into HIS design teams. Others have taken continuing education courses or have taught themselves the essential skills and taken on new roles. Each new specialty must have a beginning, but this varied approach makes it difficult to achieve and perpetuate consistencies across practice settings.

An individual nurse may find it difficult to see the larger scope of influence that informatics embraces. Identifying the essential role that individuals play in helping create and deliver a nursing informatics' agenda may be even harder. Each individual contribution is unique and important—all are considered "pioneers." Let us stay focused on the fact that our need for standardization exists—not to constrain, but to help empower us as we practice nursing in a variety of roles.

■ *References*[1]

America Online. (1999, July 29). [On-line]. Available: http://www.aol.com/corp/profile.

American Medical Informatics Association Nursing Informatics Workgroup (1999, July 29). *Roles in nursing informatics.* [On-line]. Available: http://amia-niwg.org/.

American Nurses Association. (1994). *The scope of practice for nursing informatics.* Washington, DC: Author.

American Nurses Association. (1995). *Standards of practice for nursing informatics.* Washington, DC: Author.

American Nurses Association. (1998). *Nursing minimum data set.* Washington, DC: Author.

American Nurses Association. (1999, October 19). *Nursing information and data set evaluation center.* [On-line]. Available: http://www.nursingworld.org/nidsec/.

Appleby, C. (1995). Health Plan Employer Data and Information Set (HEDIS)—Managed care's emerging gold standard. *Managed Care, 4*(2), 19–24.

Averill, C. B., Marek, K. D., Zielstorff, R., Kneedler, J., Delaney, C., & Milholland, D. K. (1998). ANA standards for nursing data sets in information systems. *Computers in Nursing, 16*(3), 157–161.

Badgett, R. G., & Lawrence, J. C. (1998). Internet health rating systems: Knowledge vs Babel. *Journal of the American Medical Association, 280,* 697–699.

Brennan, P. F. (1999). Harnessing innovative technologies: What can you do with a shoe? *Nursing Outlook, 47*(3), 128–132.

Brennan, P. F. (1998). *What is nursing informatics?* Video interview. Baltimore: The University of Maryland. [On-line], October 10, 1999. Available: http://amia-niwg.org/.

Graves, J. R., & Corcoran, S. (1989). The study of nursing informatics systems. *IMAGE: Journal of Nursing Scholarship, 21*(4), 227–231.

Heinrich, G., & Hinte, G. (1999). Emerging technologies. In M. J. Ball & J. V. Douglas (Eds.), *Performance improvement through information management: Health care's bridge to success* (pp. 162–172). New York: Springer-Verlag.

Hern, M., Weitkamp, T., Haag, D., Trigg, J., & Guard, J. R. (1997). Nursing the community in cyberspace. *Computers in Nursing, 15*(6), 316–321.

Internet2. (1999, July 30). [On-line]. Available: http://www.internet2.edu.

Iowa Outcomes Project. (1997). In M. Johnson & M. Maas (Eds.), *Nursing outcomes classification (NOC).* St. Louis: Mosby.

Jadad, A. R., & Gagliardi, A. (1998). Rating health information on the Internet: Navigating to knowledge or to Babel? *Journal of the American Medical Association, 279,* 611–614.

Kleinbeck, S. V. M. (1996). In search of perioperative nursing data elements. *AORN Journal, 63*(5), 926–931.

[1]Note: All Web addresses were current as indicated in the entries. Should you receive an addressing error message, use one or more of the various search engines now available with Web browsing software to locate the source desired.

Linberg, D. A. B., Humphreys, B., & McCray, A. T. (1993). The Unified Medical Language System. *Methods of Information in Medicine, 32,* 281–291.

Martin, K. S., & Scheet, N. H. (1992). *The Omaha System: Applications for community health nursing.* Philadelphia: W. B. Saunders.

McClosky, J. C., & Bulechek, G.M. (Eds.). (1996). *Nursing interventions classification (NIC)* (2nd ed.). St. Louis: Mosby-Year Book.

McCormick, K. (1997). Nursing in the 21st century—Guideposts in an information age. In V. D. Ferguson (Ed.), *Educating the 21st century nurse: Challenges and opportunities* (pp. 1–17). New York: National League for Nursing Press.

National Library of Medicine. (August 2, 1999). *Fact sheet: Unified medical language system.* [On-line]. Available: http://www.nlm.nih.gov/pubs/factsheets/umls.html.

North American Nursing Diagnosis Association. (1996). *NANDA nursing diagnoses: Definition and classification, 1997–98.* Philadelphia: Author.

Ozbolt, J. G. (1999). *The patient care data set: Profile.* Unpublished manuscript, Vanderbilt University Center, Nashville, Tennessee.

Rogers, E. (1995). *Diffusion of innovations* (4th ed.). New York: Free Press.

Saba, V. K. (1992). *Home health care classification (HHCC) of nursing diagnoses and interventions* (rev. ed.). Washington, DC: Author.

Silberg, W. M., Lundberg, G. D., & Musacchio, R. A. (1997). Assessing, controlling, and assuring the quality of medical information on the Internet. *Journal of the American Medical Association, 277,* 1244–1245.

Toffler, A., & Toffler, H. (1995). *Creating a new civilization: The politics of the third wave.* Atlanta: Turner.

Weiner, B. E., & Trangenstein, P. A. (1999). The third wave of information technology. In E. J. Sullivan (Ed.), *Creating nursing's future: Issues, opportunities, and challenges* (pp. 106–115). St. Louis: Mosby.

Werley, H. H., & Lang, N. M. (Eds.). (1988). *Identification of the nursing minimum data set.* New York: Springer.

ZoomTown. (1999, July 29). Unified Medical Language System® (UMLS®). [On-line]. Available: http://company.zoomtown.com.

■ Editor's Questions for Discussion

How may informatics facilitate databases and effective evaluation of nursing interventions, as discussed by Deets and Choi (Chapter 34)? How might data modeling occur? What advantages would data modeling have for nursing practice and systematic research studies? What strategies may reduce barriers in integrating automated information systems? What difference is there between nursing informatics and nursing information technology?

How has information technology changed nursing practice? How do Stevens and Weiner address telehealth implications presented by Schroeder and Long (Chapter 47)? How can information technology improve research studies concerning evidence-based practice? What information technology suggestions may apply to improve findings in the review by Deets and Choi (Chapter 34)?

How do D. Jones' (Chapter 31) and Sills and Anderson's (Chapter 77) discussions about nursing language address Stevens and Weiner's plea for a common language in nursing? To what extent are the language needs identified by those authors different? Given Deets and Choi's (Chapter 34) concerns about research quality, to what extent may standardized nursing information systems improve quality? How likely is it that evidence-based practice knowledge will become part of health information systems? What challenges must be addressed, by whom, and how? To what extent do present standardized language systems meet needs identified by D. Jones (Chapter 31), and Sills and Anderson (Chapter 77)?

Discuss ethical issues related to informatics. How might nursing as a profession have an impact on consumer access to high-quality health and illness information? What assurance can be provided for client information security in telehealth and network systems? How should electronic consumer information service sites be evaluated? What role should nursing have in the development, delivery, and evaluation of health care information Web sites? Who should provide that role in nursing for Web sites and how? What standards should be developed for informatics practice?

39

The Critical Importance of Faculty Practice

Michael A. Carter, DNSc, RN, FAAN

rofessional nursing is a practice discipline. In common with other practice disciplines, becoming a nurse requires that the aspirant be guided by expert practitioners in learning the craft. Learning the knowledge of the profession has great value, but the craft comes into its own in the acquisition of skills that distinguish the practitioner. These skills must be learned at the elbow of the clinician-teacher. This necessity was a problem for nursing education in the latter part of the 20th century, with faculty giving up their clinical practice responsibilities when moving into the university. Thus students were required to learn clinical skills in situations where their role models were not faculty, but nursing staff.

More recently, the idea has developed that faculty should resume responsibility for patient care as a part of their usual work—faculty practice. Key issues have emerged in the area of faculty practice, including how time is to be allocated among the competing demands of teaching students, conducting research, serving the organization and community, and the new expectations of practice.

Another issue is determining what constitutes faculty practice. Does it include activities undertaken to maintain skills? What is the role of student supervision? Must faculty practice constitute direct services only, or do indirect services such as consultation and administration also represent faculty practice? How should scholarship in practice be evaluated and rewarded? None of these are easy questions, and each has a number of different interpretations, based on goals of the parent institution and the nursing program.

■ History of Faculty Practice in Nursing

In the United States, professional nursing education developed within the hospital in the late 1800s, when faculty were sparse. A substantial part of teaching was done by the more advanced students training the less advanced students. The faculty that did exist were responsible for nursing care in the hospital first and the training of students second. Students tended to view these few faculty as expert clinicians as they were the only graduate nurse role models available. Over the past century, the locus of nursing education has moved from the hospital to the university. This movement was greatly accelerated in the latter part of this century and was not without controversy. Of great concern was the removal of faculty from the direct care of patients and a realization that the clinical skills of faculty might no longer be maintained.

Along with the move from hospital to university came substantial changes in the educational level and role of nursing faculty. The idea that faculty would be trained as generalists and have responsibilities for care of those patients involved in students' learning was lost with migration to the university. Faculty became specialists, with added research abilities, rather than generalists. Little about faculty characteristics for preparation of new nurses was clear.

A separation developed between how and where faculty taught students and how and where students learned the skills necessary to become nurses. Faculty became visitors in the clinical arena, rather than expert clinicians

responsible for care of patients. Faculty were responsible to the university and not to the hospital or other nursing service. This change was appropriate in that earlier approaches to nursing education had placed the student in the role of staffing nursing service first and learning second. Movement to the university meant that the student's learning came first and staffing of nursing service was not even a part of the student's role.

More recently, a movement developed in which nursing faculty have responsibilities for the care of patients as part of their expected faculty role. Beginning in a few nursing educational programs primarily located in academic health science centers, there has been a growing call for faculty to reclaim their historical role and move toward development of scholarship standards for this practice (Christman, 1982; Grace, 1981).

An important component of the evolution of faculty practice in the United States has been the concomitant evolution of advanced practice nursing. Today, almost all states recognize advanced practice nurses and provide some form of prescriptive ability for them. The federal government through its Medicare program provides for direct payment to advanced practice nurses for services to Medicare recipients. In order to teach their students, faculty in schools that prepare advanced practice nurses need to model these activities. That means the schools, or at least some faculty, hold the expectation that services provided by faculty should be reimbursed by the federal government and other third-party payers (Taylor, 1996).

■ Models of Faculty Practice

A number of arrangements are possible under which faculty may engage in clinical practice. The entire faculty in a particular school may not be practicing under the same set of agreements. The models in which faculty practice varies by the amount of role integration that is expected of them. In some models, faculty perform all customary faculty duties during the usual work day and then engage in practice on weekends, school breaks, or during the summers. This form of faculty practice does not integrate the role of teacher with the role of clinician and seldom are students a part of faculty practice. This model does little to demonstrate scholarship and, in essence, reflects two different jobs.

Another model allows faculty to practice one or more days per week, but again there is little integration here with other faculty responsibilities. This form of practice is usually covered under the provisions that many universities offer for faculty consultation. In this model, students do not have an opportunity to learn with faculty when faculty are practicing.

Some schools of nursing are organized in a manner that includes the Dean as Chief Nursing Officer for the health system. Faculty share teaching, practice, and research roles within the organization. This model has been called a unification model in that the expectation exists for full integration of all faculty responsibilities. Students learn in the faculty's practice. Faculty are the primary clinicians and have a great deal of control over patient outcomes and, thereby, student learning opportunities. In earlier times, these models existed in health science centers that had large hospital operations. As health care has changed, these models have also changed in that health science centers have now become health systems including hospitals, home health agencies, day surgery centers, long-term centers, and many other product lines as groups of service providers. New financial demands for these emerging health systems have placed challenges on the full unification models.

An additional model for faculty practice is built on a set of practice arrangements between the nursing school and a number of agencies for services of faculty. These arrangements may include a variety of options such as nursing centers and faculty practice organizations that accept capitation for services from managed care organizations, traditional fee for service practices, or contracted services. Some of these arrangements may share economic risk. This model is characterized by a high degree of entrepreneurship in the school and among faculty. In this model students learn in the faculty's practice and also learn the intricacies of practice management, quality outcome measures, and business savvy.

No one model will serve all faculty practice needs, and some schools may even blend several to achieve the school's goals. In all these models, however, two cultures often collide. On the one hand, practice is focused on the current situation that exists among the nurse, client, and delivery system, on achieving the desired outcome—usually in the very short term. On the other hand, education is focused on preparing students for the long-term future. The desired outcome is building basic learning, skills, and abilities that will serve students for a lifetime of practice. Practice is often entrepreneurial, whereas education is not. Practice focuses on doing, whereas education focuses on becoming. Resolving these differences is not always easy, but doing so falls squarely on faculty practice. It is the nexus of education, patient care, and scholarship and must stand as an exemplar for student learning.

■ Challenges of Faculty Practice

Developing the faculty practice program for a school of nursing presents a number of challenges. They can be viewed as related to the mission of the organization, changes in faculty responsibilities, and management of the nursing unit.

Mission of the Organization

Most nursing schools reside in parent colleges or universities that list their missions as teaching, research, and service. Placing a faculty practice program in this context is not an easy fit. The service mission is often used to relate to faculty practice, but community service was meant when the university set this mission. Seldom did it mean income generation through sale of professional services by faculty and staff. The nursing school may be the only professional school within the university, and demand by faculty for support of their practice activities can create tensions not only among various schools, but also between the school of nursing and university administration.

In addition to disparity with the university's mission, problems with the mission of the nursing school itself exist. Crafting new nursing school mission statements to reflect faculty practice is not easy and may conflict with the values of other faculty. However, schools of nursing in land grant universities can often draw analogies between their desired faculty practice activities and the traditional land grant mission of service to the population of the state.

Faculty

Tensions exist among faculty when a practice program is initiated. Perhaps no issue is more important to faculty members than how their work time is to be allocated. The funding of many schools is based on a formula built around generation of credit hours per student. Faculty time in these schools is assigned on the basis of the expected generation of credit hours. Faculty time is also assigned for scholarship and for service to the school or university. If new expectations for practice are added to this allocation formula, the assumption is that less time is available for the teaching, research, and service responsibilities. Few faculty believe

that they have available time to be allocated to any other activity, including practice. If some faculty are provided patient care assignments, it means that other faculty must increase their teaching and service commitments (Barger & Bridges, 1987).

Assigning faculty to practice is built on the assumption that faculty are clinically competent. Even more desirable is that faculty would be clinically expert, yet there is little evidence that such is the case. Faculty receive advanced practice education as a part of their master's degree. Few receive any clinical education as a part of their doctoral degree. If faculty are clinically competent, it is generally not because of their education. Clinical practice changes rapidly, and faculty who have not maintained current practice quickly become outdated. Time and training may have to be provided to bring faculty to a level of acceptable clinical functioning.

Another tension grows from the attempt to define practice for faculty (Potash & Taylor, 1993). Some faculty believe that clinical activities in which they engage for the purpose of maintaining their skill levels should be considered faculty practice, even if they do not receive payment for these activities. Other faculty believe that these activities are professional responsibility and should not be considered faculty practice. Other faculty believe that the time spent supervising students in clinical agencies should be considered faculty practice. Still other faculty argue that such activity is not faculty practice because the faculty member has not entered into a nurse–patient relationship and cannot expect to bill for these services.

Some faculty disagree about whether indirect service delivery such as administration and consultation constitutes faculty practice. Historically, only direct services in which faculty provided clinical services to clients were considered practice. With emergence of new and complex systems of care delivery, new services by nursing faculty are needed. These include (a) designing systems of care for organizations, (b) developing and managing quality-improvement programs, (c) defining and measuring care outcomes, (d) structuring and conducting clinical research programs, (e) providing staff educational programs, and (f) designing and monitoring case management product lines for managed care organizations.

Nursing School Operations

Development of faculty practice programs has created new issues for operations of nursing schools. One of the central issues concerns how to value faculty practice in the consideration of promotion and tenure. Few policies and procedures of the university occupy such an important prominence as promotion and tenure of faculty. Universities have had in place traditional understandings of the performance requirements of faculty in teaching, scholarship, and service; yet practice does not fit within these time-honored traditions. Adequate performance in teaching, scholarship, and service has never been sufficient for promotion or tenure. Faculty members are expected to move beyond adequacy and instead demonstrate excellence in these traditional areas. The forms of evidence of such performance are well understood, not only by the nursing program, but by the university at large. Faculty practice, however, is not usually well understood by either the nursing program or by the larger university. Fortunately, Boyer (1990) provided a framework by which scholarship in practice can be considered for promotion and tenure. Many schools of nursing have adopted this standard, and Boyer's work served as the foundation for statements of scholarship in practice adopted by the American Association of Colleges of Nursing (1999).

Distribution of income earned from faculty practice also challenges nursing schools. The university provides base salaries for faculty. Seldom is there a direct relationship between the activities of faculty and increased income to the nursing program. Faculty practice has changed this relationship because it generates income and in so doing requires reconsideration of just how the nursing school should value the work of faculty. Faculty practice plans (varying from rather simple to very complex) have been developed in schools of nursing, with some schools even developing new and separate corporations to deal with income concerns. Schools of nursing in academic health science centers often looked to the practice plan of the school of medicine to develop a model. Nursing faculty practice plans that have been developed tend to focus on the distribution of income earned by the practice and account for how time devoted to practice is paid. Beyond these two characteristics, there are few other similarities among nursing faculty practice plans.

An additional area that requires new policy formulation concerns the overall administrative, legal, and political support for faculty practice activities. Included are issues such as (a) liability insurance, (b) mandatory continuing education for practice, (c) billing and collection of patient fees, (d) quality assurance, (e) Medicare and Medicaid provider numbers, (f) credentialing, and (g) political activities to advance the practice. Few schools had in place policies and procedures to deal with these issues prior to initiation of a faculty practice program. These cited issues emerged even when the majority of care provided by faculty was through contract.

■ Vision for the Future

Creation and acceptance of a preferred vision for future faculty practice will bring with it a number of fundamental changes in how nursing schools operate. Evolution of traditional academic culture may be expected to continue along with addition of new values, beliefs, language, and relationships that are not a part of today's nursing school.

Faculty Practice Programs

Schools that offer advanced practice education in nursing will be required to develop and maintain cost-effective faculty practice programs. Faculty competent to teach advanced practice students must be based in current clinical practice as well as in theory and methods. To retain national certification, faculty will be required to engage in practice a significant portion of their work time. An integrated practice program is required to prevent pulling faculty in opposite directions. Schools that cannot achieve a viable practice program for their advanced practice faculty will soon lose them, or at best will lose the credentials of these faculty. Students are discerning consumers and quickly will know which faculty are clinically competent and which are not. Little need exists today for students to enroll in a program that does not maintain a clinically competent faculty, and there will be even less need for them to do so in the future.

In addition, there will be increased pressures for practice agencies to become more cost-effective than is the case today. Supervising students does not increase cost-effectiveness, as students are slower than experienced clinicians, require additional room, and often learn by making mistakes. Thus agencies not having some funding for teaching will be less and less able to perform teaching functions. As a result, schools of nursing must create faculty practice programs to meet teaching needs of new students. These practices must be of sufficient size and complexity to ensure quality learning. All these factors require a different type of resource than currently exists. In addition, schools of nursing often create new and innovative roles

for nursing. They should include faculty practice laboratories in which current boundaries are stretched and at times broken. Innovative new roles are very difficult to create in traditional organizations and often only faculty have the social and legal mandates to make them happen.

Future Funding

Future funding of nursing schools will be different from the past. Pressures will continue to mount for (a) providing cost-effective educational models, (b) conducting more costly research with limited budgets, (c) increasing demands on philanthropy for support, and (d) increasing reliance on funds from practice to contribute to profitability of the school. These pressures will increase tensions among the various roles and functions of faculty.

Future Integration of Roles

Successful schools of the future will be those in which there is true integration of multiple faculty roles. Teaching, research, and patient care must occur at the same time and in the same location if maximum efficiency is to be achieved. Integration will not be easy in that clinicians and scientists currently lead different professional lives and are educated in very different ways. Current PhD programs prepare graduates for a career as scientists and members of scientific teams, although seldom is there any focus in the program on advanced practice knowledge and skills. Current advanced practice programs are at the master's level and do not have sufficient time or focus to prepare the graduate, except for beginning advanced practice. What will be required in the future is development of clinical doctorates of rigor similar to that of PhD programs. These new programs will need to be of sufficient length and depth to produce graduates for leadership in health care delivery. In some cases, students will want combined clinical and research doctorates similar to those in other health related fields, such as the MD/PhD (Doctor of Medicine and Doctor of Philosophy), DDS/PhD (Doctor of Dental Surgery and Doctor of Philosophy), and PharmD/PhD (Doctor of Pharmacy and Doctor of Philosophy).

Patient Care Business

Schools of the future will need to develop abilities to understand the complex business of patient care in a way that has not been required in the past. Patient care is business and often big business. Understanding ways of capturing and maintaining market share, adjusting payor mix of patients to ensure financial viability, and constantly improving quality while decreasing the costs of care are elements of care that few nursing schools currently are prepared to achieve. Yet, these and many more areas are critical to the survival of nursing schools. Faculty will have to learn to be cost-effective, not only in teaching and research but also in patient care. Managed care organizations will profile each individual practitioner and likely disenroll those who do not meet cost and quality standards. Just what this oversight will mean is not clear when the practitioner is a faculty member whose salary in part is derived from patient care income that is no longer available.

Shift of Educational Costs

In the future, nursing schools will need to shift more of the costs of students' education to patient care dollars. This requirement will occur at the same time that payors for care will be attempting to decrease their costs of care.

That is, demands will increase to demonstrate satisfactory patient care outcomes at the lowest costs. Nursing can lead in this area. For example, patients in the future with the highest costs for care likely will be those with chronic illnesses and, particularly, with acute exacerbation of these chronic illnesses. Faculty in many nursing schools are reporting new knowledge concerning just how to prevent these exacerbations or, when they occur, how best to minimize effects. Research by nursing faculty in the future increasingly will be directed at these areas. The integrated teaching, research, and patient care practices of faculty are the best laboratory for discovery of the knowledge needed to improve patient outcomes at the possible lowest cost. An important fundamental shift in the thinking of many faculty will be required.

Future Faculty Appointments

The current, traditional understanding of tenure likely will undergo substantial evolution in the future. Tenured faculty enjoy a protected position concerning continued appointment and pay, with little that can be done to alter appointments short of gross misconduct. This protection may not be the case in the future. Salary of the tenured faculty member may not be assured beyond a minimum base. Year-to-year changes in faculty income may occur when total compensation consists of contributions from teaching, research, and practice. Tenured faculty unable to generate income from these various sources may have a continued appointment but at a very limited or no salary. In the future, the number of individuals who hold faculty appointments, but do not fit today's concept of a faculty member, is likely to increase. Such faculty may not be tenured, may not desire tenure, and may not even be eligible for tenure consideration. The value of faculty likely will reside in their ability to generate funds in excess of costs from research and practice.

■ Concluding Statement

Evolution of the faculty role in nursing schools during the past century has been dramatic. In some ways, this development reflects the similar evolution of professional nurses' roles in practice settings. Crafting a future vision for the faculty practice role likely will see an even greater acceleration in the evolution of faculty, schools, and universities.

Schools of the future cannot hope to be successful unless faculty engage in an economically viable, high-quality practice program. Such programs will be the safe learning environments for future practitioners. They also will be the idea incubators for research and clinical innovation. What will be required is the courage and commitment of faculty and administration to bring this vision to reality.

■ References

American Association of Colleges of Nursing. (1999). *Position statement of defining scholarship for the discipline of nursing.* Washington, DC: Author.

Barger, S., & Bridges, W. C. (1987). Nursing faculty practice: Institutional and individual facilitators and inhibitors. *Journal of Professional Nursing, 8*(5), 263–270.

Boyer, E. (1990). *Scholarship reconsidered: Priorities for the professorate.* Princeton, NJ: The Carnegie Foundation for the Advancement of Teaching.

Christman, L. (1982). The unification model. In A. Marriner (Ed.), *Contemporary nursing management* (pp. 91–95). St. Louis: Mosby.

Grace, H. K. (1981). Unification, re-unification: Reconciliation or collaboration-bridging the education-service gap. In J. C. McCloskey & H. K. Grace (Eds.), *Current issues in nursing* (pp. 626–643). Boston: Blackwell-Scientific.

Potash, M., & Taylor, D. (1993). *Nursing faculty practice: Models and methods.* Washington, DC: National Organization of Nurse Practitioner Faculties.

Taylor, D. L. (1996). Faculty practice: Uniting advanced nursing practice and education. In A. B. Hamric, J. A. Spross, & C. M. Hanson (Eds.), *Advanced nursing practice: An integrative approach* (pp. 469–495). Philadelphia: W. B. Saunders.

■ Editor's Questions for Discussion

Identify significant issues of faculty practice. How should faculty practice be defined? Who should define it? Should there be consensus regarding definition for faculty practice in schools of nursing and for universities? What difference does it make in faculty workload expectations and assignments or whether there is consensus regarding definition, if faculty practice is conducted outside academic assignments? What variables influence how faculty practice is implemented? Does the setting or time for faculty practice make a difference as to who or how faculty practice is defined or implemented?

Where faculty practice is implemented in the university setting or considered part of the faculty role, should it be an option or requirement? What criteria should exist for faculty in choosing faculty practice?

Debate the pros and cons of different faculty practice models. What alternative models can you suggest? Describe a step-by-step process in planning, developing, implementing, and evaluating a faculty practice model. Address each challenge presented concerning the faculty practice model. How should disagreements among faculty be resolved concerning workload, assignments, and faculty practice?

How might faculty practice change in the future? How does Barger's discussion (Chapter 52) apply to faculty practice models? Propose an "integrated practice program" as a future model. Indicate specific examples of how faculty can demonstrate patient care outcomes at low costs. What evidence exists concerning faculty research and patient care outcomes? How is integration of research and patient care addressed by Shaver (Chapter 76), Lindsey (Chapter 29), Kasper (Chapter 30), and Titler (Chapter 35)?

To what extent should faculty be expected to be expert clinicians prior to assuming a faculty role in teaching students and have time allocated for faculty practice? What part of Gray's presentation (Chapter 42) may be applied to faculty practice? How may faculty practice labs be developed? What other options exist or may be developed to maintain faculty clinical expertise? What type of collaborative relationships with clinical agencies facilitate faculty practice?

How are Carter's predictions about faculty role supported by Lindeman (Chapter 63)? What planning is essential to alter thinking of faculty and prepare for future changes?

40

Partnerships for the New Millennium

Development of Clinical Decision-Making in a Practice Profession

Kathleen M. McCauley, PhD, RN, CS, FAAN

Maureen P. McCausland, DNSc, RN, FAAN

Partnerships between nursing education and nursing practice can be traced to the beginning days of professional nursing (Nightingale, 1860/1992). The earliest preparation of nurses took place in hospital-based diploma programs, which used student nurses as a major portion of the hospital labor force delivering direct patient care. (Ashley, 1976). As nursing moves into the new millennium, lessons of the past and the current state of nursing education, practice, and research at the University of Pennsylvania set the stage for visionary nursing leadership.

■ Historical Settings for Partnerships

In the early 1960s, Schlotfeldt and Mac-Phail (1969a, 1969b, 1969c) and their colleagues at Frances Payne Bolton School of Nursing at Case Western Reserve University and the University Hospitals of Cleveland initiated "an experiment in nursing" (Schlotfeldt & MacPhail, 1969a, p. 1020). The experiment sought to capitalize on strengths of academic nursing in a university medical center while recognizing that differences between education and service exist. These innovators recognized that the primary missions of each organization differed but that each institution was responsible for promoting the goals of the other. The experiment was characterized by the creation of a new relationship between the school of nursing and the hospitals and a change in the method of operating in the two institutions. The interdependence and need to effect mutually beneficial change were recognized by the board of trustees of both institutions.

The experiment was complex and the changes substantive. Schlotfeldt and colleagues realized that (a) "expert practitioners who provide sophisticated nursing care to patients in the hospital need and want intellectual stimulation from colleagues in an academic environment"; and (b) "if faculty members are to have the opportunity to retain and further develop their specialist practitioner skills and engage in clinical inquiry, they must have identity and involvement in a setting in which they have practice and research privileges" (Schlotfeldt & MacPhail, 1969a, p. 1020).

This experiment in nursing has continued and evolved at the Frances Payne Bolton School of Nursing and University Hospitals of Cleveland. Outcomes of the relationship are many. The (a) introduction of research utilization, (b) creation of clinical nurse specialists and their role as master teachers, (c) creation of the first reported clinical advancement program in 1969, and (d) an integrated administrative structure with chairpersons from the school of nursing providing administrative leadership in the hospitals are simply a sample of their innovations. University Hospitals of Cleveland was one of the original magnet hospitals (McClure, Poulin, Sovie, & Wandelt, 1983) and continues to be recognized as an excellent practice environment.

Sovie (1981a, 1981b) described the University of Rochester unification model. A major distinction between the Frances Payne Bolton School of Nursing and the University of Rochester is organizational. Whereas University Hospitals of Cleveland is a separate corporate entity from Case Western Reserve University, the Strong Memorial Hospital is part of the University of Rochester Medical Center and owned by the university. Use of the unification model began in 1972. Ownership of the hospital by the university resulted in the school of nursing assuming complete responsibility for practice, education, and research at the hospital. Unified leadership for both practice and education was achieved through development of the clinical chief role. Thus the senior nursing management team of both the medical center and the school include the associate dean for practice and the clinical chiefs in collaboration with the dean of the school of nursing.

Sovie (1981b) reported that unification resulted in clear accountability and no scapegoating between nursing education and practice. Accountability for the practice abilities of nursing school graduates rested clearly with the joint leadership. It was empowered to make curricular revisions or alterations in practice learning experiences where needed to improve the students' knowledge base and skills. Similarly, the same group of leaders was accountable for nursing practice in the medical center. Outcomes of the unification model were (a) strong patient satisfaction with nursing care, more than 90% of patients reporting that nursing care was excellent or good; (b) strong physician satisfaction with nursing care; and (c) strong staff nurse recruitment and retention statistics.

■ *The Partnership Model*

In the early 1980s, University of Pennsylvania School of Nursing faculty and Hospital of the University of Pennsylvania nursing administrators and clinicians met to design a new, shared future. The goal was to link the research and educational missions of the school of nursing with the practice mission of the hospital, thereby strengthening the commitment of both groups to the tripartite mission of research, education, and practice. By formalizing relationships and building new ones (a) faculty and clinicians developed joint programs of research, (b) students learned from expert clinicians, and (c) research-based practice programs were implemented. See Table 40.1.

Efforts to strengthen linkages between the University of Pennsylvania School of Nursing and nurses in practice at the hospital were needed, in part, because of the structure of the university. The School of Nursing is a separate entity from the hospital and the Dean reports directly to the President and the Provost. The Hospital of the University of Pennsylvania is owned by the university. The Dean of the School of Medicine and Chief Executive Officer also reports directly to the President and the Provost. This structure (see Figure 40.1) has strengthened the presence of nursing on the campus and has made the efforts to link education, research, and practice extremely important.

The Partnership in Nursing Vision Statement (Hospital of the University of Pennsylvania, 1993) describes the mission and goals of the partnership as being directly influenced by the larger university. A major focus of the university is generation of new knowledge, new insights, and new forms of expression. With Benjamin Franklin as founder of the university, the focus always has been on applied and professional knowledge, as well as theoretical knowledge. Consequently, the partnership in nursing strives to connect the research expertise of the faculty with nurses in practice to achieve excellence in the care of patients and families, education of students, and advancement of knowledge.

Clinician Educator

Implementation of this kind of program at the University of Pennsylvania was possible because of existence of the Clinician Educator faculty role. In 1983, the University approved the Clinician Educator appointment for both the Schools of Nursing and Medicine. Clinician educators are members of the standing faculty with full faculty rights and responsibilities, except for voting rights on any decisions related to tenure (University of Pennsylvania Almanac, April 12, 1983). Faculty appointed to Clinician Educator roles are required to generate a percentage of their salary through practice efforts. This percentage is negotiated during the initial appointment process and can be renegotiated, but continued appointment is contingent on generation of practice salary support. Clinician Educator roles are not tenured positions; a separate tenure track exists. Reappointment of Clinician Educators and promotion of faculty to these roles are dependent on scholarly productivity, which is defined broadly to include not only clinical practice, but also research publications and leadership in national organizations and practice panels. Clinician Educators may have their own funded research programs or serve as members of research teams with tenured faculty. For purposes of this discussion, the term *faculty* is used to describe only those roles such as Clinician Educator or tenure positions where a doctorate and formal appointment by the University is required. Other positions such as instructor, preceptor, and master teacher are open to nurses with baccalaureate or master's degrees but are not formal faculty appointments.

Clinical practice, broadly defined, includes a wide range of clinical and administrative roles. In the early stages of the University of Pennsylvania partnership, doctorally prepared nursing administrators were recruited to lead

TABLE 40.1 University of Pennsylvania Roles, Titles, and Definitions
School of Nursing and University of Pennsylvania Health System

Term	Definition
Advanced Practice Nurse	An umbrella term that includes these specialty roles :
	Clinical Nurse Specialist, Nurse Practitioner, Certified Registered Nurse Anesthetist and Certified Nurse-Midwife. Advanced Practice nurses have met educational and clinical practice requirements beyond the 2 to 4 years of basic nursing education required by all registered nurses. (*American Association of Critical Care Nurses,* 1995, p. l)
Chief Nursing Executive and Associate Dean for Nursing Practice	The Chief Nursing Executive for the University of Pennsylvania Health System and the Associate Dean for the Nursing Practice at the School of Nursing
Chief Nursing Officer	The Chief Nursing Officer of a University of Pennsylvania Health System–owned hospital
Clinical Advancement and Recognition Program	A program that recognizes the expertise of the nurses in direct patient care through a system of promotion, salary increases and increased leadership opportunities
Clinical Director of Nursing	The Clinical Director of a group of specialty units or programs who is accountable for the nursing practice and the human and financial resources of the service
Clinical Nurse	A registered nurse who provides direct patient care
Clinician Educator	Members of the standing faculty with full faculty rights and responsibilities, with the exception of voting rights for any decisions related to tenure. A clinical component of the role is required.
Hospital of the University of Pennsylvania	A 725-bed teaching hospital that is part of the University of Pennsylvania Health System
Master Teacher	A master's-prepared nurse who serves as the official instructor for one to two undergraduate nursing students and supervises their clinical experience during her/his regular clinical practice
Nurse Manager	The nurse manager of a nursing unit or program with accountability for clinical practice and the human and financial resource management. The nurse manager is typically accountable to a Clinical Director of Nursing.
Preceptor	A nurse in clinical practice who actively participates in the education of nursing students by sharing the care of a caseload of patients with the student. The preceptor assists in the supervision of student learning and collaborates with the clinical instructor in the evaluation of student performance.
University of Pennsylvania Health System	A fully integrated health system that includes primary care practices, specialty practices, four owned hospitals, three home care programs and a school of medicine.

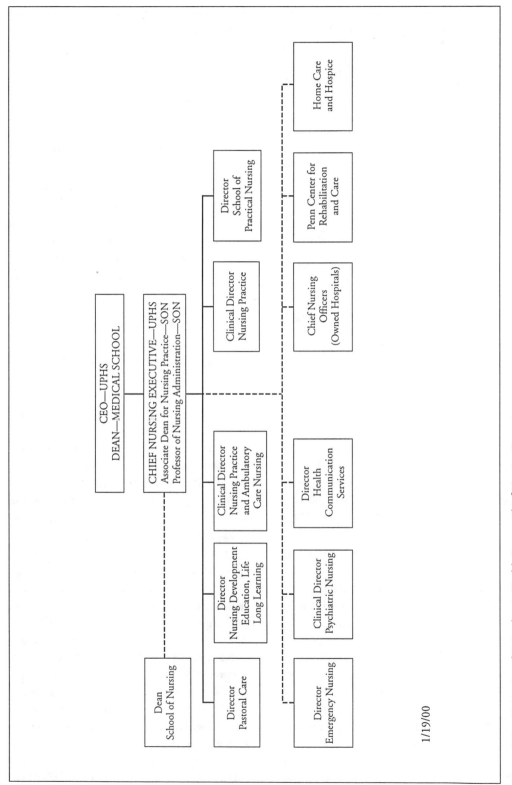

Figure 40.1 University of Pennsylvania Health System Chief Nursing Executive.

major departments within the nursing service while jointly holding faculty appointments; and the Chief Nursing Officer of the Hospital of the University of Pennsylvania served as an Associate Dean for Practice. Other faculty served as advanced practice nurses. These appointments resulted in numerous benefits, including

- priority access for University of Pennsylvania students to superb clinical sites;

- improved access to patients for faculty research;

- improved collaboration among faculty, nursing administrators, advanced practice nurses, and staff nurses for design, implementation, and evaluation of research based practice initiatives;

- faculty access to the business and management skills of seasoned nursing administrators for consultation and collaboration; and

- clinically relevant teaching efforts, lead by faculty with current and ongoing practice programs.

The full actualization of shared leadership was first achieved by recruitment of an expert clinician with strong administrative and teaching background in psychiatric mental health nursing. This faculty member served as Associate Professor of Psychiatric Nursing and Clinical Director of Psychiatric Mental Health Nursing in the Hospital and Division Head for that division of the faculty. Responsibilities in this role included (a) clinical care of patients in the hospital, (b) mentoring and development of staff and faculty, and (c) service as a full member of the administrative teams in both settings. Adjunct activity entailed participation in doctoral student education and direction of a graduate course. Positive outcomes of this role included ability to influence directly the practice models guiding care of patients and the general approach to education of students within this specialty. The specific faculty member recruited was well positioned to succeed in this combined role because of expertise as clinician and administrator and previous success in a prior faculty role.

■ The University of Pennsylvania Health System

The University of Pennsylvania Health System was created in 1993. (See Figure 40.1.) The health system currently encompasses the University of Pennsylvania School of Medicine, four hospitals, a nursing home, three home care agencies, numerous primary care practices, and a large number of specialty practices.

Several doctorally prepared advanced practice nurses hold Clinician Educator appointments and practice in expert generalist, population-based, and administrative roles within the University of Pennsylvania Health System, including those at the Hospital of the University of Pennsylvania. Many of these faculty also direct major clinical courses within the school. For example, an Assistant Professor of Gerontological Nursing directs the Nursing Care of the Older Adult course, which is an undergraduate clinical and theory course with content flowing directly from practice.

As an advanced practice nurse within the hospital, the Assistant Professor of Gerontological Nursing consults broadly, helping nursing and physician colleagues integrate clinical scholarship with the care of frail, vulnerable patients and their families. This care has included leadership in nursing's efforts to move the institution from use of patient restraints to the least restrictive alternative. This implementation of research findings of faculty colleagues (Evans & Strumpf, 1990; Evans, Strumpf, Allen-Taylor, Capezuti, Maislin, & Jacobson, 1997) has truly operationalized the tripartite mission within the school and the hospital. The efforts of this Assistant Professor of Gerontological Nursing were strongly supported by colleagues in nursing administration, who also hold faculty appointments, providing further evidence that research-based practice changes are achievable with administrative support.

The work of this gerontological nurse, in challenging practice related to restraint usage, was expanded by another colleague with a clinician educator appointment as Assistant Professor of Geropsychiatric Mental Health Nursing. In the role of psychiatric consultation liaison nurse specialist, this second Assistant Professor–Clinician Educator was able to work with colleagues to analyze care practices of patients with delirium, educate managers and staff, and ultimately reduce both restraint usage and the need for constant observation of these high-risk patients. As an alternative to restraint usage, the nursing service implemented a program of constant observation where patients, who are at risk to themselves, are individually attended by a trained staff member, usually a nursing assistant. While costly, this program enabled the use of restraints to be reduced considerably. However, all concerned recognized that the root causes of delirium were unaddressed by the observation program.

The Geropsychiatric Mental Health–Clinician Educator co-led a task force that designed an award-winning research utilization program. Using cost and quality data collected during the prior year, this faculty member knew the categories of patients who used the greatest numbers of resources and who were at greatest risk for poor outcomes, such as falls. All patients requiring constant observation were followed, and functional status data were collected, using a standardized instrument. Findings revealed that significant functional impairment accompanied delirium. Work ensued individually with the patient's primary nurse and other members of the health care team to improve functional status and minimize treatable causes of delirium. Patients benefitted enormously from having a consistent primary care nurse, and the functional status of patients improved with progressive ambulation and judicious use of physical therapy.

Nurse managers, in particular, were interested in the data-driven approach to resolving this problem. The salubrious effect from employing a clinical nurse for patient continuity and patient improvement was clear. Such nurses were more confident that the patient would do well with constant observation but it was needed only at key, high-risk times. This program demonstrates that an expert clinician with well-defined research skills can design, implement, and evaluate a program in a manner that improves outcomes and reduces cost.

■ Professional Nursing Practice in an Integrated Health System

As the University of Pennsylvania moved to become a health care system, the need for senior nursing leadership at the corporate level became apparent. The School of Nursing was influential in working with the senior leadership of the emerging health system. It became clear that a Chief Nurse Executive and Associate Dean for Nursing Practice would be a critical voice at the table as hospitals, home care agencies, and physician practices were acquired or expanded. This particular role ensures that both the School of Nursing and the health system take advantage of every opportunity to enhance the partnership. This Executive has brought a vision of scholarly nursing practice that provides extraordinary care to patients, is professionally satisfying to professional nurses, and embraces the education and research mission of the University of Pennsylvania.

Charge and Support of Senior Management

The professional practice model adopted when the Chief Nurse Executive arrived at the University of Pennsylvania provided the blueprint for nursing at the University of Pennsylvania Health System and all its practice areas. The theoretical base of the model builds on the seminal work of Henderson and Nite (1978), Manthey (1980), Clifford and Horvath (1990), and Benner and colleagues (1999). The professional practice model advances the University of Pennsylvania Health System values of easy access to patient care characterized by great quality, service, and value.

The following are the major elements of this professional practice model.

1. Primary nursing is the care delivery system; accountability and responsibility for professional nursing practice with strong continuity among nurse, patient, and family are essentials of primary nursing.

2. Interdisciplinary collaboration is a second building block of the professional practice model; a strong partnership of nurses, physicians, and hospital administrators is essential for excellent patient care, teaching, and research.

3. Clinical and nonclinical supports are an integral part of the practice model; emphasis on the systems that support patient care are constantly evaluated and improved.

4. Advancement, recognition, and compensation programs provide the mechanism for recognizing and regarding excellence in clinical practice. The goal of this component of the model is to retain professionally satisfied, expert nurses in direct patient care roles throughout their careers. Retention of nursing staff is a major goal. A major commitment is made to the preparation and socialization of future professionals.

5. Professional activities by professional nurses throughout the organization and in external arenas are encouraged and celebrated.

6. The environment for practice is created by a clinically focused nursing management team and is essential to the practice model.

This professional practice model aims to nurture a spirit of inquiry and integrate scholarship into the practice of all nurses. The nursing service at the University of Pennsylvania Health System enthusiastically supports the partnership with the school of nursing at the University of Pennsylvania. The discovery of new knowledge, evidence-based nursing practice, and preparation of future nurses are areas of synergistic activities. The clinician educator role is a key advantage of the partnership.

Enhancement of the Professional Practice Model Through the Partnership

Evaluation of the professional practice model includes the measurement of nurse-sensitive variables across all practice sites in the health system. The University of Pennsylvania was successful in recruiting a third Assistant Professor of Gerontological Nursing, who also served as the Director of Gerontological Nursing Practice at the health system. Leadership thus was afforded for defining, measuring, and improving the performance of these variables. Additionally, this position provided (a) chairmanship of the health system nursing practice committee, (b) active involvement in promoting research utilization and evidence-based practice, and (c) integration of undergraduate students into the Penn Center for Rehabilitation and Care. That nursing home is owned by the health system, and the presence of University of Pennsylvania nursing students creates an opportunity for intergenerational conversation. Students are encouraged to confront stereotypical beliefs about the aging and nursing homes, as residents share their experiences and wisdom. Residents describe the students as a pleasant diversion and value the opportunity to contribute to student learning.

Research Utilization

An outstanding example of a faculty member influencing the practice of the clinical nurse at the patient's side, through research utilization, is the work of an Assistant Professor of

Health Care of Women Nursing in improving skin care practices for infants in the Intensive Care Nursery. She is also an advanced practice nurse in the obstetrical and neonatal nursing department at the Hospital of the University of Pennsylvania. Through her service for the Association of Women's Health, Obstetrical and Neonatal Nursing (AWHONN) at the national level, this faculty member was aware of a new set of practice guidelines designed to bring best practice in skin care to intensive care nurseries nationwide. She served as a mentor for a clinical nurse who applied to be a test site coordinator for implementation of these recently developed practice guidelines.

Once selected, this clinical nurse participated in an AWHONN sponsored training program that included both implementation and evaluation of the guidelines. With continued mentoring, this nurse educated a core group of clinical nurses who revised skin care practices in their unit, influenced the care practices of all primary nurses, and coordinated the evaluation program.

An added benefit was the evaluation and revision of skin care practices for all infants, including those in the normal newborn nurseries, and improved collaboration between members of the health care team. This program was so successful that, with the faculty member's continued mentoring, the University of Pennsylvania Health System has become the first "super site" where AWHONN practice guidelines will be implemented across an integrated health system. This vignette demonstrates the powerful effect of expert nursing practice by a clinician educator in implementing a research utilization program. Nurturing a spirit of inquiry in clinical nurses, a goal of the professional practice model, was achieved.

Career Development of Clinical Nurses

An important component of both the University of Pennsylvania Health System profes-

sional nursing practice model and the partnership is a commitment to the career development of clinical nurses. All practice sites of the health system will participate in the University of Pennsylvania Health System clinical advancement and recognition program. Based on the work of Benner et al. (1999), Boyer (1990), and Schon (1983, 1987), the clinical advancement and recognition program aims to recognize and reward nurses in the mainstream of direct patient care. Benner et al. helped shape our thinking to one of career development, rather than simply a series of "jobs" in our system. Boyer, in his seminal work, states that the scholarship of integration requires practitioners to live in many neighborhoods. Clinical nurses must be consumers of research findings from a variety of disciplines. Clinician educators in clinical and administrative roles are jointly accountable with clinical nurses to meet this goal.

Recognizing that nurses' skill acquisition and clinical wisdom do not develop in a linear or sequential manner, programs and strategies are created to support clinical nurses throughout their careers. One of the earliest programs, initiated by the Chief Nurse Executive of the University of Pennsylvania's Health System and Associate Dean for Nursing Practice at the School of Nursing, was a two-pronged career development system. A 2-year residency program for new graduates of baccalaureate nursing programs welcomes new professional nurses and socializes them to the profession. The Professional Excellence for New Nurses (PENN) Program uses the strategy of a relationship between the resident and a sponsor (an experienced nurse on the unit) to coach and support the resident. Several faculty with Clinician Educator appointments were involved actively in implementation of this program. The intimacy of the sponsor–resident relationship mirrors the nurse–patient relationship and is characterized by continuity, accountability, and responsibility. Two other career transition programs were created to support development of the clinical nurse with 2 or more years of experience who wants to practice in critical care or perioperative nursing. Again, a goal of thinking in terms of a career transition to a new practice area, rather than a "transfer," reinforces professional nursing practice.

■ Role of the Partnership in Education of Students

The strong commitment of the nurse at the patient's side to education of students has been influenced by the partnership model and has influenced its growth. Prior to development of the partnership, nurses in the hospital welcomed students and also served as excellent role models. The partnership extended the teaching roles of staff in a number of ways. Master's-prepared nurses in clinical roles serve as clinical instructors for undergraduate students. The school of nursing supports their salaries for the time devoted to teaching. This routine has provided the faculty course director with a consistent group of instructors and has been a source of satisfaction for these expert clinicians as they stay in their direct care nursing roles.

Clinical nurses serve as preceptors for undergraduate students, and those prepared at the master's level serve as preceptors for graduate students. The hospital receives no additional compensation as these nurses incorporate working with the student into their own clinical practice. The actual accountability for learning and evaluation of student performance rests with the clinical instructor or faculty member who collaborates with the preceptor in the education and evaluation of students.

The roles of preceptor and clinical instructor have been combined in a unique role termed the "master teacher." Selected master's-prepared nurses in practice have been given official instructor positions for a semester and work with one or two students as part of their regular clinical roles. This policy has been most effective in accommodating a student's preference for a specific clinical area. For example, in the undergraduate senior leadership course, Advanced Clinical Practicum in Nursing, every effort is made to match a student's preference for clinical placement with the actual assignment. At times, these requests have been difficult to accommodate via the usual instructor and student clinical group arrangement. Master's-prepared clinicians in areas as diverse as the inpatient psychiatric unit and the emergency department have served as master teachers. The success of this program is based on close mentoring by the faculty course director to ensure that the student experience meets course objectives and that any difficulties that arise are handled appropriately.

Education That Is Relevant

Full integration of faculty into practice has presented unique opportunities for educating students, both inside and outside the classroom. Clinical scenarios used to illustrate content are highly reflective of the realities of today's health care challenges. When faculty are able to connect class content to a real and recent patient experience, the challenges and benefits of implementing true research-based practice become evident. For example, the Assistant Professor of Gerontological Nursing frequently serves as a preceptor for students in the gerontological nurse practitioner graduate program. These students actively participate in the management of this faculty member's personal caseload of patients. Undergraduate students seeking additional content in nursing management of frail patients and patients with complex wounds often join on rounds. Such practices result in multiple levels of learning under the guidance of a superb clinician who fully understands the learning objectives of all of the nursing programs.

Clinician Educator Role

Similar connections between practice and teaching are evident in the way that an Associate Professor of Cardiovascular Nursing has implemented the Clinician Educator role. As a longstanding clinical specialist in the care of the cardiology patients at the hospital, this faculty member has, with a physician colleague, directed the hospital's quality-monitoring efforts in cardiac resuscitations. This work requires that the faculty member collaborate with clinical colleagues, as well as key hospital support staff as diverse as maintenance and repair experts, telecommunications specialists, and attorneys, to resolve systems problems, improve staff performance, and improve quality outcomes. This faculty role entails direction of the senior undergraduate clinical leadership course, Advanced Clinical Practicum in Nursing—where content related to role transition, implementation, and evaluation of change and quality management is taught. Current experience with these issues in a complex health care system directly informs teaching in this role. Similarly, practice related to clinical care and quality management of patients suffering a cardiac arrest has presented opportunities for undergraduate students to participate in resuscitations.

Curriculum Development

The partnership model has provided unique opportunity for leaders in nursing service to actively participate in curricular development. The Chief Nursing Officer of the Hospital of the University of Pennsylvania holds a faculty position as an Assistant Professor of Nursing Administration. As such, this role has led to classroom discussions concerning management content, delegation, and team building in the Advanced Clinical Practicum course. As pressures to deliver higher quality care at lower costs increase,

preparing new graduates to succeed in practice roles within and outside hospitals becomes more challenging. Having the Chief Nursing Officer, as part of the faculty for the Advanced Clinical Practicum course, participate in both the planning and teaching of course content serves to enlighten students and faculty about the current realities of health care. This process also provides the Chief Nursing Officer with current information on the capabilities and needs of new graduates.

The Chief Nurse Executive is actively involved in the leadership of both the health system and the school of nursing. This role encompasses (a) participation in the strategic planning of the school of nursing, (b) financial oversight of clinical practices, and (c) provision of input for curricular design. Examples of recent activities of this executive at the University of Pennsylvania include (a) leading the strategic planning process for redesign of the preparation of future nurse executives, (b) participating in the redesign of the Doctor of Philosophy in Nursing (PhD) curriculum, and (c) teaching the doctoral course Issues of Nursing Leadership in Planning and Policy Making.

■ Concluding Statement

The new millennium brings with it significant challenges and opportunities for both the health care sector generally and nursing specifically. The decade of the 1990s was characterized by rapid and at times chaotic change. Patient care delivery systems frequently were redesigned and reengineered, using industrial rather than professional models. Professional nursing practice was often not the driving force in design decisions. Enrollment in baccalaureate nursing programs declined 6.6% in 1997 and 5.5% in 1998 (American Association of Colleges of Nursing, 1999). The registered nurse workforce is aging faster than other professional groups, and a significant shortage is projected as the members of the baby boom generation retire and ultimately require care.

Our vision for the next century is hopeful, despite the themes just discussed. The need exists for nursing leaders to step back and strategically assess core values and priorities, in conjunction with those of the institutions in which they practice. For nursing to make its optimum contribution, development of clinical wisdom in the nurse at the patient's side must be nurtured and actively fostered. Academic environments are rich repositories of knowledge wherein the expertise of the researcher, expert teacher, and committed practitioner can be brought together—so that the talents of each can inform the others. In some settings these nurturing relationships can happen without a system designed to support them. However, it makes much more sense to design communication strategies and work systems that will enable this growth to happen naturally.

Four areas of concentration are recommended.

1. *Systematized mentoring of clinical staff to foster development of clinical wisdom:* Ongoing experience in the direct care of patients, coupled with strategies to bring current research findings to the patient, can result in the nurse's growth—in both the art and the science of nursing.

2. *Linkages created between practice and research:* Such linkages make the spirit of inquiry the norm. When the nurse at the patient's side constantly asks "Why?" and "Is there a better way to care for this patient?" and has direct access to scholars with skills to frame the solution, true professional practice can be achieved.

3. *Strengthening of integrated roles that enable faculty to maintain clinical or administrative practice expertise:* Integration ensures that teaching in the classroom and at the patient's side is relevant, current, and meaningful to practitioners and the new generation learning to be nurses. Nursing administration, education, and practice is similarly well informed.

4. *Creating integrated roles for nursing executives that enable the tripartite mission of practice, education, and research to be inexorably linked within an institution:* Establishing this mission as part of the institution's culture facilitates translation of research into real and lasting changes in practice.

Health and illness care will only become more complex. Patients and their families need nurses who have developed clinical wisdom and research-based practice skills that will define the new care strategies necessary for promotion of health and management of illness.

■ References

American Association of Colleges of Nursing. (1999, April). *Issue bulletin.* Washington, DC: Author

American Association of Critical Care Nurses. (1995). *Advanced nursing practice: Facts and strategies for regulation, reimbursement and prescriptive authority.* Aliso Viejo, CA: Author.

Ashley, J. (1976). *Hospitals, paternalism and the role of the nurse.* New York: Teachers College Press.

Benner, P., Hooper-Kyriakidis, P., & Stannard, D. (1999) *Clinical wisdom and interventions in critical care: A thinking in action approach.* Philadelphia: W. B. Saunders.

Boyer, E. (1990). *Scholarship revisited: Priorities of the professoriate.* Trenton, NJ: Carnegie Endowment for the Advancement of Teaching.

Clifford, J., & Horvath, K. (1990). *Advancing professional nursing practice: Innovations at Boston's Beth Israel Hospital.* New York: Springer.

Evans, L. K., & Strumpf, N. E. (1990). Myths about elder restraint. *IMAGE: Journal of Nursing Scholarship, 22*(2), 124–128.

Evans, L., Strumpf, N. E., Allen-Taylor, S., Capezuti, E., Maislin, G., & Jacobson, B. (1997). A clinical trial to reduce restraints in nursing homes. *Journal of the American Geriatrics Society, 45*(6), 675–681.

Henderson, V., & Nite, G. (1978). *Principles and practice of nursing* (6th ed.). New York: Macmillan.

Hospital of the University of Pennsylvania. (1993, May). University of Pennsylvania: A partnership in nursing. *Nursing Organization, Information, and Position Description Manual* [Section of Manual: Partnership]. Philadelphia: Author.

Manthey, M. (1980). *The practice of primary nursing.* St. Louis: Mosby.

McClure, M., Poulin, M., Sovie, M., & Wandelt, M. (1983). *Magnet hospitals: Attraction and retention of nurses.* Kansas City, MO: American Nurses Association.

Nightingale, F. (1992). *Notes on nursing.* New York: Lippincott, Williams & Wilkins. (Original work published 1860)

Schlotfeldt, R. M., & MacPhail, J. (1969a). An experiment in nursing: Rationale and characteristics. *American Journal of Nursing, 69*(5), 1018–1023.

Schlotfeldt, R. M., & MacPhail, J. (1969b). An experiment in nursing: Introducing planned change. *American Journal of Nursing, 69*(6), 1247–1251.

Schlotfeldt, R. M., & MacPhail, J. (1969c). An experiment in nursing: Implementing planned change. *American Journal of Nursing, 69*(7), 1475–1480.

Schon, D. (1983). *The reflective practitioner.* New York: Basic Books.

Schon, D. (1987). *Educating the reflective practitioner.* San Francisco: Jossey-Bass.

Sovie, M. D. (1981a). Unifying education and practice: One medical center's design. Part 1. *Journal of Nursing Administration, 11*(1), 41–49.

Sovie, M. D. (1981b). Unifying education and practice: One medical center's design. Part 2. *Journal of Nursing Administration, 11*(2), 30–32.

University of Pennsylvania Almanac. (April 12, 1983). Clinical educator track in the school of nursing. *Almanac,* 7–8.

■ *Editor's Questions for Discussion*

How is the partnership model at the University of Pennsylvania the same as or different from models at Case Western Reserve University and the University of Rochester? How applicable is the University of Pennsylvania partnership model for other combined clinical and education settings? What factors contribute to success of education, clinical practice partnerships?

Discuss issues concerning the professional practice model. How can a similar model be implemented in other care settings? What impact does managed care have on professional practice models? How is the clinician educator role at the University of Pennsylvania similar to roles in other health care institutions?

Propose strategies for career development of clinical nurses. What elements are essential to development of specific programs? At what stage in career development of clinicians may faculty in nursing programs contribute? How might mentoring between clinicians and educators occur for development of partnerships? What goals of the residency program at University of Pennsylvania and that discussed by McClure (Chapter 62) for New York University (NYU) may be similar?

To what extent does the master teacher role exist in other health care settings? What organizational factors are essential for clinicians to participate in curriculum development and design? How may constraints be reduced and inducements increased to promote partnerships between education and practice settings?

41

Nursing Practice Reimbursement Issues in the 21st Century

Karen R. Robinson, PhD, RN, FAAN
Hurdis M. Griffith, PhD, RN, FAAN
Eileen M. Sullivan-Marx, PhD, RN, FAAN

In the 21st century, the health care industry will become even more consolidated, with many organizations united in integrated delivery systems. Quality and outcomes of care delivered will become a crucial determinant of individuals selecting health plans (Buerhaus, 1996). How well these systems survive will depend on their ability to compete for capitated contracts and then deliver quality care at the least cost. As the nursing profession enters the arena of integrated delivery systems, it becomes of upmost importance that monitoring of clinical outcomes, costs, and quality adequately capture nurses' activities and interventions. If this information is not measured to reflect nurses' actions, their contributions will be less visible and therefore less val-

ued by the organization and the consumer. As a consequence, nurses could be allocated fewer resources.

Direct reimbursement of nurses for their services is certainly an important, but sensitive issue (Fagin, 1987). On the one hand, it is an important issue because it increases the autonomy, visibility, image, and value of the profession. It allows nurses an opportunity to be recognized for their contributions as patient care providers and important members of interdisciplinary teams. On the other hand, reimbursement is a sensitive issue because it can be a threat to physicians as well as payors. The question to be asked of the nursing profession is "Should nurses campaign to be directly reimbursed for their services?" This question is further complicated by changes in reimbursement patterns within a system of evolving health care.

■ Background

Historically, nurses were not paid directly for their services, but rather this cost was "lumped in" with the overhead that facilities and medical providers charged their patients. In the 1940s, insurance companies paid for follow-up home nursing visits to new mothers and babies for the purpose of providing education and reducing complications. In time, this private reimbursement for maternal child health care shifted to public funding (Cherry, 1991).

Medicare began to reimburse home care agencies for skilled nursing services in the 1960s. Physician orders were required to initiate services, but reimbursement was specifically for nursing care. Medicaid also started to reimburse nursing for well-child examinations (Cherry, 1991).

In the early 1980s, even though 25 states had enacted legislation enabling direct reimbursement for specific groups of nurses and the profession acclaimed direct reimbursement as a goal, little data existed regarding implementation of these laws. A case study of implementation of legislation providing direct third-party reimbursement to nurse practitioners (NPs) in Maryland and Oregon was conducted in 1983 (Griffith, 1986). The study investigated the degree to which NPs in these two states were receiving direct third-party reimbursement and how it affected health care costs. The study's findings revealed that, 4 years after legislation was passed in Maryland, 2% of NPs were being reimbursed on a fee-for-service basis, and less than 1% of eligible NPs had received direct third-party reimbursement. In Oregon, 7 years after enactment of the legislation, only 13% of the NPs were being reimbursed on a fee-for-service basis, and 21% had received direct

third party reimbursement. In addition, the findings indicated that NPs reimbursed on a fee-for-service basis or receiving direct third-party reimbursement or both charged less for their services than salaried NPs.

Congress adopted the Prospective Payment System in 1983 and then, in 1986, created the Physician Payment Review Commission (PPRC) to advise it on reforms of the methods used to pay physicians under Medicare (Part B). Nursing groups lobbied PPRC to consider their contributions as it came up with proposals for revising the payment system. In 1989, Congress, incorporating the PPRC recommendations, passed legislation that changed physician payment from the reasonable charge payment method to a Medicare fee schedule based on a resource-based relative value scale (RBRVS). In response to the lobbying done by nurses, the legislative package as proposed by Congress included a recommendation that the PPRC study the effect of the Medicare Fee Schedule on nonphysician providers (Griffith & Robinson, 1993; Physician Payment Review Commission [PPRC], 1991). At this time it is uncertain whether further study has been conducted.

Medicare consists of two parts. Part A includes payment to hospitals, nursing facilities, home health agencies, and hospice services. Part B provides payment to physicians (MDs, DOs, dentists, and podiatrists) and "nonphysician providers" (nurse practitioners, clinical nurse specialists, certified nurse midwives, certified registered nurse anesthetists, physician assistants, psychologists, physical and occupational therapists, and others). Part B also covers laboratory services, outpatient hospital care, and supplies (PPRC, 1997).

Payment to clinical providers under Medicare fee-for-service or managed care is categorized in the Current Procedural Terminology (CPT) coding system, developed by the American Medical Association (AMA) in 1966. More than 7,000 procedures are listed in the CPT system, which predominantly describes physician procedures (American Medical Association [AMA], 1999a). The CPT has been criticized for confining codes to physician's services, thus limiting its usefulness to the current health care system that utilizes multiple providers, many of whom are now directly reimbursed by Medicare. The AMA is currently reviewing the next version of the coding system, CPT-5, and is discussing including other types of health care professionals. The CPT is used extensively by payors for fee-for-service reimbursement and tracking services in managed care.

In 1989, the resource-based relative value scale (RBRVS) was implemented by the Health Care Financing Administration (HCFA) to establish a Medicare fee schedule for Part B physician payment. This system now extends to payment for services provided by advanced practice nurses, physician assistants, psychologists, clinical social workers, and other Part B providers. In this system, a total relative value that incorporates work, practice expense, and malpractice insurance is established for each CPT code. The total relative value for a code is multiplied by a standard dollar amount and adjusted geographically to determine the allowable Medicare charge for that code (AMA, 1999b).

CPT codes are established by the CPT Editorial Panel of the American Medical Association. Relative values for work and practice expense are developed by the Relative Value Update Committee (RUC) of the American Medical Association. They are then referred to the HCFA, which establishes relative values for CPT codes, following a period of internal review and public comment (AMA, 1999b). The American Nurses Association (ANA) has been represented on advisory committees to both of these processes since 1993 and has been active in the review of commonly used evaluation and management codes in primary care and mental health services (Sullivan-Marx & Mullinix, 1999).

In its report to Congress, PPRC stated that nonphysician providers should be paid at a percentage of physician payment levels reflecting differences in physicians' and nonphysicians' resource costs—work as well as practice and malpractice expense. ANA disagreed, stating that nurses should be paid the same for the same service as physicians (Mittelstadt, 1991). The only nurse serving on the Commission, Carol Lockhart, PhD, RN, FAAN, expressed concern about lack of nursing data available to the PPRC. As cited in Griffith and Fonteyn (1989), she stated:

> Nursing's role in the delivery of Medicare Part B services is undocumented. We have little or no data showing how much of a particular service, now billed by a physician, is done by a nurse, or how many services are delivered by the nurse and billed under the physician's name. (p. 1051)

In an attempt to identify whether CPT codes might explain nursing work and therefore provide needed data requested by Lockhart, studies were conducted to look at how many billable CPT activities were done by nurses (Griffith & Robinson, 1992, 1993; Griffith, Thomas, & Griffith, 1991; Robinson & Griffith, 1997). Questionnaires returned by RNs showed that 12 of the 63 CPT codes identified on the survey instrument covered work performed by 75% of the respondents and that all 63 were performed by at least 6% of the respondents (Griffith et al., 1991). Another study surveyed nine nurse specialist groups and found that 493 CPT codes covered work performed by these nurses (Griffith & Robinson, 1993)—after elimination of duplications resulting from overlapping of services provided by these specialties. Of the 236 different codes included on the questionnaire for family nurse practitioners, 232 were performed by the respondents (Griffith & Robinson, 1993).

Results of a study comparing the frequency with which nursing activities could be categorized under the Nursing Interventions

Classification (NIC) and the Current Procedural Terminology (CPT) codes revealed that NIC was superior to CPT; the study involved 201 AIDS patients hospitalized for pneumocystis carinii pneumonia. Nursing activities were categorized as 80 NIC interventions across 22 classes and in 15 CPT codes. All terms in the data set were classifiable under the NIC system, and 60% of the terms were classified under 14 NIC intervention categories, compared to only 6% classified under CPT codes. These findings support the importance of nursing-specific classifications for health care interventions to demonstrate nursing's contribution to quality and cost outcomes (Henry, Holzemer, Randell, Hsieh, & Miller, 1997). However, another way to address the issue is to introduce nursing services into CPT if they are not otherwise described in a CPT code (Sullivan-Marx & Mullinix, 1999).

The Balanced Budget Act of 1997 (Public Law 105-33), effective January 1, 1998, amended the Social Security Act to grant direct Medicare reimbursement to nurse practitioners, clinical nurse specialists, and physician assistants in all geographic areas and health care settings at 85% of the prevailing physician rate. Enactment of Medicare reimbursement for nurse practitioners (NPs) prompted a study of the RBRVS payment system for this group of providers (Sullivan-Marx & Maislin, 2000). An objective of the study was to compare relative work values established for NPs and family physicians for selected primary care evaluation and management services. Findings from the study suggested that services provided by NPs could be reliably valued in the Medicare Fee Schedule. In addition, findings indicated that (a) the work value is similar for both groups for common primary care CPT codes, (b) practice expense relative value is based on resources used and time to perform services, which are similar for NPs and family physicians, and (c) the principle of RBRVS is to base payment on work and resources used, not specialty or type of provider. Investigators concluded that differential payment for services provided by NPs *may not be* justified, according to the RBRVS principles by which payment is based on work and resources used.

As the nursing profession moves into the 21st century, different types of nursing classifications are being used (e.g., the Nursing Interventions Classification and the Nursing Minimum Data Set). Moreover, different methods are being used to record nursing workloads (e.g., Current Procedure Terminology codes, International Centers for Disease Procedure codes, and the Resource-Based Relative Value Scale). Thus no common language or workload recording method exists. If nurses want to be directly reimbursed, their challenge must be to accurately document the contribution of nursing practice to patient and program productivity and effectiveness through workload analysis. Nurses must be able to provide useful and meaningful data to consumers, policy makers, and payors.

■ *Nursing Practice Reimbursement*

Several authors emphasized the importance of direct payment to advanced practice nurses but did not discuss reimbursement for the entire profession; however, many of their thoughts and discussions can be applied to all of nursing (Cohen, Mason, Arsenie, Sargese, & Needham, 1998; Haber, 1997; Lang, Sullivan-Marx, & Jenkins, 1996; Mittelstadt, 1993; Oberst, 1997; Pearson, 1995; Sullivan-Marx, 1998; Sullivan-Marx & Mullinix, 1999). Direct practice reimbursement would recognize nurses as unique providers in the health care system and places a value on their services, legitimizing the significant contributions that nurses make to health care. Ability to bill directly for services would allow nurses (e.g., advanced practice nurses) to be self-employed or to enhance the revenue of their employers. It also would improve their ability to conduct research on the costs and outcomes of nursing care. As a result, nurses would no longer just be members of a team receiving reimbursement for nursing's contribution.

In recent years, advanced practice nurses have celebrated passage of legislation providing direct reimbursement for their care. They can now provide quality, effective health services to their respective populations without requiring direct supervision of a physician. However, Oberst (1997) cautioned the nursing community to be aware of the obligations that go along with direct reimbursement. Evidence-based practice will probably be a reimbursement criterion for the 21st century, as certain payor groups are already moving in that direction. Malpractice insurance rates will increase as members of the nursing community receive direct reimbursement for care; nurses will be called to account for the quality of service they provide in a way that was not possible in the past. To meet the challenge, Oberst urged development of research studies that focus on outcomes of nursing practice.

Direct reimbursement of nurses for services is certainly an important topic, but it can be considered a threat to physicians as well as payors. In her study, Griffith (1986) responded to an unsubstantiated charge that providing direct third-party reimbursement for nursing services would increase health care costs. Her findings indicated that nurses who were being reimbursed on a fee-for-service basis or received direct reimbursement or both, charge less for their services than salaried nurses. Griffith concluded with an interesting point: "When the billing for the nurse's services is done under the physician's or employer's name (a middleman), charges may be greater than when the reimbursement is made directly to the nurse" (p. 304).

The Primary Care Health Practitioner Incentive Act (part of the Balanced Budget Act

of 1997), signed by President Clinton on August 5, 1997, allows nurse practitioners (NPs) and clinical nurse specialists (CNSs) to bill Medicare and receive reimbursement for their services in all settings at 85% of prevailing physician rates (Sullivan-Marx, 1998). Prior to enactment of this law, Medicare reimbursement for NPs was cumbersome and payment for CNSs was nonexistent. Where do we go from here?

Currently, the ANA has representatives on the AMA's and HCFA's committees that establish relative work values and relative practice expense values for the Medicare Fee Schedule. Current practice expense values include all nurses employed in Part B payment settings (e.g., hospital outpatient clinics, physician offices, and nurse managed centers). What about other nurses in the profession (e.g., school nurses, nurse anesthetists, orthopedic nurses, nephrology nurses, critical care nurses, primary care nurses, and emergency room nurses)? Should the profession continue to lobby for direct reimbursement for all nurses? As part of the discussions in the AMA and HCFA committees, direct payment to nurses for services has been considered, but only informally so far. If reimbursement is obtained for all nurses, will that be a threat to other members of the interdisciplinary team such as social workers, dietitians, physicians, occupational therapists, pharmacists, physical therapists, and so on? These are important questions that must be addressed by the nursing profession.

Reimbursement Barriers

Barriers imposed by external forces and those created by nurses themselves could very well impede direct practice reimbursement.

1. *Organized physician opposition.* Lobbying efforts to persuade policy makers to reimburse nurses directly can be very expensive because,

in most cases, they are coming up against well-funded, organized campaigns of medical societies that are attempting to prevent nurses from receiving direct reimbursement. From the perspective of physicians, reimbursement to a group other than their own would create a substantial change in their economic position—and one that is not positive; therefore their strategy is to block groups such as advanced practice nurses or other nursing groups from receiving direct reimbursement. Additionally, when nurses provide care for the "whole" person, aspects of this care can overlap with accountability and authority of other professions, mainly physicians, which then create feelings of noncollaboration and competition.

2. *State and national legal and regulatory inconsistencies.* Taking the advanced practice nurse group as an example, we see that multiple inconsistencies currently exist between roles and within the same role, depending on the state in which an individual practices. Additionally, there is variation among the states in terms of titles, scope of practice, use of protocols, practice agreements, prescriptive practice authority, educational preparation, and credentialing standards. In contrast, physicians generally can travel from state to state and know what procedures they may legally perform, what medications they may prescribe, and, with the exception of some managed care situations, whether or not an insurer will pay for their services (Fox-Grage, 1996; Sekscenski, Sansom, Bazell, Salmon, & Mullan, 1994).

3. *Exclusion from managed care organization provider panels.* Three focus groups comprising 27 nurse practitioners in New York and Connecticut revealed a lack of interest in being on provider panels (Cohen et al., 1998). Some in the group were concerned about job security and did not want to disrupt arrangements with their employers. Those in institutional settings did not want to disturb the status quo. There was also a sense that managed care was not their problem, as reflected by the statement, "I

get my salary and I get treated real well by the doc." Workman (1998), in a letter to the editor, stated "If NPs think that being on a managed care panel is unnecessary, or that correct completion of an application is unimportant, they will be in for a great surprise" (p. 11). The message is clear: If nurses hope to compete in a managed care market, they must become educated about applying for provider panels.

4. *Lack of understanding about capitation and other financial arrangements.* Nurses have little understanding of health care finance and accounting. Many do not realize that the goal is to stay in business, achieve a positive profit margin, but yet decrease overall costs of health care and improve quality of care. Nurses have difficulty in thinking of health care as a "business"; but it is a term payors and corporations understand and expect health care professionals, including nurses, to discuss when they come to the "table." From the payor's point of view, the only two relevant issues when deciding to provide coverage for a treatment are whether the market demands the treatment and whether the treatment is indeed effective (Lilienfeld, 1998).

5. *Lack of unity within the profession.* The nursing profession has been plagued by special interest groups that divide nursing and individually do not have enough funding or voting blocks to have any significant power or influence. Territorial barriers that exist between roles and groups prevent nursing from speaking with one voice to consumers, policy makers, and third-party payors. As the largest group of health care providers, nurses must learn to influence political decisions (O'Malley, Cummings, & King, 1996).

6. *Lack of uniform educational requirements.* A profession is defined by its common body of specialized knowledge, which is based on uniform educational requirements. Unlike nursing, the medical profession has created an extremely powerful socialization process by having standard educational requirements.

Not having such standard requirements places the nursing profession at a disadvantage in functioning as a cohesive profession (Hadley, 1996). At the present time, North Dakota is the only state in the Union that requires a baccalaureate degree in nursing for entry into practice. Additionally, the nursing profession's failure to standardize educational requirements and specialty certification for advanced practice nursing has slowed the process of state practice act reforms, thus creating vulnerability of advanced practice nursing to concerns about the quality of care provided (Aiken & Salmon, 1994).

7. *Inability to articulate contributions that nurses make to improve quality and cost-effectiveness of care.* Contributing to this barrier is lack of practice-based data. The majority of practicing nurses have no idea of the revenue they generate for their employers, nor do they have cost or outcome data on their clients. More studies similar to one by Aiken, Smith, and Lake (1994) need to be conducted. They investigated whether hospitals known for good nursing care, identified in the study as "magnets," had lower Medicare mortality than hospitals that are otherwise similar, with respect to a variety of nonnursing organizational characteristics. Findings revealed that the "magnet" hospitals had a lower mortality rate of approximately 5 per 1,000 Medicare discharges. This rate corresponded to a reduction in "excess mortality" of 5%.

Strategies Needed for Reimbursement to Become a Reality

If nurses want direct reimbursement in the 21st century, they must come together as a profession and implement certain strategies to make it a reality.

1. *Development of public policy at local, state, and national levels.* Nurses must develop personal contacts with elected local, state, and national elected officials. Contacts should include personal office visits, telephone calls, letters, and involvement in political campaigns. Nurses should be familiar with the process of giving public testimony and be willing to do so when requested. An increasing number of nurses are being elected to public office where they can be influential in drafting and voting on bills created for reshaping the payment system. However, in order to be considered effective and powerful, the number needs to increase. Through these political activities and participation on committees and boards, nurses have an excellent opportunity to influence legislation that will shape reimbursement of health care services in the 21st century.

2. *Unity within the profession.* Territorial barriers that currently exist between nursing roles and groups need to come down. Presently, nursing is viewed by legislators, consumers, and other health care professionals as being a fragmented profession in which individuals have their own personal agendas (Camp-Sorrell & Spencer-Cisek, 1995). To be successful in obtaining direct reimbursement, nurses and their professional organizations must speak with one voice. To accomplish this task, nurses must first become actively involved in their professional organizations. These groups must then come together with shared agenda for action with practice-based data if they are going to be a major player in reimbursement reform discussions. It can be done: After all, the Berlin Wall did come down! Currently, ANA is represented with the National Organization Liaison Forum (NOLF) organizations on AMA committees that are establishing work and practice expense values for Medicare Fee Schedule. ANA is also active in dialogues with AMA on inclusion of nursing work in CPT-5, with three ANA representatives serving on AMA work groups of the project.

3. *Marketing strategies.* The nursing profession needs to market what it does, how well it does it, and why it is an important member of

the interdisciplinary team. If it does not do so, it cannot expect to become a major player in the reform discussions or receive direct reimbursement. Being good at the services nursing provides is not enough. Consumers, payors, and policy makers need to know the strengths and positive patient outcomes achieved by the care that nurses deliver.

4. *Conduct outcomes-based research to demonstrate effectiveness and productivity of nurses.* A top priority must be to conduct research that not only focuses on measurable and improved outcomes for patients, but also demonstrates cost-effectiveness. Nurses must document their unique contributions and demonstrate—through research similar to a study conducted by Naylor et al. (1999)—that benefits achieved with those contributions exceed incurred costs in providing nursing care. That study demonstrated that advanced practice nurse-centered discharge planning and home care intervention for at-risk hospitalized elders (a) reduced readmissions, (b) lengthened the time between discharge and readmission, and (c) decreased the costs of providing health care. If nurses do not conduct these important research studies, others will and nurses will then have to live with the results. Prior to developing a research agenda to provide the necessary data, Buerhaus (1998) emphasized anticipating questions that may be on the minds of legislators, committee staff members, and others who are interested in changing Medicare payment policy or reimbursement for health care in general.

5. *Role clarification.* In many settings, nursing roles are not fully understood. For example, advanced practice nurses are not always identified by the public as primary care providers (O'Malley et al., 1996). In fact, when questioned, the majority of nurses in the profession are not able to distinguish between the clinical nurse specialist and nurse practitioner roles. Taking it one step further, nurses

often are unable to describe or explain their own particular roles and contributions in caring for patients. As stated by Gladys Campbell, past president of the American Association of Critical-Care Nurses, at the 1998 National Teaching Institute: "Our mothers don't even know what we do" (McKinley, 1999, p. 2). If nurses want public and legislative support for direct reimbursement, they will need to do a better job of defining and clarifying their roles so that the impact of their unique contributions are fully understood and supported.

6. *Establish relationships with various third-party payors.* When establishing relationships with payors, the nursing profession needs to present outcome data to demonstrate effectively how nurses make a difference in the cost and quality of patient care delivery. To do so, nurses must develop a uniform approach to demonstrating their contributions to patient outcomes. Jones (1997) recommended designing and implementing a network information system that describes nurses' contributions to health care systems across the United States. Basic components of the infrastructure would include standard nursing language, data capture, and transmission technology.

7. *Seek support from nursing's number one fans—patients and their families.* Developing partnerships with patients and their families is key to achieving direct reimbursement. Nurses comprise the one group of health care professionals able to identify patient needs and positively effect changes that will benefit them.

8. *Ensure competent patient care providers.* In an effort to protect consumers better from incompetent health professionals, the Pew Health Professions Commission, which was chaired by former Senator George Mitchell, urged Congress and the states to adopt more rigid standards to regulate the health care workforce. The Commission reported that the current professional regulation system has "serious shortcomings" and that nurses should

pay close attention to the recommendations and use them to their advantage. Specifically the Commission recommended that (a) health care practitioners demonstrate specific competencies throughout their careers; (b) health professional boards must be more accountable to the public by increasing significantly representation by public, nonprofessional members; (3) states should enact scopes of practice that are nationally uniform for each profession; and (4) practice authority should be shared among the various health professions (Finocchio, Dower, Blick, Gragnola, & the Taskforce on Health Care Workforce Regulation, 1998).

9. *Possess business skills.* Nurses must develop and apply proficient business skills to take advantage of opportunities in tracking revenues they generate and in establishing salaries based on fee schedules (Sullivan-Marx, 1998). Adding business courses to the nursing curriculum at both the undergraduate and graduate levels is critical.

10. *Be proactive in dealing with managed care environment issues.* The managed care concept is based on issues of prevention and health screening in contrast to the past model of curing illness. Managed care focuses on wellness; efforts are made to keep individuals out of hospitals and manage them elsewhere, such as an ambulatory care clinic, a community-based clinic, or the home. At the same time, consumers of health care are demanding high-quality care, choice of who provides the care, and appropriate length of care to meet their needs (Paladichuk, 1997). It now appears that managed care will continue to be around in the 21st century; therefore nurses can play a key role in its further development. In the hospital setting, the nurse is the most capable individual to be case manager and thus determine when, how, and what resources are used for the patient. In the community, the nurse can direct care, provide necessary screening and educa-

tion, and, if an advanced practice nurse, be a primary provider of care.

■ Directions for Future Research

The nursing profession believes that quality care has a positive effect on patient outcomes and that it also is generally cost-effective and can contribute to achieving the goals of a competitive health care system. However, outcomes-based research must be conducted to demonstrate that these services have a positive impact on both client outcomes and costs of providing health care. Florence Nightingale recognized more than 100 years ago the importance of measuring health outcomes with good data, a profound and timeless insight (Hadley, 1996). Additionally, nurses of today must keep in mind that, if they don't develop and conduct these important studies, others will—and then nurses will have to live with the outcomes.

There is need for research studies similar to that of Aiken et al. (1994) and Naylor et al., (1999). Aiken's research concerned improved Medicare mortality rates in "magnet" hospitals that are recognized for the quality of care they provide. Naylor's study dealt with advanced practice nurse-centered discharge planning and home care intervention. Additional study questions that need to be answered to demonstrate cost-effectiveness, while at the same time making a difference in quality patient care and outcomes, include the following.

1. Does direct Medicare reimbursement of advanced practice nurses increase access to their services? What are the benefits to older adults?

2. Is differential Medicare reimbursement to advanced practice nurses cost-effective?

3. Are outcomes improved for models of care using teams of reimbursable providers, such

as nurse practitioner–physician collaborative models, compared to physicians alone or nurse managed practices?

4. In capitated systems of care, to what degree does case or disease management by nurses or nurse practitioners reduce the overall cost of care in high-risk patients by preventing complications, hospitalizations, and emergency room visits?

5. Has direct reimbursement of nurse practitioners at 85% of the physician rate reduced the hiring of nurse practitioners by physicians?

6. How many nurses have applied to be on provider panels for managed care? How many were actually accepted?

7. How many nurse practitioners are still being reimbursed under the physician's name and provider number?

8. When nurse practitioners receive 85% of the physicians' rate and spend more time with patients during a clinic visit, how much less income is generated by nurse practitioners per average workday? In a collaborative practice with physicians, to what degree is the lower income generated by nurse practitioners offset by the lower salary of nurse practitioners and improved patient outcomes?

9. In managed care and capitated systems, to what degree are services performed by nurse practitioners tracked using CPT codes? In systems where nurse practitioners services are tracked using CPT codes, can outcomes of nurse practitioner care be more readily demonstrated on an ongoing basis?

■ Concluding Statement

As we move through the 21st century, rapid change will continue in the health care marketplace, thus creating opportunities and challenges for the nursing profession. The public—consumers of care that nurses deliver—will become even more interested in cost, accessibility, and quality. Because nurses have the skills and ability to deliver in all three of these areas, shouldn't they be directly reimbursed for these services? Reimbursement would certainly increase the autonomy, visibility, image, and value of the profession; however, it could be viewed as a threat to other members of the health care interdisciplinary team as well as to third-party payors.

Nursing is the one professional group capable of taking on the challenge of direct reimbursement for all its members; therefore "let's go for it." To meet this challenge, the profession must first find an acceptable cost-accounting system to track nursing productivity. Additionally, nurses must document their interventions and costs to provide necessary data to third-party payors of nursing care in every setting.

■ References

Aiken, L. H., & Salmon, M. E. (1994). Health care workforce priorities: What nursing should do now. *Inquiry, 31,* 318–329.

Aiken, L. H., Smith, H. L., & Lake, E. T. (1994). Lower medicare mortality among a set of hospitals known for good nursing care. *Medical Care, 32,* 771–787.

American Medical Association. (1999a). Physicians' current procedural terminology (4th ed.). Chicago: Author.

American Medical Association. (1999b). *Medicare RBRVS: The physicians' guide.* Chicago: Author.

Balanced Budget Act of 1997. (P.L. 105–133) (1997, August). HR3426—Medicare and Medicaid Health Insurance Act. *U.S. Statutes at Large* (Volume III, pp. 251–788). Washington, DC. U.S. Government Printing Office.

Buerhaus, P. I. (1996). Creating a new place in a competitive market: The value of nursing care. *Nursing Policy Forum, 2*(2), 13–20.

Buerhaus, P. I. (1998). Medicare payment for advanced practice nurses: What are the research questions? *Nursing Outlook, 46,* 151–153.

Camp-Sorrell, D., & Spencer-Cisek, P. (1995). Reimbursement issues for advanced practice. *Oncology Nursing Forum, 22*(8), 31–34.

Cherry, N. (1991). The evolution of nursing reimbursement in the USA. *Washington Nurse, 21*(4), 14–15.

Cohen, S. S., Mason, D. J., Arsenie, L. S., Sargese, S. M., & Needham, D. (1998). Focus groups reveal perils and promises of managed care for nurse practitioners. *The Nurse Practitioner, 23*(6), 48–76.

Fagin, C. M. (1987). The visible problems of an "invisible" profession: The crisis and challenge for nursing. *Inquiry, 24,* 119–126.

Finocchio, L. J., Dower, C. M., Blick, N. T., Gragnola, C. M., & the Taskforce on Health Care Workforce Regulation. (1998, October). *Strengthening consumer protection: Priorities for health care workforce regulation.* San Francisco: Pew Health Professions Commission.

Fox-Grage, W. (1996). States study scope of practice and reimbursement. *Issues: A Newsletter of the National Council of States Boards of Nursing, Inc., 17*(2), 1–5.

Griffith, H. (1986). Implementation of direct third party reimbursement legislation for nursing services. *Nursing Economic$, 4,* 299–304.

Griffith, H., & Fonteyn, M. (1989). Let's set the payment record straight. *American Journal of Nursing, 89,* 1051–1058.

Griffith, H., & Robinson, K. R. (1992). Survey of the degree to which critical care nurses are performing current procedural terminology-coded services. *American Journal of Critical Care, 1,* 91–98.

Griffith, H., & Robinson, K. R. (1993). Current procedural terminology (CPT) coded services provided by nurse specialists. *IMAGE: Journal of Nursing Scholarship, 25,* 178–186.

Griffith, H., Thomas, N., & Griffith, L. (1991). MDs bill for these routine nursing tasks. *American Journal of Nursing, 91,* 22–27.

Haber, J. (1997). Medicare reimbursement: A victory for APRNs. *American Journal of Nursing, 97*(11), 84.

Hadley, E. H. (1996). Nursing in the political and economic marketplace: Challenges for the 21st century. *Nursing Outlook, 44,* 6–10.

Henry, S. B., Holzemer, W. L., Randell, C., Hsieh, S., & Miller, T. (1997). Comparison of nursing interventions classification and current procedural terminology codes for categorizing nursing activities. *IMAGE: Journal of Nursing Scholarship, 29,* 133–138.

Jones, L. D. (1997). Building the information infrastructure required for managed care. *IMAGE: Journal of Nursing Scholarship, 29,* 377–382.

Lang, N. M., Sullivan-Marx, E. M., & Jenkins, M. (1996). Advanced practice nurses and success of organized delivery systems. *The American Journal of Managed Care, 2,* 129–135.

Lilienfeld, D. E. (1998). How data influence third party payers. *ASHA, 40*(2), 12.

McKinley, M. G. (1999). The power of nursing: Be clear about what you do. *American Association of Critical-Care Nurses News, 16*(2), 2.

Mittelstadt, P. (March 1, 1991). PPRC recommends payment levels for non-physician providers. *Capitol Update.* Washington, DC: American Nurses Association, 7–8.

Mittelstadt, P. (1993). Federal reimbursement of advanced practice nurses' services empowers the profession. *The Nurse Practitioner, 18*(1), 43–49.

Naylor, M. D., Brooten, D., Campbell, R., Jacobsen, B. S., Mezey, M. D., Pauly, M. D. & Schwartz, J. S. (1999). Comprehensive discharge planning and home follow-up of hospitalized elders. *Journal of the American Medical Association, 281,* 613–620.

Oberst, M. T. (1997). Direct reimbursement: Implications for research (editorial). *Research in Nursing & Health, 20,* 375.

O'Malley, J., Cummings, S., & King, C. S. (1996). The politics of advanced practice. *Nursing Administration Quarterly, 20*(3), 62–72.

Paladichuk, A. (1997). Managing transitions: A proactive approach. Interview with Susan Odegaard Turner. *Critical Care Nurse, 17*(3), 94–99.

Pearson, L. J. (1995). Annual update of how each state stands on legislative issues affecting advanced nursing practice. *The Nurse Practitioner, 20*(1), 13–18.

Physician Payment Review Commission (PPRC). (1991). *Annual Report to Congress.* Washington, DC: U.S. Government Printing Office.

Physician Payment Review Commission (PPRC). (1997). *Annual report to Congress.* Washington, DC: U.S. Government Printing Office.

Primary Care Health Practitioner Incentive Act (1997). (Part of P.L. 105–33, Section 4511). HR 3426. Medicare and Medicaid Health Insurance Act. *U.S. Statutes at Large.* (Volume III, pp. 251–788). Washington, DC: U.S. Government Printing Office.

Robinson, K. R., & Griffith, H. M. (1997). Identification of current procedural terminology-coded services provided by family nurse practitioners. *Clinical Excellence for Nurse Practitioners, 1,* 397–404.

Sekscenski, E. S., Sansom, S., Bazell, C., Salmon, M. E., & Mullan, F. (1994). State practice environments and the supply of physician assistants, nurse practitioners, and certified nurse-midwives. *New England Journal of Medicine, 331,* 1266–1271.

Sullivan-Marx, E. M. (1998). Medicare reimbursement for advanced practice nurses: In the front door! *Nursing Outlook, 46*(1), 40–41.

Sullivan-Marx, E. M., & Maislin, G. (2000). Comparison of nurse practitioner and family physician relative work values. *Journal of Nursing Scholarship, 32*(1), 71–76.

Sullivan-Marx, E. M., & Mullinix, C. (1999). Payment for advanced practice nurses: Economic structures and systems. In: M. D. Mezey & D. O. McGivern (Eds.), *Nurses, nurse practitioners* (3rd ed., pp. 345–368). New York: Springer.

Workman, L. (1998). Third-party reimbursement (letters to the editor). *The Nurse Practitioner, 23*(5), 11, 111.

■ *Editor's Questions for Discussion*

What strategies are essential for recognition and reimbursement of services provided by nurses for procedures listed in the CPT coding system? Should nursing language be correlated with physician language in the CPT coding system? What advantages or disadvantages for nursing may result? Would correlation of nursing and physician language facilitate relevance of nursing-specific classifications for categorization of health care interventions and reimbursement? In the studies reported by Robinson, Griffith, and Sullivan-Marx about billable CPT activities, were all CPT code items listed on the questionnaires? How does inclusiveness of all CPT items affect study validity and reliability?

What factors have inhibited workload analysis and outcomes measurement in nursing practice? How have those factors previously been addressed? What forces exist now for research and evidence-based outcomes? How can these forces be capitalized on for action?

Respond to the questions posed by Robinson, Griffith, and Sullivan-Marx regarding direct reimbursement for all nurses. Provide arguments in defense of your answers. What impact may direct reimbursement have on collective bargaining for nurses? Discuss reimbursement barriers presented by Robinson, Griffith, and Sullivan-Marx. Should nursing be satisfied with 85% reimbursement for nursing services? Identify the most critical barrier to reimbursement for nursing practice. Which factor if addressed may diminish the importance of other barriers? Design specific approaches to resolve each obstacle cited by Robinson, Griffith, and Sullivan-Marx. What outcome measures will indicate overcoming of barriers?

What impact might reimbursement have on interdisciplinary education, research, and collaborative practice? Propose strategies to diminish the barriers. Identify means to diffuse potential conflict in interdisciplinary approaches. Refer also to the discussions by Yocom and Thomas (Chapter 3), Fitzpatrick (Chapter 18), Lindsey (Chapter 29), and Alexander (Chapter 44) for reimbursement implications.

42

Advanced Practice Roles in Nursing

Preparation and Scope of Practice

Mikel L. Gray, PhD, RN, CUNP, CCCN, FAAN

The evolution of clinical nurse specialists and nurse practitioners over the past two to three decades has focused a great deal of attention on issues surrounding advanced nursing practice. However, it is important to remember that nurses have engaged in advanced practice for nearly 100 years. Nonetheless, recent progress in graduate education has changed our views and increased the number of nurses in advanced practice roles. Another equally important factor in producing this dramatic shift has been the legislative and economic pressures for high quality and cost-effective alternatives in health care delivery. In this chapter, current definitions of advanced practice are reviewed, the evolution of advanced practice roles and their effect on current practice are discussed, and strategies to strengthen the impact of these roles are considered as we enter the new millennium.

Bishop and Scudder (1991) provide a sound philosophical basis for conceptualizing nursing as a practice, rather than a science or an art. They define a practice as use of science and technology to bring about positive outcomes. Taken from this perspective, nursing practice becomes more than the generation and application of science or technology, as the value of practice previously was detached from scientific experiment results. Instead, nursing practice is inextricably linked with outcomes that nurses strive to produce and with decisions concerning the relative worth of pursuing various outcomes. This philosophy of nursing is inherent in the American Nurses Association (ANA) Social Policy Statement (1995) that identifies four critical characteristics of nursing: (a) inclusion of the full range of human responses to health and illness, (b) practice based on integration of objective and subjective experience, (c) ability to apply scientific and technologic knowledge to processes of diagnosis and treatment, and (d) ability to provide a caring relationship that facilitates health and healing. Based on this understanding, the nursing profession can appreciate the value of expanding the scope of nursing practice to maximize its impact on the patient's physical, mental, and spiritual health. This desire to strengthen the full force of nursing care is at the core of the endeavor to identify and promote models of advanced nursing practice.

To define advanced nursing practice, it is necessary to distinguish it from specialty or expert nursing practice. Specialty nursing practice can be defined as a nurse whose practice is based on detailed knowledge of a specialized area, such as rehabilitation or urologic nursing. The specialty practice nurse typically obtains and demonstrates this knowledge by a combination of additional education, practical experience, and certification. A specialty practice nurse may engage in either generic or advanced practice nursing (Gray, 1994). Expertise in nursing practice can be defined as a hybrid of practical and theoretical knowledge (Benner, 1984). Development of expertise in nursing practice follows a predictable pattern that can be observed in generic and specialty practice nurses. Similarly, advanced practice nursing requires significant knowledge and skills; and just as for generic or specialty practice, expertise is based on the combination of practice and theoretical knowledge, and its development requires significant experience.

When compared to specialty or expert nursing practice, the primary and unique aspect of advanced practice (AP) nursing is its autonomy (Hamric, 1996). According to the ANA Scope

and Standards of Advanced Practice Registered Nursing (1996), advanced practice requires a high level of expertise in assessment, diagnosis, and treatment of complex responses to actual or potential health problems. AP nurses continue to perform many interventions used in generic nursing practice, but they also engage in practices unique to their new role. These practices are learned through additional formal education at the master's or doctoral level, through continuing education, and through supervised and ongoing clinical experiences. AP nurses may use these skills in a specialty practice setting; expertise in this practice is developed by a combination of theoretical and practical knowledge for nurses who engage in generic or specialty practice. Currently, four advanced practice roles—clinical nurse specialist, nurse practitioner, nurse anesthetist, and nurse midwife—are recognized in the ANA Scope and Standards of Advanced Practice Registered Nursing (1996).

■ Evolution of Advanced Practice Nursing Roles

Origin of the term *advanced practice* is not known (Bigbee, 1996). Curiously, in a review of *Medline* and *Nursing and Health* databases dating back to 1966 and 1982, respectively, the key words "advanced practice" and "nursing" reveal no articles earlier than 1985 (Durham & Hardin, 1985; Young & Shamansky, 1985), long after advanced practice roles were well established in nursing. However, the concept of advanced practice nursing is known to be far older. The first AP role, the nurse anesthetist, traces its history to the late 19th century; and the term nurse specialist was used by Dewitt in 1900 to describe nurses who achieved a more autonomous practice, based on additional training following their basic education. Similarly, although the origin of the term *clinical nurse specialist* also remains unclear, Peplau

(1965) asserted that the concept was conceived in 1938. In contrast, Norris (1977) attributed origin of the clinical nurse specialist role to proceedings of a National League for Nursing (NLN) committee that was commissioned to study postgraduate clinical nursing in 1944. Whichever source is accurate, these recollections demonstrate that the idea of advanced practice nursing is far older than the recent resurgence of interest in it.

Each of the four current advanced practice nursing roles have evolved separately, but all share essential characteristics. These include (a) high degrees of autonomy in decision-making, (b) direct accountability to patients or other members of the health care team or both, and (c) advanced theoretical and practical knowledge gained at the graduate and postgraduate level. Nonetheless, important differences in education, self-perception, and scope of clinical practice of clinical nurse specialists, nurse practitioners, nurse midwives, and nurse anesthetists exist and have an impact on their current practice; these differences must be viewed within a historic context.

Nurse Anesthetists

The nurse anesthetist is the oldest advanced practice nursing role. With introduction of nitrous oxide, ether, and chloroform in the mid 19th century, skills required for surgery changed dramatically and the need for a team of professional care providers to support the patient undergoing an operation became apparent. Initially, anesthesia was delivered by surgeons whose interest was not focused on this aspect of the procedure; such surgeons soon were replaced by nurses whose attention clearly centered on safe and effective administration of anesthesia. Sister Mary Bernard, who practiced in the 1870s, has been identified as the first nurse anesthetist (Becker, 1998; Bigbee, 1996). A chapter on anesthesia delivery appeared in Robb and Adams' (1893) *Nursing:*

Its Principles and Practice for Hospital and Private Use. By the late 1800s, Sisters of the Third Order of St. Frances had established a network of hospitals where nurses administered anesthesia. In one of these hospitals at the Mayo Clinic, Alice Magaw reportedly accumulated more than 14,000 cases of anesthesia administration without a single death (Thatcher, 1953). Magaw, who is now acknowledged as the "mother of anesthesia" (Becker, 1998; Bigbee, 1996), advised that anesthesia services (comprising only nurses at that time) remain independent of the department of nursing. Although the full scope of her arguments is not known, she reasoned that this separation was desirable because the education and recognition needed by these nurses could not be ensured if they remained under the general nursing department.

During the early 20th century, physicians also began specializing in anesthesia, their interest increasing greatly during World War I (Garde, 1996). An Association of Anesthesia was established in the 1920s, and conflict between physician and nurse anesthetists evolved rapidly. The intensity of this historic disagreement is illustrated by McMechan (1915) who urged states to pass medical practice acts that removed the "menace" of the nurse anesthetist. This rhetoric led to a statement in 1911 by the New York State Medical Society declaring that nursing anesthesia practice violated the law and a 1912 resolution by the Ohio Medical Society that only physicians could administer anesthesia. Both attempts to eradicate nursing anesthesia ultimately failed; more than 25,000 nurse anesthetists currently practice in the United States (Garde, 1996).

Two issues—separation of nurse anesthetists from the nursing department and their relationships with medical anesthesiologists—are particularly significant to contemporary practice. The professional society for nursing anesthesia, the American Association for Nurse Anesthetists (AANA), was formed in 1931, and its current name was adopted in 1939 (Becker, 1998). At its first annual meeting in 1933, members of the AANA voted to merge with ANA, but the ANA rejected this proposal. The reason for this rejection is not fully known, but Thatcher (1953) argued that this rejection was based on fear that the ANA would be forced to assume responsibility for a group of colleagues who could be charged with practicing medicine. The impact of Magaw's argument to separate nursing anesthesia from the nursing department and of ANA's decision to decline a merger with the AANA continues today. For example, although nurse anesthetists acknowledge that education in this specialty practice builds on prior nursing knowledge and experience, many nurse anesthesia programs are based in colleges of allied health sciences and schools of medicine (Garde, 1996).

Strained relationships between nurse and physician anesthetists also affect contemporary practice patterns. For example, no official communication between the AANA and the American Society of Anesthesiologists (ASA) occurred between 1947 and 1963. In addition, in 1976, the ASA withdrew support of a joint statement that the two associations had released in 1972, advocating the concept of a multidisciplinary team approach to anesthesia. Anesthesiologist plaintiffs have attacked nurse anesthetists' practice in court actions as recently as 1982 and 1986 (Bigbee, 1996; Mannino, 1996).

Nurse Midwives

Whereas the nurse anesthetist represents the oldest advanced practice nursing role, lay midwifery traces its origins to the ancient civilizations of Greece and Egypt (Bigbee, 1996). Prior to the 1700s, the lay midwife was treated typically as a respected member of the community. This role fell from favor during the 1800s, however, owing to replacement by physicians, by religious views, and by inadequate training—when compared to the growing knowledge base of physician obstetricians (Capitulo, 1998). During the early part of the 20th century, Varney-Burst (1988) reports that lay midwives within the United States were accused unfairly of poor outcomes with regard to maternal and infant mortality. In reality, these outcomes were affected by a number of variables, including inadequate resources for dealing with high-risk deliveries, inadequate prenatal care, poor physician training, and a complete lack of midwife training. As a result, the Children's Bureau was established; and legislation supportive of prenatal care was passed in 1921, although it was allowed to lapse soon afterward. In addition, the Maternity Center Association was established in 1918, based on a report from the New York City Health Commissioner's Office that found an unacceptably high maternal–infant mortality rate and that advocated improved prenatal care, including midwife education and training.

Organization of this Maternity Center Association, combined with the professionalization of midwifery under a nursing model in England, led to establishment of the nurse midwife role in the United States. Several key midwifery programs characterized these efforts in the United States, including a training program at the Lobenstein Clinic in New York City and the Frontier Nursing Service in Kentucky, both established by Mary Breckenridge (Rooks, 1997). These programs obtained excellent outcomes with respect to maternal and infant mortality, even when compared with physician supervised births.

Despite documentation of excellent outcomes for women and infants cared for by nurse midwives and support from individual university settings, opposition to midwifery persisted well into the late 1960s (Capitulo, 1998). In 1958, only six nurse midwife training programs existed, including three that granted a certificate and three based in a master's curriculum. During this period of time, nurse midwives delivered care primarily to indigent patients, although a few nurse midwives established successful practices that relied on affluent patients. Nonetheless in 1960, more than 99% of all births in the United States occurred in hospitals; and nurse midwives delivered less than 1% of all recorded births in the United States. In addition, only 23% of certified nurse midwives were practicing in their chosen clinical area in 1967. Fortunately, the low value placed on nurse midwifery dramatically improved in the 1970s. Several factors, including the feminist movement and an increased demand for natural child-birthing practices, caused a reevaluation of the nurse midwife role (Capitulo, 1998; Varney-Burst, 1998). As a result, the number of nurse midwives trained in the United States has increased, and the proportion of nurse midwives who engage in direct patient care has risen to more than 50%.

The distinct identities of midwifery and nursing continues to influence contemporary practice patterns. Unlike nurse anesthetists, clinical nurse specialists, or nurse practitioners, nurse midwives see their role as a merger of midwifery with that of professional nursing. This attitude is reflected in the American College of Nurse Midwives' decision to license midwives who are not registered nurses, and in philosophical statements reflecting clear distinction between the "nursing" and "midwife" aspects of their role. This dual professional identity is reflected also in regulations of 14 states who allow licensure of midwives, provided they hold a bachelor's degree, complete an educational program for midwifery, and pass a certification examination.

Clinical Nurse Specialists

Unlike nurse midwives or anesthetists, the clinical nurse specialist role was conceived by nurses, and it evolved primarily within the framework of a hospital-based nursing service and a university-based school or college of nursing. As the name implies, this role contains elements of both advanced and specialty practice. As a result, the role of clinical nurse specialist cannot be defined as easily as the nurse anesthetist or midwife. Felder (1983) defined the clinical nurse specialist role according to its functional aspects as clinician, educator, researcher, consultant, manager, advocate, and change agent. This functional definition of the role also was emphasized by Schuurmans (1996) when she described the clinical nurse specialist role in the Netherlands where it has existed only for the past 11 years. Hamric (1996) and Field (1983) defined the clinical nurse specialist practice according to outcome and asserted that the role exists primarily to improve quality of care delivered to patients.

The first graduate curriculum designed solely for preparing clinical nurse specialists for advanced practice was established in 1954 at Rutgers University. This program prepared clinical nurse specialists in psychiatric nursing, owing in large part to scholarly contributions of Hildegard Peplau (Bigbee, 1996). Acceptance of clinical nurse specialists in the practice setting grew rapidly during the 1960s to early 1980s, and the number of nurses practicing in this role grew dramatically. However, by the late 1980s, concerns over health care costs led to a reduction in the number of clinical nurse specialists positions, and many of these specialists sought other positions in administration or education. Currently, clinical nurse specialists comprise the largest single group of advanced practice nurses, totaling more than 58,000 as of 1993 (American Nurses Association [ANA], 1993). Nonetheless, given the significant number of these individuals who practice in nursing administration, education, or who have combined their role with nurse practitioner credentials, it is more difficult to determine how many currently practice in the clinical specialist role.

This variability of practice settings and role demands of the clinical nurse specialist continues to have an impact on current practice. Unlike nurse anesthetists or midwives, no single organization truly represents the voice of clinical nurse specialists in the United States. In addition, less than 14% of these highly educated nurses are certified (ANA, 1993), compared to 100% of nurse anesthetists, 66% of nurse midwives, and 58% of nurse practitioners (Bigbee, 1996). Thus, although clinical nurse specialists probably represent the largest single advanced practice group in nursing, their role identity is also multifaceted. This complexity in role identity leads many clinical nurse specialists to associate their identity more closely with a particular specialty practice or with one component of the clinical nurse specialist role, such as manager, administrator, researcher, or educator.

Nurse Practitioner

The nurse practitioner (NP) role traces its origins to the vision of Loretta Ford and Henry Silver in the 1965 establishment of the pediatric NP educational program at the University of Colorado (Silver & Ford, 1967). Similar to the nurse anesthetist role, the NP role was criticized initially because it was perceived as a physician substitute. However, Ford (1991) asserted later that the NP role ultimately survived because of its obvious value to nursing practice. Additionally, it survived its early days because of statements of support from health policy groups (Bigbee, 1996). During this period, NP practice expanded when a family practice program was opened at the University of Washington (Marchione & Garland, 1997). As the number of family and pediatric programs increased, others were added, including adult health, women's health, and geriatric programs. A number of recent events have contributed to an explosion of interest in NP ser-

vices and the rapid expansion of practitioners from 30,000 in 1993 to 48,000 only 5 years later. The most important event for NP practice was the 1997 Balanced Budget Act, which made payment for advanced practice (AP) nursing services a reality. Combined with health care reform and the current emphasis on seeking cost-effective primary and specialty care providers, the current demand for NPs is significant, and their impact on health delivery in the United States continues to grow.

Several historically significant events have had an impact on contemporary NP practice, including creation of the physician's assistant, the 1997 Balanced Budget Act, and changes in clinical nurse specialist practice patterns. Significance of the physician's assistant (PA) credential is best understood within the historical context of its origin. The first PAs were trained at Duke University in a program that began at about the same time as the pediatric NP center at the University of Colorado (Andreoli & Stead, 1967). Both programs came into existence amid a shortage of primary care physicians and during a time of rapidly rising health care costs. The PA program was designed to meet needs of the busy medical practitioner, whereas the NP was designed to expand the nursing role in primary care delivery. In retrospect, it is regrettable that these goals were not merged into an NP role acceptable to both physicians and nurses. However, given the historical context—when physicians perceived an acute need for a "practice extender" and nurses feared the creation of a "subphysician" role—the outcome does not seem particularly surprising. Although conflicts have existed between these groups, they also have found common ground, particularly in light of recent legislative developments. As a result, joint membership NP and PA groups exist (on a state level) and their numbers are growing (Herrick, 1999).

Reimbursement under the Balanced Budget Act of 1997 has had a profound and positive impact on NP practice in the United States. In addition to attracting nurses to obtain NP education, resulting in many postmaster's and postdoctoral students, by 2002 the Health Care Financing Administration (HCFA) is to promulgate a policy requiring NPs to hold a master's degree and certification from a nationally recognized certification board. These requirements will have an impact both on currently practicing NPs and those entering the field.

Recent trends in clinical nurse specialist utilization patterns also affect current NP practice. Although the NP traditionally focused on primary care, NP practice has expanded into acute care (hospital) settings. For example, the acute care NP has rapidly evolved from a popular concept among AP critical care nurses into a well-organized role. The first acute care NP program was offered in 1995, yet 1,200 individuals had been certified by 1998 (Kelinpell, 1998). This acute NP role is particularly interesting, because of its focus on acute and critical inpatient care settings and because of its close relationship to the role of the critical care clinical nurse specialist (Ackerman, 1997). Indeed, overlap between the role of the nurse practitioner (NP) and clinical nurse specialist (CNS) has led several authors to speculate whether these roles should be combined into a single advanced practice (AP) nurse credential (Chafetz, Collins-Bride, & Lego, 1998; Deane, 1997; Shuren, 1996).

■ Preparation, Certification, and Scope of Practice

In the previous section, the unique aspects of AP nursing roles were emphasized, using historical perspective. In the following discussion, focus is on shared aspects of these roles but also their unique aspects are acknowledged. This review is used as a basis for suggesting strate-

gies to strengthen the impact of AP nursing roles and increase the number of nurses engaged in direct patient care.

Although educational preparation and certification for each of the AP nursing roles vary significantly when viewed from a historical perspective, educational, legislative, and social factors have led to common standards. As of 1998, the right to practice each of the AP nursing roles requires a nurse to hold an earned master's degree (Bigbee, 1996). In addition, based on passage of the Balanced Budget Act of 1997, HCFA will require that AP nurses hold national certification in order to receive reimbursement.

All AP nursing roles are based on mastery and application of specific clinical skills. Certain tasks are unique to a single role, but the majority of skills are shared by all AP nurses (ANA, 1996). These shared skills include (a) physical and psychosocial assessment; (b) diagnosis of specific diseases, disorders, and the presence of expected physiologic process (e.g., progression of labor and delivery and occurrence of menopause); and (c) prescription of a treatment plan, followed by evaluation of outcomes. Unique aspects of AP nursing roles are more apparent when the type of therapies provided by each clinician is considered. For example, all nurse anesthetists prescribe and administer specific pharmacologic (anesthetic) agents, and NPs are allowed to prescribe certain medications in 48 of the 50 states and the District of Columbia (Pearson, 1998). In contrast, clinical nurse specialists and nurse midwives are less likely to have prescriptive authority, and they may face local barriers to these privileges, even when legislatively granted (Baltimore & Gilett, 1998; Kaas, Dahl, Dehn, & Frank, 1998). Although AP nurses share many characteristics with regard to direct patient care, it is primarily the clinical nurse specialist who provides indirect patient care. Activities such as (a) revising policies; (b) altering the physical environment to promote care; or (c) educating other care providers, including nursing staff, assistants, and therapists are more likely to be carried out by the clinical nurse specialist than the NP (Felder, 1983).

Traditionally, NP practice has been perceived as occurring in primary care settings, the clinical nurse specialist and nurse anesthetist are assumed to practice in the hospital, and the nurse midwife in the home or birthing center. However, studies have shown that each of the AP nursing roles is practiced in a variety of settings. For example, in addition to practice in a hospital or ambulatory surgery center, nurse anesthetists also have a significant and increasing presence in the private clinic and office setting (Garde, 1996). Similarly, whereas the majority of NP practice in outpatient settings, a growing number of acute care and specialty care practitioners deliver care in acute care, inpatient settings (Hravnak, Rosenzwig, Rust, & Magdic, 1998). Nurse midwives also practice in a variety of settings, including the home, hospital, clinic, or private office (Brown & Grimes, 1993).

■ Strategies for Success

When contemplating the future of AP nursing, it is important to consider the lessons of history, the current setting, and the stated desires of AP nurses and the public they serve. Perhaps the clearest historical lesson is the lasting division caused by failures of professional nurses to communicate continuously among themselves and collaborate with colleagues. Lack of communication has affected the historical evolution of each AP nursing role; it has produced clearly negative consequences for the nurse anesthetist, nurse midwife, and NP. Professional relationships between AP nurse associations and the American Nurses Association

now are clearly more cordial and open than in earlier decades. However, these lessons must be considered as we, as nurses, seek to promote and maintain the legislative momentum enjoyed during the past several years. With the combined voices of AP nurses, we are in an excellent position to protect recently granted privileges and to seek further power in influencing policy decisions that affect AP nursing practice and the health of all Americans. Yet, to realize this goal, we must change the legitimate perception that AP nursing lacks a unified voice for most issues. No one organization (including the ANA) can provide this unified voice; instead, collaboration among all key players is demanded to ensure that our combined influence is brought to bear on all public policy issues affecting AP nursing.

Collaboration with other disciplines remains a challenge for AP nursing and for all nurses. History has demonstrated the dangers of failing to communicate with other care providers (including lay providers). History also has shown that such collaboration depends on genuine willingness of groups to discuss issues and to tolerate diversity in health care delivery. In the current setting, collaborative efforts by nurse and lay midwives and by NPs and PAs represent a positive effort to form mutually beneficial coalitions that will enhance AP nursing practice. Nonetheless, we must remain vigilant, lest others influence public policy and legislation in a manner that hinders the scope or independence essential for effective AP nursing practice.

Addressing the relationship between clinical nurse specialist and NP and arguments for blending these roles also is necessary. Several authors have reviewed arguments for and against this type of blended role (Chafetz et al., 1998; Deane, 1997; Shuren, 1996), and these arguments must be considered carefully. Regardless of the outcome of this debate, that these roles significantly overlap is apparent.

Given the requirement for master's education for both roles and growing realization that we must prepare nurses for "career security" versus "job security," graduate nursing programs must include education for both roles. Indeed, given the rich historic tradition enjoyed by each role, it seems more and more futile to spend time attempting to educate the public about yet another new AP nursing role when we can prepare AP nurses with skills needed to practice both.

■ Concluding Statement

During the 1990s, AP nursing evolved from a perceived aberration to a well-developed, multifaceted alternative for the motivated nurse. The last two decades, in particular, have seen rapid evolution in education, credentialing, and scope of practice for all AP roles. These changes provide a realistic sense of excitement for health care and professional practice in the 21st century.

■ References

Ackerman, M. H. (1997). The acute care nurse practitioner: Evolution of the clinical nurse specialist? *Heart and Lung, 26*, 85–86.

American Nurses Association. (1993). *Nurse practitioners and certified nurse-midwives: A meta-analysis of studies in nurses in primary care roles.* Washington, DC: Author.

American Nurses Association. (1995). *Nursing's social policy statement.* Washington, DC: Author.

American Nurses Association. (1996). *Scope and standards of advanced practice registered nursing.* Washington, DC: Author.

Andreoli, K. G., & Stead, E. A. (1967). Training physician's assistants at Duke. *American Journal of Nursing, 67,* 1442–1443.

Balanced Budget Act of 1997. (P.L. 105–33) (August 1997). HR 3426–Medicare and Medicaid Health Insurance Act. *U.S. Statutes at Large.* (Volume III, pp. 251–788). Washington, DC: U.S. Government Printing Office.

Baltimore, J. J., & Gilett, P. (1998). Clinical nurse specialist prescriptive authority and the legislative process. *Advanced Practice Nursing Quarterly, 4,* 78–82.

Becker, K. T. (1998). A brief history of nurse anesthesia practice. *Seminars in Perioperative Nursing, 7,* 80–85.

Benner, P. (1984). *From novice to expert.* Menlo Park, CA: Addison-Wesley.

Bigbee, J. L. (1996). Historical and developmental aspects of advanced nursing practice. In A. B. Hamric, J. A. Stross, & C. H. Hanson (Eds.), *Advanced practice nursing: An integrative approach* (pp. 3–24). Philadelphia: W. B. Saunders.

Bishop, A. H., & Scudder, J. R. (1991). *Nursing: The practice of caring.* New York: National League of Nursing Press.

Brown, S. A., & Grimes, D. E. (1993). *Nurse practitioners and certified nurse-midwives: A meta-analysis of studies on nurses in primary care roles.* Washington, DC: American Nurses Publishing.

Capitulo, K. L. (1998). The rise, fall and rise of nurse midwifery in America. *Maternal Child Nursing, 23,* 314–321.

Chaftez, L. , Collins-Bride, G., & Lego, S. (1998). Merging the CNS and NP roles in advanced psychiatric nursing: Pro and con. In A. B. Burgess (Ed.), *Advanced practice psychiatric nursing* (pp. 1–13). Stamford, CT: Appleton & Lange.

Deane, K. A. (1997). CNS and NP: Should the roles be merged? *Canadian Nurse, 93,* 24–30.

Dewitt, K. (1900). Specialties in nursing. *American Journal of Nursing, 1,* 14–17.

Durham, J. D., & Hardin, S. B. (1985). Promoting advanced nursing practice. *Nurse Practitioners, 10,* 59–62.

Felder, L. A. (1983). Direct patient care and independent practice. In A. B. Hamric & J. Spross (Eds.), *The clinical nurse specialist in theory and practice* (pp. 59–71). Orlando: Grune & Stratton.

Field, L. (1983). Current trends in education and implications for the future. In A. B. Hamric & J. Spross (Eds.), *The clinical nurse specialist in theory and practice* (pp. 237–256). Orlando: Grune & Stratton.

Ford, L. (1991). Advanced nursing practice: The future of the nurse practitioner. In L. H. Aiken & C. M. Fagin (Eds.), *Charting nursing's future: Agenda for the 1990s* (pp. 287–99). Philadelphia: Lippincott.

Garde, J. F. (1996). The nurse anesthesia profession: A past, present and future perspective. *Nursing Clinics of North America, 31,* 567–580.

Gray, M. (1994). Specialty practice and the allure of advanced practice. *Journal of Wound, Ostomy and Continence Nursing, 21,* 133–134.

Hamric, A. B. (1996). A definition of advanced practice nursing. In A.B. Hamric, J. S. Spross, & C. M. Harrison (Eds.), *Advanced nursing practice: An integrative approach* (pp. 42–56). Philadelphia: W. B. Saunders.

Herrick, T. (1999). NPs/PAs forge new partnerships. *Clinician News, 3*(1), 32, 34.

Hravnak, M. , Rosenzwig, M. Q., Rust, D., & Magdic, K. (1998). Scope of practice, credentialing and privileging. In R. M. Kelinpell & M. R. Piano (Eds.), *Practice issues for the acute care nurse practitioner* (pp. 41–66). New York: Springer.

Kaas, M. J., Dahl, D., Dehn, D., & Frank, K. (1998). Barriers to prescriptive authority for psychiatric/mental health clinical nurse specialists. *Clinical Nurse Specialist, 12,* 200–204.

Kelinpell, R. M. (1998). Acute care nurse practitioner: Reports from the practice setting. In R. M. Kelinpell & M. R. Piano, *Practice issues for the acute care nurse practitioner* (pp. 1–9). New York: Springer.

Mannino, J. M. (1996). Legal aspects of nurse anesthesia practice. *Nursing Clinics of North America, 31,* 581–589.

Marchione, J., & Garland, N. (1997). An emerging profession: The case of the nurse practitioner. *IMAGE: Journal of Nursing Scholarship, 29,* 335–337.

McMechan, F. H. (1915). (editorial). Anesthesia supplement. *American Journal of Surgery, 29,* 120.

Norris, D. M. (1977). One perspective on the nurse practitioner movement. In A. C. Jacox & C. Norris, *Organizing for independent nursing practice* (pp. 21–33). New York: Appleton-Century-Crofts.

Pearson, L. J. (1998). Annual update of how each state stands on legislative issues affecting advanced nursing practice. *Nurse Practitioner, 23*(1), 14–66.

Peplau, H. E. (1965). Specialization in professional nursing. *Nursing Science, 3,* 268–287.

Robb, I. A. H., & Adams, H. (1893). *Nursing: Its principles and practice for hospital and private use.* Philadelphia: W. B. Saunders.

Rooks, J. (1997). *Midwifery and childbirth in America.* Philadelphia: Temple University Press.

Schuurmans, M. J. (1996). The clinical nurse specialist in geriatrics in the Utrecht, the Netherlands. *Nursing Clinics of North America, 31,* 535–548.

Shuren, A. W. (1996). The blended role of the clinical nurse specialist and the nurse practitioner. In A. B. Hamric, J. A. Spross, & C. M. Hanson (Eds.), *Advanced nursing practice: An integrative approach* (pp. 375–394). Philadelphia: W. B. Saunders.

Silver, H., & Ford, L. (1967). The pediatric nurse practitioner at Colorado. *American Journal of Nursing, 67,* 1443–1444.

Thatcher, V. S. (1953). *A history of anesthesia: With emphasis on the nurse specialist.* Philadelphia: Lippincott.

Varney-Burst, H. (1998). History of nurse midwifery in reproductive health care. *Journal of Nurse-Midwifery, 43,* 526–529.

Young, K. J., & Shamansky, S. L. (1985). Taking a stand: Public health nursing is advanced practice. *Public Health Nursing, 2,* 193–194.

■ Editor's Questions for Discussion

Discuss the criteria for advanced practice (AP). Which is more relevant, expert knowledge and skills or autonomy? How similar were issues related to development of the nurse anesthetist specialty, the forerunner for all AP roles? To what extent have strained relationships with physicians resulted in all AP roles? How might positive change occur?

How do dual professional identities inherent in AP affect the profession of nursing? Discuss the disparate views and beliefs about each AP role that are held by nursing, other disciplines, and the public. Identify the most significant issue that must be resolved in each AP role. What impact does variability in practice settings and role demands have for each AP role, the profession, interdisciplinary relationships, and the public?

How important is it for the nursing profession to have consensus regarding AP role functions? To what extent do "lines" exist for nurses between practicing medicine versus practicing advanced nursing? How should disagreement regarding practice roles best be resolved within the profession and other disciplines? Given the historical conflicts with medicine about AP roles, what has nursing learned about conflict prevention and resolution?

Debate the pros and cons of combining the nurse practitioner (NP) and clinical nurse specialist (CNS) roles? What are some shared and unique aspects of each role? To what extent do NPs and CNSs diagnose disease? According to state Nurse Practice Acts, how acceptable is diagnosing disease? How do states differ regarding prescriptive privileges for advanced nurse practitioners? How could graduate education programs prepare students for shared or distinctive roles? What content should all AP roles require at the graduate level? How may the views of Snyder, Kreitzer, and Loen (Chapter 43) affect AP roles?

How should the nursing profession collaborate with other health care providers? Should there be a unified voice for AP roles. If so, provide specific strategies for how "one voice" may be achieved.

43

Complementary and Healing Practices in Nursing

Mariah Snyder, PhD, RN, FAAN
Mary Jo Kreitzer, PhD, RN
Marilyn Loen, PhD, RN

Much attention is being given to complementary therapies. In a national survey, Eisenberg et al. (1998) found that 42.1% of Americans had used one or more complementary therapies during the past year. The majority of persons (58.3%) had paid "out-of-pocket" for these treatments. Reasons that persons have given for using complementary therapies, either singly or in conjunction with biomedical therapies, include (a) the recognition that pharmaceuticals and surgical procedures often do not "heal," (b) a desire to be a partner in the healing process, and (c) a wish to receive care from professionals who are caring and concerned with patients' total selves.

Numerous terms have denoted these "new-old" therapies, many of which have a long history of use in other cultures: complementary therapies, alternative therapies, healing practices or therapies, nontraditional therapies, and nonallopathic care. Initially, the term *alternative* was used because these therapies were viewed as substitutes for biomedical or Western therapies. However, in many instances these "new-old" therapies are used concurrently with biomedical therapies. Thus the term used most frequently is *complementary therapies.* The terms *healing therapies* or *healing practices* are used less often. However, the use of *healing therapies* helps to convey that healing is a care outcome and not necessarily cure, which is the prime difference between "new-old" therapies and current biomedical practices.

Many practitioners and authors refer to these "new-old" therapies as complementary and alternative medicine. Nurses and other practitioners have objected to the word "medicine" per se, as many of these therapies have a long history in nursing and other professions.

Several definitions of complementary and alternative therapies exist. Following discussions at a national interdisciplinary conference sponsored by the Office of Alternative Medicine, the *Panel on Definition and Description of CAM Research Methodology (1997)* proposed the following:

> Complementary and alternative medicine (CAM) is a broad domain of healing resources that encompasses all health systems, modalities, and practices and their accompanying theories and beliefs, other than those intrinsic to the politically dominant health system of a particular society or culture in a given historical period. CAM includes all practices and ideas self-defined by their users as preventing or treating illnesses or promoting health and well-being. Boundaries within CAM and between the CAM domain and the domain of the dominant system are not always sharp and fixed. (p. 50)

This definition does not ascribe administration of therapies to any one profession, but rather it conveys the wide scope of therapies and practices used in healing across cultures.

The multitude of complementary therapies can be classified in various ways. The classification system proposed by the National Institutes of Health contains seven fields of practice: (a) alternative systems of medical practice, (b) mind–body interaction, (c) manual healing practices, (d) pharmacological and biological treatments, (e) herbal medicine, (f) diet and nutrition, and (g) bioelectromagnetics applications in medicine (National Center for Complementary and Alternative Medicine [NCCAM], 1999). Acupuncture, ayurvedic medicine, homeopathy, chiropractic, naturo-pathic, and traditional Chinese medicine are some alternative systems of medical practice. Many of the mind–body therapies have a long tradition of use in nursing: biofeedback, counseling, guided imagery, humor therapy, meditation, music, prayer therapy, relaxation techniques, and support groups. Therapies included in the manual healing category include osteopathy, massage, and biofield techniques. Chelation therapy and use of cartilage products are several of the therapies in the pharmacological and biological category. Herbal preparations have been used for centuries; currently more than 80% of the world's inhabitants use herbal preparations. Diet supplements and nutritional practices are used to prevent illnesses and to cure diseases. Examples of bioelectromagnetic therapies include Blue-Light treatment, electromagnetic fields or magnets, and neuromagnetic stimulation devices.

Complementary therapies are in the national spotlight. Because of the public's interest, health care systems are rushing to make these a part of their "menu of services." What is often missing is an understanding of the underlying philosophy of care that is critical to the success of these therapies. Merely adding more therapies that can be prescribed without altering the perspective within which they are administered or taught is deluding the recipient.

■ Underlying Philosophy of Complementary Therapies

Four concepts underlie the philosophy that is crucial to the success of complementary therapies: holism, caring, patient as healer, and healing. These have been an integral part of nursing for centuries. Likewise, nurses have used many of the complementary therapies in integrating this underlying philosophy in care of patients.

Providing holistic care has been held as one of nursing's hallmarks. According to the American Holistic Nurses' Association, "Holism involves studying and understanding the interrelationships of the bio-psycho-social-spiritual dimensions of the person, recognizing that the whole is greater than the sum of the parts" (as cited in Dossey, Keegan, Guzzetta, & Kolkmeier, 1995, p. 7). In an interview for *Alternative Therapies,* Barbara Dossey noted that holistic nursing is not a specialty in nursing, but rather a philosophy that encompasses the mind–body–spirit of the patient and nurse (Horrigan, 1999). Many individuals in today's society are demanding that health professionals listen to their concerns and address the total person, particularly spiritual concerns, in providing care. The American Holistic Nurses Association has identified 24 complementary therapies that nurses, operating from a holistic philosophy, frequently incorporate into their practice.

Perception of the caring and concern of the professionals administering complementary therapies has been cited as one of the key reasons for continuing to seek complementary care (Eisenberg et al., 1998). Caring has been identified as a key component of nursing. Swanson (1991) defined caring as "a nurturing way of relating to a valued other toward whom one feels a personal sense of commitment and responsibility" (p. 165).

Two interventions that nurses incorporate into administration of complementary therapies are presence and active listening. McKivergin and Daubenmire (1994) identified three levels of presence: physical, psychological, and therapeutic. In physical presence, the nurse is "there" for the patient, whereas in psychological presence the nurse focuses on "being with" the patient to provide support and comfort. Therapeutic presence is the nurse being with the patient as whole being to whole being. In this relationship the nurse uses her personal resources of body, mind, emotions, and spirit.

A nurse cannot be an active listener unless she or he is present for the patient. Active listening involves more than hearing the words spoken. The nurse is attuned to (a) not only how words are spoken but also "listens" for what is not said, (b) the nonverbal communication used, and (c) the inner spirit of the patient.

Remen (1996) noted that "the most basic and powerful way to connect with another person is to listen. Just listen. Perhaps the most important thing we give each other is our attention. And especially if it is given from the heart" (p. 143). Presence and active listening go hand in hand and allow the nurse to begin to grasp what the health experience means to the patient.

In such a climate the nurse recognizes that it is the patient who is healer and nursing's role is to put the patient in the best possible condition so that nature can act upon him or her (Nightingale, 1859/1992). One tenet of the American Holistic Nurses Association is that nursing care includes therapies that enable the patient to achieve the wholeness inherent within himself or herself (Dossey et al., 1995). According to Fulder (1998), self-healing is a paramount part of complementary therapies, with practitioners respecting and recruiting the natural healing process within each person. Many professionals who use complementary therapies recognize the active role of the client in the healing process. Dossey et al. (1995) noted that the human spirit is a major healing force.

Western medicine has focused on curing illnesses. However, with the increase in chronic illnesses for which no "cure" has been discovered, other outcomes and therapies are needed. Eisenberg and colleagues (1998) reported that complementary therapies were used most frequently by individuals with chronic conditions such as back problems, anxiety, depression, and headaches. Derivation of the word "heal" is from "haelen," which conveys the meaning of a movement toward wholeness. Thus to heal is to be made whole. Healing is an active process in which a person examines his or her attitudes, memories, and beliefs so as to release all negative patterns that are interfering with recovery (Myss, 1996). Many complementary therapies used within the holistic paradigm have potential to help individuals heal themselves.

■ Use of Complementary Therapies in Chronic Illness

The prevalence of chronic illness is increasing dramatically worldwide. Approximately one in seven persons has an illness that limits activities. Minority populations, those with lower socioeconomic status, and elders experience a disproportionately higher number of chronic illnesses (Institute of Medicine, 1991). Lubkin and Larsen (1998) defined chronic illness as "the irreversible presence, accumulation, or latency of disease states or impairments that involve the total human environment for supportive care and self-care, maintenance of function and prevention of further disability" (p. 6). This definition is aligned with nursing's focus of caring for the whole person within the context of his or her environment.

Management of symptoms becomes a major focus of care for patients with chronic illnesses, and promotion of comfort is a desired outcome. Many patients find the side effects of medications to be worse than the treatment. Thus many with chronic illnesses have sought relief of symptoms by using complementary therapies. The use of herbal preparations, one of the most popular therapies currently, is being tried as a method of avoiding negative side effects of biomedical pharmaceutics (Eisenberg et al., 1998).

Pain is the most prevalent symptom for individuals seeking health care. Numerous complementary therapies have been used to relieve pain and promote comfort: music, imagery, therapeutic and healing touch, heat and cold, biofeedback, and humor (Snyder &

Lindquist, 1998). Research findings have demonstrated that nonpharmacological nursing interventions are effective in management of pain (Johnson, Fuller, Endress, & Rice, 1978; Levin, Malloy, & Hyman, 1987; Mandle, Domar, & Harrington, 1990; Mogan, Wells, & Robertson, 1985). However, certainty of the findings remains somewhat in question due to the small sample sizes of many studies. The increasing number of research studies being conducted on complementary therapies is exciting to see, particularly in the area of pain reduction. For example, studies are being conducted now to examine the effectiveness of therapeutic touch in reducing musculoskeletal pain and anxiety and to determine the efficacy of static magnetic fields in reducing symptoms in individuals with fibromyalgia (Taylor, 1998). The University of Virginia School of Nursing is one of 11 centers nationwide funded by the National Institutes of Health to study the efficacy of complementary therapies. The purpose of the center is to evaluate the effectiveness, safety, and cost of selected complementary therapies in relieving pain and suffering (Taylor, 1998).

Another symptom commonly found in persons with chronic illnesses is stress. One of the greatest problems facing persons in Western culture is how to reduce stress—an essential skill for health promotion, improvement in the quality of life, and preventing illness. Some early research on the use of complementary therapies such as meditation, Benson's relaxation response, and biofeedback was to reduce stress. Numerous nursing studies have demonstrated the efficacy of complementary therapies in reducing stress (Snyder, 1993).

Because nurses are grounded in a caring model of healing, they are in pivotal position to manage the care of persons with chronic illnesses. With emphasis on the patient as healer and the nurse as one who facilitates that healing, it is essential that nurses be knowledgeable about the most effective healing practices for a wide array of health problems, particularly chronic illnesses. In contrast to the role established by the biomedical paradigm, the caring paradigm of nursing provides the context in which complementary therapies can be used to enhance the quality of life of patients and to reclaim a patient-centered approach in nursing practice.

■ Complementary Therapies and Cultural Diversity

The increasing diversity of the U.S. population makes it imperative that nurses be knowledgeable about health care practices and therapies around the world. According to the definition of complementary therapies proposed by the Office of Alternative Medicine (Panel on CAM, 1997), therapies classified as complementary in one culture may be considered mainstream health care in another culture. Culturally congruent health care facilitates patient satisfaction and is a powerful healing force for health (Marriner-Tomey, 1994). Western medicine, in its attempt to provide scientific-based health care, often has suppressed health practices commonly used in other cultures. Recently, however, society has begun to recognize the value of healing practices other than those found in the Western biomedical model. For example the sweat lodge, which is part of many of their tribal practices, is again becoming a part of health care for many Native Americans. Struthers (1999) reported that non-Native Americans are seeking the services of women Objibwe and Cree healers.

■ Scientific Basis for Complementary Therapies

One main objection to acceptance of complementary therapies and their incorporation into biomedical practice has been the apparent lack of a "scientific basis" for the efficacy of these therapies. This objection may have some basis, but research on complementary therapies, much of which has been conducted by nurses, has demonstrated the efficacy of a number of therapies such as imagery, therapeutic touch, and music.

The scientific community would like to have the effectiveness of all complementary therapies validated through double-blind study designs. The study of these therapies, however, suggests that indeterminate nonphysical and nonlinear relationships are significant to outcomes and to patient satisfaction (Bessinger, 1996). Kiene and von Schon-Angerer (1998) discussed the uselessness of a double-blind design in the case of complementary therapies that are open to psychological influence. They argued instead for development of methodologies that give merit to individualistic judgment and that answer the question, how well does this particular therapy work for this individual? The single-case causality assessment, for example, is a methodology that does not require randomization, comparison, or large sample sizes for study. A car drives across a field and leaves tracks that have the same surface imprint as the tires. A person can be certain that it is the tire movement that caused the tracks and that no further proof will be gained by driving the car over numerous fields (comparing the surface with untouched fields), nor with randomization of the experiment. Thus there are designs, other than the conventional double-blind research method, that can be used to determine the therapeutic efficacy of complementary therapies (Kiene & von Schon-Angerer, 1998).

Caring by the health professional is a key component of the underlying philosophy of complementary therapies. It is difficult to separate this component from the therapy when measuring outcomes. The "connectedness" of the health professional with clients is significant to treatment outcomes and patient satisfaction. The practitioner's attitudes and beliefs are communicated to the patient and have a profound impact on the healing process (Novack et al., 1997).

■ Regulation of Complementary Therapies

Regulatory issues surrounding complementary and healing therapies are complex. In contrast to disciplines with clearly defined scopes of practice, the field of complementary and alternative therapies is very interdisciplinary and boundaries of practice have considerable overlap. For example, nurses, chaplains, psychologists, physicians, and other health care providers—both licensed and unlicensed—widely incorporate imagery into their practice. No one discipline owns this practice. Acupuncture is a therapeutic modality within traditional Chinese medicine. Acupuncturists are licensed to practice in 34 states and in most states a 3-year postgraduate course of study is required to meet minimum licensure requirements. However, in many states the practice of acupuncture is not limited to licensed acupuncturists. Physicians and chiropractors may practice acupuncture legally under their medical or chiropractic licenses, exempted from additional licensure requirements. Homeopathy is an example of a field that is unregulated in most states. Practitioners of homeopathy may be licensed health care professionals, graduates of formal homeopathic programs, or lay practitioners with no formal training. One state (Arizona) has a separate medical board to license physicians who practice homeopathy. However, in most states, homeopathy is not regulated in any way and has no title protection. In other words, virtually anyone can use the title of homeopathic practitioner.

Regulation by state authority is imposed to protect public safety. According to Cohen (1996), the aims of regulatory mechanisms are to (a) protect the public from dangers of unskilled practitioners and unsound treatment or advice, (b) protect the public from reliance on unskilled practitioners, and (c) direct the public to proper medical care. Some would argue for regulation, from the premise that consumers are unable to distinguish between competent and incompetent practitioners. Others view this contention to be paternalistic and suggest that medical care is open to interpretation. Another view of regulation is that it is imposed not in the interest of the public, but rather to protect the self-interests of various occupational groups; public protection may be a secondary or incidental benefit.

Where it is imposed, regulation is a continuum from registration to certification (less restrictive regulatory mechanisms) to licensure (a highly restrictive regulatory mechanism). Under systems of registration (in some states referred to as issuing of a permit), any person may engage in an occupation as long as he or she is registered with a regulatory agency. This type of regulation most often is used when the threat to life, health, safety, and economic well-being is relatively small. Certification is an ambiguous term. It is often used by private credentialing organizations to connote a level of competence or attainment of specialized training. In some states, however, legislatures have enacted certification systems to regulate occupations in a manner that is similar to licensure. Licensure is the most restrictive form of regulation. In states with licensure laws, it is illegal for anyone to engage in an occupation without a license and only those who meet certain qualifications are licensed. Licensure most often is imposed where the unlicensed practice of an occupation poses a serious risk to public safety or economic well-being or both. Licensing laws frequently are referred to as practice acts, which grant authority to those who are licensed to engage in certain practices within a profession. As the scope of practice is established by law or statute, it is illegal for anyone without a license to perform an activity covered by the practice act.

The regulation of complementary and alternative therapies has significant implications for the practice of nursing. Many of these therapies have been within the domain of nursing practice for centuries. For example, massage has been taught in schools of nursing and has been practiced widely by nurses. To have regulation imposed that would restrict in any way nurses' ability to incorporate massage into their practice would be highly undesirable. In states where massage therapists are licensed or registered, title protection may be offered. Thus nurses, although free to incorporate massage into their practice as nurses, cannot call themselves massage therapists unless they also meet the requirements for that occupation.

Medical practice acts in many states are very broad, and nonphysician practitioners who offer complementary or alternative therapies may be at risk for charges of unlicensed practice of medicine. In contrast to broad medical practice acts, statutes defining other health professions, including nursing, often are narrowly defined and specifically prohibit the practice of medicine. To maximize nurses' ability to practice complementary and alternative therapies independently, it is critical that nurse practice acts be written broadly, so as to not limit nurses' practice in this area. Likewise, crucial modalities falling under the broad umbrella of complementary and alternative therapies should not be categorized or defined as belonging solely to medicine.

To address the multitude of complex issues that have arisen with growth in the use of complementary and alternative therapies, several states have passed provider freedom of practice acts. This type of legislation allows practitioners to continue providing services as long as service is not shown to be dangerous or harmful.

■ Reimbursement

Third-party reimbursement for complementary and alternative therapies varies considerably by modality and practitioner. In general, the vast majority of patients who seek complementary and alternative therapies pay for them out-of-pocket. According to recent estimates, in 1997 consumers spent more than $21.2 billion out of pocket on complementary and alternative therapies (Eisenberg et al., 1998). This is more than persons expended out of pocket on hospitalizations.

Two trends in reimbursement are apparent. In states where practitioners are licensed to provide complementary and alternative therapies, the likelihood that services provided by the practitioner will be reimbursed appears greater. For example, chiropractors are licensed in all 50 states, and there is a growing trend for third-party payors to provide coverage for chiropractic care. In some states, insurance coverage is mandated if practitioners are licensed. Reimbursement also is closely tied to research evidence. As evidence accumulates indicating that complementary and alternative therapies are safe and effective, the likelihood of reimbursement increases. Acupuncture, one of the most well-researched of the complementary and alternative therapies, is now reimbursed by many third-party payors for patients with chronic pain.

■ Concluding Statement

Because many complementary therapies have a long history of use in nursing and fit with nursing's holistic philosophy, it is important that nurses "claim" these therapies. Both the philosophy undergirding complementary therapies and the content about specific therapies need to permeate nursing curricula. Both are important so that nursing students are prepared to continue the tradition of incorporating these therapies into patient care. Nurses need to assess whether patients are using complementary therapies. As noted earlier, Eisenberg et al. (1998) found that more than 42% of Americans used some type of complementary therapy. For each nurse to be competent in administering myriad complementary therapies is impossible. Having knowledge about resources to consult to obtain additional information about specific therapies (Web sites are a good resource) and being aware of practitioners in the community will enable nurses to assist patients in using complementary therapies. Nurses also must publicize that many of the complementary therapies are a part of nursing's tradition.

Although considerably more research on complementary therapies is needed to provide a basis for evidence-based practice, nurses have been testing the efficacy of therapies such as imagery, music, therapeutic touch, and massage (Snyder & Lindquist, 1998). Researchers have noted the challenges of (a) conducting research in clinical settings (Snyder, Egan, & Burns, 1995), (b) having appropriate and adequate outcome measures (Sidani & Braden, 1998), and (c) identifying an appropriate design (Quinn, 1989). Because of its past efforts in conducting research, nursing has the opportunity to assume a leadership role in research on complementary therapies.

■ References

Bessinger, C. D. (1996). Reflections on reality, healing, and consciousness. *Alternative Therapies, 2*, 40–45.

Cohen, M. H. (1996). Holistic health care: Including alternative and complementary medicine in insurance and regulatory schemes. *Arizona Law Review, 38*, 83–164.

Dossey, B. M., Keegan, L., Guzzetta, C. E., & Kolkmeier, L. G. (1995). *Holistic nursing: A handbook for practice.* Gaithersburg, MD: Aspen.

Eisenberg, D. M., Davis, R. B., Ettner, S. L., Appel, S., Wilkey, S., Von Rompay, M., & Kessler, R. C. (1998). Trends in alternative medicine use in the United States, 1990–1997: Results of a follow-up national survey. *Journal of the American Medical Association, 280*, 1569–1575.

Fulder, S. (1998). The basic concepts of alternative medicine and their impact on our views of health. *The Journal of Alternative and Complementary Medicine, 4*(2), 147–158.

Horrigan, B. (1999). Barbara Dossey, RN, MS, On holistic nursing, Florence Nightingale, and healing rituals. *Alternative Therapies, 5*(1), 79–86.

Institute of Medicine. (1991). *Disability in America: Toward a national agenda for prevention.* Washington, DC: National Academy Press.

Johnson, J. V. H., Fuller, S., Endress, P., & Rice, V. (1978). Altering patient's responses to surgery: An extension and replication. *Research in Nursing and Health, 1*(3), 111–121.

Kiene, H., & von Schon-Angerer, T. (1998). Single-case causality assessment as a basis for clinical judgment. *Alternative Therapies, 4*, 41–47.

Levin, R., Malloy, G., & Hyman, R. (1987). Nursing management of postoperative pain: Use of relaxation techniques with female cholecystectomy patients. *Journal of Advanced Nursing, 12*, 463–472.

Lubkin, I. M., & Larsen, P. D. (1998). *Chronic illness: Impact and interventions.* Boston: Jones and Bartlett.

Mandle, C., Domar, A., & Harrington, D. (1990). Relaxation response in femoral angiography. *Radiology, 174*, 737–739.

Marriner-Tomey, A. (1994). *Nursing theorists and their work.* St. Louis: Mosby.

McKivergin, M., & Daubenmire, J. (1994). The essence of therapeutic presence. *Holistic Nursing, 12*(1), 65–81.

Mogan, J., Wells, N., and Robertson, F. (1985). Effects of preoperative teaching on postoperative pain—A replication and expansion. *International Journal of Nursing Studies, 22,* 267–280.

Myss, C. (1996). *Anatomy of the spirit.* New York: Three Rivers Press.

National Center for Complementary and Alternative Medicine. (1999, April 1). Fields of practice: What is CAM? [On line]. Available: http://altmed.od.nih.gov/nccam/.

Nightingale, F. (1992). *Notes on nursing: What it is, and what it is not.* Philadelphia: J. B. Lippincott. (Original work published 1859)

Novack, D. H., Suchman, A. L., Clark, W., Epstein, R. M., Najberg, E., & Kaplan, C. (1997). Calibrating the physician: Personal awareness and effective patient care. *Journal of the American Medical Association, 278,* 502–509.

Panel on Definition and Description of CAM Research Methodology. (1997). Defining and describing complementary and alternative medicine. *Alternative Therapies, 2*(2), 49–57.

Quinn, J. F. (1989). Therapeutic touch as energy exchange: Replication and extension. *Nursing Science Quarterly, 2*(2) 79–87.

Remen, R. N. (1996). *Kitchen table wisdom.* New York: Riverhead Books.

Sidani, S., & Braden, C. J. (1998). *Evaluating nursing interventions: A theory-driven approach.* Thousand Oaks, CA: Sage.

Snyder, M. (1993). The influence of interventions on the stress–health outcome linkage. In J. S. Barnfather & B. L. Lyon (Eds.), *Stress and coping: State of the science and implications for nursing theory, research, and practice* (pp. 159–170). Indianapolis: Sigma Theta Tau International.

Snyder, M., Egan, E. C., & Burns, K. R. (1995). Efficacy of hand massage in decreasing agitation behaviors associated with care activities in persons with dementia. *Geriatric Nursing, 16,* 60–63.

Snyder, M., & Lindquist, R. (1998). *Complementary/alternative therapies in nursing.* New York: Springer.

Struthers, R. (1999). *The lived experience of Ojibwa and Cree women healers.* Unpublished doctoral dissertation, University of Minnesota, Minneapolis.

Swanson, K. M. (1991). Empirical development of a middle range theory of caring. *Nursing Research, 40,* 161–166.

Taylor, A. G. (1998). A nurse-directed interdisciplinary center for the study of complementary therapies. *Journal of Emergency Nursing, 24,* 486–487.

■ *Editor's Questions for Discussion*

Discuss complementary therapies used in nursing practice. To what extent have evaluation studies been conducted regarding complementary therapies? Why is "holism" now emphasized, as it has been integral to nursing care for centuries? How have chronic illness and lifespan contributed to complementary therapy?

Discuss the efficacy of therapeutic touch (TT) and research findings on its outcomes. How do you reconcile the statements concerning TT by Snyder, Kreitzer, and Loen with the findings presented by Deets and Choi (Chapter 34)? What is essential in research design and methodology for such studies? What is essential in evaluation of complementary or alternative therapies for valid research? How valid is the example of tire tracks made by a moving car for justifying single-case causality assessment in evaluation of complementary therapies? How generalizable are findings of single-case causality assessment? If generalization is not possible, what value do such assessments have? What intervening variables may be involved in therapeutic efficacy of complementary therapies?

Debate the pros and cons of regulating the use of complementary and alternative therapies in nursing. What impact would regulation of complementary and alternative therapies have for the consumer, health care system, reimbursement, and the profession of nursing? What does nursing need to do to promote the legitimacy in health care of historical nursing practices?

How can the profession of nursing increase acceptance of complementary and alternative therapies in nursing practice? How does Snyder, Kreitzer, and Loen's discussion apply to parish nursing (McDermott, Chapter 49), palliative care (Corless, Chapter 46), home health care (Schroeder and Long, Chapter 47), community health care (Alexander, Chapter 44), rural health care (Pullen, Chapter 50), and health care for the underserved (Todero, Chapter 51)? How does Kriteks' discussion (Chapter 74) apply to content presented by Snyder, Kreitzer, and Loen?

44

Community Health Service

Now and in the Future

Judith W. Alexander, PhD, RN, CNAA

The U.S. health care delivery system encountered drastic changes toward the end of the 20th century. What the system will look like in the 21st century is still uncertain. Community health services will have an important role in shaping and providing services in this system. Community settings will be the site for the delivery of many health services, but services provided may not be under the umbrella of community or public health. In this chapter, I outline the turmoil that community and public health face in meeting the challenges of improving the health of Americans within the constraints of shrinking resources. The future calls for public health practice to return to its core functions by forming partnerships with community leadership.

Community-service organizations, whether official public health, private, voluntary, or nonofficial agencies, will render community-focused care, managing individuals, aggregates, and populations while preparing people to build and maintain healthy communities. New models of community health service delivery will evolve to accomplish these goals. In this chapter, I provide a framework for the role of nursing during this evolutionary process.

■ Background

As a first step in describing community health nursing services of the future, a foundation of definitions, roles, and settings is needed.

Clearly, much confusion surrounds these concepts. What is clear is that the purpose of community and public health is to improve the health of the public by promoting healthy lifestyles, preventing disease and injury, and protecting the health of communities (Berkowitz, 1995). This section provides a description of this confusion over the past 15 years to lay foundation for the current situation, particularly related to the role of nursing.

In 1988, the Institute of Medicine (IOM) indicated the U.S. public health system was in disarray. This report indicated that the mission of public health is to fulfill society's interest in ensuring conditions in which people can be healthy. To achieve this mission, the core functions of public health are assessment, policy development, and assurance. Assessment involves systematic data collection on the population, monitoring the population's health status, and making this information available. Policy development includes providing leadership in policies that support the health of the population, using a scientific knowledge base. Assurance is ensuring that essential communitywide health services are available. The IOM study recommended that public health practice return to these core functions.

These recommendations—along with changes in health care reimbursement systems, managed care, and budgetary cuts—have led to the change in community health practice from being predominately clinic-based. Concurrently, professional nursing produced several statements on community health nursing practice (American Nurses Association [ANA], 1986; American Public Health Association [APHA], Public Health Nursing Section, 1996; Association of Community Health Nurse Educators [ACHNE], 1995). Each statement clarifies nursing roles in community settings, but each defines community health nursing differently. What is common in these statements is that community nurses provide services in a variety of locations, including public health, homes, schools, employment sites, primary care centers, and other ambulatory settings (Stanhope & Lancaster, 1996).

Nurses in public health are providing fewer direct care services while nurses in other settings are filling in this gap. However, all community health nurses face the challenge of providing a broad range of high-quality clinical services while strongly emphasizing the health of the entire community and population and working with multidisciplinary teams (Helvie, 1998). This switch from promoting and preserving the health of individuals to care of families, aggregates, and populations has created additional stress for community health practitioners (Berkowitz, 1995; Gebbie, 1999). Many policy analysts believe that the current workforce may not be prepared adequately to meet these challenges. Numerous reports have been issued that address the preparation and needs of the community and public health workforce in the 21st century (O'Neil, 1993; Pew Health Professions Commission, 1995: U.S. Department of Health and Human Services [USDHHS], 1997).

Finally, *Healthy People 2000* focuses on health promotion, health protection, and preventive services that community health nurses provide. Objectives are outlined in 22 priority areas that address determinants of health: human biology, environment, lifestyle, and health care (USDHHS, 1990). *Healthy People 2010* is scheduled to be released in 2000 (USDHHS, 1998) with similar determinants. These factors are essential to community health nursing practice, and the objectives have had a major influence on delivery of community health services. Often these objectives have become the foundation for program planning within community health nursing practices.

■ Current Community Health Practice

As society moves into the 21st century, many forces are influencing community health practice. These forces are focusing on community-based care rather than community-focused care, managed care, emphasis on outcomes of care, or privatization of public health services.

Focus of Community Health

Much discussion has ensued and consternation has been expressed about the focus of community health nursing practice. Community-based nursing care is a philosophy of providing care for individuals, families, and groups wherever they are located, by developing partnerships with clients and having an appreciation of community values (Baldwin, Conger, Abegglen, & Hill, 1998: Zotti, Brown, & Stotts, 1996). Using this definition, health practitioners often provide traditional acute care and primary care services in community settings, such as outpatient surgery centers, health education classes at congregate feeding centers for the elderly, and prenatal clinics in high schools. These settings define community as location. Such programs provide needed services to individuals, families, and groups in a culturally sensitive manner, but they do not comprise the true locus and vision of community-focused care. Community-focused care encompasses community-based care, but it also adds the full scope of primary health care (Shoultz & Hatcher, 1997), including community and population assessments.

According to Zotti et al. (1996), primary health care is "essential health care made accessible universally to individuals and families within a community, made available to them with their full participation, and provided at a cost that the community and country can afford" (p. 211). Population assessment focuses on a target population and the environment in which the population is located. Thus population-focused care emphasizes health promotion and disease prevention regardless of geographical location (Baldwin et al., 1998). Community health nursing practice embraces community-focused care and defines community as client, using a population-focused approach (Stanhope & Lancaster, 1996).

Managed Care

During the 1990s, the dominant model for organization and financing of health care services was managed care. Some see this model as an opportunity for community health agencies and professionals to work together. Collaboration with managed care organizations (MCOs) could improve not only the care of "covered" populations, but also the health of society as a whole (Levy, 1998). The managed care industry may emphasize all levels of prevention (primary, secondary, and tertiary), reach out to populations, and use community health nurses as an alternative to institutionally based care (Bauman, 1998). With changes in reimbursement systems, clients are being discharged from acute care facilities earlier, sicker, and often without appropriate follow-up care (Brennan & Cochran, 1998). This situation led to growth in the home care portion of community health nursing.

Others are concerned that a market-driven system will overemphasize cost containment and increase the number of uninsured (Levy, 1998). This more pessimistic view purports that hospitals and other traditional providers may try to recapture lost revenues and provide community-based services (Bauman, 1998). A change in the reimbursement system, not directly related to managed care, was a result of the Balanced Budget Act of 1997 and implementation of the Interim Payment System (IPS) for Medicare Home Health Clients. This change in Medicare funding, through limits on reimbursement, cut funds to reimburse community health services (Harris, 1998). In the spring of 1999, the IPS conditions were suspended. However, the outlook is that reimbursement for all community health services will remain tight.

Outcomes

Because of the presence of managed care systems, all health care providers are becoming increasingly concerned with outcomes of care, which demonstrate the quality of care provided. As part of outcomes analysis, providers must justify the effectiveness of interventions and systems of care and evaluate the costs of treatment alternatives. Within community health, identifying outcomes is difficult due to the many factors (environment, socioeconomic forces, access issues, family dynamics, and the physiology of health and illness) that influence the results of care. However, community health nurses must address the measurement and achievement of outcomes. Attempts to identify community nursing outcomes involve the use of nurses' perspectives through classification systems of clients' status, clients' perspectives though satisfaction measurement, or nurses' perceptions of the implementation of the nursing process. Only recently have researchers attempted to measure client and nursing outcomes simultaneously across all settings in which community health is delivered (Alexander & Kroposki, 1999).

The Agency for Health Care Policy Research (AHCPR) (1998) legitimized emphasis on outcomes. It developed numerous clinical practice guidelines and, since 1997, has sponsored development of evidence-base practice (EBP) guidelines (AHCPR, 1998). EBP focuses on health care, using research findings, expert consensus, or both to direct the provision of care. The intent of the guidelines is to foster effective care and positive client outcomes. Use of EPB in community health nursing is just beginning to appear (Madigan, 1998; Strohschein, Schaffer, & Lia-Hoagberg, 1999), but will grow in the new millennium.

Privatization of Community Health Services

Several factors have led to the private sector providing community health services that they were unwilling or unable to provide after implementation of Medicaid and Medicare. These factors include (a) the returning of governmental agencies to core public health functions, (b) managed care organizations increasing the competition among health care providers, and (c) the willingness of private providers to deliver care to underserved, vulnerable populations. The Committee on Medicine and Public Health (Lasker et al., 1997) produced a monograph about medicine and public health collaboration. Nineteen case illustrations demonstrated where private sector medicine delivered services in the 1990s across the United States. Services ranged from free clinics to "one-stop" centers to provision of services in public health facilities to the acceptance of Medicaid clients by private practices. Nursing had a vital role in establishing and maintaining these private initiatives. This trend, as well as trends toward community-focused care, managed care, and emphasis on outcomes, will continue.

■ Transition to the 21st Century

For community health services to be effective in the 21st century, community providers will need to continue their positive gains from the recent past. Community health nurses should not only reclaim the traditional territory of early visiting nurses and health departments, but they should also discover new opportunities for independent practice and specialization (Bauman, 1998). Community health providers need to (a) hone their skills in community and population assessment and program planning, (b) work in integrated and interdisciplinary teams, (c) recognize and use alternative and complementary forms of health care, and (d) acknowledge interface of the environment with health.

Community and Population Assessment

As mentioned earlier, the use of community and population assessment differentiates community-based from community-focused health care. Community health providers, especially nurses, need to obtain resources quickly to complete these assessments. Data needed for such assessments include (a) population demographics, including age and educational levels; (b) morbidity and mortality statistics; (c) information on health care facilities and providers; (d) economic indices, including educational and recreational facilities, communication resources, and transportation systems; (e) involvement of religious institutions; and (f) environmental quality indicators. Assessment tools are readily available in community health texts (e.g., Helvie, 1998). In addition to collecting these data, the community health practitioner must analyze the information in collaboration with interdisciplinary teams and consumers from the populations and/or community.

Program Planning

Program planning is essential for the establishment of services to meet the needs of com-

munities and vulnerable populations. Planning should involve regional, state, local, and agency levels. In community health, program planning is the orderly process of assessing health needs, defining health problems, and developing, implementing, and evaluating health programs to meet those needs (Fairbanks & Wiese, 1998).

Community health practitioners must use the planning approach to ensure that the services provided are both appropriate to and cost-effective in achieving health outcomes. Many planning models have proven successful. A comprehensive model, at the health problem level, is the Health Analysis and Planning of Preventive Services (HAPPS) (Centers for Disease Control [CDC], 1989). Some models have been successful at the community level, particularly when community involvement and coalitions empower citizens to continue planning for health promotion. Three such models are the Planned Approach to Community Health (PATCH) (CDC, 1994); Predisposing, Reinforcing, and Enabling Constructs in Educational and Environmental Diagnosis and Evaluation (PRECEDE); and Policy, Regulatory, and Organizational Constructs in Educational and Environmental Development (PROCEED) (Green & Krueter, 1999). Models of entire communities coming together with a goal of establishing an infrastructure and coalition building for community change are the Healthy Cities Model (Flynn, 1992) and the Community Health Improvement Process (ICHIP) model (Durch, Bailey, & Stoto, 1998).

Community health nurses use these models to assess needs and trends, using available data and information sources, and then develop innovative action plans and evaluate outcomes. Especially important is the evaluation component, to ensure that outcome data are available to demonstrate to policy makers and financiers of health care that services are effective in meeting community health needs (Stanhope & Lancaster, 1996).

Interdisciplinary Teams

The Institute of Medicine (IOM) (1988) study reconfirmed that the practice of public health is a team effort consisting of partnerships between the public and committed professionals. To plan population-based programs, community health nurses will be required to possess interdisciplinary knowledge, ability to work on multidisciplinary teams, and skills in interagency collaboration (Misener et al., 1997). Multidisciplinary teams consist of nurses, physicians, social workers, nutritionists, economists, health educators, epidemiologists, demographers, and researchers, as well as community leaders.

Alternative and Complementary Health Care

More than a third of the U.S. population uses health products such as minerals and vitamins and health services such as chiropractic and acupuncture (Levy, 1998). Community health practitioners need to be aware of these treatment modalities and evaluate them the same as any mainstream modality. If community health is truly going to provide culturally sensitive, community-focused care, traditional provision of community health services needs to integrate these practices. Additionally, as more emphasis is placed on community empowerment and coalition building, community health providers can learn much from these practices.

Environmental Interface with Health

The last major consideration for community health practitioners as they transition into the 21st century is to promote the environment as an important component of health. Environmental health is concerned with those forms of life, substances, forces, and conditions in people's surroundings that may affect their health and well-being. Community health providers must consider all aspects of the epidemiological triangle (host, agent, and environment) (Stanhope & Lancaster, 1996). Issues include environmental pollution, safety and health in the workplace, and hazards in daily life. Pope, Synder, and Mood (1997) supported the idea that community health practitioners should view the environment as an integral part of health and proposed methods to strengthen the environment–health relationship to improve community health. Community health nurses have a vital role in this process (Neufer, 1994). This movement must continue, as environmental hazards will increase with population growth and industrial technological advances.

■ Model for Direction of Community Health Services

Emerging trends and directions reflect the evolution of community health services and their current status. Community health practitioners must capitalize on lessons learned and initiatives begun while developing a model to continue the proud tradition of ensuring the health of the U.S. population. The model for directing community health services in the 21st century should include formation of partnerships across the continuum of health care providers, community involvement with health strategies, leadership competencies, and sociotechnical system (STS) elaboration. Using Contingency Theory in classical organizational theory posits that four interacting variables (task, technological, structural, and human) determine the effectiveness of organizations

(Leavitt, 1965). The model presented here for community health services delivery is based on that approach.

Task variables represent the jobs that must be performed to achieve desired outcomes. In community health care, one of the main tasks relates to the formation of partnerships between traditional acute care and community health organizations. Empowering communities to become healthy through consistent health promotion, education, and prevention strategies is another task. Developing coalitions and interdisciplinary teams, using community and population assessment skills, and developing program plans are other essential tasks.

Leadership competencies represent the human variables. Levy (1998) stated that public health needs to have leadership to translate public health values and visions into actual policies and programs. This leadership is both internal and external to an organization. Through a national Delphi study, Misener et al. (1997) concluded that nursing and public health leaders must be equipped with broadly based competencies from a variety of disciplines. These competencies fall into four domains: political skills, business acumen, program leadership abilities, and management capabilities.

The proposed model includes examination of technological and structural variables within an STS framework. In this framework, every organization consists of people and how they are organized (the social system) to use tools, techniques, and knowledge (the technical system) to produce goods or services valued by customers (outcomes) (Pasmore, 1988). The proposition of the model is that, when a proper fit exists between organizational technology and structure, organizational outcomes improve. Typically, lay people relate machinery and equipment to technology (Jones & Alexander, 1993). However, examination of the literature from philosophy, organizational theory, and nursing indicates that technology is somewhat broader, encompassing dimensions of instability, variability, and uncertainty. In contrast, structure is the allocation of work roles and administrative mechanisms to control work activities—for example, how a unit divides and assigns patient care. This perspective views structure along three dimensions— vertical participation, horizontal participation, and formalization (Alexander & Bauerschmidt, 1987; Alexander & Randolph, 1985).

Measurement of the outcomes in this model is necessary to determine whether "things are being done right" (process evaluation) and whether "the right things are being done" (outcome evaluation). Earlier discussions in this chapter presented the progress of community health in measuring outcomes. Two studies using the model being discussed have begun such an evaluation. In the first study, Cumbey and Alexander (1998) used the STS model to examine the relationship of organizational variables to job satisfaction (the outcome) among public health nurses. They found that the critical variable for predicting job satisfaction among public health nurses was organizational structure.

In the second study, Alexander and Kroposki (1999) divided nurse-sensitive outcomes in a variety of community health settings into four domains: (a) the client's psychosocial components of care, (b) the client's physiological components of care, (c) nursing intervention, and (d) implementation, environmental, and community safety components of care. Community health practitioners need to conduct more research on outcome measurement, but this study is a beginning.

This proposed community health services delivery model purports that, when an appropriate mix of variables are present, tasks will be accomplished and outcomes achieved. One variable is the level of leadership skills and competencies possessed by community health practitioners. A second variable is the fit between technology (tools, techniques, and knowledge) and structure (people and how they are organized) within an organization. Community health leaders need to test this model, using the mechanisms discussed.

■ *Concluding Statement*

The stage is set for community health services to be in the forefront of the U.S. health care system in the 21 century. Nursing has always been a leader in the community health setting and the provider of the majority of services. Let us continue this proud tradition.

■ *References*

Agency for Health Care Policy Research. (1998). AHCPR *Overview*. [On-line, April 19, 1999]. Available: http://www.ahcpr.gov/about/overview.htm.

Alexander, J. W., & Bauerschmidt, A. D. (1987). Implications for nursing administration of the relationship of technology and structure to quality of care. *Nursing Administration Quarterly, 11*(4), 1–10.

Alexander, J., & Kroposki, M. (1999). Outcomes for community health nursing practice. *Journal of Nursing Administration, 29*(5), 49–56.

Alexander, J. W., & Randolph, W. A. (1985). The fit between technology and structure as a predictor of performance in nursing subunits. *Academy of Management Journal, 28*, 844–859.

American Nurses Association. (1986). *Standards of community health nursing practice.* Washington, DC: Author.

American Public Health Association. Public Health Nursing Section. (1996). *The definition and role of public health nursing.* [On-line, December 5, 1997]. Available: http://www.apha.org/science/sections/phnrole.html.

Association of Community Health Nurse Educators. (1995). *Perspectives on theory development in community health nursing.* Louisville: Author.

Balanced Budget Act of 1997. (P.L. 105–33) (August 1997). HR 3426—Medicare and Medicaid Health Insurance. *U.S. Statutes at Large* (Volume III, pp. 251–788). Washington, DC: U.S. Government Printing Office.

Baldwin, J. H., Conger, C. O., Abegglen, J. C., & Hill, E. M. (1998). Population-focused and community-based nursing—Moving toward clarification of concepts. *Public Health Nursing, 15*, 12–18.

Bauman, M. K. (1998). Community health nursing: Exploring new frontiers while reclaiming old territory. In E. O'Neil & J. Coffman (Eds.), *Strategies for the future of nursing* (pp. 144–168). San Francisco: Jossey-Bass.

Berkowitz, B. (1995). Health system reform: A blueprint for the future of public health. *Journal of Public Health Practice, 1*(1), 1–6.

Brennan, S. J., & Cochran, M. (1998). Home health care nursing in the managed care environment, Part II. *Home Healthcare Nurse, 16*, 281–287.

Centers for Disease Control. (1989). *Program management: A guide for improving program decisions.* Atlanta: Author.

Centers for Disease Control. (1994). *Planned approach to community health.* Atlanta: Author.

Cumbey, D. A., & Alexander, J. W. (1998). The relationship of job satisfaction with organizational variables in public health nursing. *Journal of Nursing Administration, 28*(5), 39–46.

Durch, J. S., Bailey, L. A., & Stoto, M. A. (1998). Improving health in the community: A role for performance monitoring. *American Journal of Preventative Medicine, 14,* 372–373.

Fairbanks, J., & Wiese, W. H. (1998). *The public health primer.* Thousand Oaks, CA: Sage.

Flynn, B. C. (1992). Healthy cities: A model of community change. *Family and Community Health, 15*(1), 13–23.

Gebbie, K. M. (1999). The public health workforce: Key to public health infrastructure. *American Journal of Public Health, 89,* 660–661.

Green, L. W., & Krueter, M. W. (1999). *Health promotion planning: An educational and environmental approach* (3rd ed.). Mountain View, CA: Mayfield.

Harris, M. D. (1998). The impact of the Balanced Budget Act of 1997 on home care agencies and nurses. *Home HealthCare Nurse, 16,* 435–437.

Helvie, C. O. (1998). *Advanced practice nursing in the community.* Thousand Oaks, CA: Sage.

Institute of Medicine. (1988). *The future of public health.* Washington, DC: National Academy Press.

Jones, C. B., & Alexander, J. W. (1993). The technology of caring: A synthesis of technology and caring for nursing administration. *Nursing Administration Quarterly, 17*(2), 11–20.

Lasker, R. D., & the Committee on Medicine and Public Health. (1997). *Medicine & public health: The power of collaboration.* New York: New York Academy of Medicine.

Leavitt, H. J. (1965). Applied organizational change in industry: Structural, technological and humanistic approaches. In J. G. March (Ed.), *Handbook of organizations* (pp. 1144–1170). Chicago: Rand McNally.

Levy, B. S. (1998). Creating the future of public health: Values, vision, and leadership. *American Journal of Public Health, 88,* 188–192.

Madigan, E. A. (1998). Evidence-based practice in home healthcare: A springboard for discussion. *Home Healthcare Nurse, 16,* 411–415.

Misener, T. R., Alexander, J. W., Blaha, A. F., Clarke, P. N., Cover, C. M., Felton, G. M., Fuller, S. F., Herman, J., Rodes, M. M., & Sharpe, H. F. (1997). National Delphi study to determine competencies for nursing leadership in public health. *IMAGE: Journal of Nursing Scholarship, 28,* 47–51.

Neufer, L. (1994). The role of the community health nurse in environmental health. *Public Health Nursing, 11,* 155–162.

O'Neil, E. H. (1993). *Health professions education for the future: School in service to the nation.* San Francisco: Pew Health Professions Commission.

Pasmore, W. A. (1988). *Designing effective organizations.* New York: John Wiley & Sons.

Pew Health Professions Commission. (1995). *Critical challenges: Revitalizing the health professions for the twenty-first century.* San Francisco: USCF Center for the Health Professions.

Pope, A. M., Synder, M. A., & Mood, L. H. (1997). *Nursing, health, and the environment: Strengthening the relationship to improve the public's health.* Washington, DC: National Academy Press.

Shoultz, J., & Hatcher, P. A. (1997). Looking beyond primary care to primary health care: An approach to community-based action. *Nursing Outlook, 45,* 23–26.

Stanhope, M., & Lancaster, J. (1996). *Community health nursing: Promoting health of aggregates, families, and individuals.* St. Louis: Mosby.

Strohschein, S., Schaffer, M. A., & Lia-Hoagberg, B. (1999). Evidence-based guidelines for public health nursing practice. *Nursing Outlook, 47,* 84–89.

U.S. Department of Health and Human Services, Public Health Service. (1990). *Healthy People 2000: National health promotion and disease prevention objectives.* Washington, DC: Author.

U.S. Department of Health and Human Services, Public Health Service. (1997). *The public health workforce: An agenda for the 21st century.* Washington, DC: Author.

U. S. Department of Health and Human Services, Public Health Service. (1998). *Healthy People 2010 draft objectives.* Washington, DC: Author.

Zotti, M. E., Brown, P., & Stotts, R. C. (1996). Community-based nursing versus community health nursing: What does it mean? *Nursing Outlook, 44,* 211–217.

■ Editor's Questions for Discussion

To what extent have Healthy People 2000 objectives been basic for community health content in nursing programs? How are those objectives operationalized in health care services for communities and in public health programs?

What has contributed to confusion about content of community health practice? What is the difference between public health and community health? What is the difference between community-based and community-focused health care? How have predictions about managed care become a reality? What effects result from market-driven systems in terms of cost for care and quality care? How may outcomes in care be measured in terms of cost, patient satisfaction, and nursing outcomes? Provide examples of outcomes for care expected in managed care and community health care.

How might privatization of community health services increase via nurse-managed centers and entrepreneurship (see Barger, Chapter 52; Duffy, Chapter 53)? How can faculty and nursing students be involved with assessment of community health needs? What type of learning experiences should be provided for nursing students to develop leadership potential in community health care? What leadership skills and competencies are essential for future development of health care in communities? How may relationships be developed among parish nursing (McDermott, Chapter 49), nursing centers (Barger, Chapter 52), mobile nursing centers (Todero, Chapter 51), community partnerships (Hollinger-Smith, Chapter 45), and home health care (Schroeder and Long, Chapter 47) to facilitate community health services?

45

Building and Sustaining Community Partnerships

Models for Nursing Practice

Linda Hollinger-Smith, PhD, RN

The 21st century will mark dynamic changes in health care. Community partnerships represent a growing movement whereby health care responsibility shifts from the hands of health care professionals as "authority" to a "partnership" of health care providers, community residents, and organizations. As strong supporters of client advocacy and health promotion, nurses will be at the forefront of this partnership evolution. Concomitant with new health paradigms modeled after wellness behaviors, nursing faculty will need to integrate experiences that facilitate community participation in curricula, research, and practice. Developing community partnerships is a long-term investment, but it

is well worth the effort for both health care providers and the community.

■ Community Partnerships in Health Care: A Changing Paradigm

Revolutions in health care during the next several years will signify a reengineering of health care models from the traditional focus on disease prevention to a wellness model centering on health promotion. Consumers of health care will influence this new direction in many ways. The degree of consumer participation in health care, perceived quality and value of health, cultural diversity, and growth in information technology are some of the factors driving consumers to seek a more active role in health care. With the evolution of a health promotion model, the nursing profession will need to develop strategies and seek new opportunities as primary health care providers.

To see that health care models continue to stress disease prevention, all you need to do is examine the distribution of health care expenditures. In 1994, the U.S. Public Health Service determined that 99% of all health care expenses paid for medical management and only 1% supported public health programs (U.S. Public Health Service [USPHS], 1993). Considering that public health initiatives targeting health promotion could have a greater impact on preventing premature deaths then medical treatment alone does not seem a sagacious allocation of resources.

Reengineering the Provision of Health Care

Prevention or eradication of disease at the individual or population level is at the core of traditional health care models. The Health Belief Model, first proposed in the 1960s, explains individual health-seeking behaviors as a result of (a) the degree to which the problem is perceived to be a threat, (b) the extent to which the health behavior is believed to be beneficial, and (c) the extent to which barriers or costs are perceived to produce the health behavior (Becker & Maiman, 1975). Many years of research have led to the conclusion that perceived barriers and susceptibility to particular diseases most strongly predict health-seeking behaviors (Janz & Becker, 1984). With its emphasis on health behaviors as a way to avoid or counterbalance disease, the Health Belief Model is considered to be a disease-prevention rather than a health-promotion framework.

From a population-based perspective, the epidemiologic approach focuses on the occurrence of disease in population cohorts. Although more of a method than a health care model, it was described in earlier community nursing textbooks as a process for counseling families about ways to cope with health care problems (Leahy, Cobb, & Jones, 1977). Community health nurses based health education programs on diseases with high incidence in a given population. They identified common risk factors (i.e., physical, psychosocial, cultural, and environmental) with the goal of reducing unhealthy behaviors.

In application to wellness models, the epidemiologic approach tends to be limited in two ways. The underlying reason for development of the epidemiologic method was to study the incidence and prevalence of communicable diseases in populations; thus its premises follow a disease-prevention framework. Additionally, the epidemiologic method is based on the reductive-objective paradigm which the researcher determines the "objective truths" from a methodology under the researcher's control. A population-based wellness model challenges health care providers and researchers to go beyond traditional scientific methods and paradigms, centering on key components of community participation and the community's socioenvironment.

Adopting a wellness model for health care supports the World Health Organization's (WHO's) definitions of health and health promotion (Turner, 1986). Health is defined as the presence of complete physical and psychosocial well-being. Health promotion expands that definition to encompass healthy environments and lifestyles for individuals, families, and communities. Additionally, WHO recommends that health promotion be at the center of public policy to improve environmental health issues.

Wellness is not a new concept, and models of wellness have been reported in the literature for almost 40 years. Dunn (1961) proposed a high-level wellness model that describes health as the integration of body, mind, and spirit along developmental stages of increasing function. Health promotion behaviors serve as the catalyst to achieve wellness in all aspects of life. Greenberg (1985) refined the model, considering wellness as the state of balance among five segments of health: physical, mental, social, emotional, and spiritual. Such a model is useful in describing why an individual, in the absence of disease, may feel full of life and active one day but fatigued or moody the next.

The Health Promotion Model (HPM) was derived from Dunn's work in the early 1980s and has been widely tested and revised during the past 15 years (Pender, 1996). The HPM takes a biopsychosocial perspective of health promotion and is based on both nursing and behavioral theories. The individual has an active role as the central decision-maker for health promotion behaviors. Individual, interpersonal, and environmental factors influence health behaviors both directly and indirectly in the HPM. For instance, socioeconomic status and other demographic variables tend to have an indirect impact on health promotion behaviors such as exercise. Factors such as prior history of exercise or local accessibility to exercise programs have a direct influence. The strength of the HPM lies in its flexible application to a wide range of cultural groups allowing for integration of individual health beliefs that may fall outside defined health care norms.

The evolution of a new paradigm in public health has expanded population-based approaches to what is termed "participatory eco-epidemiology" (Schwab & Syme, 1997). This paradigm supports the practice and study of wellness from the community's perspective, with the community and health care providers acting as equal partners. A "participatory" approach views the community as the central decision maker, and an interdisciplinary team is assembled to collaborate with the community to establish common health goals. The "ecological" viewpoint indicates that public

health care, education, and research takes place as lived experiences in the community.

Focusing on a wellness model requires that the current health care system and providers share responsibilities inherent in health promotion. Health care systems can do so in three specific ways by (a) reducing the barriers to community health care, (b) increasing community involvement in health care, and (c) promoting the value of health care. Barriers to community involvement in health care have the overall effect of reducing the community's access to needed services. External barriers may include (a) limited community health resources, (b) inadequate support networks, and (c) reluctance of health care providers to shift decision-making power to community members. Internal barriers, such as lack of community motivation, insufficient knowledge about healthy behaviors, or certain cultural beliefs, may impede the community's involvement. With the numerous daily stressors faced by medically underserved communities, the motivation to give health care a high priority is sorely lacking. Thus health care providers need to focus on fostering community involvement in health care through wellness models and participatory roles.

Changing Roles for Nurse Practitioners

A health care paradigm focusing on wellness and community participation will require health care providers to establish new roles. Nurse practitioners (NPs) are prepared to provide comprehensive health care to their patients with an emphasis on health promotion. Contemporary roles for NPs must support both autonomy as advanced practice nurses and collaboration as members of interdisciplinary teams.

Demographic trends will also have an impact on developing roles for NPs. Growth in racial and ethnic diversity, population aging, chronic disease, poverty, and environmental problems have implications for community health care (Cox, 1997). *Life care partners* may be a future role for NPs in primary care settings. In such a position, the NP is culturally sensitive to the community's needs, establishes long-term relationships, and develops supportive health programs across all ages. In many cases, the NP may be the sole provider to underserved communities, and so must be prepared to access scarce resources creatively. In acute settings, advanced practice nurses are developing new roles as case managers in the evolving managed care environment, functioning in collaborative relationships with other health care team members. As third-party reimbursement is being established for NPs, many hospitals and specialty units are employing them as case managers. Reports of high patient satisfaction and reduced costs support the expansion of these roles (McGee, 1995).

■ Community Empowerment Strategies

Facilitating community participation is considered to be the foundation of a two-step process. The first step is promoting community empowerment, which leads to the second step, that of establishing community partnerships. The benefits of empowerment as a social intervention process that strengthens community bonds form the basis of community partnership development.

Models of Community Empowerment

The Cornell Empowerment Group (1989) defined empowerment as "an intentional, ongoing process centered in the local community, involving mutual respect, critical reflection, caring and group participation, through which people lacking an equal share of valued resources gain greater access to and control over those resources" (p. 2). Empowerment models are described in terms of a particular level or group (i.e., individual, organizational, or community). Regardless of the level, empowerment connotes that decision making shifts from one participant to another.

The *interactive model* of community empowerment focuses on the individual level. Characteristics such as cultural background, social supports, intrinsic motivation, cognition, and previous experience with health care systems influence the patient–caregiver relationship. The interactive model of empowerment centers on supporting the individual's right to self-determination, accepting cultural and social norms that affect health behaviors, and ensuring informed choice through information and education.

The *reciprocal model* of community empowerment is usually described at the organizational level. Human service organizations typically utilize "professional-centered" rather than "consumer-centered" delivery models (Salzer, 1997). Such organizations view the professional as the expert, and programs are subsequently developed from a "top-down" perspective (i.e., the expert professional designs the "best" services for the community). Services are underused if the community does not feel a part of the process or does not consider its relationship with experts as reciprocal. In a "consumer-centered" model, service organizations place values on the community's contributions in developing and evaluating human services. In some cases, community members are invited to function as equal voting board members of community service organizations (Bond & Keys, 1993).

A *community capacity model* for empowerment takes a unique perspective of community involvement. Rather than stressing problems faced by a community, the model centers on the assets and strengths inherent in the community. In many cases, health promotion programs are based solely on health risks and disease rates identified in a particular group. Some cultures hold fatalistic views of diseases, such as cancer. A program focused on breast cancer screening might garner community support, but recruiting those who could benefit most from preventive services might be difficult. A community capacity model assesses "enablers" or indicators of community readiness and potential to develop program initiatives. Community capacity is evaluated on several dimensions, including (a) participation and leadership, (b) group process skills, (c) community resources, (d) community networks, (e) sense of community belonging, (f) community history, (g) community power, (h) common values, and (i) ability to self-evaluate (Goodman et al., 1998). Unique to this model is the *idea* that empowerment grows from within the community. Through the process, the community builds on its own assets rather than from the "top-down" models described. The role of the outside agency shifts from "leader" or "expert" to that of "consultant" for the community.

Empowerment as a Social Intervention Process

By its very nature, empowerment is a social process, involving participation and cooperation between a community and outside resources, to improve residents' daily lives. The degree of participation will always be dynamic because communities themselves are continuously evolving. Empowerment also builds social relationships within communities. Social roles evolve as some members surface as "informal leaders" or "bridge builders" for the community. Habermas (1984) remarked that equality in dialogue is achieved only when participatory capacity is balanced among community and outside members. Implied in relation to health promotion is that communities and health care professionals perceive their relationship as an equal partnership in developing, implementing, and evaluating preventive services.

■ Establishing Community Partnerships

Collaboration is the key to establishing community partnerships. Cahill (1996) conceptualized collaboration as the foundation for community participation leading to the development of partnerships. Constructing partnerships or alliances between a community and outside agencies (i.e., a health care system, university or academic medical center, or a service organization) takes time to nurture and be responsive to the community's assets and needs. Through collaboration, the partners come to realize the interdependent nature of their relationship. For some professionals, who see their role primarily as "expert" and the community as "passive" recipients of their assistance, this point is often difficult to grasp and accept. In this case, the "partnership" may be from the perspective of the health care professional rather than from the community's viewpoint. Milio (1989) contrasted this narrow view, predicting that a future health care system needs to be based on "interdependence among nations, communities, and groups; between environments and individuals; between policies and patterns of action. . . . It is time that health be viewed within this ecological perspective, one in which health is a balance between people and their environments" (p. 315).

Apparent across efforts focused on the development of health promotion programs is that the community's willingness to participate and its degree of active involvement is not a given. Partnership development is contingent on a host of factors that may differ among communities and even among a community's subcultures. Gaining an appreciation for diverse values and priorities facilitates the process of partnering.

Examples of Community Partnerships

The *Consortium for the Immunization of Norfolk's Children* (CINCH) was designed as a coalition-building approach to improve rates of childhood immunizations in Norfolk, Virginia (Butterfoss et. al., 1998). The effectiveness of the program in targeting community capacity was mirrored in the comment of one resident, who stated that the CINCH program "helped families help themselves to better health," p. 214). One of the greatest challenges was recruiting and maintaining the involvement of parents whose children were at greatest risk. Education of the community on the importance of immunizations and ways to increase access for the underserved facilitated development of collaborative relationships within the community. Work groups consisting of CINCH health care providers, community members, and service agencies were formed to maintain the program after external funding ended. CINCH had a positive impact in several ways: (a) immunization rates for 2-year-olds significantly increased, from 46% to 66% (pre- to postimplementation), (b) 86% of community respondents surveyed were satisfied with the program, (c) use of social networks through volunteerism promoted access to underserved groups, and (d) the majority of community participants felt that they had an active role in program decision-making.

The *Resource Sisters/Compañeras Program* focused on developing community empowerment through peer support mechanisms (Lugo, 1996). With private and public funding, the March of Dimes Foundation's Florida Chapter partnered with communities in Orange County that had high incidences of infant mortality and low-birth-weight new-

borns. Community women were trained and hired as peer counselors to provide support and education to at-risk mothers. Home visits were a critical part of the outreach program, thereby overcoming many access barriers. Development of trusting relationships with peer counselors encouraged mothers to attend community support group meetings. Topics identified by the group dealt with issues affecting daily life in the community (e.g., violence, housing and transportation problems, and lack of family supports). Although attendance at support groups was not at the level hoped for, participants viewed the project as an important education and information link to needed resources.

A large-scale project establishing community health promotion partnerships is North Carolina's *Project ASSIST* (Kegler, Steckler, McLeroy, & Malek, 1998). Ten community partnerships were formed throughout the state, combining the expertise of schools, employers, health care agencies, and communities. A crucial aim of the project was implementation of sustainable, long-term health promotion programs according to community-designed action plans. To implement and maintain activities, members of community partnerships identified the need for (a) open communication channels, (b) feelings of belonging, (c) community leader development, (d) time allocated to develop partnerships, and (e) task force groups to target specific program objectives.

The *Healthy Neighborhoods Project* (HNP) in Contra Costa County, California (in the San Francisco Bay area) partnered the local health department and community residents to design a preventive health care agenda (El-Askari et al., 1998). Fundamental to the program was the agreement that the health department function as a resource and equal partner to residents. A community capacity model (McKnight & Kretzmann, 1990) gave structure to the program, as residents had the opportunity to identify assets and priorities in their urban environment. Initial interviews with community residents had a positive slant, asking them about skills, community involvement, perceptions of their neighborhood, and lay advising roles to friends and families. Interestingly, the tone of the interviews revitalized community involvement. The community initiated several public health and safety programs, and some residents expanded their participation at the city and regional levels in outreach endeavors to improve the quality of life for the inner-city neighborhoods.

The final program described makes use of the lay health advisor (LHA) model. The LHA model involves selection and training of individuals trusted by the community and deemed "natural helpers" by family and neighbors. Detroit's *East Side Village Health Worker Partnership* (Parker, Schulz, Israel, & Hollis, 1998) integrates collaborative, community-based prevention, and LHAs, targeting women's and children's health. Identifying LHAs from the community was a great challenge. Due to the social complexities inherent in urban areas, community groups and organizations had their own agendas that influenced recommendations for program participants and interventions. LHAs have been effectively utilized in community health promotion programs focusing on breast cancer screening (Eng, 1993) and sexually transmitted diseases (Thomas, Eng, Clark, Robinson, & Blumenthal, 1998).

Preventive Services Facilitated Through Community Partnerships

Establishing health promotion programs in the community occur as community-level interventions or through clinical preventive services. Advanced practice nurses may participate at all levels and thus need to be aware of the common prevention strategies for both average-risk and high-risk communities. The *Put Prevention Into Practice* (PPIP) initiative, developed by the Office of Disease Prevention and Health Promotion of the U.S. Public Health Service, serves as one framework for delivery of health promotion programs. A major strength of this program is that recommendations for screening services, immunizations, and counseling are based on findings from a wide gamut of expert authorities and researchers. Designed for the PPIP program, the *Clinician's Handbook of Preventive Services,* 2nd edition (USPHS, 1998) presents guidelines for the development of health promotion and preventive programs.

Community partners aid in targeting specific risk factors for health promotion and preventive services. As high-risk areas represent a subsector of a community, examining city or community statistics on disease morbidity or mortality rates may not be sensitive enough to identify high-risk groups in the community. For example, when the Chicago Department of Public Health (CDPH) reported a decrease in the incidence of lead poisoning in inner-city school districts, a group in the North Lawndale area on Chicago's west side looked into the situation in its area. The *Homan Square Community Project* represents a partnership of local businesses, community, and civic leaders in North Lawndale. The Shaw Company (community redeveloper), Family Focus Lawndale (social services), the Rush Primary Care Institute of the Rush System for Health, and the Rush University College of Nursing (CON) work with the community to enhance its capabilities in addressing all aspects of daily life (Hollinger-Smith, 1998). Under guidance of NP faculty from the CON, nursing students perform community assessments and plan health promotion programs in collaboration with the community. One of these programs targeted lead screening in several North Lawndale elementary schools. A significant number of children were found to have elevated blood lead levels in a school that did not participate in the citywide screening. The CDPH immediately performed an environmental assessment of the school, and the parents received counseling regarding lead poisoning. Home safety assessments were then performed by CON nursing students as follow-up from the CDPH. These assessments were more inclusive, such as for fire safety and prevention of poisoning.

Screening services may be categorized by age and gender. Common screening for children and adolescents include vision and hearing, tuberculosis, blood pressure and cholesterol, lead poisoning, depression and suicide, and anemia. For adults and the elderly, screening programs typically include cancer detection, blood pressure and cholesterol, vision and hearing, tuberculosis, anemia, depression, sexually transmitted diseases, pap testing, mammography, and cognitive/functional testing. Immunizations represent an important part of preventive services. Childhood immunizations include vaccination against diphtheria, tetanus, and pertussis (DTP); haemophilus influenzae type B; hepatitis B; measles, mumps, and rubella (MMR); poliomyelitis; and varicella-zoster virus. Adult immunizations include vaccinations against hepatitis B, influenza, pneumococcus (for at-risk groups), rubella (for women of childbearing age without proof of immunity), and tetanus and diphtheria (TD booster).

Health counseling and education reach a wider audience as a community-based program, but they are also important preventive services offered in clinic settings. Health promotion education for all ages include topics such as alcohol and drug abuse, nutrition, oral health, exercise, safety, sexually transmitted diseases, HIV infection, tobacco use, and violence prevention. For older adults, polypharmacy is also an important area for education.

Developing health promotion programs and preventive services should be done in col-laboration with the community. As a resource to the community, advanced practice nurses and other health care providers bring knowledge and education into the planning process. Community residents also need to play an active role and be willing to make health promotion a meaningful part of their daily lives.

■ Strategies for Nursing Practice: New Opportunities for Community Partnerships

Preparing nurses and other health care providers for a new paradigm based on health promotion and collaboration requires changes in how education and research are developed, conducted, and evaluated within community partnership models. Nursing has the unique opportunity to lead the way in this regard, not being restricted to practice solely under a medical model. Thus health promotion and community partnership concepts should be integrated into nursing education and research to achieve what Mundinger (1994) considered as "a promising redirection for nursing" (p. 28).

Implications for Nursing Education

A new paradigm centered on wellness and community partnerships means that nursing faculty and students will function in an interactive environment requiring creativity and critical thinking skills (Gauthier & Matteson, 1995). Educators and students will need to develop understanding and sensitivity about a culture's health beliefs. They will need to know how to deal with incongruity when differences arise between the norms of a cultural group and the expectations of health care providers.

Nursing curricula also need to expand their current focus on health promotion as the individual's responsibility, with standards being set by the health care professional as "role model."

For example, undergraduate nursing students are frequently taught about health by assessing their own lifestyles. Although that is an important learning experience, it fails to take into account socioenvironmental factors affecting lifestyles in other cultures or underserved communities. Unrealistic expectations about health promotion may be set in the student's care plan, given the client's situation. Learning situations whereby students participate in community coalition building and collaborate with residents and leaders in planning community-based health programs encourage students to examine the social, cultural, and political factors affecting a community's health. Clinical experiences become shared learning encounters between the nursing college and the community. As partners in learning, faculty, students, and the community share values and knowledge in establishing health promotion activities congruent with a community's lifestyle and available resources.

Implications for Nursing Research

For nurse researchers, working in an environment of community partnerships provides opportunities to increase residents' levels of involvement in all aspects of research studies. Researchers studying vulnerable populations are often confronted with feelings of mistrust on the part of these groups. Residents in high-risk areas may feel that providing information to researchers has a negative impact on the residents' situation. Additionally, they may perceive that research participation has no long-lasting effect on their daily lives. Entwistle, Renfrew, Yearley, Forrester, and Lamont (1998) outlined a framework for facilitating lay participation in research and recommended ways to recruit key contributors from the community, based on the research questions posed.

Community-based research tends to fall into three main categories: (a) population-focused clinical studies, (b) participatory action research, and (c) program evaluation. Population-focused clinical studies target topics such as family violence, teenage pregnancy, substance abuse, and homelessness. Gaining access to these high-risk populations is often hampered if researchers are considered "strangers." Through community partnerships, researchers work with community leaders, both formal and informal, to identify recruitment strategies. Avoiding "research" terminology, offering incentives, and developing a sense of trust can strengthen the quality of population-based studies and increase the value of study results for both the researchers and the community.

Participatory action research is both a research methodology and a means of encouraging collaboration among researchers and communities, focusing on joint problem solving. Part of the process may include community education to develop problem-solving abilities. In turn, researchers may need to engage in a process of "cultural immersion," thereby gaining a sense of understanding and respect for problems faced by the community from its perspective.

Program evaluation methods are integral to development of any health related program established in the community. The design of evaluation instruments should be done in collaboration with community residents. Residents may recommend questionnaire wording to clarify information being sought. In the ideal situation, the community as the user of health services should design evaluation instruments to assess the program's quality and effectiveness from its perspective.

■ Future of Community Partnerships

The evolution of community partnerships is in its early stages in many areas. In this regard, opportunity for nursing's involvement in developing sustained community partnerships is immense. Growth of information technology, movement of health promotion into community settings, and increasing incentives for community partnering are some of the primary factors having an impact on the future of these coalitions. By increasing their knowledge and involvement in these areas, nurses can be the leaders in community-based partnerships for health promotion.

Information and Health Care

The "information age" is making a definitive impression on health care by empowering consumers with "health online" computer Web sites. The growth of online consumer health information has been exponential over the past few years. More than 25% of all Internet searches are by people seeking health information (Ferguson, 1997). A system of virtual health care management also is evolving. Consumers will be able connect to a Web site to obtain the latest health care information, communicate online with health care professionals, and participate in live chat rooms with other consumers about their health experiences. Nurses and lay health advisors can collaborate in establishing online health networks that provide accurate information, with the nurse functioning as a partner in care.

Settings for Health Promotion in the Future

Along with increased computer usage, health promotion will continue to move into the community, and health care providers will need to go where the residents are. Trained lay health advisors and home visitors from the community can facilitate this movement, bringing health promotion into homes to reach families and into schools to target children and educators.

Incentives for Community Partnerships

A final consideration in the future of community partnership development is that of incentives to support health promotion programs. Earlier in this chapter, I discussed issues related to the lack of public health funding for wellness programs. Federal grant programs that support studies on effectiveness of preventive services and the ability of health promotion interventions to facilitate healthy behaviors are growing. Insurers have been slow to provide reimbursement for preventive services, but this reticence appears to be changing in some areas. Grants or loans to foster community partnerships between academic institutions and underserved communities should also be promoted at the federal and state levels.

■ Concluding Statement

Community partnerships sustaining health promotion are at the cutting edge of changing health paradigms. With its focus on comprehensive care and collaboration, nursing is in position to expand its roles. As partners in care, nurses work with the community, building on inherent assets to develop educational, research, and service initiatives. With communities seeing roles as active and equal participants in health care decisions, community partnerships can continue to flourish.

References

Becker, M., & Maiman, L. (1975). Sociobehavioral determinants of compliance with health and medical care recommendations. *Medical Care, 13*(1), 10–4.

Bond, M., & Keys, C. (1993). Empowerment, diversity and collaboration: Promoting synergy on community boards. *American Journal of Community Psychology, 21*(1), 37–57.

Butterfoss, F., Morrow, A., Rosenthal, J., Dini, E., Crews, R., Webster, J., & Louis, P. (1998). CINCH: An urban coalition for empowerment and action. *Health Education and Behavior, 25*(2), 212–225.

Cahill, J. (1996). Patient participation: a conceptual analysis. *Journal of Advanced Nursing, 24*(3), 561–571.

Cornell Empowerment Group (1989). Empowerment and family support. *Networking Bulletin, 1*, 1–23.

Cox, R. (1997). Family health care delivery for the 21st century. *Journal of Obstetrics, Gynecology and Neonatal Nursing, 26*(1), 109–118.

Dunn, H. (1961). *High level wellness.* Thorofare, NJ: Charles B. Slack.

El-Askari, G., Freestone, J., Irizarry, C., Kraut, K., Mashiyama, S., Morgan, M., & Walton, S. (1998). The Healthy Neighborhoods Project: A local health department's role in catalyzing community development. *Health Education and Behavior, 25*(2), 146–159.

Eng, E. (1993). The Save Our Sisters Project: A social network strategy for reaching rural black women. *Cancer, 72*(3, supp.), 1071–1077.

Entwistle, V., Renfrew, M., Yearley, S., Forrester, J., & Lamont, T. (1998). Lay perspectives: Advantages for health research. *British Medical Journal, 316*(7129), 463–466.

Ferguson, T. (1997). Health online and the empowered medical consumer. *Journal on Quality Improvement, 23*(5), 251–257.

Gauthier, M., & Matteson, P. (1995). The role of empowerment in neighborhood-based nursing education. *Journal of Nursing Education, 34*(8), 390–395.

Goodman, R., Speers, M., McLeroy, K., Fawcett, S., Kegler, M., Parker, E., Smith, S., Sterling, T., & Wallerstein, N. (1998). Identifying and defining the dimensions of community capacity to provide a basis for measurement. *Health Education and Behavior, 25*(3), 258–278.

Greenberg, J. (1985). Health and wellness: A conceptual differentiation. *Journal of School Health, 55*(10), 403–406.

Habermas, J. (1984). *Theory of communicative action* (Vol. 1). Boston: Beacon Press.

Hollinger-Smith, L. (1998). Partners in collaboration: The Homan Square Project. *Journal of Professional Nursing, 14*(6), 344–349.

Janz, N., & Becker, M. (1984). The health belief model: A decade later. *Health Education Quarterly, 11*(1), 1–47.

Kegler, M., Steckler, A., McLeroy, K. & Malek, S. (1998). Factors that contribute to effective community health promotion coalitions: A study of 10 Project ASSIST coalitions in North Carolina. *Health Education and Behavior, 25*(3), 338–353.

Leahy, K., Cobb, M., & Jones, M. (1977). *Community health nursing* (3rd ed.). New York: McGraw-Hill.

Lugo, N. (1996). Empowerment education: A case study of the Resource Sisters/Compañeras Program. *Health Education Quarterly, 23*(3), 281–289.

McGee, D. (1995). The perinatal nurse practitioner: An innovative model of advanced practice. *Journal of Obstetrics, Gynecology and Neonatal Nursing, 24*(7), 602–606.

McKnight, J., & Kretzmann, J. (1990). *Mapping community capacity.* Evanston, IL: Center for Urban Affairs and Policy Research.

Milio, N. (1989). Developing nursing leadership in health policy. *Journal of Professional Nursing, 5*(6), 315–321.

Mundinger, M. (1994). Health care reform: Will nursing respond? *Nursing and Health Care, 15*(1), 28–33.

Parker, E., Schulz, A., Israel, B., & Hollis, R. (1998). Detroit's East Side Village Health Worker Partnership: Community-based lay health advisor intervention in an urban area. *Health Education and Behavior, 25*(1), 24–45.

Pender, N. (1996). *Health promotion in nursing practice.* Stamford, CT: Appleton & Lange.

Salzer, M. (1997). Consumer empowerment in mental health organizations: Concept, benefits, and impediments. *Administration & Policy in Mental Health, 24*(5), 425–434.

Schwab, M., & Syme, S. (1997). On paradigms, community participation and the future of public health. *American Journal of Public Health, 87*(12), 2049–2051.

Thomas, J., Eng, E., Clark, M., Robinson, J., & Blumenthal, C. (1998). Lay health advisors: Sexually transmitted disease prevention through community involvement. *American Journal of Public Health, 88*(8), 1252–1253.

Turner, J. (1986). Health for all: Some critics less critical. *Lancet, 2*(8510), 818–819.

U.S. Public Health Service. (1993). *Health care reform and public health: A paper on population-based core functions.* The Core Function Project, Public Health Foundation, Washington, DC: Author.

U.S. Public Health Service. (1998). *Clinician's handbook of preventive services* (2nd ed.). McLean, VA: International Medical Publishing.

■ Editor's Questions for Discussion

Because promotion must be focused on by all participants, how should nursing education programs further address the need for community partnerships? What suggestions by Boland (Chapter 71) might apply? What strategies in developing health policy might facilitate emphasis on high-level wellness? Apply content from Heinrich and Wakefield (Chapter 8) in formulating responses.

What roles should nursing centers play for providing care as discussed by Todero (Chapter 51) and Barger (Chapter 52)? How can faculty practice (Carter, Chapter 39) reinforce community health? What legal and ethical concerns exist in utilizing nursing students at nursing centers? Apply content about cultural competence presented by Purnell (Chapter 37) to community learning situations for students.

How are advanced practice nurses in key roles to influence heath promotion? See Gray (Chapter 42) and Gerber (Chapter 57). How are Hollinger-Smith's suggestions for community models reinforced by Alexander (Chapter 44)?

Can nursing advance community health care without decreasing resources and energy in illness care? What strategies and plans must be employed to prevent gaps in providing care?

How may community partnerships facilitate interdisciplinary research suggested by Lindsey (Chapter 29) and that emphasized by Grady (Chapter 73)? Identify applications of technology presented by Stevens and Weiner (Chapter 38) in developing community partnerships.

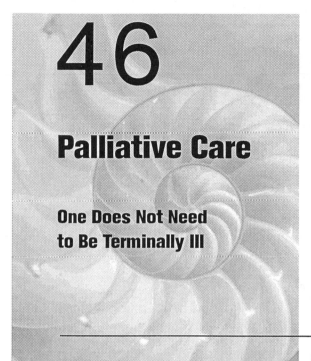

46

Palliative Care

One Does Not Need to Be Terminally Ill

Inge B. Corless, PhD, RN, FAAN

P alliative care, and in particular end-of-life care, is receiving attention as an important component of health care (Block & Billings, 1998; Block, 1999). Impetus for this attention is, in part, the Support study (Support Principal Investigators, 1995) and the findings that patients were not ending their lives in comfort or in the place of their choosing. This situation was shown to be due largely to a failure of physicians to discuss these vital issues with their patients in a timely manner (Solomon, 1995). The response to the Support study by philanthropic organizations has been to generate renewed interest in the delivery of palliative care.

What precisely is meant by palliative care and when to initiate such care is still being debated, however. Further, the similarities and differences between palliative care, end-of-life care, and hospice have yet to be elucidated. This lack of closure provides an opportunity for a reconceptualization that incorporates nursing's contribution to what is becoming specialization in a medical practice. In this chapter, some of the creative projects funded by philanthropic organizations, particularly those involving the integration of palliative care into nursing and nursing education are reviewed. Barriers to palliative care and implications for practice and education are also

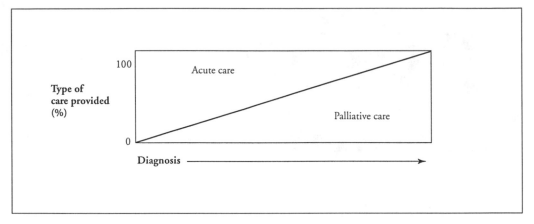

Figure 46.1 Chronic Disease Trajectory (Saunders Paradigm).

explored. The thesis of this chapter is that a person does not need to be terminally ill to receive palliative care.

■ Palliative Care Explicated

Palliative care is not a new concept. From the start, Dame Cicely Saunders incorporated palliative care into her vision of end-of-life care (Saunders, 1999). In the conceptualization of the relationship of acute and palliative care presented by Saunders, a rectangle is bisected into two triangles with acute care occupying the triangle on the left and palliative care dominant on the right, as shown in Figure 46.1. Note that acute care and palliative care are always in juxtaposition with one another, creating a dynamic whereby, when there is more of one, there is less of the other. The concept of acute care has some common understanding, but precisely what is meant by palliative care is still under discussion.

A definition frequently cited is that of the World Health Organization (WHO) (1990) and the Department of Palliative Care, King's College (1998):

Palliative care is the active total care of patients whose disease is not responsive to curative treat-

ment. Control of pain, of other symptoms, and of psychological, social and spiritual problems is paramount. The goal is achievement of the best possible quality of life for patients and their families. (WHO, p. 11; Dept. of Palliative Care, p. 1)

In explicating their theory on end-of-life, Ruland and Moore (1998) emphasized quality of life. Key concepts in their theory are "not being in pain, experience of comfort, experience of dignity/respect, being at peace, and closeness to significant others/persons who care" (p. 174).

As is evident, these concepts address the physical and psychosocial aspects of care. An interview with Ira Byock elicits other aspects of care (Rabinowitz, 1998). Byock is concerned with incorporating the preferences of the patient into care and with the notion that palliative care is more than a set of medical methods. At the same time, with the advances in the health care armamentarium, health care providers are confronted with utilizing this technology appropriately, which is no easy task. Providers are challenged to see and respect the person, not only to provide care to the body (Quill, 1993).

That attention is being given at all to palliative care is a hopeful sign. For too long, too little attention has been paid to palliative care other than for a fortunate few and those who

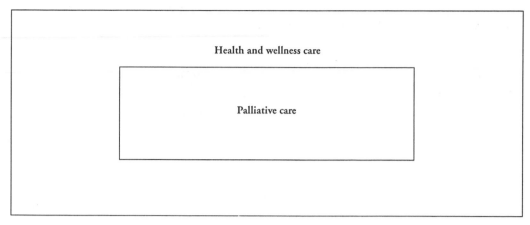

Figure 46.2   Integration of Palliative Care into Health Care.

received hospice care. The emphasis currently is on integrating quality end-of-life care into health care. See Figure 46.2. This focus on quality end-of-life care as part of mainstream medicine is a new phenomenon but one hoped for by hospice pioneers (Corless, 1983).

The WHO (1990) noted that "many aspects of palliative care are also applicable earlier in the course of the illness in conjunction with anti-cancer treatment" (p. 12). This assertion has led to debate on precisely when to initiate such care, with some calling for palliative care upon onset of symptoms and before diagnosis of disease. Agreement that palliative care is not necessarily synonymous with, nor coincident with, end-of-life care is heartening. The question is no longer "if" but "when" to provide palliative care. The "when" is yet to be clarified.

Palliative care does not rule out the delivery of active therapy for underlying pathology. Ferris (1994) formulated a definition of palliative care that encompasses the possibility of active and palliative care being given together at any point in the disease trajectory.

In this sense, palliative care is different from hospice care. Hospice admission includes acknowledgment by the patient of 6 months or less to live and a foreswearing of aggressive "active" therapies aimed at cure. This bedrock of hospice care has been modified in recent years to accommodate therapies of persons living with the human immunodeficiency virus (HIV) and acquired immunodeficiency syndrome (AIDS). These individuals have made use of a variety of therapies both active and supportive from formal and informal providers. When these therapies are successful, hospice clients are discharged—alive.

The continuum of palliative care formulated by the Canadian Palliative Care Association accommodates both approaches to care by incorporating comfort and supportive treatment at an earlier point in the disease trajectory (Ferris & Cummings, 1995). In fact, comfort care is initiated after "disease, distress, discomfort, and dysfunction" occur and prior to diagnosis (p. 13). With diagnosis, the bulk of treatment is disease-specific, although comfort and supportive care are present. Ferris and Cummings differ from Saunders in initiating palliative care prior to diagnosis. In other respects their conceptualization is similar to that of Saunders, with an inverse relationship between acute and palliative care. Palliation treats the patient; acute care treats the disease. This stark distinction is inherent in a conceptualization of acute care and palliative care.

The statement by Ferris (1994) that "palliative care may be combined with therapies

---

TABLE 46.1 Barriers to the Provision of Quality Palliative Care

Lack of discussion about death in society	Paucity of volunteers
Reimbursement	Multiple demands on caregiver
Gaps in payment systems	Expertise of caregiver
Capitation of hours for care delivery	Provider attitudes
Family structure	Provider behavior

---

aimed at reducing or curing the illness, or it may be the total focus of care" (p. 12) is truly revolutionary. It is a change in the concept of palliative care, as practiced in the first two decades of hospice care in the United States and at the Palliative Care Service of the Royal Victoria Hospital in Montreal, Canada, where the focus was on palliative care alone. As impressive as this change in thinking is, namely, that palliative care and acute care can be provided simultaneously, much remains to be accomplished. Barriers to the inclusion of palliative care in health care remain, as enumerated in Table 46.1.

Sociocultural Barriers to Providing Palliative Care

A sociocultural barrier to the availability of palliative care is the lack of discussion about disease-related death in society. The "stiff upper lip" still prevails in an era when letting it all hang out occurs in lifestyle and couture. An example of this lack of discussion has occurred at least twice in the history of the HIV and AIDS pandemic. In the 1980s, when death from AIDS occurred with greater regularity in countries of the North than it does today, there was a noticeable lack of interest in what the death and dying field could offer to those involved in HIV and

AIDS care. Now, once again, in the era of triple and quadruple antiretroviral combination therapy, when some are failing to achieve the Lazarus-like return to life and health, this information along with "failures" are hidden from view lest they spoil the pretty picture of rejuvenation. Maintaining a stiff upper lip, these individuals are dying to scream out that all is not well, but such behavior is not acceptable in the "politically correct" world of AIDS care politics.

Both in the make-believe motion picture world and the real world of the front pages of newspapers, death is more usually associated with violence. And the violence depicted both horrifies and fascinates. What is repeated again and again on television is the violence of the act and the sorrow of the survivors. Violence-related death offers little preparation for death's earthy appearance from chronic disease. Such preparation also is not routine in most medical facilities. However, it is part of hospice and palliative care—for patients and their caregivers—both formal and informal.

Political and Financial Ramifications

Palliative care and end-of-life care are accepted by some health care providers as synonymous terms and concepts. The question of how to define palliative care and its parameters—that is, the appropriate time in the illness trajectory to initiate such care—is part of the current discussion of palliative care. It is a discussion with political and financial ramifications and repercussions. For example, palliative medicine and care will require reimbursement. The source of the monies and whether funding for palliative care will mean a reduction in funding for other modalities is not at all clear. The assumption, as with hospice, is that palliative care will be if not cost-saving then cost-neutral. The excellent Institute of Medicine report (Field & Cassel, 1997) indicates the need to "revise mechanisms for financing care so that they encourage rather than impede good end-of-life care and sustain rather than frustrate coordinated systems of excellent care" (p. 8).

A practice that has implications for finance and care, for example, is the refusal to refer to hospice in a timely manner. Often referrals to hospice are made literally at the end of life, at which time providers—in particular nurses—are stressed to produce the hospice miracle of grace and resolution. Although refusal to make timely hospice referrals may be steeped in the caregiver's belief of doing everything possible and not giving up or abandoning the patient, such thinking also may have a more mundane derivation—concern about income and its loss. The result is a failure to initiate hospice care in a timely manner. Although the suggestion that hospice care be initiated earlier in the illness cycle entails sociocultural and financial considerations, the assumption of active versus palliative mitigates against inclusion of both.

Parenthetically, hospice programs in the United States have also engaged in this dualistic thinking—if hospice care, then no acute care. Part of the concern has been that hospice not be added to the costs of acute care, thereby increasing the overall costs of care. Whether such concerns were philosophical, financial, or governmental in origin—or some combination thereof—the opposition on the part of various stakeholders to integration of hospice care earlier in the disease trajectory remains. This barrier creates difficulties for those providers, who in recommending hospice or palliative care for patients, are concerned about symptom relief as well as attention to end-of-life issues.

An impediment to hospice care is also related to the structure of the health care benefit that shapes the type of care given. The benefit as outlined in an insurance plan indicates which services will be reimbursed, thereby influencing the care delivered.

Other economic constraints include the prospective payment system that may result in a gap in health care coverage from one level of care to another. This gap occurs when a patient is discharged from home care and is not ready for hospice care. Care may be needed during the interim but is not provided for under current funding mechanisms. Furthermore, capitation of the number of hours provided under the traditional home care benefit limits both the type and amount of care available. These gaps could be breached were a funding mechanism for palliative care developed.

Lack of Expertise

Funding is not the only obstacle to effective care. Palliative care requires expertise. Some patients continue to experience pain that an experienced palliative care clinician would be able to address (Elshamy, 1998). Nursing expertise is also needed when it is said that "nothing more can be done." For example, during the early years of the HIV and AIDS pandemic prior to discovery of Zidovudine (or AZT as it is still called), care for HIV-infected patients was largely nursing care (Lewis,

1989). It was the provision of comfort care (Tsoukas, 1986). Human immunodeficiency virus disease was and still is a major challenge for nursing, whether in adherence to medications or in palliative care when antiretroviral medications are no longer effective. When antiretroviral drugs fail and there is no salvage regimen, care is focused on comfort and quality of life.

Unfortunately, many nurses like other health care providers do not feel confident in the skills necessary for comfort, such as pain management, symptom control, and knowledge about the psychosocial implications of dying. Many providers are also uncomfortable with dying patients. Concern about increasing the flow rate of a morphine drip in patients with pain or respiratory difficulties may be related to a fear of hastening death and to underlying discomfort with a patient dying on their shift. The ethical concept of double effect is not understood or accepted by all nurses and leaves some professionals challenging an approach that, as a consequence of reducing discomfort, may shorten life.

Interdisciplinary Challenges

On an interdisciplinary level, nurses are in possession of what might be termed "hidden knowledge." It is a concept reminiscent of Weisman's "middle knowledge" (Kastenbaum, 1993). In this instance, nurses know that a patient is dying but the physician does not acknowledge the situation. These circumstances are particularly tricky when the patient is receiving an experimental protocol and the physician is concerned about collecting data end points. What is especially dismaying about this scenario is that what is heard from colleagues today has not changed from the same observations made decades earlier. Shannon (1997) examined the basis for interdisciplinary conflict and noted that "con-

flict around decisions about the use of life-sustaining therapies is inevitable, but interdisciplinary collaboration is inescapable if one is committed to quality ethical decision making" (p. 26).

Other interdisciplinary challenges include failure to establish "code" status, that is, written communication regarding what to do or not do upon cessation of a patient's vital functions. In a tertiary care facility such discussions remain the purview of the physician, although the literature suggests the need to enhance provider–patient–family communication (Hofmann et al., 1997; Tulsky, Fischer, Rose, & Arnold, 1998).

Challenges Intrinsic to Palliative Care

One of the most difficult challenges for all caregivers is making the transition from aggressive to comfort care. The timing of this transition is both science and art. Whatever the focus of care, clear communication with patient and family is essential in planning goals of care. Patient and family need to know that their care providers will be as aggressive in approaches to palliative care as they have been to curative care.

Another clinical challenge is the use of intravenous (IV) hydration—an issue that is still unresolved. Some caregivers insist on its use and consider it a pain reduction modality. Others prefer to substitute artificial saliva, tears, and the use of ice chips. Although IV hydration is perceived by some as a comfort measure, it may also increase secretions, cause pooling of fluids, and prolong life or prolong dying. Indeed, refusal of food and fluids is considered a means by which a patient can control his or her dying. Such refusal has been discussed as an alternative to assisted suicide (Eddy, 1994).

Integration into Health Care

The most significant challenge remains—that is, integration of palliative care into health care. Some movement to this end has occurred but is conceptualized as palliative medicine. There is some concern that other characteristics of hospice care will be omitted in the drive to make palliative medicine a credible part of medical care (O'Connor, 1999). These characteristics include the focus on the interdisciplinary team (i.e., nursing, social work, chaplaincy, physical therapy, art therapy, pharmacy, and the use of volunteers). Volunteers, the hallmark of hospice, have not been mentioned in most of the writings about palliative medicine. Moreover, interdisciplinary often means another medical specialty to physicians and not another discipline altogether.

■ Funding for Change

Nonetheless, we are in a remarkable period of change during which attention to integration of palliative care into medicine has been enhanced through funding of a number of projects in medical and nursing education. Funding has been provided, as well, for projects that will increase awareness of citizens about attitudes regarding palliative care; a review of some of these projects is as follows.

The Project on Death in America, funded by the Soros Foundation, has two foci: to finance innovative projects and to fund key medical personnel, primarily physicians, as Project on Death in America (PDIA) scholars (Field & Cassel, 1997). Scholars are engaged in projects at home sites as well as participating in PDIA meetings.

The Robert Wood Johnson (RWJ) Foundation has also made a major commitment to improving end-of-life care. The Support study (Support Principal Investigators, 1995) men-

tioned at the beginning of this chapter was funded by RWJ. Another project supported in part by RWJ is the Missoula Demonstration Project: Quality of Life's End (MDP) (Field & Cassel, 1997). Ira Byock and his colleagues are attempting to change the way people die in a discrete community by changing attitudes not only of health care providers but expectations of the populace.

Other major projects initiated by various organizations are the following.

- The Center to Improve the Care of the Dying in Washington, D.C., which has sponsored a number of initiatives, including a tool kit to measure quality of end-of-life care, a "Sourcebook on Dying," and an investigation of the impact of a new policy "medicaring" that might serve as the prototype for funding for palliative care (Sherman, 1999).

- The Institute of Medicine (IOM) report Approaching Death: Improving Care at the End-of-Life, funded by the Soros Foundation, which concludes its thorough and thought-provoking analysis with recommendations for each of the health professions (Field & Cassel, 1997).

- The American Medical Association, which initiated an effort to improve end-of-life care by educating physicians. The project is appropriately named Education for Physicians in End-of-Life Care (EPEC) and provided 2-day educational sessions held regionally in late 1998 and early 1999 (Solomon, 1998).

Nursing Discipline–Focused Projects

A number of projects have been developed to improve end-of-life care by nurses. The American Association of Colleges of Nursing (AACN) sponsored a 2-day meeting in November 1997, at which a small group of educators, researchers, and clinicians (expert in

TABLE 46.2 Competencies Necessary for Nurses to Provide High Quality Care to Patients and Families During the Transition at the End-of-Life

1. Recognize dynamic changes in population demographics, health care economics, and service delivery that necessitate improved professional preparation and end-of-life care.

2. Promote the provision of comfort care to the dying as an active, desirable, and important skill, and an integral component of nursing care.

3. Communicate effectively and compassionately with the patient, family, and health care team members about end-of-life issues.

4. Recognize one's own attitudes, feelings, values, and expectations about death and the individual, cultural, and spiritual diversity existing in these beliefs and customs.

5. Demonstrate respect for the patient's views and wishes during end-of-life care.

6. Collaborate with interdisciplinary team members while implementing the nursing role in end-of-life care.

7. Use scientifically based standardized tools to assess symptoms (e.g., pain, dyspnea, constipation, anxiety, fatigue, nausea/vomiting, and altered cognition) experienced by patients at end-of-life.

8. Use data from symptom assessment to plan and intervene in symptom management using state-of-the-art traditional and complementary approaches.

9. Evaluate the impact of traditional, complementary, and technological therapies on patient centered outcomes.

10. Assess and treat multiple-dimensions, including physical, psychological, social and spiritual needs, to improve quality at the end-of-life.

11. Assist the patient, family, colleagues, and one's self to cope with suffering, grief, loss, and bereavement in end-of-life care.

12. Apply legal and ethical principles in the analysis of complex issues in end-of-life care, recognizing the influence of personal values, professional codes, and patient preferences.

13. Identify barriers and facilitators to patients' and caregivers' effective use of resources.

14. Demonstrate skill at implementing a plan for improved end-of-life care within a dynamic and complex health care delivery system.

15. Apply knowledge gained from palliative care research to end-of-life education and care.

American Association of Colleges of Nursing. (1998). *Peaceful Death: Recommended Competencies and Curricular Guidelines for End-of-Life Nursing Care* (pp. 2–3).

care of the terminally ill) met and agreed on competencies necessary for "Nurses to Provide High Quality Care to Patients and Families During the Transition at the End-of-Life" (see Table 46.2). The 15 competencies cover a range of abilities including communication, symptom control, physical, psychological, social, and spiritual care (American Association of Colleges of Nursing [AACN], 1998).

Stating that "the literature indicates that nursing programs, as a whole, offer little systematic preparation for dealing with the inevitable experiences of death and dying, or for more advanced training in providing end-of-life care" English and Yocum (1997) developed *Guidelines for Curriculum Development on End-of-Life and Palliative Care in Nursing Education.* The guidelines were developed to provide an outline of materials on "The Human Response to Dying (Approaching Death)" and "The Human Response to Life Threatening Illness (Palliative Care)." This project was developed and completed by the National Council of Hospice Professionals of the National Hospice Organization (English & Yocum, 1997). The authors shared these guidelines with AACN for its November 1997, meeting.

Supported by a grant from the Project on Death in America, Ferrell, Virani, and Grant (1998) developed and implemented a Home Care Outreach for Palliative Care Education (HOPE) curriculum. The five training modules developed were provided to home health agencies.

Ferrell et al. (1999) have also been funded by the Robert Wood Johnson Foundation to achieve the following goals:

1. To improve content regarding pain and end-of-life care included in major textbooks used in nursing education.

2. To ensure adequacy of content regarding pain management and end-of-life care as tested by the national nursing licensure examination, the NCLEX.

3. To support key nursing organizations in efforts to promote nursing education and practice in the areas of pain management and end-of-life care.

Wouters (1994) raised questions about the qualifications of nurse trainers because it is important that nurse educators bring both theoretical and clinical knowledge to the classroom. The Tool Kit Project for Nursing Excellence at End-of-Life transitions (TNEEL), headed by Diana Wilkie (1999) and funded by

the Robert Wood Johnson Foundation, will support nurse educators in the classroom by development of computer-based teaching materials.

Medical Discipline Focused Projects

Block and Billings (1998) argue for importance of palliative care education for medical students. As noted previously, a number of projects are directed at medical students and physicians. Palliative Care Centers have been funded at Harvard and Stanford by the Robert Wood Johnson Foundation. The Harvard Palliative Care Center will provide short courses to medical and nursing faculty. Other efforts include those by Bascom (Christopher, 1998) at Oregon Health Sciences University, who developed a self-guided curriculum for medical students. Other educational programs are directed at clinical staff in order to change the way in which palliative care is delivered (Adelstein & Burton, 1998).

Internet Education

Changes are also occurring in the manner in which educational programs are delivered. Palliative care courses are advertised over the internet. Grant McEwen Community College (1998) provides course descriptions, objectives, and outlines for a number of palliative care courses. As demonstrated by the College, this area is ripe with potential for distance learning.

Community-Focused Projects

The community as venue for education was identified in the Missoula Demonstration Project and in the Community and State Partnership initiative (Long, 1998). The latter project seeks to stimulate and link projects within a state. Another effort, the Last Acts campaign with which more than 330 organizations are affiliated, including major nursing organizations, is also working to improve end-of-life care through a variety of initiatives, including online chat rooms (Solomon, 1999). A separate initiative, Americans for Better Care of the Dying (ABCD), is headed by Joanne Lynn (Lynn, 1998). The goals of this organization are "effective pain and symptom control, protection of families from financial distress, social support systems to limit emotional distress of patients and families, continuity of care and care providers, (and) clear communication between patients and providers" (p. 7). All these efforts will provide momentum for change in professional education, in palliative care, and in end-of-life care that individuals demand and receive.

■ Concluding Statement

The purpose of this chapter was to explore the thesis that someone does not need to be terminally ill to receive palliative care. The definition of palliative care has been explicated and barriers to provision of palliative care noted. Finally, projects that address need for educated providers have been described. Looking to the future, Stanley (1998) suggests the following approaches:

- Restructure health care education by including palliative care in the standard curriculum.

- Educate current health care practitioners from multiple disciplines in the art and science of palliative care.

- Create a cadre of palliative care experts who can provide consultation and serve as role models for other practitioners.

Efforts to implement these approaches are currently underway.

If the conceptualization of palliative care proposed in this chapter becomes accepted, health care providers will move from the dichotomy of care discussed in the literature to unity of palliative with acute and chronic modalities. No longer will texts in acute care discuss treatment of the disease in isolation of the person. Nor will palliative care texts be able to claim special honors for treatment of the person. Once this artificial duality has been removed, contribution of special knowledge from both sources will be welcomed in service to the patient. When a person does not need to be terminally ill to receive palliative care, all patients will be relieved of unnecessary suffering, and health care will have taken a giant step forward—one appropriate for a new millennium. In so doing, philanthropies and caregivers will have achieved their shared goal, namely, to change end-of-life care in America for the better.

■ References

Adelstein, W., & Burton, S. (1998). Palliative care in the acute hospital setting. *Journal of Neuroscience Nursing, 30*(3), 279–289.

American Association of Colleges of Nursing. (1998). Competencies necessary for nurses to provide high-quality care to patients and families during the transition at the end-of-life. *Peaceful Death: Recommended Competencies and Curricular Guidelines for End-of-Life Nursing Care* (pp. 2–3). [On-line]. Available: http://ar/endlife/deathfin.

Block, S. (1999, March 26). Medical education and training. Plenary Presentation at Meeting of *Community–State Partnership*, Virginia Beach, VA.

Block, S., & Billings, J. A. (1998). Nurturing humanism through teaching palliative care. *Academic Medicine, 73*(7), 763–765.

Christopher, M. (1998, June). Survey data support change in curriculum and clinical practice. *State Initiatives in End-of-Life Care (issue 1),* 6–7.

Corless, I. (1983). The hospice movement in North America. *Hospice care principles and practice.* New York: Springer.

Department of Palliative Care and Policy. (1998). A definition. *King's College School of Medicine and Dentistry and St. Christopher's Hospice.* [On-line]. Available: http://www.Kcl.ac.UK/Kis/schools/palliative/Who/weare.html.

Eddy, D. M. (1994). A conversation with my mother. *Journal of the American Medical Association, 272*(3), 179–181.

Edmonton Palliative Care. (1998). *Defining palliative care.* Author. [On-line]. Available: http://www.palliative.org/pc_defining.html.

Elshamy, M. (1998). Needs of patients and caregivers at the end-of-life: Insights from recent research. *Innovation in Breast Cancer Care, 4*(1), 13–17.

English, N., & Yocum, C. (1997). *Guidelines for curriculum development on end-of-life and palliative care in nursing education.* Arlington, VA: National Hospice Organization.

Ferrell, B. R., Virani, R., & Grant, M. (1998). Hope home care outreach for palliative care education. *Cancer Practice, 6*(2), 79–85.

Ferrell, B. R., Virani, R., & Grant, M. (1999). Analysis of end-of-life content in nursing textbooks. *Oncology Nursing Forum, 26*(5), 869–876.

Ferris, F. D. (1994). Working definition of the CPCA standards committee 1995. (A paper originally presented at the Canadian Palliative Care Association in 1994.) In F. D. Ferris & I. Cummings (Eds.), *Palliative care: Towards a consensus in standardized principles of practice* (p. 12). Canadian Palliative Care Association.

Ferris, F. D., & Cummings, I. (Eds.). (1995). *Palliative care towards a concensus in standardized principles of practice.* Edmonton, Alberta, Canada: Canadian Palliative Care Association.

Field, M. J., & Cassel, C. K. (Eds.). (1997). *Approaching death-improving care at the end-of-life.* Washington, DC: National Academy Press.

Grant McEwen Community College. (1998). *Introduction to palliative care.* Edmonton, Alberta, Canada: Author. [On-line]. Available: http://www.gmcc.ab.ca/users/hcs/pcare/ courses/NE737.3.html.

Hofmann, J. C., Wenger, N. S., Davis, R. B., Teno, J., Connors, A. F., Desbiens, N., Linn, J., & Phillips, R. S. (1997). Patient preferences for communication with physicians about end-of-life decisions. *Annals of Internal Medicine, 127,* 1–12.

Kastenbaum, R. (1993). Avery D. Weisman: An Omega interview. *Omega Journal of Death and Dying, 27,* 97–104.

Lewis, A. (1989). Development of AIDS awareness: A personal history. In I. B. Corless & M. Pittman-Lindeman (Eds.), *AIDS—principles, practices and politics* (pp. 331–336). New York: Hemisphere.

Long, K. (1998). Communities become focal points for success. *Last Acts* (summer), 1.

Lynn, J. (1998). *Annual activities report: 1998.* Americans for Better Care of the Dying.

O'Connor, P. (1999). Hospice vs. palliative care. *The Hospice Journal, 14*(2 & 3), 123–137.

Quill, T. E. (1993). *A midwife through the dying process.* Baltimore: Johns Hopkins University Press.

Rabinowitz, B. (1998). Integrating palliation into end-of-life care. An interview with Ira Byock. *Innovations in Breast Cancer Care, 4*(1), 18–21.

Ruland, C. M., & Moore, S. M. (1998). Theory construction on standards of care: A proposed theory of the peaceful end-of-life. *Nursing Outlook, 46,* 169–175.

Saunders, C. (1999). Origins—International perspective, then and now. *The Hospice Journal, 14*(2 & 3), 1–7.

Shannon, S. E. (1997). The roots of interdisciplinary conflict around ethical issues. *Critical Care Nursing Clinics of North America, 9*(1), 13–26.

Sherman, D. W. (1999). End-of-life care: Challenges and opportunities for professionals. *Hospice Journal, 14*(2 & 3), 109–121.

Solomon, M. Z. (1995). The enormity of the task-support and changing practice. *Hasting Center Report, Special Supplement* (November–December), 528–532.

Solomon, M. Z. (Ed.). (1998). AMA trains MD's on end-of-life issues. *Last Acts, 5* (summer), 4.

Solomon, M. Z. (1999). A campaign of more than 330 organizations to improve end-of-life care. *Last Acts, 6* (spring), 1.

Stanley, K. J. (1998). End-of-life care: Where are we headed? What do we want? Who will decide? *Innovations in Breast Cancer Care, 4*(1), 3–8.

Support Principal Investigators. (1995). A controlled trial to improve care for seriously ill hospitalized patients: The study to understand progress and preferences for outcomes and risks of treatment (support). *Journal of the American Medical Association, 274,* 1591–1598.

Tsoukas, C. (1986). AIDS: Future implications for palliative care. *Journal of Palliative Care, 2*(1), 35–38.

Tulsky, J. A., Fischer, G. S., Rose, M. R., & Arnold, R. M. (1998). Opening the black box: How do physicians communicate about advance directives? *Annals of Internal Medicine, 129*(6), 441–449.

Wilkie, D. (1999). Tool-kit for nursing excellence at end-of-life transition. *Prospectus proposal to the Robert Johnson Foundation.* Unpublished.

World Health Organization. (1990). *Cancer pain relief and palliative care.* (Technical report series 804). Geneva, Switzerland.

Wouters, B. (1994). Teaching palliative care: A challenge to nurse trainers. *European Journal of Palliative Care, 1*(4), 178–183.

■ Editor's Questions for Discussion

What is the difference in nursing practice between palliative and acute care? Discuss the distinction made by Corless: "Palliation treats the patient; acute care treats the disease." What implications exist for nursing practice with regard to palliation, health maintenance, and prevention of illness? How does care differ in palliation and hospice?

What financial considerations must be resolved for palliative care? How might strategies be developed to influence change in reimbursement of health and illness care? How might the most appropriate type of care for a patient be an option in structuring health care benefits? Propose mechanisms for funding palliative care.

Discuss the ethical and legal implications for nursing practice in palliative and hospice care. Refer particularly to the discussions by Davis (Chapter 6), Kopala (Chapter 5), and Lane and Paterson (Chapter 7). How might professional nurses resolve personal and interdisciplinary conflicts regarding life-sustaining therapies? Discuss alternatives to assisted suicide that may be considered palliative care.

Suggest strategies for nursing curriculum development in palliative care? What content is appropriate for undergraduate versus graduate students? How might palliative care concepts and content be integrated into curriculum regarding acute, chronic, and community care? What implications exist for palliative care in home care (Schroeder and Long, Chapter 47), care in the community (Alexander, Chapter 44; and Hollinger-Smith, Chapter 45), parish nursing (Schroeder and Long, Chapter 47), and rural health care (Pullen, Chapter 50)?

47

Impact of Home Health Care on Clinical Practice and Education

Mary Ann Schroeder, PhD, RN, FAAN
Carol O. Long, PhD, RN

Home health care is the component of a continuum of care provided to individuals and families in their places of residence (home, nursing home, or assisted living facility) for the purpose of promoting optimum health. The home health care structure refers to licensed and Medicare-accredited agencies that provide professional and ancillary health care in the place of residence. Services requested can be for skilled, nonskilled, or hospice care.

■ Types of Home Care

Various types of home care systems exist. They are classified according to ownership and tax status, as determined by the Internal Revenue Service, and may be either public or private. There is also a classification system within public and private and profit and nonprofit categories. Public agencies may be official agencies (e.g., supported by government and tax dollars) or voluntary (e.g., Visiting Nurses Association). Private agencies may be free-standing organizations in the community. Home health agencies can be hospital-based, hospice-based, independent, or part of a large alliance or network. Hospital-based agencies are part of a hospital's organizational structure, and authority rests with the hospital's Board of Directors. Referrals to other agencies generally are patients being discharged from hospitals.

575

Home health agencies may or may not be Medicare- or Medicaid-certified. They are dependent on government or nongovernment third-party reimbursements to defray the costs of services provided. Managers administer the programs of these agencies and oversee their day-to-day operations. Large home health agencies may have several branches. Demand for home health care can be for basic custodial, skilled, or hospice care. Basic custodial care is rendered to clients who are unable to perform personal care activities, such as bathing and grooming. Skilled professional care is provided by nurses or therapists when medically necessary to treat the client's injury or illness. Hospice involves delivery of palliative and supportive care to clients with life expectancies of 6 months or less. The focus is on quality of life for the dying client and family.

Home health care can precede or follow acute care, long-term care, or an outpatient episode. Home health care may also stand alone as a distinct entity, providing services in the residence of a client who is considered "homebound." Coordination with other health care delivery systems such as hospice, community waiver programs, and outpatient clinic services may be involved. Home health care often is an alternative to the more expensive hospital care. It also may be an adjunct to health care in the home that is needed to maximize client independence and autonomy or to deter entry into long-term care settings.

■ History of Home Health Care

Organized home health care had its historical beginnings in about 1885 to 1889 and flourished until about 1930. During this period, the most seriously ill were cared for in the home, which was the workplace for most nurses (Marrelli, 1994). Under the direction of nurses, agencies provided skilled nursing care to patients with both chronic and acute health care problems. Sponsorship was provided by "voluntary" philanthropically financed organizations. Agency services focused on a model of health promotion and illness prevention. Health was the general theme for services.

Transition to Hospital Care

The growing centrality of the hospital from 1930 to 1965 resulted in fewer sick patients being cared for at home, with care being transferred to hospitals and staffs of trained nurses. Then, coordinated community-based nursing services began to evolve. Between 1955 and 1964, the home as a site for provision of health care regained popularity because of (a) rising hospital costs, (b) increasing incidences of chronic illness, and (c) a rapidly growing elderly population (Home Health Information, 1997). Interestingly, it was not appropriate for physicians to direct home care prior to 1965 (Rice, 1995).

Impact of Legislation

Introduction of Medicare and Medicaid legislation in 1965 shifted the focus of health care from a health promotion, disease prevention model to a medical model. Physicians ordered home health care, but nurses had a great deal of latitude in planning the actual delivery of care. Home health care continued to grow, with increasing numbers of Medicare patients being discharged to the home—from 9.1% in 1981 to 17.9% in 1985 (Home Health Information, 1997).

An estimated 5.9 million (2.5%) of the U.S. population received formal home care services in 1989; this number increased to 8 million (4%) in 1997 (Home Health Information, 1997). Introduction of diagnosis-related groups (DRGs) in 1983 stimulated the shift of Medicare patients being discharged from acute care facilities to home care and fostered "high-tech" care at home. The impact of managed care on the health care industry portends significant consequences for the future of home health care.

Organization for Home Care

Eventually, an organization was formed to represent the interests of home health care providers and clients alike. The National Association for Home Care (NAHC) was founded in 1982. The mission of this organization is to promote quality care for home care and hospice patients; preserve the rights of caregivers; and represent all home care and hospice providers (Home Health Information, 1997).

■ Benefits of Home Health Care

Home health care has contributed to reduction in health care expenditures; it provides hospital patients with an opportunity for early discharge, followed by more economical care in the home. One of home health care's greatest appeals is, in fact, its cost-effectiveness. Traditionally, home care services are delivered at a cost 30% to 70% below hospital or nursing home costs. However, providers will be challenged to continue to provide quality care at even lower cost in the future as federal reimbursement shifts from a cost-based model to a prospective pay system (PPS), designed by Medicare to reduce home health expenditures.

Costs of Care

Positive outcomes are usually measured in terms of cost-effectiveness first, and quality of care second. In most cases, home health care is cost-effective when hospital and home health charges per visit are compared. The NAHC (1999) reported that, in 1997, hospital charges per day were $2,121 compared to an average charge of $88 for a home health care visit. Even with multiple visits, charges for home health care are significantly less than a hospital stay for a day. These savings are even more evident in the case of a specific diagnosis. For example, for congestive heart failure (CHF), the NAHC (1999) reported average per-patient, per-month hospital costs of $1,758 compared to $1,605 for home care costs—a per-patient, per-month saving of $153.

Quality of Care

One of the most positive impacts of home health care is the quality of care achieved by patients and families. Home health care quality has been measured in terms of (a) enhancement of quality of life for the client by being cared for in a familiar and loving environment, (b) more rapid achievement of health improvement, (c) reduction in level of family stress, and (d) improve appropriateness of care by matching individual care needs with the appropriate level of care.

■ Growth of Home Care

The growth of home care services has again increased dramatically during the past several years, after sluggish growth during most of the 1980s. Recent growth has been stimulated by implementation of DRGs, increased managed care, and patients' preference for care in a familiar, caring environment—the home. Total home care spending is difficult to estimate due to lack of consistent data. Payments to providers other than Medicare and Medicaid hospital-based agencies are difficult to track. Nevertheless, the distribution of payments for services is estimated as follows: Medicare (40%), Medi-

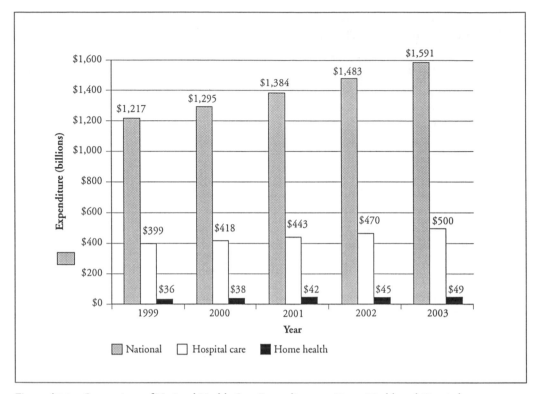

Figure 47.1 Comparison of National Health Care Expenditures to Home Health and Hospital Expenditures, Calendar Years 1999–2003.

U.S. Department of Health and Human Services, Health Care Financing Administration. (1999). *A profile of Medicare home health chart book* (DHHS Publication No. HCFA-10138). Washington, DC: U.S. Government Printing Office.

caid (15%), private health insurance (11%), other private funds (12%), and out-of-pocket payments (2%) (U.S. Department of Health and Human Services [DHHS], 1999). The Health Care Financing Administration (HCFA) (1998) projected total, hospital, and home health care expenditures for the period 1999 through 2003, as illustrated in Figure 47.1. It also projected the growth of home health expenditures (dollars versus percentage change) for the same period, as shown in Figure 47.2.

Home health care continues to capture a growing share of the health care market—now 4%. The NAHC (1999) reported that the number of Medicare-certified home health agencies almost doubled, from 5,676 in 1989 to 9,120 in 1995. In 1997, an estimated 20,215 home health organizations provided care to more than 7 million Americans (Home Health Information, 1997). Part of this demand for home health care can be attributed to the prospective payment system, resulting in earlier discharge of patients from hospitals. Again, in most instances, caring for patients in an acute care setting is much more costly than providing community-based home health care. For example, a study conducted by Kornowski et al. (1995) supported the effectiveness of home care surveillance for congestive heart failure patients. They found that hospitalizations declined from 3.2 to 1.2 per year and that length of stay decreased from 26 to 6 days per year.

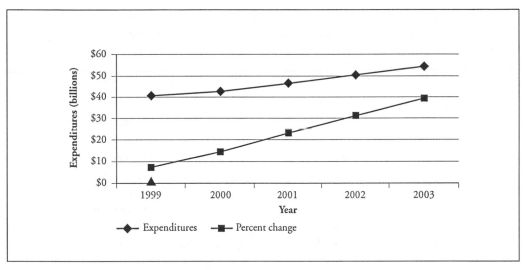

Figure 47.2   Medicare Home Health Expenditures.

U.S. Department of Health and Human Services, Health Care Financing Administration. (1999). *A profile of Medicare home health chart book* (DHHS Publication No. HCFA-10138). Washington, DC: U.S. Government Printing Office.

Growth Factors

Contrary to public opinion, the growth of Medicare home care programs is not a consequence of fraudulent activities on the part of some hospital and physicians' associations. Rather, growth can be attributed to the (a) increased numbers of the elderly and disabled, (b) earlier discharge of acutely ill hospital patients (related to DRGs and managed care), (c) decline in nursing home utilization, (d) greater awareness of home care services, (e) third-party reimbursement for home care, (f) increased availability of home-bound medical technological innovations, and (g) public preference for health care services in the home. The Census Bureau reported that, between 1995 and 2000, the U.S. population 65 years of age and older was expected to increase by 10% and those 85 years of age and older was expected to increase by 42% (U.S. Bureau of the Census, 1996). These data also support the likelihood of continued growth of home health care services.

■ *Financial and Technological Effects on Home Health*

Recently, the number of home health care agencies has declined. The situation was caused by changes in HCFA's Medicare home health reimbursement plan, the Interim Payment System (IPS) enacted as part of the Balanced Budget Act of 1997. The introduction and implementation of the IPS by HCFA will have profound effects on home health care reimbursements—in effect, resulting in numerous additional closings of independent home health agencies.

Closures and Inaccurate Data

A 1998 General Accounting Office (GAO) report indicated that 554 voluntary and 206 involuntary health agency closures occurred between October 1997 and June 1998, for a total of 760 closures (Scanlon, 1998). Branch closures have a great impact on patients living in rural areas. But the GAO report did not consider the extent of patient access problems caused by agency closings in rural areas.

Medicare Reimbursement

The home health care industry has been affected seriously by Medicare fraud. Medicare lost approximately $20.3 billion in fiscal year 1997 due to fraud and waste (Scanlon, 1998). The Balanced Budget Act of 1997 was passed in part in response to this loss. Medicare currently reimburses home health agencies on a cost basis, subject to limits. The Balanced Budget Act provides for reductions in existing cost limits and changes in reimbursement, with the establishment of a new per beneficiary cost limit, followed by a prospective payment system (PPS) very much like that of the DRGs in 1983. Under the PPS system of reimbursement, a predetermined payment per unit of service (adjusted by case mix) was to be implemented as of October 1, 2000. Until the PPS can be realized, an interim payment system (IPS) has been implemented. The IPS limits per beneficiary annual reimbursement to 105% of the medical cost per visit, based on the facility's cost reporting year ending in federal fiscal year 1984 (Scanlon, 1998).

Possible effects of the PPS system may be that home health agencies may become selective in the types of patients accepted, number of visits per beneficiary may be reduced, and less prepared personnel may be substituted for professional caregivers. However, reduced reimbursements may create impetus for home health agencies to develop streamlined care protocols further to achieve cost reductions and increase the quality of care. The per beneficiary limit will also introduce a new element of care—utilization management. Care and data systems will have to be developed and implemented; data will need to be collected, managed, and analyzed.

Outcome and Assessment Information System

The Outcome and Assessment Information System (OASIS) (1999) was developed by the Center for Health Services and Policy Research at the University of Colorado Health Sciences Center under contract with the HCFA. The OASIS is a patient assessment system that can be used to measure outcomes in home health agencies (Shaughnessy, Crisler, Schlenker, & Hittle, 1998). These outcomes then will be used to improve quality of care and ultimately be linked to the reimbursement system. The OASIS was not developed to be a complete assessment tool, but rather it is to be used in conjunction with the assessment tool currently in use by home health agencies. However, all Medicare-certified home health agencies are required to complete the OASIS as a prerequisite for meeting Medicare conditions of participation. Home health agencies that do not comply with this requirement will not be able to receive Medicare certification. Data from the OASIS is transferred electronically to a database established by HCFA in each state.

In the *Federal Register* of January 25, 1999, HCFA estimated the total start-up costs nationwide for implementation of OASIS to be $30 million (Medicare and Medicaid, 1999). Potential contributions of the new data to cost containment and quality of care apparently justify a favorable cost-benefit ratio. However, the home health care industry has not been able to collect, analyze, maintain, and manage home health data in the past. Now, agencies that cannot afford the expense of OASIS implementation are being forced to close if their funding depends on Medicare patients. The HCFA has made available to home health agencies (at no charge) a software program, Home Assessment

Validation and Entry (HAVEN), that can be used to enter OASIS-generated data into the system. HCFA later had to announce that the effective date for transmission of OASIS data would be July 19, 1999.

■ Impact of Electronic Technology

The HCFA's requirement to transfer data from OASIS assessments electronically is only one example of the impact of electronic technology on the home health care industry.

Clinical Practice

Computer technology is changing the way that some health care services are provided (Computer Technology, 1995). For example, computers are used by the Visiting Nurse Association of Los Angeles to monitor congestive heart patients receiving treatment for congestive heart failure (CHF).

Computers also are being used in two home health care projects developed by Dr. Patricia Brennan of Case Western University. ComputerLink projects provide interactive electronic connections among patients and caregivers to facilitate sharing of information for patients with AIDS and caregivers of patients with Alzheimer's disease (Computer Technology, 1995). The three supportive functions of this link include (a) an electronic encyclopedia, (b) a decision support system, and (c) a communication pathway to peers and health care providers.

Nightingale Tracker™ System

Education of nurses to furnish quality care in the community has included the challenge of providing and supervising nursing students in home health care. Experts agree that the 1,500 undergraduate nursing programs in the

United States will need to evaluate integration of community health care experiences into nursing curricula further. The Nightingale Tracker™ System, developed by FITNE, provides the instructor with data management and communication tools in delivery of safe care (FITNE, 1999). The device's software facilitates interactive communication between an instructor, who may be at an academic center, and a student, who is giving care in the home. Documentation of the student's visit—process and practice—is recorded and transmitted to the instructor. Thus the System facilitates (a) assignments, (b) preplanning for patient visits, (c) patient–student visit, and (d) postvisit evaluation. The System represents a technological advance that not only permits an instructor to evaluate a greater number of students more effectively, but it also enhances the educational process by giving students immediate feedback for clinical performance.

The Nightingale Tracker™ System is an excellent example of telecommunications use. "Store and forward" technology generates, stores, and transfers digital images from one location to another. Telecommunication also has been used in home health care settings by nurses—for example, using video equipment to transfer a digital image of a clinical condition, such as a wound, to a physician at another location. This feature is particularly important in rural areas where homebound patients do not have access to medical care. Home health care could be a booming part of the telecommunication field. A program in Japan has patients communicating with physicians, nurses, and physical therapists (Cooper, 1996).

■ Impact of Home Health Care on Clinical Practice and Education

With the changing nature of the home health care industry, service providers, educators, and researchers will need to be both responsive and proactive in evaluating the delivery of high-quality, low-cost services in the home. This challenge can be met only if caregivers fully understand the needs of home health care clients and how agencies and nursing can be effective in the context of the revolution that is occurring in home health care.

Opportunities for Nursing Students

Schools and colleges of nursing must develop opportunities for nursing students to have clinical experiences in community-based settings. Clinical practice opportunities, ranging from community health experiences to home health care and hospice, can expose new nurses to potential career opportunities. In addition, home-based experiences can expand students' understanding of effective discharge planning from hospital to home, use of community resources, and efforts to maximize independence and wellness for clients beyond the institutional walls of a hospital or nursing home.

Competencies

Continuing education in home health care or hospice agencies must be directed at meeting competency-based standards of practice for nurses new to home-based care (i.e., new graduates or nurses transitioning from acute care to home health care settings). Continuing education for nurses currently employed in home health care or hospices also is important, as more clients are now acutely ill at home with complex medical–surgical problems. Because home health care nurses tend to be isolated in their practice, ensuring ongoing competency must center on addressing the new ways to meet client needs and on updates in health care advancements.

Additional Skills

Beyond clinical management competencies, survival skills are needed in today's home health care environment. Case management, assessment and teaching strategies, and critical thinking are needed to augment the nursing process aimed at producing desired client outcomes within time limitations. Nurses and agencies will be called upon to participate in educational programs directed at meeting these needs. Other essential skills for the home health care nurse include (a) communicating effectively, (b) mastering techniques to maximize client adherence to plans of care, (c) establishing and maintaining effective interdisciplinary coordination and collaboration, (d) applying advocacy approaches, (e) developing ways to discover and utilize community resources, and (f) managing time and finances effectively.

Not to be forgotten are educational sessions aimed at acquiring new knowledge, not merely clinical techniques. Basic gerontological nursing concepts for home health care nurses—who generally have a large caseload of older adults—may assist in broadening sensitivity and basic understanding of needs for this population group. Merging educational tracks aimed at meeting basic clinical and management skills for nurses new to or continuing to practice in home health care will allow home health agencies to progress.

■ The Future of the Home Health Care Industry

The home health care industry may be expected to rebound from the impact of the mandated prospective payment reimbursement system, which replaces the past fee-for-service reimbursement system. Need for home health care exists, given the expected significant increase in elders and those who are medically disabled in the United States. Structure, process, and reimbursement for home health must be evaluated critically for quality to increase and costs to decrease.

Needed Response

Smaller, independent "mom and pop" home health agencies, especially in rural areas, may be forced to close. Networking will result in larger home health corporate organizations. If home health agencies are to remain financially solvent, home care must capture a larger market share of the health care industry. Cost-effectiveness and quality benefits of home health care need to be further marketed to obtain a greater numbers of referrals from various sources. An analogy is the health maintenance organization (HMO) industry, with fixed beneficiary costs, which has had to increase its member volume to remain financially solvent. In addition, technology will promote greater access to care by those in rural areas. Educators will need to respond in the transition of nurses from acute care settings to the home health care environment. For example, the College of Nursing at Arizona State University has responded to the growing field of home health care by designing and implementing an undergraduate course in home health care, which is required in the final year of the curriculum (Long, 1995).

Final Challenge

A very real challenge for the PPS and HCFA is to develop a case-mix adjuster that reflects costs of providing services to various types of patients. The Medicare Home Health Prospective Payment Demonstration (Goldberg & Schmitz, 1994) is a small example of the benefits of creating a valid prospective per-beneficiary reimbursement system. Concerns about the sample size also were voiced when DRGs were introduced in 1983. The DRGs, however, have not caused financial distress in health care but have provided opportunities for cost savings and quality enhancements. The same result will occur in home health care.

■ Concluding Statement

Change challenges any system. Often, change requires alterations in process and structure to achieve stated goals, but change is usually productive. Challenges to home health care are no different. The home health care industry will step up to this challenge and continue to provide appropriate and necessary health care to those in homes, nursing homes, and hospices. In a world of greater "tech" than "touch," health care providers have the opportunity to offer quality and compassionate care in a familiar and comfortable environment. The home health care industry can best provide this type of care.

■ References

Balanced Budget Act of 1997. (P.L. 105–33) (August 1997). HR3426—Medicare and Medicaid Health Insurance Act. *U.S. Statutes at Large* (Volume III, pp. 251–788). Washington, DC: U.S. Government Printing Office.
Computer Technology. (1995). *Delivering health care through computer technology.* [On-line]. Available: http://www.ev.net/FITNE/tracker/deliver.htm.

Cooper, J. (1996). *Telemedicine is coming of age.* [On-line]. Available:
http://www.atsp.org/basics/comingOFAge.html.

FITNE. (1999). *The Nightingale tracker system.* Athens, OH: Author.

Goldberg, H. B., & Schmitz, R. J. (1994). Contemplating home health PPS: Current patterns of Medicare service use. *Health Care Financing Review, 16*(1), 109–130.

Health Care Financing Administration (HCFA), Office of the Actuary. (1998). *National health care expenditures projections.* [On-line]. Available:
http://www.hcfa.gov/stats/NHE-Proj/tables/default.htm.

Home Health Information. (1997). *History of home health care.* [On-line]. Available:
http://www.indian-river.fl.us/health/homecare/history.html.

Kornowski, R., Zeeli, D., Averbuch, M., Finklestein, A., Schwartz, D., Moshkovitz, M., Weinreb, B., Hershkovitz, R., Eysal, D., Miller, M., Levo, Y., & Pines, A. (1995). Intensive home-care surveillance prevents hospitalization and improves morbidity rates among elderly patients with severe congestive heart failure. *American Heart Journal, 129*(4), 762–766.

Long, C. (1995). Home healthcare—The curriculum mandate. *Home Healthcare Nursing, 13*(6), 46–50.

Marrelli, T. M. (1994). *Handbook of Home Health standards and Documentation Guidelines for Reimbursement* (2nd ed.). St. Louis: Mosby.

Medicare and Medicaid. (1999, January 25). Medicare and Medicaid programs: Reporting outcome and assessment information set (OASIS) data as part of the conditions of participation for home health agencies and comprehensive assessment and use of the oasis as part of the conditions of participation for home health agencies. *Final Rules, 64 Fed. Reg. 3783.*

National Association of Home Care. (1999). Basic statistics about home care 1996. *Consumer Information.* [On-line]. Available: http://www.nahc.org.

Outcome and Assessment Information Set (OASIS). (1999). *HCFA announces the mandatory use of OASIS (regulations).* [On-line]. Available: http://www.hcfa.gov/medicare/oasis/hhregs.htm.

Rice, R. (1995). *Home health nursing practice, concepts and application* (2nd ed.). St. Louis: Mosby-Year Book.

Scanlon, W. J. (1998, August 6). *Interim payment system for home health agencies.* (GAO Publication Number T-HEHS-98-234). Washington, DC: U.S. Government Printing Office. [On-line]. Available: http://www.gao.gov/reports/html.

Shaughnessy, P., Crisler, K., Schlenker, R., & Hittle, D. (1998). *Medicare's OASIS standardized outcome and assessment information set for home health care, June 1998.* Denver: Center for Health Services and Policy Research.

U.S. Bureau of the Census. (1996). *Resident population of the United States: Middle series projections, 1996–2000, by age and sex.* (Current Population Reports, Series P25-1130, Population Projections of the United States by Age, Sex, Race, and Hispanic Origin: 1995 to 2050). [On-line]. Available: http://www.census.gov/population/projections/nation/nas/ npas9600.txt.

U.S. Department of Health and Human Services, Health Care Financing Administration. (1999). *A profile of Medicare home health chart book* (DHHS Publication No. HCFA-10138). Washington, DC: U.S. Government Printing Office.

■ *Editor's Questions for Discussion*

How has managed care affected the home health care industry? What future legislation may be predicted that will have an impact on home care? What evidence is available regarding cost-effectiveness and quality of care pertaining to home health care? Given that home care and demand has increased, why have the number of agencies providing health care declined? What factors may result in developing more agencies? How does Schroeder and Long's definition of hospice differ from Corless' (Chapter 46)?

How can learning experiences be provided for nursing students in home health care, given agency restrictions? With changes in sites for nursing practice, what implications exist for nursing program curriculum development? Propose ways to integrate community health experiences into nursing curricula. Should community-based experiences and home health care be required at each level of a 4-year nursing program? How might such a requirement alter nursing students' perceptions, the definition of nursing, and nursing values? How can nursing students safely and adequately be supervised by faculty in home care and community health experiences? Propose strategies to increase student interest in home health care and community health nursing. What ethical and legal issues may increase in the future in home care and community health care? See Kopala (Chapter 5), Davis (Chapter 6), and Lane and Paterson (Chapter 7).

How can clinical competencies be developed and evaluated in home health care and community health care? Discuss the application to home health care of the discussions of Jones-Dickson (Chapter 4), Buerhaus (Chapter 10), Purnell (Chapter 37), Stevens and Weiner (Chapter 38), McCausland and McCauley (Chapter 40), Snyder et al. (Chapter 43), Alexander (Chapter 44), Sefcik and Jones (Chapter 48), McDermott (Chapter 49), Pullen (Chapter 50), Barger (Chapter 52), Gerber (Chapter 57), and Conger (Chapter 58).

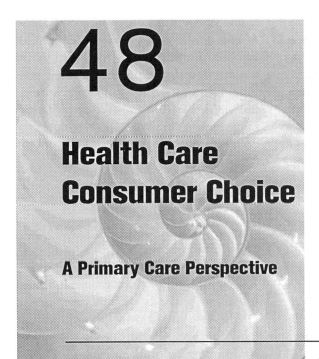

48

Health Care Consumer Choice

A Primary Care Perspective

Elizabeth Sefcik, PhD, RN, CS
Rebecca A. Patronis Jones, DNS, RN,
CNAA

As the health care system becomes more complex, the consumer is faced with an increasing number of product choices and with these choices have come changes in primary health care perspectives. These developments involve increased dissemination of information through health care education materials and one-on-one nursing intervention about medications, activity, exercise, and nutrition.

By making choices about health care the consumer either moves forward on the continuum of being healthy, or if moving away from a healthy lifestyle, the consumer contributes to escalating health care costs while reducing his or her number of productive years. The consumer then contributes to ever-growing pressures on the health care and treatment systems and resources that are available to maintain health.

One focus of the primary care nurse is to evaluate the patient in terms of "Objectives of the Nation" developed by the Office of Disease Prevention and Health Promotion for attainment by the year 2000 (U.S. Department of Health & Human Services [USDHHS], 1992). A summary of these objectives follows. No more than one in five adults and less than 15% of teenagers should be overweight. More than 90% of adults should know the risk factors for cardiovascular disease that can be controlled (i.e., high blood pressure, high blood cholesterol, smoking [the most preventable], and obesity). At least 90% of adults should

587

know their blood pressure reading and have had it checked within the past 2 years. At least one half of all households should purchase foods low in sodium, prepare foods without salt, and not add salt at the table. More than three quarters of overweight people aged 12 or older should adopt weight loss plans combining diet and exercise. At least 85% of teens should link cigarette smoking with great risk to health and also with social disapproval. The exercise goal is three times per week minimum for 20 minutes at a moderate pace. The rationale for this objective is that exercise is of major aid to losing weight, maintaining calcium in bones, and physically benefiting the cardiovascular system.

Progress was made toward achieving these objectives, but fell short. Objectives for 2010 (Maiese & Fox, 1998) now are being formulated. Feedback and suggestions developed from the successes of previous objectives and directions have been provided by all groups of health care professionals in the United States. Healthy People objectives form the basis for primary care nursing practice. Nursing interventions are designed to promote health education and prevention as pertain to nutrition, healthy life styles, and smoking cessation.

This chapter is designed to help both provider and consumer understand that choices made and way of life do make a difference in the quality of life—and in how long a person lives. If the information is convenient and the support system is adequate for the foundation of health and wellness, the consumer is encouraged to make choices for optimum health that will become part of a typical daily routine. The consumer's voice is getting louder, and demands for provider responsiveness will increase. Expectations for better service from insurers will rise as the desire for choice and availability grows. Alternative therapies will be sought in greater numbers, and more information will be accessed electronically. As the shift accelerates from more costly

health delivery settings to home and noninstitutional care, choices will increase further. The purposes of this chapter, therefore, are to review (a) consumer decision-making processes, models, and theories; (b) the technology that supports that decision-making; and (c) the relationship of these two topics to primary care decisions.

■ Decision-Making Models

Several processes and models describe consumer decision-making: (a) the traditional process, (b) nurse assisting a patient in the process, (c) patient decision to change a behavior, and (d) the consumer decision-making process. Jones and Beck (1996) provide a complete review of decision-making models and processes. You should consider each model for its fit with a specific situation before making a selection.

Traditional Decision-Making Process

Readers may be familiar with the five-step process that an individual normally uses to make everyday decisions. First, a problem is identified by analyzing the situation, gathering pertinent facts, and choosing criteria that support achievement of a goal. Next, lists of alternatives or potential solutions are generated. The third step involves selecting one of these alternatives and then, fourth, implementing it. Finally, the outcome is evaluated to assess whether the goal was met.

Assisting a Client with Decision-Making

We have synthesized a five-step client decision-making model from the work of Corcoran (1988) and Gadow (1980) in Jones and

Beck (1996). First, the nurse ensures that information relevant to the situation is available. Next, the client selects items from the information that would help in the decision-making process. Third, the nurse discloses his or her view (i.e., shares personal views and opinions). Fourth, the patient is assisted in determining values for possible alternatives. Last, the nurse helps the client attach personal meaning to the decision. The development of a decision tree with options, the likelihood of events associated with each option, and outcomes of options (considering the client's individual values) helps further clarify the process as the nurse and client work though each step.

Client Decision to Change a Behavior

Often, decision-making in primary care involves the client changing existing behavior. Donatelle, Snow, and Wilcox (1999) assert that, for the majority of people, changing existing behaviors can be a challenge that is met with systematic use of practical strategies. That is, a person must take steps to "own" a behavior after having made a decision to change. They propose the following general steps for helping a person change.

- Set realistic goals.
- Prioritize.
- Identify resources.
- Analyze barriers or potential problems.
- Make a plan.
- Take action and continuously reevaluate.
- Reward small successes and acknowledge setbacks.

By taking these steps, a client may make choices in behaviors that lead to achievement of an optimum balance among the physical, psychological, social, environmental, intellectual, and spiritual domains.

Consumer Decision-Making

Other authors describe a consumer decision-making model (Leemans & Stokman, 1992; Mowen, 1997). It is similar to the traditional decision-making process and involves the following steps: (a) problem recognition, (b) information acquisition, (c) alternative evaluation, (d) choice, (e) purchase, and (f) postacquisition.

Factors Influencing the Decision-Making Process

Several factors may influence the decision-making process. Determinants include lifestyle, society, culture, reference groups, family, and family life cycle (Mowen, 1997). Lifestyle, such as the frequency of travel, would influence the type of personal care products purchased. For example, a housewife might purchase a heavy-duty, bulky hair dryer, whereas the traveling saleswoman might settle for one with less wattage, a lightweight compact style, and battery power. Social groups such as a person's church, corporation, club, fraternity, or sorority might influence choice of clothes. Culture also includes religious beliefs and values, food preferences, language, and views on health. If a culture accepts that obesity is a sign of health, it is difficult for health care providers to influence healthful food choices and consumer eating habits. Family members may be influential in the type of purchases. In some families, both husband and wife work full time outside the home. If the spouse who has less concern for nutrition shops for groceries at lunch time, healthy food choices may not always be made because of time limitations. The family life cycle also may influence decision-making. Families in the child-rearing phase are more likely to purchase certain safety products for the home to prevent toddlers from entering potentially dangerous areas, where elder couples might invest their dollars in improved lighting. The consumer decision-making model influenced by various factors follows a series of sequential steps or stages.

Problem Recognition

In the first phase, the consumer recognizes that a need exists by identifying a discrepancy between the actual and desired state of being. Various situations may cause a need including hunger, poor health, running out of a product, or having a product wear out or break.

Information Acquisition

The second phase consists of searching for information, which may be extensive or limited, depending on the degree of the consumer's involvement. An internal search involves the consumer's attempting to retrieve from long-term memory information about products and services, which may involve brand awareness. An external search involves seeking information from friends, family, advertisements, and written literature about products and services. Searches may be deliberate and occur prepurchase or ongoing to build a store of information for future use.

Alternative Evaluation

The third phase involves evaluating potential solutions to solve the problem or potential purchases that might satisfy a need. During this phase consumers identify specific attributes for a product or service and rank their importance. These rankings are then applied to each alternative. Some consideration would be given to the degree of positiveness or negativeness of each attribute and its potential outcome.

Choice and Purchase

In the fourth phase, the consumer makes a choice about whether to buy or save the money. If the decision is to buy, the decision involves which brand to buy and from what store to buy the product. Then the consumer makes the purchase.

Postacquisition

In the final phase, the consumer uses the product or service purchased and evaluates outcomes based on expectancies. Depending on the nature of the outcomes, the consumer may be satisfied or dissatisfied, leading to brand loyalty and repeat buying behavior if satisfied or to brand avoidance and complaints if dissatisfied. Brand loyalty may advance to brand commitment if emotional or psychological attachment exists. Brand commitment usually occurs with a product that relates to consumer values or needs. The final phase of the postacquisition process is product disposition, in which case the consumer might keep the product for later use, get rid of it permanently, or get rid of it temporarily by renting or loaning it out.

Technology in Consumer Decision-Making

Technology includes modern machines that assist in the primary care decision-making process. Examples are telephones that access prerecorded information and the Internet (Kopf, 1996), cards with magnetic metallic strips similar to credit cards, fax machines, televisions, computers, and audio and video players. Use of the Internet via both computers and television enables clients to (a) communicate with their health care providers, (b) access health information, (c) purchase the latest health care products, (d) check on their latest laboratory tests, (e) fill a prescription, or (f) even locate a health care provider (Federwisch, 1999; Gross, Edmonson, Brull, & Shine, 1995; Menduno, 1998). Imagine placing your thumb on your computer screen and having a pop-up display relay your temperature, heart rate, and blood pressure! Or envision your health maintenance organization (HMO) card containing your health history, diagnoses, current medications, and latest health care provider—all in the magnetic metallic strip on the back of your card! Such information could be available to you (and even updated) at the swipe of the card in a magnetic metallic strip reader.

The trend in technology today is to merge text, images, audio (comprising sound effects, music, and voice), video clips, graphics, and animations into integrated multimedia programs (Jimison & Sher, 1995). Multimedia products can be used to compile, store, and disseminate health care information and instruction programs. The following are examples of such technology. Analog video disk systems store video and still frames and may be purchased as stand alone units or connected to a microcomputer. Some of these systems have interactive components. Compact discs (CDs), audio disks, compact disk read only memory (CD-ROM), and compact disk interactive (CD-I) serve as storage media for databases and textbooks. Photo CDs are used to record photographic images on a compact disk that can be displayed on a television system or used with a CD player or CD-ROM drive on a computer.

The following types of health care information may be available in one of those technological forms. Software products for use on computers and audio and video disk players cover health promotion, health-risk appraisal, emergency and first aid advice, assessment of risks for disease, health care benefits and planning, and nutrition analysis. Many health reference books now are available on disks.

Libraries have computerized databases specifically for health promotion and prevention topics. Other forms of technology are available to assist patients with decision-making concerning treatment options and risky behaviors associated with chronic diseases.

Nurse–Consumer Interaction

"Ask a nurse" may become a popular recommendation for clients needing assistance with decisions concerning the use of technology. Nurses can provide patients with a wealth of information about Internet and prerecorded telephone information on a number of health promotion and education topics. Nurses are involved on a day-to-day basis in assisting the patient, family members, and friends through the decision-making process—whether it is deciding to change a risky behavior or to purchase or learn how to use a new piece of technology to access health information.

Often, patients may access health information and still need further clarification by a nurse or other health care professional. Approximately one of every five clients is functionally illiterate and reads at a fifth grade level or below (Jimison & Sher, 1995). Thus the nurse must be available to assist the patient in the learning process. The nurse also needs to assess the client's understanding of the material presented.

Technology certainly has enhanced the convenience and accessibility of patient information. However, effective patient education also requires interventions by the nurse (Jimison & Sher, 1995). It is not enough simply to provide the client with information. The nurse must include in the care plan activities to encourage the client to participate actively and appropriately in promoting and maintaining health or achieving an optimum level of rehabilitation for a chronic health problem.

■ *Decision-Making in Primary Care*

The methods of delivering primary care are changing rapidly, and there is an urgency to evaluate and adapt to circumstances as they unfold. The most current Institute of Medicine (IOM) (1994) definition of primary care is "the provision of integrated, accessible health care services by clinicians who are accountable for addressing a large majority of personal health care needs, developing a sustained partnership with patients, and practicing in the context of family and community" (p. 4). The public health nurse usually is employed by the local health department and delivers prenatal care and well-baby care, adult primary care, immunizations, health counseling, and home visits. The nurse practitioners in public health deliver antenatal classes, primary care in clinics, and the prescriptive care that is covered by their practice act. In addition, the community health advanced practice nurse specialist delivers primary care to families and the community.

Nutrition and Obesity

Food industry changes have offered the consumer increased choices among both fresh and packaged foods. Perhaps it is now time for the restaurant industry to offer more nutritional food to their public. In an attempt to attract health conscious purchasers, the food industry is making more products available that are low in fat, calories, or sodium. The best exchange of nutritional information occurs in a meeting of experts. Although a registered dietician (RD) admittedly is the nutrition expert, the nurse clinician is an on-site expert with a role in discretionary referral and advancement of recommended nutrition practices. The client is the self-expert in life history, needs, experiences, and barriers to health (Tucket, Boultos, Olson, & Williams, 1985).

Optimal nutrition prevents or delays the onset of many chronic illnesses and serves as therapeutic treatment for others (Harvard Medical School Publications Group, 1994). The American Dietetic Association (ADA) has been in the forefront of nutritional education, but large numbers of clinicians from all disciplines have begun to offer nutritional education; several public health campaigns have been developed around the importance of dietary modification to prevent disease.

A higher prevalence of obesity exists among U.S. women than among men, and despite public health efforts, the incidence of obesity among women has increased in recent years. Data for 1988 through 1994 (Centers for Disease Control [CDC], 1997) showed that 35% of all women aged 20 through 74 were overweight. The prevalence of overweight is highest among younger women, with 8.4% of women aged 25 through 34 gaining more than 30 pounds during a recent 10-year period. There is solid evidence that morbidity increases as weight increases. Statistics also show that the proportion of U.S. men who are overweight rose from 24% in 1988 to 32% in 1991 (Harvard Group, 1994).

In surveying ethnic groups, the prevalence of overweight was highest among African American, non-Hispanic, and Hispanic women and adolescents (CDC, 1997). Overweight adolescents aged 12 through 19 rose from 15% in 1976 to 24% in 1994, an increase of 60%. The Healthy People 2000 target was 15% (USDHHS, 1992).

Exercise

A majority of children in grades 1 through 12 should participate in daily physical education classes. Schools are a key setting to reach children and adolescents, but, unfortunately, no states currently require daily physical education as part of the curriculum and the number of children who participate in daily physical education has declined in recent years. One approach to help increase participation in school physical education might be to broaden the concept of comprehensive school health to include physical education. The proportion of students in grades 9 through 12 who participated in daily physical education declined from 42% in 1991 to 25% in 1995, a decrease of 40% (U.S. Public Health Service [USPHS], 1995a).

Risk Factors

About 30% of the adult population still smoke and many of these people began smoking while teenagers or earlier. Hence involvement of parents is crucial to controlling smoking (Donatelle et al., 1999).

The Community Hypertension Evaluation Clinic Study evaluated 1 million people. It found that hypertension in those who were overweight was 50% to 300% higher than in those who were of normal or low weight (Stamler, 1991). It is estimated that prevention or reversal of obesity would result in a 48% reduction of hypertension among whites and a 28% reduction among African Americans (Slater et al., 1991).

Cholesterol

A Healthy People 2000 recommendation was to reduce blood cholesterol levels of 240 milligrams per deciliter or greater for 20% of adults (USDHHS, 1992). Baseline prevalence for 1976 through 1980 showed that 29% of women had cholesterol levels of 240 or greater (USDHHS, 1992). Only one in four youths met dietary recommendations to reduce fat to 30% or less of total calories consumed and saturated fat to less than 10% of total calories consumed.

Primary sources of cholesterol in diet intakes are meats and dairy products. Consumers need information on how to replace consumption of medium- and high-fat beef and pork with lower fat beef, pork, poultry, and fish. Restaurant menus need to contain number of calories and saturated fat information.

Other Risk Factors

Certain risk factors are associated with increased susceptibility to illness and premature death, such as obesity, smoking, and lack of exercise, which already were discussed. These conditions and behaviors also interfere with a high level of wellness. Each American needs to assess the likely consequences to these conditions and behaviors and decide whether to make lifestyle changes to overcome them.

External Factors

Individuals who are educationally, socioeconomically, or otherwise disadvantaged often have difficulty adopting a primary care lifestyle. Mortality rates for the working poor, for minority groups, and for the elderly on fixed incomes in comparison to white middle- and upper-class Americans demonstrate that the United States has an unequal system for promoting health and wellness (USDHHS, 1995b).

All these external factors play a significant role in determining whether a person is predisposed, reinforced, or enabled to make positive behavioral changes; however, the client's own actions or lack of actions represent perhaps the single greatest influence on overall health and wellness.

■ Scenario

The following scenario illustrates an application of decision-making models. Mr. M. is a 50-year-old Hispanic and the owner of a small business—a corner grocery store in his community in south Texas. He smokes two packs of cigarettes per day, drinks a six pack of Carolla beer every two days, has no exercise or leisure sports in his daily lifestyle, and eats three meals per day that are high in cholesterol and calories. Mr. M is 25 pounds over his ideal body weight. Both of his parents died in their sixties from cardiovascular disease. His wife, Mrs. M, works by his side in the grocery business as accountant and bookkeeper. Both value health and long life and are aware that their lifestyle may not reflect those values. Mr. M wants to consult the neighborhood "curandisimo" (folk medicine man) for a quick cure. Mrs. M talks him into keeping his appointment with the nurse at the family practice clinic to discuss his health.

Nurse N helps the family, using the following decision-making processes and models. In exploring factors contributing to hypertension, Nurse N and the Ms agree that Mr. M needs to change his smoking and exercise behavior and develop a diet plan. The model for client decision-making is used. Mr. M sets a goal to decrease smoking to one pack per day in the next month and zero packs per day by the end of 6 months. His exercise goal is to exercise for 30 minutes three times per week in the first month and take up golf, using a rolling cart, as a leisure sport one time per week by the end of 6 months. Stopping smoking is prioritized as the primary goal. Nurse M provides the Ms with a videotape, containing weekly exercise ideas, and a prescription for nicotine patches along with a referral to a support group for people who trying to quit smoking. Barriers identified include the grocery store hours. The Ms create a plan for a worker to cover 30 minutes in the morning so that they may have exercise time and one evening per week for attendance at the smoking support group. Nurse N schedules a return visit in 2 weeks to help them evaluate this plan. If the goals for Month 1 have been achieved, Mr. M's reward will be to buy a new set of golf clubs.

Next, the team (nurse and family) uses the consumer decision-making process to develop a diet plan. As there is a discrepancy between a desired state, healthy lifestyle, and the actual state, hypertension, they move to the information acquisition phase. Nurse N helps the Ms search for information about the disease on the Internet. First, they visit the American Heart Association (AHA) Web site on hypertension and print out information about hypertension and client self-help with regard to risk factors. Either the American Dietetic Association (ADA) Web site or referral for a Registered Dietician (RD) consultation might well be selected as a resource regarding diets. Three diet plans were reviewed and the producers were contacted.

The M's contacted Hearty Heart of Healthy Heart. They evaluated three facsimile type of diets that could be called: Life Choice, Susy Slim, and Calorie Counters. In evaluating the three alternatives, the Ms used cost, time involved, and social support, weighted in that order. The Life Choice plan was lowest in price because Mr. M received a grocery owner's discount and no extra time was involved so they selected that plan. Time saved in food preparation could be spent on exercise. The Calorie Counters plan included a social support group, but Nurse N explained that some support would also be available through the smokers support group. Thus the social support attribute was less important in the decision. The Ms' satisfaction with the Life Choice plan was so great that they agreed not only to continue the plan for weight maintenance, but also to include a special display in the grocery store, featuring Mexican food meal plans. At the end of 6 months, Mr. M had stopped smoking. Exercise and the Life Choice food plan had become a part of the Ms' daily routine. Mr. M had lost 15 pounds and was able to go on a lower dose antihypertensive medication. Both the Ms and Nurse N were pleased with their implementation of the consumer decision-making process in controlling Mr. M's hypertension.

■ Concluding Statement

Consumer decision-making and the role of the nurse in relation to individuals and families making decisions regarding primary care issues have been presented. Factors influencing the decision-making process were addressed. The influence of technology on the availability of health care information is prevalent. Adequate nutrition and exercise are dominant concerns for Healthy People 2000. The nurse, as viewed in the scenario presented, may facilitate consumer goals for health far beyond 2000.

■ References

Centers for Disease Control. (1997). NHANES III, Third National Health and Nutrition Examination Survey—Update: Prevalence of overweight among children, adolescents, and adults—United States, 1988–1994. *MMWR Morbidity & Mortality Weekly Report, 46*(7), 199–202.

Corcoran, S. (1988). Toward operationalizing an advocacy role. *Journal of Professional Nursing, 4*(4), 242–248.

Donatelle, R., Snow, C., & Wilcox, A. (1999). *Wellness: Choices for health and fitness* (2nd ed.). Boston: Wadsworth.

Federwisch, A. (1999). Clickscriptions: Are online pharmacies ethical. *Health Week, 4*(3), 1, 8.

Gadow, S. (1980). Existential advocacy: Philosophical foundation of nursing. In S. Spikes and S. Gadow (Eds.). *Nursing images and ideals* (pp. 79–101). New York: Springer-Verlag.

Gross, N., Edmonson, G., Brull, S., & Shine, E. (1995, November 20). Payoff time at Thompson? *Business Week,* 110, 114.

Harvard Medical School Health Publications Group. (1994). Losing weight: A new attitude emerges. *Harvard Heart Letter, 4*(7), 1–6.

Institute of Medicine. (1994). *Defining primary care: An interim report.* Washington, DC: National Academy Press, 1994.

Jimison, H. B., & Sher, P. P. (1995). Consumer health informatics: Health information technology for consumers. *Journal of the American Society for Information Science, 46*(10), 783–790.

Jones, R. A. P., & Beck, S. E. (1996). Decision making in nursing. Albany, NY: Delmar.

Kopf, D. (1996). Emerging technology. *America's Network, 100*(12), 108, 110, 114.

Leemans, H., & Stokman, M. (1992). A descriptive model of the decision-making process of buyers of books. *Journal of Cultural Economics, 16*(2), 25–50.

Maiese, D. R., & Fox, C. E. (1998). *Laying the Foundation for Healthy People 2010—The First Year of Consultation.* [On-line]. Available: http://web.health.gov/healthypeople/2010article.htm.

Menduno, M. 1998. Prognosis: Wired. *Hospitals & Health Networks, 72*(21), 28–35.

Mowen, J. C. (1997). *Consumer behavior.* Upper Saddle River, NJ: Prentice-Hall.

Slater, E. E., Dustan, H. P., Grimm, Jr., R. H., Kotchen, T. A., Landsberg, L., McCarron, D. A., Oberman, A., Reed, J., Stamler, J., & Tobian, L. (1991). Metabolic and nutritional factors in hypertension. *Hypertension, 18* (1 suppl), 1–21.

Stamler, J. (1991). Blood pressure and high blood pressure: Aspects of risk. *Hypertension,* *18*(1 suppl), 95–107

Tucket, D., Boultos, M., Olson C., & Williams, A. (1985). *Meeting between experts.* New York: Tavistock.

U.S. Department of Health and Human Services, Public Health Service. (1992). *Healthy People 2000: National health promotion and disease prevention objectives.* Boston: Jones & Bartlett.

U.S. Department of Health and Human Services, Public Health Service. (1995a). *Healthy People 2000: Midcourse review and 1995 revisions.* Hyattsville, MD: Author.

U.S. Department of Health and Human Services, Public Health Service. (1995b). *United States health and preventive profile.* Hyattsville, MD: Author.

■ Editor's Questions for Discussion

Identify common consumer health problems that require decisions made by the health care consumer (client). Apply decision-making models presented by Sefcik and Jones to formulate a decision about health behavior for each identified problem. What factors influenced your decision-making process? Apply decision-making models to consumers making decisions about obtaining primary health care and services. Which decision-making model may be more effective than the others and why?

Discuss the use of technology in consumer decision-making. What ethical implications exist in using technologies described by Sefcik and Jones? How can consumers be assured that accessed health information is valid, reliable, and appropriate for their needs? How do consumers evaluate health information? What type of patient education is essential for the diverse and multiple technologies available?

Discuss the role of nurses in providing health education. Provide strategies to reach large numbers of consumers, increase consumers' knowledge of risk factors, and promote compliance with health education suggestions. How can positive changes in health behavior be maintained and sustained? Discuss strategies to increase motivational variables. Which motivational variables are most effective for long-term change? Which factor is the best predictor?

49

Parish Nursing

When the Population Served Is a Congregation

Mary Ann McDermott, PhD, RN, FAAN

The focus of practice for parish nursing is the faith community and its health ministry. The health promotion and disease prevention role of the parish nurse does not regularly include invasive practices. The promotion of whole person health is conducted through seven role activities, most recently referred to in the literature as functions: health educator, personal health counselor, referral agent, trainer of volunteers, developer of support groups, health advocate, and the most distinctive function—integrator of faith and health (McDermott & Burke, 1993; Solari-Twadell, 1999).

■ The History of Parish Nursing

The history of nursing, Donahue (1985) states, "first becomes continuous with the beginning of Christianity" (p. 93). The roots of parish nursing are entwined quite specifically with those of deacons and deaconesses in the early church, later with monks and nuns who cared for the sick and the poor, and then with Lutheran deaconesses in the United States (Egenes, 1999). The individual most influential in developing and promoting the concept of whole person health, facilitated by nurses in churches, was the late Granger Westberg. An ordained Lutheran minister, Westberg and a group of colleagues in the Department of Preventive Medicine and Community Health at the University of Illinois College of Medicine, in a project cosponsored with the W. K. Kellogg Foundation, developed a number of holistic health centers in churches during the late 1960s (Westberg, 1999). Physicians, nurses, and clergy worked collaboratively to render care to the whole person. Although the 10-year evaluation of this project was quite favorable, inflation dictated a new, less costly, model of care delivery. The spiritually oriented nurse was seen as the bridge, the translator, who assisted the physician's and minister's communication with the patient.

In 1984, Westberg approached the leadership of Lutheran General Hospital, Park Ridge, Illinois, a northwest suburb of Chicago, with a plan to initiate the first institutionally based parish nurse program. Six congregations (four Protestant and two Roman Catholic) were sought out and agreed to participate in a trial that held the churches increasingly financially responsible for the nurses' 20-hour a week salary over a 3-year period. The preparation and ongoing professional development of these first six parish nurses is described by Westberg (1999).

The idea of nurses working in congregations, salaried or as volunteers, grew rapidly in Chicagoland and spread through the Midwest. The National Parish Nurse Resource Center and an Advisory Board were established and sponsored by the Congregational Health Partnership Program of the Lutheran General Health System. Ann Solari-Twadell was named Director of the Center, which also served to educate interested congregations from across the United States about the idea of parish nursing and to orient prospective or newly employed parish nurses to the role. The Center has continued to monitor and enhance the growth and development of the movement, studying organizational models, functions,

educational preparation, and denominational affiliations of parish nurses (Lloyd & Solari-Twadell, 1994).

A large number of congregations in rural Iowa committed to this new nursing role soon after hearing presentations by Westberg. Well documented by Striepe (1990) are the work of (a) Jan Burg, RN; (b) St. Luke's Regional Medical Center in Sioux City, Iowa; (c) development of a rural parish nurse network and a Kellogg 3-year parish nurse grant project, under the leadership of nurse Jan Striepe and the Northwest Aging Association; and (d) initiation of a Minister of Health Education and Intern program under direction of Chaplain David Carlson of Iowa Lutheran Hospital in Des Moines.

Some 100 nurses, clergy, and others interested in this new ministry attended the second Annual Westberg Parish Nurse Symposium held in September 1988 at Lutheran General Hospital. The Parish Nurse Resource Center Advisory Board sponsored a session to explore establishment of a separate membership organization. Open to all those interested in Health Ministry—nurses, clergy, educators, social workers, physical therapists, and others—the Health Ministries Association was born.

■ The Current Practice of Parish Nursing

The individual practicing in the Parish Nurse role may be referred to in a specific congregation as Health Minister, Congregational Health Nurse, Pastoral Nurse or Faith Community Nurse. Congregation Nurse, Kallilah (Community) Nurse, or Shul Nurse are terms deemed more appropriate in Judaism (Chase-Ziolek & Holst, 1999). The original institutionally based, salaried group of six parish nurses practicing in Chicagoland has expanded to approximately 3,000 institutionally or congregationally based salaried or unpaid parish nurses internationally (personal communication with Center Staff Person, International Parish Nurse Resource Center [IPNRC], April 6, 1999). The change in name from National Parish Resource Center to International Parish Resource Center in 1996 came about for good reason! The concept of parish nursing had been introduced in Alberta, Canada, in 1993. A major commitment to an interdisciplinary approach to parish nursing education was initiated at the University of Alberta (Olson, Clark, & Simington, 1999). However, North America's experience of parish nursing in its entirety was not transferable to Australia. Van Loon (1999) described her work in establishing an ongoing relationship with the IPNRC in 1995. She adapted the parish nursing concept in establishing a Faith Community Nursing demonstration project with 10 congregations, developing an association of Australian Faith Community Nurses and offering basic educational preparation courses for nurses. Moreover, nurses from Korea, England, and Ireland interested in initiating parish nursing, have attended the Westberg Symposium in recent years.

The practice of the parish nurse is a collaborative one. The nurse collaborates with the congregation as a whole and with parishioners individually. Parish nurses collaborate with other parish nurses in small geographic areas and, more recently, throughout the world. Members of each Health Cabinet are collaborative partners with all members of the parish staff and physicians in the community (Joesten, 1999; Kirschner, 1999; Lloyd & Ludwig-Beymer, 1999; Ludwig-Beymer & Sarran, 1999; Nelson, 1999). An outstanding contribution to the parish nurse's understanding of the parish as a system—with all the challenges of communication, power, and conflict that tend to frustrate collaborative efforts—are described by Fite (1999) in *The Congregation as a Workplace*.

Functions of the Parish Nurse

Seven functions constitute the parish nurse role: health educator, personal health counselor, referral agent and liaison with congregational and community resources, trainer of volunteers, developer of support groups, health advocate, and integrator of faith and health.

Health Educator

Health education is carried out both formally and informally with individuals and groups, with young children, adults, and seniors. Teaching of the congregation and wider community is done in church, in the nurse's office, in the parish school, at Rotary Club meetings, at Area Agency on Aging Seminars, on grocery store bulletin boards, at homeless shelters, at meal sites for the elderly, and in weekly or monthly parish bulletin articles submitted by the nurse or members of the health cabinet or advisory committee. Education accompanies all planned health promotion and disease prevention activities.

Personal Health Counselor

Individual health counseling often is conducted in conjunction with health education, health promotion, and screening activities. Requests for assistance with a very specific mental, physical, or spiritual health concern, however, are often initiated by individual parishioners or their families. Coping with and managing chronic illness, medication regimes, postpartum depression, acceptance and reconciliation with an adult child with HIV, crisis intervention, grief, decision-making about long-term care for an elderly parent, and loss of a pregnancy are among requests received by the parish nurse.

Referral Agent and Liaison with Congregational and Community Resources

The parish nurse is likely to be involved in numerous activities. Among them are assistance with transportation to church or a doctor's appointment, a request for a friendly visitor from the congregation or meals on wheels from the city; connecting and coordinating with other church sponsored ministries (i.e., Stephen, Elizabeth, or BeFrienders); referral to home health or hospice care; and offering church facilities as a site for a 12-step program or an after school care service.

Trainer of Volunteers

The parish nurse often collaborates in training sponsored by other congregations or community volunteer groups. In addition, the nurse serves as a consultant and support to volunteers and helps them to reflect on their gifts and on their service as an avenue to spiritual growth.

Developer of Support Groups

A wide variety of support-group offerings are evident in parish nurse practice. Caregiver support groups are described most often in the literature. Others include, but are not limited to, bereavement, breast cancer survivors, sexual abuse, and chronic pain support groups.

Health Advocate

Evident early in development of the parish nurse role but only recently specifically addressed in literature is the parish nurse function of health advocate. Linked initially with activities of the referral agent and community resource liaison, the health advocate function has expanded and incorporated its activities on behalf of the entire congregation and of the larger community. These advocacy activities are in addition to those that are more traditionally associated with individuals and their families.

Integrator of Faith and Health

Both the Old and New Testaments reflect health and healing as a central ministry of the faith community. Congregations that commit to parish nursing, for the most part, see their church as a "health place" in the community. The most distinctive function of parish nursing is to help parishioners recognize and link their faith and health. The parish nurse works in a context where certain meanings are not only allowed, but are expected to be articulated explicitly. The parish nurse contributes to the sacramental and liturgical life of the faith community, which has the potential to enhance a deeper understanding and integration of faith and health.

Summary: Diversity

Diversity in implementation of these seven functions is evident in current practice. A review of the recent literature on parish nursing suggests that only one or two of the functions often are being emphasized in an individual parish nurse practice rather than the entire array (Biddix & Brown, 1999; McDermott & Burke, 1993; Solari-Twadell, 1999). Needs and expectations of the congregation, the education and experience of the nurse, and the amount of time (hours per week) allotted to the position appear to contribute to variation in practice.

Education

One of the variables affecting practice, education of the parish nurse, has changed considerably during the past decade. Because of the autonomy inherent in this community health role, a minimum requirement of a baccalaureate degree in nursing for the position has been recommended for some time (McDermott & Burke, 1993). Studies conducted periodically suggest that individuals practicing in this role have a variety of formal educational backgrounds—diploma through doctoral degree. The level of preparation has continued to increase, however, not always with an emphasis on a degree in nursing. Coursework in education, theology, and pastoral care is evident.

First attempts at orienting interested individuals (nurses, clergy, and lay leaders) to the parish nurse role were made by the Lutheran General Health System. Its Resource Center originally began offering both educational programming and consultation. Two and one-half day "Orientation to Parish Nursing" continuing education programs for nurses, which included a half-day accompaniment with a parish nurse, comprised the initial offering. Today, the system's International Parish Nurse Resource Center (IPNRC, 1999) makes available a wide variety of educational opportunities throughout the United States for those interested in becoming a parish nurse. Most are sponsored by health care institutions—others through regional parish nurse networks, congregational, or denominational sponsors at the national level. An increasing number of programs are university-based, primarily through schools of nursing, but several are based in or linked with a seminary. Prior to 1998 no educational program existed to prepare parish nurse coordinators, a management role that has emerged, which serves as a liaison between congregations and cosponsoring institution(s) in the community

The increase in university credit-bearing offerings is due primarily to an IPNRC–sponsored project that began in 1994, with an invitational colloquium on the development of guidelines for parish nurse education (Solari-Twadell, McDermott, Ryan, & Djupe, 1994).

Following this event was a series of surveys of parish nurses and parish nurse coordinators, who identified essential content for parish nurses and for a coordinator role. Recommendations for content experts from across the United States to develop curriculum modules on identified topics also were subsequently solicited. This assessment served as basis for a 3-year collaborative development and implementation project among Marquette University, Loyola University–Chicago, and the IPNRC (McDermott, Solari-Twadell, & Matheus, 1998). In April 1997, experts, who had developed curriculum modules in their respective content areas and who had reviewed the modules developed by other experts, were invited to a second colloquium. The content experts were joined by representatives from the American Nurses Association and the National League for Nursing, several leading nurse educators from the United States, and parish nurse coordinators from Canada and Australia. The assembled group validated and endorsed both a basic parish nurse and a parish nurse coordinator curriculum. These curricula were then evaluated in pilot programs over the following 12 months. To ensure a measure of uniformity in teaching this content and experiencing the process dimensions of such coursework, a week-long preparation session for university or university-linked faculty was offered initially in June 1998 and repeated in June 1999—both enthusiastically received. Participants received copies of the curricula and, in turn, could market their offering of coursework as that endorsed by the Resource Center.

Accountability

Accountability for parish nurses should be the same for those who are unpaid as for those who are paid. There should be no distinctions in this regard. When a congregation enters into an agreement to place a nurse on parish staff, the position description should address the important matter of accountability: for what, of what, to whom, and the manner in which the nurse will be accountable. However, that is not now always done (McDermott, 1999; McDermott & Burke, 1993).

Documentation of parish nursing practice is an essential component of accountability. Although acknowledging that documentation is a professional responsibility, both parish nurses and clergy often struggle with perceived value versus legal imperative. Many feel that documentation is constraining and takes valuable time away from providing services.

The Lutheran General Health System (LGHS) in collaboration with Trinity Regional Health System (Trinity) of Moline, Illinois, was awarded a large "Partners in Health and Healing" W. K. Kellogg grant in 1994 to develop an infrastructure for parish nursing that included a documentation system. These two systems, serving a primarily urban and suburban population (LGHS) and a mainly rural population (Trinity), together supported 77 paid and unpaid parish nurses. A decision was made by the nurses and grant staff to adopt a record-keeping system that reflects the North American Nursing Diagnosis Association (NANDA) and Nursing Intervention Classification (NIC) languages. Computer software was identified and purchased to facilitate this form of documentation in both the LGHS and Trinity health care systems. Descriptions of the project, detailed accounts of the process, and reports of the lessons learned from the experience are reported elsewhere (Burkhart & Kellen, 1999; Johnson, Ludwig-Beymer, & Micek, 1999). Those publications also included proposed spiritual, religious, community, and interpersonal diagnoses and interventions unique to parish nursing. These proposals were forwarded to the University of Iowa's NDEC and NIC teams for inclusion in their respective national classification systems and the identification of Core Parish Nurse Interventions.

■ Parish Nursing in the 21st Century: Challenges and Opportunities

Infrastructure

Will parish nursing be not only viable but vital during the 21st century? Interest continues to grow in alternative and complementary health care practices and systems of care, and credibility of many of their outcomes is being recognized. In addition, attention given in the media and by curricula in respected nursing and medical schools to whole-person health bodes well for development and expansion of parish nursing. With increasing national concern for health care costs, focus on wellness and toward limited in-patient stays, and creation of integrated delivery systems, it appears parish nurses have potential for a prominent role in the changing health care system. Maybe!

Creation of an infrastructure to support parish nursing in an organization and in the community will be vital to success. The basic necessities are (a) appropriate placement and reporting relationships within an organization; (b) leadership, sponsorship, and advisory staff that are committed to the program; (c) financial support for salaries and operating budgets that are fair and just; and (d) educational resources including an interdisciplinary faculty and legal assistance. For parish nursing to flourish, information systems that support access to patient and parishioner information across sites in an integrated delivery system will need enhancement. Assistance with public relations and community outreach, as well as facilitation by a foundation or development fund-raising staff, will become crucial elements to ongoing success of a parish nurse program.

How will parish nursing be funded? Volunteer, unpaid nurses are contributing professional services in generous fashion at the turn of the century. Is this just? Should other professionals be expected to donate their services to their congregations? Certainly, but usually on a sporadic rather than on a regular daily or weekly schedule. Even those parish nurses who practice on a part-time paid basis admit that they often are actually working a full-time position.

Will health care institutions, especially those with church sponsorship or a church-related heritage, come forward and recognize parish nursing as an excellent example of "Mission in Action" or at least a way to maintain their community benefit, 501-C-3 Not For Profit status? Could a source of endowment for parish nursing come from gains realized from the sale of a hospital in a community? Are foundations that already have been formed to distribute monies from these sources aware of parish nursing? What would happen if large congregations or even denominations on a citywide or national level formed their own health maintenance organizations and employed parish nurses as care and case managers?

Differentiated Nursing Practice

As already noted, there is diversity in parish nursing and how its seven functions are implemented in practice settings. As positive as this diversity might at first appear, disparity potentially may create confusion in the public as to the nature of the parish nurse's role. Are all nurses who contribute time to their church in effect parish nurses who assist parishioners in acknowledging the relationship between faith and health in their lives? Many nurses, paid or unpaid, may provide several hours a month to blood pressure screening or 20 to 40 hours a week educating, counseling, coordinating volunteers, developing support groups, making numerous referrals, and advocating system change. Are they then to be classified "parish

nurses"? What about the nurse practitioner who starts a practice in a church setting?

Different levels of education bring different and unique gifts. There is plenty of God's work to do! All should be welcome; however, to stimulate thinking, Solari-Twadell (1999) suggested that now is the time to explore differentiation of nursing practice in the context of the faith community, and she proposed seven different role descriptions and titles.

Credentialing Issues

Parish nursing was designated a specialty at the American Nurses Association's Congress for Practice in February 1997 (American Nurses Association [ANA], 1997). This action was closely followed by approval of a "Scope of Practice" statement and acknowledgment of the "Standard of Parish Nursing Practice" in February 1998, as developed in 1996 and forwarded by the Health Ministries Association as a professional organization representing parish nurses (ANA & Health Ministries Association [HMA], 1998). Although there is difference of opinion as to appropriateness of their action, the scope and standards statements are now widely available and, for the most part, have been accepted.

Accreditation of educational offerings and certification, as a voluntary credential, appear to be the next steps in credentialing of parish nurses. The cost of developing and administering a valid, reliable test and maintaining test security for a specialty exam is estimated by the American Nurses Credentialing Center (ANCC) to be $100,000 (personal communication, C. K. Lewis, director, August 20, 1999). At present, credentialing does not appear to be a priority of the ANA, HMA, or IPNRC. Small (1999) urges parish nurses to seek certification in other specialties for which they might qualify, to demonstrate commitment to excellence and to provide consumer and employer with a benchmark of provider competency.

The relationship of the IPNRC to other professional organizations will be a challenge and an opportunity to move forward. The Health Ministries Association, as a multidisciplinary organization, has its roots in the center. The Director of the Center, Solari-Twadell, has served on its Advisory Board for some time; however, the relationships have been strained. The Advisory Board has seldom been consulted on major issues, such as the process used for development and subsequent submission of the "Scope and Standards" to the ANA. Some believe that the HMA is not the professional organization for parish nurses, but no alternative exists at this time. Representatives of the ANA and NLN attended the endorsement colloquium for Basic Parish Nurse and Parish Nurse Coordinator curricula. What did their signing an endorsement document signify? Which organization will or should facilitate accreditation of parish nurse curricula in the future? How might the Center and parish nursing relate to associations, organizations, and interest groups of Community Health and Ambulatory Care Nurses, as well as to the American Public Health Association?

Scholarship

The need for research and publication in the area of parish nursing practice is widely acknowledged. Several dozen master's theses and doctoral dissertations, primarily descriptive studies of parish nursing, have been completed in recent years. The W. K. Kellogg Foundation has been a generous funder of many start-up projects and demonstration grants to congregations and health systems throughout the United States. Articles describing the concept of parish nursing, parish nurs-

ing education, or a particular parish nurse practice have appeared in nursing and religious studies literature and in other health-related journals. How will the book on *Parish Nursing* published recently by Sage (Solari-Twadell & McDermott, 1999) be received and used in nursing programs? Does the book have a future in seminary education in this country and abroad? Scholarship that addresses making a difference and accountability is sorely needed. The increase in attention to documentation of interventions and outcomes on a national level, using a common nursing language, will facilitate the collection of data.

How can the concept of parish nursing be implemented in other countries throughout the world? The Canadian and Australian experiences (Olson, Clark, & Simington, 1999; Van Loon, 1999) provide evidence that, with certain modifications, the practice can be adapted culturally in other countries. This progress needs to be documented systematically. The literature contains descriptions of how parish nursing is implemented in different locales in United States (urban, suburban, and rural), by several different denominations, and with different ethnic populations. However, comparative studies have not commenced, and these would provide a rich avenue for future research.

■ Concluding Statement

The future viability and vitality of parish nursing depends on, and resides in, the ability of parish nurse practitioners to implement and articulate distinctiveness in their "integrator of faith and health" role. At the turn of this new century, both the profession and society appear receptive. It will be up to the parish nurse to deliver the promise!

References

American Nurses Association. (1997, February). *Congress for Practice Meeting.* Washington, DC: Author.

American Nurses Association & Health Ministries Association. (1998). *Scope and standards of parish nursing practice.* Washington, DC: American Nurses Association Publications; Ramona, CA: Health Ministries Association.

Biddix, V., & Brown, H. N. (1999). Establishing a parish nursing program. *Nursing and Health Care Perspectives, 20,* 72–75.

Burkhart, L., & Kellen, P. (1999). Proposed diagnoses and interventions. In P. A. Solari-Twadell & M. A. McDermott (Eds.), *Parish nursing, promoting whole person health within faith communities* (pp. 258–267). Thousand Oaks, CA: Sage.

Chase-Ziolek, M., & Holst, L. E. (1999). Parish nursing in diverse traditions. In P. A. Solari-Twadell & M. A. McDermott (Eds.), *Parish nursing, promoting whole person health within faith communities* (pp. 195–204). Thousand Oaks, CA: Sage.

Donahue, M. (1985). *Nursing: The finest art.* St. Louis: Mosby.

Egenes, K. (1999). *"Reasonable service" in a divided community: The work of Lutheran deaconess nurses in the Norwegian immigrant community of Chicago, 1891–1930.* Unpublished manuscript.

Fite, R. C. (1999). The congregation as a workplace. In P. A. Solari-Twadell & M. A. McDermott (Eds.), *Parish nursing, promoting whole person health within faith communities* (pp. 123–133). Thousand Oaks, CA: Sage.

International Parish Nurse Resource Center. (1999). Available: 205 Tuohy Avenue, Suite 104, Park Ridge, IL 60068.

Joesten, L. (1999). Team ministry in the congregation. In P. A. Solari-Twadell & M. A. McDermott (Eds.), *Parish nursing, promoting whole person health within faith communities* (pp. 135–143). Thousand Oaks, CA: Sage.

Johnson, B., Ludwig-Beymer, P., & Micek, W. T. (1999). Documenting the practice. In P. A. Solari-Twadell & M. A. McDermott (Eds.), *Parish nursing, promoting whole person health within faith communities* (pp. 233–245). Thousand Oaks, CA: Sage.

Kirschner, G. (1999). Parish nurse and physician relationship in serving the congregation. In P. A. Solari-Twadell & M. A. McDermott (Eds.), *Parish nursing, promoting whole person health within faith communities* (pp. 145–150). Thousand Oaks, CA: Sage.

Lloyd, R., & Ludwig-Beymer, P. (1999). Listening to faith communities: Collaboration with those served. In P. A. Solari-Twadell & M. A. McDermott (Eds.), *Parish nursing, promoting whole person health within faith communities* (pp. 107–121). Thousand Oaks, CA: Sage.

Lloyd, R., & Solari-Twadell, P. A. (1994). Organizational framework, functions and educational preparation of parish nurses: National survey 1991 and 1994. In *Proceedings of eighth annual Westberg symposium: Ethics and values: A framework for parish nursing practice* (pp. 105–115). Park Ridge, IL: National Parish Nurse Resource Center.

Ludwig-Beymer, P., & Sarran, H. S. (1999). Parish nurse–physician partnership: A continuum of care. In P. A. Solari-Twadell & M. A. McDermott (Eds.), *Parish nursing, promoting whole person health within faith communities* (pp. 151–160). Thousand Oaks, CA: Sage.

McDermott, M. A. (1999). Accountability and rationale. In P. A. Solari-Twadell & M. A. McDermott (Eds.), *Parish nursing, promoting whole person health within faith communities* (pp. 227–232). Thousand Oaks, CA: Sage.

McDermott, M. A., & Burke, J. (1993). When the population is a congregation: The emerging role of the parish nurse. *Journal of Community Health Nursing, 10*(3), 179–190.

McDermott, M. A., Solari-Twadell, P. A. & Matheus, R. (1998, January-February). Promoting quality education for the parish nurse and parish nurse coordinator. *Nursing and Health Care Perspectives, 19,* 4–6.

Nelson, G. (1999). Pastoral reflections. In P. A. Solari-Twadell & M. A. McDermott (Eds.), *Parish nursing, promoting whole person health within faith communities* (pp. 161–167). Thousand Oaks, CA: Sage.

Olson, J. K., Clark, M. B., & Simington, J. A. (1999). The Canadian experience. In P. A. Solari-Twadell & M. A. McDermott (Eds.), *Parish nursing, promoting whole person health within faith communities* (pp. 277–286). Thousand Oaks, CA: Sage.

Small, N. R. (1999). Professional credentialing for parish nurses. *Connections, Information & Contacts for The Health Ministries Association, 99*(2), 6.

Solari-Twadell, P. A. (1999). Nurses in churches: Differentiation of the practice. In P. A. Solari-Twadell & M. A. McDermott (Eds.), *Parish nursing, promoting whole person health within faith communities* (pp. 249–256). Thousand Oaks, CA: Sage.

Solari-Twadell, P. A., & McDermott, M. A. (1999). *Parish nursing, promoting whole person health within faith communities*. Thousand Oaks, CA: Sage.

Solari-Twadell, P. A., McDermott, M. A., Ryan, J. A., & Djupe, A. M. (1994). *Assuring viability for the future: Guideline development for parish nurse education programs*. Park Ridge, IL: Lutheran General Health System.

Striepe, J. (1990). The developing practice of the parish nurse: A rural experience. In P. A. Solari-Twadell, A. M. Djupe, & M. A. McDermott (Eds.), *Parish nursing: The developing practice*. Park Ridge: IL: Lutheran General Health System.

Van Loon, A. M. (1999). The Australian concept of faith community. In P. A. Solari-Twadell & M. A. McDermott (Eds.), *Parish nursing, promoting whole person health within faith communities* (pp. 287–298). Thousand Oaks, CA: Sage.

Westberg, G. (1999). A personal historical perspective of whole person health and the congregation. In P. A. Solari-Twadell & M. A. McDermott (Eds.). *Parish nursing, promoting whole person health within faith communities* (pp. 35–41). Thousand Oaks, CA: Sage.

■ Editor's Questions for Discussion

Define parish nursing and parish nursing practice. How does differentiated practice in nursing apply? What planning, development, and implementation are necessary for parish nursing to be established? How are parish nursing centers evaluated? Propose systematic research that should be undertaken. Identify distinctive ethical issues that may be of concern in parish nursing. What criteria should exist for members of a parish health cabinet or advisory committee? What distinctive infrastructure and accountability issues exist in parish nursing? What should be the educational preparation for a parish nurse? Identify specific curricula essential for parish nursing. How does advanced practice addressed by Gray (Chapter 42) apply? What accreditation criteria may be distinctive for evaluation of parish nursing programs?

How might parish nurses collaborate with nurse entrepreneurs and nursing centers? Apply content from Barger (Chapter 52) and Duffy (Chapter 53). Address questions raised by McDermott about funding for parish nursing. What impact may parish nursing HMOs have for health care delivery systems?

What parish nurse applications may be made to rural and underserved health care areas as described by Todero (Chapter 51) and Pullen (Chapter 50). What alterations or accommodations may be necessary in roles of parish nurses for areas where health care services are limited? How may integrated care systems as presented by Pinkerton (Chapter 56) apply to parish nursing? What informatics issues (Stevens and Weiner, Chapter 38) should be of particular concern to parish nurses?

What is the relationship between the IPNRC and the ANA? What lessons have previously been learned by professional nursing organizations in developing relationships with other interested organizations? How should those experiences be applied to affiliations between the IPNRC, ANA, and HMA?

50

Issues in
Rural Health Care

Carol H. Pullen, EdD, RN

Many rural areas have for years experienced problems in obtaining adequate health care. Various strategies have been employed to address the issues of health care, along with related problems of economics and geographic access. As the Office of Technology Assessment (OTA) (1991) pointed out, "Although often isolated and remote, America's rural communities do not exist in a vacuum. They will inevitably change as the world around them changes" (p. 5). Understanding the characteristics of rural populations and communities will provide a backdrop for rural nurses to provide leadership at the local, state, and national levels in efforts to ensure that health care is available, acceptable, and accessible. Recent and emerging technological advances will play a dramatic role in changing the way rural residents live and work, and the way health care is provided and received.

■ The Rural Setting

Defining Rural

There is no single definition of *rural*. Which definition is used can make a significant difference in the way demographic and health data are presented. I begin this chapter with some common and widely used definitions. Definitions developed by the U.S. Bureau of the Census (1991) and the OTA

(1990), respectively, are (a) a community population under 2,500 people, and (b) nonmetropolitan, meaning the absence of a central city of 50,000 or more in population. The latter definition is most commonly used in discussions of rural health.

The designation *frontier* is used to denote sparsely populated counties, with a population density of less than six people per square mile (Elison, 1986). Still another definition is used by the U.S. Department of Agriculture (USDA), which classifies counties according to their primary economic enterprise, such as farming, manufacturing, or mining (Cordes, 1989).

Characteristics of Rural Populations

Rural populations are diverse, but certain commonalities have been identified. In most areas, rural economic factors lag behind the rest of the nation in growth, income, and employment (Korczyk, 1994). Nationally, goods-producing industries are giving way to service-producing industries, but more than one third of the rural economy is still tied to the goods-producing sector. Many rural communities are poorly positioned to compete in the services sector. Rural employment grew only 6.9% between 1979 and 1986, compared to the national rate of 10.8% (Korczyk, 1994).

Rural residents have lower average incomes, higher rates of poverty, and less access to Medicaid coverage than their urban counterparts. Significant numbers of rural residents are uninsured or underinsured (Summer, 1991). Poverty rates among nonelderly rural residents are more than 16% higher than among urban residents. Rural poverty differs in character from urban poverty, as the rural poor are more likely to be employed than the urban poor (Norton & McManus, 1989).

Two population groups with special needs, people over 65 and under 17, reside in greater proportion in rural areas, compared to urban communities (Cordes, 1989). The elderly are more likely to require a wide array of services due to the chronic illnesses that typically afflict this population. Rural elderly residents are less likely than urban residents to have access to or use preventive and health promotion services (Bergman-Evans & Walker, 1996). A higher rate of infant mortality exists in rural areas, a fact attributed to the lack of health care services. All these groups, along with an increasing minority population in many rural areas, strain an already overwhelmed health care system.

Rural residents tend to be less healthy than urban residents. People in rural areas are more likely than those in urban areas to be (a) without a regular source of health care, (b) in fair or poor health, and (c) contending with a chronic or serious illness (Norton & McManus, 1989). More rural than urban residents evaluate their health as poor. Rural residents are more likely to be injured at work, and rural persons are more likely to die from injury resulting from lightning, natural disasters, machinery, and the like (Norton & McManus, 1989).

■ Health Care Delivery in Rural Areas

Factors Affecting Rural Health Care Delivery

Health care in rural areas should be available, affordable, and accessible. Availability has improved somewhat in recent years. Many rural communities have hospitals and health care providers; however, numerous rural hospitals have closed, and those hospitals that have survived face severe financial problems. In addition to disparity in reimbursement, rural hospitals are not able to compete with urban hospitals in the range of services offered.

In many states, the health professional shortage continues to be a major problem and is the focus of concern about rural health activities. More than 70% of the primary care shortage is in rural areas (Korczyk, 1994). Some rural advocates take the position that available health care should be within 30 minutes or 30 miles of a provider. However, in frontier areas, such proximity may not always be feasible or even practical, as there may be only one ranch within a 30-mile area. In a study of rural frontier areas where distance to providers averaged 47 miles, Thorson and Powell (1992) found that residents did not perceive distance as a barrier and reported high levels of satisfaction with the level of health care available. An interesting anecdotal example concerned a resident who drove 120 miles to a physician that he preferred seeing rather than go to the closest physician; Thorson and Powell (1992) called this the "drive by phenomenon" (p. 252).

Affordable health care exists when the client has money to pay for health care services or has service paid for by another means such as private insurance, Medicaid, or Medicare. Having Medicaid or Medicare does not necessarily mean that health care services are affordable. Many individuals with Medicare coverage have out-of-pocket expenses that make health care unaffordable for them. Rural residents are more likely to lack health care coverage than urban residents and more likely to have difficulty meeting out-of-pocket expenses (Korczyk, 1994). Even when health care is available, it is not necessarily accessible to certain populations. Adequate public transportation, even in well-populated rural areas, is lacking. For elderly persons who no longer are able to drive or for the poor who do not own cars, health care becomes inaccessible. Health care facilities do not always provide flexible hours; that is, they are not open when the consumer can come. Language and cultural barriers experienced by minority populations make health care unacceptable and therefore not accessible to many.

Rural Health Care Delivery Systems

Rural health care delivery has focused on rural hospitals; however, closures occurred at a rapid rate in the 1980s and continue today. Hospital finances have been affected by a variety of factors including (a) a declining rural economy, (b) outmigration of rural residents, (c) inadequate reimbursement for service, (d) uncompensated care burden, and (e) declining inpatient admissions (American Hospital Association [AHA], 1992). Rural hospitals most vulnerable to closure are those with fewer than 25 beds, which represent about one third of rural hospitals (Mohr, Blanchfield, Cheng, Evans, & Franco, 1998). Decreases in Medicare and Medicaid reimbursement are particularly difficult for rural hospitals to absorb because most depend on those sources for much of their revenue. With passage of the Balanced Budget Act of 1997 and redesigned payment systems for Medicare, rural facilities faced new financial problems (Greene, 1998).

Managed care penetration has been greater in urban areas than rural; however, limited data are available about rural availability and enrollment in health maintenance organizations (HMOs). Although Krein and Casey (1998) found that the number of rural counties served by HMOs had continued to increase, managed care organizations in rural areas will most likely differ from urban models, having to adapt to meet rural needs better.

Rural hospitals have shifted their focus to ambulatory care, community-based clinics, and emergency care services, including stabilization and transport to a major medical center. Long-term care and home health centers often are owned by a hospital and may even be housed in the same building. Physicians and other health care providers from medical centers periodically provide counseling, conduct specialty clinics, and perform selected medical procedures and surgeries. Use of mobile technology units helps to keep patients in the local community for screening services (Hartley & Moscovice, 1996); however, these units may be more cost-effective when used as part of a regional network. Nurse-managed clinics for primary care and school-based clinics provide valuable services; the number of these clinics is increasing, but they are not the norm for most rural areas. Two innovative rural projects at the University of Nebraska Medical Center are the College of Nursing Mobile Nursing Center and the College of Pharmacy Drug Information Network. Mobile nursing services have provided assessment, screening, and teaching about health promotion and prevention to rural populations within a specified rural area. The Drug Information Network enables rural community pharmacies to become health education centers that provide drug information and health care resources to local practitioners and rural residents via computerized databases.

Telehealth

Telehealth, as defined by the Health Resources and Service Administration, is "the use of telecommunications and information technologies to share information and to provide clinical care, health professions education, consumer health education, public health and administrative services at a distance" (U.S. Department of Commerce, 1997b). *Telemedicine,* a more common term but narrower in scope, is limited to providing or supporting clinical care at a distance. Telemedicine gives rural providers access to newer medical technologies in use at urban facilities, enabling providers to offer more services and follow-up care locally. Thus the rural client whose health status is already compromised does not incur stress or costs of travel. For the financially troubled rural health facility, use of telemedicine can decrease use of urban facilities.

By the end of 1996 nearly 30% of rural hospitals were using telemedicine to deliver patient care; 68% of the usage involved telera-

diology (Office of Rural Health Policy, 1997). Other common clinical applications were in cardiology, orthopedics, dermatology, and psychiatry. Small rural hospitals have the greatest need for services and, in federal demonstration projects, had the most teleconsults; however, these hospitals usually have the least ability to pay for equipment and services. Despite the early promise of telemedicine, several key issues have emerged: (a) lack of hard evaluation data to demonstrate that telemedicine provides cost-effective services; (b) lack of clinical practice guidelines; (c) limited coverage by third-party payors, including Medicare, Medicaid, and private payors, and lack of procedures for cross-state licensure of professionals (U.S. Department of Commerce, 1997a).

Telehealth has great potential for improving health care services and the quality of life in rural communities. Applications have provided not only health care services, but also health professions education, and rural development. Several states, including Georgia, North Dakota, South Dakota, Iowa, Nebraska, and Kansas, have initiated telehealth applications that include concentration on distance education across the state (Witherspoon, Johnstone, & Wasem, 1993). Distance education initiatives make it possible for place-bound rural residents to obtain initial degrees or higher levels of education. Health professions education delivered to a rural community increases the potential that rural residents enrolled in it will remain to practice in that community after graduation. The delivery of continuing education to rural health providers helps them remain current in their disciplines and should reduce professional isolation.

An exciting application for telehealth is the delivery of home health care (Adams, 1997/1998). Demands for home-based care have increased considerably, encompassing patients with acute and chronic illnesses, permanent disabilities, and terminal illnesses. Kenney (1993) found that rural counties are less likely to have home health care agencies and have fewer agencies per square mile and provide a narrower array of services than urban counties. However, advances in telecommunications and the emergence of affordable, user-friendly desktop multimedia applications have made it possible to deliver home health care at a distance. Recent studies have demonstrated that, with a telehealth system, a single nurse can serve as many as 20 patients in a day rather than the 4 to 7 typical for home health agencies (Allen, 1996, p. 27).

■ *Rural Nursing*

Brief History

Rural nursing is not a new phenomenon. In the early 1900s, community-based practice was the norm because there were no rural hospitals. As early as 1912, the Rural Nursing Service established by the Red Cross began offering formal health care services in some rural areas (Kelly, 1992). The service provided nurses for illness care and health teaching, but it was not totally successful, as many communities did not participate, either due to a lack of finances or an unwillingness to work with a national organization. Eventually, Red Cross involvement declined; however, the Metropolitan Life Insurance Company started offering such services to its policyholders. In the 1940s, federal Hill-Burton funds led to establishment of hospitals in many rural communities, which considerably changed the number and type of jobs available to rural nurses.

Rural Nursing Theory

A theory base for rural nursing has been developed, which should ultimately help nurses in rural areas provide better health care (Long & Weinert, 1989). Qualitative and quantitative methods were used to assess the health of residents in the frontier areas of Mon-

tana. Key concepts of rural nursing that emerged from this work are (a) work beliefs and health beliefs, (b) isolation and distance, (c) self-reliance, (d) lack of anonymity, (e) outsider and insider, (f) old-timer and newcomer.

Three relational statements are currently being tested in various research projects.

1. Rural residents define health as the ability to work or do usual tasks.

2. Rural residents are self-reliant and resist receiving help or services from those seen as outsiders or agencies, such as national or regional "welfare" programs. Rural residents tend to seek help through an informal rather than a formal system.

3. Health care providers in rural areas must contend with lack of anonymity and greater role diffusion than providers in urban settings.

As more is learned about rural residents, health care can be planned and adapted to meet their special needs. With health professional shortages in rural areas, information about the challenges that health care providers face is particularly important, especially in recruitment of urban professionals to the rural setting.

Characteristics of Rural Nursing

The registered nurse (RN) to population ratios are lower in rural than in urban areas. The ratio of RNs per 100,000 population in 1988 was 675 for urban areas but only 385 in rural counties (Kindig, Movassaghi, Juhl, & Geller, 1990). In a survey of RNs, Moses (1990) found that 82% were located in urban areas and that urban RNs were more likely to be employed in nursing than rural RNs. In rural areas the population of nurses was generally older, but the proportion of nurses working after age 54 tended to be lower. In addition, rural nurses have the lowest educational levels; only 20.1% of rural nurses have baccalaureate degrees, compared to 29.5% of urban nurses. Only 2.5% of rural nurses have graduate degrees, compared to 6.7% of urban nurses (Kindig et al., 1990).

Skills of nurse practitioners (NPs) are well suited to the needs of rural areas. Nurse practitioners provide health promotion and disease prevention services, manage clients with chronic disease, and provide services to women, children, and elderly clients (American Nurses Association [ANA], 1996). They can provide most of the primary care needed in rural communities, are assuming a greater role in rural health care delivery, and are more likely than physicians to practice in rural communities (Korzcyk, 1994). However, the proportion of NPs practicing in rural areas has declined slightly (Bigbee, 1993). The movement of NPs to urban areas may be due to better employment opportunities there. In responses to surveys, the most frequently cited barrier to practicing in rural areas was the lack of physician backup and support. In fact, in some areas of the United States, physicians still do not support the use of advanced practice nurses. Political, legislative, and financial barriers to nursing practice in many rural areas have not been completely addressed or resolved.

Positive and Negative Aspects

Rural nursing has both positive and negative aspects. Interestingly, what one nurse may perceive as a positive aspect of rural nursing, another nurse will identify as a negative factor. Rural nurses are often described as generalists, with broad background and a wide range of skills (Bigbee, 1993). These nurse-generalists function in a variety of practice areas within inpatient settings and may even have responsibilities for outpatient and community nursing. It is not unusual for a nurse in a small rural hospital in a single day to work in medical, surgical, obstetric, and pediatric areas—and even in the emergency room. Some nurses find work-

ing as a generalist to be exciting and an opportunity to use the many skills they possess; other nurses may find responsibilities as a generalist to be daunting because of the need to be prepared and remain up-to-date in so many areas. For the new graduate and even the experienced nurse, these responsibilities may be overwhelming, particularly in terms of legal liability.

Rural nurses are described as having close community relationships as they care for friends, neighbors, and family members (ANA, 1996). These close ties may lead to role diffusion—that is, difficulty in separating their personal and professional lives. These nurses are called on frequently when "off duty" and lack personal anonymity. The blurring of roles may lead to inadvertent breaches of confidentiality even though the nurses try to maintain both their own and their clients' privacy.

Typically, rural nurses are regarded as valuable community members, and many assume positions of leadership within the community. The respect they receive leads to greater self-esteem and a sense of being valued. Nurses often have the opportunity to influence local health policy (Turner & Gunn, 1991).

Greater interdisciplinary collaboration seems to exist among rural health professionals, particularly in areas of shortage where they may have to assume roles of various allied health workers. Greater cohesiveness among nursing staff tends to lessen professional fatigue despite heavy responsibilities and practice demands (Fuszard, Slocum, & Wiggers, 1990).

Advantages and Disadvantages

Rural nursing is characterized by independence and self-direction, which can be a predictor of job satisfaction. However, independence also can lead to isolation, as there is less opportunity for backup and consultation from nursing colleagues and other health professionals. Technology may prove to be instrumental in decreasing the isolation of rural nurses. With opportunities to engage in continuing education via interactive television or the Internet, a nurse can interact with other nurses and other health care professionals. The wide range of resources available on the Internet provides information at any time of day. Many nurses find Internet chat rooms to be a valuable method of networking, both as an opportunity to gain more information and to receive support for the unique demands of rural nursing.

Possible disadvantages of working as a rural nurse compared to urban nurses include lower salaries and less opportunity for advancement as fewer positions are available. Rural nurses also may be asked to work longer hours, including more evenings and weekends. Frequently, there are fewer full-time than part-time positions, for which nurses do not receive benefits. The social climate in a rural community, with limited recreational events and cultural activities, may be a negative aspect of rural nursing for some, especially nurses who have lived previously in an urban area. Another area of concern may be lack of opportunities for family members, such as job choices and adequate schools (Bigbee, 1993).

■ Future Challenges in Rural Health Care

To meet the challenges of providing health care in rural areas, consumers, practitioners of all disciplines, educators, and policy makers must work collaboratively.

Needs and Services in Rural Areas

Changes in national and state reimbursement rarely bode well for rural areas, as an urban model is frequently applied to the rural setting. The Balanced Budget Act of 1997 has had negative consequences for rural hospitals, nursing homes, and home health agencies because of the altered reimbursement structure for Medicare and Medicaid. The reforms in the Balanced Budget Refinement Act of 1999 have focused on temporary, short-term solutions to complex problems (National Rural Health Association, 2000).

An additional challenge for rural facilities is keeping up with regulatory changes that require upgraded computer systems and accounting programs. However, the act also contains positive aspects for rural areas. An extension of a federal program aimed at assisting rural hospitals creates a new class of "critical access hospitals"; however, many policy analysts are fearful that this new classification will help only remote, small, and financially strapped hospitals.

A new structure for organizing resources has appeared in rural areas and is expected to continue. An integrated rural health network is a "formal organizational arrangement among health care providers (and possibly insurers and social service providers) that uses the resources of more than one existing organization" (Moscovice et al., 1996, p. 4). These networks may be effective in overcoming the fragmentation of health services delivery in rural areas. Clearly, small rural communities can no longer afford to provide a wide array of services; in fact, effective networks may mean the survival of health services in these communities.

Political advocates must continue to inform legislators of the special needs of rural areas. When rural is defined as nonmetropolitan, rural populations account only for about 23% of the total population; therefore rural needs are in the minority and may be overlooked in the political arena. Information about rural needs must be based on solid empirical evidence; thus the need for health services research is evident and critical.

Implications for Nursing Practice

Advanced practice nurses are well positioned to provide care in underserved rural areas, even in areas of physician shortages. Increasing numbers of NPs are expected in states where laws relating to independent practice are least restrictive (Grandinetti, 1999). Many rural consumers and physicians still need to be better informed about the merits of advanced practice nursing and the independent scope of practice, but simply providing information about NPs may not be sufficient; observation of actual practice may also be needed. Ideally, NPs demonstrate the benefits of a holistic approach to health care combined with the diagnostic and curative aspects in rural area practice. Educational programs provide just that opportunity by placing a student NP with a physician preceptor. The preceptorship often leads to a job opportunity for an NP as the physician recognizes the NP's potential benefits to the practice. Cejka (1999) cites benefits of an NP to a physician's practice as (a) expansion, (b) cost-effectiveness, and (c) improved patient access to the practice. Studies have provided ample evidence of client satisfaction with NP practice (ANA, 1992). A survey by Grandinetti (1999) showed that the most likely employers of NPs are younger physicians, female physicians, managed-care practices, and services in rural areas (23%) rather than urban areas (19%).

Implications for Nursing Education

Nursing education in rural areas face many challenges. Educational programs in states with large rural populations, or graduates who will be working with rural populations, have a responsibility to prepare nurses for rural practice and the special needs of rural residents. Numerous projects designed to increase the number of health professionals in rural areas have shown that educational programs would do well to consider the following strategies (National Rural Health Association, 1992): (a) incorporate the preparation of health professionals for rural practice into academic pro-

grams, (b) target rural students for recruitment efforts, (c) combine both rural orientation in both didactic and clinical instruction, (d) utilize well-qualified rural preceptors who understand the objectives of rural health care components and allow time for role modeling in the clinical and sociocultural aspects of rural practice, (e) present sociocultural and ethnographic information about the rural population prior to and concurrent with rural clinical placements, and (f) allow rural students to remain in their communities for as much of their education as feasible.

Rural areas typically have larger numbers of diploma and associate degree graduates. The importance of baccalaureate and master's-prepared nurses in meeting the critical, complex needs of rural communities must be conveyed with sensitivity to practitioners in rural areas. It is not always easy to convince employers of the need for a higher level of nursing, particularly if the experienced nurse administrator is at a lower educational level.

■ Concluding Statement

Health care in rural America faces many challenges and, in many rural areas, a somewhat uncertain future. Rural areas have health care issues that are similar to those in urban areas but also other health care issues that are unique to the rural setting. Rural populations have poorer health and less access to available and affordable health care than urban populations. Rural nurses have many opportunities to play a valuable role in provision of health care to rural areas, but these nurses encounter geographic, economic, and political barriers. Recent advances in telehealth hold promise for addressing many barriers encountered in rural areas. An interdisciplinary health care model that includes consumers and policy makers is essential for devising timely solutions to long-term problems of rural areas.

■ *References*

Adams, D. L. (1997/1998). Home healthcare: A new venue for telemedicine. *World Medical Technology Update,* 226–228.

Allen, A. (1996, January/February). Telemedicine in home care, 1996 trends. *Remington Report, 4,* 26–27.

American Hospital Association. (1992). *Environmental assessment for rural hospitals 1992.* Chicago: Author.

American Nurses Association. (1992). *A meta-analysis of process of care, clinical outcomes, and cost effectiveness of nurses in primary care roles: Nurse practitioners and nurse-midwives.* Washington, DC: Author.

American Nurses Association. (1996). *Rural/frontier nursing: The challenge to grow.* Washington, DC: Author.

Balanced Budget Act of 1997. (P.L. 105-33) (August 1997). HR 3426—Medicare and Medicaid Health Insurance Act. *U.S. Statutes at Large* (Volume III, pp. 251–788). Washington, DC: U.S. Government Printing Office.

Bergman-Evans, B. F., & Walker, S. N. (1996). The prevalence of clinical preventive services utilization by older women. *Nurse Practitioner, 21*(4), 88–106.

Bigbee, J. (1993). The uniqueness of rural nursing. *Nursing Clinics of North America, 28*(1), 131–144.

Cejka, S. (1999). You and midlevel providers—A good fit? *Medical Economics, 76*(3), 159–163.

Cordes, S. M. (1989). The changing rural environment and the relationship between health services and rural development. *Health Services Research, 23*(6), 757–784.

Elison, G. (1986). Frontier areas: Problems for delivery of health care services. *Rural Health Care, 5,* 1–2.

Fuszard, B., Slocum, I., & Wiggers, D. (1990). Rural nurses, part II: Surviving the shortage. *Journal of Nursing Administration, 20*(5), 41–46.

Grandinetti, D. (1999). Midlevel providers: Making their mark in doctors' offices. *Medical Economics, 76*(3), 141–155.

Greene, J. (1998, November). A stormy season for rurals. *Hospitals & Health Networks, 72*(22), 28–30.

Hartley, D., & Moscovice, I. (1996). The mobile hospital technology industry: Focus on the computerized tomography scanner. *Journal of Rural Health, 12*(3), 225–234.

Kelly, L. Y. (1992). *The nursing experience: Trends, challenges, and transitions* (2nd ed.). New York: McGraw-Hill.

Kenney, G. M. (1993). Is access to home health care a problem in rural areas? *American Journal of Public Health, 83*(3), 412–414.

Kindig, D., Movassaghi, H., Juhl, N., & Geller, J. (1990). *Characteristics of nonmetropolitan nurses: Results from the 1988 survey of registered nurses.* Grand Forks, ND: University of North Dakota Rural Health Research Center.

Korczyk, S. M. (1994, Spring). *The NRECA report on health care needs, resources and access in rural America.* Washington, DC: The National Rural Electric Cooperative Association's Retirement, Safety and Insurance Department.

Krein, J. S., & Casey M. (1998). Research on managed care organizations in rural communities. *Journal of Rural Health, 14*(3), 180–199.

Long, R., & Weinert, C. (1989). Rural nursing: Developing the theory base. *Scholarly Inquiry for Nursing Practice: An International Journal, 3*(2), 113–127.

Medicare and Medicaid, and SCHIP Balanced Budget Refinement Act of 1999. (Incorporated into P.L. 106-113), November 29, 1999, HR 3426.

Mohr, P. E., Blanchfield, B. B., Cheng, M., Evans, W., & Franco, S. (1998, December). The financial dependence of rural hospitals on outpatient revenue. *Policy analysis brief.* Bethesda, MD: Walsh Center for Rural Health Analysis.

Moses, E. B. (1990, June). *The registered nurse population: Findings from the national sample survey of registered nurses, March 1988.* Washington, DC: U.S. Department of Health & Human Services.

Moscovice, I., Wellever, A., Christianson, J., Casey, M., Yawn, B., & Hartley, D. (1996). *Rural health networks: Concepts, cases and public policy.* Rockville, MD: Office of Rural Health Policy.

National Rural Health Association. (1992). *Study highlights: Study of models to meet rural health care needs through mobilization of health professions education and services resources, 2.* Kansas City, MO: Author.

National Rural Health Association. (2000). Roadmap to a healthy rural America. [On-line], June 20, 2000. Available: http://www.NRHrural.org/dc/roadmap.html.

Norton, E., & McManus, M. (1989). Background tables on demographic characteristics, health status, and health services utilization. *Health Services Research, 23*(6), 725–755.

Office of Rural Health Policy. (1997, February 1). *Exploratory evaluation of rural applications of telemedicine.* Rockville, MD: Office of Rural Health.

Office of Technology Assessment. (1990). *Health care in rural America.* Washington, DC: U.S. Government Printing Office.

Office of Technology Assessment. (1991). *Rural America at the crossroads: Networking for the future.* Washington, DC: U.S. Government Printing Office.

Summer, L. (1991). *Limited access: Health care for the rural poor.* Washington, DC: Center on Budget and Policy Priorities.

Thorson, J. A., & Powell, F. C. (1992). *Health care perceptions of Nebraska's urban and rural aged.* (Report 92-1). Omaha: University of Nebraska at Omaha, College of Public Affairs and Community Service.

Turner, T,. & Gunn, I. (1991). Issues in rural health nursing. In A. Bushy (Ed.), *Rural nursing* (pp. 105–110). Newbury Park, CA: Sage.

U.S. Department of Commerce, Bureau of the Census. (1991). *Census of population 1990: Preliminary counts.* Washington, DC: U.S. Government Printing Office.

U.S. Department of Commerce. HRSA. (1997a). *Telemedicine report to Congress.* Washington, DC: U.S. Government Printing Office.

U.S. Department of Commerce. HRSA. (1997b). Office for the Advancement of Telehealth (OAT). [On-line]. Available: http://telhealth/hrsa.gov.

Witherspoon, J. P., Johnstone, S. M., & Wasem, C. J. (1993, September). *Rural Telehealth: Telemedicine, distance education and informatics for rural health care.* Rockville, MD: Office of Rural Health Policy.

■ *Editor's Questions for Discussion*

Identify health care issues unique to rural areas. What data are needed for planning rural health care? Propose systematic health services research in health care and nursing practice for rural areas. Discuss challenges and opportunities for nursing centers in rural areas. Apply content from Carter (Chapter 39), Schroeder and Long (Chapter 47), Todero (Chapter 51), and Barger (Chapter 52) in addressing rural health care issues.

What ethical and legal issues may arise in rural health care? How does content by Kopala (Chapter 5) and Lane and Paterson (Chapter 7) address challenges in rural health care? How will mutual recognition in nursing practice facilitate care as described by Yocom and Thomas (Chapter 3)? What additional resources may be necessary to provide distance education for large rural areas? Recalling the discussion of Yeaworth et al. (Chapter 14), what adaptations may need to be made for effective distance health education in rural areas?

Propose recruitment strategies to attract professional nurses to rural areas. What relevance does advanced practice as examined by Gray (Chapter 42) have for rural areas? What qualifications should exist for preceptors in rural areas? Propose strategies for increasing educational preparation of nurses in rural areas. How may barriers be reduced and benefits increased?

Define the theory base for rural nursing. How does theory for nursing differ from other nursing theory? Based on the definition of health by rural residents, how will health education needs differ from those for urban residents? Suggest strategies for providing health education in rural areas.

51

Mobile Nursing Center for Vulnerable Populations

Catherine M. Todero, RN, PhD

A nursing center can be considered as both a place and a concept (Frenn, Lundeen, Martin, Riesch, & Wilson, 1996). By definition, nursing centers make nursing care directly accessible to clients, families, and communities in a practice that is controlled by nurses. Although centers without walls can exist (Walker, 1994), space and place often become defining characteristics of a center. These properties determine such things as services offered or populations served. Space may dictate whether groups or individuals are served, location determines who is served, and physical layout or equipment available may define other service parameters.

The University of Nebraska, College of Nursing, Mobile Nursing Center (MNC) is a 36-foot motor home configured and furnished to look like a typical clinic. The vehicle has a waiting area, lab area, and examination room. Mobility of the Center and its equipment afford opportunities to provide consistent, high-quality, and diversified services to varieties of populations whether in urban or rural locations. The mission of the MNC is to improve the health and quality of life of individuals, families, and communities through primary health services to diverse populations. The well-equipped mobile center supports the MNC nursing model, which is characterized by mobility, flexibility, and connection to the communities served.

■ Establishing a Nursing Center

Building Faculty Support

Building faculty support for a nursing center operation is critical for supporting the health educational goals of the center. As with any new endeavor, there were some faculty at the University of Nebraska Medical Center (UNMC) who immediately embraced the learning value of a mobile nursing center. They worked to develop and establish services and formed a steering committee for the MNC. Regular steering committee meetings throughout the academic year were used to discuss issues, strategic plans, policies, standards, and clinic or educational procedures. The steering committee gave needed advice and direction for recruitment and for inclusion of additional faculty to provide student learning experiences. Methods for keeping the total faculty and interested others informed of MNC activities included publishing a periodic newsletter, writing columns in other agency newsletters, making verbal reports at general faculty meetings, and publishing an annual report. Personal contacts with selected faculty and invitations for students to participate in scheduled activities that closely matched the level of their learning needs also served as effective strategies to ensure faculty and student involvement. For example, when the MNC provided a flu immunization clinic, undergraduate students who were learning basic skills were invited to participate. When annual physical examinations were needed for employees, nurse practitioner students were targeted for participation.

Partnership Development

The MNC is a partnership between the College of Nursing and the Cornbelt Federation of Cosmopolitans. Cosmopolitans International is a community service organization that has a particular interest in diabetes and related health care. In Nebraska the group comprises approximately 15 local clubs, which together pledged support for the health related activities of the MNC. The partnership allows the group to be part of a project that directly benefits their community. A major advantage to this partnership is the sharing of the workload and financial burdens involved in providing services.

The MNC vehicle was purchased by the Cosmopolitans and given to the College of Nursing to use for nursing services. The Cosmopolitans assume responsibility for the maintenance, cleaning, storage, and operating expenses of the vehicle. The group also provides a driver and covers expenses associated with the driver's travel. The drivers, some of whom are trained emergency medical technicians (EMTs), assist nursing staff insofar as their training and abilities allow. Club members are kept abreast of MNC Center activities and provide other types of assistance as needed. The publicity gained from involvement has allowed clubs to increase their membership, an outcome they were seeking.

True partnerships involve issues of shared decision-making, which must be addressed. Differences related to philosophy or culture may create challenges for all concerned. Riesch (1992) reported that all definitions of nursing centers included, as the dominant theme, that nurses control the professional practice and patient care. This concept is one that may require frequent reinforcement when center resources are dependent on funding from organizations that have agendas of their own. Blending an altruistic or academic culture with one that is entrepreneurial or business oriented also challenges traditional nursing ways of thinking. But nursing centers must develop alliances with businesses, more traditional health care systems, and other institutions if they are to survive. Such alliances may mean surrendering some operational control.

■ Comunity Support

Community Development Strategies

A mobile center has multiple and various communities to consider. Providing care in rural underserved communities creates a very different scenario than when care is provided in urban minority populations. Barriers to care in rural communities may include distance or lack of health care providers. Barriers to adequate care in urban minority populations may involve poverty, language, or cultural issues. An understanding of the issues with which each population must deal is essential to the provision of adequate nursing care. A community assessment of health care needs and resources available typically precedes the decision to provide services in a community. Some populations served were identified as needy by the MNC staff, but others identified themselves as needy and invited the MNC to provide service. Regardless of how a community is chosen, cultivating a relationship with a community champion who understands the needs of constituents and is willing to serve as contact, advisor, ally, spokesperson, and remote worker is an important element in the process of providing successful service.

Because mobile health care services are provided on a rotational outreach basis, well-developed referral networks are essential. Problems discovered that may need specialty care or follow-up before the MNC returns to the community must be referred for follow-up treatment. Vulnerable populations frequently have no money to pay for services and therefore a referral for specialized care may not be possible or appreciated by the provider to whom the referral is made. Therefore collaboration with other health care providers who are willing to accept responsibility for referrals is essential and must be negotiated. Case management of complex clients has been referred to local student nurses serving the community, greatly expanding the resources of the MNC and providing excellent learning opportunities for the students in community-based care. Creative use of all resources available often requires insider knowledge of the community, and it is here that the role of the community champion becomes critical.

Advisory Groups

One way to determine health care needs of a community is to ask its members. Knowledgeable insiders may help identify overall community needs. But, if actual consumers of care have an opportunity for a say-so in the selection of services, they may feel a sense of ownership and have greater impetus for participation. This principle was evident when a cholesterol screening and monitoring program was implemented by the MNC at request of the adults and elderly clients served in several rural communities. Client encounter numbers were consistently higher when this service was offered along with the usual service options. Satisfaction surveys assist providers to gain insight into services desired, but frequently individual comments are focused on satisfaction with care already received and not on potential options for care. Focus groups, when directed to think about unmet needs, are generally more beneficial in providing guidance for the design of potential services. Community-based focus groups can advise and help set priorities for important and urgent health care needs of the community. In the urban African American population served, asthma management was deemed the most important problem by the community advisory board. The MNC now offers an active home-based asthma disease management program in this community.

Community Barriers

Despite considerable time and attention to community development activities, providers of nursing services nonetheless may encounter barriers. Even in areas determined to be underserved, issues of competition may arise. Physician providers in the area may not see the benefit of nurse practitioner services in their communities and may only see the potential for competition and erosion of their patient base. Even when the services provided are complementary and not directly competitive, some physician providers may be threatened. In one rural community, when reasons were sought to explain a dramatic drop in MNC encounters, community representatives reported that town residents were made to feel guilty if they used the services of the MNC. They perceived that local physicians would deny them future medical services if they were seen at the MNC.

Gate-keeping issues also have arisen due to organization of health care agencies into systems. The unique and mobile nature of MNC services is attractive to many needy groups. The MNC has been approached to contract for services, then blocked from negotiating requested services by local hospital or provider organizations that would rather try to establish their own mobile services and keep the "Medical Center's system" out of their communities. The perception that the MNC is owned and operated as an outreach clinic by the Medical Center and that an agenda for service is to garner more patients for Medical Center physicians is incorrect. Here the MNC must battle historical realities of patients who sought specialty care and then never returned to their home town primary care physicians. The MNC's operating philosophy is to refer or coordinate care with the client's identified primary care provider. This collaborative rather than competitive approach is one that must be frequently reinforced to cautious and suspicious providers.

■ Advantages of a Mobile Center

Access to Varieties of Vulnerable Populations

Providing health care to vulnerable persons always has been a special concern of nurses. Historical perspectives that trace the roots of nursing centers to the work of such nursing pioneers as Lillian Wald, Margaret Sanger, and Mary Breckenridge reflect this long-standing desire to address inequities of health care for poor and underserved populations (Walker, 1994). Vulnerable populations are those groups that have limited economic or environmental resources and therefore are highly susceptible to adverse health outcomes. Groups recognized as vulnerable typically include women and children, ethnic people of color, immigrants, gay men and lesbians, the homeless, and the elderly (Flaskerud & Winslow, 1998). In rural states, lack of access to health care providers in the community creates vulnerability for all residents.

The MNC has identified vulnerable groups in both urban and rural communities. One advantage of a mobile center is its ability to bring health care services directly to these groups. Barriers of transportation and travel are eliminated when care is provided where people live, work, worship, and play. Several communities in central Nebraska, federally designated as medically underserved areas, were targeted for services. The MNC travels regularly to these communities and provides health care at work sites and community or senior centers. The elderly and working middle-aged adults are typical consumers of MNC health care services in these communities. Providing care to rural populations presents a unique set of challenges, considerations, and issues, such as available resources for referral and follow-up, which must be addressed.

Minority populations usually are accessed in urban locations where groups gather. The MNC visits to a traditionally African American church and a Hispanic church are a regular Sunday activity. Cultural appropriateness is emphasized and translators are used as needed. Parking lot clinics for Hispanics after Sunday Mass emulate plaza gatherings and activities in Mexico and Central America.

Affiliation and collaboration with other agencies to expand services they offer to minorities is another effective strategy for improving care to these groups. One example of this approach is the relationship that the MNC established with the Intertribal Treatment Center (ITC) in Omaha. This facility is a residential treatment center for Native American substance abusers. As clients recover from their addictions they become aware of numerous health conditions that need treatment. The ITC staff focus on substance abuse issues and staff of the MNC focus on all other health concerns, thereby providing a more comprehensive and holistic service.

The MNC provides services to children and their families at school sites. Schools selected for services are those with large populations of Hispanic and African American students. Hours of service are chosen to accommodate both students and parents. For example, if the service is directed at the family, the hours of MNC operation would be planned for evening to coincide with a Parent Teacher Association meeting or some other event that is likely to draw parents or families to the school.

Opportunities for Multicampus, Distant Learner Participation

A second advantage of a mobile nursing center is the ability to provide learning opportunities in community-based nursing with diverse populations for different levels of stu-

dents at more than one campus location. The University of Nebraska has a multicampus nursing program that spans the state. Students, like patients, frequently have transportation or travel barriers that would prevent their participation in a nursing center located only in one community. When the MNC establishes a service site, students and faculty from the closest campus participate in the care. Because clinical resources and equipment are consistent and reliable, the structure, efficiency, and planning for services is facilitated. Nursing services are planned around specific needs of the community and resources of the center.

Public Visibility

A third advantage of a mobile nursing center is the public visibility that is promoted. The MNC vehicle is clearly marked and serves as a moving billboard, advertising nursing services as it rolls down the highway and into a community. The image of nurses providing services with state-of-the art resources is powerful. The public perceives access to quality care, and the reputation of advanced practice nurses as effective providers of primary care services is promoted.

■ Providing Community-Based Nursing Services

Providing Customer-Driven Services

The MNC is a health care delivery system characterized by mobility, flexibility, and connection to the community. The MNC provides a core of health services that include health promotion, disease prevention, screening and case finding, physical examinations, behavioral and lifestyle modification counseling, chronic illness management, minor acute illness and injury care, home and community interventions, and referral. Determining the quantity and types of services in each community is done through community assessment and negotiation with community leaders or spokespersons. The MNC has developed a reputation for successful outreach to difficult populations. Often, its services are requested to assist other agencies in some particular event. Expanding its services beyond those traditionally offered by nursing is possible through collaboration and connections with the larger resources of the UNMC. For example, the MNC has successfully facilitated physical therapy, medical nutrition, and dental services to needy groups.

"Selling" Nursing Services

Most academic nursing centers are developed to provide patient care, serve as faculty practice sites, and create direct linkages between service and education. Financial gain or viability is frequently at issue because these centers often focus on providing services to those who are uninsured and cannot afford to pay for services unless they are provided at a highly discounted rate. Targeting vulnerable people is a way of obtaining access to primary care populations for advanced nursing practice while avoiding direct competition with other providers of primary care services. The strategy is helpful for meeting educational objectives of many nursing centers but is not likely to be very beneficial in helping nursing centers meet their financial objectives. Developing product lines that capitalize on the resources and strengths of nursing center staff can provide much needed income, allow outcomes of nursing services to be showcased, and help establish a reputation as an expert provider of certain services.

It is critical that health care delivery systems focus on primary prevention and tertiary prevention interventions, if health care costs related to acute care and institutionalization are to be controlled (Walker, 1994). Nurses routinely provide or coordinate health promo-

tion, disease prevention, or disease management interventions. Nurses generally are considered providers of choice because of a holistic approach and skill in helping clients manage disease in complex environments. Packaging these services and selling them directly to a health maintenance organization (HMO), employers, physicians, and the general public not only provides revenue for the nursing center but can also reinforce the value of the services rendered. Careful program development and standardization of service protocols are necessary to ensure quality control, especially if a variety of nurse providers or students are involved. Having a clearly delineated product or package of services also allows for ease in marketing. Customers then are clear about what nursing interventions will include and what must or will be referred.

Interdisciplinary collaboration is a hallmark of many services marketed by the MNC. Home disease management programs in asthma, chronic obstructive pulmonary disease (COPD), and heart failure are funded by a contract with an HMO but rely on referrals from physicians. Close collaboration with these physician providers is critical for prevention of medical crises requiring more expensive modes of care. Collaboration with school or occupational nurses, physical therapists, and social workers helps create environments where symptoms of disease are more easily avoided.

Innovative uses of technology can be employed to facilitate interdisciplinary collaboration or monitor and support patients in their homes. Telemedicine consultations from remote sites or homes to physician offices can be accomplished through laptop computers, small portable video cameras, and Internet connections. A less complicated and less expensive method of supporting patients at home is use of the Health Buddy system. The Health Buddy is a small electronic device that hooks into the patient's telephone line. It transmits data to a database accessible by the provider and sends information and advice from the provider back to the patient. This technology can be used to monitor and manage patient symptoms and behavior better, as well as to educate and motivate patients to manage their own conditions.

Measuring Nursing Outcomes

The competitive nature of health care makes it imperative that nursing centers focus efforts on generating outcome data and initiating cost-effective methods (Hoffman, 1997). Both qualitative and quantitative data are necessary to truly appreciate the impact that nursing services make in patients' lives. Ability to collect, sort, analyze, and disseminate information about outcomes of nursing services in an efficient manner is essential to long-term survival of nursing centers (Hoffman, 1997). The MNC uses the Omaha System, which comprises nursing diagnoses, nursing interventions, and an outcomes rating scale; this system is particularly suited for use in community-based settings. The Omaha System taxonomy was used to organize the files, but the only way to retrieve the data in an efficient manner was to computerize the database. This task was accomplished by using Access software.

The computerized record was a challenge to implement in the practice setting. Several problems had to be solved to permit effective use of the system at point-of-service. The mobile nature of the service meant that laptop computers had to be linked to each other through a mobile local area network (LAN). Proper setup and tear-down of the LAN system required a certain amount of technologic savvy of staff. Additionally, electronic charting at point-of-service and printing of referrals slowed the provision of NP services. Because of a desire to avoid waiting-time for clients, charting often was done at the end of the day from notes taken earlier. Thus documentation of patient care became a major task to be completed after all clients had been seen, creating dissatisfaction among MNC providers. Making a quick, written note in a paper chart would have been easier, but with thousands of records, the computer allowed much quicker access to patient records at each site. Faced with the choice of a few laptop computers or numerous boxes of paper records to transport, the advantages of a computer record quickly became obvious to the providers and staff.

Computer technology in rural and remote locations allows linkages to resources at the College of Nursing and UNMC. With appropriate software, Internet connections can be made through phone lines even in communities without an Internet service provider. A satellite dish mounted atop the MNC allows television downlinks to educational programming.

■ Integrating Service and Education and Research

Learning Opportunities and Issues for Undergraduate Students

The MNC provides wonderful learning opportunities for students at all levels. However, scheduling students when clients need services rather than when students want classes is an issue. Nursing centers that operate for only a few midday hours on weekdays most likely are not meeting the health needs of vulnerable groups. But scheduling students for evening and weekend hours is difficult and a constant challenge. The complexity of clients encountered creates a second issue. Often even advanced practice, well-experienced nurses can be overwhelmed with the level and number of needs of some individuals. Undergraduate students need excellent faculty role models to appreciate the full scope of holistic nursing services required. Careful mentoring of students to provide adequate nursing care is essential but can tax available faculty resources.

Despite the most careful planning of staff and faculty and client ratios anticipated at each site for various services, consumer demand has on occasion overwhelmed or underwhelmed the staff. Predicting client no-show rate, especially in rural communities, is difficult when the MCN leaves home base on a sunny day, only to encounter snow, wind, or rainstorms 200 miles away. Special events in a community may prompt additional visitors to the Center, which operates on a walk-in basis. Constant effort is required to try to balance staff resources that meet both clients' needs for care and students' needs for learning.

Graduate Student Learning Opportunities

Opportunities for graduate student learning go beyond providing primary care nursing services to patients. Students have engaged actively in the design of clinical programs, tool development, analyses of MNC systems, outcomes research, quality improvement process management, and case management. The synergy and creative energy of graduate students has helped the MNC evolve into a dynamic project.

■ Sustainability and Other Business Issues

Funding Challenges

Altruism and desire to provide services to vulnerable people, must be tempered with the realism that someone must pay for services when clients cannot. Nurses may recognize the value of their interventions but typically have no idea of the cost of services. Faculty, relatively new to the practice arena, are passionate in their desire to provide the highest quality care and may assume, because there is a client need, it must be met. But the desire to provide services to vulnerable populations must be balanced with efforts to provide services that are

likely to generate income. Many nursing centers have a mandate that they must be self-sufficient. Few meet this goal.

A major problem to overcome in quest for self-sufficiency is the cost of the nursing model. Working with multiple communities of vulnerable populations is both labor and time intensive. Additionally, active and substantial student participation adds to the cost. Methods must be designed to keep costs down, and cost containment in health care must extend to nursing centers. Lack of reimbursement for services that focus on health promotion and disease prevention, hallmarks of the nursing model, make it unlikely that clinic revenue alone could support an endeavor based primarily on these services. Community support and donations or state and local grants are likely to be necessary to help cover the costs of services to vulnerable people.

Nursing Centers and Managed Care Contracts

As managed care extends into Medicaid and Medicare populations, opportunities for nursing centers to negotiate contractual services in these groups increase. Managed care vendors will be looking for ways to control costs in groups consuming the most expensive health care resources. Disease management programs are one strategy being used to cut utilization and costs while improving care and outcomes. These programs often focus on health education and health promotion, secondary prevention, and case management and are ideal products for nursing centers to develop and market. In the managed care environment, with capitation or discounted fees-for-service, primary care providers are unlikely to have the time or resources to give complementary components of care, even in clients with serious chronic illness.

The MNC has negotiated contracts with an HMO to provide disease management services in patients with asthma, congestive heart failure (CHF), and COPD. The HMO seeks referrals from physicians by scanning utilization data, markets service as a benefit to their members, and pays for it from their risk pools.

Risk Taking and Entrepreneurial Spirit

Professional nurses generally receive little education in the business aspects of delivering health care. Nurses have a long history of giving away their services; Mackey, Adams, and McNiel (1994) asserted that the attitude of "nurses will do it for free" is perpetuated by services that target nonpaying groups, such as the homeless or welfare groups. Why do nursing centers target these types of populations? Reasons may include (a) the general disposition of nurses who are motivated by a desire to help people; (b) nursing education that teaches the values of the professional nurse, including altruism and social justice; and (c) perhaps, a reluctance to compete with other, more established and resource rich providers for the same market. Collaboration and teamwork, rather than competition, are behaviors that professional nurses have emphasized. Financial negotiating skills, proprietary thinking, business savvy, marketing, development of an entre-

preneurial spirit and risk-taking behaviors, and a quid pro quo philosophy are not part of the typical nursing curricula. Perhaps those topics should be, for future nursing centers may be more dependent on these skills than those currently taught in advanced nursing programs.

■ Concluding Statement

Mobile nursing centers are ideal for meeting the needs of vulnerable populations and support of nursing educational goals as well. Advantages include (a) ability to target diverse populations of needy groups, (b) flexibility to meet a variety of service requests because of access to a well-equipped clinic, (c) learning opportunities in locations that are convenient for students, (d) opportunities for collaboration and partnerships with a variety of community or health care agencies, and (e) high public visibility. Mobile nursing centers face the same issues of competition, lack of financial reimbursement, outcomes generation, and proof of cost-effectiveness as other nursing centers. Innovative technology, greater emphasis on business and negotiation skills, and a shift in nursing and academic models of thinking may be necessary for survival.

References

Flaskerud, J. H., & Winslow, B. J. (1998). Conceptualizing vulnerable populations health-related research. *Nursing Research, 47*(2), 69–78.

Frenn, M., Lundeen, S. P., Martin, K. S., Riesch, S. K., & Wilson, S. A. (1996). Symposium on nursing centers: Past, present and future. *Journal of Nursing Education, 35*(2), 54–62.

Hoffman, S. E. (1997). Nursing centers—Models of professional practice. *Journal of Professional Nursing, 13*(6), 335.

Mackey, T. A., Adams, J., & McNiel, N. O. (1994). Nursing centers: Service as a business. *Nursing Economics, 12*(5), 276–282.

Riesch, S. K. (1992). Nursing centers: An analysis of the anecdotal literature. *Journal of Professional Nursing, 8*(1), 16–25.

Walker, P. H. (1994). Dollars and sense in health reform: Interdisciplinary practice and community nursing centers. *Nursing Administration Quarterly, 19*(1), 1–11.

■ *Editor's Questions for Discussion*

Discuss the types of planning and development that are essential prior to implementing and establishing a mobile nursing center (MNC). Apply suggestions from chapters by Carter (Chapter 39), Barger (Chapter 52), and Duffy (Chapter 53). Describe different types of MNCs, such as school-based, screening, and health education mobile units. How might issues be different, depending on the types of MNC provided and whether they are based in rural rather than urban areas?

Identify advantages and limitations of MNCs. Describe ethical and legal concerns unique to MNCs. Apply the discussions by Yocom and Thomas (Chapter 3), Davis (Chapter 6), Kopala (Chapter 5), Lane and Paterson (Chapter 7), and Purnell (Chapter 37) to MNCs. What qualifications are essential for RNs practicing in MNCs? Describe advantages and limitations of nursing students' experiences in these centers. How may advantages be capitalized upon and limitations minimized? How may nursing students be supervised in MNCs? Propose strategies to resolve issues and meet challenges.

What criteria should be considered in choosing advisors for the development of MNCs? Describe methodologies for assessing health care needs of a community. How can accurate information about MNCs be disseminated and misperceptions corrected? Discuss application of informatics technology and knowledge essential for MNCs. What advances described by Stevens and Weiner (Chapter 38) will benefit nursing centers, in particular?

Discuss cost containment and income producing strategies for MNCs. What role may nursing education programs and alumni play in resolving funding challenges?

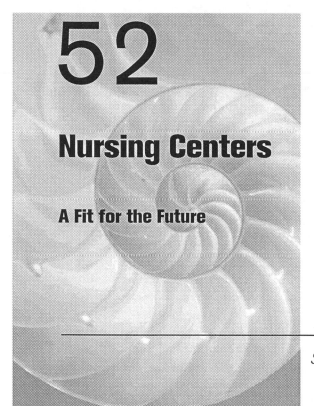

52

Nursing Centers

A Fit for the Future

Sara E. Barger, DPA, MN, RN, FAAN

The final two decades of the old millennium saw unprecedented change in health care delivery—in what care was delivered, where it was delivered, and how it was financed. It is within this maelstrom of change that nursing centers were born, flourished, and either expanded or died. The foundation built by nursing centers during the 1980s and 1990s became their launching pad to the new millennium. In this chapter, those two decades of nursing centers' performance are reviewed to project their fit for the future. The O'Neil and Pew Health Professions Commission's (1998) predictions of challenges and trends for health care delivery in the new century provide the framework for examining how nursing centers will fare in that expected environment. Finally, a prototype of the nursing center positioned for a preferred future is proposed.

■ Overview of Nursing Centers

Definition

As growing numbers of nursing centers began appearing in the 1980s, particularly in schools of nursing, the American Nurses Association (ANA) convened a task force to define and describe these centers. The resulting publication, *The Nursing Center: Concept and Design,* by Aydelotte et al. (1987) provides one of the most comprehensive and frequently cited definitions of nursing centers in the literature.

> Nursing Centers—sometimes referred to as community nursing organizations, nurse managed centers, nursing clinics and community nursing—are organizations that give the client direct access to professional nursing services. Using nursing models of health, professional nurses in these centers diagnose and treat human responses to actual and potential health problems, and promote health and optimal functioning among target populations and communities. The services provided in these centers are holistic and client-centered and are reimbursed at a reasonable fee level. Accountability and responsibility for client care and professional practice remain with the professional nurse. Overall accountability and responsibility remain with the nurse executive.
>
> Nursing centers are not limited to any particular organizational configuration. Nursing centers may be freestanding businesses or may be affiliated with universities or other service institutions such as home health agencies and hospitals. The primary characteristic of the organization is responsiveness to the health needs of the population. (p. 1)

Past Performance

Throughout the 1980s and 1990s a number of surveys were conducted in an attempt to identify existing centers. Although these surveys generally focused on centers run by schools of nursing (Barger, 1986; Barger & Bridges, 1990; Boettcher, 1989; Higgs, 1988; Roehrig, 1989), several studies focused on a broader profile of nursing centers, regardless of their institutional affiliation.

The first such study was conducted by the National League for Nursing (NLN) with funding from the Metropolitan Life Foundation (Barger & Rosenfeld, 1993). Investigators in this study had identified a total of 170 centers for inclusion in the study, but only 80 surveys contained sufficient data for analysis. The profile that emerges from this study is a center

that is less than 5 years old, affiliated with a parent organization, and serving a disproportionate share of the economically disadvantaged, including the very young and the very old. Predominant services include primary care, assessment, and screening. Reimbursement for services is from out-of-pocket—private pay—(30%); uncompensated (20%); Medicaid (14%); private insurance (13%); Medicare (10%); and other (11%) (Barger & Rosenfeld, 1993).

In a more recent study, Watson (1996) surveyed centers identified through the NLN's Council for Nursing Centers and through the National Rural Health Association. From a distribution of 234 surveys, 57 (or 49%) of 117 returned surveys reported having a nursing center. Again, most centers were affiliated with a larger organization, and the majority (54%) were established in the past 5 years. The sample included 31 academic centers and 26 centers affiliated with other organizations. Centers continued their pattern of reporting multiple funding sources but identified grants as the single most significant source of funding, followed by private pay, Medicaid, community support, Medicare, and private insurance. Persons aged 65 through 84 comprised the age group most served by nursing centers. Forty-two percent of the centers reported that 61 to 100% of those receiving services were indigent. Services included health teaching and nutrition counseling, physical exams, treatment for minor health problems, immunizations, and maternal and infant care. This second study corroborates the profile of nursing centers described in the 1993 NLN study, as the centers are relatively new and depend on multiple funding sources to serve age- and income-vulnerable populations.

These aggregate studies are supported by more than two decades of literature replete with many descriptions and case studies of operating nursing centers. A review of articles finds a significant number of centers targeting their services to the elderly (Arlton & Miercort, 1980; Bear, Brunell, & Covelli, 1997; Fielo & Crowe, 1992; Gresham-Kenton & Wisby, 1987; Haq, 1993; Pulliam, 1991; Smith & Sorrell, 1989; Taira, 1991; Taylor, Resick, D'Antonio, & Carroll, 1997; Thibodeau & Hawkins, 1987). Other vulnerable populations being served by these centers include the homeless (Scholler-Jaquish, 1996; Testani-Dufour, Green, Green, & Carter, 1996; Turner, Bauer, McNair, McNutt, & Walker, 1989) and residents in low income neighborhoods (Clark, 1984; Lundeen, 1993; McNeal, 1996; Ossler, Goodwin, Mariam, & Gillis, 1982). Centers also serve community residents, including many who live in rural areas (Barger, 1991; Lenz & Edwards, 1992).

As the nurse practitioner movement gained momentum during the 1990s and grant opportunities provided strong incentives to offer primary care services, more and more nursing centers expanded their earlier focus on health promotion and health maintenance to include increased emphasis on primary care and treatment of illnesses. Throughout descriptions of these centers is woven a thread of constant financial vulnerability, which is particularly ironic in that these centers frequently target services to an already vulnerable population.

Perhaps then it is not surprising that the literature in the 1990s documents growing emphasis on the financial aspects of running a nursing center. Elsberry and Nelson (1993) urged nursing centers to diversify their revenue streams by using multiple sources of financial support including fee-for-service, third-party reimbursement, contracts, charities, and grants. At the same time, others explored opportunities to maximize nursing center income (Walker, 1994). Centers also turned to the business literature for guidance in establishing themselves as viable businesses (Stark, Mackey, & Adams, 1995).

Thus, at the end of the 1990s, nursing centers faced the new millennium from a position of instability and vulnerability, despite increased attention to the business aspects of their operations. Studies since 1986 consistently showed the majority of centers to be less than 5 years old (Barger, 1986; Barger & Bridges, 1990; Barger & Rosenfeld, 1993; Watson, 1996). These findings suggest that a steady stream of new centers have been opening as others have closed, leaving the most vulnerable populations once again without health care. Moreover, although the need for research to measure outcomes of these centers and analyze effectiveness, efficiency, and quality of care has been recognized (Riesch, 1992), evidence suggests that research in these areas remains inadequate.

■ Forecasting the Future for Nursing Centers

At the end of the 1990s, nursing centers were in a state of flux—in a health care system that itself continued to be in constant state of almost revolutionary flux. While becoming more efficient in its use of resources, that system had disenfranchised more than 43 million people who had no health insurance (O'Neil & Pew Health Professions Commission, 1998). It is from this very population that nursing centers have frequently drawn the majority of their clientele. Thus the Commission's challenges for this century present very real threats to nursing center survival, much less their ability to thrive.

O'Neil and the Pew Health Professions Commission (1998) suggest a future that will require health care to respond to five challenges.

1. *Balancing the interests of the individual and society.* In a system that has traditionally focused on the individual, providers will be required to embrace a new outlook that

focuses on health of the whole population. This change will limit consumer choice.

2. *Introducing accountability to the system.* Performance standards for both internal benchmarking and external marketing are critical. Although reliable measurements of health improvement have not yet been developed, they will be adopted, albeit unevenly, across insurance markets. As plans subcontract with other providers to meet goals, the set of accountable relationships will widen.

3. *Truly managing care.* Managed care is defined by the commission as "those processes that work to rationalize the use of health care resources at the lowest possible cost and the highest possible quality" (p . 6). For managed care systems to demonstrate that they can lower costs and improve quality, management tools will be used that require increased scrutiny of individual providers by much broader networks of purchasers and plans.

4. *Making consolidation work.* Integrated delivery systems are evolving phenomena. It is believed that adequate size is needed to ensure long-term survival.

5. *Responding to demands of the emerging health care market.* Market forces are reorienting health care toward the culture of finance and big business. Four key constituencies shaping the emerging health care market are purchasers of care, insurance companies, providers, and individual consumers.

It is within context of these challenges of the commission that future risks for nursing centers are considered.

Future Risks

The nursing center in this century will be found in consolidated delivery systems. Although nursing centers in the past frequently were located in organizations, often nursing academic units, these centers usually operated independently with little organizational oversight. Their future existence will require that they merge into regional delivery systems, with the potential loss of identity for individual centers. The term *nurse-managed,* which has been a defining characteristic of these centers, may no longer be relevant as these centers become more oriented toward business. Thus health care will require leadership that has business and marketing expertise while maintaining its focus on quality of care. These requirements will decrease the likelihood of nurses as executives in these centers, unless nurses obtain additional business knowledge and skills.

Nursing centers also will be expected to participate in accreditation and to collect data for standardized evaluations, processes that will be new to most centers. Although an accreditation process for nursing centers similar to that used for home health agencies was developed by the NLN in the 1980s, centers did not seek accreditation. Most center directors cited cost and extensive allocation of resources to the process as reasons for not pursuing accreditation. In fact, there were no incentives for centers to pursue accreditation because there was no link between accreditation and reimbursement. However, this lack of experience with service accreditation will increase risks for these centers.

It will no longer be possible for centers to avoid accreditation for several reasons. Although centers have had a high degree of autonomy and have been insulated from outside scrutiny, the emerging health care system will require more accountability at all levels. Purchasers of care, managed care companies, insurers, and consumers themselves are demanding aggregated data on quality measures. Centers can expect to participate in an extensive process focused not only on measuring cost and patient satisfaction but also on outcomes in terms of health improvement. Moreover, as part of larger systems, centers will be required to conform to the same processes of data collection and accreditation used by larger systems. Many system institutions are accredited by the Joint Commission on Accreditation of Healthcare Organizations (JCAHO), which has required monitoring of a number of outcome measurements, using a system called Oryx (Moore, 1997). Thus nursing centers also can be expected to be monitored on outcome measures. Again, centers' lack of experience with these measures in a larger system that has experience may increase their levels of risk. How centers carry out their work will be of interest to a broader network of purchasers of care, insurance companies, and other providers than ever before.

It is clear that challenges for health care identified by O'Neil and the Pew Health Professions Commission actually may be viewed as threats by nurses in nursing centers. In fact, such fears are probably well founded. Therefore it is incumbent on those who would like to ensure the survival and even the success of these centers to capitalize on opportunities provided by this changing environment.

■ Positioning Nursing Centers for a Preferred Future

Nursing centers have long prided themselves on being on the "cutting edge" of health care delivery. Thus nine trends identified by O'Neil and the Pew Health Professions Commission (1998) that "will play a major role in the future of health care in the United States" (p. 11) provide opportunities for nursing centers. These trends create opportunities for nursing centers.

Trend #1—Continued Pressure on Costs

Although managed care has slowed the rate of growth in health care expenditures, it is predicted that health care costs soon will be rising as health plans are forced to raise their premiums. However, employers and government, as

major payors of care, are unwilling to pay more for health care. At the same time, providers are resisting reductions in compensation and consumers are demanding more choices. This conflict will require additional realignment in the health care system (O'Neil & Pew Health Professions Commission, 1998).

Nursing Centers have touted themselves as cost-effective health care providers for more than two decades. The expected continuing pressure on costs provides opportunities for centers to design more cost-effective ways to offer existing services and even expand into new service areas that are of high quality and modest cost. Because labor costs are the major contributor to the total cost of health care, centers have opportunities to keep costs low by using the lowest credentialed provider who can accomplish the task while maintaining quality. Frequently, nurse practitioners rather than physicians have been the provider of choice in these centers. Other, less-skilled providers can be used for tasks not requiring the expertise of a nurse practitioner. This task reallocation will include nurses at all educational levels as well as unlicensed assistive personnel.

Trend #2—Oversupply of Resources

A result of a system that historically reimbursed by cost, the oversupply of providers, hospitals, and technology existed because providers were able to generate demand for their services. This supply-driven resource market first began to be curbed in the 1990s, but it will take several decades for it to balance out because of resistance of communities to the closure of hospitals and of providers to reduction in numbers or income (O'Neil & Pew Health Professions Commission, 1998).

As the pressure to control costs continues, consolidated systems will have to face the inevitability of closing more hospitals. The history of locating nursing centers in underserved areas and serving "medically underserved populations" increases the probability that they will be located in areas affected by hospital closures. Because physician practice has traditionally been tied to the presence of a hospital, it is hard to imagine many physicians remaining in these areas, regardless of the predicted oversupply. Expected closure of hospitals and subsequent departure of physicians will require nursing centers to reexamine existing services in relation to potentially new demands and markets. These centers may need to expand both their hours and services to cover deficits in health care left by departing providers. These deficits are likely to be most extensive in both rural and inner city areas.

To have necessary access to both the referral mechanisms and technology that will be required, centers must be integrated into larger systems with providers and facilities located distally from the nursing center. The technology of telehealth will provide necessary linkages to specialists without the risks to safety and quality that result from excess capacity. Such risks occur when there are too many specialists or providers who do not have adequate numbers of clientele to maintain their expertise. Thus, in tele health clients will find themselves "connected" to specialists with adequate breadth and depth of experiences with specific diagnoses to be highly competent in their field.

Trend #3–Aging Population

A dramatic increase in the number of seniors during the next three decades will mean that roughly 20% of the population will be 65 or older by 2030. The number of seniors aged 85 and older will grow at an even faster rate. This population is more likely to have greater incidences of chronic diseases and mental and physical disabilities (O'Neil & Pew Health Professions Commission, 1998).

Nursing centers already serve more seniors than any other age group, so they are well positioned as important providers for this fastest growing age group. Moreover, instead of focusing on expensive treatment for this age group, nursing centers traditionally have directed services for seniors toward prevention, including health education and early detection. The growing incidence of chronic diseases in this population suggests that nursing centers should routinely include case management in their service inventory, since it can be used to lower costs and improve quality (Cesta & Falter, 1999). The fact that greater numbers of seniors are living in locations distant from their grown children makes case management an even more valued service. Regardless of the authorization of payment for case management services from established insurance or payor systems, it is likely that distant children will contract willingly with nursing centers for case management services for their aging parents.

Trend #4–Information Technology

Availability to the consumer of information on health and disease through information technology, specifically the Internet, has changed the knowledge base of consumers about not only disease, but also treatment choices. More will use this resource to obtain more and better information (O'Neil & Pew Health Professions Commission, 1998).

Since nursing centers have been viewed as valuable educational resources for consumers, they will be able to assist clients in sorting out options and choices. Nursing centers can continue to assist consumers in both obtaining the information and then making sense of it, thus extending the role of counselor and consultant.

Trend #5–Advances in the Treatment of Disease

Technological advances in treatment of disease are expected to continue with better imaging, less invasive surgery, and micromachines that travel inside the body. Payors will be assessing new technologies relative to cost and effectiveness (O'Neil & Pew Health Professions Commission, 1998).

Nursing centers, consistently operating at the low end of technology, may be able to capitalize on advances in a particular technology (e.g., screening for a specific chronic disease) to meet a special need. However, the cost-benefit ratios of these advances for centers will have to be analyzed carefully in order to incorporate only those technologies that allow centers to maintain their low-cost, high-effectiveness niche in the health care market place.

Trend #6–Improving Quality

Whereas, in the past, measurements of quality in health care have focused on structural and process measures, there are increased efforts to focus on results or outcomes. These efforts are made more productive by advances in information management. Continuous Quality Improvement (CQI) also has expanded its focus to the entire process of care, including tracking of results. Moreover, consumers will demand quality measures and information, thus changing accountability in professional practice (O'Neil & Pew Health Professions Commission, 1998).

Nursing centers have documented clients' satisfaction with services through numerous surveys (Haq, 1993). Nevertheless, movement toward a standard set of outcomes measures will enable nursing centers to collect data that will facilitate comparisons across providers and service delivery sites. It will be important for centers to have management information systems that allow data collection and analysis consistent with national systems for tracking quality. System requirements include a computerized medical record with complete flexibility in outputs, allowing centers to analyze various data elements for outcomes. These

systems will yield new opportunities for documenting quality previously unknown to centers.

Trend # 7–Changing Role of the Health Care Consumer

With increased out-of-pocket costs and more knowledge about the impact of lifestyle choices, consumers are expected to make more informed decisions about health care utilization, considering factors of quality and cost. Increased access to information technology along with advances in quality measurement certainly will empower tomorrow's consumer (O'Neil & Pew Health Professions, 1998).

Nursing centers have never really taken patients for granted and have focused many services on health promotion and disease prevention strategies. Hence they already are prepared for a role in changing individual attitudes and empowering consumers to take charge of their health and their health care. Centers need to ensure that information about their services and providers is available online and that they submit data to systems collecting it across a range of standardized criteria.

Trend #8–Disparities in Population

Improvements in health care are not available to all. The future could see two distinct groups of patients: the wealthy with information and health care, and the poor without either. As the income gap between rich and poor is the most important predictor of a nation's health—as measured by life expectancy—and that gap is expected to increase, the overall health of the nation is expected to decline. Moreover, rural and inner city populations will continue to suffer from lack of health care resources and providers available to those in other areas (O'Neil & Pew Health Professions Commission, 1998).

Nursing centers, already in inner city and rural areas, have a rich history of serving disproportionate numbers of disenfranchised populations, a finding well documented in the literature. Professionals in nursing centers understand this reality and are equipped with skills to manage the health care of these populations. With recognition by national policy makers of the impact of these disparities on morbidity and mortality measures of the nation's health, nursing centers are well positioned to take a leadership role in moving "organizations, systems and policies toward strategies that can change the reality" (O'Neil & Pew Health Professions Commission, 1998, p. 23). Despite the oversupply of resources identified in Trend #2, O'Neil and the Pew Commission do not suggest that resources and providers will redistribute themselves to inner city and rural areas. Because nursing centers historically have been the providers of record in many of these areas, nurses in these centers must use their knowledge to influence policy makers. Needed are legislation and administrative policies that provide adequate compensation to providers with capabilities for changing morbidity and mortality data with respect to these vulnerable populations.

Trend #9–Broadening the Definition of Health

Beginning steps that the managed care industry has taken toward a more population-based approach to health management will be expanded in the future. Tracking prevalence and effectiveness of preventive care is included in that approach. "As providers and plans manage larger groups under capitation, and as our aging population presents with more chronic illness, we will see a greater emphasis on the prevention and management of disease" (O'Neil & Pew Health Professions Commission, 1998, p. 23).

Nursing centers from the very beginning have focused a major component of their services on health promotion and disease prevention. Despite adding a broader array of services over the years, most centers continue to have health promotion as their central core of services. A few centers have even focused on alternative treatment such as therapeutic touch. Therefore nursing centers can capitalize on a health care environment with greater emphasis on prevention.

However without major policy changes, nursing centers will be unable to continue providing these services because, generally, they have been uncompensated. Nevertheless, when those in nursing centers help policy makers understand the relationship between the problem of health disparities in the population (Trend #8) and the solution of the effectiveness of preventive care (Trend #9), new approaches to financing these services will be found.

■ A Nursing Center That Fits the Health Care System of the Future

Since the hospital closed several years ago, the nursing center will be the gatekeeper and maintenance provider of health care for people living in the area. Many people will find that the center meets almost all their health care needs and that, when additional services and expertise are needed, the nursing center is tied into a multilevel network of other providers. Due to the many telehealth technologies available, people usually will find their health care needs met without leaving their communities. The center will have a cadre of case managers who follow clients who have expensive chronic diseases. In addition, the center will provide case managers to others who request them on a fee-for-service basis. Over the years the average age of those using the center will increase.

The center will increase its information technology in order to network with other providers and collect data needed for the national total quality assessment system required of all providers. With centers being paid on a capitation basis, and earning bonuses when individuals are managed entirely by the center, centers will expand their disease prevention services and focus even more on healthy lifestyles.

The center's providers will become very involved in influencing policy and regularly discuss issues with elected officials at the state and national levels. They also will work with administrators in state and local offices who have oversight functions for the quality of services offered in the center. The center will monitor carefully the health care environment for trends that require modification in service or direction.

■ *Concluding Statement*

O'Neil and the Pew Health Professions Commission provided the framework to assess threats and opportunities for nursing centers in the new millennium. Results of this assessment indicate that nursing centers must retain their core values while learning new survival strategies.

The prototype of a successful center for the next century will be found in an inner city or rural area as an integrated component of a large managed care system. The center's leaders will recognize that success of the center is predicated on continuous and timely assessment of the goodness-of-fit between needs of the population, quality and availability of services, and the availability of resources.

References

Arlton, D., & Miercort, O. (1980). A nursing clinic: The challenge for student learning opportunities. *Journal of Nursing Education, 19*(1), 53–58.

Aydelotte, M. K., Barger, S.E., Branstetter, E., Felving, R. J., Lindgren, K., Lundeen, S., McDaniel, S., & Riesch, S. K. (1987). *The nursing center: Concept and design.* Kansas City, MO: American Nurses Association.

Barger, S. E. (1986). Academic nursing centers: A demographic profile. *Journal of Professional Nursing, 2*(4), 246–251.

Barger, S. E. (1991). The nursing center: A model for rural nursing practice. *Nursing & Health Care, 12*(6), 290–294.

Barger, S. E., & Bridges, W. C. (1990). An assessment of academic nursing centers. *Nurse Educator, 5*(2), 31–36.

Barger, S. E., & Rosenfeld, P. (1993). Models in community health care: Findings from a national study of community nursing centers. *Nursing & Health Care, 14*(8), 426–431.

Bear, M., Brunell, M. L., & Covelli, M. (1997). Using a nursing framework to establish a nurse-managed senior health clinic. *Journal of Community Health Nursing, 14*(4), 225–235.

Boettcher, J. H. (1989). Nurse practice centers and faculty job satisfaction. *Nursing Connections, 2*(3), 7–17.

Cesta, T. G., & Falter, E. J. (1999). Case management: Its value for staff nurses. *American Journal of Nursing, 99*(5), 48–51.

Clark, M. J. (1984). Nursing leadership in a shoestring clinic. *Topics in Clinical Nursing, 6*(1), 56–62.

Elsberry, N., & Nelson, F. (1993). How to plan financial support for nursing centers. *Nursing & Health Care, 14*(8), 408–413.

Fielo, S. B., & Crow, R. L. (1992). A nursing center in Brooklyn. *Nursing & Health Care, 13*(9), 488–493.

Gresham-Kenton, L., & Wisby, M. (1987). Development and implementation of nurse-managed health programs: A problem-oriented approach. *Journal of Ambulatory Care Management, 10*(3), 20–29.

Haq, M. B. (1993). Understanding older adult satisfaction with primary health care services at a nursing center. *Applied Nursing Research, 6*(3), 125–131.

Higgs, Z. (1988). The academic nurse-managed center movement: A survey report. *Journal of Professional Nursing, 4*(6), 422–429.

Lenz, C. L., & Edwards, J. (1992). Nurse-managed primary care: Tapping the rural community power base. *Journal of Nursing Administration, 22*(9), 57–61.

Lundeen, S. P. (1993). Comprehensive, collaborative, coordinated, community-based care: A community nursing center model. *Family & Community Health, 16*(2), 57–65.

McNeal, G. L. (1996). Mobile health care for those at risk. *Nursing and Health Care: Perspectives on Community, 7*(3), 134–140.

Moore, J. D. (1997, December 15). JCAHO's fix for ORYX: Ease provider rules. *Modern Healthcare,* 16.

O'Neil, E. H., & Pew Health Professions Commission. (1998, December). *Recreating health professional practice for a new century.* San Francisco: Pew Health Professions Commission.

Ossler, C., Goodwin, M., Mariam, M., & Gillis, C. (1982). Establishment of a nursing clinic for faculty and student clinical practice. *Nursing Outlook, 30*(7), 402–405.

Pulliam, L. (1991). Client satisfaction with a nurse-managed clinic. *Journal of Community Health Nursing, 8*(2), 97–112.

Riesch, S. K. (1992). Nursing centers. *Annual Review of Nursing Research, 10,* 145–162.

Roehrig, M. J. (1989). Nursing centers: State of the art—Survey results. In *Nursing centers: Meeting the demand for quality health care* (pp. 61–77). New York: National League for Nursing Press.

Scholler-Jaquish, A. (1996). Walk-in health clinic for the homeless. *Nursing and Health Care: Perspectives on Community, 17*(3), 119–123.

Smith, J. M., & Sorrell, V. (1989). Developing wellness programs: A nurse-managed stay well center for senior citizens. *Clinical Nurse Specialist, 3*(4), 198–202.

Stark, P. L., Mackey, T. A., & Adins, J. (1995). Nurse-managed clinics: A blueprint for success using the Covey framework. *Journal of Professional Nursing, 11*(2), 71–77.

Taira, F. (1991). Teaching independently living older adults about managing their medications. *Rehabilitation Nursing, 16*(6), 322–326.

Taylor, C. A., Resick, L., D'Antonio, J. A., & Caroll, T. L. (1997). The advanced practice nurse role in implementing and evaluating two nurse-managed wellness clinics: Lessons learned about structure, process, and outcomes. *Advanced Practice Nursing Quarterly, 3*(2), 36–45.

Testani-Dufur, L., Green, L., Green, R., & Carter, K. F. (1996). Establishing outreach health services for homeless persons: An emerging role for nurse managers. *Journal of Community Health Nursing, 13*(4), 221–235.

Thibodeau, J., & Hawkins, J. (1987). Evolution of a nursing center. *Journal of Ambulatory Care Management, 10*(3) 30–39.

Turner, S. L., Bauer, G., McNair, E., McNutt, B., & Walker, W. (1989). The homeless experience: Clinic building in a community health discovery-learning project. *Public Health Nursing, 6*(2), 97–101.

Walker, P. (1994). A comprehensive community nursing center model: Maximizing practice income—A challenge to educators. *Journal of Professional Nursing, 10*(3), 131–139.

Watson, L. J. (1996). A national profile of nursing centers: Arenas for advanced practice. *Nurse Practitioner, 21*(3), 72–81.

■ *Editor's Questions for Discussion*

Identify implications and applications from Barger's presentation to the writings of Titler (Chapter 35), Carter (Chapter 39), Robinson, Griffith and Sullivan-Marx (Chapter 41), Sefcik and Jones (Chapter 48), Hollinger-Smith (Chapter 45), McDermott (Chapter 49), Pullen (Chapter 50), Todero (Chapter 51), Gerber (Chapter 57), and Boland (Chapter 71). Based on the known financial aspects of nursing centers, what factors have kept nursing centers from responding effectively to those issues? Propose viable strategies for addressing financial concerns. How can nursing successfully strategize to resolve financial dilemmas in nursing centers?

What criteria and resources are essential for planning and developing a nursing center? Identify the minimal professional resources that are essential. How does a Center's Director or Board entice larger organizations or universities to endorse or commit resources for nursing centers? To what extent should nursing centers be interdisciplinary in providing services? What negotiating considerations are essential for the administration and control of nursing centers by nursing?

Why has research concerning nursing centers been inadequate? Identify specific research questions that must be addressed for nursing centers to be viable. How can nursing executives plan for nursing centers in consolidated delivery systems? What may ensure that nursing executives are allowed to perform a leadership role in consolidated systems? How should nursing education programs prepare students for such systems?

Discuss the pros and cons of accreditation for nursing centers. How is accountability addressed now and expected to be addressed in the future? To what extent should the nursing profession focus on accountability as a priority in nursing centers? How might such a focus be a key to the effectiveness and resolution of numerous issues? Propose specific strategies for resolving conflicts between provider compensation and consumers' choices in health care. How might case management lower costs and improve quality in nursing centers?

In positioning nursing practice for the future, propose specific strategies that the nursing profession could adopt to address the Pew Health Professions Commission's nine trends, as presented by Barger. Identify specific implications for nursing education programs and other practice settings regarding these trends. To what extent do the discussions of Pullen (Chapter 50) and Todero (Chapter 51) address Barger's concerns for the future? How does Boland's (Chapter 71) health emphasis as a nursing education concept align with Barger's view?

53

Nursing Entrepreneurship

Potential, Plausibility, and Prospects

Virginia J. Duffy, PhD, RN, CS, NP

Changes in the health care system and the practice of nursing are astonishing. At times we hardly recognize ourselves or our profession. As a result, we are concerned, frustrated, and angry about many important issues. Short staffing, floating, use of unlicensed personnel, increased acuity of patients, increased responsibility, decreased respect, autonomy and job security, managed care obstacles, compromised patient care, and a change of focus from patients to profits are all taking their toll. Nurses everywhere are experiencing a crisis of personal and professional identity, often feeling powerless, due to low status in the hierarchy and yet responsible for handling many of the problems in the health care system. We have been near burnout but have still managed to care for others. These feelings have led us to take a long, hard look at ourselves and our profession, where we have been, and where we want to be. The same factors that are causing so much upheaval are also impetus for remarkable changes in our profession and ourselves.

In the long tradition of nursing, we have rallied our resources and called on our creativity and skills to deal with upheaval. Self-reliance, adaptability, caring, decision-making, and innovation have allowed us to think beyond traditional roles and create myriad opportunities for ourselves. We understand that we have worked independently for a long time in many situations and have not been recognized for it. We have fought for our patients but less so for ourselves. In addition to providing outstanding patient care, nurses have developed, executed, and administered successful programs that have kept health care systems viable. We have taken on enormous responsibilities while the financial rewards and recognition have gone to others. Some of these realizations have angered and astounded us—and ultimately forced us to consider alternatives to what we have been doing for so long. There must be a better way!

To some, entrepreneurship came as a surprise. The first time someone referred to me as an entrepreneur, I was startled. Sometimes, circumstances compel us to seek other means of professional and financial survival. There is nothing like losing your job to make you an entrepreneur! Many of us are beginning to realize that they do not need parental systems to manage their careers. We do not need to be directed in how we should practice as health care providers or what our philosophy should be. We can make our own decisions about career matters without administrators and physicians telling us what to do or be.

The "deinstitutionalization" of nursing is in full swing. The force of this change has sometimes left us frightened, but it has also energized us to look beyond the safety of the institution. The opportunities for nursing entrepreneurship both inside and outside the system are many, and more continue to be discovered every day. They seem to be limited only by our imagination. These opportunities offer increased independence and autonomy, further realization of talents, skill building, and, yes, even increased financial rewards. At the same time that nurses are developing business skills, they are also increasing their confidence and self-esteem.

Who are these nurses who are venturing out on their own? What are they like? What do they do and how do they do it? How do they learn what it takes to become an entrepreneur? They are nurses who enjoy freedom and a change of routine. They are independent decision makers. They love what they are doing, but they also expect both personal and financial compensations. These are nurses with superb clinical skills who are able to identify their own strengths and weakness. They are sometimes bored or suffocated in their jobs or feel a strong desire to undertake a project or offer a needed service. They are risk-takers and leaders (either formal or informal) to whom others look for advice. They have self-discipline, and they plan ahead. Nurse entrepreneurs are realistic in determining what skills they need, are willing to develop them, and seek knowledge wherever it is available. They read and conduct the necessary research, attend conferences and meetings, hire consultants, take formal and informal classes, seek out professional mentors, network regularly, and ask many questions. They capitalize on personal characteristics important for entrepreneurship, and strengthen those that need work. They practice thoughtful risk taking, engage in confidence building, and allow themselves mistakes.

■ Business Possibilities for Nurses

Independent practice is more and more enticing, not only to advanced practice nurses but also to all registered nurses (RNs). Nurses as licensed professionals have the ability not only to work independently in their areas of expertise, but also to contract themselves out to large institutions. The day is fast approaching when many nursing services will be contracted. Some ingenious nurses are developing groups, partnerships, and corporations that offer a variety of nursing services directly to clients at home, clinics, hospitals, schools, jails, adult homes, and other agencies. In general, consultation in many fields, including nursing, has grown tremendously with the move from an industrial to an information society. Nurses are offering services or consultation in their areas of expertise, such as specialized health care, home health care, health teaching, gerontology, emergency and trauma, management of chronic illness, rehabilitation, research, and quality management and improvement. The incredible growth of health maintenance organizations (HMOs) has offered a variety of opportunities for nurses to become case managers and quality assurance providers. These positions are sometimes open for employees but also are frequently offered on a contractual basis. Nurses are also becoming "intrapreneurs," remaining within the system but carving out a niche for themselves over which they have more control.

What ventures are nurse entrepreneurs engaged in? *Everything* seems to be the most appropriate response. They are consultants in many areas, private practitioners, educators, salespersons, and business owners. Nurses are publishers, writers, therapists, holistic practitioners, motivational speakers, home health care agency owners, case managers, inventors, medical–legal consultants, coaches, and geriatric specialists. They are consultants to HMOs, attorneys, nursing homes, hospitals, insurance companies, businesses, and other places that need and appreciate the expertise and experience they offer.

Nurses are using their keen awareness of patient and system needs to become inventors of everything from health care products to systems processes, such as scheduling care planning and quality monitoring. They are selling products of interest to, and needed by, the public and health care professionals. Education and seminar presentation can be a rewarding way for nurses to prosper, using their skills in teaching and their broad nursing knowledge. Nurses are being creative for profit and fun. They are writing for magazines, publishing books, developing videos, and often marketing them themselves. Publishers recognize the potential of nurse writers,

and nurses themselves are starting publishing companies.

■ *Successful Nurse Entrepreneurs*

Let me tell you my story and that of two other nurse entrepreneurs. For me, becoming an entrepreneur started many years ago with a part-time private practice of psychotherapy. I longed to be independent and wished to have control over my own destiny. I am a risk-taker and an innovator, tend to be outspoken, and like to be in control. (These same attributes have at times caused me to be labeled as "difficult.") I was motivated to turn part-time work into a full-time career about 5 years ago when I finally accepted what I had long suspected. In the system where I was employed, I did not have the power to change the things I believed needed changing. I also was not receiving the recognition or financial reward I believed I deserved. I finally admitted to myself that this was not likely to change. I decided to market myself on a contractual basis as a psychiatric nurse practitioner.

I developed a business and collaborating agreement with a physician colleague. Within a year I had enough offers that I was able to choose among them. In time I have become respected, valued for my skills, and pursued. Over time, I expanded my business, gave it a name (PsychSense), and now offer seminars and educational materials on a variety of mental health topics and on nurse entrepreneurship. I market myself as offering practical, psychological seminars that are affordable and applicable to daily living. One of my selling points is that I strive to make things understandable without making them too simple. I have my own Web site (www.notjustyourdoctor.com) to help market my products and myself. It is fun and exciting!

Along the way I have encountered obstacles, but they have not been insurmountable.

As a nurse I have needed to market myself and educate others about my skills. I have had to convince others that I have something special to offer. I started with very few business skills and even less understanding. Learning to advertise myself has been a struggle. Women and nurses have been discouraged from self-acclaim. I have negotiated methods of reimbursement that, for the most part, have been self-payment; however, I have used sliding scales and occasionally have billed under the collaborating physician. I have also fought to gain admission to as many HMO panels as possible. The greatest barriers for me, and I believe for most nurse entrepreneurs, are psychological.

As women and nurses we have been taught to care for others, minimize financial rewards, and avoid competition. The things that have helped me the most have been my tenacity, willingness to take risks, and perhaps most of all, finding supportive people who have similar ideals and goals. I am no longer afraid to ask for advice and mentoring when I need it. I encourage other nurses dreaming of becoming entrepreneurs to network, develop their business skills, and hire consultants as needed. Get involved with other women and nurses in business, but most important do what you really love and believe in.

Having personal freedom and time are my highest priorities. I have decided to work less and spend more time with the people and things I care about. I try to take care of myself and to keep my life relatively simple. Due to these choices, my business remains small, my income is less than it could be, but I am attaining my goals and enjoying success. Keeping a balance in my personal, professional, and spiritual life, although challenging, is critical.

Vergie Seymore, RN, MA, is President and Chief Executive Officer (CEO) of VSWAN Corporation. She is an inventor and manufacturer and owner of Vergie's Manor residential care facilities for the elderly in Carson, California. She remembers vividly her motivation to start her own business (V. Seymore, personal communication, February 15, 1999). Vergie had been visiting a convalescent hospital and what most affected her was the overwhelming smell of urine. Thus began her lifelong personal quest to eradicate that smell from her memory. She states that she has always wanted to be her own boss, be a leader, and be a mentor to others. Her incontinence product, The Dignity Apron, is a combination of function and self-respect. It is currently in the process of review by Medicare. Vergie's adult residences provide high-level care and individualized attention in a homelike atmosphere, with no smell of urine! She has a long waiting list and her homes are widely recognized for excellence.

Seymore emphasizes how important it is to believe in yourself, even when others may not. Like many of us, she has not always received the support and encouragement from others that she would have hoped. As a black woman in business, she has had to prove herself more than once. The qualities that have helped her most are believing in herself, being a self-starter and motivator, and being able to take risks. Entrepreneurship has brought her independence and self-satisfaction. Most important, it has allowed her to help others by caring for the elderly in a honorable and dignified way and providing satisfying employment opportunities for others. Sometimes, she says, she "feels married" to her business, but she has decided that the rewards have been worth it.

Vergie Seymore strongly urges aspiring entrepreneurs to develop a concrete plan and stick to it and to commit to long-term and short-term goals and call them to mind often. She encourages others to "strive to reach the top, as the bottom is crowded."

Laura Gasparis Vonfrolio, PhD, RN, is a nurse entrepreneur extraordinaire! She is the President and Chief Executive Officer of three companies: Education Enterprises, Power Publishing, and Revolution Design on Staten Island, New York. Education Enterprises specializes in seminars, particularly vacation seminars for nurses. Laura has made presentations to more than 60,000 nurses. She publishes books on a wide variety of nursing topics. Revolution Design specializes in graphic design and advertising. Laura is also the president of the National Nurses in Business Association. She has been a mentor to countless nurses interested in entrepreneurship.

Laura became a nurse entrepreneur because she felt that the traditional work environment expected too much conformity from nurses and was often degrading to them (L. G. Vonfrolio, personal communication, February 15, 1999). She thought that being her own boss would reward her with increased self-esteem and a sense of power. She was right! Laura's biggest challenge was finding staff who had the same vision that she has. She suggests that you work with those whose strengths complement your own.

Vonfrolio believes that her greatest strength is her ability to rise and try again if she stumbles or falls. She describes herself as stubborn and persistent, with ample stamina. Vonfrolio truly views obstacles as challenges but recognizes that she sometimes works too hard. She states she has succeeded financially and delights in using her resources to help others, especially nurses. Vonfrolio has been a mentor and cheerleader for many new entrepreneurs. Her advice for those interested in following the path of entrepreneurship is to "just go for it." She encourages nurses to trust themselves and try to get beyond their fear of failure.

■ Barriers to Entrepreneurship for Nurses

If things are so positive, why aren't more nurses becoming entrepreneurs? There are many barriers for nurse entrepreneurs to overcome; they may be legal, financial, or psychological.

Although nurses are already licensed and may be self-employed as independent practitioners, the concept of entrepreneurship often goes unrecognized by many in the profession. As Catherine Welch (1986) pointed out:

> Prior to the Depression nursing, like medical practice, was predominantly private-duty independent contractor service. It is important to emphasize that nursing's shift from the entrepreneurial to the employee role was not planned, designed or directed as a strategy to develop professional autonomy or extend public access to our services. Rather as a profession, nursing was swept along and shaped by the social and economical voices of the times. (p. 2)

Questions about scope of practice arise continually, particularly in light of new technology, the rapidly changing field, and nursing's base of responsibility. License endorsement processes used by the states are confusing, but the expanding field of telemedicine is increasing awareness of this issue and forcing nurses to negotiate. Planning for implementation of a mutual recognition system of nurse licensure to facilitate practice across state lines is underway. Questions about advanced practice can also be confusing, and the laws vary from state to state. The necessity of physician collaboration is a barrier for many advanced practice nurses. Finding competent collegial physicians willing to collaborate in a business relationship can be a challenge.

Many areas remain fraught with unanswered questions and are without legal precedent. Legal consultation is critical but sometimes results in contradictory or vague advice.

Nurses usually have little formal education in business; it is rarely addressed in undergraduate nursing curricula. Unfamiliarity with business issues such as tax laws, liability, and accounting practices can seem overwhelming to a new entrepreneur. Lack of business knowledge and skills can be a significant barrier to nurses seeking self-employment or business ownership. Many nurses have not learned to think in business terms, have few skills in marketing, and little experience with money management or the corporate world. When starting a business, you must often do everything yourself, while at the same time develop all the new skills necessary for success. This can be extremely stressful. Most of us have avoided acquiring business skills, partly because we view them as being opposed to what nurses "do," that is, nurturing and caring for others for altruistic reasons.

Nurses rarely have the capital to become self-employed and often are unfamiliar with financial matters. Financial issues are complex, and start-up costs are high. It is necessary to have personal and business operating funds for at least a year to allow the business time to be successful. Expenses need to be projected and anticipated accurately. The initial outlay of money can be daunting and is usually underestimated. In developing a budget, payment of taxes, purchase of malpractice, health, and disability insurance, allowing for sick and vacation time, and savings for retirement need to be anticipated. On the one hand, overspending can result in debt that is difficult to eliminate. On the other hand, trying to be too frugal can limit success. Raising capital can be a challenge. Seeking business loans can cause much anxiety, and they may be difficult to obtain if the applicant is not an astute business person.

Nurses have a history of mediocre salaries. Often, nurses have accepted low salaries and high expectations without question. Those who have tried to demand better salaries and working conditions have sometimes been accused of being unprofessional or uncaring.

Many nurses are uncomfortable asking for financial compensation in providing service. Determining fees is difficult. Skills should be priced fairly, but not underpriced. Reimbursement for nursing services continues to be difficult to obtain. This issue is vexatious, and its seriousness varies by insurance company, location, and credentials. However, nurses have begun to make improvements in this area.

Money is not the only factor that determines success, even though many believe that failure is due to low capital. More often, however, failure is due to lack of skill, poor management strategies, or lack of commitment or confidence. Money will not substitute for creativity, perseverance, and self-esteem.

Psychological barriers may be the most difficult to overcome. Business knowledge can be acquired and business skills can be developed, but personality traits most helpful to entrepreneurs may be impossible to attain. As women and nurses we have been enculturated to think and behave in certain ways. We avoid seeking rewards for ourselves and tend to be hypercritical and hesitant to tell others about our skills and talents regardless how proficient we may be. Asking for money has been an unthinkable idea for many.

The competitive behavior necessary for survival in the business world is something that nurses have avoided. Traditionally, we have been encouraged to be quiet and follow the orders of physicians, hospitals, and administrators. From them, we have experienced insufficient interest in our personal or professional welfare. We struggle within ourselves and our profession about many of these issues, sometimes handicapping ourselves. As a result, other health care professionals may be encouraged to believe that nurses should remain in traditional roles—and express that preference. We as nurses often do not support other nurses who venture beyond traditional roles, perhaps out of fear, envy, or simply resistance to change. Change however, is inevitable, both for women and for nurses, even though at times it can seem slow indeed.

■ Overcoming Barriers: Where to Start

Although there may appear to be innumerable obstacles to overcome, there are resources to help, and ways to help oneself. Be honest with yourself about what you want from your business. Is it money? More freedom? The ability to change things or have an impact on a system? Take an honest look at your personal characteristics. Identify your strengths and those areas in which you must grow if you are to succeed as an entrepreneur. These characteristics, although difficult to change, can be nurtured and broadened by enhancing self-awareness, seeking out mentors, and by trial and error. Make specific plans to address your limitations. Take classes, read journals and books, and attend workshops and lectures. Concentrate on personal growth, practice communication skills, improve your professional image and engage in self-confidence building.

Support is critical. Surround yourself with likeminded persons who can offer support and honest feedback. Avoid naysayers! Join organizations of entrepreneurs and enlist friends and family to support you. You can learn and develop the required skills yourself, but you also can, and should, consult and collaborate with those who have expertise in your areas of need.

Consultation and networking will aid success and facilitate support. Networking is natural to some people, but others have to force themselves to do it. It becomes easier in time, but starting is the key. Trying to anticipate and solve all possible problems before they occur will only impede progress. It is better to find a consultant than spend precious hours floundering. Qualified and effective consultants may not be easy to find—and they don't come cheap. Often consultants are needed in more than one area and the right consultant may not be the first one you contact. Discernment and intuition are invaluable in choosing a consultant.

For questions regarding the practice of nursing, you should consult the Nurse Practice Act in your state. The American Nurses Association Standards of Clinical Practice (1998) and its Ethical Code for Nurses (1985) can be help-

ful. The U.S. Small Business Administration (SBA) (1999) has development centers that offer free consultation in many states. The Service Corps of Retired Executives (SCORE) is a group that volunteer their time to help aspiring entrepreneurs (National Score Office, 1999).

Nurses must be able to compete in the marketplace. As nurses, we must be comfortable dealing with CEOs and speaking the language of both health care and business. Formal classes and degrees in business are possible but not necessary. Nurse entrepreneurs should be reading business journals, especially those related to health care. Business shrewdness will make us more comfortable when negotiating with those in power. We must know what administrators need, what their priorities are, and be able to persuade them that nurses are capable to meet those challenges. We do not need to know it all, but we must know what we need and where to find it! Table 53.1 is a guide for attaining that essential knowledge.

Develop a business plan, put it in writing, and refer to it often. It does not need to be complicated, but it should be well thought out. Be clear about your goals and set a time frame for each. Describe clearly your product or service and target audience. Know what the demand is for your product or service, who your competitors are, what they offer, and what they charge. Develop a budget and organizational and staffing plans. Have a contingency plan.

To be an independent contractor you must meet certain criteria set by the Internal Revenue Service (IRS). These include defining your own hours and whether you will be working for more than one firm. This information is available from the IRS. Many nurses start off using sole proprietorship as the legal structure for their business. Partnerships, profit, and nonprofit corporations are other alternatives. If you want to give your business a name other than your own, you need to register it with the local county clerk and get a doing business as

TABLE 53.1   What You Need to Know!

Money management	Start-up costs, raising capital, budget, and accounting procedures
Business legal structures	Sole proprietorship, partnership, or corporation
Business plan	Mission, goals, objectives, internal analysis, action plan, organization, staffing, and contingency plan
Legal issues	Regulations, nurse practice act, public health laws, business law, and tax law
Market analysis/strategies	Market needs, competition, definition of product or service, or both, and target population
Records management	Accounts, sales, and expenses
Insurance	Liability, malpractice, personal, disability, and reimbursement
Marketing	Advertising strategies and networking

(DBA) certificate. Registration is inexpensive and protects the name of your business, so no one else can use it.

■ Marketing

Marketing is a world in itself. You can hire a publicist or marketing specialist, but doing so will certainly be costly for a new business. Developing good public relations is an excellent marketing strategy. Offering something to the community at no cost, serving on boards and committees, and arranging for press releases are all ways to market yourself at no cost. Because such activities take time, try to think of ways to combine efforts and accomplish more than one thing at a time. For example, a press release may be used as a short article or in a brochure. Use every public contact to market yourself. Never expect all your business or revenue to come from one source or from one type of marketing tool.

Market what is unique about you. Be clear about what you have to offer that is unique and try to be slightly less expensive or offer more for the fee. Be flexible with fees and suggest ways for prospective customers to obtain funding or cut their costs. The most effective advertising is first in terms of what you can do for the customer and then in terms of your product or service and credentials. Aim for a specific market and keep overhead down. Know your competition, their missions, their prices, and their products or services.

In addition to acquiring new clients, relationships with current clients should be nurtured; keep in touch with those you have. Small inexpensive giveaways or simple contacts help your clients believe that their business is important to you and promotes loyalty. In addition, significant new business is often obtained through referrals from satisfied customers.

As your business grows, it is easy to forget to take care of yourself. Some entrepreneurs burn out due to self-neglect and set themselves up for failure. Many entrepreneurs will say that you must be willing to work innumerable hours a week and make significant personal sacrifices to succeed. That may be the case, but how much time and energy you spend also depends on your individual goals. Each entrepreneur must make these decisions for herself or himself. Being able to enjoy your success is important. Life changes quickly, and things that were once important can suddenly become meaningless. These changes are often unpredictable; you must know yourself and your priorities well and be flexible enough to manage these changes. Learn from your mistakes and be able to say "no," even to people you like. No one way is the right way, and new ideas often come from unexpected places. Keep your goals in mind!

■ Future Directions

What does the future hold for nurse entrepreneurs? The health care scene and workforce are changing so fast that predictions are difficult. The only certainty is change! Wilson (1998) estimated that

> by the year 2000 half of all working Americans, some 60 million people, will have joined the ranks of freelance providers of skills and services. (p. 4) The concept of pay for position is fading away replaced by pay for performance. (p. 2)

Information is key. Having information and being able to communicate it to the right people in the most efficient manner will be the path to success. The potential of the Internet is only just beginning to be realized. Nurses need to adapt and advance with it. Telehealth will be a major part of health care in the future and the opportunities for nurses will expand as it does. More nurses will be working in independent practice as contractors and in groups and partnerships with nurses and others.

Political power is vital, and we realize that we need to speak up and be heard. Unity will help us all. Internal struggles weaken us and are barriers to the success of our profession, whether we are entrepreneurs or not. Changes are needed in nursing that we must be able to discuss, debate, and disagree about without dividing. Unity will enable us to pave the way, not just follow the path.

■ Concluding Statement

I hope that this chapter has sparked interest in the marvelous opportunities for nurses as entrepreneurs. New experiences can enrich our quality of life, expand our minds, enhance our confidence, and offer possibilities of financial and professional success.

References

American Nurses Association. (1998). *Standards of clinical practice* (2nd ed.). Washington, D.C.: Author.

American Nurses Association. (1985). *Code for nurses with interpretive statements.* Kansas City, MO: Author.

National Score Office. SCORE (1999). Washington, DC: Service Corps of Retired Executives.

U.S. Small Business Administration. (1999). Washington, DC.

Welch, C. (1986). New York State Nurses Association Task Force. *Entrepreneurship in New York State.* New York: New York State Nurses Association, 2.

Wilson, C. K. (1998). Mentoring the entrepreneur. *Nursing Administration Quarterly, 22*(2), 1–12.

■ *Editor's Questions for Discussion*

Identify the characteristics of successful entrepreneurs. What content should nurses be taught for entrepreneurship in nursing education programs? Is entrepreneurship a skill that can be developed? Identify opportunities for nursing entrepreneurship. Provide examples of entrepreneurship. What influences affect the development of intrapreneurship in a system?

Indicate strategies for nurses to use in developing supportive behaviors with each other. How might subversive behavior be prevented or curbed in a business or profession? What clues may be evidence of saboteur behaviors? How does an entrepreneur develop trusting relationships for a successful business? What role does discernment have in entrepreneurship?

What marketing strategies facilitate successful entrepreneurship? What competencies must entrepreneurs have? Is graduate school education and certification essential? Discuss the education preparation for a nurse entrepreneur.

What specific content from Yocom and K. Thomas' (Chapter 3) apply to the licensure issues raised by Duffy? What specific ethics content covered by Kopala (Chapter 5) and Davis (Chapter 6) and legal concerns raised by Lane and Paterson (Chapter 7) apply to entrepreneur practice?

54

Genetics

New Directions for Nursing and Health Care

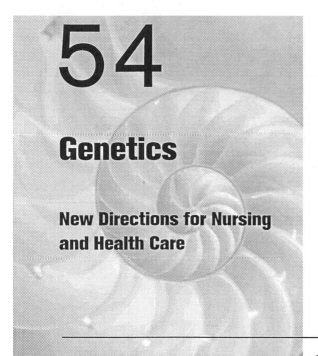

Jean F. Jenkins, PhD, MSN, RN

I nnovators have the potential to make a difference in creating tomorrow's vision. Innovators are those who perceive change as a challenge and an opportunity (Kirton, 1976). One such challenge results from recognition of the contribution of genetics to health and illness. This recognition has progressed rapidly over the past 10 years as result of a centralized research focus, the Human Genome Project (Collins, 1997a). This federally funded basic research project has provided a wealth of scientific information, biotechnological capabilities, and a foundation of genetics data that expand possibilities to improve on options available for health care services. Nursing innovators have an opportunity to create the desired future for health care through understanding, designing,

and implementing services and programs that integrate the genetics discoveries of today with the delivery of health care.

■ The Human Genome Project

The Human Genome Project (HGP) began in 1990 as a 15-year international program to decipher the complete set of genetic instructions held within the human genome (U.S. Department of Energy [DOE], 1997). This basic scientific information of the structure of genes will provide important tools to be utilized by researchers, health care providers, and society to enhance understanding of the contribution of genetics to the diagnosis, prevention, and treatment of illness. The Project's new goals for 1998–2003 expand the focus to include exploration of the relationship of genetic variation to the risk of disease (see Table 54.1).

Availability of basic science discoveries is enabling a new approach to (a) the interpretation of the function of DNA (deoxyribonucleic acid) within genes, (b) the interaction of external influences such as the environment with DNA, and (c) ultimately the impact of these factors on disease occurrence. Because of the complex issues that arise as a result of potentially having genetic knowledge about individuals, families, and communities, the HGP also includes goals that focus on the ethical, legal,

TABLE 54.1   Goals of the Human Genome Project

Focus Area	Goal	Status
Genetic maps	Develop new markers and technology that facilitate rapid genotyping. Complete the 2–5 centimorgan (cM) resolution map.	1cM map published 9/94. Plans to complete by 2003.
Physical maps	Map 30,000 *STS of the human genome.	52,000 STSs mapped as of 10/98. Plan to complete by 2003.
DNA sequencing	Develop efficient approaches and technological capability to sequence 80 Mb for all organisms by 1998.	180 Mb human plus 111 Mb non-human sequenced as of 10/98. Finish 1/3 of human sequence by 2001; complete by 2003.
Gene identification	Incorporate known genes onto physical maps to facilitate scientists studying the role of the gene in disease. (Functional genomics)	30,000 *ESTs mapped 10/98. Full length *cDNAs desired by 2003.
Human sequence variation	Basic information about types, frequencies, and distribution of polymorphisms in the human genome and human populations.	Not a goal initial plan. Goal for 2003 is to have 100,000 *SNPs mapped; to develop technology.
Technology development	Automation and robotics to improve efficiency, cost, and effectiveness of genome research. Cost of 90Mb/year capacity at ~$0.50 per base for sequencing technology.	Automate to achieve 500 Mb/year at <$0.25 per base for sequencing.
Model organisms	Completion of other species genetic maps to facilitate modeling and understanding of the human genome. (Comparative genomics)	*E. coli* complete sequence published 9/97; yeast 4/96; *C. elegans* 80% complete 10/98—done by 12/98; *Drosophila* 9% done 10/98—complete by 2005. Mouse map 12,000 STSs mapped; working draft by 2005
Informatics	Efficient data management, data analysis, and data distribution access.	Continue focus on software, tools for analysis, and databases for bioinformatics.

and social implications of these discoveries (Colby, 1998). In addition, the predictions of how potential genetic research outcomes will be viewed from philosophical, theological, and ethical perspectives has necessitated inclusion of funding within the HGP for research and education regarding these important issues (Collins et al., 1998). Genetic discoveries will require nurses to incorporate this new knowledge rapidly and determine how best to utilize it in providing holistic patient care (Lea, Anderson, & Monsen, 1998). The first step in incorporating such knowledge into nursing education and practice is awareness of its existence and potential. Introducing nurses to this knowledge is the beginning of the innovation

---

TABLE 54.1 *continued*

Focus Area	Goal	Status
ELSI program	Focus on issues that require policy discussions and recommendations such as privacy of genetic information and genetic testing.	Continue focus on implications of genetics for the individual and society, including: implications of completion of human DNA sequence and study of human variation; integration of information into clinical, nonclinical, and research settings; interaction of this information with philosophical, theological, and ethical perspectives; and impact of socioeconomic factors, race, and ethnicity.
Training	Encourage development of scientists and interdisciplinary researchers.	Focus on educational support to nurture scientists skilled in genomic research.
Technology transfer	Encourage transfer of discoveries into and out of genome research labs and centers.	This truly is an international effort Recognition of contributions of both public and private sector to progress in goal attainment.
Outreach	Share all information and materials within 6 months of development.	Continued policy for human sequence data: 1–2 kb in size should be released into public databases within 24 hrs of generation and that finished sequence should be released on a similarly rapid time scale.

*STS: Sequence tagged sites
ESTs: Expressed sequence tags
cDNAs: Complementary DNA
SNPs: Single nucleotide polymorphisms

Source: Collins, F., & Galas, D. (1993). A new five-year plan for the Human Genome Project. *Science, 262,* 43–46; Collins, F., Patrinos, A., Jordan, E., Chakravarti, A., Gesteland, R., Walters, L., and members of the DOE and NIH planning groups. (1998). New goals for the U.S. Human Genome Project: 1998–2003. *Science, 282,* 682–689.

diffusion process developed by Everett Rogers (1995) and illustrated in Figure 54.1. Nurses have a responsibility to take that first step and become aware of their potential to influence the outcomes from utilization of genetics in the care of individuals.

■ Diffusion of Innovation

Everett Rogers' theory of diffusion of innovations provides a theoretical framework for viewing the process of adoption and diffusion of genetics knowledge. He defines an innovation as an idea, practice, or object perceived as new by the individual, group, or organization (Rogers, 1995). When confronted with an innovation, the individual can decide to adopt the innovation, reject it, or defer a decision until later. Factors influencing this decision are important, as they influence the rate of an individual's progression through the stages of accepting an innovation and putting it into practice.

Introduction of the individual to knowledge about genetics is only the beginning (Rogers, 1995). Characteristics that affect how an individual receives and uses knowledge include prior experience, personality, cultural factors (including socioeconomic status), and the work environment. Most people selectively choose what knowledge is relevant to or needed by them. Awareness of an innovation then can motivate a person to obtain more information. Knowing does not mean using, as the individual must be persuaded that the innovation is worthy of adoption. The decision to adopt or reject an innovation is influenced by its characteristics, such as its relative advantage, compatibility, complexity, trialability, and observability (Rogers, 1995). If a decision is made to adopt the innovation, implementation and confirmation of outcomes of the decision are the next steps.

Although genetics knowledge is increasing, use of that knowledge may not be. Getting a new idea accepted, even when it appears to have advantages, is difficult. Not often do people have the luxury of envisioning the future and the time to begin to prepare for the ideal way that they'd like that future to evolve. But that future is coming—sooner than initially projected—with the HGP goal of having a working draft of the human genome sequence by the spring of 2000, rather than the original goal of having it by 2005 (Human Genome Project, 1999). Potential implications of genetics knowledge will offer nurses background information to consider when assessing the importance of this innovation in both personal and professional terms and deciding how to ensure that genetic discoveries can be translated appropriately to those they serve.

■ Implications for Health Care Practice

All diseases are now thought to have a genetic component (Collins & Jenkins, 1997). Medical genetics is now poised to uncover these genetic predispositions, opening the possibility of highly sophisticated diagnostic and therapeutic strategies. Genes that contribute to common polygenic conditions, such as diabetes, hypertension, most forms of cancer, heart disease, and major mental illnesses will be identified (Beaudet, 1999). These genetic discoveries will lead to molecular insights that will revolutionize the treatment of disease, using generalized gene therapy or individualized, tailored treatments (Regalado, 1999). All health professionals eventually will be required to distill this evolving body of knowledge and utilize genetic information to facilitate consumer decision-making about health care options (Collins, 1997b).

Infrastructure and Resources

When administrators realize that all care settings will be affected by genetic discoveries,

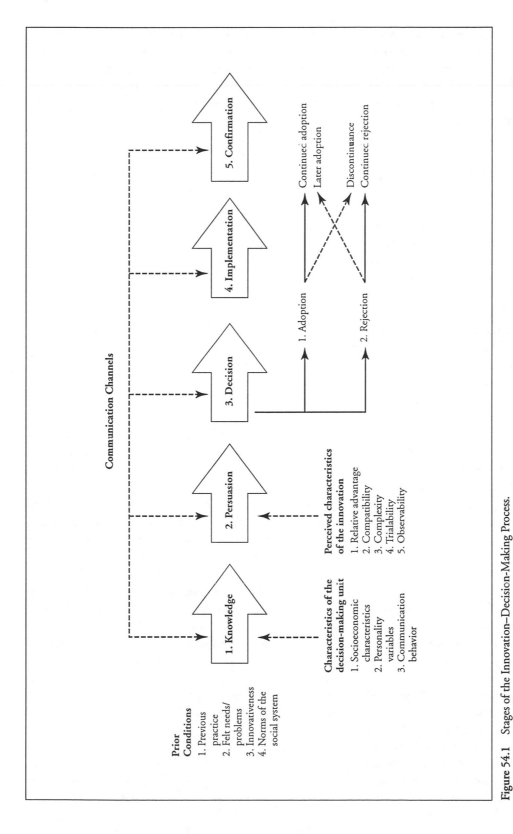

Figure 54.1 Stages of the Innovation–Decision-Making Process.

Source: Rogers, E., *Diffusion of innovations* (4th ed.). (p. 163). New York: Free Press. Copyright © 1995 by E. Rogers. Copyright © 1962, 1971, 1983 by the Free Press. Reproduced with the permission of the Free Press, a Division of Simon & Schuster, Inc.

enhanced availability of access to quality services will become a goal. Provision of collaborative teams to offer services in diverse settings will require economic investment to prepare staff to offer knowledgeable, cost-effective, and efficient care. Guidelines for care that integrate genetics into professional responsibilities will be developed.

Economics

Administrators of funding agencies that offer grants to develop genetics education, clinical services, and research will facilitate diffusion of this innovation. Education about genetics should prepare administrators to recognize the importance of planning for the future and considering economic investments in genetics services now.

Currently offered medical and clinical genetics services often are considered preventive and may therefore not be covered by insurance. Ability to provide equitable and effective application of this powerful technology will offer challenges to access, cost, and payment mechanisms. As genetic services expand to the general population, significant attention must be paid to economic issues related to health care resources and the costs of these services.

Models of Care

Traditionally, genetics services were provided in genetics clinics or centers (Forsman, 1994). The new genomic medicine offers the promise of opportunities for expanded services. Delineation of where the services are to be provided, who will provide them and to whom, and how genetics will be integrated into the health care delivery system offers challenging choices. What types of service should be available? Does specific space need to be designated for genetics services and clinics or are genetics services to be integrated

with ongoing services? What professional team members are needed to offer those services—genetics nurses, genetic counselors, and geneticists? How much time will be needed by staff to prepare individuals adequately to make informed decisions about the use of these services, such as predisposition genetic testing? The focus of genetics services is not only on the individual, but also has implications for families (ASHG Social Issues Subcommittee on Familial Disclosure, 1998). These and many other questions need to be considered when future models of care are being designed.

Balancing Act

There is a need to balance the excitement about genetic technologic innovation with responsiveness, reality, and sensitivity. As genetics technologic capabilities enhance diagnostic predictions, for a time scientists will be able to predict risks for illness, but health care providers will not be able to do much about preventing them (Scanlon & Fibison, 1995). Current health care philosophy does not emphasize individual responsibility for wellness. Nor does society in general value preventive care. As a result, effective early diagnosis, monitoring, and intervention for most diseases are lacking. Also, genetic knowledge could be used against the individual or family if insurance companies or employers decide that the risk for illness has potentially negative implications for them (Hudson, Rothenberg, Andrews, Kahn, & Collins, 1995). These issues create a dilemma for nurses in terms of discussing and providing a balanced view of available information that could facilitate consumers' health, well-being, and decision-making.

Dilemmas

The implications of genetic testing for health care practice have the potential to create ethical dilemmas for the nurse. For example, a genetic mutation has been identified in individuals who have a hereditary predisposition for colon cancer. Members of a family with hereditary nonpolyposis colorectal cancer (HNPCC) syndrome can have a genetic test to determine whether their DNA signals the possibility of an increased lifetime risk of developing colon, uterine, or other types of cancer (Glaser, 1998). Genetic testing services are to be offered at a local community hospital, and staff need to be hired to provide these services. The administrator is assessing the type of professional that can best offer education and counseling and do the blood test. Additionally, the administrator is concerned about the potential market for these services. Even if marketing provides excellent visibility for this facility, individuals may not avail themselves of these services because the costs are not covered by insurance companies or out of fear of discrimination. How can nurses best prepare to make a difference in creating tomorrow's vision in such a scenario?

■ Implications for Nursing Practice

Nurses will influence how genetic information is used and interpreted (Touchette, Holtzman, Davis, & Feetham, 1997). One problem is that not all nurses recognize the implications of genetics discoveries for their practice. Or, some may fear new terminology, concepts, or meaning of the genetic information being made available to them that limits integration of genetics into practice. In reality, genetics offers new challenges and opportunities for all nurses. The profession of nursing now has the opportunity to develop a plan to prepare all nurses to translate genetics research into practice.

Role Ambiguity

Opportunity, however, also creates uncertainty. How do nurses begin to envision genet-

ics as part of their role? Baseline understanding of genetics by all nurses is needed. Perhaps, depending on the setting, advanced roles need to be developed within nursing that enhance translation of genetics research findings into practice.

Scope of Practice

The American Nurses Association (ANA) (1998), in conjunction with the International Society of Nurses in Genetics (ISONG), has developed a statement on the scope and standards of genetics clinical nursing practice. Current role ambiguity within nursing was addressed: "All licensed registered nurses, regardless of their practice setting, have a role in the delivery of genetic services and the management of genetic information" (p. 2). Nurses at the basic level must be prepared to incorporate knowledge of genetics into their assessments of, plans of care for, interventions with, and evaluations of outcomes for clients who are affected with or at risk for conditions having clear genetic components. Advanced nursing practice in genetics requires specialty knowledge that enables the nurse to provide leadership, education, expanded practice skills, research, and consultation in meeting identified standards of care related specifically to genetics (ANA, 1998).

Gaps

Current gaps in knowledge diminish the influence of nurses on the use and interpretation of genetic information. Schools of Nursing need to address the inadequate preparation of nurses with regard to genetics science and ethical issues arising from genetics discoveries (Anderson, 1996). The numbers of faculty, continuing education offerings, textbooks, and other publications that can enable nurses to understand genetics are insufficient (Lashley, 1999; Lea, Jenkins, & Francomano, 1998).

Partnerships

Opportunities exist for nurses to join with others to foster the scientific and professional growth of nurses in the area of human genetics. The ISONG (1999) promotes such networking and knowledge building. Other professional nursing organizations are beginning to create special interest groups in genetics, provide educational opportunities at annual meetings for learning about genetics, and publish articles pertaining to genetics research and applications of research findings. Another partnership of health care providers that includes nurses is the National Coalition for Health Care Professional Education in Genetics (NCHPEG) (Collins, 1997b). This coalition encourages partnerships among health care disciplines to identify competencies needed by all health care professionals that relate to genetics and to improve the quality of care through certification or credentialing in genetics. The coalition also provides visibility for and access to genetics information on its Web site (NCHPEG, 1999). Nurses need to be open to such partnerships, which can be brought about through individual mentoring, via professional organizational efforts, and with national initiatives.

Dilemmas

The implications of genetic discoveries may well create dilemmas for the practicing nurse. For example, nurses have been trained to focus on the individual within the context of family and community. Nurses possess knowledge about developmental stages, counseling, and educational concepts. Nurses advocate for the patient. As colleagues and team players, nurses have a solid foundation for influencing the translation of genetics science and knowledge to practice. However, the sheer pace of progress in biomedical research poses a serious threat to the future competency of nurses. How can

quality knowledge and skills related to genetics be assured for nurses? How can nurses further prepare themselves to make a difference in creating tomorrow's vision in this scenario?

■ Implications for Nursing Education

The knowledge and skills repertoire of future nurses rests in the hands of educators. Unfortunately, recognition of the importance of genetics to the future of nursing has been limited (Jenkins, 1999).

Academia

Genetics courses, or even basic science courses, in nursing curricula are minimal (Hetteberg, Prows, Deets, Monsen, & Kenner, 1999). Only recently did the American Association of Colleges of Nursing (AACN) (1998a) recognize that nurses will be faced with ethical dilemmas created by research advances such as the human genome project. The new AACN "Essentials" that define core standards for bachelor's-degree nurse education recognize that in the future an important component of the professional nursing role will be the focus on health promotion and risk reduction. As scientific discoveries allow prediction of health problems, nurses will be called on to design and implement interventions to modify risk factors and promote healthier lifestyles (AACN, 1998b). Genetics was identified as one of the newly evolving aspects of health care that will require specific academic preparation. Schools of Nursing are beginning to explore methods of integrating genetics and its implications into curriculum design to prepare all nurses to deal with this new knowledge appropriately.

Advanced nursing preparation in genetics currently is offered in five schools of nursing. Several schools are assessing the possibility of developing master's or doctoral programs with a focus on genetics nursing. Although to date demand has not been overwhelming for such programs, that is expected to change soon.

Continuing Education

Although preparation of future nurses is crucial, the need to address genetic knowledge gaps for currently practicing nurses is even more challenging. Sixty-eight nursing spe-cialty organizations were surveyed to deter-mine whether their current and future contin-uing education plans included genetics. Only 30% indicated plans to offer content in genet-ics in future programming (Monsen & Ander-son, 1999). Jenkins (1999) identified a start-ing point for inclusion of genetics content in such programs, and ranked content items by importance for their inclusion (see Table 54.2).

TABLE 54.2 Those Items Seen As Most Important to Include in Genetics Education of Nurses (highest to lowest priority)

1. Item: Knowledge of basic human genetics

   Competency: Demonstrates increased knowledge of basic human genetics and current applications to practice

2. Item: Relevance of genetics to practice

   Competency: Able to identify relevance of genetics to nursing practice

3. Item: Indication for a genetic referral

   Competency: Recognizes indications for a genetic referral

4. Item: Genetic evaluation and counseling

   Competency: Describes the essential components of genetic evaluation and counseling

5. Item: Psychological impact of genetics

   Competency: Describes the psychological impact of genetic information and technology on the individual and family

6. Item: Ethical and societal issues of genetics

   Competency: Able to identify ethical and societal issues related to genetic information and technology

7. Item: Awareness of own attitudes and values

   Competency: Evaluates effects of one's own attitudes, self awareness, and values related to genetic science and services

8. Item: Identify appropriate resources

   Competency: Able to identify appropriate resources (professional and patient)

9. Item: Awareness of new genetic methods

   Competency: Demonstrates an increased awareness of the new genetic methods and technologies

10. Item: Ethnocultural differences

    Competency: Recognizes the effects of ethnocultural differences as they relate to genetics

---

Source: Jenkins, J. (1999). Innovation diffusion: Genetics nursing education. Unpublished doctoral disserta-tion, George Mason University, Fairfax, Virginia, p. 55.

This ranking provides direction for themes, competencies, and content as a foundation of both continuing education programs and academic courses. Through its use, professional organizations and educators can design programs for all nurses. Reinvention of educational materials on genetics by different specialty nursing organizations thus may be prevented. Rather, tailoring content to specialty practice can provide effective use of resources while providing specific guidance for specialty application.

Educational Resources

Opportunities for dissemination of such materials include plenary sessions on genetics within nursing specialty organization meetings, incorporation of genetics into licensure and certification exams, and development of Web sites featuring genetics material. As more nurses have access to computers, the possibilities for computer-assisted education expand. Applications such as CD-ROM, Web sites, and computer-assisted instruction offer avenues for creative, timely, and continuing genetics education. A variety of methods to provide such education undoubtedly will be developed.

Dilemmas

The implications of genetics discoveries will create dilemmas for nursing education. For example, a nursing specialty organization recognizes that its membership needs to hear about progress of the human genome project and its potential implications for nurses. There are currently insufficient knowledgeable nurses in the organization to provide the program. The speakers' bureau of the ISONG has a list of available nurses who could offer genetics expertise. How might the specialty organization tap that resource to begin to prepare its leaders and membership to assume an active role in genetics education? How can nurses best prepare to make a difference in creating tomorrow's vision in this scenario?

■ Implications for Nursing Research

Opportunities for nursing research related to application of genetics information is wide open. The focus of research to date has included consumer interest in genetic testing, impact of genetic testing for individuals and families, and educational methods for instruction in genetics (Sigmon, Grady, & Amende, 1997). Outcomes of nursing research have the potential to influence the development of policy, evaluate the quality of services, and assess the adequacy of nursing to ensure safe and ethical applications of genetics science.

Funding Opportunities

The National Institutes of Health (NIH) (1999) and other federal agencies have recognized the importance of nursing to the application of genetics findings to practice, education, and research. Examples include available funding for postdoctoral training at the National Institute for Nursing Research; grants for ethical, legal, and social implications research through the National Human Genome Research Institute; and genetics services offered through a Cancer Genetics Network as funded by the National Cancer Institute.

■ Future Directions

Nursing now has an entree into new opportunities and new markets for service—genetics. As genetics becomes more central to an understanding of health and disease, preventive services will become the key to health maintenance. An expanded role for the nurse will offer new opportunities for collaboration as a knowledgeable team member and as an entrepreneur (Poste, 1998).

Diffusion of Innovation

As technology enhances the ability of genetic information to be utilized in practice, education to understand genetics will be important. The nursing profession has begun to recognize that genetics education is needed and has gained an increasing awareness of future implications of this knowledge. The diffusion of genetics education will be influenced by personal attitudes and knowledge about the innovation, characteristics of the innovation, and the social process.

Knowledge

Educational preparation is a beginning step in ensuring that all nurses will be able to translate new genetic knowledge and skills into deliberations about health care decisions and actions. As more is learned about the structure of the human genome, this enhanced understanding will offer greater possibilities for early diagnosis, risk reduction, and intervention on the basis of genetic profiles. (Regalado, 1999).

Tools

Tools that permit faster and less costly identification of the genetic code will enhance researchers' ability to study the structure and actions of multiple genes. Data from analyses must be stored, analyzed, and manipulated through massive bioinformatic data systems. Understanding of gene chips and other methods of genetic analysis will be important for recognition of the benefits and limitations of each (Watson & Akil, 1999). Other tools need to be developed by health care providers that facilitate both patient and nurse education about genetics technology and methods.

Opportunities

Opportunities for nurses to assume leadership in this new direction for nursing and health care are limitless. Recognition that genetics is essential to the care provided to individuals, families, and communities has the potential for opening up many new possibilities for nurses who are administrators, educators, researchers, and care providers. Nurses can make a difference in creating tomorrow's vision.

Obligations

Nurses have an obligation to fulfill with respect to genetics. This technology offers interesting, personal, and potentially damaging information about each of us. Nurses as individuals and as professionals must become knowledgeable about genetics to ensure that neither individuals nor societies are damaged by abuse of these scientific advances. Only then can a positive direction for nursing and health care be assured.

■ Concluding Statement

Nurses must take time to reflect on what genetics discoveries and information mean, how to lead in translating genetics science into practice, and how to integrate genetics into a vision for tomorrow. Only through using their hands and hearts can nursing ensure that it is in touch with the discoveries that will have a dramatic impact on those served.

References

American Association of Colleges of Nursing. (1998a). Educational mobility. *Journal of Professional Nursing, 14,* 314–316.

American Association of Colleges of Nursing. (1998b). *The essentials of baccalaureate education for professional nursing.* Washington, DC: Author.

American Nurses Association. (1998). *Statement on the scope and standards of genetics clinical nursing practice.* Washington, DC: American Nurses Association and the International Society of Nurses in Genetics.

Anderson G. (1996). The evolution and status of genetics education in nursing in the United States 1983–1995. *IMAGE: Journal of Nursing Scholarship, 28,* 101–106.

ASHG (American Society of Human Genetics). Social Issues Subcommittee on Familial Disclosure. (1998). ASHG statement: Professional disclosure of familial genetic information. *American Journal of Human Genetics, 62,* 474–483.

Beaudet, A. (1999). 1998 ASHG presidential address. Making genomic medicine a reality. *American Journal of Human Genetics, 64,* 1–13.

Colby, J. (1998). An analysis of genetic discrimination legislation proposed by the 105th Congress. *American Journal of Law & Medicine, 24,* 443–480.

Collins, F. (1997a). Sequencing the human genome. *Hospital Practice, 32,* 35–53.

Collins, F. (1997b). Preparing health professionals for the genetic revolution. *Journal of the American Medical Association, 278,* 1285–1286.

Collins, F., & Galas, D. (1993). A new five-year plan for the Human Genome Project. *Science, 262,* 43–46.

Collins, F., & Jenkins, J. (1997). Implications of the Human Genome Project for the nursing profession. In F. R. Lashley (Ed.), *The genetics revolution: Implications for nursing* (pp. 9–13). Washington, DC: American Academy of Nursing.

Collins, F., Patrinos, A., Jordan, E., Chakravarti, A., Gesteland, R., Walters, L., and members of the DOE and NIH planning groups. (1998). New goals for the U.S. Human Genome Project: 1998–2003. *Science, 282,* 682–689.

Forsman, I. (1994). Evolution of the nursing role in genetics. *Journal of Obstetric, Gynecologic, and Neonatal Nursing, 23,* 481–486.

Glaser, E. (1998). Inherited predisposition to colon cancer. *Cancer Nursing, 21,* 377–383.

Hetteberg, C., Prows, C., Deets, C., Monsen, R., & Kenner, C. (1999). National survey of genetics content in basic nursing preparatory programs in the United States. *Nursing Outlook, 47,* 168–180.

Hudson, K., Rothenberg, K., Andrews, L., Kahn, M., & Collins, F. (1995). Genetic discrimination and health insurance: An urgent need for reform. *Science, 270,* 391–393.

Human Genome Project aims to finish working draft next year. (1999). *Nature, 398,* 177.

International Society of Nurses in Genetics. (1999). [On-line]. Available: http://www.nursing.creighton.edu/isong.

Jenkins, J. (1999). *Innovation diffusion: Genetics nursing education.* Unpublished doctoral dissertation, George Mason University, Fairfax, Virginia.

Kirton, M. (1976). Adaptors and innovators: a description and measure. *Journal of Applied Psychology, 61,* 622–629.

Lashley, F. (1999). *Clinical genetics in nursing practice* (2nd ed.). New York: Springer.

Lea, D., Anderson, G., & Monsen, R. (1998). A multiplicity of roles for genetic nursing: Building toward holistic practice. *Holistic Nursing Practice, 12,* 77–87.

Lea, D., Jenkins, J., & Francomano, C. (1998). *Genetics in clinical practice: New directions for nursing.* Boston: Jones & Bartlett.

Monsen, R., & Anderson, G. (1999). Continuing education for nurses that incorporates genetics. *The Journal of Continuing Education in Nursing, 30,* 20–24.

National Coalition for Health Care Professional Education in Genetics. (1999). [On-line]. Available: http://www.nchpeg.org.

National Institutes of Health. 1999. [On-line]. Available: http://www.nih.gov.

Poste, G. (1998). Molecular medicine and information based targeted healthcare. *Nature Biotechnology, 16,* 19–21.

Regalado, A. (1999). Inventing the pharmacogenomic business. *American Journal Health-System Pharmacists, 56,* 40–50.

Rogers, E. (1995). *Diffusion of innovations* (4th ed.). New York: Free Press.

Scanlon, C., & Fibison, W. (1995). *Managing genetic information: Implications for nursing practice.* Washington, DC: American Nurses Association.

Sigmon, H., Grady, P., & Amende, L. (1997). The National Institute for Nursing Research explores opportunities in genetics research. *Nursing Outlook, 45,* 215–219.

Touchette, N., Holtzman, N., Davis, J., & Feetham, S. (1997). *Toward the 21st century. Incorporating genetics into primary health care.* New York: Cold Spring Harbor Laboratory Press.

U.S. Department of Energy. (1997). *The Human Genome Project program report: Overview and progress.* Germantown, MD: Author.

Watson, S., & Akil, H. (1999). Gene chips and arrays revealed: A primer on their power and their uses. *Biological Psychiatry, 45,* 533–543.

■ Editor's Questions for Discussion

Discuss the ethical, legal, and social implications of discoveries resulting from the Human Genome Project for nursing education and professional nursing practice. How may nurses best be prepared to distill and use evolving genetics knowledge? How might nurses influence care outcomes using knowledge of genetics? What strategies and mechanisms need to be developed to facilitate the diffusion of genetics into education programs, professional practice, and research protocols?

Provide examples of genetics integrated into curriculum design for nursing programs. How might nursing students obtain learning experiences in genetics? At what level in nursing programs should such experiences be offered or required or both? How should faculty be prepared to transmit evolving genetics knowledge and implications in nursing programs?

Propose guidelines for nursing care that integrate genetics into the professional nursing role. What planning needs to be done and by whom for economic issues related to health care resources and genetics services to be addressed? Respond to the questions raised by Jenkins about models of care. Provide examples of dilemmas that nurses may face in balancing views about available genetics information for consumers. Propose means for resolving the dilemmas presented by Jenkins for education programs and in nursing practice.

Address implications for diffusion and application of genetics knowledge through nursing research. What applications related to genetics knowledge are apparent in the discussions by Stevens and Weiner (Chapter 38), Lindsey (Chapter 29), Titler (Chapter 35), Froman and Owen (Chapter 33), and Grady (Chapter 73)?

PART VI

Nursing Administration–Service

". . . Yet knowing how way leads on to way,
I doubted if I should ever come back . . ."

Perhaps no greater challenge, as well as opportunity, for leadership is more wide open than that of providing direction as a nurse administrator for the delivery of health care services. The nursing practice "travelers" of the profession need leaders and administrators who see far down the road through all obstacles along the paths of providing care and service. Nurse administrators are required to assess quickly how one decision may lead to another and understand how that one action may affect other persons and consequent management decisions. Such leaders must have integrity and courage, as well as management knowledge, in guiding routes and actions, understanding well that once a pathway is chosen there is seldom an option to retreat.

Prospective and future leaders and managers of health care services will do well to contemplate the writings of the authors in this Part. It is the responsibility of such nursing professionals to anticipate, plan, and create healthy environments for providing high-quality care. Further, because of the constant change in the health care scene, nurse executives will need to be flexible in adapting and creating new environments, structures, and integrated systems for care. How can such individuals best be prepared so that they will not be daunted in the process of leading others in paths for service? The chapters that follow offer direction for the beyond.

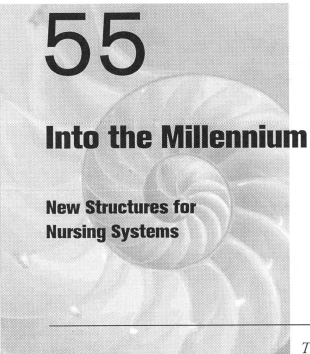

55

Into the Millennium

New Structures for Nursing Systems

Timothy P. Porter-O'Grady,
EdD, PhD, RN, FAAN

I t's a new age for health care. The convergence of sociopolitical changes, economic reconfigurations, and technological invention have together created conditions that have altered the provision of health care services forever. Newer structures and relationships will emerge in the health care system, requiring intersections, relationships, and practices different from those generated in the past.·Newer models of work organization and structuring for health care will require different behaviors and patterns of work in health care, resulting in further innovation, creativity, and decentralization of health care services. In this chapter, I explore these considerations and challenge providers to confront the impact of health system changes on their own clinical practices.

Never before has so much change in nursing systems occurred in such a short period of time. Three converging signposts of change—sociopolitical, economic, and technological transformations—have converged to create conditions for a shift in the social reality, in short, an age change. Only serendipitously related to the forthcoming millennium, this age change has created conditions that require a shift in human thinking, social response, and individual action. Accompanying this shift is the impact on social institutions and organizations within which the work of society unfolds (Blendon & Brodie, 1994).

■ Implications for the Future

As social, political, economic, and technological constructs reconfigure, they create overwhelming implications for building the future. These implications include the following.

- Complexity of conjunctive changes (those changes occurring all at one time) creates conditions that result in inability to cope. The sense of being overwhelmed by complexity and the number of changes occurring concomitantly overwhelms and incapacitates the individual, preventing the individual from responding.

- Highly organized and orderly organizational structures cease to address effectively the intensity of issues, problems, and concerns confronting ordinary activities associated with accomplishing work.

- Ability to predict with any clarity the next steps or stages of change diminishes radically when conditions for change and understanding it operate under the influence of emerging unfamiliar sets of rules.

- Technology has converged to so change human experience that it is creating new reality before people are able to understand its implications and actions on their lives. As a result, they feel out of control and intimidated by the force and power of a technology they have not yet come to fully understand.

- Sustainability has come to require different balancing of the economic equation. For so long Western society has been able to live on credit it generated through high levels of growth, manufacturing, and productivity. As the paradigm shifts to technology and service, characteristics of growth, health, and economic advancements operate under a different set of conditions. Balancing the economic value equation is required if social and political sustainability is ever to be ensured in an increasingly global economic equation.

Finally, out of an age where the primary international social concern was viability and sustainability of those born into the world, issues of social concern at the other end of the age spectrum are generated. Health care and good public health have created conditions leading to a significant increase in longevity and societal impacts not experienced since the beginning of human history (Coile, 1994).

Signposts of Real Change

These and a host of other circumstances are signposts of the radical nature of change being experienced in this generation. Several components of this change are altering life experiences.

- Age change prevents a shift not only in experience but also in reality. People are now dealing with a reality they neither asked for consciously nor are prepared to handle (Handy, 1998).

- People's understanding of reality has moved into a quantum mechanics context, altering forever their view of the world and how it works, as well as their role in giving form to change (Wheatley, 1996).

- The United States has a primarily "fix-it," late-engagement service structure. It needs sickness to thrive. All the structures of both payment and service are founded on treating the sick and fixing problems late in their development (American Nurses Association & Endorsers, 1991).

- Good public health has had more to do with the health of the nation than many of the advances in medicine (Barnes et al., 1995).

- Focus on illness as the core of health system service has ultimately wrung resources from society at a rate that is untenable, cripples society, and keeps it from addressing other problems related to social needs (Gustafson, Helstad, & Hung, 1995).

- Because of the burden of health costs, inappropriate attention has been focused on controlling costs, and thus decisions have been based on resource use rather than better ways to provide efficient, effective, and sustainable health service (Pauly, 1995).

- As a result of the untenable focus on cost, little progress has been made in service reconfiguration. Reductions in key service providers, such as nurses, has resulted in poorly prepared service personnel replacing more broad-based, high-utility professionals. Now that the need for their decision-making skills is clear, these professionals are no longer available where they are needed (Brown, 1995).

• Moving the tremendous infrastructure of the health system to a more user-friendly, early-engagement service system is now a major task, creating much structural, economic, and service noise for every participant in the change (Editors, 1996).

Changing Context for Health Service

Fortunately, forces are converging to create conditions and circumstances that will require restructuring and retooling of the entire framework for delivery of health care services (Lathrop, 1994). These forces, working in concert, create conditions requiring necessary responses in the delivery of health care services. On top of the need for change is evidence, driven through research and technology, suggesting mechanisms and applications that will be necessary if operating in this new frame of reference is to be successful. The following are several such considerations.

• Controlling the cost of current services and service configurations only temporarily halts spiraling increases in costs. Simply addressing the issue of cost, and better managing those costs, is only a temporary solution to a structural problem.

• Tremendous cost is associated with managing information flow from multiple methodologies related to documenting, sharing, and billing for services. Health care systems and providers are now almost completely overwhelmed by multiple requirements of payors for clinical information, documentation, and billing.

• Technology increasingly has created conditions that require less use of residential, bed-based, sickness-driven services. Perhaps the most significant technological impact in the past 30 years has been the tremendous movement of health care services from predominately inpatient activities to outpatient, non-resident, and highly decentralized activities.

• Due to television and other media, the consuming public is becoming increasingly aware of options, choices, and expectations for health care. Additionally, understanding of the need for personal life management and control over personal choices is growing. The secondary result of this awareness is the changing and deepening expectation in the health care system for a different relationship and growing perception (albeit small) of options and choices in personal health care management.

• As the bulk of Americans age, a change in focus from acute intervention to chronic care management requires a shift in infrastructure. This transition calls for services entirely different from the highly institutional, interventive, and acute care–oriented system currently well established. The health care system thus needs to refocus and retool its infrastructure in a way that addresses a growing population of essentially healthy, better educated, highly mobile, and longer living American citizens (Coile, 1993).

Demand for Restructuring

Increasingly the consolidation, linkage, and integration of health care delivery has created an orientation that is moving service away from institutional to system structures. At this stage, it is important to recognize that health care systems of the future must restructure the delivery and infrastructure of health care services. Health care professionals will work predominately within multifocal, horizontally delineated health delivery systems for the foreseeable future (D'Aunno, Alexander, & Laughlin, 1996).

From Institution to System

Working within a health system is different from working within incremental, nonaligned,

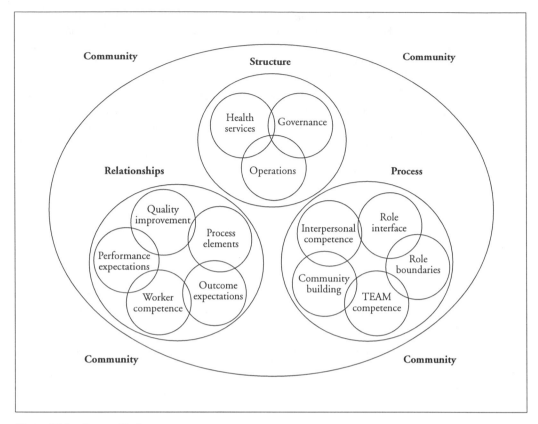

Figure 55.1   System Design.

and compartmentalized institutional structures. Systems require different insight, understanding, and knowledge. Operating a system changes conditions and circumstances of both structure and process in fundamental ways. Systems challenge the historic view of work and raise issues about emerging formats for service delivery (Contributors, 1997).

Systems also change the basic constructs of professional work. In old organizational structures, each discipline operated within its own frame of reference, had its own job descriptions and performance expectations, and dealt with control processes that attempted to manage its own members. In a system, all these unilateral and discipline-specific barriers lose relevance (see Figure 55.1).

Increasingly, the relationship between providers and impact of their work on that of others and the composite for those they serve moderate the structure and relationships built. Characteristics of a discipline—such as self-direction, self-ownership of process, self-management, unilateral standards of service, discipline specific work patterns, behaviors, performance expectations, and so forth—are no longer viable. In their place, comprehensiveness, integration, mutual performance factors, outcomes orientation, interdisciplinary relationships, and horizontal communication patterns emerge as predominating characteristics of professional practice.

This new framework threatens existing structures and the synthetic sense of independence and nonaligned ownership that has emerged over the past 100 years in the major professions of health care. Old animosities, antagonisms, uncertainties, and lack of meaningful relationships are not compatible with the integrated model now necessary. The system now requires a different relationship for every provider. That requirement raises all the unresolved issues and organizational barriers that have hitherto been part of the modus operandi of health service delivery (Porter, Van Cleave, Milobowski, Conlon, & Mambourg, 1996).

A New Health Care Relationship

In the initial stages of restructuring health care, the reaction to a different health care relationship creates tremendous negative response from almost every component of the health care system. Providers claim loss of control and independence. Patients claim lack of sensitivity to needs. Leadership claims lack of commitment on the part of providers and workers to the need for change. Policy-makers strive to hold onto their service saddles and do not welcome the inevitable requirements for fundamental systems and performance change. Policy-makers have a rationale that makes sense to them and justifies lack of engagement with inherent challenges. To accept would mean to embrace the work involved in changing the underpinnings of both the system and its disciplines (Lipman-Blumen, 1996).

In time, of course, none of these reactions endure. Each is simply the first step of a series of stages necessary to participate fully in the reconstruction of health care. Each leader is called to address changes in ways that create a different orientation to provision of service. Out of this demand comes an alteration to the structure of the professions and to the relationship between provider and public that will drive much of the reorientation of health care during the next two decades.

■ Structural Changes

Some structures have already changed. Through mergers, alliances, partnerships, and amalgamation of services, whole new arrangements for the delivery of health care have emerged (Zuckerman, Kaluzny, & Ricketts III, 1995). Although it is yet unclear as to how these systems will operate over the long term, their reconfiguration is already a certainty.

- The shift from process-oriented, incremental, and vertical orientation to thinking of care, planning, outlining, and delivering service has already occurred. The strategy for care has moved from patient-based to population-based thinking (Lamb & Zazworski, 1997).

- There is movement away from notions of cost control. Efficiency and effectiveness—historically nonaligned with performance, product, or outcome—now are intricately linked in a growing process–outcome relationship. Focus on outcome has changed the emphasis on design. Historically, process, performance, and function were the critical indicators of effectiveness.

- Orientation to outcomes radically alters the role, activities, and mental models of disciplines from excellence in work, emphasis on activity, and function to clarity of results of action and activity and the meaning and value provided in the work (Zander, 1995).

- The new focus on outcomes does not diminish the argument that nurses make regarding value of relationship and caring, but it does create an additional obligation on the part of the profession to indicate more clearly the impact of relationship and caring on results and sustainability in the system (Redmond, 1995).

- Today, in every option in clinical decision-making cost is included as a part of the decisions about the quality and service provided by any discipline or work group (Waress, Pasternak, & Smith, 1994).

- In the future, a nurse will not be able to make a clinical decision without recognizing the

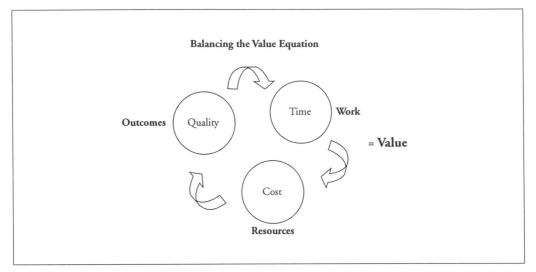

Figure 55.2   Creating Sustainable Value.

implications of its value. As a result (see Figure 55.2), instead of making the "best choice" for patients, the nurse will have to make the "wisest choice" for patients (Sullivan, 1996).

- Lines of demarcation that are discipline-specific or institutionally delineated have less and less meaning in a systems orientation. Work is increasingly identified in interdisciplinary terms (Coffey, Stagis, & Fenner, 1997).

- Design and structure of a health care system now focuses on life management of populations rather than intervention of specific diseases (Herzlinger, 1998).

- Organization of service now relates around specific populations, their needs and characteristics and joins together the requisite disciplines necessary to adequately address the scope of needs of that population (Porter-O'Grady & Wilson, 1997).

- The system now has an obligation to ensure the convergence and configuration of the disciplines necessary mutually to serve defined populations and to meet the specific demands generated by population-driven configurations (Porter-O'Grady, 1997).

New Models for the Disciplines

No longer orienting the design of health care delivery around discipline-specific structures raises serious considerations about how disciplines address specific issues. Leadership in the system involves promulgating the goodness-of-fit between and among disciplines in the context of specific population driven design. Each discipline is obligated to identify for itself its unique issues and concerns and to develop mechanisms and processes that address them, prior to playing a role in multidisciplinary relationships.

Emerging is the system's lack of emphasis on discipline-specific issues, concerns, or processes. It is this loss that perhaps creates the greatest noise within each discipline. Historically, the organization or institution acted as the locus of control in an organized way for the discipline's decision-making. As a result, the institution was the frame of reference for discipline-specific decision-making. Within a system, that format disappears. The discipline no longer has a structure that specifically addresses its unique characteristics. It now must address issues of the discipline, speak for its members, and promulgate its agenda (Evans, Hawkins, Curley, & Porter-O'Grady, 1995). The discipline must articulate its concerns, obligations for service, social mandates, and professional standards, in a way that can be translated into interdisciplinary relationships.

This reality carries over to differentiation within disciplines between roles and functions. In the past, community health, outpatient services, acute care services, intensive care services, school health, and so forth were all perceived as independent and nonrelated services provided by nurses and others. The focus of each was its own service and development of caregivers unique to its particular operation. In the systems approach, comprehensiveness becomes the framework for delivery of service. As a result, the relationships between and among each of these previously distinct clinical services becomes an important consideration for sustainability of service (see Figure 55.3).

Because population now drives service, integration of services is required across the life span continuum of defined patient populations (Shoultz & Hatcher, 1997). For example, elderly care that moves from highly intensive and acute to community and home health, and perhaps residential services, may need to be linked. Each of these previously distinct services now must have a relationship that indeed may be a part of the same continuum of services for specific and designated populations. Creating this relationship across the life span now is part of good life management of a population of patients, rather than simply intervention based on procedures or to treat acute illnesses—the focus of the old nonaligned system.

Aligning Service Pathways

The impact on the structure of life span services may require that these services be aligned within services that may have multiple provider arrangements.

- These pathways may be distinct configurations within the system made up of multiple disciplines and service structures and managed by a wide variety of professionals (Schneller & Ott, 1996).

- A nurse specialist or other practitioner, because of the nurse's particular skills, will often lead this service team (Doerge & Hagenow, 1996).

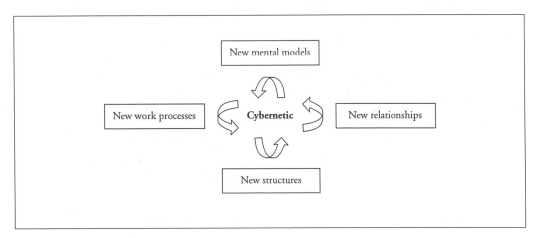

Figure 55.3   Future Positioning.

The future of health care service will be delineated by the information infrastructure (Duncan, 1994).

Building on the Information Infrastructure

The information infrastructure is like a river of data that flows through all of the activities and functions that exemplify the purpose of the system. The primary role of the system is to make sure that these functions and activities are linked and that the information necessary to success of these activities is generated in seamless and effective way (Milio, 1996).

It is clear that, today, seamlessness is more dream than reality. However, it is only a matter of time before the flexibility and fluidity of information generated is available to everyone in the system. Creating this seamlessness is the primary work of the health care system at this time. During the next two decades, more than 50% of capitalization resources for health care will go toward creating the information infrastructure for decision-making of the future (Beckham, 1996).

The purpose of the information infrastructure is to make possible wise and appropriate decisions that result in sustainable action at the point of service. Increasingly, in decentralized, multifunctional, horizontally oriented systems, point-of-service decision-making becomes crucial to the system's ability to survive. That is, providers must have information in a format that is meaningful at the time desired in a way that is useful and capable of being applied immediately (Dertouzos, 1997). Building this infrastructure and creating the structural support for it is the essential work of leadership today.

Transferring Skill Sets

What is important for the provider is recognition that the information infrastructure will increasingly create increasing portability of clinical work. In the industrial age, work systems and structure were fixed and site-specific. In the information age, work will be fluid, flexible, and highly mobile. The professional will be required to move from a historic emphasis on fixed skill sets to increasing emphasis on mobile skill sets. The challenge for every professional is recognition of those fixed skill-set activities that must be given over, transferred, or given up and replaced by mobile skill-set activities that can be applied in a variety of settings across the continuum of care (Schraeder & Britt, 1997).

The most significant characteristic of the health system of the future will be the high fluidity and mobility of professionals in providing services in a variety of settings. Because population will more clearly define the characteristics of service, population also will define fundamental activities of that service. Nurses, physicians, and other health professionals must adjust to specific functions based on population characteristics, technologic structures available, and service demands created. As more information becomes available and more technology is created to reduce intensity of intervention, the entire character of service provision will be altered. Factors likely to have a significant impact will be the increasingly mobile population and demands for more chronic care. Nurses and other providers will have to become ever more flexible and depend increasingly on the information system, the outcomes of services rendered, and the sustainability of the clinical actions undertaken. This dependence, combined with continual growth of microtechnology and noninvasive interventions, will create a different professional role for every nurse (Negroponte, 1995).

The Structure of Mobility

Much of the structuring and management of health care services in this framework will facilitate the mobility of the nurse. No longer will a nurse need to be located in particular fixed sites to render service. Clearly, there will always be fixed-site intervention for acute care services. However, the need for it will be lessened, as technology and system infrastructure make possible the delivery of effective health care services in a decentralized and mobile society (Gage, 1998).

Increasingly, information-age notions of modularity and structure will have a greater impact on the design and provision of health care systems. Because the population will be highly mobile and have needs moving between acute and chronic care, modularity in design will be critically important. Although modules of care may focus on specific needs, they will be integrated into broader comprehensive methods of meeting the needs of both individuals and populations.

Module designers will array clinical approaches as bases for design. For the health care industry, computer technology and the technology of service provision will provide a context for structuring health care services. As technology becomes more "micronized," individuals will carry their health histories on chips and will have communicating devices for linkage with health care any place the consumer may be located. Therefore mobility and modularity create a goodness-of-fit in the health care system and provide an opportunity to address systematically the unique needs of individuals, as well as those of populations, regardless of where that demand may be created (Griffith, 1998).

Three Major Elements of Change

In final analysis, nurses and other health care professionals will have to incorporate three major elements of change in their understanding of clinical practice for the foreseeable future. These indicators are signposts of the radical shift in emphasis, design, and structuring of health care that will occur during the next two decades.

1. *Movement from institution to system.* Sociopolitical decision-making, economics, and technology have converged to create conditions making it possible for systems management and horizontal linkage of health services to occur across the continuum of care. The major emphasis of health care will be on building health prescriptive, proactive, integrated, and linked services in a systematic way. A focus on linkage, integration, and continuum will have tremendous impact on disciplines—their relationship to each other, to the consumer, and to the health care system. Each discipline will be obligated to reconfigure itself. Each discipline will have to define the unique characteristics it brings to relationships with other disciplines. The team approach thus will characterize delivery of health care services within the context of life management and across the continuum of care.

2. *Technology increases portability of service.* Nursing and other disciplines must recognize that health care is becoming less institutional, incremental, and intensive in its intervention processes. Increasingly, health care is becoming more mobile, population based, proactive, and health driven. The major shift in clinical practice will be away from incremental, interventive, and disease-driven constructs. Conversely, health care will be more health script–driven, integrated, and focused on management's clinical knowledge and the demand of populations and individuals intersecting with the health care system. This shift is a long-term consideration, requiring significant alteration in application and resource use, but such adaptation is fundamental and inevitable. Nurses need to begin to retool the discipline's emphasis on incremental, event-based, disease-driven, institutional, and fixed-site models of clinical practice to address more broadly based issues of life management in a highly flexible and mobile health environment.

3. *The information infrastructure is the new architecture for the future of health care.* Perhaps the most dramatic and traumatic shift in the context and structure of health care is that being driven by the emerging information infrastructure. Nurses and other health care professionals must become competent and proficient in the use of information, as it has important impacts on the design, structuring, and management of clinical services across the health care system in each and every community. Linkage, interface, integration, collaboration, and goodness-of-fit all will become cornerstones of the clinical environment. Understanding, applying, and managing this technology as part of the clinical structuring and delivery of health care services will be essential components of all nursing and clinical practice in the future. The hardware, software, processes, and technological interfaces being created further decentralizes and mobilizes the nurse for action in more fluid, flexible, and focused models of clinical practice in health care delivery.

■ Concluding Statement

Structures and formats for delivery of health care services will be much more integrated, fluid, and flexible than at any time in the history of humankind. The major work of the involved disciplines is to build into professional development, education, and management an ability to understand and translate realities of the future into guiding and leading the professions' work in a population-based, highly distributed health care system. The influence of economics, social, and technological shifts have created a requisite for professional change. Structures of health care that will emerge will be able to link a wider variety of people across a broader framework of service in much more flexible and mobile ways. To deal with inevitable change is and will be the sustaining work of nurses and other health care leadership today and for the foreseeable future.

■ References

American Nurses Association, & Endorsers. (1991). *Nursing's agenda for health care reform.* Washington, DC: American Nurses Association.

Barnes, D., Eribes, C., Juarbe, T., Nelson, M., Proctor, S., Sawyer, L., Shaul, M., & Meleis, A. (1995). Primary health care and primary care: A confusion of philosophies. *Nursing Outlook, 43*(1), 7–16.

Beckham, D. (1996). Hearing the tidal wave. *Healthcare Forum Journal, 39*(2), 68–78.

Blendon, R., & Brodie, M. (1994). *Transforming the system: Building a new structure for a new century.* (Vol. 4). New York: Faulkner & Grey.

Brown, M. (1995). The economic era: Now to the real change. *Health Care Management Review, 19*(4), 73–82.

Coffey, R., Stagis, S., & Fenner, K. (1997). *Virtually integrated health systems.* San Francisco: Jossey-Bass.

Coile, R. (1993). *Revolution: The new healthcare system takes shape.* San Francisco: Grand Rounds Press/Wittle Books.

Coile, R. (1994). Transformation of American healthcare in the post reform era. *Healthcare Executive, 9*(4), 8–12.

Contributors. (1997). *Integrated delivery systems.* Chicago: Health Administration Press.

D'Aunno, T., Alexander, J., & Laughlin, C. (1996). Business as usual? Changes in health care's workforce and organization of work. *Hospitals & Health Services Administration, 41*(1), 3–18.

Dertouzos, M. (1997). *What will be: How the new world of information will change our lives.* Cambridge, MA: MIT Press.

Doerge, J., & Hagenow, N. (1996). Integrating care delivery. *Nursing Administration Quarterly, 20*(2), 42–48.

Duncan, K. (1994). *Health information and health reform: The need for a health information system.* San Francisco: Jossey-Bass.

Editors. (1996). All our tomorrows: The economics of ageing. *The Economist, 338*(7950), 1–16.

Evans, K., Hawkins, M., Curley, T., & Porter-O'Grady, T. (1995). Whole systems shared governance: A model for the integrated health system. *Journal of Nursing Administration, 25*(5), 18–27.

Gage, M. (1998). From independence to interdependence: Creating synergistic healthcare teams. *Journal of Nursing Administration, 28*(4), 17–26.

Griffith, J. (1998). *Designing 21st century healthcare.* Chicago: Health Administration Press.

Gustafson, D., Helstad, C., & Hung, C. F. (1995). The total costs of illness: A metric for health care reform. *Hospital & Health Services Administration, 40*(1), 154–171.

Handy, C. (1998). *Beyond certainty: The changing world of organizations.* Boston: Harvard Business School Press.

Herzlinger, R. (1998). *Market driven health care.* Boston: Harvard Business School Press.

Lamb, G., & Zazworski, D. (1997). The carondelet experience. *Nursing Management, 28*(3), 27–28.

Lathrop, P. (1994). *Restructuring health care: The patient focused paradigm.* San Francisco: Jossey-Bass.

Lipman-Blumen, J. (1996). *The connective edge: Leading in an interdependent world.* San Francisco: Jossey-Bass.

Milio, N. (1996). *Engines of empowerment: Using information technology to create healthy communities and challenge public policy.* Chicago: Health Administration Press.

Negroponte, N. (1995). *Being digital.* New York: Knopf.

Pauly, M. (1995). When does curbing health care costs help the economy? *Health Affairs, 14*(2), 51–67.

Porter, A., Van Cleave, B., Milobowski, L., Conlon, P., & Mambourg, R. (1996). Clinical integration: An interdisciplinary approach to a system priority. *Nursing Administration Quarterly, 20*(2), 65–73.

Porter-O'Grady, T. (1997). Process leadership and the death of management. *Nursing Economic$, 16*(6), 286–293.

Porter-O'Grady, T., & Wilson, C. (1997). *Whole systems shared governance: Architecture for integration.* Gaithersburg, MD: Aspen.

Redmond, G. (1995). "We don't make widgets here": Voices of chief nurse executives. *Journal of Nursing Administration, 25*(2), 63–66.

Schneller, E., & Ott, J. (1996). Contemporary models of change in the health professions. *Hospitals & Health Services Administration, 41*(1), 121–136.

Schraeder, C., & Britt, T. (1997). The care clinic. *Nursing Management, 28*(3), 32–34.

Shoultz, J., & Hatcher, P. (1997). Looking beyond primary care to primary health care: An approach to community based action. *Nursing Outlook, 45*(1), 23–26.

Sullivan, S. (1996). Meeting the value test. *Healthcare Forum Journal, 39*(2), 57–59.

Waress, B., Pasternak, D., & Smith, H. (1994). Determining costs associated with quality in health care delivery. *Health Care Management Review, 19*(3), 52–63.

Wheatley, M. (1996). *A simpler way.* San Francisco: Berrett-Koehler.

Zander, K. (1995). *Managing outcomes through collaborative care: Care mapping and case management.* Chicago: American Hospital Publishing.

Zuckerman, H., Kaluzny, A., & Ricketts III, T. (1995). Alliances in health care: What we know, what we think we know, and what we should know. *Health Care Management Review, 20*(1), 54–64.

■ Editor's Questions for Discussion

What signposts of change presented by Porter-O'Grady are addressed by Boland (Chapter 71), Robinson, Griffith, and Sullivan-Mark (Chapter 41), Alexander (Chapter 44), and Pinkerton (Chapter 56)? What service providers have replaced professionals with less-skilled workers? What evidence should be available regarding such service providers? Discuss considerations for restructuring the delivery of health care services. What data are available regarding relevance of conditions for reframing structures?

How does Pinkerton (Chapter 56) provide a response to Porter-O'Grady's demand for restructuring? How do discipline-specific frames of reference lose relevance in restructuring? What does Porter-O'Grady reinforce regarding integrated design structures as described by Pinkerton (Chapter 56)? Specify how the restructuring advocated by Porter-O'Grady differs from previous designs.

Discuss structural changes that have already occurred in the delivery of health care. Provide specific examples of those changes cited by Porter-O'Grady. Identify discipline-specific issues and concerns related to new structural models that are emerging. What implications about structural models affect community relationships, as advocated by Alexander (Chapter 44), Hollinger-Smith (Chapter 45), Schroeder and Long (Chapter 47), Barger (Chapter 52), Gray (Chapter 42), and Robinson et al. (Chapter 41)? How may content provided by Stevens and Weiner (Chapter 38) address the information infrastructure concerns raised by Porter-O'Grady?

How does Porter-O'Grady's discussion about transferring skill sets apply to faculty practice (Carter, Chapter 39), rural health care (Pullen, Chapter 50), mobile nursing centers (Todero, Chapter 51), nursing centers (Barger, Chapter 52), and nursing entrepreneurship (Duffy, Chapter 53)? Address the three elements of future change described by Porter-O'Grady. What evidence exists that nurses must address these elements? How may nursing prepare for the changes predicted by Porter-O'Grady? What outcomes measures may be developed concerning change resulting from these three elements?

56

Organizing Nursing in an Integrated Delivery System (IDS)

SueEllen Pinkerton, PhD, RN, FAAN

The integrated delivery system (IDS) has become the structure of choice for health care systems. Although various forms of the IDS have been around since the 1970s, their specific cost and efficiency benefits are still unclear.

Reorganizations of this magnitude have an impact on nursing services because nursing has historically been the largest single department in the hospital, with the most full-time equivalents and the highest budgeted salaries and wages (Clifford, 1998). However, the impact of changes on nursing and other clinical departments in the move to an IDS is rarely discussed as hospitals reposition themselves for reorganizations of this type and continued resource restraints (Clifford, 1998).

In this chapter I will focus on nursing in an IDS. Although an IDS potentially can have a negative impact on the organization of nursing services, it also presents an opportunity to try new models and new organizational structures. Taking advantage of these opportunities can have a positive impact on the profession, professional strength, and development, and hence patient outcomes.

■ History of Integrated Delivery Systems

Integration of health care services began in the 1970s with formation of multihospital systems, nursing home chains, and physician group practices (Burns & Thorpe, 1995). This is referred to as horizontal integration, which is pursued to gain economies of scale and an increased market share. It involves the joining of two or more organizations that are providing similar services to become one organization or entering some type of partnership (Conrad & Shortell, 1996).

In the 1980s, vertical integration of health care services began, following a strategy pursued by large corporations. It was aptly referred to as "corporate restructuring" and involved hospitals integrating backward by acquiring or developing a supply of patients through ambulatory care centers and physician practices. Hospitals also integrated forward by acquiring and developing distribution outlets for patients, such as home care agencies and nursing homes (Burns & Thorpe, 1995).

Vertical integration involves combining separate organizations having products that are inputs to or outputs from the production of one another's services. Primary reasons for vertical integration are to lower transaction costs between separate production processes, such as hospitals and home care, and to reduce average production costs by sharing common inputs, such as physician and nurse practices (Conrad & Shortell, 1996). Two forms of vertical integration exist: (a) the classical form, in which a single organization has ownership; and (b) the virtual form, which an organization operates under long-term, exclusive contracts, affiliations, and operating agreements with any number of other organizations (Conrad & Shortell, 1996).

Integrated delivery systems are combinations of vertical and horizontal integration. These systems contract with managed care plans to provide a full range of services, including physician practices, hospitals, and ambulatory, long-term, and wellness care. The ultimate goal of an IDS is to enter into a contract to manage the total health of a specific population for a specific amount of money for a specific time period of time (Burns & Thorpe, 1995).

Fully integrated health organizations (IHO) combine an IDS and ownership of a financing element, such as a health maintenance organization (HMO) (Burns & Thorpe, 1995). The IHO is intended to provide better quality, satisfaction, and price than an IDS is able to provide without ownership of an HMO.

Outcomes of the IDS related to efficiencies and costs have not yet been clearly defined (Burns & Thorpe, 1995). Preliminary data from Shortell, Gillies, Anderson, Erickson, and Mitchell (1996) demonstrate that IDSs performed better financially than their competitors. There is general agreement, however, that IDSs need more time to mature before their benefits can be accurately measured and better understood.

As IDSs gain experience, some are taking steps to eliminate ownership (referred to as deintegration) of physician practices due to the high cost of operating practices. Other IDSs are moving to virtual integration and leaving ownership, governance, and operations that are not their core services to those with experience and success in those areas. Still others (mainly IHOs) are relinquishing ownership of the financial elements (HMOs or PPOs, preferred provider organizations) because an IHO, by owning an HMO, competes with other managed care companies whose business they are trying to obtain for the IHO.

Despite their relative newness and unclear benefits (which are still being measured and tested), the IDS has become the structure of choice for health care. Nursing, however, is essentially absent from network development discussions despite the fact that hospital restructuring efforts have had an impact on nurses and have begun to reshape the nature of nursing services (Clifford, 1998).

■ Connecting Nursing Practice in an IDS

Nursing practice may exist at any point along the continuum of care in an IDS. Nursing practice may be part of the input to an IDS—in clinics, independently, or as part of a group. In this instance, they would be expected to refer patients to component organizations of the IDS (in either the classic or virtual systems). Other practice arenas for nurses in the IDS would be hospitals, nursing homes, skilled nursing facilities, rehabilitation facilities, and home care agencies. The Chief Nursing Officer (CNO) of an IDS is challenged to integrate nursing practice at numerous points of service delivery.

Commonly, there is a system-level CNO who may or may not have line authority for nursing leaders in the component organizations of an IDS. But, in some instances, no nursing leader is designated in component organizations, mostly due to the product or service line structure. In this case, coordinating and connecting nursing points of delivery is more complex, and the naming of nursing leader for each component organization should be pursued by the CNO. A CNO can achieve this objective by negotiating with the appropriate administrator at the system or component organization level.

A successful structure that coordinates and connects all points of nursing delivery in an IDS is a Chief Nursing Officer Council (CNOC). Its members are the designated leaders of each component organization of an IDS, including the College of Nursing if the IDS has a relationship with one. The chair of the group is the CNO for the system or a designate of the CNO.

The CNOC can develop concepts to support a structure, including a vision statement, such as the one adopted by Shands HealthCare (SHC) (1998): "To set a new standard of excellence for autonomous, accountable nursing practice, committed to patient advocacy and innovative patient care in a climate of trust and collaboration" (p. 2). The CNOC can also state a purpose, such as the one also adopted by SHC (1998): "To develop and implement strategic planning and to act as the official spokesperson for Shands HealthCare nursing"

(pp. 2, 3). In addition, SHC adopted the definition of nursing from the American Nurses Association Nursing's (ANA's) (1995) Social Policy Statement: "The diagnosis and treatment of human response to actual or potential health problems" (p. 6).

A final component of the SHC's CNOC structure was the development of goals (SHC, 1999):

- Provide systemwide input on resource allocation.

- Provide oversight and evaluation of nursing practice standards and performance standards.

- Monitor quality of care trends.

- Plan and implement a research program.

- Identify opportunities to share resources and joint ventures.

- Provide educational opportunities and avenues for professional development.

Strategies were developed on the basis of the system's needs and goals. The following are examples of systemwide strategies to meet one of the CNOC's goals.

Goal: Monitor quality of care trends
Strategies:

- Review system risk management cases; track trends related to nursing practice; discuss corrective actions taken and plans to avoid future cases.

- Review quality committee reports from all component organizations of the system including nursing quality indicators and plan actions, as appropriate.

- Review patient satisfaction data and plan interventions as appropriate.

Other functions of the CNOC include focusing on the ANA's Scope and Standards for Nurse Administrators (1995). These standards are the basis for the Magnet Nursing Services Recognition Program (American Nurses Credentialing Center [ANCC], 1998). Magnet Nursing Services Recognition, in itself, is a worthy goal and can be pursued by a system, depending on some organizational or CNO structural criteria (ANCC, 1998). In addition to acute care, long-term care, and home care, recognition can be pursued to achieve the goal of Magnet Nursing Services Recognition for an IDS.

Adopting a governance system for an IDS is also a laudable goal. Although shared governance, a model used in nursing and extended hospitalwide for the last 15 to 20 years, has been organization-specific, it is also being supported to span an IDS (Porter-O'Grady, Hawkins, & Parker, 1997).

Clearly, any of numerous concepts, goals, and structures (many not mentioned here) may be used as a focus in organizing a CNOC in an IDS. A focus can

- enhance consistency in patient outcomes,
- unify nursing practice,
- help move individuals from "silo" thinking to systems thinking,
- develop system-level leadership skills in individuals, and
- structure succession planning for leadership.

■ Outcomes From Integrating Nursing in an IDS

Currently, there is much concern for value in health care. Shortell et al. (1996) stated that "more integrated systems will demonstrate their value when more markets across the United States move to emphasizing quality, patient satisfaction and outcomes and not just price" (p. 51). Organizing and connecting nursing practice in an IDS can lead to increased value in several ways.

Cuddeback and Gaintner (1997) presented a simple value equation:

$$Value = \frac{Quality}{Cost} \times Efficacy$$

In this equation, quality is related to outcomes and satisfaction. Efficacy relates to the appropriateness of care (acquiring, transmitting, and using knowledge). Therefore value is expressed as quality at a reasonable cost in a milieu of efficacy. Figure 56.1 depicts a model for this equation that translates it into everyday practice.

This equation and model demonstrate the underlying process of defining, measuring, and rewarding for value—points made by Shortell et al. (1996)—which are important as outcomes in an IDS.

The top part of the model addresses quality.

- *Did we satisfy the customers' needs and expectations?* This question can be answered in part by using the Nursing Quality Indicators (ANA, 1999) to measure four patient satisfaction areas—pain management, educational information, overall care, and nursing care. In addition, other areas to measure are access (lack of barriers) and meeting community needs.

- *Did we achieve the desired results?* This question addresses outcomes and can be measured against outcomes identified in clinical pathways or, again, those identified in the Nursing Quality Indicators (ANA, 1999) related to pressure ulcers, patient falls, and nosocomial infections. As mentioned in the goals of the CNOC, patient outcomes can be tracked and reported for the system through existing data collection. This capability affords the CNOC an opportunity to enhance patient outcomes in component organizations of the system, as needed. It also provides an opportunity to ensure that comparable standards for nursing practice and patient care are in place throughout the system, by measuring what exists against what should exist or what is needed and expected.

- *Did we do it well?* This measure can be accomplished by collecting data in any of the areas previously mentioned (patient satisfaction and outcomes). Certainly, meeting patient satisfaction expectations is a prime component of making the determination of whether we did it well. "Perception is everything."

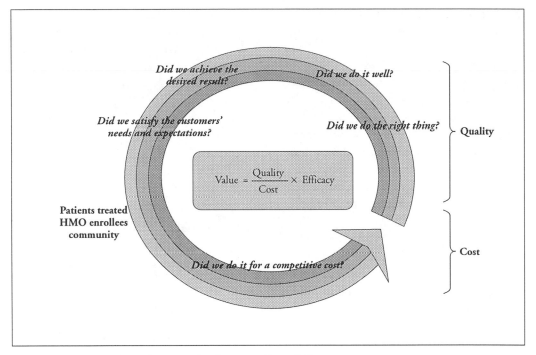

Figure 56.1   Process for Evaluating Value Outcomes for an IDS.

- *Did we do the right thing?* This question refers to the efficacy portion of the value equation. As stated, efficacy is acquiring, transmitting, and using knowledge in care delivery. In nursing, using benchmarks to set best practices is part of doing the right thing. Also included is participation in research and the use of research findings to direct nursing practice. Because of the variety of component organizations in an IDS, nursing has ample opportunity to contribute to research development and knowledge generation, especially if there is an extensive and all-inclusive continuum of care in an IDS. These opportunities give nursing researchers access to a large number of potential patients to serve as participants in research activities.

The bottom part of the model addresses the cost component of the value equation.

- *Did we do it for a competitive cost?* Again, there are benchmarks that can be used to measure cost. Balancing quality and cost is a skill constantly being improved by nurse administra-

tors. Opportunities exist for reducing expenses through economies of scale in an IDS. For example, some IDSs have central education, so efforts are not duplicated by each component organization. Central education is used for courses such as intensive care unit orientation, basic life support, and advanced life support. Other IDSs may have a central staffing office (CSO) so that this function also is not duplicated. Obviously, geographic distance would be a factor in whether a CSO sends staff to a number of facilities.

Although every organization in health care addresses value, it can be enhanced through an IDS. Component organizations have the opportunity to share experiences, successes, and missed opportunities without the competitive threat often cited by organizations that are not bound by a relationship such as an IDS. Enhancing value is a challenge to nursing for growth, and organizing nursing in an IDS is an opportunity to do so.

■ *Maintaining Professional Integrity While Organizing Nursing Services*

In an IDS where the CNO of the system has no line authority over the designated nurse leaders of the component organizations, how can the CNO influence nursing practice and patient outcomes? How will nursing's professional integrity be maintained? Who will be responsible for the development, growth, and continued contributions of the nurses? How can the CNO be effective without budgetary authority and responsibility?

Lasswell and Kaplan (1959) in their enduring and classic works describe eight resources of power: power (which can be a resource for more power), respect, moral standing, affection, well-being, wealth, skill, and enlightenment. The CNO has differing access to these resources and can effect change, using a variety of power bases, without a traditional structure of line authority. For example, a CNO who is respected can be of significant influence in maintaining professional integrity without having to have line authority.

The CNO is responsible for integrating the goals of professional nurses with the mission and goals of the organization or system. The intent of this integration is to maximize the quality of patient care, professional satisfaction of the nurse, and cost-effectiveness of the system (Clifford, 1998, p. 5).

The corporate-level nursing position of the CNO has several functional components that need to be kept in mind as nursing services are organized. First, the geographic area that the system covers is a factor in being able to affect nursing practice. It may be easier to organize a nursing effort in an urban area that contains all the component organizations. Difficulty increases as component organizations are scattered throughout a state, several states, nationally, or internationally.

Organizing the nursing effort is also complicated by the number and types of practice sites served by the IDS. Nursing practice may take place in an independent practice, clinic, nursing home (or a variety of skilled nursing facilities), home care, and numerous acute care settings wherein the level of acute care that is practiced varies. The CNO then is challenged to find common ground and interests for discussions at CNOC meetings.

Discussion Topics

The following are some topics that may help unite the component organizations' nursing leaders (who often possess different levels of nursing preparation and professional experience).

- Present and discuss individual opinions on the need for access to expert nurses and how access might be accomplished in the system. For example, can home care nurses have access to acute care nurses for information in their particular areas of expertise (e.g., wound care and ventilator care)? If so, how can that be accomplished? Should one resource person channel all such requests or should a resource directory be available?

- Is there a difference in professional socialization between different specialty hospitals, geographic locations, or different levels of educational preparation? How should professional socialization be achieved? For example, videotapes on professional behavior could be developed and shared throughout the system. This effort could be a project staffed and led by nurses from the component organizations. Will involvement of these nurses in such an effort lead to greater nurse satisfaction?

- How can we together efficiently manage our resources, both human and financial? This topic gives the CNO an entrée for involvement with the nursing leader of each component organization. Standing meetings with component organization administrators and component organizations' nursing leaders (together and separately) are an effective way to outline how the CNO may be helpful. And any help with the budget is usually welcomed and provides for ongoing dialogue.

- How can we properly orient newly appointed component organization nursing leaders? The CNO can set the stage for continued relationships by helping newly appointed nursing leaders relate to the CNOC's purpose, goals, and definition of nursing, and prepare presentations for nurses and department heads outlining plans for the component organization.

- How do the CNO, who usually has extensive experience, and the other nursing leaders in the system create an environment for sharing experiences and stories? That can be done to a limited extent at CNOC meetings. Perhaps a better way is to have periodic retreats to focus on vision and purpose and, in doing so, to share stories and to get to know the contributions others may make. Envisioning everyone coming together as separate colors that form a quilt, or each as separate instruments that form an orchestra, is a powerful way to celebrate the separateness of everyone while becoming aware of opportunities for synergy (Kritek, 1997). Reporting a history of the system is also enlightening, as is having guest speakers who were leaders of the component organizations but are now retired.

Shared Governance

Nurses have made a paradigm shift to shared governance, which essentially is a transformation in their way of thinking. It is more than a change in organizational structure; it is a supportive system that encourages nurses to be responsible for their actions (Krejci & Malin, 1989). Shared governance in itself is a base that can be used to maintain integrity of the nursing discipline. Many shared governance–based nursing departments have long-standing councils organized around patient care (standards), quality, research and evaluation, management systems, and nursing staff development. Integrity of the nursing discipline revolves around having (a) requisite knowledge to evaluate the quality of patient care and (b) management systems to support nurses' efforts. Therefore, no matter where nurses report in

the organization or system, the profession can grow and thrive by having such councils and governance (Pinkerton, 1998).

Nurturing the Soul of Nursing

One last important focus for maintaining the integrity of the discipline of nursing is to take an active role in nurturing its soul. Caring is the soul of nursing practice. Caring is the core element of humans, and nurses are charged with caring for that core element. What a wonderful responsibility to have. What a wonderful opportunity to see what impact a nurse can have on the wholeness of human beings. And what wonderful rewards nurses have when they see the human spirit rally. Nurses often influence the human spirit to overcome what many may have said were insurmountable odds. But the human spirit won. Nurses are privileged to be witnesses to and part of such achievement. We need to foster the continuing of such nursing practice and not let it be lost to reorganizations, criticisms, and theft of the spirit of nursing.

■ Barriers to Maintaining the Integrity of the Nursing Discipline

Not surprisingly, there are barriers to maintaining the integrity of the nursing discipline in an IDS. One such barrier is the lack of skilled nursing leaders to implement integration (Arista Associates and Modern HealthCare, 1998). The IDS is a relatively new form of health care organization and not many nurse administrators have had experience leading nursing in such a system. A CNO should be aware of this lack and do appropriate succession planning. The CNO can delegate system-level functions to qualified others and participate in preceptorships and mentoring. The CNO should also share experiences with colleagues at CNOC and local and national meetings. Writing for publications is also a great way to share.

Conrad and Shortell (1996) identified additional barriers. The first mentioned is a resource barrier, which refers to information systems, especially in connecting points of service along a continuum of care. Well-developed information systems enable nursing services to be organized effectively. They also enable evaluation of nursing and patient outcomes to identify better performing practitioners for possible use as resources.

Mental models and organizational culture are the second identified barrier. To overcome them, system members need to eliminate "silo" thinking, which may be limiting them to one point of care on the continuum; instead, they need to consider what might be best for the patient as he or she moves along the continuum. It is a shift to whole-person, systems thinking. There is also no longer a place for discipline-centered thinking. Having such governance models as whole-system shared governance will help nursing to move from provincial thinking to systems thinking, while keeping nursing focused on maintaining integrity of the discipline.

The barrier of conflicting incentives has adverse impacts on nursing when incentives to contain total cost conflict with quality of care and services. Nursing must be diligent at the local and system levels in tracking outcomes and monitoring trends. Negative impacts on nursing and patient outcomes are serious, and although cost control may not be the reason, any threat to nursing and patient care outcomes threatens the integrity of the discipline. All outcomes must be thoroughly examined and corrected. Good patient outcomes that are supported by valid data are readily accepted by other conscientious individuals as sound reasons for negotiating resources.

■ Preparing for the Future

The most important component of integration is defined as clinical, or the extent to which patient care services are coordinated in an IDS (Devers et al., 1994). How are the nursing components connected along the continuum of care? Organizing a CNOC is a proven model, especially when identified goals for the CNOC complement system goals.

A second way to position nursing, especially to maintain integrity of the discipline, is to seek a CNO for the system who has experience at the system level or has been mentored by such a CNO. This need reinforces the advisability of succession planning, to teach people to be system thinkers, and to develop system leaders.

As an IDS is organized, adequate and secure information systems that will provide data to monitor patient outcomes must be installed. Clinical information system installations have typically lagged behind installation of management information systems. Such delays have created vacuums in monitoring some aspects of nursing and patient care. But a much more difficult situation has been created by the lack of information systems support to the continuum of care, which should be pursued as IDSs are developed.

■ Concluding Statement

Needless to say, nursing can best be served in an IDS by having a system-level CNO. This puts nursing at the system's deliberation, discussion, and negotiating table. It also gives nursing access to resource discussions and an opportunity for early intervention when unintended patient care outcomes arise.

A CNO also begins to address the issue of potential impacts of the changes an IDS brings to the management and administration of nursing and other clinical services (Clifford, 1998). Nursing, in many discussions, is the only clinical discipline represented and can enhance discussions by wearing a multidisciplinary hat.

Leading an IDS involves leading a system that is a fuzzy compilation of a medley of components (Greene, 1998). What is best for the system has to be kept at the forefront, and a team has to be built around this vision. Good leadership in an IDS requires the ability to manage the people side of the equation, as well as the balance sheet; the IDS must be recognized first as a social entity and then as an economic one. This focus is a particular strength that the CNO, who typically has valuable experience in process negotiation, can bring to the table.

Many suggestions have been made for organizing nursing in an IDS. Nursing presence is important in an IDS, as is organization of the nurses in an IDS. Nursing has the skills and opportunity to support and enhance the IDS, contributing to its achievement of outcomes of high quality, great satisfaction, and low cost.

■ References

American Nurses Credentialing Center. (1998, November). *The magnet nursing services recognition program for excellence in nursing service acute care.* (Instructions and Application Process). Washington, DC: American Nurses Publishing.

American Nurses Association. (1995). *Nursing's social policy statement.* (Booklet). Washington, DC: Author.

American Nurses Association. (1995). *Scope and standards for nurse administrators.* [Booklet]. Washington, D.C.: Author.

American Nurses Association. (1999). *Nursing facts.* [Brochure]. Washington, DC: Author.

Arista Associates & Modern HealthCare. (1998). *1998 Survey of integrated delivery systems.* Fairfax, VA, & Northbrook, IL: Author.

Burns, L. R., & Thorpe, O. P. (1995). Managed care and integrated health care. *Health Care Management State of the Art Review, 2*(1), 101–108.

Clifford, J. C. (1998). *Restructuring: The impact of hospital organization on nursing leadership.* Chicago: American Hospital Publishing.

Conrad, D. A., & Shortell, S. M. (1996). Integrated health systems: Promise and performance. *Frontiers of Health Services Management, 13*(1), 3–40.

Cuddeback, J., & Gaintner, J. R. (1997). *Quality model and value equation.* Gainesville, FL: Shands HealthCare. (Unpublished manuscript).

Devers, K. J., Shortell, S. M., Gillies, R. R., Anderson, D. A., Mitchell, J. B., & Morgan Erickson, K. L. (1994). Implementing organized delivery systems: An integration scorecard. *Health Care Management Review, 19*(3), 7–20.

Greene, J. (1998). Coaching the entire team: Do you have what it takes to manage an integrated delivery system? *HealthCare Executive* (January/February), 16–19.

Krejci, J. W., & Malin, S. (1989). A paradigm shift to the new age of nursing. *Nursing Administration Quarterly, 13*(4), 40–45.

Kritek, P. B. (1997). *Special consultation at the chief nursing officers council.* Gainesville, FL: Shands HealthCare.

Lasswell, H. D., and Kaplan, A. (1959). Power and society: A framework for political inquiry. *Yale Law School Studies* (Vol. 2). New Haven, CT: Yale University Press.

Pinkerton, S. E. (1998). The ties that bind. *Journal of Professional Nursing, 14*(2), 66.

Porter-O'Grady, T., Hawkins, M. A., & Parker, M. L. (1997). *Whole-systems shared governance: Architecture for integration.* Gaithersburg, MD: Aspen.

Shands HealthCare. (1998, May 5). *Vision and Purpose(s)*. Chief Nursing Officer Council Presentation to Management Executive Committee. Gainesville, FL: Author.

Shands HealthCare. (1999, March 16). *Goals and Strategies*. Chief Nursing Officer Council Presentation to Management Executive Committee. Gainesville, FL: Author.

Shortell, S. M., Gillies, R. R., Anderson, D. A., Erickson, K. M., & Mitchell, J. B. (1996). *Remaking health care in America: Building organized delivery systems*. San Francisco, CA: Jossey-Bass.

■ Editor's Questions for Discussion

Identify the advantages and limitations of integrated delivery systems (IDS). How can IDS affect patient outcomes? What evidence exists that horizontal and vertical integration lowers costs? What other benefits may result from IDS? How do IDS models differ from previous models for delivery for health care? Why has nursing been absent from network development discussions for IDS? How can nursing be more influential in the development of IDS?

Propose an IDS vision statement and state how it could be implemented. How might shared governance systems span an IDS? What impact does shared governance have on quality care? What additional measures for quality might be used in the shared governance IDS model? How does the shared governance IDS model lend itself to future outcomes research as identified by Deets and Choi (Chapter 34) and Titler (Chapter 35).

What preparation is essential for the position Chief Nursing Officer (CNO)? What statements by M. Fisher (Chapter 17), McCausland and McCauley (Chapter 40), Kerfoot (Chapter 75), Porter-O'Grady (Chapter 55), and Dienemann, Campbell, and Agnew (Chapter 59) have particular relevance to the CNO and the IDS?

Respond to the discussion questions posed by Pinkerton concerning the CNO. What data are needed to address the questions and issues? What impacts do collective bargaining units have in shared governance structures? How does Felton (Chapter 1) reinforce Pinkerton's emphasis on the role of nursing?

How do Stevens and Weiner (Chapter 38) address barriers concerning information systems in IDS? Provide examples of whole-person systems thinking versus discipline-centered thinking. How can conflicts between costs and quality of care be reduced?

57

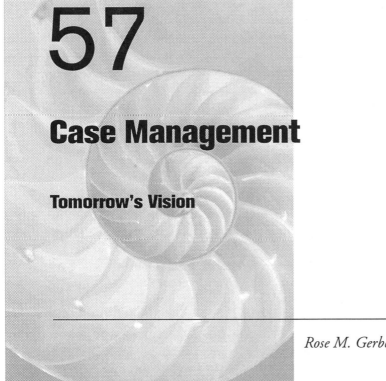

Case Management

Tomorrow's Vision

Rose M. Gerber, PhD, RN

S ince the mid 1980s, case management has exploded as a form of professional nursing practice in the United States and is gaining momentum in a growing number of other countries. Nurses for many years have used the case management process within community health nursing and other segments of the profession. However, tremendous growth in the number and variety of nurse case managers (NCMs) has occurred primarily in response to new and unmet needs for the delivery of high-quality, cost-effective health care. In the United States, multiple environmental factors have influenced development of nursing case management significantly. Causes include but are not limited to movement from fee-for-service to prospective payment meth-ods for obtaining health and illness care, technological advances, and demographic changes in society. Today, the concept of nursing case management, although not well defined, is accepted as an essential nursing role within the health care delivery system.

When we as nurses think about the future of case management, three questions come to mind. Where are we now? Where are we going? And, how in the world do we get there? Although case management practice is inter-disciplinary in nature and is practiced by mul-tiple disciplines, in this chapter I focus on case management within nursing. First, I define nursing case management within the context of current practice. Then, believing that on-going change is a necessary condition and expecting that the future can be shaped proactively, some thoughts are offered about the future of nursing case management.

■ Nursing Case Management: Context and Definition

Historically, case management has been recognized as an interdisciplinary field of practice within the health care delivery system, with the majority of case managers having educational and experiential backgrounds in social work, rehabilitation, occupational health, psychiatric–mental health and the like. With the advent of prospective payment for health services in the 1980s and the growth of managed care that followed, nurses have become an increasingly large part of the evolving case management industry and nursing case management has become a specialty within nursing (Mullahy, 1998).

Professional nurses have a unique knowledge and skill set that has added value to provision of quality care in a cost-contained and resource-constrained environment. Hence the unanticipated demand for nurse case managers escalated very quickly; they have been employed in large numbers, far beyond the reasoned expectations of nurse administrators and educators. As a result of the unexpected and generally unplanned expansion of the NCM role, almost any nurse today can be called a "nurse case manager" and nursing case management is practiced in nearly as many forms as there are nurse case managers. An axiom within the field of case management is: "If you have seen one case manager, you have seen one case manager." The same is generally true within the practice of nursing case management.

Over time, nursing case management has been described as a system, role, technology, process, and service (Bower, 1992); strategy (Flarey & Blancett, 1996); care delivery innovation (Lynn & Kelley, 1997); and practice structure (Smith, 1993), among others. The Case Management Society of America (CMSA), the nation's largest case management association, has defined case management as "a collaborative process that assesses, plans, implements, coordinates, monitors and evaluates options and services to meet an individual's health needs through communication and available resources to promote quality, cost-effective outcomes" (Case Management Society of America [CMSA], 1995, p. 8). Today consensus is developing whereby nursing case management is considered a process (Cesta, Tahan, & Fink, 1998; Mullahy, 1998; Rossi, 1999).

As a process, case management is a recognizable force that makes the current health care system operational, ensuring that the patient or client receives the appropriate level of care at the right time and encouraging the highest quality care possible at the right price (Rossi, 1999). Patient advocacy always has been one of the hallmarks of case management. This function of NCM practice has become critical as care delivery systems have become more complex and, at times, less responsive to individuals in systems of care.

In nursing today, a movement to refocus practice to include care of aggregates and communities is evident. More nurses are working with groups of clients who share a common characteristic, such as a specific disease or clinical disorder, or who have come together in a particular health-related or clinical setting. Increasingly nurses are practicing within complex organizations. Hospitals are becoming ever more complex and are emerging into large, comprehensive systems of care delivery. More than ever before, providers of care and direct care givers must be knowledgeable about payor systems and health care economics.

Smith (1993) suggested that the term *case management* may be an aphorism for the ideal structure of professional nursing practice: "The common values of nursing that affirm human dignity, freedom, and wholeness must be foundational to any nursing case management practice" (p. 8). The idea proposed was that nursing case management practice must be based on nursing theory and values reflecting a caring relationship that facilitates health, healing, and quality of life. Smith further suggested that, when the nursing perspective is missing, nursing case management is little more than nursing practiced with either a medical focus on cure or a financial focus on cost-containment, neither of which meets the ideals of professional practice. Therefore any definition of nursing case management necessarily must integrate the essence of case management and professional nursing as it now occurs in a complex, business-focused environment.

When CMSA's (1995) definition of case management is integrated with Smith's (1993) concern that nursing case management incorporate the values and perspective of professional nursing, a unique definition of nursing case management emerges. *Nursing case management,* then, can be defined as

> the application of the collaborative and interdisciplinary case management process by professional nurses to promote the delivery of high-quality, holistic, cost-effective health and illness care to individuals and groups within communities and complex organizational systems through patient advocacy, communication, and effective management of available resources.

Nursing case management, then, is a process—a case management process that (a) has much in common with the traditional nursing process; (b) is used for the purpose of delivering high-quality and cost-effective professional care to those who are served; and (c) achieves care outcomes through patient advocacy and the effective management of resources.

■ *Nursing Case Management: State-of-the-Art*

Although efforts are underway to establish a stronger science base for nursing case management practice, the actual body of knowledge available to guide the practice of nurse case managers remains fairly limited (Lamb, 1995). Historically, many of the earlier studies (a) lacked theoretical support, (b) had no clear operational definition of case management, (c) focused on cost savings in terms of increased efficiency in the organization in which case management was practiced, (d) included heterogeneous samples, and (e) used a variety of outcome indicators that were not sensitive to case management intervention (Lamb, 1995). By necessity, NCM practice has been based on an organizational need to save money, conserve human and physical resources, and enhance the efficiency of patient care systems. Financial risk-sharing arrangements have required care providers to manage the cost of care and to remain competitive in a volatile market. Therefore the more urgent need for the practice as an art has outpaced the ability of either the case management industry or the nursing profession to develop the desired science base for practice. Thus today's reality is that professional nursing case management tends to be practiced more as an art than as a science.

Voluntary Control Mechanisms

Another current characteristic of case management in general, with implications for nursing case management as a specialty, is the use of voluntary control mechanisms to regulate both the practice and the practitioner. When carefully developed and properly implemented, voluntary control mechanisms established through professional associations can be quite effective. Today, accepted standards of practice exist for case managers (CMSA, 1995) and are applicable to the role of nurse case manager. Standards of practice establish guidelines for excellence, as well as provide a framework that can be used to guide public policy, education, and research.

Documentation of case management expertise is now available through voluntary certification by examination. As might be expected, employers eagerly seek case managers who are credentialed. Likewise, certified case managers are more marketable and can command higher salaries (Strickland & Mullahy, 1997). Currently at least seven *multidisciplinary* certification examinations are available to RNs (Levin, 1999; Mullahy, 1998; "Scrambling for," 1997). Additionally, in 1997, the American Nurses Credentialing Center (ANCC) introduced a module for certification of registered nurses in case management. Nurses now have an opportunity and an obligation to select appropriate certification as case managers, based on a systematic assessment of their own clinical experience, practice setting, eligibility criteria, and content domain of each test (Levin, 1999).

In 1996, CMSA developed the Center for Case Management Accountability (CCMA) to provide a mechanism for measurement, evaluation, and reporting of case management outcomes. Accountability is about demonstrating the value of case management services, helping others make informed decisions about purchasing and using case management services, and stimulating widespread improvement in the processes and outcomes of case management (Center for Case Management Accountability [CCMA], 1997). CCMA addresses a spectrum of accountability through identification of *key direct outcomes* of case management, including patient knowledge, patient involvement in care, patient empowerment, patient adherence, and coordination of care. Other end outcomes of the larger health system also are addressed by CCMA and include *health* outcomes, quality of care, and cost of care. The premise of

CCMA is that the value of case managers must be measured where they have direct influence. That is, the true value of case management can be demonstrated most clearly by identifying those interventions that are within the scope of the case manager's control. Again, the CCMA mechanism is a voluntary effort to self-regulate the practice of case management.

Accreditation of case management services and agencies is now gaining momentum (Carneal, 1998; D'Andrea & Hamill, 1999; Whitaker, 1999). In January 1998, the American Accreditation HealthCare Commission and Utilization Review Accreditation Commission (URAC), a nonprofit charitable organization founded to establish standards for the managed care industry, voted to develop accreditation standards for case management programs in managed care organizations (Gerson, 1998). The primary goal for URAC's accreditation program is to enhance the quality of case management services through the voluntary process of accreditation. Although many case managers welcome the proposed standards, some concern has been expressed about the unknown effect of standard setting on independently owned small businesses (Whitaker, 1999). The types of standards being developed include such considerations as scope of case management programs, staff qualifications, quality management requirements, program accessibility, confidentiality and patient rights, dispute resolution, legal/regulations compliance, and the like (D'Andrea & Hamill, 1999; Gerson, 1998). Whereas case manager certification has become the benchmark for individuals performing the case management role, accreditation is expected to become the benchmark for case management programs (Carneal, 1998).

Case Management Education

Interestingly, despite strong commitment to case management accountability, very little regulation or oversight of case manager education has occurred. Historically, NCMs have been educated through on-the-job training, in-service education programs, continuing education conferences and workshops, publications and journals, and even the "see one, do one" visitation program approach. In nursing, case management education currently consists of (a) a few formal certificate programs, (b) increasing integration of case management content into academic programs, and (c) some specialized programs at the graduate level that also include emphasis on leadership knowledge and skills relative to case management (Cesta, Tahan, & Fink, 1998). The variable educational preparation of NCMs is due largely to the (a) explosive need for people to perform the NCM role, (b) lack of a clear definition of the role to be performed, and (c) lack of a responsive and organized approach to guide educational programming. Achieving consensus on educational requirements for case management in general has been difficult, considering the variability in the case management practice. Some case management functions, such as insurance claims adjustment or utilization review, can be performed legitimately by laypersons or by those who are minimally licensed to do so within another discipline. However, consensus that the baccalaureate degree should be the minimal preparation for basic case management practice is evolving (American Nurses Association [ANA], 1988; Chan, Leahy, McMahon, Mirch, & DeVinney, 1999). For advanced case management practice and leadership positions, the master's degree is desirable (Anderson-Loftin, 1999; Llewellyn & Moreo, 1998).

Although ethical considerations always have been a concern in case management, greater emphasis is being placed on the need for ethical case management practice, particularly in these times when case managers frequently serve as the link between payor and provider. When case managers are not cognizant of their personal value systems, they unwittingly may be drawn into situations in which core values such as patient advocacy or quality care can be compromised. For example, although payment incentives may be a useful and appropriate tool for enhancing efficiency in care giving, care providers must not lose sight of core values and need for ethical behavior. As health care resources and financing become more limited, the opportunity for fraud and abuse increase. Unfortunately, all case managers today are faced with ethical dilemmas on a regular basis.

During the past 10 years of intense growth in the case management industry, much progress has been made in the professionalization and regulation of case management in general. Case management, as an interdisciplinary process, is here to stay for the foreseeable future. As case management becomes a clinical specialty in nursing, support is growing for regulation of NCM practice through voluntary certification and placement of more emphasis on formal education as preparation for the role.

■ The Future of Case Management Practice

With regard to case management in general, Steinhauser (1999) has suggested that "accreditation, outcomes measurement, technology, globalization and patient advocacy will help determine case management's place in the [future] health care system and the role case managers will play" (p. 18). When asked to identify the greatest opportunities in the future of case management (Strickland & Mullahy, 1997), leaders in the industry spoke of such things as "tremendous opportunities to create specialized practices within the community" (p. 73) such as elder care, health promotion, health care counseling and teaching, and "geriatric home care case management" (p. 73). These same leaders suggested that, by 2002, the case manager's job will be affected greatly by advances in telecommunications and other forms of communication technology; that, as brokers and synthesizers of information, case managers will benefit from having better information on which to base decisions (Strickland & Mullahy, 1997).

Case Management Roles

Mullahy (1998) has proposed that case management shift in the direction of disease management. This change will mean 24-hour coverage, use of more "carve outs" of certain elements or special services within health benefit plans, and more "outsourcing," whereby selected activities such as utilization review and record keeping are purchased. Many such functions are already being obtained from outside the health care system to avoid the cost of an in-house systems upgrading.

An unknown source has wisely suggested that "the best way to predict the future is to create it." Perhaps the best approach to designing the future of nursing case management is to (a) build on the strengths of the past, (b) identify likely needs and opportunities in the future, based on what is known about the larger field of case management and trends in health care delivery, and (c) move forward with haste.

Accountability-Based Practice

Clearly, treating case management as an accountability-based practice has been a strength that can and should be carried forth into the future. NCMs would do well to (a) continue to refine the functions of their practice, (b) document the direct outcomes of their practice, and (c) relate the direct outcomes of practice to the more general outcomes of the health care delivery system. Such activities require considerable expertise in data collec-

tion, analysis, and reporting. NCMs cannot practice in a professional vacuum, but they must be able to document unique contributions of nurses and nursing knowledge in the delivery of health care. In the future, NCMs must continue to be accountable for the process and outcomes of the services they provide.

Patient Advocacy

Client-focused care and patient advocacy is another aspect of future NCM practice. Establishing therapeutic and helping relationships with clients within complex bureaucracies is an art and science that needs to be explicated clearly. Every client needs assurance that someone cares about him or her as a unique individual with unique needs for information and service. As health care delivery systems become more complex, requirement for assisting clients to obtain needed care through establishment of caring connections and partnerships will increase. Need for financial and medical terms to be translated into understandable lay language will continue, and positioning NCMs organizationally to fulfill an enhanced patient advocacy role in the future will be important.

High-Quality Care and Work Life

Providing quality care is an essential component of future NCM practice, particularly since all stakeholders in health care delivery must continue to work with limited resources in the years to come. Llewellyn (1998) pointed out that case management (CM) and utilization management (UM) are the main processes that have successfully controlled health care spending in recent years and suggests that UM programs must be clearly linked to CM programs. "Both UM and CM professionals strive to eliminate fragmentation in the health care system by removing barriers to timely care and avoiding duplication" (p. 51). Together these professionals share a passion for excellence and a determination to achieve quality, cost-effective care delivery through appropriate utilization of limited resources. Increasingly, UM and CM professionals need to come together and work collaboratively.

Quality of work life for NCMs is an important issue that must be considered now and in the coming years. Mullahy (1998) aptly stated that "case management is not for the faint at heart" (p. 3). According to Mullahy, because the case manager usually is found in the center of the confusion in today's health care delivery system, there is tremendous potential for NCMs to become stressed and overextended as they negotiate a very complex system filled with multiple opposing forces. Although Anderson-Loftin (1999) and Lynn and Kelley (1997), among other researchers, have found that NCMs report job satisfaction, Cook (1998) uncovered inconclusive evidence of such satisfaction associated with inpatient case management models. As the NCM role continues to evolve, managers of case management services would do well to monitor the quality of work life and NCM responses to the work environment so that appropriate management interventions can be planned and implemented as needed.

Action Research

Systematic study of the structures, processes, and outcomes of nursing case management need to be continued for the foreseeable future. However, traditional research methodologies tend to produce knowledge rather slowly in an environment in which expediency and efficiency are needed if findings are to be utilized effectively. Although coordination of targeted programs of research is one useful approach (Lamb, 1995), the time may have arrived to use other approaches, such as action or reflexive research—a divergence from the traditional scientific research paradigm. Action research is a way of generating knowledge by introducing changes and scientifically observing the effects of those changes on a process. Practitioner involvement and immediate local application of findings are attractive characteristics of action research, particularly in the face of the rapid changes that are occurring in the delivery of health care. Other, creative scholarly activities will be needed to expand the knowledge base of case management.

Developing a Knowledge Base and Competency

Finally, the competency and educational preparation of future case managers must be addressed, especially as "basic" and "advanced" levels of case management are being identified (Llewellyn & Moreo, 1998). Raiff (1993) suggested that "a program or practice may be characterized as 'advanced' if it displays innovative behavior on five possible dimensions: client, practitioner, organization, model of service delivery, and/or attention to quality assurance" (p. 14). Llewellyn and Moreo (1998) identified common attributes and skill levels of advanced case managers. Chan et al. (1999) systematically examined job activities and knowledge areas deemed essential for effective case management practice and have identified essential knowledge areas for performance as a case manager. The results from this Delphi study of a panel of experts suggest that the foundational knowledge and practice domains of case management remain constant despite changes in the environment (Chan et al., 1999). They further stated that experts have provided only a general framework for conceptualizing work role behaviors and knowledge requirements of case managers. They also suggested that work roles and knowledge dimensions of case management and differences in emphasis among various professional groups, such as nursing, must be further delineated.

Mundt and Cohen (1999) have identified six emerging competencies for NCMs, relative to the history and traditions of nursing: (a) active engagement with consumers; (b) integration of broader, increasingly global perspectives into health approaches; (c) reframing of leadership to ask unpopular questions; (d) practice that is rooted in ethical principles and values; (e) mastery of information technology and communication; and (f) political savvy, system know-how, and conflict resolution. Nurse educators have the opportunity and obligation to develop programs of study that prepare nurses to function as an integral member of an interdisciplinary team while simultaneously promoting the values and unique function of nursing.

■ Concluding Statement

In summary, modern nursing case management, born of need in a rapidly changing health care delivery system, has become an integral part of the larger case management industry, and is likely to flourish in the years to come. Significant steps have been taken during the past 10 years to enhance the quality of case management services. However, the future of nursing case management clearly depends on defining the specialty practice, building the knowledge base of practice, preparing competent practitioners, establishing effective partnerships and alliances, and remaining flexible and creative in the delivery of quality care.

■ References

American Nurses Association. (1988). *Nursing case management.* Kansas City, MO: Author.

Anderson-Loftin, W. (1999). Nurse case managers in rural hospitals. *Journal of Nursing Administration, 29*(2), 42–49.

Bower, K. A. (1992). *Case management by nurses.* Kansas City, MO: American Nurses Publishing.

Carneal, G. (1998). Getting accredited. *Continuing Care, 17*(10), 18–20, 23–24, 42.

Case Management Society of America. (1995). *Standards of practice for case management.* Little Rock, AR: Author.

Center for Case Management Accountability. (1997). *A framework for case management accountability* [Deliverable number one of five]. Little Rock, AR: Author.

Cesta, T. G., Tahan, H. A., & Fink, L. F. (1998). *The case manager's survival guide: Winning strategies for clinical practice.* St. Louis: Mosby.

Chan, F., Leahy, F. J., McMahon, B. T., Mirch, M., & DeVinney, D. (1999). Foundational knowledge and major practice domains of case management. *The Journal of Care Management, 5,* 10, 13–14, 17–18, 26–28, 30.

Cook, T. H. (1998). The effectiveness of inpatient case management. *Journal of Nursing Administration, 28*(4), 36–46.

D'Andrea, G., & Hamill, C. T. (1999). Case management organization accreditation under way. *The Case Manager, 10*(1), 53–61.

Flarey, D. L., & Blancett, S. S. (1996). *Handbook of nursing case management.* Gaithersburg, MD: Aspen.

Gerson, V. (1998). Case management accreditation: Setting the standards. *The Case Manager, 9*(5), 79–82.

Lamb, G. (1995). Case management. In J. J. Fitzpatrick & J. S. Stevenson (Eds.), *Annual review of nursing research, 13* (pp. 117–136). New York: Springer.

Levin, L. M. (1999). Countdown to certification. *The Case Manager, 10*(2), 65–68.

Llewellyn, A. (1998). The utilization and case management connection. *The Case Manager, 9*(6), 49–52.

Llewellyn, A., & Moreo, K. (1998). Transitioning from basic to advanced case management. *Nursing Case Management, 3,* 63–65.

Lynn, M. R., & Kelley, B. (1997). Effects of case management on the nursing contest— Perceived quality of care, work satisfaction, and control over practice. *IMAGE: Journal of Nursing Scholarship, 29,* 237–241.

Mullahy, C. M. (1998). *The case manager's handbook* (2nd ed.). Gaithersburg, MD: Aspen.

Mundt, M. H., & Cohen, E. L. (1999). Emerging competencies for nurse case managers. In E. L. Cohen & V. DeBack (Eds.), *The outcomes mandate: Case management in health care today* (pp. 86–91). St. Louis: Mosby.

Raiff, N. R. (with Shore, B. K.). (1993). *Advanced case management: New strategies for the nineties.* Newbury Park, CA: Sage.

Rossi, P. (1999). *Case management in healthcare: A practical guide.* Philadelphia: W. B. Saunders.

Scrambling for CM certification? Here's what to know about 6 choices. (1997). *Case Management Advisor, 8*(1), 1–5.

Smith, M. C. (1993). Case management and nursing theory-based practice. *Nursing Science Quarterly, 6*(1), 8–9.

Steinhauser, E. K. (1999). Gaining momentum for the next century. *Continuing Care, 18*(1), 18–20, 22–23, 29.

Strickland, T., & Mullahy, C. (1997). Forecasting the future of case management. *The Case Manager, 8*(6), 69–76.

Whitaker, C. (1999). Commission/URAC's new case management program standards. *The Case Manager, 10*(2), 28–29.

■ Editor's Questions for Discussion

Discuss the history of case management in nursing. What factors contributed to the term becoming less known and used in public health nursing? What factors contribute to developing nursing case management in acute case and other settings? Is case management a management and leadership function or clinical specialty in nursing or both? Provide reasons and examples in your answers.

What content is essential for case management programs in nursing? What is the difference between basic case management practice in nursing and advanced case management practice? How does case management pertain to integrated delivery systems?

To what extent do case managers serve as links between payors and the providers? What ethical issues come into play? How can case managers balance focus on patient's individual needs with the environment and the total care providing system? What is the difference between case management and utilization management? Specifically, what does a case manager do in practice? What role must nursing case managers fulfill in interdisciplinary terms? How can nurse educators best prepare case managers for that role?

58

Managed Care Health Organizations

Implications for Nursing

Margaret M. Conger, EdD, RN, CM

Delivery of health care in the United States has undergone a paradigm shift from fee-for-service to a capitated managed care system during the past 20 years. With this shift has come increased emphasis on delivery of quality care that is cost-effective. These changes are credited with significantly reducing the rate of health care cost increases; but at the same time, they have engendered anger among consumers who perceive that their choices in care options have eroded. In response to this anger, managed care organizations are again altering strategies used for the delivery of health care. It is within this ever-changing system that nurses are seeking to envision their future and gain a clear understanding of managed care organizations.

Managed care is a term used to describe both organizational structures that provide for health needs of an enrolled population and various techniques used by health care organizations to control the costs of providing health care. Managed care organizations use many different forms of organizational structure. Perhaps the best known is the health maintenance organization (HMO), which has a variety of permutations. Differences among HMOs are usually based on the type of relationship between physicians and other health care services such as laboratories, outpatient facilities, and acute care hospitals. In this chapter these issues are explored.

■ Health Maintenance Organization (HMO) Revenue

Capitation is the payment method used by an HMO. In a capitated payment system, an employee or an employer pays a set monthly fee that covers most health care services. Based on the plan contract, the enrolled member may be charged a copayment for services such as an office visit or a prescription. However, these copayments tend to be less than charges in the typical fee-for-service contract. The HMO member's prepayment for services without regard to type or number of services rendered, with the HMO assuming full risk for care, gives the member a great deal of financial security. If the cost of the member's care exceeds the total of fees paid, the HMO must absorb the difference. If the cost of the member's care is less than the total of fees paid, the HMO keeps the difference. This type of arrangement provides an incentive for the HMO to focus on preventive care so that enrolled members remain healthy.

The capitated payment system is a radical departure from the more familiar fee-for-service system that has been the primary health care payment structure since the 1940s. In the fee-for-service arrangement, payment is made by either the patient or the insurer for each visit or service provided. In such a system, an increase in services provides increased revenue, thus promoting overuse of services. With health care services largely paid by third parties, such as the government or insurance companies, the consumer has no reason to limit the amount of service sought. However, the third-party payor is very interested in setting limits because each increase in health service represents a loss. Thus, payors and providers are driven by opposing motivations (Bodenheimer & Grumbach, 1995).

In a capitated system, providing services in areas with a concentration of people is an economic advantage. This advantage has led to heavy penetration by managed care organizations in urban areas. To maintain a fully integrated system in which the organization is able to provide the majority of needed services requires a population of 450,000 enrolled members. Just to establish a semi-independent HMO, using some shared services, requires an enrolled population of 180,000. Such numbers are not available in rural areas. Even an HMO that provides only primary care services requires a population of 10,000 members. Thus growth of HMOs in rural areas has been slow (Christianson, 1998). Counties adjacent to metropolitan areas tend to have a higher penetration of HMO services than do more rural counties.

HMOs also differ in terms of the source of primary funding. Many older HMOs are not for profit; that is they do not sell shares of stock or respond to the needs of shareholders. As such, they pay no taxes but must turn profits back into service to consumers. During the 1980s, the for-profit health care organization began to dominate the scene. This type of organization is responsible for returning part of its profit to its shareholders. Further, a for-profit organization is required to pay taxes and has little obligation to provide services to meet community needs. As of 1996, it was estimated that more than 50 million Americans belong to some type of managed care health plan (Bodenheimer, 1996). A large proportion of these plans—62%—were investor owned (Kuttner, 1999). However, the days of high profits from investor owned companies appear to be on the wane. Perhaps this trend is a response to public outcry from perceived imbalances between delivery of service to enrolled members and profits earned by shareholders (Kuttner, 1999). The health care system may again be entering a new era.

■ *Relationship of a Provider to an HMO*

HMOs also differ in terms of the relationship of a provider, usually a physician, with the HMO. Some older HMOs directly employ the provider. Others contract with physicians to supply health care to enrolled members at discounted prices.

Staff Model HMO

In the staff model, physicians and other health care providers are employed directly by the HMO and see only patients who are enrolled members. This arrangement often is referred to as a "closed panel" model and provides for close control over utilization of services because of the tight arrangement between the physicians and the HMO. If the HMO does not have a specific service within its organizational structure that a member requires, referral is made to an outside physician with the HMO picking up the cost. Utilization review practices are effective because physicians, as employees of the organization, are closely regulated. Incentives such as bonuses for meeting performance and productivity standards often are provided to increase buy-in among the physicians in exchange for their submitting to tight control (Wagner, 1997).

One problem with this model is that, if the physician panel is limited, the HMO may have difficulty attracting potential members. Consumers who have a prior relationship with a physician who is not a member of the HMO would not be inclined to choose it. Of course, freedom of selection is only possible if it is the individual who is choosing the HMO. When the HMO is selected by an employer as the only option, such individual preferences do not matter. The staff model also can have problems in maintaining cost-effectiveness if the array of specialty practice is too limited. Use of extensive referrals outside the HMO reduces its ability to control costs.

Group Model

A less restrictive type of physician arrangement with an HMO is the group model. In the group arrangement, the HMO contracts with groups of doctors who provide care on a capitation basis for enrolled plan members. The physicians remain employed by their group practice rather than by the HMO. In the closed model type of organizational structure, physicians can see only members of the HMO. However, some contracts also allow physicians to see private patients.

In the group model, the HMO is able to control costs quite effectively because of its close control over the physicians. Another advantage of this model is that the HMO does not have to provide capital for salaries and to set up physician's offices. These outlays are the responsibility of the physician group. A disadvantage of this type of HMO is similar to the staff model if provider choice is too limited.

Network Model

The network model is similar to the group HMO. In the network arrangement, the HMO contracts with physicians to provide medical services for HMO members. A multi-specialty group of physicians is sought, particularly because of the broad health care coverage it provides. Cost control is maintained by the HMO by providing to the physician group a set amount of money per HMO member. If referrals need to be made to physicians outside the contracted group, the physician group must pick up the cost.

Independent Practice Association

The least restrictive arrangement between physicians and HMOs is the Independent Practice Association (IPA), in which individual physicians contract with an HMO to provide services to enrolled members. Each physician practices in an independent office, either singly or in a small group, and has the freedom to see both HMO patients and fee-for-service patients. The HMO pays the physician either by means of a discounted fee-for-service arrangement or a capitated plan that is based on number of members for which the physician is responsible.

The IPA format is attractive to potential HMO members due to the breadth of possible physician choices. However, looseness of the connection between the HMO and the individual physician makes it difficult for the HMO to maintain control over cost and utilization of services. The IPA type of HMO was thought originally to be a stepping stone toward development of a fully integrated system. In contrast to other HMO types, the IPA format is used in rural areas in which the population is not sufficient to support a full-service HMO. Overall, the IPA format was the fastest growing type of HMO arrangement in the late 1990s; this development is thought to be due to backlash against the tight restrictions of other HMO practices (Bodenheimer, 1999b).

■ Alternative Types of Managed Care Arrangements

In addition to HMOs that use capitation, other more traditional health insurance plans also use cost containment strategies that have been developed in HMO practices. One example is the preferred provider organization (PPO), the most common form of a fee-for-service organization available today.

Preferred Provider Organization

In a PPO, the insurance company contracts, at a discounted rate, with health care providers—both physicians and other health services, such as laboratory, physical therapy, occupational services, and hospitals. This arrangement provides more choices to enrolled members than do typical HMO organizations but results in less coordination of care and thus less control over costs. This type of structure currently is gaining in popularity with consumers because of wide range of provider choices available (Bodenheimer, 1999b). Providers accept discounted contracts, based on the belief that increased patient loads will result from the access to them provided to enrolled members. The PPO also benefits by being able to provide health care services at less than the going rate for the community.

Enrolled members in the PPO receive discounted prices as long as they use providers approved by the agency. If an enrolled member goes outside the approved provider list, a higher copayment is required. This higher copayment is used by organizations with "point-of-service" plans, which are becoming popular and are growing rapidly (Bodenheimer, 1999b). Because of the loose arrangement between the PPO and the physician group, intensive utilization of management practices are needed to control costs. Both preauthorization for services and management of acute care hospital stays and outpatient services are used.

Physician–Hospital Organization

The physician–hospital organization (PHO) is an alliance of physicians and hospitals that contracts with either a managed care organization or large employer group, using a capitation payment system. Physician membership in the organization can be either open or closed. In an open situation, virtually all physician members of the hospital's medical staff may join. In a closed arrangement, physician membership is limited by either specialty practice or a proven record of cost and quality effectiveness.

The advantage of a PHO is an increased strength of position when negotiating with managed care organizations and thus being able to obtain a more lucrative contract than physicians could achieve independently. This advantage, of course, could backfire if the managed care organization can get contracts with other groups at better rates. Both employers and large employee unions have used this type of arrangement in an effort to control administrative costs charged by HMOs. PHOs also have been developed in rural areas where the potential population for membership in a managed care organization is limited (Wagner, 1997). The success of PHOs though may be limited due to their inexperience with managed care strategies that are necessary for survival in today's health care market.

Physician Network

A physician network is an arrangement whereby a group of doctors accept financial risk for covering enrolled persons without going through an intermediary such as an insurance company. This arrangement avoids the cost of paying the insurance company and provides for greater autonomy for physicians. Movement into such groups has escalated, as backlash against some of the tight fiscal controls of HMOs has increased and physicians attempt to regain control over medical decision-making.

■ Demand for Quality Health Care

As part of the backlash against managed health care organizations, the American public has been vocal in demanding new standards for measuring the quality of health care received. This demand has been addressed both through new legislation and development of agencies designed to measure quality of care. The legislative process has been used to increase consumer access to emergency and specialty care. Issues such as providing for 48-hour postpartum care, use of emergency services for situations that a "prudent person" would deem necessary, and continued ability to maintain physician–patient relationships even when an HMO drops a physician from its panel have all been resolved through legislation (Bodenheimer, 1996).

The number of agencies that scrutinize health care delivery by HMOs also is on the rise. Both procedural practices and client outcomes are under review. One organization actively involved in such review is the National Committee for Quality Assurance (NCQA). It provides accreditation services for HMOs and has developed performance measures—the Health Plan Employer Data and Information Set (HEDIS). Included are more than 50 performance standards related to outcomes such as patient satisfaction rates, access to care, and immunization and health screening rates (Bodenheimer, 1999b). Data collected by this group have been provided mainly to employers who seek information regarding selection of an HMO plan for their employees. Some HMOs with high scores have publicized their scores for the general public. To be expected, HMOs with low scores have not so freely published such information.

The Health Care Financing Administration (HCFA)—the coordinator of Medicare and Medicaid programs—also has developed standards to measure quality of care. The HCFA data on both hospital and provider care are expected to be released to the public for review. Another organization involved in developing quality standards is the Foundation for Accountability (FACCT). It disseminates standards for other organizations to use in assessing quality health care (Bodenheimer,

1999a). As significant quality indicators are developed and as businesses that provide health insurance for employees use these data, improved quality of care is anticipated. The unknown, of course, is the financial cost to achieve improved quality of care.

Tarlov et al. (1989) suggested a number of outcomes measures that should be developed and used in a quality management program. Physiological and clinical parameters that demonstrate control of a chronic illness need to be identified. Functional status that a client should achieve at the specified end point of care should be determined. Other factors to measure include the person's perception of health, energy level, pain level, and life satisfaction. Finally, customer satisfaction, including satisfaction with access and convenience of care and adequacy of financial coverage provided by the health plan, need to be measured.

Measures of Quality of Nursing Care

Traditional quality indicators of mortality, morbidity, and length of stay (LOS) have questionable relevance to nursing care. Mortality is more closely related to the patient's age, severity of illness, and extent of comorbidities than to specific nursing interventions (Newell, 1996). Some aspects of morbidity, such as hospital-acquired infections, do have a direct relationship to nursing care. However, the complexity of conditions that lead to increased morbidity reduce its use as a measure of the quality of nursing care. Likewise, LOS is often an event over which nursing has little control. Thus new indicators are needed.

Nurse-Sensitive Indicators

Various nurse-sensitive indicators (see Table 58.1) have been proposed. Some are related to the traditional indicators of mortality and morbidity; others focus on new areas. Prevention of infection has historically been the province of nursing (Bonadonna & Johnson, 1992). Practices related to use of universal precautions, intravenous and urinary catheter management, and dressings techniques are controlled directly by nurses. Thus these indicators are appropriate for evaluation of nursing care. Other nurse-sensitive indicators include risk-management perspectives such as rates of patient falls, development of pressure ulcers, and medication errors.

Patient quality of life is another area for consideration. Papenhausen (1996) suggests direct relationship between a person's ability to manage symptoms of illness and nursing care received. Nurses also have an impact on the ability of a person to carry out self-care such as grooming, dressing, bathing, and ambulation, as well as household activities. As the nurse works with patients and their families to find ways of managing each of these tasks, quality of life is enhanced.

Other nurse-sensitive quality issues are concerned with the patient's psychosocial status. One measure is the person's stress level at a specified point in care (Brooten & Naylor, 1995). Another is the person's social satisfaction, that is, the ability to participate in social activities with family and friends. Nurses help patients work through these issues and find strategies that enhance their quality of life. Finally, measurement of caregiver burden can be used to evaluate the quality of nursing care (Girouard, 1996). Nurses are often involved in helping families manage the demands of caring for a chronically or terminally ill family member or providing assistance to sort through caregiver options (Gold, Reis, Markiewicz, & Andres, 1995).

■ Nursing's Role in Achieving Managed Care Organization Objectives

New opportunities for nursing are emerging in this new era of managed care. Many strategies

---

TABLE 58.1 Nurse-Sensitive Quality Indicators

Morbidity	Grooming
Practices related to use of universal precautions	Dressing
Intravenous site infections	Bathing
Urinary catheter infections	Ambulation
Surgical dressing sites	Household activities
Risk management	**Patient psychosocial status**
Patient falls	Stress level
Development of pressure ulcers	Social satisfaction
Medication errors	
	Caregiver burden
Patient quality of life	
Symptom management	
Ability to perform self-care activities	

---

required for achieving the cost reduction and quality enhancement goals of managed care are based on skills and roles that have long been part of nursing practice. Some of these nursing roles need to be reemphasized; others need to be developed further. Nursing is well positioned to have a positive impact on health delivery systems involving managed care organizations.

Delegation to Unlicensed Assistive Personnel

Nursing care in acute care hospitals has undergone significant changes under the constraints of managed care. A large number of unlicensed caregivers have been introduced into the workforce, leading to new responsibilities for the RN. Nurses must learn to delegate nursing tasks to less skilled workers, using both legally sound and safe decision-making. Staff educators must develop programs to teach delegation strategies that maintain and promote quality care.

Introduction of unlicensed caregivers into the health care system has occurred with little or no research to measure outcomes of this practice. It is imperative that nurses participate in research to measure such outcomes. Is this practice really a cost-saving mechanism? Or does it lead to increased lengths of stay or other costly and inefficient outcomes? Until research documents current outcomes from this practice, it should not continue. The need for nurse researchers to become involved in this arena is imperative.

Health Promotion and Disease Prevention

Emphasis in managed care organizations must shift to primary concern for services designed to help enrolled members remain healthy from illness management common in the traditional fee-for-service structure. A capitated health care organization needs to keep its members healthy. Often a ratio of 80 well members to 20 ill members is considered to be a cost-effective balance. Strategies to promote health among enrolled members include focusing on health education and screening programs to detect disease in its early stage. Many chronic diseases such as hypertension, respiratory disease, heart disease, and diabetes can be managed at low cost, if identified early. Disease prevention measures such as programs to increase immunization rates among children and reduction of risk behaviors such as smoking are an important part of the managed care organization strategy. These are activities in which nurses have long been active

Community-Based Care

Another cost-saving strategy used by managed care organizations is to provide care in low-cost community settings rather than in acute care hospitals. This policy has resulted in increased use of outpatient services such as day surgeries, laboratory testing, and diagnostic services (Venegoni, 1996). It also has led to increased use of subacute care settings such as rehabilitative centers and nursing homes. This movement into the community has led to enormous growth of the home health industry, which is reported to be the fastest growing segment of health care (Olsten Health, 1997). With the transition of health care into community settings, nurses increasingly are finding employment outside acute care hospitals, and this trend is expected to continue. Nursing education must be responsive to this shift and develop educational programs to prepare future nurses for these new roles.

Coordination of Care

Another strategy needed to meet cost goals of a managed care organization is coordination of services for enrolled members. Avoiding overuse of testing, treatments, and specialty care is important. One way to do so is to require prior approval for all medical procedures. The health care organization also will control when a member is allowed to use hospital, home health care agency, or other outpatient services. The goal is always to provide needed service at the most appropriate level of care. To help persons find their way through the maze of a managed care organization, the role of nurse case manager (NCM) has emerged. The NCM integrates in-depth clinical knowledge, familiarity with community resources, and financial strategies to coordinate patient care (Wunderlich, Sloan, & Davis, 1997). Outcomes of such coordination are improvements in both the financial picture for the organization and the quality of care received by the patient. To be successful in managing the complexities of this role, NCMs need advanced education similar to that provided for advanced practice nurses (Harrington & Estes, 1997).

Leader of Teams to Develop Outcome Measures

Quality and cost-effective care goals can be achieved only when all health care providers have clear outcome goals. As a result, a number of structured care methodologies, such as treatment algorithms and clinical pathways, have been developed. Advanced practice nurses working in multidisciplinary teams have been in the forefront of developing such clinical management tools. As the need for such tools increases, employment opportunities for nurses in this area also increase. Skills gained in graduate nursing education (e.g., negotiation, team building strategies, and clinical knowledge) are important to the success of this role.

Primary Provider Roles

The advanced practice role of nurse practitioner (NP) has been demonstrated to be a cost-effective provider of care in community settings and, more recently, in the acute care hospital. Many NPs function in a "gatekeeper" role, controlling access to utilization of health services. All requests for treatment are funneled through this person. The gatekeeper also is responsible for coordinating care so that duplication of services is avoided.

Acceptance of the NP as a primary care provider in an HMO has been mixed. Some make extensive use of NPs; others have restricted the practice of NPs by refusing to place them on provider panels. Securing a role for NPs in the managed care environment is a goal toward which nurses must strive actively. One way of doing so is to support adoption of "any willing provider" legislation that requires managed care organizations to open provider panels to NPs (Sochalski, Jenkins, & Auth, 1999).

Advocate Access to Care for Everyone

Another political action area for nurses is to advocate universal access to health care. An undesirable outcome of managed care is the increase in the number of individuals and families without health care coverage. Kuttner (1999) stated that Americans without health insurance has risen from 14.2% in 1995 to 16.1% in 1997. This percentage translates into 43.4 million people without health insurance. In addition, a significant number of those with health insurance are underinsured, thus requiring large payments for services not covered

under their policies. The most significant group of underinsured are the elderly, with Medicare coverage and Medigap plans that do not cover out-of-hospital pharmaceutical costs. An estimated 19 million elderly persons have no coverage for prescription drugs (Kuttner, 1999).

One approach to providing better health coverage is through development of community health centers. A number of nurse managed health care centers have demonstrated cost-effective outcomes in providing care to people who either do not qualify for publicly funded health programs or have health insurance through an employer.

■ Concluding Statement

The health care delivery system is changing radically and rapidly. Nurses need to view changes that managed care is bringing with excitement for new opportunities, rather than with alarm. Nurses can have a great impact on providing care to the entire population. Until the goal of accessible care for all is met, maintaining a health care system that is cost-effective cannot be achieved. Nurses have a stake in this future.

■ References

Bodenheimer, T. (1996). The HMO backlash—Righteous or reactionary? *New England Journal of Medicine, 335*(21), 1601–1604.

Bodenheimer, T. (1999a). The movement for improved quality in health care. *New England Journal of Medicine, 340*(6), 488–492.

Bodenheimer, T. (1999b). The American health care system: Physicians and the changing medical marketplace. *New England Journal of Medicine, 340*(7), 584–588.

Bodenheimer, T. S., & Grumbach, K. (1995). *Understanding health policy: A clinical approach.* Norwalk, CT: Appleton & Lange.

Bonadonna, I. A., & Johnson, J. U. (1992). Integrating infection control into a nursing quality program. *Journal of Nursing Care Quality, 6*(4), 75–80.

Brooten, D., & Naylor, M. D. (1995). Nurses' effect on changing patient outcomes. *IMAGE: Journal of Nursing Scholarship, 27*(2), 95–99.

Christianson, J. (1998). The growing presence of managed care in rural areas. *Journal of Rural Health, 14*(3), 166–168.

Girouard, S. A. (1996). Evaluating advanced nursing practice. In A. B. Hamric, J. A. Spross, & C. M. Hanson (Eds.), *Advanced nursing practice: An integrative approach* (pp. 567–600). Philadelphia: W. B. Saunders.

Gold, D. P., Reis, M. F., Markiewicz, D., & Andres, D. (1995). When home caregiving ends: A longitudinal study of outcomes for caregivers of relatives with dementia. *Journal of American Geriatrics Society, 43*(1), 10–16.

Harrington, C., & Estes, C. L. (1997). *Health policy and nursing.* Boston: Jones & Bartlett.

Kuttner, R. (1999). The American health care system: Wall Street and health care. *New England Journal of Medicine, 340*(8), 664–668.

Newell, M. (1996). *Using nursing case management to improve health outcomes.* Gaithersburg, MD: Aspen.

Olsten Health. (1997). *21st century home care—Back to the future.* [On-line]. Available: http://www.olstenhealth.com/indepth/homecare.htm.

Papenhausen, J. L. (1996). Discovering and achieving client outcomes. In E. L. Cohen (Ed.), *Nurse case management in the 21st century* (pp. 257–268). St. Louis: Mosby.

Sochalski, J., Jenkins, M., & Auth, R. L. (1999). Dynamics of public policy: Community-based practice meets managed care. In D. J. Mason & J. L. Leavitt, *Policy and politics in nursing and health care* (pp. 160–172). Philadelphia: W. B. Saunders.

Tarlov, A., Ware, J. E., Greenfield, S., Nelson, E. C., Perrin, E., & Zubkoff, M. (1989). The medical outcomes study: An application of methods for monitoring the results of medical care. *Journal of the American Medical Association, 262,* 925–930.

Venegoni. S. L. (1996). Changing environment of healthcare. In J. V. Hickey (Ed.), *Advanced practice nursing: Changing roles and clinical application* (pp. 77–90). Philadelphia: Lippincott.

Wagner, E. R. (1997). Types of managed care organizations. In P. R. Kongstved (Ed.), *Essentials of managed health care* (2nd ed., pp. 36–48). Gaithersburg, MD: Aspen.

Wunderlich, G. S., Sloan, F. A., & Davis, C. K. (1997). Nursing staff in hospitals and nursing homes: Is it adequate? In C. Harrington & C. L. Estes (Eds.), *Health policy and nursing* (pp. 142–156). Boston: Jones & Bartlett.

■ Editor's Questions for Discussion

HMOs are designed to focus on preventive care as a financial incentive, but do they? What evidence is available? What staff models of HMO structures are available in the United States? What examples of HMO group models exist? Does it make a difference for nursing practice as to the type of HMO model that is available for providing care? Discuss.

Discuss the advantages and disadvantages of HMOs versus alternative types of managed care arrangements. What implications do the various types of care arrangements have for nursing practice? What role does nursing currently have versus what role it should have in developing standards for measuring quality of health care provided under managed care arrangements?

What nursing indicators for high-quality care should be implemented in managed care in addition to those proposed by Conger? Why has nursing not systematically documented outcomes related to employment of unlicensed caregivers? What forces are necessary for nursing administration and the profession to become proactive regarding high-quality care and new types of personnel in care settings? What high-quality research evidence is available regarding utilization of unlicensed assistive personnel?

What implications are evident regarding coordination of care, as addressed by Conger for the role of nurse case managers (NCMs) and portrayed by Gerber (Chapter 57)? How does Gray's discussion (Chapter 42) about advanced practice apply to Conger's views of primary provider roles?

59

Incorporating Interventions for Social and Environmental Risk Factors into Nursing Services

Jacqueline A. Dienemann, PhD, RN, CNAA, FAAN
Jacquelyn C. Campbell, PhD, RN, FAAN
Jacqueline Agnew, PhD, RN, FAAN

Conflict always has existed in the United States between the organization of health care on an entrepreneurial basis and recognition that many citizens cannot afford the cost of good health. Resolution of this conflict is needed.

■ Historical Separation of Health, Social, and Environmental Services

Historically this conflict has been resolved by development of private clinics for charity care and provision of government health services to protect the public's health. Traditionally, government-sponsored public health departments also have included maternal and child health

services, as society's values did not justify withholding prenatal care that would compromise the health of newborns. The purpose of these programs was to improve the physical health of the "deserving poor" or those perceived as being innocent, particularly young women and children. Access to these services was subject to federal, state, and local budget vagaries, and frequently benefits were cut back in times of economic difficulty.

These services, as well as traditional primary and acute care, have used an individual patient presenting–problem approach that views social and environmental factors as "external factors" not directly addressed by nursing or medical services. Public health nursing included prenatal and well-child clinics with both this focus and prevention and surveillance activities. Ambulatory care nursing also utilized this approach.

This artificial separation of health and social problems from services stemmed from the American values of rugged individualism and independence from government. One consequence is that, although it is well established that social factors such as poverty, are responsible for the largest proportion of variance in health status, the U.S. health care system historically has addressed only physical health problems (Callahan, 1998). Public health reports identify the impact of social, environmental, and psychological conditions or processes on health status, but health care does not directly address these underlying causes of ill health.

Separate branches of government at the federal, state, and local levels address problems in the environment, issues of violence, social welfare, and health—even though they all have a direct impact on health status. For instance, despite significant health problems incurred by the public as the result of the "social" issue of violence, not until 1985 was violence officially declared a public health problem and 1990 when violence was included in the *Healthy People 2000* official health objectives (U.S. Department of Health and Human Services [DHHS], 1986, 1990). The health care system did not address child abuse—the group for whom the society feels most responsible—until 1962, even though child abuse had been addressed by official "social welfare" departments of the government since 1910 (Gordon, 1988). Interestingly, the official health care system first became interested in domestic violence when it was established that women were abused during pregnancy and therefore the health of children could be affected.

Not only are social and health services separate, but mental and physical health care services are also separate. Insurance reimbursement is defined separately for mental and physical health. The entrepreneurial and government health care systems carefully have avoided reimbursement for "social services" and provide much lower rates of reimbursement for mental health care. This history demonstrates that Americans, as a society, are willing to pay for the diagnosis and treatment of physical symptoms and conditions for its citizens but are generally unwilling for health services to address the underlying causes.

Health Care for the Public

Traditional American values of individualism and personal responsibility have been the cornerstone of health care for the public, with a concentration on providing individuals with information and skills (Callahan, 1998). Individuals are held responsible for their own health promotion and for obtaining professional health care services as needed. Even so, nurses have long pointed out the need to take into account environmental and social contexts within which individuals and families are more or less facilitated in health promotion (Butterfield, 1990; Milio, 1983). The health system, in which they work, has not been responsive.

The historical tradition of public health nursing is an advocacy model that includes environmental and social factors as part of the nurse's scope of practice (Reverby, 1987). However, government-supported public health nursing practice included ambulatory care in clinics, family-based home visits for health assessment and teaching, school nursing, and surveillance of communicable diseases. Advocacy for families was done informally through liaison with other departments such as environmental health or social services. In recent years, the service delivery function of local health departments has been curtailed severely, and public health nursing is an endangered species.

Although the most fundamental inequalities in health care relate to socioeconomic status, factors such as race and gender also limit access to and the effectiveness of health care (Bunting, 1996; Funkhouser & Moser, 1990). Even though the most egregious racial and gender disparities have been corrected through changes and challenges in the legal system, subtle stigmas and structural inequalities remain that restrict both access and treatment. For instance, long waiting time in clinics attended by people of color reflects a lower valuing of their time and creates a barrier to full utilization. Women also experience subtle barriers to access; their gender is a liability in seeking low-cost health insurance due to their having more longevity and higher utilization of health care than men. This problem occurs despite the fact that the purpose of health care is greater longevity and some of women's longevity may be due to higher appropriate utilization of health care. The impact of power relationships within communities to define rules for access to care and the degree to which it is paternalistic is an important social risk factor to the health of low power individuals (Jones & Meleis, 1993; Shields & Lindsey, 1998).

Managed Care and Integrated Care

During the last decade, health care delivery has been redesigned to use a gatekeeper system that limits choice for most Americans having health insurance. This system, referred to as managed care, is intended to lower costs through (a) reducing inappropriate use of services, (b) providing services by the lowest cost qualified provider, and (c) capping physician and hospital fees through contracting and risk sharing. Managed care has been successful in reducing the rate of increase in costs, sometimes at the expense of the degree of coverage for individuals (Wassel, 1995). Although one objective of its cost-containment strategy is better integration of programs and services, managed care's actual effect sometimes has been to fragment control and impede exchange of information.

Another outcome has been the privatizing of charity care, in the hope of achieving the same savings. In many cities this move has meant (a) closing or selling the city hospital, (b) closing city or county health clinics, and (c) requiring those receiving medical aid (Medicaid) health insurance to join a managed care company that has contracted with the government to deliver health services. After receiving contracts and working with these populations, many companies discover that the contracts are not profitable and then decline to bid for renewal. Recent reports about many Medicare patients losing coverage reflects this trend.

Despite extensive writings predicting that managed care would lead to integration of care, increased emphasis on entrepreneurial care has not resulted in an increase in integrated care. Managed care does control a client's choice through limiting reimbursement to services of a panel of physicians, contracted hospitals, pharmacies, and medical device vendors. Managed care does not bring acute and primary care together within *one* system, with *one* set of health care professionals providing care using *one* set of practice standards. So, payment is integrated and standardized through contracts, but services are still fragmented and separated by each health care professional.

Nursing Services and Integrated Care

Nursing services are organized to fit into this loosely connected, integrated care system as adjuncts to each type of facility that delivers services. Nurses continue to work as employees of hospitals, physician's offices, clinics, home health agencies, and public health departments. Although recent trends have been that hospitals vertically integrate and be renamed as health care systems (because they own home care agencies, nursing homes, and other related facilities), increase in integration of nursing care does not result. Each facility is operated with separate patient records, staff, and billing systems. Health care remains divided among distinct entities, each responsible for an episode of care to an individual patient.

Additionally, reengineering within hospitals has introduced more allied personnel and increased complexity of health care. Clinical pathways do standardize care for specific episodes, but do not provide accountability by one nurse or one physician. Patients remain in hospitals for less time and are more acutely ill when there, thus reducing opportunities for nurses and other providers to become aware of social and environmental factors affecting their health. This situation has reduced, not increased, integration of care for individuals.

Nurses are taught that the nursing process is the foundation of nursing practice. For each patient nurses should assess, diagnose, intervene, and evaluate. Recently, changes in health care have encouraged addition of consideration for cost and desired patient outcomes to nursing practice. Nurses are aware of the importance of viewing the patient holistically—a person with a culture, lifestyle, health history, and other personal factors. However, this view still focuses primarily on the individual patient within an episode of care.

Many factors are converging to make this approach obsolete. People are living longer and, as they age, are more likely to have several chronic conditions that require lifestyle adaptations and continuous symptom management. New technology also allows people with disabilities not only to live longer but to be able to marry, work, travel, and otherwise be active members of society with certain technological assistance. Medical scientists are discovering new information about the interaction of genetic characteristics and the environment, which people can influence through informed decision-making. Health care professionals are recognizing the importance of social norms and mores in the health of entire populations. Nursing needs to move from focusing on a patient and that patient's primary diagnosis during an episode of care to the underlying factors affecting that patient's health over time.

Nursing is moving toward integrating care for individuals, as shown by development of case management for a population of patients as a nursing role within acute care. This process is carried out through standardizing care, using practice standards, clinical guidelines, and clinical pathways. A newer development is continuum clinical pathways for patients with chronic conditions, which follow them beyond a specific episode of care. Another development is case managers for specific complex individual cases employed by both the insurance company and hospital. Yet, case managers for occupational illness or injury or mental health frequently are social workers or technicians with no education in pathophysiology or the linking of physical, social, and mental health (Parker-Conrad, 1997). None of these approaches necessarily provide inclusion of context of health for the individual or integration of care across time, place, and medical condition.

Nursing and the Environment

Health care still remains separate from social welfare, the environment, the workplace, and other social institutions outside traditional health care. For example, the State of Maryland has separate departments of Health and Mental Hygiene, Human Services (social welfare), and the Environment. This fragmentation leads to ineffective interventions when someone is harmed by an environmental exposure.

For example, lead is one of the oldest recognized environmental toxins, but its identification as a cause of illness may take an unreasonably long time. In part, that may be because signs and symptoms of lead poisoning are insidious—ranging from altered behavior to disturbed gastrointestinal function. However, other reasons include failure to ask about environmental sources of toxic exposure during health assessment, isolation of episodes of care, reliance on office visits for patient care, and lack of follow-up of household members when environmental toxic exposure is diagnosed. A school nurse who observes a child's vague complaints and mood changes may not be aware of the child's weekend visit to an emergency department with gastrointestinal symptoms. Furthermore, the nurse probably has never seen the child's home environment and the potential it presents for lead dust exposure from lead paint in substandard housing, lead-contaminated soil in the yard, or the dusty work clothes of a family member who works in a battery plant. Even if elevated blood lead levels are detected in the child, the provider may or may not initiate health surveillance for others who share the home environment. This lack of integrated care and inclusion of environmental risk factors in health assessment neglects opportunities for primary or secondary prevention.

Health education in the United States typically has omitted emphasis on, or even mention of, environmental risk factors associated with where people work, play, and learn. Nurses have acknowledged this deficiency only recently (Pope, Snyder, & Mood, 1995). This gap can lead nurses to overlook risk factors that pose immediate danger. It also may be a barrier to nurse participation in multidisciplinary efforts aimed at prevention. For example, coordinated programs to alert employers and workers to the need to protect family members from work-generated home contamination are still needed (Whelan et al., 1997). Nurses need to join collaborative efforts with other health professionals, families, landlords, environmental engineers, and other public health officials, to identify children at high risk for lead poisoning and to increase lead abatement efforts.

Awareness that disadvantaged populations bear a disproportionate burden of environmental health risks in their communities and workplaces is increasing. Evidence that class and race are linked with degree of toxic exposures has, during the past decade, prompted the emergence of "environmental justice" or "environmental equity" as a national priority, and public health officials are struggling to address this public health issue (Sexton, Olden, & Johnson, 1993). Populations affected often are those without political clout to oppose location of potential sources of toxicity near their homes and work sites. Solutions will require convergence and coordination of efforts by professionals in health policy, environmental safety, social welfare, and health care. Until solutions can be achieved, nurses must be alert to assessing patients for the potential risks associated with residing near sources of toxicity, such as polluted rivers where they may swim or catch and eat contaminated fish.

Nursing and Social Causes of Ill Health

When presented with a patient, nurses and physicians focus on the individual's physiological function when assessing injuries and symptoms. Such focus may lead to misdiagnosis of the root cause of a health problem and ineffective intervention. For instance, a woman who is pregnant and has small children at home may come for a primary care appointment complaining of fatigue and feeling low. The nurse assessing her will ask about the severity of depression, how long it has been present, and assume that it is related to the burden of child care. The underlying cause may be domestic violence, which the woman will not volunteer unless asked. Even if this facility does have routine screening for abuse, the nurse may not screen for it because this is not the patient's initial visit.

If health care integrated social causes and had more of a family focus, the nurse would be aware that pregnant women are at high risk for domestic violence and should be screened for it at each visit. The nurse also would consider the community and family in which a woman lives and presence or absence of supports for her. Norms in some communities support male prerogatives such as wife beating. Some religious groups sanctify marriage, regardless of partner behavior. What are the police attitude and local laws regarding domestic disputes? Do courts provide ex parte and no fault divorce? Are shelters and counseling services available for women and their children experiencing domestic violence? Does a woman have family and friends who know about the situation and support her? To help this woman be safer and healthier, the nurse needs to look beyond bedside or even the health care system to be part of a coordinated community response to domestic violence. By working to create a social climate that condemns domestic violence and empowers the woman to be safe, the nurse will have more options to offer this client as she helps her work through her problem.

Often, health care providers express frustration with patients experiencing domestic violence because there is no "quick fix." This threat to a woman's health is inextricably linked to her community and family. Interventions to increase effectiveness need to go beyond the individual. New links among health care, justice, social welfare, and clergy are needed to potentiate nursing interventions for this population.

Nursing in the Workplace

The practice of occupational health nursing illustrates several of the points just raised. With roots in public health nursing, the earliest models included advocacy for workers and their families. In fact, in late 1800s Ada Mayo Stewart was employed by Vermont Marble Company to do inpatient hospital injury care, home visits for follow-up, and well-baby, and provide school health, company infection control, and employee health education services (Parker-Conrad, 1988). This broad scope of work was based on the belief of her industrial employer that employees would work more safely and productively if not distracted by their own and their family's health problems. One century later we typically do not incorporate the value of health care for reducing indirect costs of stress, uncertainty, and job dissatisfaction into calculations of worker productivity.

It is interesting to note that treatment and prevention are often separated in health care to the point that they do not benefit the individual patient. For example, a case manager may follow a worker with carpal tunnel syndrome in a managed care system, but that may not trigger evaluation of the workplace to eliminate serious and persistent risk factors related to job design.

Evolution of Nursing Role

As nurses expand assessment of patients to include lifestyle, family, and community factors, nursing care can have an impact on patient outcomes beyond the immediate episode of care. Such assessment will require changes in delivery of nursing services to follow the patient over time and across locations to measure the actual impact of nursing interventions. For this to happen, nurses must move primary nursing to a new level. Patients could have a nurse, as well as a physician who is their primary provider. The nurse would assess the patient, family, and community for impact on health and well-being. An alternative would be transitional nursing care for high-risk patients extending beyond an episode of care, such as that reported by Naylor et al. (1999) in successful clinical trial to improve health outcomes and reduce health costs.

Another alternative is expansion of community nursing centers (CNOs). Four CNOs for the elderly have demonstrated increased continuity and coordination of care, cost containment, and consumer satisfaction (American Nurses Association [ANA], 1999). This model also has been developed for other populations. Nurse managed occupational health centers have been shown to integrate treatment and prevention (Wachs, 1997). Examples of services include early disease detection, primary care delivery, case management, risk-reduction education, injury prevention, stress reduction, and worksite analysis. Emphasis is on continuity of care for workers, and sometimes their dependents, who are followed as groups over time.

Presently the nursing profession is talking about increased accountability for nurses regarding cost of care and the health-related outcomes of their actions. Through this chapter the nurse is asked to be accountable for knowing risk factors in the environment, society, and family and incorporating them into the nursing process. Nursing is asked to advocate for the equitable health care system described by Callahan (1998), whereby all have access to a population-focused, evidence-based, health care system aimed at reduction of premature death and disability—rather than the limited access, high-tech, high-cost, disease-specific care available today. Nursing interventions may focus on an individual patient or family, local community, workplace, or larger geographic or political boundary. This focus fits with recent developments in health policy such as the Violence Against Women Act of 1994 and the Americans with Disabilities Act of 1990 that mandate coordinated community responses to health risk factors. Nursing interventions should reach beyond the health system to other relevant social institutions to assist clients in leading healthier lives (Drevdahl, 1995; Kendall, 1992).

■ Concluding Statement

Nursing roles have expanded in scope and variety. Nurses now work at all levels of health prevention, including hazard identification and control in the environment. Nurses identify vulnerable individuals, families, and communities and intervene to promote and protect their health. This expanded perspective requires educators and health care administrators to help nurses look beyond the patient to the context in which the patient lives. Sometimes intervening with those outside traditional health care, such as the police or housing inspectors, may have greater impact on patient outcomes than direct patient care. Nursing in an advocacy, emancipatory, empowerment mode that partners with patients to reduce health risks in their homes, schools, workplaces, and communities is needed (Kendall, 1992; Moccia, 1988; Rodrigues-Trias, 1995).

■ References

American Nurses Association. (1999). *Managed care: Challenges and opportunities for nursing*. Washington, DC: Author.

Americans with Disabilities Act (1990). 42 U.S.C. §§ 12101.

Bunting, S. (1996). Sources of stigma associated with women with HIV. *ANS (Advances in Nursing Science), 19*(2), 64–73.

Butterfield, M. J. (1990). Thinking upstream: Nurturing a conceptual understanding of the societal context of health behavior. *ANS (Advances in Nursing Science), 12*(2), 1–8.

Callahan, D. (1998). *False hopes: Why America's quest for perfect health is a recipe for failure.* New York: Simon & Schuster.

Drevdahl, D. (1995). Coming to voice: The power of emancipatory community interventions. *ANS (Advances in Nursing Science), 18*(2), 13–24.

Funkhouser, S. W., & Moser, D. K. (1990). Is health care racist? *ANS (Advances in Nursing Science), 12*(2), 47–55.

Gordon, L. (1988). *Heroes in their own lives: The politics and history of family violence.* New York: Viking/Penguin.

Jones, P. S., & Meleis, A. (1993). Health is empowerment. *ANS (Advances in Nursing Science), 15*(3), 1–14.

Kendall, J. (1992). Fighting back: Promoting emancipatory nursing actions. *ANS (Advances in Nursing Science), 15*(2), 1–15.

Milio, N. (1983). *Primary care and the public's health.* Lexington, MA: Lexington Books.

Moccia, P. (1988). At the faultline: Social activism and caring. *Nursing Outlook, 36*(1), 30–33.

Naylor, M. D., Brooten, D., Campbell, R., Jacobsen, B. S., Mezey, M. D., Pauly, M. V., & Schwartz, L. (1999). Comprehensive discharge planning and home follow-up of hospitalized elders: A randomized clinical trial. *Journal of the American Medical Association, 281*(7), 656–657.

Parker-Conrad, J. E. (1988). A century of practice: Occupational health nursing. *Occupational Health Nursing, 36,* 156–161.

Parker-Conrad, J. E. (1997). Nurse managed occupational health centers: Quality nursing care by occupational health nurses. *AAOHN Journal* (American Association of Occupational Health Nursing), *45*(10), 475–476.

Pope, A. M., Snyder, M.A., & Mood, L. H. (Eds.). (1995). *Nursing, health, and the environment: Strengthening the relationship to improve the public's health.* Washington, DC: National Academy Press, National Academy of Sciences, Institute of Medicine, Division of Health Promotion and Disease Prevention, Committee on Enhancing Environmental Health Content in Nursing Practice.

Reverby, S. (1987). A caring dilemma: Womanhood and nursing in historical perspective. *Nursing Research, 36,* 5–11.

Rodriguez-Trias, H. (1995). Promoting women's rights to promote women's health. *Journal of the American Medical Women's Association, 50*(3, 4), 73.

Sexton, K., Olden, K., & Johnson, L. (1993). Environmental justice: The central role of research in establishing a credible scientific foundation for informed decision making. *Toxicology and Industrial Health, 9*(5), 685–727.

Shields, L. E., & Lindsey, A. E. (1998). Community health promotion nursing practice. *ANS (Advances in Nursing Science), 12*(4), 23–36.

U.S. Department of Health and Human Services. (1986). *Surgeon General's workshop on violence.* Washington, DC: Author.

U.S. Department of Health and Human Services. (1990). *Healthy People 2000: Health objectives for the nation.* Washington, DC: Author.

Violence Against Women Act (VAWA). (1994). *Title IV of the Violent Crime Control and Law Enforcement Act of 1994* (P. L. 103–322).

Wachs, J. E. (1997). Nurse managed occupational health centers: An overview. *AAOHN Journal* (American Association of Occupational Health Nursing), *45*(10), 477–483.

Wassel, M. L. (1995). Occupational health nursing and the advent of managed care: Meeting the challenges of the current health care environment. *Journal of the American Association of Occupational Health Nurses, 43*(1), 23–28.

Whelan, E. A., Piacitelli, G. M., Gerwel, B., Schnorr, T. M., Mueller, C. A., Gittleman, J., & Matte, T. D. (1997). Elevated blood lead levels in children of construction workers. *American Journal of Public Health, 87*(8), 1352–1355.

■ *Editor's Questions for Discussion*

Provide examples of the profession's pointing out the need to address environmental and social factors related to health promotion. Do you agree with Dienemann, Campbell, and Agnew that public health nursing is an "endangered species"? Provide justification or evidence for your response. How accepted is public health nursing as a role to provide integrated care? Should public health and school nurses address environmental issues in care? Is there a difference between public health nursing and community health nursing? How may these roles be integrated? Discuss how socioeconomic status makes a difference in the quality of care provided. Suggest ways in which health care inequalities can be resolved.

Debate the pros and cons of managed care. What data are available to support your responses? How does Pinkerton's (Chapter 56) addressing of integrated delivery systems apply to Dienemann, Campbell, and Agnew's advocacy of integrated care? What relationship exists between integrating care and case management? How may Gerber (Chapter 57) agree with your response? What risks to individual care needs may be involved in integrated care?

How is health education best provided—for whom and by whom? Give examples in your response. Apply the discussions by Sefcik and Jones (Chapter 48), Alexander (Chapter 44), Todero (Chapter 51), and Barger (Chapter 52) in your answers concerning health education. To what extent do Dienemann, Campbell, and Agnew and the authors just mentioned advocate that nurses be primary providers of care? How does transitional care, as presented by Corless (Chapter 46), address evolution of the nursing role advocated by Dienemann, Campbell, and Agnew?

60

Climbing Out of the Crab Bucket

Strategies for Resolving Conflict Among Nurses

Sandra P. Thomas, PhD, RN, FAAN

I t has been said that nurses are like a bucket of crabs: You do not need to put a lid on a bucket of crabs because when one crab gets to the top, the others will pull it back down. The metaphor of the crab bucket is useful for introducing this chapter on conflict resolution in nursing practice. First, I explore the causes of infighting among nurses and then present strategies for climbing out of the crab bucket. Effective methods of resolving conflict are essential, given research evidence that interpersonal conflict is one of the major sources of stress for nurses (Grout, 1980; Hipwell, Tyler, & Wilson, 1989). Nursing's work of assisting human beings in life crises is stressful enough without augmentation by excessive internal strife. Although there is ample documentation

of conflict between nurses and other members of the health care team, especially physicians, in this chapter I focus on nurse-to-nurse conflict. Getting nursing's house in order is imperative if nurses are to meet successfully the challenges of the 21st century.

■ Genesis, Manifestations, and Consequences of Nurses' Anger and Conflict

What Nurses Are Angry About

In an anger study that involved more than 500 women, nurses and other human service workers were found to score highest among occupational groups on overall anger proneness (S. P. Thomas, 1993). This intriguing research finding led my research team to undertake subsequent studies of both female nurses (Smith, Droppleman, & S. P Thomas, 1996) and male nurses (Brooks, S. P. Thomas, & Droppleman, 1996) because we wanted to know what nurses were so angry about. The research team interviewed RNs who worked in intensive care, coronary care, behavioral health, orthopedics, neurology, oncology, medical–surgical, home health, primary care, long-term care, maternity, public health, and nursing education. The predominant theme of nurses' anger was their *powerlessness.* Violations of nurses' values, rights, and beliefs fueled impotent anger that was most often expressed in *horizontal hostility toward coworkers* rather than being directed upward in the hierarchical system, toward management or physicians. The phenomenon of horizontal hostility is evident in all oppressed, lower status groups that are forbidden to express anger toward dominant, higher status groups. Manifestations of horizontal hostility in our data included fault-finding, back-biting, needling, and name-calling (i.e., referring to other nurses as "dizzy lizzies," "bad apples," and "dingbats"). More subtle forms, such as unkind gossip, were also prevalent.

Geary (1982) attributed nurse-to-nurse friction to diverse educational preparation of RNs and to the predominantly female gender composition of the profession. She alleged that women's early socialization to compete with other women for men's attention caused nurses' subsequent failure to help and mentor their colleagues. But it was clear from our study of male nurses that horizontal hostility is not confined to females. We saw many instances of it in our sample of male RNs. Horizontal hostility does not occur just because most nurses are women. It occurs because all nurses—male and female—have been oppressed (S. P. Thomas, 1998).

Thus, although conflict among nurses is not new, it escalated during the radical restructuring of the health care system in the 1990s. New care delivery models were introduced without empirical evidence of effectiveness. Organizational downsizing was undertaken without recognition of its devastating effects on the productivity and psychological well-being of the remaining work force. Experienced bedside nurses, clinical specialists, and managers were shocked at the receipt of pink slips, and their colleagues who survived cuts wondered who would be next. Nurses affected by downsizing no longer trusted the organization or the people who were making the decisions (Schilder, 1997). In addition to pervasive mistrust, nurses exhibited high levels of anxiety about forced cross-training and floating, unsafe staffing patterns, and mandatory overtime. In this climate of fear, employee complaints about other employees increased dramatically (Curtin, 1995). By 1999, Kritek asserted that 50% of staff nurses' time and 75% of administrators' time was being spent in conflict.

Nurses whom we interviewed described their workplaces as hostile, a virtual war zone in which they were frequently under assault. No two of the study participants worked in the same institution, yet the hostile climate was common to all. Military metaphors abounded in the data: "I become very fatigued by having to do all these battles"; "There is character assassination": "I was getting flak"; "I went in with loaded guns"; and "We feel sabotaged." Adversarial relationships were particularly evident between nurses "in the trenches" and their supervisors, who were perceived to have "deserted the troops." For example, a staff nurse told us that nurse administrators "sell you down the tubes. They have totally lost sight of the nursing side. And you shouldn't be at sides or at war." Studies other than our own have also found nurses' work environments depicted as battlefields (Brandi, 1998). An embattled nurse executive in Brandi's study reported asking herself, "Is this the hill I want to die on today?"

Application of Conflict Theories to Typical Situations in Nursing

Numerous theories about conflict have some relevance to nurses. Simmel (1955) proposed that desire, hate, need, and envy were the causes of human conflict. He held a rather dark view of human nature, contending that interpersonal hostility is more likely to occur than closeness. Simmel's factor of envy also appears to be a causative factor in Rodgers' explanation of conflict in the nursing profession. Rodgers (1982) dates the origin of human envy to the early relationship of infant with mother: The breast is the first object of envy and therefore woman is the first person envied. According to Rodgers, nursing, as a predominantly female profession, evokes the image of the nursing mother, triggering envy in colleagues (although there may not be conscious awareness of its source). Conflict fueled by envy is often observed in the workplace when a nurse achieves advanced degrees or promotions. Colleagues seek to disparage or undermine upwardly mobile nurses, rather than taking pride in their accomplishments.

Several theorists (e.g., Sumner, 1963; Weber, 1968) have proposed that a common precursor of conflict is scarcity of resources. When valued objects or goods are in short supply, competitive struggles ensue. This theory seems particularly relevant to contemporary conditions of hospital downsizing, as widespread elimination of middle-management positions leaves staff nurses few avenues for advancement. The scarcity of tenure slots in many nursing schools likewise fuels intense competition and horizontal hostility among faculty members. And many nurses are just plain job-scared.

Corwin (cited in Sexton, 1986) pointed out that specialization accentuates differences between individuals. Perhaps disunity within the profession increased as the once-simple division of nurses into categories of "general duty" and "private duty" gave way to today's plethora of clinical specialties and subspecialties. An interesting hierarchy of nursing's specialties was revealed in our study (Smith et al., 1996), wherein critical care nursing was viewed as a higher status specialty than psychiatric or maternal-child nursing. This hierarchical ranking was related to the amount of technology required for giving patient care.

Although not offering a theory of conflict, Umiker (1998a) provided a useful list of six major causes: unclear expectations, poor communication, lack of clear jurisdiction, incompatibilities of temperament, individual or group conflicts of interest, and operational or staffing changes. However, he pointed out that the etiology of a conflict is not always readily apparent, nor can conflict always be attributed to a single etiology.

Finally, the conflict-prone context in which nurses practice must be considered. Conflict is inevitable when professionals (who expect to have autonomy in practice) are employed in bureaucratic institutions (which have multilayered administrative hierarchies and numerous rules and regulations). But in the 1990s, patient-focused values of nurses clashed even more sharply with the cost-cutting emphasis of profit-focused corporations. According to Stokols (1992), conflict-prone organizations are characterized by an absence of shared goals, rigid ideologies, competitive coalitions, nonparticipatory organizational processes, and prospects of unemployment because of economic changes. Unfortunately, this list of characteristics exemplifies the current practice setting of many nurses.

Some organizational cultures are dysfunctional. Many health care organizations are, in fact, unhealthy places to work. Among the "neurotic organizations" described by deVries and Miller (1984) are organizations that are paranoid (characterized by managerial suspiciousness), compulsive (wedded to ritual), dramatic (impulsive and dangerously uninhibited), depressive (passive), and schizoid (led by distant, uninvolved leaders). My own career experience in nursing includes all of these types. Such organizational cultures lessen likelihood of free and honest communication and create considerable psychosocial distress in workers.

Resolution of conflict is complicated when an organization is threatened by the presence of conflict and tries to pretend that it does not exist. Problems that are denied cannot be resolved, and workers eventually become demoralized. Likewise, conflict is difficult to resolve when accompanied by too much angry emotionality. Nurses often personalize conflicts, taking too personally colleagues' opposition to their views. Their resultant anger is not managed effectively. How then is nurses' anger expressed?

How Anger Is Expressed by "Onion" Types and "Garlic" Types

In a satirical and very funny article, Osmun and Naugler (1998) proposed a progressive taxonomy of workplace anger, sulk–tantrum–snit–hissy fit–riot, and urged that methods of hissy fit prophylaxis and treatment (perhaps sublingual Ativan) be instituted in all health care settings. Workshops that I conduct across the country have convinced me that nurses usually manage their anger in one of two ways: suppression or outbursts. Nurses do not feel good about either. I use the simple typology of "onion people" and "garlic people" to explain the dynamics of the two styles. "Onion people" swallow most of their anger, and just as individuals who eat onions suffer later, so do anger suppressors. The anger seems to keep trying to come back up. In contrast, "garlic people" freely spread their anger around, causing others to suffer although they themselves

are unaware of the lingering stench created by their outbursts.

The anger suppressor ("onion") often stews about grievances in silence, unwilling or unable to confront the offender. If the suppressor is female, she may consciously or unconsciously conform to rules she learned for anger display during childhood gender role socialization. She may have been taught that direct anger expression is unfeminine, unattractive, and detrimental to relationships. She may have observed female role models who conveyed their feelings indirectly through sulking, sighing, or withdrawing. Healthier anger management for the "onion type" involves (a) giving oneself permission to express anger assertively rather than suppressing it, and (b) decreasing anxiety and guilt about being angry. Contrary to popular myth, anger is neither maladaptive nor sinful, and in many cases actually serves as a protective mechanism. Anger can be a useful signal that one's rights or values are being violated and, therefore, corrective action is in order. Thus the habitual anger suppressor needs encouragement to be more outspoken about injustices.

Whereas overt anger expression can be a healthy way to defend oneself from injustices, the "garlic" person is too verbal and too prone to overreact to minor provocations. Our research showed that blowups accompanied by screaming and crying left nurses feeling embarrassed and unprofessional. Furthermore, their volatility caused coworkers to avoid them. Improved anger management for the "garlic type" involves (a) decreasing reactivity to anger-producing stimuli, (b) using calming techniques such as deep breathing, and (c) decreasing the amount of ventilation.

Anger management pointers that may benefit everyone, regardless of expression style, include (a) taking constructive action on precipitants of anger whenever possible; (b) finding a healthy way to discharge high physiological arousal through exercise, laughter, or meditation; and (c) avoiding useless, no-win arguments and fruitless bickering sessions. Exiting gracefully from a conflictual situation is sometimes a rational decision, not a cop-out.

Consequences of Mismanaged Anger and Conflict for Individual Nurses and the Profession

Much of nurses' anger is understandable. But there is abundant evidence that it is mismanaged. The anger is too frequent, too intense, and too prolonged. Its manifestations are personally as well as professionally destructive. For example, some nurses in our studies used alcohol and drugs to medicate negative emotion. This remedy has the potential for grave consequences. Incidence of chemical dependency is 50% higher in nurses than in the general population (Kabb, 1984). Use of other mood regulators, such as cigarettes and food binges, was acknowledged by many nurses in our sample. However, masking negative emotion does not make it go away. For some nurses, chronic anger proliferates like a malignant growth that eventually chokes the love of nursing out of them (S. P. Thomas, 1998). Nurses with the highest scores on a burnout questionnaire reported the greatest amount of conflict with other nurses (Hillhouse & Adler, 1997). Frequently, nurses change shifts or leave their jobs to escape the conflict. Some leave nursing altogether—a tragic loss that the profession can ill afford.

■ Promoting Healing Dialogues with Colleagues

For the nursing profession to advance, collegial cooperation and mutual respect must replace ubiquitous conflict. Nurses are often excluded from policy debates because they are regarded as divided (Davies, 1995). Although nurses deplore the inability of their national leaders

and organizations to achieve consensus, healing actually begins at the level of the work unit, whether that is a hospital floor, an outpatient clinic, or a department in a nursing college. That is where a nurse's work life is spent, 40 (or more) hours per week, week after week. Quality of interaction with peers in this workplace is a vital element in personal well-being. Research shows that group cohesion strongly influences nurses' job satisfaction (Lucas, Atwood, & Hagaman, 1993).

Creating a culture of cooperation requires the ability to engage in dialogue. Dialogue involves sharing honest opinions and listening respectfully to the opinions of others. All views must be accepted as legitimate. Open-ended questions elicit more information than questions that can be answered with a simple yes or no. Creative strategies for problem solving can only be generated when members of a team can freely share perspectives. In meetings with nurse colleagues, I am often struck by our vastly different perceptions of a situation. A Charles Shultz "Peanuts" cartoon is illustrative: Lucy, Linus, and Charlie Brown are lying on the ground watching clouds. Lucy asks Linus, "What do you see in the clouds up there?" Linus replies, "That cloud on the left looks like a map of British Honduras. The cloud in the center reminds me of a bust of the famous artist Thomas Eakins. The cloud on the right shows the stoning of Stephen. You can see St. Paul standing there." Lucy then asks Charlie Brown what he sees. Charlie's answer? "I was going to say that I saw a horsie and a duckie, but I've changed my mind."

Each nurse must make greater effort to understand coworkers' points of view and motives. In a study by Baumeister, Stillwell, and Wotman (1990), participants in conflict were asked to provide narratives about their anger experiences. Angry people nearly always insisted that the other person's point of view was wrong but that their own was justified. Offenders were characterized as unreasonable, arbitrary, selfish, and even malicious. In contrast, offenders held a much more benign view of things, providing reasonable explanations of their behavior. Taking an "I'm right-and-they're-wrong" stance prevents resolution of conflict.

Many nurses hold irrational beliefs that produce conflict (e.g., "Other nurses should do work the right way, the way that I would do it"; "Good nurses should work until they drop and do overtime PRN"; and "The day shift should have finished all of that work instead of leaving part of it for us"). Irrational beliefs can be identified by looking for explicit or implied "shoulds" or "oughts" regarding behavior of other people. Other prevalent cognitive distortions among nurses include blaming, overgeneralizing, dichotomous "all-or-nothing" thinking, focusing almost exclusively on the negative, and catastrophizing. A careful self-analysis of the triggers of work-related anger can reveal recurrent themes or patterns in a person's thoughts. Discarding these irrational cognitions can defuse much nonproductive anger at coworkers (S. P. Thomas, 1998).

What Managers Can Do to Improve Relationships with Staff

Turbulence created by hospital reengineering has created nightmarish dilemmas for many nurse managers, particularly those in middle-management positions. Mid-level administrators interviewed after organizational redesign at two midwestern hospitals expressed feelings of powerlessness, unpreparedness, and being caught in the middle (Cook, Ingersoll, Fogel, & Wagner, 1999). Similarly, an ICU manager whom I interviewed also spoke of being "caught" and becoming the brunt of staff anger to boot: "I'm caught between understanding my nurses' anger regarding staffing and justifying my budget to upper management." Another manager said that she saw her job as "continu-

ally in this sandwich of making peace with all." Serving as a lightning rod for staff anger is distressing and often tends to evoke defensive responses that subsequently worsen manager–staff relationships.

What can managers do to improve relationships with staff? I believe that provision of support must be the number one priority of managers (S. P. Thomas, 1998). Staff nurses who participated in our studies longed for support from their managers. Too often nurses related incidents when they had called to ask for help and received a sarcastic retort, such as this response from a night supervisor: "Well, where do you think I'm going to get these nurses, cut out paper dolls?" Supervisory personnel must remember to give positive feedback. Nurses were always being told what they were doing wrong, but no one ever told them what they were doing right. A male nurse we interviewed described his autocratic nurse manager walking through the unit "like a stick stirring up rattlesnakes," getting all the nurses "in a uproar and tense . . . pointing out these small things." Tensions between management and staff can often be reduced by giving staff greater control. For example, self-scheduling eliminates one source of staff resentment.

Managers must create a climate in the work unit that facilitates conflict resolution. It is a manager's responsibility to serve as the third-party manager of conflict that has been observed among staff members. Too often the manager's attitude toward conflict is avoidance rather than mediation. Conflict does have some positive functions, such as getting a troubling matter on the table for open discussion and stimulating a search for new facts. Problems can be reframed as goals to be attained. Brainstorming for alternative solutions should be encouraged. Parties to conflict should be apprised that compromise will probably be necessary for goal attainment.

Some staff members are carriers of the workplace negativity virus. Managers should realize that individuals with personality disorders (e.g., passive–aggressive, borderline, or obsessive–compulsive) use defense mechanisms that prevent them from seeing their own contributions to conflictual situations. Rather than becoming involved in power struggles with these individuals, managers should help them to decrease inappropriate behaviors and become more productive team members (Trimpey & Davidson, 1994). Chronically angry, disruptive staff members should be referred to a counselor or employee assistance program.

What Staff Can Do to Improve Relationships with Managers

Staff nurses in our studies were often resentful because their managers did not rescue them: A subtheme of powerlessness in the interview data was "waiting for rescue" (by those perceived to have the power). Typical exemplars of this theme included: "We don't seem to have the leadership"; "My lifesaver was not in town"; and "I think it's out of my hands." Staff nurses thought that managers should magically know what they wanted and needed. However, managers are not clairvoyant; it is incumbent on staff to communicate requests and grievances directly. Silent resentment and passive–aggressive tactics do not bring about improved working conditions. Even if a manager cannot take remedial action, staff members will feel better about themselves when they have clearly articulated their concerns.

A first step in alleviating the global powerlessness felt by many staff nurses is selecting one specific issue or problem to bring to management's attention—in other words, "narrowing the focus" (M. D. Thomas et al., 1999). State hospital nurses studied by M. D. Thomas' team did find ways to exert power by using this approach, focusing concern on a particular patient or policy and taking a stand.

As one study participant put it, "To survive one must pick the battles, plan to move slow . . ." (p. 57).

■ Projecting Toward Nursing's Future

Empowering Every Practicing Nurse

Because the crux of nurses' anger is *powerlessness*, the solution must be *empowerment*. Empowerment means enhanced ability to take action and resolve problems. As noted by Ward and Mullender (1991), empowerment is an empty concept unless it is linked to commitment to challenge oppression. Although nurses' mismanaged anger has negative consequences, *assertively* expressed anger is empowering—and commands attention to one's concerns. Florence Nightingale knew how to use anger to get results. In an 1864 letter, she revealed her strategy for getting the British War Office to improve conditions for Army doctors: "You may think I am not wise in being so angry. But I assure you, when I write civilly, I have a civil answer—*and nothing is done.* When I write furiously, I have a rude letter—*and something is done* (not even then always, *but only then*)" (cited in Nash, 1931, p. 240). Repetition, usually in a spate of letters, was a key element in Nightingale's strategy and remains just as useful today. Getting the attention of individuals who can act on one's concerns may require several conversations, written reports, and presentations of data. Enlisting nurses' associations, politicians, and the media may be necessary.

It is an old truism that the powerful do not give away power. Nurses must make an effort to acquire it. No one benefits when nurses continue to acquiesce to the status quo. Thus nurses must decide that they want power, about which they traditionally have been ambivalent (Valentine, 1992). Unfortunately, nurses have seen power as antithetical to caring (Rafael, 1996). I do not use *power* here in the negative sense of becoming exploitive or manipulative to "win" in conflictual situations. A powerful nurse is one who outlines a position confidently but then interacts with peers respectfully during negotiations. Nurses must become more skillful in persuading, bargaining, and negotiating—skills that are not taught in nursing schools. Effective negotiators prepare carefully, marshalling data to support their proposals. Graphs and charts depicting supporting data are presented. Benefits of various options are pointed out, and points of agreement are sought. Ultimatums are avoided (Umiker, 1998b).

To address workplace issues such as unsafe conditions, inadequate resources, and ill-conceived policies, nurses must form coalitions. For example, nurse colleagues in one agency, exhausted because of staff cutbacks, began to keep statistics and used them to argue for relief. The group met regularly to develop strategy, even creating its own stationery (Rafael, 1998). Another group of nurses successfully challenged institutional norms that limited their autonomy, transforming a "fiercely patriarchal and autocratic hospital culture" (Breda et al., 1997, p. 77). After similarly successful coalition-forming had produced positive outcomes, one of our study participants proudly reported: "We feel like we have our unit back in control again, which is the way it should be" (Smith et al., 1996).

Characteristics of Empowered Individuals

Feeling in control is characteristic of empowered individuals. Such individuals are effective change agents because they are assertive, knowledgeable, and exhibit positive self-esteem. They do not ruminate about old grievances. Conflictual anger issues are dealt with promptly, not allowed to fester. A study of

women who coped via assertive action showed that they actually experienced *less anger* (Wells, Hobfoll, & Lavin, 1997).

Climbing Out of the Crab Bucket and Working Cooperatively Toward Solving Problems and Achieving Mutual Goals

If the nursing profession is distinctive because of its caring, as Jean Watson, Margaret Newman, Madeleine Leininger, and others have claimed, then nurses must climb out of the crab bucket and start caring for each other. Conflict will never be completely eliminated, but its negative impact can be minimized with open, ongoing discussion of issues. Collegial support and empathy must be substituted for antagonism and mistrust (S. P. Thomas, 1998). Among its many benefits, collegial support is a proven preventive measure for burnout: The more a nurse perceives support from colleagues, the less he or she burns out (Duquette, Kerouac, Sandhu, & Beaudet, 1994). Nurses reporting high support from their coworkers also have a stronger sense of personal accomplishment than nurses with few sources of support (Ogus, 1990). Each nurse must make a commitment to supportive, caring colleagueship. And if a nurse is to have sufficient energy to devote to the care of colleagues, commitment to proper self-care is essential too. A burned-out, cynical nurse is not likely to be a caring colleague.

■ Concluding Statement

Solving workplace problems in the new millennium must begin with a new mindset. Although it has been said that no one really likes change except a baby with a wet diaper, the only certainty as we enter the 21st century is continued change. Vicenzi, White, and Begun (1997) suggested that nurses abandon expectations of job security, control, and stability and become comfortable with chaos, complexity, and change. No nurse can rely on an institution to provide security. Reliance on the empowered self and on coalitions of colleagues with mutual goals will be the key to successful adaptation. Power built through strong collegial relationships must supplant destructive conflict that has hampered nursing's progress.

■ References

Baumeister, R., Stillwell, A., & Wotman, S. (1990). Victim and perpetrator accounts of interpersonal conflict: Autobiographical narratives about anger. *Journal of Personality and Social Psychology, 59,* 994–1005.

Brandi, C. L. (1998). A typology of women nurse executives on the managed care battlefield. *Journal of Nursing Administration, 28*(5), 13–16.

Breda, K., Anderson, M., Hansen, L., Hayes, D., Pillion, C., & Lyon, P. (1997). Enhanced nursing autonomy through participatory action research. *Nursing Outlook, 45*(2), 76–81.

Brooks, A., Thomas, S. P., & Droppleman, P. (1996). From frustration to red fury: A description of work-related anger in male registered nurses. *Nursing Forum, 31*(3), 4–15.

Cook, J., Ingersoll, G., Fogel, S., & Wagner, L. (1999, February). *Mid-level nurse administrators' role responsibilities and reactions to major organizational redesign.* Paper presented at the Southern Nursing Research Society, Charleston, South Carolina.

Curtin, L. (1995). To see ourselves... *Nursing Management, 26*(9), 7–8.

Davies, C. (1995). *Gender and the professional predicament in nursing.* Philadelphia: Open University Press.

deVries, M. K., & Miller, D. (1984). *The neurotic organization.* San Francisco: Jossey-Bass.

Duquette, A., Kerouac, S., Sandhu, B., & Beaudet, L. (1994). Factors related to nursing burnout: A review of empirical knowledge. *Issues in Mental Health Nursing, 15,* 337–358.

Geary, P. G. (1982). Toward androgyny. In J. Muff (Ed.), *Women's issues in nursing: Socialization, sexism, and stereotyping* (pp. 248–254). Prospect Heights, IL: Waveland Press.

Grout, J. W. (1980). Occupational stress of intensive care nurses and air traffic controllers: Review of related studies. *Journal of Nursing Education, 19*(6), 8–14.

Hillhouse, J., & Adler, C. (1997). Investigating stress effect patterns in hospital staff nurses: Results of a cluster analysis. *Social Science and Medicine, 45,* 1781–1788.

Hipwell, A. E., Tyler, P. A., & Wilson, C. M. (1989). Sources of stress and dissatisfaction among nurses in four hospital environments. *British Journal of Medical Psychology, 62,* 71–79.

Kabb, G. (1984). Chemical dependency: Helping your staff. *Journal of Nursing Administration, 14*(11), 18–23.

Kritek, P. (1999, February). *Research 2000: Negotiating the turn.* Paper presented at the Southern Nursing Research Society, Charleston, South Carolina.

Lucas, M., Atwood, J., & Hagaman, R. (1993). Replication and validation of anticipated turnover model for urban registered nurses. *Nursing Research, 42,* 29–35.

Nash, R. (1931). *A short life of Florence Nightingale.* New York: Macmillan.

Ogus, E. D. (1990). Burnout and social support systems among ward nurses. *Issues in Mental Health Nursing, 11,* 267–281.

Osmun, W. E., & Naugler, C. (1998). The impact of hissy fits in primary care. *Canadian Medical Association Journal, 159,* 1457–1459.

Rafael, A. R. F. (1996). Power and caring: A dialectic in nursing. *Advances in Nursing Science, 19*(1), 3–17.

Rafael, A. R. F. (1998). Nurses who run with the wolves: The power and caring dialectic revisited. *Advances in Nursing Science, 21*(1), 29–42.

Rodgers, J. A. (1982). Women and the fear of being envied. *Nursing Outlook, 30,* 344–347.

Schilder, E. (1997, June). *The impact of organizational downsizing and restructuring on the worklife of nurses on acute medical wards in a tertiary care hospital.* Paper presented at the Eighth Congress of the International Council on Women's Health Issues, Saskatoon, Saskatchewan, Canada.

Sexton, D. L. (1986). Organizational conflict: A creative or destructive force. In E. C. Hein & M. J. Nicholson (Eds.), *Contemporary leadership behavior: Selected readings* (pp. 299–306). Boston: Little, Brown.

Simmel, G. (1955). *Conflict and the web of group affiliations.* New York: Free Press.

Smith, M., Droppleman, P., & Thomas, S. P. (1996). Under assault: The experience of work-related anger in female registered nurses. *Nursing Forum, 31*(1), 22–33.

Stokols, D. (1992). Conflict-prone and conflict-resistant organizations. In H. S. Friedman (Ed.), *Hostility, coping, and health* (pp. 65–76). Washington, DC: American Psychological Association.

Sumner, W. G. (1963). *Social Darwinism.* Engelwood Cliffs, NJ: Prentice-Hall.

Thomas, M. D., Hagerott, R. J., Hilliard, I. A., Kelly, J., Leichman, S., Osborne, O., & Thurston, J. (1999). Meanings of state hospital nursing II: Coping and making meaning. *Archives of Psychiatric Nursing, 13*(1), 55–60.

Thomas, S. P. (1993). Anger and its manifestations in women. In S. P. Thomas (Ed.), *Women and anger* (pp. 40–67). New York: Springer.

Thomas, S. P. (1998). *Transforming nurses' anger and pain: Steps toward healing.* New York: Springer.

Trimpey, M., & Davidson, S. (1994). Chaos, perfectionism, and sabotage: Personality disorders in the workplace. *Issues in Mental Health Nursing, 15,* 27–36.

Umiker, W. (1998a). Collaborative conflict resolution. In E. C. Hein (Ed.), *Contemporary leadership behavior* (5th ed., pp. 259–263). Philadelphia: Lippincott-Raven.

Umiker, W. (1998b). Negotiating skill for health professionals. In E. C. Hein (Ed.), *Contemporary leadership behavior* (5th ed., pp. 264–269). Philadelphia: Lippincott-Raven.

Valentine, P. (1992). Feminism: A four-letter word? *The Canadian Nurse, 85*(12), 20–23.

Vicenzi, A. E., White, K., & Begun, J. W. (1997). Chaos in nursing: Make it work for you. *American Journal of Nursing, 97*(10), 26–31.

Ward, D., & Mullender, A. (1991). Empowerment and oppression: An indissoluble pairing for contemporary social work. *Critical Social Policy, 11*(2), 21–30.

Weber, M. (1968). *Economy and society.* New York: Bedminster.

Wells, J. D., Hobfoll, S. E., & Lavin, J. (1997). Resource loss, resource gain, and communal coping during pregnancy among women with multiple roles. *Psychology of Women Quarterly, 21,* 645–662.

■ Editor's Questions for Discussion

What additional factors contribute to anger among nurses than those presented by Thomas? How might nurses in early career development learn positive means for expressing hostility? What interventions are critical for changing a climate of fear to trust? How might strategies be effectively implemented for environments of trust?

Identify characteristics of dysfunctional organizations. What type of leadership is essential to create healthy environments? How might individuals who are "onion" or "garlic" types learn healthier anger management methods? What positive reinforcement strategies may be deployed in anger management? How are suggestions advocated by Pesut (Chapter 70) regarding inner work applicable for anger management?

Should accountability be established with empowerment in organizations? If so, how? How may staff nurses assess sincerity and support for another? How may nurses best facilitate strong collegial relationships?

61

Creating Healthy Work Environments for Nursing Practice

Joanne M. Disch, PhD, RN, FAAN

Creating a therapeutic environment for patients is a fundamental responsibility of nursing practice. Moreover, when the environment itself becomes dangerous to nursing staff who practice in it, action must be taken. In this chapter, trends are described in society and health care related to violence and abuse and strategies are presented not only for decreasing these rates and their consequences, but also for moving beyond them to create healthy work environments.

■ *Violence in the Workplace*

Prior to 1986, when 13 postal workers were shot in Edmonton, Oklahoma, violence in the workplace was rare in this country. However, between 1980 and 1992, there were 9,937 homicides in the workplace (Jenkins, 1996). Moreover, a study sponsored by Northwestern National Life Insurance (Lawless, 1993) reported that one in four full-time workers was the victim of workplace violence between July 1992 and June 1993.

I would like to gratefully acknowledge the invaluable assistance of two colleagues, Dayle Stubbs, RN, MSN, and Karen Whiley, RN, BSN, nurse managers at Fairview-University Medical Center, who created both the Case Study and the healthy work environment described herein.

Study results showed that an estimated 2.2 million workers are physically attacked, 6.3 million are threatened, and 16.1 million are harassed annually. This growth in workplace violence mirrors the increased violence in the United States in general where the homicide rate is 10 times higher than in England, and 25 times higher than in Spain (Simonowitz, 1996).

Definition

The definition of workplace violence varies greatly. The Occupational Safety and Health Administration (OSHA) (1996) defines it as any physical assault, threatening behavior, or verbal abuse occurring in the work setting. Warshaw and Messite (1996) add that individuals are victims whether they be intentional targets or innocent bystanders involved only accidentally. As an alternative framework, Neuman and Baron (1998) suggest that workplace violence should be limited to instances involving direct physical assault and that *workplace aggression* should be used to describe all forms of behavior by which individuals attempt to harm persons at work or their organizations. Other authors have further expanded the concept of aggression to address specifically verbal threats (Cole, Grubb, Sauter, Swanson, & Lawless, 1997); assaults that produce not only physical but also psychological harm (Lawless, 1993); personal or motor vehicle theft at work (Bachman, 1994); and self-directed violence (e.g., suicide) (Center for Mental Health Services [CHS], 1994). Finally, some agencies count as violence only those physical attacks which result in one day away from work (Bureau of Labor Statistics [BLS], 1994).

Underreporting

Inconsistency in defining violence poses several problems. First, underreporting occurs due to (a) lack of consistent terminology, (b) lack of reporting systems, (c) the practice of only counting episodes that result in lost work time, (d) the fact that workers' compensation data do not include self-insured employees, (e) the assumption that violence is just part of the job, (f) pressure from peers not to report, (g) cultural variability in accepting violence, (h) lack of employer interest, and (i) fear of blame or reprisal. Estimates vary, but 50% underreporting is not uncommon, and one study described a 25-fold greater incidence than reported (Bensley, Nelson, Kaufman, Silverstein, & Kalat, 1993).

Second, depending on the definition, examination of predisposing factors and development of effective prevention or treatment strategies obviously will differ. Additionally, costs to the individual and organization will vary (e.g., workers' days lost, workers' compensation payments, and replacement workers).

Third, the extent to which an organization views violence as a pervasive problem, or minor inconvenience, and establishes it as a priority for action will depend on the data describing it.

The Victims

Individuals who are particularly vulnerable to workplace violence are employees who are (a) involved in the exchange of money; (b) working alone or in small numbers, especially if the periods of isolation are predictable; (c) working late at night or early in the morning; (d) working in high crime areas; (e) guarding valuable property; (f) working in community settings; (g) providing care to people who are distressed, fearful, ill or incarcerated; (h) dealing with people who are very angry, resentful, have feelings of failure, or have unreasonable expectations of what the organization or worker can provide; (i) working under great stress; and (j) experiencing plant closings and downsizings (Warshaw & Messite, 1996).

Some industries or job categories are inherently high risk (e.g., firefighters, police officers, and correctional officers); high risk when robbery is the primary motive (e.g., restaurants, armored cars, taxis, and convenience stores); or high risk because the employees can be assaulted by physically or mentally disabled students, clients, or patients (Nelson & Kaufman, 1996). Health care workers are at high risk of experiencing assaults by patients, either deliberate or unintentional (Lipscomb & Love, 1992). This will be covered in more detail in a later section. An emerging area of violence in the workplace relates to victims of domestic violence: In one study, 75% of women in domestic violence relationships reported being harassed by their abuser at work by telephone or in person (Fitzgerald, Dienemann, & Cadorette, 1998).

The Aggressors

Whereas most homicides in the community are committed by acquaintances and family members, homicides at work are more likely to be committed by strangers (BLS, 1994). Alternatively, nonfatal violence is more likely to be committed by coworkers and supervisors (Cox, 1991b; Lawless, 1993). Situational variables contributing to aggression include a workplace where the environment is strained and competitive, with poor managerial practices (CMHS, 1994; Cole et al., 1997); work group harmony is lacking (Cole et al., 1997); and the physical environment is unsupportive (e.g., high humidity, heat, and poor lighting) (Neuman & Baron, 1998).

The American Psychiatric Association (APA) (1994) notes that most workplace violence is not committed by a criminal or a psychotic, but rather by a basically normal person who has an outburst related to stress. The source of the stress can be work-related, or personal. Nonetheless, some personal factors have been linked with workplace violence (e.g., a

history of certain psychiatric disorders and prior criminal activity) (APA, 1994; Neuman and Baron, 1998; Warshaw & Messite, 1996) or abuse of alcohol or drugs (Warshaw & Messite, 1996).

The Impact

Violence in the workplace is costly. For the individual, the cost can take the form of psychological complaints, physical symptoms, job dissatisfaction and burnout, and, for some, a form of post-traumatic stress disorder (PTSD). For the organization, it can mean reduced productivity and morale, absenteeism, turnover and increased costs. The Bureau of Labor Statistics (1994) reported that victims of physical attack commonly require an average of 5 days away from work to recuperate.

The Workplace Environment

The American workplace environment has become increasingly stressful, as reflected in the factors just cited that are associated with violence. Petry, Mujica, and Vickery (1996) conducted a cross-sectional study of 5,000 U.S. workers and found that 60% felt a substantial amount of pressure on the job, with 56% feeling some pressure to act illegally or unethically. Employees in manufacturing (26%) and health care (24%) felt the highest levels of pressure. Examples of unethical or illegal activities included (a) cutting corners on quality, (b) covering up incidents, (c) abusing or lying about sick days, (d) falsifying numbers or reports, (e) withholding important information, and (f) discriminating against coworkers. The researchers found that factors contributing to pressures in the workplace included (a) balancing of work and family (52%), (b) poor leadership (51%), (c) poor internal communication (51%), (d) workload hours (51%), (e) lack of management support (48%), (f) little or no recognition for achievements (46%), (g) insufficient resources (40%), (h) job insecurity (35%), (i) downsizing effects (33%), (j) technological advances (31%), and (k) increasingly diverse workforce (23%).

■ Violence in Health Care Settings

Between 1980 and 1990, 106 health care workers suffered violence-related deaths. In that period of time, at least 69 registered nurses were killed at work (Goodman, Jenkins, & Mercy, 1994). Workers' compensation data from the state of Washington showed that the six occupations with the largest number of assault-related claims were health and social services–related: nursing aids, health aids, health technicians, social workers, licensed practical nurses, and registered nurses (RNs) (Nelson & Kaufman, 1996). Nursing homes had the highest rate of any industry in assaults by people (Felton, 1997). Table 61.1 lists risk factors in the health care setting associated with work-related assaults.

A number of studies have focused on violence in nursing, finding that as many as 59% of nurses have reported being victims of physical abuse and as many as 97%, verbal abuse (Cox, 1991b; Felton, 1997). In one study, one of every three nurses in the sample had experienced some form of abuse during the previous 5 days (Graydon, Kasta, & Khan, 1994).

Verbal Abuse

This particular form of aggression is the most common and also most underreported in national statistics on workplace violence, largely because it does not result in physical harm or lost days from work. Defined as any communication that a person perceives to be a harsh, condemnatory attack on herself or himself, profes-

sionally or personally (Cox, 1991a), it is experienced by many hospital workers; but nurses experience it more often and from more sources. Braun, Christle, Walker, and Tiwanak (1991) found that 25% of nurses reported being verbally abused six or more times per month.

Verbal abuse comes from patients, their families, physicians, peers, and supervisors. Cox (1987, 1991b) found that physicians were the greatest source of verbal abuse for nursing staff, and Braun et al. (1991) reported that patients were the greatest source. Nurses in some clinical areas seem to be at particular risk for verbal abuse and violence: long-term care (Felton, 1997; Gates, 1998); critical care (Drury, 1997; Williams & Robertson, 1997); emergency rooms (Barlow & Rizzo, 1997; Robinson, 1998); psychiatric facilities (Warshaw & Messite, 1996); operating rooms (Larson & Martinson, 1990).

The impact of verbal abuse is significant. At one medical center, 96% of respondents had experienced verbal abuse and 20% said that it had caused them to resign from a previous job (Braun et al., 1991). In addition, nurses have reported that care has been compromised, errors have increased, productivity has declined, and nurses themselves have become physically ill (Cox, 1991b).

Violence and the Medical Staff

Reports of medical staff and students being abused are emerging in the literature. Silver and Glicken (1990) found that, by senior year, 81% of students had experienced abuse in medical school (e.g., verbal humiliation, intentional neglect, sexual harassment, and physical abuse). According to Barlow and Rizzo (1997), 59% reported having witnessed one or more physical attacks, and 38% reported having been attacked. Of 475 respondents, 470 reported having carried a gun themselves or knew someone in the hospital environment who did (staff, security, and students).

TABLE 61.1   Violence Risk Factors in Health Care

- Increased number of weapons being brought into health care facilities
- Police using hospitals to care for disturbed and violent individuals
- Increased number of mentally ill patients being released from hospitals and placed in community long-term or residential facilities
- Availability of money and drugs
- Unrestricted movement of the public
- Increased presence of gangs and drug or alcohol users
- Distraught family members
- Long waits in emergency rooms, admitting areas, or clinics
- Low staffing levels
- Isolated work during examinations and treatment
- Solo work outside the facility, especially when there is no back-up or ready assistance
- Lack of training to recognize and manage aggressive individuals
- Poorly lighted areas, especially parking areas
- Acceptance of violence as "part of the job"

Note: Adapted from *Guidelines for Preventing Workplace Violence for Health Care and Social Service Workers* (OSHA 3148-1996). Washington, DC: U.S. Department of Labor; and "Preventing Violence in Health Care Settings," by D. M. Gates, 1998, *Journal of Healthcare Safety Compliance and Infection Control*, p. 260.

■ Today's Health Care Environment

Challenges for Nursing

Today's health care workers are vulnerable not only to factors associated generally with workplace violence but also to increasing financial and performance pressures on organizations brought about by managed care. In addition, nurses encounter several other potentially life-threatening dangers on a daily basis: (a) latex allergies, (b) blood-borne pathogens, (c) back injuries, and (d) health care pollution. Nursing shortages and increased patient acuity affect nurses directly and often cause great anguish and frustration. Relationships with colleagues can be supportive or aggravating, as well. Oliver (1987) found that unacceptable

behaviors of coworkers bothered staff nurses more than any other factor in evaluating how the workday was going. Unacceptable behaviors included incompetent nursing care, use of poor nursing judgment, unwillingness to help coworkers, being uncooperative, or perceptions of unfair assignments.

In many settings, nurses are angry. Droppleman and Thomas (1996) conducted the Women's Anger Study, surveying more than 500 female participants, 75 being nurses. The nurses reported that their work environment was hostile, that working in a hospital was "like being in a war," and that they were "survivors" (1996, p. 1). Comments included that they were tired of "not being heard" (p. 2). Recent graduates described feeling unprepared for the clinical situations encountered. Relevant to the theme of this chapter, nurses described subtle and not-so-subtle forms of sabotage, ranging from cutting remarks to withdrawal of support.

According to Droppelman and Thomas (1996), many nurses turned their anger, however, into empowerment. This transition took the following forms.

1. They worked to channel their anger to develop their power.

2. They viewed anger as a protective and helpful ally, a helpful signal that their rights and values were perhaps being jeopardized.

3. They were politically active locally or nationally; they had forums for action.

4. They took action.

Opportunities for Nursing

Complete portrayal of the current health care environment must also include the fact that a number of exciting new opportunities are available to nurses. Advanced practice nurses are in increasing demand, new sites and models of care delivery are evolving, new partnerships with physicians and other health care providers are developing, and new technologies and therapies are expanding the tools by which nurses provide care. Health care is certainly no more dangerous than other settings. However, the extent of special consideration that nurses enjoyed in the past because they were caregivers may be eroding.

■ Forces for Change

For a variety of reasons, companies are finding it necessary to change and begin dealing with the issue of workplace violence. The most basic reason is that OSHA (1996), under the "General Duty Clause," of its guidelines, requires employers to provide workers with a place of employment free from recognized hazards likely to cause death or serious physical harm. However, reducing violence and danger in the workplace is not sufficient. To be viable,

organizations need to re-create themselves, provide workers with needed new skills, and establish systems for tackling workplace environment issues. These issues will have an impact on the following aspects of organizational life.

- *To be competitive:* Organizations will need to be able to connect with diverse customers, (a) partnering effectively with a wide array of constituents, (b) responding quickly to challenges and opportunities, and (c) differentiating themselves in markets.

- *To be accountable:* Organizations are expected to be socially and environmentally responsible for (a) enhancing the greater good, (b) regulatory and legal compliance, (c) promoting work–family–life balance, and (d) creating an internal community supportive of the organization and its objectives.

- *To improve productivity:* Organizations will have to find ways to (a) enhance quality while improving productivity, (b) establish internal partnerships and create effective teams, (c) achieve continuity within the workforce, (d) promote recruitment and retention of employees with key skills and knowledge, (e) manage training and recruitment costs, and (f) employ innovation as a strategic resource.

- *To address ethical issues:* DeMarco (1998) has stated that creating a new kind of an environment is an ethical issue, based on professional codes of ethics that define "the scope of activities or the nature of relationships that should exist individually between members and their clients. They also establish duties that professionals owe accountably to each other" (p. 131).

The second edition of the Standards of Clinical Nursing Practice of the American Nurses Association includes the standard: "The nurse interacts with, and contributes to the professional development of, peers and other health care providers as colleagues" (Disch et al., 1998, p. 13). Caring relates not only to patients, but nurses have an intraprofessional responsibility to communicate directly with each other in the workplace.

- *To reflect the "new spirit at work":* Leigh (1997) noted that, not only are customers demanding integrity, value, and quality, but employees also are searching for meaning in their work. "People come to work with more than their bodies and minds; they bring their individual talents and unique spirits" (p. 26).

Wheatley (1994) commented that

Our concept of organizations is moving away from the mechanistic creations that flourished in the age of bureaucracy. We have begun to speak in earnest of more fluid, organic structures, even of boundary-less organizations. We are refocusing on the deep longings we have for community, meaning and dignity in our organizational lives. (p. 13)

Although this workplace transformation appeals to many employees, it is not being embraced by all organizations. It brings disruption, expense, the unpredictability of people other than leaders being involved, and with unknowns and factors that cannot be easily controlled, which can be daunting to corporations. However, a growing body of research shows that organizations can be both good places to work and financially strong when they actively involve employees, establish channels for open communication, provide training and sufficient physical and mental resources, and develop mutual respect and trust (Good, 1998; Leigh, 1997; Miller, 1998). Whereas the old mission was "to increase shareholder wealth," M. L. Kerpan suggests that the new one should be "to produce a quality service or product that promotes the well-being of the community and to provide a working environment conducive to personal growth and creative productivity while increasing shareholder wealth" (Leigh, 1997, p. 27).

■ A Healthy Work Environment

A healthy work environment (HWE) is a work setting in which policies, procedures, and sys-

tems are designed so that employees are able to meet organizational objectives and achieve personal satisfaction in their work. Organizations approach this responsibility differently, but common elements can be found in what they do.

- *Administrative commitment:* This has to be visible, tangible, and ongoing, particularly from the Chief Executive Officer (CEO) or other leader of the group. Strategies for establishing the environment have to incorporate input from employees, but designation of this initiative as a priority within the organization has to come from senior management.

- *Opportunities for communication:* These need to be "regular, open, and candid" (Petry et al., 1996, p. 31) rather than one-way informational directives from management.

- *Employee involvement:* This can take many forms but Leigh (1997) notes that achieving a healthy work environment requires that there be worker engagement, a willingness to participate and cooperate, high levels of effort and attention to work, encouragement of improvement suggestions, and adaptability and willingness to change.

- *Training and education:* Managers and employees need new skills, among them communication, assertiveness and crisis intervention techniques. Organizations may need to help employees and leaders develop skills in treating people and their differences as assets. Miller (1998) said that embracing diversity is not enough. Diversity merely describes the makeup of a group. Inclusion is needed, which "describes which individuals are allowed to participate and are enabled to contribute fully in the group" (p. 151). Educating patients and families is seen as increasingly important so that they can contribute to a safe environment, develop realistic expectations of care, and become effective partners in the care process.

Strategies for Developing Worker-Friendly Workplaces

A growing body of literature describes strategies for developing worker-friendly workplaces (Gates, 1998; Good, 1998; Leigh,

---

TABLE 61.2   Strategies for Controlling Violence

- Communicate to employees, patients and customers that violence is not tolerated
- Develop reporting and tracking mechanisms
- Institute and train threat assessment and response teams
- Provide training for all employees and physicians
- Develop policies to decrease waiting times
- Ensure adequate staffing, especially during high-risk times, including access to back-up
- Strengthen policies for entry, access, movement of patients, families, staff throughout the institution
- Require all employees to wear name badges while on duty
- Develop a plan to treat aggressive clients and those likely to escalate to aggression
- Provide safe parking for employees, and support by security to these areas in off-periods
- Encourage and support home care employees to avoid or leave situations that appear threatening
- Conduct postincident evaluations of all situations in which employees have been abused or breaches of security have occurred

---

Note: Adapted from *Guidelines for Preventing Workplace Violence for Health Care and Social Service Workers* (OSHA 3148-1996). Washington, DC: U.S. Department of Labor; and "Preventing Violence in Health Care Settings," by D. M. Gates, 1998, *Journal of Healthcare Safety Compliance and Infection Control*, p. 260.

1997; Miller, 1998). Table 61.2 lists several strategies, adapted from OSHA's helpful publication, *Guidelines for Preventing Workplace Violence for Health Care and Social Service Workers* (Gates, 1998), that focus on minimizing violence, as a first step.

A number of nursing authors also have developed specific strategies for creating healthy work environments for nursing staff (Disch, 1996; Drury, 1997; Kreitzer, 1996; Kreitzer et al., 1997). A common premise for all these approaches is that preventing violence of any type is a necessary precursor to a healthy work environment—necessary, but not sufficient.

The Team

The impact of team effectiveness on the work setting is significant. A crucial aspect of the health care team is the nurse and physician relationship. The importance of extending the concept of a healthy work environment to medical staff cannot be overemphasized. In many health care organizations, employees are expected to function within certain institutional guidelines, whereas medical staff are exempt, the rationale being that medical staff are not employees of the organization. If the intent is to create a safe, effective work environment in which patients can receive care and where staff are respected and integrated as members of the team, medical staff must be actively included in the process. This change may mean that the medical staff has to collaborate in developing the organization's policies and practices and, necessarily are held accountable, or it may mean that the medical staff has to address the issue through medical staff bylaws.

When problems occur, staff need recourse for dealing with issues involving the medical staff. One approach is to develop something such as a Disruptive Conduct Policy. Table 61.3 presents an excerpt from a policy devel-

---

TABLE 61.3   Excerpt from the Disruptive Physician Policy

UMHC MEDICAL STAFF
DISRUPTIVE CONDUCT POLICY
DEFINITION

An occasional problem within medical staffs is the medical staff member whose conduct is so disruptive that it creates a work environment detrimental to the delivery of quality care, or has the potential to adversely affect the health or welfare of patients. Such unacceptable behavior can take many forms, e.g., tirades in the OR, abusive treatment of patients or employees, or disruption of meetings.

It is acknowledged that a hospital setting presents an especially stressful working environment, so outbursts or other misconduct that probably would not be tolerated elsewhere are often excused. That makes enforcement of a "disruptive conduct" policy particularly difficult. There are clearly limits to the tolerance, however.

That a medical staff member's behavior is unusual, unorthodox or different is not sufficient to justify disciplinary action. Unacceptable disruptive conduct can include, but is not limited to, such behavior as:

- Attacks leveled at other appointees to the medical staff which are personal, irrelevant, or go beyond the bounds of fair professional comment

- Impertinent and inappropriate comments written in patient medical records, or other official documents, impugning the quality of care in the hospital, or attacking particular medical staff members, hospital staff members, or hospital policy

- Non-constructive criticism, addressed to its recipient in such a way as to intimidate, undermine confidence, belittle, or to impute stupidity or incompetence

- Verbal abuse of employees

- Imposing idiosyncratic requirements on the hospital staff which have nothing to do with better patient care but serve only to burden the staff with 'special' techniques or procedures

- Abusive conduct, demeanor, or comments to patients or relatives of patients that cause complaint by the patient or relatives to the administration or medical staff.

Note: The balance of the policy, not included here, describes the procedure to be implemented once disruptive conduct has been identified as occurring.

Source: Fairview/University Medical Center, 1997.

---

oped by medical staff and hospital personnel at the former University of Minnesota Hospital and Clinic. The complete policy describes situations in which it would apply and the procedures to be followed; it would serve as a companion document to hospital policies that guide how employees work with each other.

Nursing Leadership

Kreitzer (1996) described special responsibilities that nurse administrators have in creating healthy work environments, among them

to (a) acknowledge the reality of the environment, (b) state and clarify expectations, (c) communicate and manage conflict, (d) provide skill-building opportunities, and (e) implement systems and structures that support a healthy work environment. These responsibilities are particularly important because, in many institutions, nursing is the profession or department that first realizes the need for improvement in the work environment and feels the keenest responsibility for bringing it about. Although a full institutional commitment greatly assists the process, the nursing leader may be the person in the organization who must launch the initiative for an area of responsibility and then work to extend it to the rest of the organization through a senior management role.

Nursing directors and managers are essential in this process. Without their active and ongoing involvement, such an initiative will fail. This task requires (a) daily modeling of desired behaviors; (b) developing their own new skills; (c) providing environments that are safe for dialogue; (d) resolving disagreements and conflict; (e) establishing effective interpersonal relationships with physicians and other department heads; and (f) being willing to learn, change, and grow as the process unfolds.

■ A Case Study

Background

On January 1, 1997, the University of Minnesota Hospital and Clinic (UMHC) merged with Fairview Riverside Medical Center (FRMC) to become Fairview-University Medical Center (FUMC), a new entity with two campuses separated by the Mississippi River. The health care environment in the Twin Cities and state of Minnesota that forced this merger is a market heavily based on managed care, overbedded, and experiencing dwindling support from state and federal government for education and research. The merger combined a tertiary research and teaching hospital with a large community hospital.

As often happens with mergers, many employees opted to leave. Members of previously stable work teams were replaced by employees who were unfamiliar with their new areas, the parent organization (Fairview Health Services), or the new entity, FUMC. For nursing, restructuring and rebidding required by union contract (FRMC had a unionized nursing staff; UMHC did not) prompted additional nurses to leave, although actual layoffs were minimal. Thus most work teams were either directly or secondarily affected by the restructuring and rebidding and by the inevitable reorganization required when two very diverse organizations integrate.

Chartering the Initiative

For many within the organization, extensive changes threatened whatever level of healthy work environment existed prior to the merger. A goal of the new organization was to become the "employer of choice" within the region, a daunting task. Building on earlier work done within UMHC and FRMC, a Healthy Work Environment Task Force was sponsored by the Vice Presidents of Patient and Family Services and Professional Services; this unit subsequently was chartered by the organization's Quality Council, an interdisciplinary oversight group whose membership included medical staff, institutional leaders, managers, and clinicians.

A key difference in this initiative was that it was to focus not only on nursing, but also on the local work team. A core assumption was that a well-functioning team was needed so that nurses could do their best work. Achieving a healthy environment for nurses within context of a dysfunctional larger group would be less successful.

Task Force Membership and Work

Members of the Task Force included a social worker, a nurse manager, the two vice presidents, an environmental services supervisor, a dietary supervisor, and two organizational learning specialists. Membership on the Task Force was selected so as to (a) be diverse, (b) represent individuals in roles that may not provide care but have a distinct impact on daily operations of a patient care area, and (c) provide ongoing involvement and support by senior management. The fundamental belief was that a work environment that assisted teams in working effectively in the new organization was crucial to achieving the organizational goal of becoming the employer of choice.

After reviewing the literature, Task Force members in groups of three visited several patient care areas within the organization. The purposes of these visits were to (a) gather input from employees on what a healthy work environment looks like; (b) obtain nonverbal cues from the work environments as to whether the work area exhibited a healthy tone and whether the individuals in it functioned as a team; and (c) enable Task Force team members to view assessments through eyes of coworkers with different perspectives (one group, for example, consisted of the Vice President of Patient and Family Services, an organizational learning specialist, and the supervisor from environmental services).

Task Force members pulled this information together, identified elements and behaviors essential to a healthy work environment, and developed criteria defining who was on the team in a patient care unit (e.g., a unit on which physical therapists (PTs) cared for many patients would consider PTs to be essential team members); another patient care area might consider those PTs to be consultants. The roles of primary physician and medical house staff in this process were discussed. It was decided, for this particular effort, that the focus first would be on engaging employees, as the project was being created as it unfolded. In addition, because of the ongoing work of integrating the organizations, FUMC already had numerous work groups in which physicians were actively involved in working with hospital staff to create meaningful change.

The Pilot

The patient care unit selected as pilot was the Neuroscience Unit on one of the campuses of FUMC. Goals were to (a) improve efficiency of the team, (b) expand the notion of who was a member of the unit, and (c) welcome new members to the unit. Feelings of isolation and lack of a cohesive sense of team could lower commitment and involvement in ensuring smooth operations of the unit. Particular attention was paid to including staff members who were crucial to effective operation of the unit but were traditionally on the periphery of former definitions of "team." For example, environmental service workers did not feel part of the hospital team and often felt anonymous. These workers were not comfortable sharing physical space that was intended for breaks or lunch in the unit, nor were they comfortable joining in celebrations or other unit events. This situation was not merely perceptual on the part of these workers; at times, nursing staff would regard the break room as their own.

Because a Neuroscience unit was moving to a newly remodeled unit within the hospital, the move date was used as the "kick-off" for Healthy Work Environment initiatives. Unit staff were surveyed regarding assessment of their current working environment in terms of the recently established goals.

- Coworkers know my name and use it.
- The work environment is welcoming.
- The work environment is respectful.
- I can share common space with rest of the unit staff.
- I feel part of the team.

On the day of the move, all unit staff, including social workers, dietary, environmental services, RNs, nursing assistants, and pharmacists were given "Move Survival Kits." The kits contained sweets for energy, a "stress indicator," tips for reducing stress, and a small toy and were well received. All team members were photographed, with photos and names being placed on a bulletin board in the corridor that welcomed patients and staff to the unit (a bulletin board formerly just for nursing staff). The phone or pager numbers for all team members were written on the unit's greaseboard, which had previously only contained numbers of the professional staff. The expectation that all staff would have clearly visible name tags was reinforced.

Using Fairview's organizational values of dignity, integrity, service, and compassion as a framework, unit's members (the team) were asked to develop their own healthy work environment principles. Being respectful, supportive, and having open communication were three that were highly valued by the team. A unit-based HWE group was formed, and the following activities were held during the next several months.

- Relaxation tapes were placed on the unit for "self-care" breaks.
- Healthy work environment issues were on the agenda of monthly staff meetings.
- Unit staff participated in "Service is the Center," workshop sessions on customer service.
- Monthly potlucks were planned, as sharing food is a highly valued way of connecting socially. This activity can be a challenge because not all employees can afford to bring in extra food; a small amount in the budget for employee activities helped offset some of these costs.
- A Kudos board was placed in the common area for team members to recognize and appreciate each other.
- Short biosketches were done on team members to help them get to know each other.

One year after the kickoff, members of the unit staff informally judged it to be a success. Commitment to each other is manifested in the smooth operation of this large surgical unit and in the positive attitudes that are visible. The unit is highly respected for its achievements within the organization: The team is seen as effective, flexible, and respectful. Next steps include resurveying staff regarding perceptions of the work environment, and rolling the concepts out to other areas of FUMC.

■ *Concluding Statement*

We cannot change the direction of the wind, but we can adjust the sails. (Anonymous)

Unrelenting pressures within health care will continue and perhaps intensify, given impending changes related to Medicare reimbursement. Furthermore, health care will continue to be influenced by forces at work within the greater society. However, administrators, nursing leaders, and staff can influence the environment where they do business and provide care. In fact, accountable leaders must find ways to do so. Eliminating negative behaviors of individuals and counterproductive systems of organizations that foster violence is an important first step. Working together to achieve organizational goals and create environments that promote health and healing for patients, their families, and the workforce is essential.

■ References

American Psychiatric Association. (1994). *APA fact sheet: Violence and mental illness.* Washington, DC: Author.

Bachman, R. (1994, September). Violence and threat in the workplace. *Exchange, 4–5.*

Barlow, C. B., & Rizzo, A. G. (1997). Violence against surgical residents. *Western Journal of Medicine, 167*(2), 74–78.

Bensley, L., Nelson, N., Kaufman, J., Silverstein, B., & Kalat, J. (1993). *Study of assaults on staff in Washington State psychiatric hospitals.* (Safety and Health Assessment and Research for Prevention). Olympia: Washington State Department of Labor and Industries.

Braun, K., Christle, D., Walker, D., & Tiwanak, G. (1991). Verbal abuse of nurses and non-nurses. *Nursing Management, 22*(3), 72–76.

Bureau of Labor Statistics. (1994). *Violence in the workplace comes under closer scrutiny.* Washington, DC: U.S. Department of Labor.

Center for Mental Health Services. (1994). *Forum report: Preventing violence in the workplace.* Rockville, MD: Substance Abuse and Mental Health Services, U.S. Department of Health and Human Services.

Cole, L. L., Grubb, P. L., Sauter, S. L., Swanson, N. G., & Lawless, P. (1997). Psychosocial correlates of harassment, threats and fear of violence in the workplace. *Scandinavian Journal of Work Environment and Health, 23,* 450–457.

Cox, H. (1987). Verbal abuse in nursing: Report of a study. *Nursing Management, 18*(11), 47–50.

Cox, H. (1991a). Verbal abuse nationwide, Part I. *Nursing Management, 22*(2), 32–35.

Cox, H. (1991b). Verbal abuse nationwide, Part II. *Nursing Management, 22*(3), 66–69.

DeMarco, R. F. (1998). Caring to confront in the workplace: An ethical perspective for nurses. *Nursing Outlook, 46*(3), 130–135.

Disch, J. (1996). Building strategic linkages for nursing. In J. Disch (Ed.), *The managed care challenge for nurse executives* (pp. 35–50). Chicago: American Organization of Nurse Executives (AONE)/American Hospital Association (AHA).

Disch, J., Ballard, K., Harkness, G. A., Huser, M., O'Connor, K., Peters, D. A., Pires, M., & Schuring, L. (Eds.). (1998). *Standards of clinical nursing practice* (2nd ed). Washington, DC: American Nurses Association.

Droppleman, P. G., & Thomas, S. P. (1996). Anger in nurses: Don't lose it, use it. *American Journal of Nursing: Contjinuing Education Series,* 1–11.

Drury, T. (1997). Recognizing the potential for violence in the ICU. *Dimensions of Critical Care Nursing, 16*(6), 314–323.

Felton, J. S. (1997). Violence prevention at the health care site. *Occupational Medicine, 12*(4), 701–715.

Fitzgerald, S., Dienemann, J., & Cadorette, M. F. (1998). Domestic violence in the workplace, *AAOHN Journal* (American Association of Occupational Health Nursing), *46*(7), 345–353.

Gates, D. M. (1998, August). Preventing violence in health care settings. *Journal of Healthcare Safety Compliance and Infection Control,* 259–265.

Good, W. A. (1998). Developing a worker-friendly workplace. *Association Management, 50,* 30–36.

Goodman, R. A., Jenkins, E. L., & Mercy, J. A. (1994). Workplace-related homicide among health care workers in the United States. *Journal of the American Medical Association, 272,* 1686–1688.

Graydon, J., Kasta, W., & Khan, P. (1994). Verbal and physical abuse of nurses. *Canadian Journal of Nursing Administration, 7*(4), 70–89.

Jenkins, E. L. (1996). *Violence in the workplace: Risk factors and prevention strategies.* (Department of Health and Human Services, NIOSH [National Institute of Occupational Safety and Health], Publication Number 96-100). Washington, DC: U.S. Government Printing Office.

Kreitzer, M. J. (1996). Creating a healthy work environment. In J. Disch (Ed.), *The managed care challenge for nurse executives* (pp. 65–74). Chicago: American Organization of Nurse Executives (AONE)/American Hospital Association (AHA).

Kreitzer, M. J., Wright, D., Hamlin, C., Towey, S., Marko, M., & Disch, J. (1997). Creating a healthy work environment in the midst of organizational change and transition. *Journal of Nursing Administration, 27*(6), 35–41.

Larson, B. A., & Martinson, D. J. (1990). Words can hurt. *AORN Journal* (Association of Operating Room Nursing), *52*(6), 1238–1241.

Lawless, P. (1993). *Fear and violence in the workplace.* Minneapolis: Northwestern National Life Insurance Company.

Leigh, P. (1997). The new spirit at work. *Training and Development, 51*(3), 26–33.

Lipscomb, J. A., & Love, C. C. (1992). Violence toward health care workers: An emerging occupational hazard. *AAOHN Journal* (American Association of Occupational Health Nursing), *40,* 219–228.

Miller, F. A. (1998). Strategic culture change: The door to achieving high performance and inclusion. *Public Personnel Management, 27*(2), 151–160.

Nelson, N. A., & Kaufman, J. D. (1996). Fatal and nonfatal injuries related to violence in Washington workplaces, 1992. *American Journal of Industrial Medicine, 30,* 438–446.

Neuman, J. H., & Baron, R. A. (1998). Workplace violence and workplace aggression: Evidence concerning specific forms, potential causes, and preferred targets. *Journal of Management, 24*(3), 391–420.

Occupational Safety and Health Administration. (1996). *Guidelines for preventing workplace violence among health care and social service workers.* (OSHA 3148-1996). Washington, DC: U.S. Department of Labor.

Oliver, N. R. (1987). *Processing unacceptable behaviors of co-workers: A naturalistic study of nurses at work.* Unpublished doctoral dissertation, New York University.

Petry, E. S., Mujica, A. E., & Vickery, D. M. (1996, Fall). Sources and consequences of workplace pressure: Increasing risk of unethical and illegal business practices. *Business and Society Review,* 25–30.

Robinson, K. S. (1998). Nurses caught in the crossfire: Assisting patients outside. *Journal of Emergency Nursing, 24*(5), 380–381.

Silver, H. K., & Glicken, A. D. (1990). Medical student abuse: Incidence, severity and significance. *Journal of the American Medical Association, 264,* 527–532.

Simonowitz, J. A. (1996). Health care workers and workplace violence. Violence in the workplace: State of the art reviews. *Occupational Medicine, 11,* 277–291.

Warshaw, L. J., & Messite, J. (1996). Workplace violence: Preventive and interventive strategies. *Journal of Occupational and Environmental Medicine, 38*(10), 993–1006.

Wheatley, M. (1994). *Leadership and the new science.* San Francisco: Berrett-Koehler.

Williams, M. L., & Robertson, K. (1997). Workplace violence: Prevalence, prevention, and first-line interventions. *Critical Care Nursing Clinics of North America, 9*(2), 221–229.

■ *Editor's Questions for Discussion*

What situational variables contribute to conflict and potential aggression in health care settings? What patterns regarding violence in the workplace exist? How might such data be predictors of abuse in health care settings? Discuss causes for assault in health care settings? How can verbal abuse be prevented or curbed among professionals and their relationships? What distinctions exist between acceptable verbal corrections and verbal abuse in health care? How have increased opportunities for nurses also increased stress and conflict? What factors increase pressures in the workplace? How effective are conflict management workshops and training for health care personnel?

When perceptions differ among personnel, how can accountability, rewards, and admonitions for behavior be equitable? What positive reinforcement can be implemented to foster equity? How do nursing leaders and administrators influence the work environment?

Discuss advantages and disadvantages of fluid, organic, and boundary-less structures in organizations. How do points made by Porter-O'Grady (Chapter 55), Pinkerton (Chapter 56), Conger (Chapter 58), Dienemann, Campbell, and Agnew (Chapter 59), and Thomas (Chapter 60) apply to creating healthy environments? What evaluation mechanisms might have been used to evaluate formally the changes described in the case study presented?

To what extent do organizations that you are most knowledgeable about have healthy work environment elements, as identified by Disch? Indicate specific suggestions for correcting or improving the organizations you cite. What additional strategies may create healthy work environments? Define your own principles for healthy work environments. Specify means to evaluate environmental "health."

62

Nurse Executive Practice for the New Millennium

Margaret L. McClure, EdD, RN, FAAN

Considering the future of nurse executive practice would be literally impossible without acknowledging that the health care world is undergoing change at a truly unprecedented rate. That fact alone makes prediction exceedingly difficult and anxiety a constant companion for most of us as nurses.

Adding to the disquiet are the following findings of a VHA (1995) study:

In working with health care organizations undergoing major change initiatives, we have discovered two important issues:

1. Organizational change—even proactive, positive change—is never easy. It requires team-

work, objectivity, and most importantly, leadership.

2. "Leading the charge" has often fallen squarely on the shoulders of two individuals: the CEO and the nurse executive (p. 7).

Such responsibility is awesome in many respects. Yet, it also carries wonderful intellectual challenges and the opportunity to help craft the shape of care delivery in the 21st century.

The idea of "leading the charge" might be addressed by examining the challenges that nursing faces at three interrelated levels: the health care system, individual organizations, and the profession of nursing.

■ *The Health Care System*

At the outset, I believe that changes in the health care system have been driven by economic conditions that have confronted the United States and, indeed, the entire world. The continuous upward spiraling of health care costs, in the face of such an environment, created a situation requiring drastic steps. Led by corporate bodies that pay the nation's medical bills, managed care was born.

Managed care entered health care markets in the United States at vastly different rates of speed. In the early 1990s, the University Hospital Consortium commissioned a study that explicated four stages of managed care development. These stages ranged from low to high penetration. Researchers were able to place all consortium members' cities within one of the stages. More important, they described this model as evolutionary and predicted that all U.S. health care would pass through these stages, moving gradually (or not so gradually) from Stage I to Stage IV.

Those involved in the continuing study of this framework readily admit that they do not know and cannot predict the stage or stages beyond Stage IV. Rather, there is a fairly widespread belief that the model may represent a transition into an entirely different system of health care financing. In keeping with that notion, a number of authorities in the field have predicted that the experience with managed care so far will inevitably lead to a national, single-payor system (Look at it this way, 1996).

A Shift in Focus

Amid all this uncertainty, the following concept emerges. Those of us who are providers increasingly will be forced to shift our focus from individual patient care to the care of populations and from episodic care to the continuum of care needed by the people we serve. It seems to me that this is the crux of the revolution occurring in health care, a revolution that

most of us in nursing should embrace with outstretched arms because it is part of a philosophy that we have long valued. With this shift in focus comes a concomitant shift to additional responsibilities outside the acute care hospital and into a variety of community settings. Why? Because responsibility for populations brings into sharp relief the serious and long-term link between cost and quality. With this recognition comes the need also to recognize that

1. populations are not homogenous, and subpopulations often have special needs that must be addressed (e.g., certain diseases are specific to particular ethnic groups, such as Mediterranean Jews, African Americans, etc.); and

2. nonusers of services often become high-cost users, over time.

What is important to understand is the fact that prevention, screening, and early detection approaches have long been valued by all health care providers, but chiefly in the abstract. We actually have very little experience in developing the strategies and incentives to deliver the goods, especially in a cost-effective manner.

Furthermore, human nature being what it is, incentives will be an important part of any strategy. We all know registered nurses who fail to have regular pap smears and mammograms. We all know physicians who smoke. Access to primary care and patient education is only the beginning of effective, quality care delivery models. As we begin to share the financial risk for populations, we will be forced to tackle these difficult issues. We are moving into new aspects of the health care business, with very new work involved.

The Role of the Nurse Executive

Within the context of this radically changing environment, an examination of the role of the nurse executive is interesting. What appears to be happening is movement in two opposite directions.

First, and foremost, is the model in which nurse executives assume added responsibilities, beyond nursing, for a variety of services. New titles reflecting this change have become commonplace (e.g., Vice President for Patient Care). In each instance the array of departments coming under the executive's purview differs, depending as we would expect, on the politics and the needs of the organization. Less common, but increasingly seen, is the model in which nurse executives retain their nursing leadership role while also serving as the chief operating officer for the organization.

I suggest two major reasons for this expansion of responsibilities. First, our backgrounds in nursing provide us with a unique and thorough understanding of the way in which hospitals operate. Elsewhere (McClure, 1991), I have labeled our overall coordinating function as "integrator," a subset of the nurse's role. Due to this integrator experience, we are particularly knowledgeable about contributions of each discipline and department as well as interfaces needed to create the totality of patient care. We are the people who make the patient care quilt out of a large array of disparate patches.

Second, we are the only clinical discipline that has systematically attempted to educate our practitioners for administration. This approach was true throughout the 20th century and occurred at virtually every level of intensity, from inservice to doctoral preparation. And many of us are very good at it!

One word of caution is necessary. We are beginning to see a trend toward the elimination of both the word *nurse* and the designation *R.N.* for many top nursing administration positions, which should give us cause for concern. It is too easy to be lulled into complacency on this issue. We need to rethink our titles so that they actually reflect our major responsibility for giving leadership to the practice of nursing. The addition of our own professional identification focuses others on the centrality of nursing within the institution or the health system. Further, it makes clear the fact that this is a *nursing* role.

I am aware that some of my colleagues believe that the word *nurse* has taken on a negative connotation within their organizations and that they can be more influential if they remain silent on the issue. I suggest that this is actually symptomatic of our substantial power and threat to others.

In stark contrast to instances of expansion of nurse executive roles are situations in which the nurse executive position has been eliminated altogether. Although these occurrences are not common, rumors persist on the grapevine that such changes are taking place. This type of restructuring is unlikely to gain in popularity or be long-lived in those instances in which it has occurred. Witness the striking example of the unfortunate set of chemotherapy incidents and errors at one of our nation's leading cancer institutes. When the state health department investigated, it discovered that the institute had been without a nurse executive for more than a year. A major part of the remedial action was the requirement to hire a nurse executive. What became apparent was that nursing leadership at the executive level ensures the provision of policies and procedures necessary to safeguard patients (Dana Farber bolsters RN leadership, 1995).

■ Individual Organizations

Cost Reduction Responsibilities

Moving from the macro level to the organizational level, we can see that the need for us to assist in cost reductions at the institutional level will continue unabated for the foreseeable future. Thus we also will continue to deliberate and experiment with the use of unlicensed assistive personnel (UAPs). Needless to say, this must be done with a rationale based on a clear definition of the role of the nurse in relation to the population of patients being served. This means that our own vision and understanding of essential, professional components of practice are identified and made explicit to nursing and non-nursing leaders alike.

There already is evidence that the use of UAPs may not succeed to the extent originally thought possible. For example, an article in the *Pittsburgh Post Gazette* reported on one Texas hospital's negative experience, quoting an administrator as saying, "We lost patients. We lost nurses. And we lost doctors. That's a catastrophe. . . . That's going to close your doors over time" (Twedt, 1996, p. 14). Eventually the hospital realized its error and began to reverse the situation by hiring more registered nurses, after which admissions increased dramatically.

Our professional literature reflects concern about the impact of UAPs, although the research to date leaves a great deal to be desired. Krapohl and Larson (1996) summarized the work as follows:

> Studies were frequently anecdotal in nature, conducted at a single institution, lacked comparison groups, used instruments of untested reliability and validity, and were of small sample size. . . . Nor were these studies sufficiently rigorous in nature to measure costs, since a number of multiple variables such as increased supervisory personnel, re-admission rates, length of stay, and training costs were not addressed. (p. 108)

Clearly we need valid and reliable data to guide our efforts so that major damage is not done to patients and their care. The cost-effectiveness of such efforts likewise needs to be demonstrated.

One of the great benefits of expanded responsibilities that most nurse executives now carry is the opportunity to influence resource utilization decisions more broadly within their institutions. Evidence exists that decreased lengths of stay create the real home runs in decreasing costs. Some of the barriers to achieving minimal lengths of stay can be found at the intersections between departments and services. Interdisciplinary teamwork is clearly the order of the day for tackling these problems and devising creative new approaches to solutions.

New Corporate Structure and Responsibilities

The foregoing represents the old work of our organizations. The new work involves movement from single to multiple institution corporations or systems. Mergers, acquisitions, and partnerships—heretofore unheard of in healthcare—are suddenly on everyone's agenda. We all are scrambling hard to determine what this means for our respective settings. With all this activity, it seems evident that very few of us will continue to work in the same corporate structure that we do today.

As these developments occur, many nurse executives will be called on to assist in the development and elaboration of their systems. Central to our contributions will be the challenge of creating a truly integrated care delivery model. We have an unprecedented opportunity to advocate for patients and their families, using our nursing-based knowledge and experience as a foundation for the design and implementation of the new systems.

Once again, we find ourselves uniquely qualified to guide this new work. Although that may seem like a highly biased statement, the same case was made by Dr. Bernadine Healy, when she was the Dean of the Ohio State University School of Medicine and former Director of the National Institutes of Health. In her keynote speech (September 18, 1996) at ceremonies marking the 10th anniversary of the National Institute for Nursing Research, Dr. Healy acknowledged nursing's special expertise in relation to the new environment. Specifically, she alluded to our tradition of concerns related to continuity of care, patients' rights and responsibilities, community and chronic care, and the area of prevention—where we have had long involvement. Definitely we have valuable contributions to make as our organizations reconfigure and redesign themselves to meet the challenges of vertical integration.

The Corporate Level Nurse Executive

In keeping with new structures, the question of a corporate role for the nurse executive will undoubtedly arise in many of our situations. This role represents an interesting opportunity, but it is also one that requires careful examination and thought.

Is there or should there be a corporate nursing role? On the one hand, my immediate reaction is to answer in the affirmative, and that may be correct. On the other hand, there are very likely definitive differences between the new corporate roles and those that we have known in the past—differences that may not be immediately apparent.

Perhaps the most important issue is the structure of the position in regard to line versus staff authority. The line approach is rarely attempted, principally because, like politics, administration works best when it is local. In successful multihospital systems, site nursing administrators report to site hospital administrators. Efforts to impose a higher authority from "headquarters"—even in a matrix form— usually have disastrous effects. Thus the corporate role for the nurse executive is likely to be a staff position. Its responsibilities most often involve general concerns such as quality oversight, continuing education, and Joint Commission on Accreditation of Healthcare Organizations (JCAHO) preparation.

Most practicing nurse executives are really line administrators at heart and do not find the transition to a staff function easy (Davidson,

1996). The latter involves using one's influence quite differently and is likely to prove more frustrating than rewarding in many circumstances. However, there is an exciting role opportunity regarding the new work of the corporation that can capitalize on our talents.

As our organizations move into health delivery systems, nurse executives have important contributions to make in structuring the components involved. First, there is the work of identifying the essential elements of a vertically integrated system. Second, appropriate nursing components for each of these elements must be devised. Third, these elements need to be coordinated so that they are both efficient and user-friendly (for the patient). And last, means by which "best practices" can be shared across sites must be devised so that quality is enhanced for patients and their families.

Work related to the elements of the system will vary in intensity, depending on the setting, what is already available in the community, and past relationships. To some extent, this task becomes a question of the traditional "buy or build" approach. For example, substantial home care services will be needed. Whether the new system will be adequately served by the services currently available will need to be assessed. Contracting with an existing agency may prove more advantageous than creating a new and separate service. Like each of the other essential elements, providing home care will involve consideration of future patient needs, geographic distribution, financial feasibility, and ability to link information systems. It is in this kind of work that the purely administrative aspects of nursing intersect with the clinical and, I would submit, where nurse executives can make critical contributions.

Another role for nurses involved in corporate positions has become apparent, namely, that of representation. As the system begins to deal with those who contract for services from the organization, nurse executives have proven to be highly valued participants. Noteworthy has been our ability to translate requirements of our customers into program and vice versa (i.e., to help the consumer understand the programs available).

Perhaps the most important work for the nurse executive at the corporate level is related to standards of practice. For a system actually to function as one corporation, physicians, patients, and families must be assured that comparable levels of nursing care will be provided across all sites. Although it is a tall order, it may, however, prove to be the most positive outcome of the merging of institutions and agencies.

Creation of networks affords new and formalized opportunities for nurses engaged in various aspects of patient care to come together. Sharing best practices permits learning from one another and developing evidence-based protocols and guidelines. This approach is particularly beneficial to small institutions with little or no access to specialists and no advanced practice nurses on their own staffs. It can provide them with a level of expertise that enhances both quality of patient care and growth and development of the nurses involved. It has the potential for a real win–win situation.

For example, patient education materials can be developed jointly and shared among agencies and sites in a system. There are enormous benefits to this approach. More and better tools can be made available because every entity does not need to create its own package for a particular disease or health need. Pooling of resources within the system also is likely to improve both process and content. That adds considerably to the quality of the products. Perhaps most important, representation of the various components across the health care continuum creates a sharing that ensures continuity of care. Thus a patient who is newly diagnosed with asthma is taught from identically the same materials in the hospital, in the home, and in the outpatient setting.

From the foregoing, it should be evident that the corporate role for nurse executives is still in its formative stages. What a wonderful time! We are more able today than we have ever been to do what role theorists would call role-making, as opposed to role-taking (Hardy & Conway, 1978). In other words, now is the time for us to seize important and influential opportunities for ourselves and for nurse executives of the future.

■ The Profession

As we nurse executives busy ourselves with this brave new world of health care, it is important that we not overlook or minimize our role in leading the profession. The future for nursing is, in my opinion, very bright. Yet we do have pessimists in our ranks who do not share my outlook. I would suggest that our differences really relate to a certain myopic viewpoint that has led many to conclude that the job market for nursing is in serious decline. The data, however, indicate that nothing could be farther from the truth.

Nursing Workforce Issues

We are, of course, experiencing continuous changes in professional nursing positions in inpatient facilities. These involve

- decreased lengths of stay in inpatient facilities,
- increased use of UAPs, and
- elimination of middle-management positions.

Most of us are keenly aware of these factors and understand both the causes and the consequences very well. Even in the mid 1990s, however, the end result was not a decrease in the number of nursing jobs available, but rather a decrease in the growth rate of jobs. We were still adding positions every year, but the slope of the upward curve was less steep (Salary slowdown, 1999). That slowing of growth turned out to be short-lived and somewhat of an anomaly.

In addition to traditional inpatient positions, enormous numbers of opportunities continue to become rapidly available in areas such as

- outpatient facilities, including surgical, oncology, and maternity centers;
- private practice; and
- managed care.

Moreover, the need for advanced practice nurses, especially nurse practitioners, is likely to skyrocket over the next few years. It will be spurred by the inexorable downsizing of residency programs for the medical profession. Obviously, nurses will be called on to fill the void. As a result, it will be difficult to supply the demand for acute care nurse practitioners prepared to serve in intensive care units (ICUs), operating rooms (ORs) as first assistants, emergency rooms (ERs), and so forth.

Preparation for Practice

This optimistic view of the future carries with it several issues that the nursing profession must confront. First and foremost, it is time for us to finally put the "entry into practice" debate to bed. The jobs that will be available to nurses in the future will require special knowledge and skills, for which the baccalaureate degree will only be beginning preparation. One vision that I would propose is two levels of nursing workers: professional nurses prepared at baccalaureate and/or higher degree levels, and UAPs, prepared in on-the-job training programs. This dichotomy would clarify roles and could be achieved through hiring practices and system design changes.

The second and also a critical issue is that of preparing new graduates for the new market-

place. We will continue to experience a terrific imbalance. We will have new graduates and we will have new jobs, but the former will be unable to fill the latter. All the newly created and expanded positions will be characterized by high degrees of independence and autonomy. Many schools are now attempting to confront this problem by infusing their curriculum with additional courses and field work in assessment, use of technology, and community nursing (Noble, Redmond, Williams, & Langley, 1996). Such efforts are certainly laudatory but probably insufficient. A cursory glance at the want ads for nurses in any periodical tells the story. Many attractive positions are offered, but they require a minimum of 1 year's experience, often with a stated preference that the experience be in medical–surgical nursing.

In an effort to deal with this twist in the supply and demand equation, the NYU Medical Center embarked on an exciting program. It created a nurse residency, which is 1 year in length and provides specific, intensive experience and education for new graduates during the course of their first year. Some of the content is clinical in nature. Some deals with such universal issues as interdisciplinary collaboration (especially with physicians), conflict management, and career planning.

Each resident works with a mentor, meeting on a weekly basis. This approach has proven central to the success of the program. The mentor is an experienced nurse assigned to the same unit and plays a role that is a combination of teacher, counselor, and confidant. In all the evaluations conducted of the residency over the years, the mentorship consistently receives the highest marks of all the elements in the program.

At the conclusion of the year, a recognition ceremony is held at which certificates are given to the residents. Most continue on the staff of the Medical Center. However, whether they pursue a career in acute care or in other settings, there is evidence that the residency has enabled them to develop beyond the novice stage. Such a strong foundation creates a safer practitioner for patients and a springboard for meaningful career opportunities for the new nurse.

Because of the success of the program, it has been suggested that such an approach might well become a national model and perhaps even a requirement in the future. Obviously the precedent is in medicine. Historically, graduates of medical schools were permitted to obtain a license and begin practice immediately upon graduation, but that has not been the case for many years. The requirement for postgraduate training for physicians prior to taking the licensing boards has been in place since early in the 20th century. Perhaps it is time that we too consider introducing our own postgraduate residency as a prerequisite to taking state boards.

Mentoring

Another developmental issue that we need to confront is more broad-scale mentoring, particularly as it relates to the concept of "career." For nearly 100 years, there has been such a plentitude of jobs that most nurses have been able to give little or no thought to designing their careers. The 21st century is not likely to provide this luxury, however, and we as leaders need to take our roles as mentors more seriously. We also need to make career counseling more widespread so that greater numbers of nurses become sensitized to their needs in this regard.

As a part of nurse executive mentoring efforts, two areas of the profession stand out as especially needy. First, we desperately require more nurses who are prepared to manage data and assist in the development of outcome measures. This need exists at the institutional level, at the system level, and at the national level. Every aspect of health care delivery today is being challenged to provide data, especially

outcome data. Many new groups and agencies, including health maintenance organizations (HMOs), are hungry for measures that will support their decision-making processes. Nursing variables cannot afford to be left out of this effort.

The second needy area is nursing administration. For a short period of time, this specialty seemed to be gaining in respect and credibility. But that was short-lived and once again we see a decline in interest in graduate work in administration. Rather, preparation in advanced practice has taken the spotlight. We need to steer our brightest and best toward careers in administration so that a leadership void is not created in an era in which leadership was never more important.

Preparation for Nursing Administration

Beyond mentoring, of course, is the question of formal preparation for tomorrow's administrators and executives. Because we will be required to be much more conceptual in our approach, this matter merits serious attention.

Many of our best potential executives are preparing in graduate programs for advanced practice roles. It is important, however, that some move into organizational leadership positions as they mature in their careers. Experience has begun to indicate that educational preparation for transition into administration will most likely occur in postmaster's or doctoral programs. A proportion of those who go into advanced practice roles should be expected and encouraged to move into managerial and executive positions.

Such an approach may ultimately serve patients and health care best. Knowledgeable clinicians are clearly well positioned to give leadership to a practice discipline. They have the credibility that comes with experience and expertise. Added to their clinical competence and credibility, graduate-level work related to finance, organizational theory, and human resources will serve to strengthen immeasurably the decisions they make at the executive level of future organizations.

In future corporate structures, as we merge our interests with those of other disciplines, many of whom may have been former competitors, we need to understand the difficulties we face in this new millennium. Because much of our knowledge comes from the world of animals, it is probably instructive to look at the behavior of lions. These wonderful felines live in packs called "prides," which are totally closed. If a lion or lioness from outside the pack attempts to join the pride, he or she will be seriously injured or even killed. The fact that they are of the same species is of no consequence.

We will undoubtedly witness a great deal of lionlike behavior in our merger experiences. The signing of legal documents is no guarantee that members of our "pride" will not attack other members. All of us in administrative positions need to consider what actions we might take to counteract the animal instincts of ourselves and others in our organizations. This may prove to be the biggest challenge that we face in the new millennium.

■ Concluding Statement

As we enter the 21st century, health care is facing a plethora of difficult issues and most experts are hard-pressed to predict the shape that the delivery system will take, even in the near future. Yet this will undoubtedly be one of the most exciting and intellectually stimulating times to be in nurse executive practice. It is a time to redefine, to reform, and to redesign ourselves so that those in the nursing profession and, more important, our patients are the beneficiaries.

■ References

Dana Farber bolsters RN leadership. (1995). *American Journal of Nursing, 95*(12), 64, 66.

Davidson, D. R. (1996). The role of the nurse executive in the corporatization of health care. *Nursing Administration Quarterly, 20*(2), 49–79.

Hardy, M. E., & Conway, M. E. (1978). *Role theory: Perspectives for health professionals.* New York: Appleton-Century-Crofts.

Krapohl, G. L., & Larson, E. (1996). The impact of unlicensed assistive personnel on nursing care delivery. *Nursing Economics, 14*(2), 99–110.

Look at it this way. (1996, July). *Hospitals and Health Networks, 70*(7), 66–76.

McClure, M. L. (1991). Differentiated nursing practice: Concepts and considerations. *Nursing Outlook, 39*(3), 106–110.

Noble, M. A., Redmond, G. M., Williams, J. K., & Langley, C. (1996). Education for the nurse of tomorrow. *Nursing and Health Care Perspectives, 17*(2), 66–71.

Salary slowdown. (1999, March). *Hospitals and Health Networks, 73*(3), 61.

Twedt, S. (1996, February 12). Tale of 2 hospitals. *Pittsburgh Post Gazette*, pp. 13–14.

VHA. (1995). *The impact of organizational redesign on nurse executive.* Irving, TX: Author.

■ *Editor's Questions for Discussion*

What implications are there for nursing education programs, nursing practice, and nursing administration with the shift in focus to care of populations and continuum of care? What new strategies must be developed to deliver high-quality care in a cost-effective manner? What evidence exists that new strategies may be effective?

Explicate nursing administration as a nursing role. To what extent must nursing administrators at every level in the health care delivery system maintain clinical nursing competencies?

How might unlicensed assistive personnel (UAPs) be utilized without compromising the *professional* components of nursing practice? How might nurse executives clearly define the role, utilization, and evaluation of UAPs?

What are the advantages and disadvantages of nurse executives assuming expanded responsibilities in their positions? What differences are there between the new corporate roles and those that nurses have known in the past? How does a nurse executive exert influence when in a staff position versus a line position? Discuss the effects, skills, knowledge, and experiences needed by a nurse executive who changes from a single to a multiple institution, corporation, or system. What preparation (education, clinical, and administrative practice) is essential for nurse executives who have increased responsibilities in corporate structures?

What planning, strategies, and programs are essential for postgraduate residencies being a prerequisite for taking the licensing nursing examination? Discuss whether differentiated practice includes two different licenses. What relationship exists between Felton's (Chapter 1) plea for clearly differentiated practice policies and McClure's suggestion for two levels of nursing workers?

What are the implications for the licensed practical nurse and associate degree nurse of the two levels of nursing personnel proposed by McClure? What strategies and policies are essential for the implementation of McClure's proposal? Propose strategies that nurse executives may employ to demonstrate high-quality, cost-effective care resulting from two levels of nursing personnel.

PART VII

Nursing Administration– Academic

" . . . And looked down one as far as I could
To where it bent in the undergrowth; . . ."

Visionary is the key adjective that best describes the academic nurse administrator now, tomorrow, and beyond—but with another qualifier. The nurse administrator and leader of academic nursing programs can look forward to enormous changes. Some definitely are occurring, as described by the authors in this Part, others are predicted, and still others are unforeseen, potential alterations in structures and processes for outcomes that lurk in the "underbrush" of academic administration. Functions and roles of academic nurse administrators and man-

agers—particularly the executive officer for nursing programs—and faculty are being affected by seen as well as hidden forces.

Whereas previously, heavy reliance on the head of nursing programs and management associates has been on being facilitators and leaders, the authors present here additional substantive new requirements. Ingenious, creative, and integrated structures and programs will be mandated. In-depth understanding of dynamics and behaviors in management processes is critical. Demands for accountability and quality, with a focus on student-centered programs, are driving forces.

The "worn" paths of various institutional structures, processes, dynamics, and outcomes of academic programs are rapidly becoming outmoded. These authors offer visionary, new paths that will enable programs to thrive in the future. The question to contemplate is: How can academic executive leaders, nurse administrators, and faculty best prepare and adapt?

63

The Changing Roles of Faculty and Dean

The Impact of Market-Driven Educational Reform

Carol A. Lindeman, PhD, RN, FAAN

I n the 1940s, U.S. colleges and universities experienced a dramatic social transformation. Almost overnight they changed from producing an intellectual elite to being the means by which every person could carry his or her education as far as native capacities permitted (Boyer, 1990). Higher education was viewed as a right, not a privilege.

■ The Educational Environment

Post–World War II

In the years that followed, new colleges and universities were built, new faculties were hired, and new programs were developed. Par-

ents who had not finished high school experienced the pride of having children who graduated from college.

For the next several decades, both the private and public sector invested increasing amounts of money in higher education. Student enrollments grew. Minorities and women became larger parts of student bodies. States developed systems of higher education to provide easy access to a broad array of academic programs, with accountability resting with the system. Quality of educational institutions was measured in terms of structure variables (e.g., academic qualifications of the faculty, number of faculty, research productivity, external grant funding, library holding, and qualifications of incoming students).

The 1980s and Reduced Resources

In the 1980s, the picture started changing. State legislators were faced with increasing demands for funding prisons, health care, and basic education. Some states were experiencing significant downward shifts in the economy. Funding for higher education started to decline. In addition, legislators and community leaders pressured institutions of higher education to provide quantifiable evidence of the quality of the education being provided. The concern was that institutions were not providing the quality of graduate needed in the current society. Some state legislators responded by micromanaging their state system of higher education. Others demanded more and more data to justify funding.

■ Today and Tomorrow

By the 1990s the situation for higher education had taken on new parameters. It, like other social institutions, was now expected to operate in the marketplace. This shift from traditional values surrounding higher education to market values reflects the contemporary view of U.S. society that free and competitive markets bring supply and demand into equilibrium and thereby ensure the best allocation of resources (Soros, 1997). Higher education has been turned into a business.

Higher Education as a Business

Although many institutions have felt the impact of reforms and restructuring associated with a competitive marketplace, the full impact lies in the near future. Sullivan (1997) described the situation for higher education as follows:

> The 19th century university model, still common today, is obsolete. This model championed scholarship over application and lecture without discussion, was professor-centered rather than student-centered, and used a cumbersome system of self-governance.
>
> The forces of change are many and complex. They include the demand for public accountability of how society's money is spent, demographic changes, student demands for relevant experiences, the impact of economics, and technological advances. All are changing the face of higher education such that it will never be the same. (p. 143)

In the short term, administrators will experience great pressure to reduce the cost of programs, provide seamless educational opportunities, and commit to a niche in the student marketplace.

Costs of Education

There isn't an administrator in higher education that doesn't have to justify the cost of each and every program offered. Even programs that are considered essential to the well-being of everyone are subjected to critical review along with all other programs. Comparison of program costs among similar institutions (benchmarking) is occurring more and more frequently. If, for example, the University of Phoenix can offer quality educational programs and report profits, why can't other institutions of higher education? The University of Phoenix (referred to from here on as Phoenix) is part of the Apollo Group, Inc., that reported profits of $21.4 million in 1996 (Strosnider, 1997). Although Phoenix is frequently criticized for its approach by some in education, it has a satisfied and growing student body and positive relationships with the business community. Also, some traditional institutions are designing programs on the Phoenix model.

Techniques used by Phoenix to reduce costs of programs are those that every institution must consider: (a) unencumbered governance structure, (b) standardized curricula, (c) emphasis on teaching, (d) more part-time than full-time faculty, and (e) a mission for a specific type of learner. Not every institution should be like Phoenix, but all administrators need to be prepared to justify why they need to be different.

Seamless Education

Those reforming higher education are committed to the principle that the education system in the United States ought to have no barriers between segments, welding education from cradle to grave into one seamless whole (Langenberg, 1997). Inherent in this principle is the assumption that education involves more than passing courses. It involves development of personal qualities and skills associated with success in the work world (e.g., initiative, persistence, integrity, effective communication, critical and creative thinking, and working in teams).

The existing educational system is based on the notion of layers, with each layer having a distinctive role. The degree associated with that layer is used as a code word for the knowledge, skills, and qualities the graduate possesses. Unfortunately, this system does not match reality on two counts. First, there is a great chasm between what schools claim they are doing and what is actually achieved in terms of student outcomes—for example, in the area of preparing critical thinkers. Second, the current layered system does not account for what we know about learning (i.e., people learn in very different ways and at very different rates).

A seamless system would emphasize student assessment and adapt delivery of instruction to the student's circumstances. It would include linkages between and among colleges and universities. Students could take classes simultaneously from an array of institutions without penalty.

Nursing certainly needs to be prepared to justify barriers that exist, or are perceived to exist within nursing education, or to remove at least some of them. Is nursing education a fossilized educational layered cake? Must it remain the way it has been for the last 40 years? Can society expect nurse educators to commit to the principle of seamless education?

Marketplace Niche

In an era of unlimited financial and human resources, schools could modify courses and schedules to meet the needs of a more and more diverse student body. For example, instead of courses offered between 8 a.m. and 6 p.m., which met the needs of the high school graduate starting college, schools could offer night or weekend classes to meet the needs of working adults.

However, the student marketplace is now so large and so diverse that no one institution can do everything for everybody and maintain any degree of cost-effectiveness. The primary market is for education that leads directly and immediately to employment, followed by additional continuing education that maintains and increases workers' skills and knowledge (Davies, 1997).

Not all existing institutions of higher education will survive the impact of the marketplace. Those that succeed in doing so will offer custom-designed programs and consumer (student)-friendly service (Davies, 1997). Traditional institutions that survive will have to offer programs that are distinctive in some way. Institutions that remain less selective in terms of a market niche will be at risk, as will those that underestimate the effect on student admissions of electronically delivered education or for-profit universities.

Many schools of nursing feel safe because they are the only school in a geographic region or because they are part of a famous institution. They believe that as long as they are there, students will come. Other schools continue to hold on to a faculty-centered approach to curriculum design and course offerings. These are the attitudes that place a school at risk in this educational reform environment.

■ The Changing Role of Faculty

Traditional Faculty Role

In the traditional university setting, the time that a faculty member devotes to teaching is distributed over direct and indirect activities.

Direct Activities

- Course designer who controls educational inputs (e.g., classroom content, required readings, and guest lecturers).

- Lecturer who delivers information amassed from research, readings, and personal experience.

- Discussion moderator who helps students understand the material from lectures and readings.

- Evaluator who writes and administers tests, and decides how well students have mastered a subject.

Indirect Activities

- Committee work to create, modify, and evaluate academic policy (e.g., admission and graduation requirements).

- Committee work to create, modify, and evaluate curriculum and course requirements.

- Committee work to fulfill internal accountability issues (e.g., promotion, tenure, and faculty welfare).

- Committee work to establish and maintain faculty's role in governance of the academic unit and institution.

Reform Drivers

Four interrelated marketplace reform drivers are affecting the role of faculty.

Technology

Technology is the systematic application of scientific or other organized knowledge to practical tasks. Two assumptions underpin reform efforts associated with technological developments: (a) the primary rationale for reform is increased productivity, and (b) the new technologies supply the tools to implement and institutionalize these reforms (Van Dusen, 1997). New instructional technologies offer both student and teacher numerous options for interaction and subject matter engagement.

Increased Competition and the Free Marketplace

As a consequence of tuition and related costs of education increasing at a rate faster than inflation and declining public confidence in higher education, higher education is under the same pressures as other businesses. Technology has opened the door for virtual universities to compete with traditional universities for students. For-profit institutions are also competing for a larger share of the market. For the public, the bottom line is what value do I receive for the dollar spent. This attitude opens the door to consider the full array of educational options.

Seamless Education and Job Preparedness

As discussed earlier, two main concerns represent public discontent with the productivity of institutions of higher education. Artificial layers of education that have been maintained by academia are not in harmony with today's rapidly changing work world. Today's work world requires lifelong learning for all workers as required competencies change and jobs emerge and disappear. Those funding higher education want assurance that completion of a program of studies means more than passing courses—that it means being prepared intellectually and personally for success in the work world.

External Accountability

Academic institutions are held in great esteem and given great freedom in the United States. Society is now demanding accountability and information regarding academic productivity. The measures used in the 1960s and 1970s to address questions regarding quality are no longer adequate for the public. Institutions must provide quantifiable evidence of quality, particularly in undergraduate education.

Faculty Role in the High Technology Educational Environment

The following is one scenario of the role of faculty in the emerging high-technology cost-conscious environment (Young, 1997).

Direct Activities

* Assess job history, academic transcripts, and career objectives for a diverse student population.

* Custom-design an educational program for each individual student.

* Lead discussions in classrooms and in on-line chat areas.

* Serve as a "guide-on-the-side," helping students learn how to analyze and synthesize information.

Indirect Activities

* Serve on ad hoc task forces operating in a total quality improvement mode.

Off-Site Activities for Selected Faculty

* Courses designed and produced by teams of technology experts and faculty, which are then marketed by publishers or "brand name" colleges and universities.

* Lectures replaced by multimedia CD-ROMs or World Wide Web sites that include video recordings of talks by world-renowned scholars.

* Grading done by independent assessment organizations, reassuring employers that evaluations are impartial and not subject to grade inflation.

Although this description of the faculty role may seem unlikely and undesirable, it does represent the changes that are occurring. Faculties in many settings are resisting change, but as market pressures increase, they will have to participate in increasing productivity while cutting costs. The challenge will be to retain humanistic values in a market-driven environment.

■ The Role of Dean in a Market-Driven Environment

Historical Perspective

In 1981, the American Association of Colleges of Nursing (AACN) sponsored a continuing education conference for nurse academic administrators (Anderson, 1981). Workshops were organized around four major roles: dean as administrator, dean as scholar, dean as colleague, and dean as person.

Typical Responsibilities of the Dean

* Obtain and allocate financial and human resources.

* Determine and modify organizational and administrative structures.

* Develop strategic plans.

- Facilitate and coordinate the work of faculty, staff, and students.

- Communicate within the school, university, and community.

- Administer interdisciplinary activities.

- Demonstrate scholarly productivity.

- Mentor and counsel faculty, staff, and students.

- Provide academic leadership.

- Perform magic!

The Impact of a Market-Driven Educational Environment

Unlike changes in the faculty role, where some activities were eliminated and others were substantially modified, changes in the role of dean will be subtler, additive, and require a reorientation in values.

Expectations of the Dean

Define outcome measures that address the issue of quality from the perspective of the public.

- Increase faculty productivity.

- Develop and maintain the databases required to address outcomes and productivity.

- Aggressively market programs designed for a specific niche in the marketplace.

- Establish cooperative relationships with leaders in the health care industry.

- Create and maintain a flexible learning organization.

- Ensure faculty competence.

- Perform spectacular magic!

The dean is the key to creation of an academic unit that is successful in the marketplace. The dean must demonstrate how traditional academic and humanistic values can coexist with the bottom-line value of the marketplace.

Discernment

Deans report a pattern in events when taking a new position (Anderson, 1981). There is usually a honeymoon period in which everyone likes the new dean and the new dean also likes everyone. Then groups form within the faculty and staff, with some supporting actions of the new dean, others disliking those actions, and still others sitting back and waiting to see what will happen. During this time, some faculty retreat to nostalgia about the good old days. This period is followed by a period of intense complaining, which is then followed by a period of forward movement.

These changing relationships with faculty are extremely difficult for a dean. As Jarratt (1981) stated:

> On the personal side, the dean's colleague relationship with faculty is the most difficult, the most complex, the most rewarding, and sometimes the most frustrating of all roles. Trying to keep the process going is one of the heaviest drains on energy and psyche, but that academic partnership is the key to quality of program and quality job satisfaction. (p. 23)

In the workshops referred to earlier, presentations about the dean as a person always produced applause, followed by an uncomfortable silence, followed by intense discussion. The project staff (Cunilio, 1981) interpreted the response to that presentation with this statement:

> People do not easily accept humanness—their own or others—especially when the subject is broached for reflection and discussion. For it is our humanness and all that it implies—values, associations, and experiences—which ultimately mark us as vulnerable to attack, admiration, love, and feelings. (p. xviii)

DeTornyay (1981) was one of the deans speaking about the dean as a person. As part of her presentation, she shared the results of a study of deans' satisfaction. The main reward was the autonomy and power imbedded in the position. Costs of the position were more numerous, with the greatest being associated with daily hassles: making unpopular decisions, experiencing loneliness in the position, considering exceptions to policies, taking undue amounts of blame, and so forth. Costs inherent in the position highlight the humanness and vulnerability of the dean.

Each time a dean makes an unpopular decision or agrees to an exception to a policy or awards salary increases on the basis of merit, the dean must rely on discernment (i.e., the ability to see clearly). Each time the dean acts as a colleague with faculty, the dean must rely on discernment. Action based on discernment requires courage and confidence in oneself. Unfortunately many administrators are more aware of their humanness than their competence. They do not trust their own intuition.

Discernment has always been an important ability of an administrator. However, in times of rapid change and the consequences of that change on relationships with faculty, it is even more important. In relatively stable circumstances a dean could hope for 50% of the faculty supporting a decision. In times of rapid change, the percentage is likely to drop. After all, what faculty would be positive about measures to increase faculty productivity while cutting costs? A dean has to accept that, as part of the job, some will want the dean to fail. As one dean commented when speaking of these issues, "Paranoia is as good a management theory as any other" (D. Diers, personal communication, 1978). That comment was made more than 20 years ago when resources were relatively more plentiful and institutions were more stable.

■ Concluding Statement

Ability to adapt to change is essential for success in the years ahead. It is as important in personal life as it is in professional life. There are no procedure manuals for coping with constant change. Each individual is the key to his or her own success. Willingness to adapt is the key factor in survival and success.

Once a person has accepted responsibility for adapting to change, these suggestions might prove helpful:

1. Be smarter collectively, reflectively, and spiritually. Collectively, smarter means staying in touch with the energy and ideas of those around you. Reflectively, smarter refers to noticing yourself noticing. Step back and see how your mind works, what you attend to, and what you overlook. Spiritually, smarter is paying more attention to your own spiritual qualities, feelings, insights, and yearnings. It means reaching inside yourself for that which is authentic—to know what you value and why.

2. Find a mentor and be a mentor. A new model of mentoring is emerging as a requirement for the 21st century (Weeks, 1997). This relationship has three characteristics:

   • Dynamic and flexible, including benefits for the mentor, mentee, and organization

   • Mentee initiated, based on self-assessment and goals

   • Variable over time, involving a diverse group of people, including some outside your own discipline

In this model of mentoring, the mentee receives thoughtful, honest feedback; a more experienced point of view; and a chance to process a new challenge, crisis, or opportunity with a trusted confidant. It is an opportunity to deal with fear. Because everyone has something to learn and something to teach, an individual might be both a mentee and a mentor at any particular time.

We live in an era when knowing and doing are not enough. It is an era where trying may be the best we can do.

■ *References*

Anderson, E. H. (1981). According to Edith H. Anderson . . . In *Have you ever thought of being a dean?* (Vol. III, pp. 1–10). Washington, DC: American Association of Colleges of Nursing.

Boyer, E. L. (1990). *Scholarship reconsidered: Priorities of the professoriate.* Princeton, NJ: The Carnegie Foundation for the Advancement of Teaching.

Cunilio, C. M. (1981). Introduction. In *Have you ever thought of being a dean?* (Vol. IV, p. xviii). Washington, DC: American Association of Colleges of Nursing.

Davies, G. K. (1997, October 3). Higher-education systems as cartels: The end is near. *Chronicle of Higher Education,* A68.

DeTornyay, R. (1981). According to Rheba DeTornyay . . . In *Have you ever thought of being a dean?* (Vol. IV, pp. 1–14). Washington, DC: American Association of Colleges of Nursing.

Jarratt,V. R. (1981). According to Virginia R. Jarratt . . . In *So you want to be a dean?* (Vol. III, pp. 18–38). Washington, DC: American Association of Colleges of Nursing.

Langenberg, D. N. (1997, September 12). Diplomas and degrees are obsolescent. *Chronicle of Higher Education,* A64.

Soros, G. (1997). The capitalist threat. *The Atlantic Monthly, 297*(2), 45–58.

Strosnider, K. (1997, June 6). An aggressive, for-profit university challenges traditional colleges nationwide. *Chronicle of Higher Education,* A32–33.

Sullivan, E. J. (1997). A changing higher education environment. *Journal of Professional Nursing, 13*(3), 143–149.

Van Dusen, G. C. (1997). *The virtual campus: Technology and reform in higher education.* (ASHE-ERIC Higher Education Report, Vol. 25, No. 5.) Washington, DC: George Washington University, Graduate School of Education and Human Development.

Weeks, D. (1997, September). 21st-century mentoring. *World Traveler,* 33–39.

Young, J. R. (1997, October 3). Rethinking the role of the professor in an age of high-tech tools. *Chronicle of Higher Education,* A26–A28.

■ *Editor's Questions for Discussion*

What quality assurance strategies and measures are appropriate in justifying nursing program costs? Discuss the advantages and disadvantages of benchmarking. What data are essential for valid and reliable benchmarking of program costs? How does the governance structure of nursing programs affect cost? What attitudes need to change for viable cost-effective nursing programs to occur? How are such attitudes changed? What viable options do faculty and nursing programs have in increasing productivity while decreasing costs?

What implications exist for multiple program entry into the profession if the principle of seamless education is followed? How might faculty and nursing programs best prepare for changing faculty roles in a high-technology environment? How may resistance to change in faculty role effectively be addressed? Given the faculty role scenario presented by Lindeman, what applications may be made from the discussions of Yeaworth et al. (Chapter 14), Billings (Chapter 15), Nichols and Renwanz-Boyle (Chapter 16), Fleming (Chapter 22), A. Fisher and Habermann (Chapter 21), Hoffman (Chapter 64), and Boland (Chapter 71)?

Discuss the import of the education reform drivers that are effecting the faculty role. How might the faculty role change because of those drivers? What change in values may occur? What impact may be felt on faculty employment and tenure requirements?

How typical is the pattern of events described by Lindeman for new deans today? How are changing relationships with faculty the most difficult challenges for a dean? Discuss factors that contribute to the difficulties of doing so. What interventions may be most effective? Which ideas presented by S. Thomas (Chapter 60), Disch (Chapter 61), Chaska (Chapter 68), and Pesut (Chapter 70) may be applicable to resolution of those difficulties? How likely might predicted changes in faculty role increase or diminish challenging relationships for a dean? Provide reasons in responding. What planning strategies will enable deans to prepare themselves and faculty for changes due to altered faculty roles?

Given S. Thomas' (Chapter 60) discussion about dysfunctional environments, how might prospective deans assess an organization? How can a dean assess potential for culture change in universities? How can someone determine whether expectations for culture change are realistic? Apply Pesut's discussion in your response. How does the dynamics of discernment and team development advanced by Lindell (Chapter 69) reinforce Lindeman's statements? What skills identified by Lindell (Chapter 69) are essential?

64

Academic Health Centers— Dinosaurs or Models for the Millennium?

Sharon E. Hoffman, PhD, MBA, RN, FAAN

Academic health centers, unique American models for educating health care professionals, have been under siege for the past decade. As the health care market continues to change, these educational, caregiving research models find themselves burdened with academic red tape, under attack for their high cost of care, and unable to be nimble players in a very competitive marketplace. Decreased federal and state funding, increased public oversight, and emphasis on the community perspective of health and illness have changed the very culture of these organizations. Their future existence is being debated internally in schools throughout the United States and in the halls of Congress. If these dinosaurs of the 20th century are to survive and prosper in the new millennium, a cultural transition needs to take place. Faculty in all health care professional schools must transcend the outdated views of their roles, survive the organizational changes and transitions, and continue to lead the world in scientific discoveries. Held in the balance is the very future of these organizations and the important health science research they conduct. This is cutting edge research that the American public has come to depend on.

■ What Are Academic Health Centers?

Academic health centers (AHCs) are sometimes called academic health science centers

(AHSCs) or academic medical centers (AMCs). Although the terms are used interchangeably, they actually characterize different organizational entities. An academic health center is defined by the Association of Academic Health Centers, as "an institution that includes either an allopathic or an osteopathic school of medicine, teaching hospital(s), and at least one other health education school or program such as a school of nursing, dentistry, or pharmacy" (1999 Directory of the Association of Academic Science Centers, p. ix). The hospital(s) may be affiliated or owned; however, some organizational control or alliance is exercised by the AHC.

Academic Health Centers may be freestanding educational, research, or care centers such as the state-supported Medical College of Georgia, Medical University of South Carolina, Medical College of Ohio, the AHCs of the University of Texas system, Louisiana State University Medical Center, Oregon Health Sciences University, and the University of Arkansas for Medical Sciences. Such freestanding state educational entities may or may not have their own boards of trustees, but they operate under higher educational coordinating councils or boards. Other freestanding AHCs may be private educational, care, or research entities such as Rush University in Chicago. Many AHCs are not free-standing but are part of a larger university structure (public or private), such as Johns Hopkins University, the University of Utah, and Big Ten schools such as Iowa, Minnesota, Michigan, Ohio, and Wisconsin. Still others are on a health campus of a large state university system such as the University of Maryland and Indiana University in Indianapolis. Although physically separate from other schools, they are governed under a structure similar to their sister schools in the system.

The term *academic health science center* is sometimes used in place of AHC to emphasize all the health professional schools and health science research conducted on campus. Most AHCs belong to the Association of Academic Health Centers. Of the members of this organization, more than 75% have three or more health professions schools, indicating a broader base than just medicine. In 1998, the Association of American Medical Colleges (AAMC) listed 125 schools of medicine in this. However, that figure will change with the addition of new schools or the merger of existing ones.

The term *academic medical center* usually includes teaching hospital(s) and affiliation with a medical school. Academic medical centers usually do not have schools of nursing but serve as clinical sites for a variety of health care professional students. They may be organized as either public or private, nonprofit or for-profit entities. They usually own large, acute care hospitals. Although these three terms—academic health center, academic health science center, and academic medical center—are used interchangeably. Understanding their distinctiveness in governance, ownership, and alliance is important.

Higher educational institutions are also categorized under the Carnegie classification system. AHCs are usually categorized as either Research Universities I, Research Universities II, or Professional Schools and Other Specialized Institutions. According to the definitions, Research I Universities are institutions that offer a full range of baccalaureate programs, are committed to graduate education through the doctorate degree, and give high priority to research. They must also award 50 or more doctoral degrees each year. In addition, they receive annually at least $40 million or more in federal support. Because of their emphasis on research, many AHCs are Research I institutions. Some AHCs are Research II Universities. They also offer a full range of baccalaureate programs, are committed to graduate education through the doctorate degree, and give high priority to research. They, too, award 50 or more doctoral degrees each year. In addition, they receive annually between $15.5 million and $40 million in federal support. AHCs that don't meet these criteria, either because they do not offer a full range of baccalaureate programs or do not confer at least 50 doctoral degrees a year, fall under the category of Professional School and Other Specialized Institutions.

Schools of Nursing Within AHCs

According to Berlin, Bednash, and Hosier (1999), only 84, or approximately 16.3%, of all baccalaureate and higher degree schools of nursing in the United States are part of an AHC. This small percentage belies the influence of AHC schools of nursing on the profession. In fact, 38.2% of all full-time nurse faculty teach in AHCs. The highest salaries for faculty and administrators are in AHCs and the graduate programs consistently rated the highest by *U.S. News & World Report* are in AHCs (Berlin et al., 1999). In the *U.S. News & World Report* (1998) annual guide, only 7 of the top 52 graduate programs (master's degrees) were not in AHCs. Academic health centers also are home to 78.5% of all students graduating with a doctoral degree in nursing (PhD or DNS), 51.3% of all master's students, 100% of all ND (Doctor of Nursing) students, and 25.8% of all baccalaureate students. There are various types of ND programs in schools of nursing, all of which differ from a PhD or DNS doctoral degree in nursing. The ND is either an undergraduate degree program, or designed similarly to an MD (Doctor of Medicine) program in medical school, or a combination of undergraduate and graduate courses for a graduate degree in schools of nursing. See Miller (Chapter 36) for a complete discussion regarding doctoral education programs in and for nursing. A majority of all the NINR-funded research goes to schools of nursing within AHCs (Berlin et al., National Institute of Nursing Research 1999). In addition to the scholarship and teaching activities of these schools of nursing, there is also an emphasis on patient care, new nursing interventions, and advanced practice. The "best" advanced practice programs listed in the exclusive rankings of *U.S. News & World Report* (1998) are in AHCs, including anesthesia, clinical specialist, midwifery, and practitioner options.

The mission of AHCs often encompasses patient care as the service part of the tripartite mission of research, teaching, and service. Health science students have ample opportunity for enriched clinical experiences due to the emphasis on the latest high-technological medical practices, as well as health services research. Interestingly, in the 1998–1999 AACN institutional data, only 40 AHC Schools of Nursing had academic nursing centers (Berlin et al., 1999). These nurse managed clinics usually focus on primary care, something that until recently has not been in the forefront of AHCs, whose focus more likely has been specialized acute care.

Schools of nursing within these enriched environments have unique forces that affect them. Balancing the roles of research, advanced practice, and teaching with the necessity to "bring in part of the monies" through faculty practice, contracts, and research requires special skills. These schools vie for the faculty from the highest ranked doctoral programs in the country and have expectations for tenure that often exceed those of less research-intensive schools. They must meet the highest standards endorsed by higher education as well as the profession of nursing. Competition among health science schools for research dollars, patients for practices, and excellent students is common. Due to the changes in the health care system, cooperation and collaboration are expected, whereas fierce competition actually exists. Increased emphasis on interdisciplinary education and multidisciplinary education from outside funding agencies and state higher education boards adds to the stresses in this environment.

Unique Organizational Models

Organizational models within AHCs vary. Some are based on historical precedence in which the Dean of the Medical School also serves as Vice Chancellor for Health Affairs. In this model all other health science school deans find themselves reporting to one of their "peer," deans who also acts as their "supervisor." This model is quickly disappearing as funding and accreditation practices change and other schools achieve independence and active professional control over their own disciplines. In AHCs that are part of a larger university system, Health Science deans may report to the campus Executive Vice President. In this typical academic model, the health science deans usually are organized into a coordinated group to deal with the unique situations inherent in clinical education and its funding. Each of these models has advantages and disadvantages, and schools of nursing can be found within both. Internal organizational structures in AHC Schools of Nursing are as varied as the organization of non-AHC Schools of Nursing. Whether there are departments, the actual numbers of departments, Associate and Assistant Deans, and nursing centers and nursing clinics vary. The history of the school and the internal models used by other disciplines seem to be factors in determining internal organizational structures. Some AHC entities of nursing are called "Schools of Nursing" and other, similarly sized units are called "Colleges of Nursing." Sometimes, internal university rules determine the title, and sometimes the title is a factor of historical relevance.

■ Goals of Academic Health Centers

The goals of AHCs are (a) to educate and train the next generation of health care professionals, (b) to produce the nation's research (bio-medical, clinical, behavioral, health services research, health promotion, and population-based prevention), and (c) to provide care to the most vulnerable and special needs populations. Clearly, AHCs cannot be burdened with the bureaucratic red tape inherent in large educational institutions. Due to the changing fiscal environment, organizational models are being reengineered to fit the health care marketplace. The emergence of managed care, reduced revenue from governmental programs, and increased restrictions and oversight have managed to decrease revenues from virtually every stream of funding formerly available to AHCs. In addition to the decline in revenues for patient care, overall federal and state funding for educational and research programs has diminished. These factors and the increase of competition in the health care arena have brought about cataclysmic changes. Pardes (1997) reports that the "greater the penetration by managed care, the slower the rate of growth of research done by an academic medical center" (p. 98). A recent article in the popular press entitled "No Time for the Poor" laments the fact that the more health care professionals depend on managed care for their income, the less likely it is that the uninsured will be cared for in free clinics (Shapiro, 1999).

These changes have resulted in a switch from viewing AHCs as profit centers to viewing them as cost centers. The outcome has been some unusual efforts by AHCs to adapt, including the selling of university hospitals and contracting out parts of the service enterprise. Some AHCs have spun off faculty clinical practice or closed schools. Unusual mergers have occurred between competitive centers, merging schools of medicine and nursing, along with the hospitals they formerly owned. Other AHCs have focused on internal reorganization to face market forces. These reorganizations have included a variety of cost saving measures, including reducing expenditures, consolidating clinical facilities, reengineering the clinical care process (e.g., shortening length of stay), and developing critical pathways. Philanthropy and an increase in aggressive marketing of all kinds of health care services have become the norm. Schools of Nursing are inextricably linked to their health professional partners in AHCs. Infrastructure support, as well as the underwriting of some educational costs of nursing education, is provided in the AHC environment. The fiscal health of AHCs directly affects the health of the Schools of Nursing within them. Academic Health Center revenue subsidizes the research and educational missions in all these schools.

■ Dean's Responsibilities in Academic Health Centers

Deans of Schools of Nursing in AHCs have special responsibilities as important stakeholders in their centers. Increased accountability for fiscal resources and increased accountability for educational outcomes are an added part of role expectations. Schools of Nursing in AHCs are looked to as leaders in new nursing interventions, informatics, and research. They serve as the role model for health promotion and disease prevention policies and practices. Deans are called on to seek partnerships actively with their nursing service colleagues to combine resources. In some settings Deans of AHCs have line responsibility for nursing services in addition to their usual educational leadership roles. Due to the organizational changes and transitions going on in the AHCs, Deans are expected to create a healthy work environment. If that weren't enough, fund raising has become a typical expectation. The School of Nursing often takes the leadership role in creating opportunities for partnerships with other health care organizations and nonprofit entities. Balancing these sometimes conflicting responsibilities requires an unusual mix of leadership skill and

experience. The Deans of AHC Schools of Nursing must, indeed, be able to walk on water.

■ Positioning Schools of Nursing in Academic Health Centers

In addition to the roles just discussed, which emphasize fiscal and educational accountability of Deans in AHSs, perhaps the most important overall responsibility is strategic positioning. As are their counterparts in other schools in an AHC, Deans of Schools of Nursing are responsible for improving the image and prominence of their programs and thus their internal and external positioning. As schools jockey for students, research funding, patients, and excellent external peer rankings, they compete internally with each other for monies and influence. Fund raising and the amounts contributed to individual schools, their investigators, and departments, are compared at the end of the fiscal year. Deans find that they are more and more involved in the new mission(s) of the school. Enrollments, external research funding, publications, and faculty prominence also are measured in one form or another and compared and contrasted with other AHC Schools. Faculty leadership in campus governance and on key committees assists in internally positioning the school, as do important internal campuswide assignments for the Dean. Positive internal imaging assists with the influence and support necessary for external positioning.

Variables

A school's position in the profession consists of a number of variables, some objective and some subjective. Objective measures may include amount of external research dollars generated, student scores on standardized tests, quality and number of faculty publications, presence of a nursing doctoral program, number and prominence of doctoral graduates, and the like. Subjective measures may include the image and ranking of the "mother" institution, faculty and dean visibility, and student satisfaction. More and more comparing one program's data to those of peers will be a normal annual occurrence. Data collection and comparison, also known as benchmarking, will provide insight for schools interested in comparing outcomes with their competitors.

Visibility of the Dean

Deans must be a visible force for their schools, becoming involved nationally in professional organizations and representing the school in important venues. State involvement in professional and governmental policy groups, as well as a definite local "presence," is expected. Internal and external leadership roles add to image and hoped-for external rankings so important to a school's reputation. The academic community often has the expectations that the dean will lead these efforts, although they are rarely verbalized or listed in position announcements (Hoffman, 1998).

Competitive Strategies

The elements of successful positioning and competitive strategy are basic for most organizations, whether they are educational, nonprofit service enterprises, or for-profit business entities. Michael Porter (1980), in *Competitive Strategy: Techniques for Analyzing Industries and Competitors,* provides a comprehensive set of analytical techniques for understanding the milieu and behaviors of one's competition. He proposed "that there are significant benefits to gain through an explicit process of formulating strategy, to insure that at least the policies...are coordinated and directed at some common set of goals" (p. xiii). In Porter's discussion of formulating strategy, he emphasized the necessity of knowing your rivals and attempting to establish a difference between you and them. In the

marketing world this uniqueness is called *differentiation.* Successful competitive strategy depends on doing many things well and being able to synthesize and integrate these activities. The "fit," or alignment, of strategies with the school's goals and mission is important. If there isn't a fit, there will not be sustainability. In higher education these strategies are formulated in a school's strategic planning document.

Differentiation

Competitive strategies may involve differentiation or focus. Creating a niche, something that is perceived as being unique or responding to a new need, allows a school to differentiate itself from others. Doing so involves anticipating shifts in the health care industry and responding appropriately to them, thereby exploiting change by choosing a strategy appropriate to the new environment before the competition recognizes it. Some schools in the United States offer unique majors, capitalizing on their environment or specific strength in their AHCs. In the past these offerings have included nursing majors in informatics, ethics, gerontology, midwifery, and the like. In the future, a whole new health care environment will provide opportunity for competitive schools to design new offerings and position themselves appropriately.

Target Population

Deans applying competitive strategies will focus or target offerings to a specific population. Some AHC schools focus on the acute care needs of a community, educating individuals with specialized skills (e.g., neonatal nurse practitioners, acute care nurse practitioners, or nurse anesthetists). Others in AHCs with strong primary care focus on promotion of health behaviors of aggregate populations. Still others in AHCs in predominately rural areas focus on rural health and community nursing centers.

Challenge for the Dean

The dean as faculty leader is responsible for benchmarking appropriate outcomes, leading the faculty community to position its offerings strategically—by differentiation and focus and by changing the institutional culture. The challenge for deans in strategic positioning is to craft new adaptive strategies that successfully position the school while retaining the core values and mission so vital to its enterprise.

■ A Culture in Conflict

Academic Health Centers are experiencing turmoil in all three of their missions. The external stressors of decreased funding, increased oversight, and change in the very delivery of health care in the United States has exacerbated the clash of values inherent in the system. The emphasis on high-level clinical care is sometimes at odds with the research mission, so teachers and administrators may have strongly conflicting perspectives. The business acumen necessary for a viable clinical enterprise is sometimes at odds with the faculty view of using the clinical enterprise only as a vehicle for teaching. Faculty bristle at increased oversight as attacks on their academic freedom.

If AHCs and the Schools of Nursing in them are to survive in this new milieu, faculty and administrators alike need to transcend old roles and patterns of behavior. Faculty must have a better understanding of the total system in which they operate and develop new skills in organizational responsibility and change. Administrators must develop public relations skills to communicate to various stakeholders the necessity of keeping AHCs viable. They also need to devote considerable time to the clinical business of the enterprise. Classical decision-making in this part of academia will have to change for organizations to be nimble and to be able to cope with rapid change.

■ Concluding Statement

The organizational reward structure needs to switch from rewarding solitary work to rewarding collaborative initiatives that emphasize teams and collaboration. Cooperative institutional efforts such as strategic planning, goal setting, and resource allocation need everyone's attention. Setting and carrying out goals that are organizationally aligned, instead of individually centered, will be difficult for the traditional faculty member. Cooperative institutional efforts often are not valued in the traditional AHC. This view must change. If AHCs are to continue to thrive in the 21st century, they will need to cast off their dinosaurs and develop organizational cultures that will enable them to continue to be one of America's greatest health care institutions.

■ References

Association of American Medical Colleges. (1998). *1997–1998 annual report.* Washington, DC: Author.

Berlin, L., Bednash, G., & Hosier, K. (1999). *American Association of Colleges of Nursing 1998–1999 enrollment and graduations in baccalaureate and graduate programs in nursing.* Washington, DC: AACN.

Hoffman, S. (1998). Strategic positioning and personal leadership. *Journal of Professional Nursing, 14*(6), 320.

1998 annual guide to exclusive rankings, America's best graduate schools (1998, March 2). *U.S. News & World Report,* 66–98.

1999 Directory of the association of academic health centers. (1999). Washington, DC: Association of Academic Health Centers.

Pardes, H. (1997). The future of medical schools and teaching hospitals in the era of managed care. *Academic Medicine, 72*(2), 97–102.

Porter, M. (1980). *Competitive strategy: Techniques for analyzing industries and competitors.* New York: Free Press.

Shapiro, J. (1999, April 5). No time for the poor. *U.S. News & World Report,* 57.

■ Editor's Questions for Discussion

Discuss the pros and cons of the present models of Academic Health Centers. What effect do those models have on nursing? What alternative designs do you foresee? What impact may other models have on nursing as a profession?

Discuss influence of AHC Schools of Nursing on the nursing profession. How do such schools exert leadership different from that of other Schools of Nursing? What strategies might further empower Schools of Nursing in AHCs to be instrumental in potent health care legislation?

What evidence exists that the AHC cost-saving measures cited by Hoffman are effective? How have such measures affected Schools of Nursing and quality of patient care?

Propose mechanisms and strategies that a School of Nursing Dean might utilize to fulfill the responsibilities in an AHC. Which of Lindell's applications (Chapter 69) are most relevant to Hoffman's discussion about a Dean's responsibilities? How do variables differ in Schools of Nursing in AHCs from those in other Schools of Nursing that affect a Dean's responsibilities? How might prospective deans best prepare themselves to assume those responsibilities? What skills are essential for a dean to achieve strategic positioning? What effect(s) might utilizing competitive strategies in nursing have on the profession? How might competitive strategies be a positive force and result in fewer negative outcomes?

Discuss the culture conflict in AHCs referred to by Hoffman. In Schools of Nursing, what cultural differences exist between AHCs and other types of state or private entities? To what extent are conflicts the same or different in Schools of Nursing regardless of the type of setting? What are the most significant type of cultural conflicts in Schools of Nursing? How might these conflicts be resolved with minimal negative outcomes? How does decision-making and faculty governance in Schools of Nursing influence the culture of a school? What cultural changes do you expect in the future of Schools of Nursing? How can cultural change be achieved for positive, lasting outcomes?

65

Schools of Nursing in Public and Private Sectors

Challenges and Opportunities

Sarah B. Keating, EdD, RN, C-PNP, FAAN

Shannon E. Perry, PhD, RN, FAAN

Schools of Nursing have existed in institutions of higher education since shortly after 1900. Two of the earliest such schools were based at the University of Minnesota, a public university, and Vanderbilt University, a private university. Esther Lucile Brown (1948) in *Nursing for the Future* noted that "preparation of the professional nurse belongs squarely within the institution of higher learning" (p. 138). Her descriptions of curricula, faculty preparation, and financing of schools of nursing are worth reading today.

■ Schools of Nursing in Public Institutions of Higher Education

Public universities consist of colleges or schools that confer the bachelor's degree and of graduate and professional schools that confer master's and doctoral degrees. From its origins of training ministers at Harvard in 1636, the university in America evolved to teaching a variety of subject areas, including science, mechanics (engineering), agriculture, practical skills and crafts, and the art of teaching. In the 1860s research was introduced into the educational system as a purpose of the university (Unger, 1996).

The mission of universities changed from education of the elite for the ministry, government, and professions (law and medicine) to the practical goal of educating industrial classes in a variety of branches of learning. This transition was facilitated in public universities by establishment of land grant colleges made possible by the Morrill Acts passed by Congress in 1862 and 1890, which opened higher education to all qualified applicants whatever their social or economic status (Unger, 1996). The result was a large network of agricultural and engineering colleges that were free and managed by the state, which formed the basis for today's public university systems.

In 1924, another innovation occurred when the College of the Pacific created a college that offered only upper division courses and awarded the bachelor's degree (Unger, 1996). This early program was a precursor of present day articulation agreements between associate degree and baccalaureate programs in nursing.

With the explosion of enrollments following World War II, the university curriculum expanded to include more than 100 majors with several thousand courses (Unger, 1996). During this time also, students changed from passive recipients to active consumers of education.

Nursing began its movement into institutions of higher learning in 1899. This change from a hospital-based apprentice model initiated development of the current model of modern university-based baccalaureate and higher degree programs. In the baccalaureate program the student enters as a freshman or transfers credits toward a Bachelor of Science in Nursing (BSN) eligibility for the licensing examination to become an RN. The first master's degree in nursing programs originated in 1923 (Creasia & Parker, 1996).

With inception of community college–based programs in the 1960s, movement of nursing education into colleges and universities accelerated. The student earns an associate degree in nursing and becomes eligible to take the licensing examination to be licensed as a registered nurse (RN). Upper division, post licensure courses and additional education work can then be completed at the baccalaureate and higher degree college or university.

■ Comparing Public and Private Institutions of Higher Education

Mission and Goals

The majority of colleges and universities in the United States have three major purposes for higher education: education (teaching and learning), community service, and research. Most identify teaching as their primary mission. However, emphases on the other two purposes may vary with the primary mission of the college or university. For example, public universities may have legislative or systemwide mandates or issues. Research institutions place a high value on developing new knowledge and testing hypotheses. Comprehensive colleges and universities may place equal value on community service and research. Other, smaller colleges, particularly those with a religious heritage, emphasize service to students and community. Some privately funded colleges are institutions with special foci on preparation for the professions—for example, health sciences or academic medical center colleges. Several single-purpose colleges have evolved, such as the transformation of diploma schools of nursing into college programs. The "New American College" is another category of private colleges that was identified previously as small liberal arts colleges. The New American Colleges have a potpourri of offerings, including extended education, professional programs, and graduate studies.

Nursing administrators and faculty must be familiar with the mission of their institution. Most accrediting bodies require that the mission of the nursing program be consistent with that of its parent institution; philosophically speaking, a match between the program and its key administrators and faculty is necessary. Some missions are one or two succinct statements patterned after a business model that explains to the consumer what it offers and expects to produce (e.g., to educate students for a life of highly skilled and compassionate service in health care). Other, traditional colleges may have long treatises explaining the mission according to the traditional threefold expectations for college education.

The mission is the philosophical underpinning for the curriculum and provides guidelines for developing goals that will serve as measures for meeting the stated mission of the institution. The missions of private schools usually are a bit narrower and more focused than those of public schools. Many private schools emphasize liberal arts as a foundation for professional education. Others may have a special focus, such as the health sciences. Large, multipurpose research universities emphasize expansion of the body of knowledge of its various disciplines. For example, a nursing program in a health sciences institution can emphasize nursing's role in the health care industry and interdisciplinary collaboration. A program in a Research I University can emphasize nursing science and, therefore, graduate education. In many ways, these focused missions create an easier task for nursing constituents as they develop the discipline's philosophy, mission, and goals that are congruent with those of the parent institution.

Nursing is an asset to many colleges, as its clinical practice readily applies to the community service mission of an institution. Nurse managed clinics and health care services that faculty and students provide during their clinical experiences are part of an institution's commitments to the community (Starck, Walker, & Bohannan, 1991). With its predominantly female faculty, a School of Nursing also contributes to overall gender equity within the university.

Academic Administration

The role of the nursing academic administrator is structured much the same in both private and public institutions. The title of the chief nursing education administrator depends on the organizational structure and size of the institution. Thus the executive nurse educator may hold the title of dean, director, or chair. The administrator must have the time necessary for program management. The time allotted preferably is full time, but should be at least 60% for programs with fewer than 100 students. Depending on size of the nursing program, its administration may consist of only the dean. In larger institutions, the administrative team may comprise Dean, Associate Dean(s), Chairs of Departments, and Directors of programs. These positions usually have pro rata appointments with release time for fulfilling administrative responsibilities. In private education where programs are tuition-driven, release time becomes a major challenge owing to costs associated with release time. However, adequate time for administration is necessary to maintain effectiveness of the program and to preserve educational quality.

It is not uncommon for the nursing administrator to hold dual responsibilities when acting as administrator of a health sciences unit that also contains a nursing program. Some deans hold dual appointments as Dean and Vice President for Patient Care Services in major privately sponsored academic medical centers. When the administrator must devote equal attention to both programs, issues related to equitability of academic and financial support decisions may arise.

Academic administrators of the future increasingly will have an external role that involves forging business and community partnerships and fund-raising. This role will be less like the chief operating officer of an academic unit and more like a university president who constantly must scan the external environment (McBride, 1999).

Faculty Governance

The form of faculty governance derives from the sponsoring institution and its fit within the structure. Depending on its mission and whether it is religious or secular, the organization of the nursing program can be influenced greatly by directions set by the Board of Regents or Board of Trustees and the administrative leadership. Both public and private universities may have faculty teaching unions and often have on-campus chapters of the American Association of University Professors (AAUP). Most academics subscribe to the AAUP principles of academic freedom and governance. Presence of a union requires compliance with the memorandum of understanding or contract negotiated between the administration and the union. Academic administrators must be cognizant of provisions of such agreements and adhere to them.

Leadership Functions for Academic Administrators

Leadership functions for nursing administrators are classic, including human resource management, strategic planning and evaluation, financial planning and budget management, curriculum and instruction supervision, fund raising, and public affairs. Although it is tempting to believe that being an administrator in a private institution allows more freedom in faculty hiring, retention, and promotion decisions, in fact human resources

policies and procedures still apply. According to fair employment practices and academic freedom protections, faculty members are entitled to due process—no matter the type of institution. Human resource issues are no less rigorous in private institutions than in public institutions.

Through hiring and retention practices and faculty development opportunities, the chief administrator ensures continued quality of faculty. Except in richly endowed colleges and universities, funds for faculty development often are limited. Bringing experts to campus for group workshops, lectures, and seminars often proves to be cost effective for programs with limited faculty development funds. Participating in consortia can enable administrators to pool resources.

Administrators usually enjoy more freedom for program development in private institutions, owing to less bureaucracy and having to negotiate with fewer levels of governance. In contrast, in state-supported institutions, multilevel groups must pass on new programs and proposals with an eye on other state colleges and universities and the competitiveness of proposals within the system. Financial planning and budget expenditures depend on the governance structure of the sponsoring institution. The administrator's role may range from active participant to interested observer in both the macro and micro budget planning stages. In private institutions where funding is tuition driven, the administrator must use creative budgeting strategies that include revenue-generating activities, such as faculty practice clinics and consulting services. In heavily endowed private institutions the burden of budget is somewhat lessened, although the administrator many times becomes active in securing endowment funds and scholarship support for students. In public institutions, obtaining external funding for support of faculty, student development, and scholarships is

TABLE 65.1   Comparison of Revenue Sources of Public and Private Colleges and Universities

Revenue Source	Public (%)	Private (%)
Tuition and fees	17.1	40.7
Federal government	10.6	15.3
State governments	38.3	2.5
Local governments	3.7	<0.05
Private gifts, grants, and contracts	4.0	8.3
Endowment income	0.6	4.8
Sales and services	23.1	23.3
Educational activities	2.9	2.6
Auxiliary enterprises	9.5	10.3
Hospitals	10.9	4.4
Other sources	2.6	4.4

Note: Data from "University Finances" by H. G. Unger, 1996, *Encyclopedia of American Education,* Vol. II. (pp. 1021–1022). New York: Facts on File.

increasingly important. Grant writing for program development and faculty research is very important to maintenance of faculty, program quality, and continued support over time.

Sources of Funding

Because of its high faculty-to-student ratio, nursing is a comparatively expensive program. Private education depends on tuition and fees for its revenues, in contrast to state-supported schools that receive appropriations from general funds. Financing of public universities has moved from "state supported" to "state assisted" to what some refer to currently as "state located." Obtaining external funding is increasing in importance. Considerable time, faculty resources, and university support are allocated to securing such funding. Concomitantly, pressure on nursing faculty and administrators to secure such funding is increasing. Table 65.1 compares the financing of private and public universities.

Endowment funds provide the foundation of financial health for private institutions. Grants, scholarships, and unrestricted gifts are important to the economic well-being of these institutions. The larger the endowment and scholarship programs, the larger are the financial aid programs available to students. Various state- and federally-sponsored financial aid programs provide assistance to needy students; these help underwrite costs of tuition for students. Thus private institutions can use these programs to build a diverse student body rather than rely only on tuition payments from wealthy parents and students. These financial aid packages include scholarships, loan programs, and outright grants. Enterprising students can be directed to hospital auxiliaries, health care systems, private donors, and charitable organizations that award smaller, privately funded scholarships. Many students aggregate these scholarships into a financial aid package that supports them throughout their educational program. To assist students, financial aid offices and nursing programs should maintain an active list of potential private scholarships for students.

Strategic Planning and Visioning

Strategic planning is a vehicle for forecasting the future and mapping future needs. These plans provide a framework for measuring program performance against the strategic plan (Merante & Ireland, 1993; Merrill, 1992). Strategic initiatives and planning focus on forecasting the market for baccalaureate and advanced practice nursing needs and the available applicant pool for the programs. Institutions granting doctorates must read the market as well. On the one hand, private institutions have a good record for graduating students on time from 4-year degree programs, owing to their ability to manage resources and costs. State-supported schools, on the other hand, must respond to the public's demand for education and the whims of state legislatures who may or may not strongly support funding for higher education. Private institutions thus have more latitude in planning for admissions, enrollments, and graduations within their prescribed curricula plans and length of programs. Thus forecasting and planning in 3- to 5-year segments become easier, and independent programs are able to respond more rapidly to changes in market supply and demand.

Private schools often have more freedom to envision the future and create innovative educational programs that meet the future needs of the nursing profession in particular and health care system in general. This advantage derives from the ability of private education to move new programs faster through the governance systems of institutions and the immunity, which private education enjoys, from statewide academic program imperatives and resource constraints. These conditions foster development of unique programs that are both innovative and attractive to potential students and respond to market demand. These incentives for enrollment, while more expensive, provide opportunities for professional preparation that meet current and future health care needs. These innovative programs can become models for professional education in both private and public institutions of higher education.

Challenges

Competitive Arena

Private Schools of Nursing and, increasingly, public Schools of Nursing find themselves in extremely competitive markets with increasing numbers of nationwide Web-based and distance education programs available to nurses seeking further education. Many state-supported public institutions have extensive infrastructure systems in place and can easily link with one another for a plethora of course and degree offerings. Private nonprofit institutions have been slower to adopt these learning strategies, owing to prohibitive costs and fierce competition from for-profit schools that have the business acumen to market their programs and realize financial profits.

In most instances, private education is at a disadvantage in distance education programs. Video telecasting and the dedicated classrooms necessary for support and the cable and wiring costs for supporting Web-based education are examples of infrastructure expenses that must be incurred in distance education. Not included are the hardware and the software packages necessary for offering the courses and the costs involved in faculty development and release time for formatting courses for distance learning.

Private educational institutions have begun to purchase services for distance learning from vendors with the expertise to initiate and maintain such programs. Until adequate numbers of students enroll in the programs, however, private institutions are forced to take financial risks when they enter technology-based education. Only through large numbers of enrolled students can private institutions enjoy a break-even or net gain in this business. Thus grants to initiate programs are crucial for start-up, and business plans must be based on accurate enrollment projections to maintain the programs. Private institutions can identify positive and negative effects from publicly supported distance education programs and benefit from their experience. Private institutions can use that information to develop the best methods and blends of strategies to meet their missions and philosophies of teaching and learning.

The other major competitive arena for private schools occurs in the marketplace for potential students. It is difficult for private schools to compete against lower tuition, state-supported schools. Marketing the private school and developing unique programs become essential to its life (Delne, 1991; Hauptman, 1994). Smaller classes, closer contact with faculty, higher retention rates, graduation on time, and earlier entry into practice are advantages that private schools can cite when marketing their programs. Private schools may offer evening and weekend programs tailored to a specific market. Using outcomes assessment and benchmarking techniques to provide additional data and comparisons with other schools is important for both public and private institutions in documenting the effects of the educational program.

■ Nursing as a Discipline in the Academy

In 1899, nursing made its first effort to move into academic institutions (Creasia & Parker,

1996). Despite more than 100 years of experience in higher education, nursing continues to find it difficult to be accepted as a discipline in the academy. Perhaps its past entry into practice through hospital-based diploma programs and the birth of associate degree programs for nursing in the 1960s prompted disdain from other disciplines in higher education. Nursing has been likened to apprentice education, in contrast to professional education at the master's or doctoral level. Dialogue in the nursing profession concerning entry into practice at the baccalaureate level continues to this day and gives mixed messages to the public about the extent of the profession's scientific knowledge base. However, for the most part, nursing is accepted by institutions of higher education as a profession, much like that of engineering and teaching.

Private Schools of Nursing—especially those in smaller, liberal arts colleges—still find themselves having to defend the profession as an academic discipline to colleagues in the humanities, arts, and sciences. However, the growing number of generic master's degree programs, the demand by industry for baccalaureate-prepared nurses, and the need for advanced practice nurses are trends that should promote acceptance of nursing as a discrete discipline in academe (California Strategic Planning Committee for Nursing [CSPCN], 1999). The recent position statement on scholarship in nursing from the American Association of Colleges of Nursing (AACN) (1999) is an excellent example of how the profession defines itself—in terms of higher education—through scholarship in discovery, teaching, application, and integration (Boyer, 1990).

Developing a Cadre of New-Age Faculty

Shortage of qualified nursing faculty is a major challenge facing nursing programs. The nursing faculty workforce is aging. For example, in California, more than 67 faculty positions in baccalaureate and higher degree programs are expected to be vacant in 2002 (CSPCN, 1999). The average age of an Assistant Professor in Nursing is 46 years, whereas in other professions the median age is 31 to 39 years (Anderson, 1998). In addition, fewer than half the faculty teaching in baccalaureate and higher degree programs in nursing are doctorally prepared, limiting their participation in the full mission of the university (Anderson, 1998). Except for heavily endowed private institutions, Schools of Nursing face major challenges in recruitment of faculty owing to competition from industry for advanced practice nurses and the lure of state-supported research universities, which can offer higher salaries and more opportunities for research funding. Many nurse educators in private schools are learning to nurture and mentor their younger master's-prepared faculty in the teaching role. Incentives for progressing into the faculty role include (a) forgivable loan programs for doctoral studies, (b) an adjunct faculty track that has fewer demands than the tenure track and provides time for doctoral study, and (c) joint appointments for practice and education. Nurse-managed clinics that generate funds for the school and individual faculty are attractive to faculty and an example of an incentive for recruiting and maintaining faculty.

Faculty development programs are essential for building a cadre of faculty prepared for the future (Kavoosi, Elman, & Mauch, 1995; Zickel, 1978). Schools with limited funds can plan relatively inexpensive faculty development programs by using their experienced master teachers to provide continuing education experiences such as planned brown bag lunches, invited guest lectures by experienced faculty and leaders in nursing, and collaborative professional development series with other Schools of Nursing. Planned ongoing orientation sessions and assignment of mentors to new, inexperienced faculty benefit the program

and lessen common frustrations encountered as new faculty develop. Owing to the need for private schools to retain a competitive edge, more opportunities and freedom for developing innovative educational programs exist. These features can be appealing to faculty who enjoy creative planning and implementation.

Recruiting and Maintaining Diverse Student Scholars

With increasing opportunities in other fields for women, recruiting students into nursing has become difficult. Owing to the relative expense of private schools compared to publicly supported institutions, recruiting students into private nursing programs is even more challenging (Riggs, 1994). Seeking foundation, scholarship, and endowment funding to provide financial aid for economically disadvantaged students must be in place to build diversity. Federal and state funding is available for these purposes and it behooves private schools of nursing to investigate programs and provide access to such aid for their students. Enrolled students and alumni are excellent sources for recruiting ethnically diverse students. Their testimony about the support they received in the program and the quality of the teachers and program are assets to recruitment and retention of a diverse student body.

Faculty representing the U.S.'s multicultural and ethnic population are excellent role models for students from underrepresented groups in nursing (Gary, Sigsby, & Campbell, 1998). Schools can build enrollments through contacts with nursing and community organizations that represent minority groups. Offering space on campus to these groups for meetings helps to build the network of support for recruiting and graduating a diverse student body. Representatives from the community can serve as sponsors of a community member in the nursing program. Having a student services unit in the institution involved in a planned program for offering support services that are culturally and ethnically sensitive to students' learning needs is important. Nursing faculty and administrators should work closely with these services and at the same time avoid stereotyping students according to cultural and ethnic groups and learning needs. These are but a few examples of conscious efforts nursing programs can take to increase student population diversity.

The Crumbling Infrastructure

As American higher education enters the 21st century, universities recognize that campus buildings are aging. At the same time, higher education is entering the era of technology-based educational programs that include virtual campuses comprising learners' homes or workplaces and faculty offices. Capital expenditures loom large as educators debate the need for improving and adding new buildings or investing in technology programs. Nursing with its clinical practice requirements needs laboratory sites to teach students skills prior to application in real settings with clients. Most institutions of higher education recognize these needs of the profession and build these costs into their budgets.

Educators in nursing education, especially those in institutions supported by tuition, commonly charge lab fees. With escalating costs of medical supplies, fees must be increased. Such increases are a burden to students, especially those in private schools who are paying higher tuition than those in publicly supported schools. Thus educators need to develop innovative ways to cut costs for practice labs. Examples of ways to cut costs include (a) soliciting donations of equipment and supplies from affiliated health care agencies, (b) recycling used supplies without imperiling aseptic technique, and (c) seeking practice sites at clinical agencies. Because nursing students represent potential buyers of equipment and supplies, durable medical equipment manufacturers, suppliers, pharmaceutical companies, and individual salespeople may be willing to defray some costs. Faculty, administrators, students, and staff should be aware of costs associated with labs. These expenses need to be as cost-effective as possible to keep costs at a reasonable level and minimize increases in student fees.

Opportunities for Nursing in Private and Public Education

Influencing Policy

Nursing educators must collaborate on issues facing nursing education in order to influence public policy. One of the major problems facing nursing educators in institutions of higher education remains the question of which level of education is appropriate for licensure (i.e., entry into practice). Arguments over this issue are old and tired, and nursing needs to move on instead of incessantly arguing among its members. Rather than continuing the same debate, it is time for the profession to admit that State Boards of Registered Nursing are mandated through legislation to define the scope of practice and safe nursing care. Beneficial effects of more education should be the theme for the profession (McBride, 1999). Although often not appreciated, additional education essential to provision of nursing must be recognized. Such knowledge includes learning regarding the community, family theory, leadership skills, basic understanding of research, economics of health care, and so forth. Nursing practice must recognize the need for additional knowledge and skills that can be obtained through further education. Job functions that recognize levels of education must be differentiated in the workplace by the health care industry, and salaries must be increased accordingly. To influence public policy, nurse educators need to collaborate with all levels of nursing education, their communities, legislators, and other health care providers to ensure that the nursing workforce is well prepared to deliver the quality of care demanded by consumers.

Collaboration among nurses means identifying common issues and working together toward their resolution. Vested interests must be put aside for the common good. Exhibiting the strength of a unified voice by nursing to the public is essential. It is important that educators meet with their counterparts in nursing practice and leaders in the professional nursing organizations to lobby legislators and ensure that health care needs of the population are met through a well-qualified nursing workforce. Working with the various nursing organizations and their lobbyists is a powerful way in which resources, people, and time can be unified and influential in bringing about change.

Nurses are vitally interested in influencing policy and legislation related to such issues as women's health, assisted suicide, and prescriptive authority for advanced practice nurses. The need for increased funding in the National Institutes of Health (NIH) for nursing research is clear. Nurses were successful in establishing the National Institute for Nursing Research (NINR), and nurses continue to lobby for adequate funding to address issues of importance to the health of the population.

■ Building Partnerships and Consortia

In today's world of mergers, megacorporations, and managed health care systems, nurse educators must work together to provide cost-effective, high-quality education. Periodic meetings among regional nursing education programs benefit educators by identifying which institution is best equipped to offer certain programs. Rather than offering redundant programs, collaboration fosters strategic plan-

ning to avoid unnecessary competition; students then receive the best education from the program(s) best qualified to offer them (Cardozier, 1988). Innovative collaboration with service settings such as offering classes on-site at a clinical agency with the agency bearing some of the cost can help meet needs of both institutions (Williams & Widman, 1998).

Setting enrollment targets is another method of collaboration. To avoid overburdening regional clinical facilities, program administrators can agree among themselves about the amount and nature of the facilities that each needs, the days and the times of year they are needed, and how the programs can work together. For example, schools can place associate degree, baccalaureate degree, or master's degree students in the same agencies and have these students function at the level of practice for which they are being prepared. This process can help socialize students in their roles and, at the same time, avoid crowding agency units. An additional benefit is that faculty can be shared for possible cost savings.

Building consortia for external funding helps to initiate new programs or sponsor faculty and student nurse-managed clinical services. Funding agencies are interested in consortia that demonstrate collaboration among programs, secure financial resources, commitment to continuing the program, save costs through efficient use of personnel, and meet overall health needs and workforce demands for the region.

Legitimizing Nursing in the Professional World

In a public opinion poll conducted by Louis Harris and Associates, Inc., in June 1999, 76% of the respondents said that "nurses need more than four years of college to perform their jobs" (Gray, 1999). When nursing education is compared to that of other health care providers and the types of highly skilled services that nurses provide, it is dismaying to recognize that nursing is so far behind other disciplines. That traditional professional education for doctors, clergy, and lawyers requires professional degrees at the doctoral level is well established. The majority of newer disciplines in health care, including therapists, require at least a master's degree for entry into practice and some are initiating entry-level doctorates. The number of "generic" master's degrees in nursing programs is increasing throughout the country. That is, students with earned baccalaureate degrees enter a nursing program, receive the nursing component of baccalaureate nursing education or its equivalent, and then move into master's-level courses. Some graduate-level work is specialized, and other work prepares students for generalist roles.

Several entry-level doctoral programs in nursing exist in the United States. Some master's and doctoral entry-level programs admit students as freshmen and move them through two-plus-four, or three-plus-three programs modeled after pharmacology and engineering professional programs. In these programs, prerequisite or preprofessional content is completed in the first 2 or 3 years, and the professional content is completed in the latter 4 or 3 years. Depending on state licensure requirements, eligibility for examination to be licensed as RNs could occur toward the end of the 6-year program or after graduation upon completion of degree requirements. Such approaches may portend the future of nursing education programs.

Health care today is complex and requires far more nursing knowledge and skills than in the past. Rather than a continual argument over entry into practice at the associate degree, diploma, or baccalaureate degree levels many believe that it is time to move into master's degree or higher preparation. Unquestionably, the need for technical providers of care in the nursing profession exists. At what level of education that should occur remains to be determined. However, the professional level needs to be moved into graduate study so that nursing becomes a credible profession respected by its peers and colleagues in health care.

Rather than seeking legislative mandates, influencing a policy change rests with educators and partners in practice who can initiate innovative programs. With support of colleagues in practice, nursing educators can meet the challenge for quality health care services in an increasingly complex health care system by preparing a well-educated nursing workforce.

International Collaboration

International collaborative initiatives among educational programs have increased as communication, distance education, and technology systems have improved. Faculty and student exchanges promote cross-cultural understanding and opportunities for teaching and learning experiences. Rich research opportunities to study health-related cultural similarities and differences are available. Participating in curriculum development and instructional strategies in another country lead to enrichment of faculty's appreciation for other cultures and potential application to their own curriculum and learning experiences.

Private institutions can use international partnerships to increase enrollments through on-campus enrollment of students or through distance education experiences. Examples include video broadcasting, Web-based courses, e-mail, and intensive courses on-site in the other country. Many opportunities exist for faculty from other nations to spend time in a host college in the United States. Charging tuition or bartering for student and faculty exchanges, including provision of room and board, are examples of ways in which these projects can be funded.

A caveat to providing learning experiences for faculty and students from other countries is the frequency of requests from participants to remain in the United States following completion of their programs. This desire presents an ethical dilemma for the host school. Most U.S.

educators who become mentors for international teachers and students are sympathetic to those who do not want to return to their home countries. However, U.S. educators are obligated to foster the visitors' return to their home countries to promote the development of nursing practice and nursing education programs in those countries.

■ Maintaining a Vibrant Curriculum to Meet Health Care System Needs

We have observed that the life of a nursing curriculum is about 7 years. Most nursing faculty develop curricula according to a conceptual framework. Using a selected framework takes several years to match the curriculum plan to that of the institution's mission and the faculty's philosophy (Duffy, Foster, Kuiper, Long, & Robison, 1995; Sohn, 1991; Sutcliffe, 1991). In contrast, the health care system changes rapidly, and to the dismay of faculty, a curriculum plan developed 2 years ago may be out of date by the time the first class is to graduate. The challenge is to find a curriculum that is responsive to change and, at the same time, envisions the future and prepares nurses who can meet future health care needs (Huston & Fox, 1998).

National, professional, and regional accrediting bodies have come to realize that rigid criteria hamper the quality of educational institutions rather than giving them freedom to respond to the needs of communities they serve and their future graduates. Most accrediting agencies now focus on assessment of learning and measuring outcomes. Many allow institutions to respond to these basic tenets in ways that match the institutions' missions and goals. Total quality management and measurement of program outcomes are now recognized as excellent ways for open systems of education to grow and develop.

Educators have much to learn from the business world about measuring quality. Focus on the student for the educational effort and learning becomes central. Nursing educators should identify quality indicators and benchmarks against which to measure their progress in providing a quality education for students. Periodic conferences relating to (a) curriculum development, (b) educational technology, (c) instructional design and strategies, and (d) student services are essential to maintenance of a vibrant curriculum. Opportunities for faculty to share with each other can contribute to the development of faculty. Jointly sponsored conferences and workshops for faculty in private and public education will promote nursing curricula that are ready to address the health care needs of the 21st century.

■ Concluding Statement

Schools of Nursing have met numerous challenges in developing high-quality professional programs in universities for more than 100 years. However, demanding tasks remain. New challenges will emerge for both state-supported and private institutions and academic administration. Nursing's history provides clues for future success far beyond the known.

■ References

American Association of Colleges of Nursing. (1999, March). *AACN position statement: Defining scholarship for the discipline of nursing.* Washington, DC: Author.

Anderson, C. A. (1998). Academic nursing: A desirable career? *Nursing Outlook, 46,* 5–6.

Boyer, E. (1990). *Scholarship reconsidered. Priorities for the professoriate.* Princeton, NJ: Carnegie Foundation for the Advancement of Teaching.

Brown, E. L. (1948). *Nursing for the future, a report prepared for the National Nursing Council.* New York: Russell Sage Foundation.

California Strategic Planning Committee for Nursing. (1999, May). Personal report to *CSPCN based on survey of Deans and Directors of the California Association of Colleges of Nursing.* Oakland: S. B. Keating.

Cardozicr, V. R. (1988). Joining forces: Public and private institutions take cooperative action. *Educational Record, 69*(3–4), 34–39.

Creasia, J. L., & Parker, B. (1996). *Conceptual foundations of professional nursing practice* (2nd ed.). St. Louis: Mosby.

Delne, G. C. (1991). How small colleges can thrive in the '90s. *AGB Reports, 33*(4), 6–11.

Duffy, N., Foster, C. D., Kuiper, R., Long, J. T., & Robison, L. D. (1995). Planning nursing education for the 21st century. *Journal of Advanced Nursing, 21*(4), 772–777.

Gary, F. A., Sigsby, L. M., & Campbell, D. (1998). Preparing for the 21st century: Diversity in nursing education, research, and practice. *Journal of Professional Nursing, 14,* 272–279.

Gray, B. B. (1999). Public opinion. Nurses rank high. *Nurseweek, 12*(14), 1, 28.

Hauptman, A. M. (1994). Are price wars coming to private education? *Trusteeship, 2*(5), 6–8.

Huston, C. J., & Fox, S. (1998). The changing health care market: Implications for nursing education in the coming decade. *Nursing Outlook, 46,* 109–114.

Kavoosi, M. C., Elman, N. S., & Mauch, J. E. (1995). Faculty mentoring and administrative support in schools of nursing. *Journal of Nursing Education, 34*(9), 419–426.

McBride, A. B. (1999). Breakthroughs in nursing education: Looking back, looking forward. *Nursing Outlook, 47,* 114–119.

Merante, J. A., & Ireland, R. C. (1993). The competitive edge: Why some small colleges succeed. *College Board Review, 69*(8–13), 28–29.

Merrill, E. B. (1992). *Planning for organizational adaptation: The relationship between strategic planning and performance in baccalaureate schools of nursing.* Doctoral dissertation. Washington, DC: George Washington University.

Riggs, H. E. (1994). Are merit scholarships threatening the future of private colleges? *Trusteeship, 2*(3), 6–10.

Sohn, K. S. (1991). Conceptual frameworks and pattern of nursing curriculum. *Journal of Advanced Nursing, 16,* 858–866.

Starck, P. L., Walker, G. C., & Bohannan, P. A. (1991). Nursing faculty practice in the Houston Linkage Model: Administrative and faculty perspectives. *Nurse Educator, 16*(5), 23–28.

Sutcliffe, L. (1991). An examination of the implications of adopting a process to curriculum planning, implementation and evaluation. *Journal of Advanced Nursing, 17,* 1496–1502.

Unger, H. G. (1996). *Encyclopedia of American education.* New York: Facts on File.

Williams, R. P., & Widman, K. A. (1998). Partners in quality. *Nursing Management, 29*(11), 22–26.

Zickel, J. N. (1978). *A consortium approach to faculty development: Use of faculty facilitators to enhance teaching performance.* Paper presented at the International Conference for Improving University Teaching, Aachen, Germany.

■ *Editor's Questions for Discussion*

Describe the differences between state, private, and academic science universities and the distinctions that affect nursing programs. How does the role of academic nursing administration differ by type of university? What issues arise when deans hold a dual appointment as dean and vice president for patient care services?

How might private schools increase enrollments without jeopardizing quality of programs and program costs? From Keating and Perry's presentation, what challenges are most difficult for academic nursing administration? How might these be addressed? How are human resource issues different in private and state-supported universities? What constraints may be more challenging in one type of school versus the other? How can a dean capitalize on the strengths of a university and school and minimize their limitations? Provide specific examples. What negotiations are essential before an academic nursing administrator accepts a position as a dean?

Suggest approaches for recruiting students into nursing programs. To what extent should university strategic plans be reflected in specific plans of action for school or college programs? How can faculty development programs be initiated in nursing programs when resources are extremely scarce? What strategies are most effective for recruitment of doctorally prepared nursing faculty? Indicate further initiatives for building collaboration rather than competition between nursing programs of universities for recruitment, clinical learning sites, and faculty. What should be the basis and source for curriculum change in nursing? What benchmarks for high-quality exist in nursing education programs?

How can the entry into practice arguments be permanently resolved? What are the advantages of master's-degree or higher preparation being required for professional practice? What level of education is essential for "technical providers" of care in nursing? How should (or will) educators provide leadership to define and insist on policy change for two levels of practice? What forces are in play that previously have not existed that may result in a clear distinction and definition of professional practice?

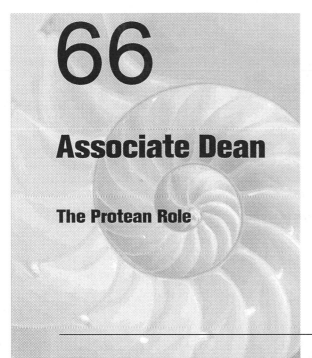

66

Associate Dean

The Protean Role

Marilyn E. Flood, PhD, RN

The Associate Dean title is a familiar feature in academic settings. But the shape of the role varies from place to place. In fact, it is unusually variable, even considering only nursing academic settings.[1] Despite this variability, some of the functions and necessary characteristics are common across institutional settings.[2] This role can contribute substantially to a unit, providing linkage at the intersection between faculty and administrative concerns. Major qualitative changes in the role are likely and essential, given the changes that are projected for higher education.

■ Factors Influencing the Shape of the Role

Commonly, the shape that the associate dean (AD) role assumes is attributed to some mixture of (a) aspirations and skills of the incumbent, (b) preference of the dean, and (c) expectations of influential, usually senior, faculty members. But additional factors also exert major influences:

• *Subunit organization within the school.* Organization into subunits is a result of the size of the school (number of students and faculty), as well as its differentiation (number of different educational programs and the extent to which faculty have responsibility for research or clinical practice). The AD role in a school with established departments, each having its own goals and budgetary authority, will be very different from the AD role in an equally large unidepartment school. Such massive single department schools may have yearly rotating Coordinators for faculty who teach in various clinical areas or years in an undergraduate program (Balderston, 1995).

- *The school's position in its organizational life cycle.* A school that is in an entrepreneurial growth spurt, whether due to its recent formation or due to a renaissance following stagnation and drift, will call for a different balance of activities and style from one that is in a mature, productive phase (Hunt, 1991).

- *Existence of other associate deans (ADs) with defined areas of responsibility.* Beyond the clarity (which can be a freedom or, conversely, a limitation) that comes with multiple AD roles, the very existence of multiple semiparallel roles influences each. This situation provides opportunity for specialization that a broad "operating officer" or "internal associate dean" role does not. If, however, the unit is not large or complex enough to require multiple AD functions, the faculty may feel overwhelmed by the number of initiatives emanating from multiple offices. Further, additional coordinating time entailed by the multiple positions will not be productive.

- *Structure of the position that includes the associate dean role.* If the AD must continue to meet promotion requirements based on instructional and research activity, the individual will, at the least, have less time to devote to AD functions; moreover conflicts of interest may exist at times between the two parts of the position.

- *Experience and capacity of persons in positions adjacent to the AD role.* As in any other organic system, boundaries of the role have to be somewhat flexible so that the system remains effective overall. For example, activities of the role will differ if year-group Coordinators or Department Chairs or other ADs are inexperienced or distracted for any number of reasons, compared to when they are experienced and fully engaged in their roles.

- *Career expectations of the AD.* In some settings, the AD responsibility is rotated among all senior faculty who have the necessary aptitude. Such assignment is not necessarily sought, and immediately after fulfilling this obligation, the incumbent expects to return to a "pure" faculty role. By contrast, the AD role may be the first official administrative experience for a mid-career faculty member who envisions becoming a dean. Thus the AD responsibility may be a stepping-stone or at least a ringside seat to the dean role. Certainly the range of career plans operating for prospective and incumbent ADs influences role performance.

Finally, seemingly minor factors may assume major importance. Just the simple availability of clerical staff to gather data, handle routine details, and serve as another conduit of information creates latitude for the role that is otherwise absent. Likewise, an information system that provides timely data decreases the number of false starts in planning.

■ Functions Fulfilled by the Role

Four of the seven functions of the AD role, (a) launching initiatives, (b) coordinating processes and activities, (c) managing "complaints," and (d) environmental scanning, are almost universal. The remaining three functions, (e) boundary spanning, (f) managing operational activities that cross subunits, and (g) providing counterbalance to strengths and weaknesses elsewhere in the organization, are of varying importance within a specific organization at a particular time. When these functions are needed or defined as part of the role, however, they may be as critical to the school as the first four.

Launching and Supporting Initiatives

The AD carries initiatives arising from groups of which she or he is a part (e.g., collective school vision development, the administrative group, the interaction of faculty groups with the AD), or the AD's own perspective. Regardless of the source, any initiative requires forethought about (a) its congruence with the external mission of the school and expectations by its publics, (b) its feasibility (i.e., availability of essential resources, both internal and external to the school), and (c) its timing (i.e., answering the question: "Given the time, energy, and dollars that will be needed to accomplish this task, is now the time to do it?").

Most major initiatives will require preliminary consultation with a number of people, if not approval by the whole faculty, who likewise weigh these critical factors. But with the exception of initiatives that arise from a whole-faculty visioning process, starting an initiative through the approval process makes no sense unless the AD herself or himself believes, on the basis of a preliminary assessment and data, that the initiative satisfies the mission, external public support or tolerance, feasibility, and timing criteria. Faculty (or staff) deliberation time is too valuable to waste on triage of unconsidered ideas.

Initiatives that have goals related to the AD scope of responsibility also will arise directly from faculty, either from individuals or groups. Support for these initiatives is also inherently a function of the AD role. Sometimes, it is merely a matter of ensuring that the proposal moves through the approval process in an orderly and timely way. At times support involves interpreting the intent of the proposal or giving clarifying detail. At other times it involves active argument on behalf of the proposal. At minimum, the AD aims for the proposal to get a fair and full hearing, whether or not the AD personally thinks it is a wise course of action. The AD certainly has the right to voice an opinion and to argue it forcefully. But once that has been done, she or he acquiesces to the collective voice of the decision-making body with some faith in the collective wisdom of the group over time. Without that faith, it is impossible to balance the "fair process" and "shared responsibility for decision outcome" responsibilities of the role.

The culture and customs of the faculty group determine the ideal style of initiative launch and the range of approaches that are effective. Unique history can make the same approach ideal in one faculty group and outrageous in another. But setting aside the occasional anomalies, consideration of the following factors helps avoid pitfalls:

- *Is the question being raised early enough to allow for full discussion?* Granted, sometimes external circumstances sharply limit the timeline, in which case everyone needs to know this at the outset. Because people vary widely in their pace of decision-making, striking a balance between "deliberators" and "early closers" is the challenge. Both ends of that spectrum reflect serious efforts to make wise collective decisions, but both also may be invoked to cover political maneuvering.

- *Is the question being brought with sufficient concreteness so that it can be considered and, paradoxically, with sufficient openness so that shaping is still possible?* Even "in principle" approval requires some specific detail in the proposal. Most major initiatives could be configured in multiple ways, so a simple "yes" or "no" question effectively forecloses many options. In some cases, a long prehistory of the initiative has shaped the formal proposal, so the openness criterion is met effectively before the question is formally brought for action.

- *Are the known implications of adoption or rejection "on the table?"* Is one of the acknowledged functions of discussion to get any other known implications out for consideration? Certainly dire predictions of risks of either adoption or rejection can be motivated politically, as can wildly exaggerated claims of benefits. But part of the purpose of discussion is to evaluate validity of the various predictions.

The academic calendar cycle is a critical consideration in introducing new initiatives. The introduction to decision to initial action process suffers the least distortion and delay if the whole process occurs within the same academic year. Multiyear consideration usually involves some change of committee membership and consequent need for rediscussion at the least, if not a total evaluation of the first year's work, before progress can be made. Even when the length of deliberation time would allow introduction of a question late in the year, it may not get thoughtful consideration if people are overwhelmed with other responsibilities. Further, some consideration should be given to the number and magnitude of changes in the recent past. Common sense requires that, if people are overwhelmed with change fatigue, nonurgent initiatives should be deferred. Given this need for pacing, it is essential to anticipate insofar as possible the likely major issues or initiatives over a 2-year period (Hunt, 1991).

■ Coordinating Processes and Activities

Everyone in a school has to be involved in coordinating relevant aspects of her or his work with that of others. But the AD role has a substantial coordinative component that, if done well, is invisible much of the time. The goal is to achieve coordinated activity by using a minimum of faculty time, but preserving faculty involvement and sense of ownership in its areas of responsibility and in the overall program of the school. Absent this AD coordinative function, a great deal of faculty energy can be dissipated in frustration, confusion, and wasted talking time.

Coordination may be done in a number of ways:

- orienting and giving background to other persons, either academic or clerical, who will have the primary responsibility for coordination;

- getting policies and practices developed for recurring activities and having them available to individuals who need them intermittently or for orientation; (Overcodification and too many written policies or practices, however, defeat the purpose. Regardless of indexing, faculty will not be able to find the relevant policy in a massive policy or practice listing. Further, the organization loses its flexibility. Resisting the temptation to codify customs in the hope that writing will "make it so" may be essential);

- identifying resource people, often nonacademic staff, who know the details of processes (that any individual faculty or staff person rarely needs) so that they serve the "ready reference" function for others;

- developing practical aids, such as flowcharts or schedules, that enable all involved to understand the reasons for deadlines and necessary sequencing of steps; and

- doing hands-on coordination, reminding, summarizing, and so forth to keep a process on track.

All the above presumes ongoing attentiveness to the situation for signs that the several processes and activities occurring simultaneously are unfolding smoothly, whether or not the AD is involved directly in the coordination. The AD has to hold a fundamental sense of final responsibility for the organization's accomplishing its goals, along with an understanding that the process belongs to everyone involved. The AD can confer, inform, remind, urge, offer support, and invoke collateral inducements, but in the end she or he must recognize that people—in this case faculty and other administrators—retain sovereignty over their own actions (Koerner & Mindes, 1997). Obviously the AD role is not one for persons with high control needs; but neither is it a role for persons with a laissez-faire approach to the task. Both extremes provoke faculty frustration and wasted activity (Rosovsky, 1990).

"Complaint" Management

The associate dean—because of the linking nature of the role, the positional authority of the role, and perhaps the identified "complaint recipient" function—will not only hear complaints, but be expected to work toward their resolution. Student complaints (up to and including a formal grievance) and faculty complaints (ranging from noting problems to explosive protest) may be part of the mix. Familiarity with work on conflict management and negotiation certainly is useful, both to keep the perspective that conflict is a normal phenomenon and also for knowledge of approaches to conflict resolution (Fisher & Ury, 1991; Weeks, 1992).

Hearing a complaint accurately is important both to the complainant and to the AD. A mental filter that either minimizes or magnifies a complaint serves neither the complainant nor an effort to resolve the situation. Minimizing may take the form of attributing clashes of fundamental values to more superficial "political," structural, or interpersonal sources, as well as overlooking the importance to the individual. Magnification creates a major moral or ethical question out of a simple disagreement and generalizes from one instance to a whole climate. On the one hand, inserting oneself directly into the resolution process may be inappropriate or rob the complainant of a sense of competence in handling the situation. On the other hand, an imbalance of power between the complainant and other person or group may argue for direct involvement. And, sometimes, the AD is in position simply to cut through some perceived barrier and resolve the situation without further pain to the complainant or anyone else. Serving as resource on relevant policies, customs, and practices allows this institutional "umpiring" framework to operate so that all parties can make their cases, taking into account the same "rules of the game."

Beyond dealing with the specifics of complaints constructively and appropriately, the AD—in a sort of "finger-on-the-pulse" way—notes the overall level of conflict in the organization and reflects on (a) why it is so now, (b) whether it is healthy, and (c) if it is unhealthy, what can be done to modify it. Sometimes, the reason for high conflict is obvious and unmodifiable; at other times, observation can be shared with others to get concerted thinking about changing the situation.

Environmental Scanning and Boundary Spanning

Environmental scanning involves the range of activities that provide critical information about the context in which the school operates. A comprehensive list of such areas is beyond the scope of this chapter. However, examples include (a) local, state, and national developments in nursing practice and nursing education; (b) extramural agency research funding priorities; (c) information on the institution in which the school is located and the institution's relevant environment; (d) organized nursing developments (local and state, at least); and (e) practicing nurse attitudes (alumni, nurse administrators in agencies, staff, and advanced nursing practice) (Ginter, Swayne, & Duncan, 1998). Without ongoing environmental information, it is impossible to do good preassessment of potential ideas for change in activities of the school. Certainly, comprehensive feasibility work done before the school's full commitment to a course of action will forestall unwise major changes. However, considerable time and other resources can be lost—and perhaps the goodwill of one or more publics, as well—if there is not a good preassessment even before the full-scale feasibility review.

Ideally every member of the faculty is involved in environmental scanning related to his or her particular interest, and at least some therefore will also have valid data to contribute to preassessment of overall school directions. Even in instances where the Dean focuses primarily on external relations and the AD attends to the internal operations of the school, the AD has to be attuned to external realities.

The focus and extent of the "boundary spanning" function varies considerably. When there is one AD and the division of responsibility is "inside and outside," the AD perhaps will interface with (a) her or his counterparts in other schools; (b) campus offices involved with students, academic programs, and facilities; (c) perhaps with clinical agencies in which students are placed; and (d) visitors to the school. In such a case there is little expectation—from the position definition at least—for wider boundary spanning. The need for the AD to do so also will be modified by the propensity of the faculty to do boundary spanning for the school. The more complex the school's relevant environment (i.e., the greater the number and interaction of factors and groups that potentially affect it), the more total boundary spanning the faculty and administration will need to do. The sheer volume of boundary spanning needed may draw an otherwise "inside AD" more heavily into this activity.

Coordinating Functions Across Subunits

Specific activities involved in this area will vary considerably by school and the particular focus of the AD's responsibility. Classroom and course scheduling is often a component; coordination of business and space-related actions of subunits is another; clinical placement planning is yet another. Organizing subunit involvement in preparation of self-studies for external reviews commonly falls within purview of the AD position, as well.

In most instances the reason a specific activity has been allocated to the AD for coordination is that (a) it is more costly or time-consuming (inefficient) for liaison representatives from subunits to fulfill the function jointly, (b) complexity of the job requires one person to integrate and order the variables to get a workable product, or (c) facilitation by the AD, and even mediation at times, is needed to get persons or units with disparate or conflicting interests to address the overarching collective project or goal.

The challenge inherent in this function is to understand and respect the cultures of the various subunits (or work styles of individuals) and nevertheless get a usable product by the deadline, using only the resources available for the task. Part of the skill involved is thinking about process from the standpoint of the subunit or faculty and fashioning it in as painless a way as possible. Another part is exercise of interpersonal skills. Some pitfalls can be avoided by engendering a preliminary set for the task, discussing time and resource limits, and pointing out consequences of delay or bad information. In egregious situations, with truly critical tasks, confrontation and threat of negative sanction can be used, but these are effective only if used rarely and judiciously.

Providing Counterbalance to Strengths and Weaknesses Elsewhere in the Organization

High-functioning organizations—particularly those involved in human services as contrasted with mass production of goods—require participants to make constant "organic" adjustments to compensate for variability in both clients (in this case students) and other participants (in this case faculty, subunit coordinators, and deans). Needed adjustments are most visible during the orientation phase, when someone new fills a position adjacent to the AD. How the newcomer will implement her or his role becomes apparent over time. Positions around the new appointee (including the AD position) gradually adjust to make the organization work. In addition to short-term change of functions in the AD position at transition and during the orientation period, long-term change is likely to be needed for the organization to remain effective. To the AD, such change may feel like a loss or an opportunity, depending on the AD's interest, characteristics, and liking for variety.

In addition to probable longer term change in the AD role for overall organizational effectiveness, various short-term, task-related flexes are required for the overall agility and capacity of the organization. Concrete examples could be (a) working out the terms of a joint service–education partnership, (b) developing data for a Task Force to advance its work, or (c) covering responsibilities of another administrator or faculty who is on leave or immersed in a major project. Although task-related flex activity does not have to fall to the AD position necessarily, it often does. At the extreme, there can be so much "flex activity" that any semblance of coherence in the position is lost and the person comes to believe the working title is "Associate Dean for Everything." Conversely, there may be enough other positions to cover the range of short-term flex needs so that this task does not become a burdensome element of the position. Whatever the extent, this aspect of the role will be somewhere on the continuum from distressing fragmentation to welcome variety.

■ Relationship to the Dean Role

One model of the Dean and Associate Dean working relationship is based on the assumption that incumbents need to have a holistic sense of the current and near-future issues of the deanship. From this comprehensive context, each takes initiative and fulfills responsibility in her or his area while maintaining continuing communication with the other. This structure might be termed the "rich context" model. An alternative model, perhaps named "specialized function," expects that each appointee will communicate necessary information for coordination to the Dean (and other ADs). However, in this model, comprehensive detail about issues with which the Dean's Office, in the aggregate, is dealing is deemed not essential and perhaps only distracting. Handling these details might be compared to singing choral music: Some use the notes as guides, but with dependence on the collective sound; others sing the notes as written, assuming that the composer and conductor are ensuring a pleasing mix of sound.

Each model has practical limits. But considering only the workable range in these approaches, the two (or more) persons involved may have very different ideas about what constitutes a desirable level of contextual background, or "necessary information" versus "distracting detail." Further, preferences of incumbents may change over time, due to experience in the role or setting. Aspiring to the goal of "no surprises" and feedback about unpleasant "surprises" may be the most practical way to strike a balance that works for all concerned. Periodic reflection on recent snags in ongoing work, with a mental search for patterns, is good preparation for conversation about preventing future problems.

At one end of the spectrum, an AD position may be established to solve a problem for which no one currently has a solution, in the hope that the new appointee will bring ideas and skills that will lead to a seemingly miraculous resolution. At the other end of the spectrum is a position onto which many people hope to transfer tasks without granting accompanying authority. If the offloading is from one person, the position takes on the character of an "Assistant to . . ." position; if it is from several, it becomes an "Assistant Dean for Miscellany" position. No organization establishes a position for hypothetical eventualities, and no appointee wants a role empty of responsibility and commensurate authority. But both the "magical solution" and "task without authority" possibilities warrant a caveat (Eble, 1978).

Depending on circumstances, the AD may want to be open with the Dean about her or his interest in eventually seeking a deanship. In the ideal world, and many times in reality, the Dean is supportive and creatively provides a range of experience and sponsorship for the aspirant. If the deanship is sought for the institution where both the AD and Dean are employed currently, the dynamics and reaction may be somewhat different than if it is a deanship "somewhere someday." Understandably, a Dean's enthusiasm about "grooming" withers if the AD is focused on the future at the expense of current contributions.

Given that the relationship between these two roles (like all organizational roles) continues to be negotiated over time, can any generalization be made about the relationship? I believe that there are three.

The Dean and Associate Dean must have somewhat corresponding positive and negative visions for the organization. That is, if the positive vision of each were represented as a circle in a Venn diagram, there must be substantial overlap. And the negative vision—what each would say the organization ought not be or do—should not appear in the positive Venn of the other. If these visions of the Dean and Associate Dean are too disparate, with few exceptions the AD needs to exit (or avoid entering) the role.

- Each can expect the other to bring energy to the role, engagement with its demands, and at least the level of aptitude displayed at the outset. Additionally, each often brings an ethical and moral engagement to the role and the issues it presents. "Loyalty" is often listed as a mutual expectation. This deserves some exploratory conversation if it is mentioned in pre-appointment or early appointment conversation. No dean, in the abstract, wants

"groupthink 'loyalty,'" and yet assured support in the fray is comforting. No one thinks "loyalty" entails agreement on small details, but sometimes "small" details are critical and therefore no longer small. Perhaps the concept of fidelity approaches what is often termed loyalty. With fidelity, the relationship is established on the bedrock assumption that the good of the school is served by the success of the deanship (among other factors) and that the Dean along with the AD are committed to that success. When the AD no longer believes this, fidelity demands exploration of issues surrounding the conflict and, if unresolvable, that the AD withdraw from the role.

- Most Associate Deans serve at the pleasure of the Dean. As a consequence, the Dean has, in a sense, a double stake in the AD's effectiveness. The Dean not only needs the work of the AD role to be done, but wants to avoid the distraction of faculty criticism of the AD appointee. From the AD's standpoint, this stake clarifies the relationship of the roles, though it can distract the inexperienced AD from attention to other significant relationships and from focus on the work itself. This "at the pleasure of" characteristic of the appointment can be compatible with a strong AD role, but it is up to both the AD and the Dean to make it so.

■ Desirable Characteristics for the Associate Dean

I am arbitrarily separating desirable AD characteristics into attitudes, skills, and actions. My bias is that attitudes are most fundamental and also are most subject to fluctuation over time.

Attitudes

Part of the challenge of remaining effective in the AD position is finding ways to renew the following attitudes.

- A hopeful, optimistic "we can do this and it's worth it" response to challenges facing the school overall, as well as to concrete project accomplishment and day-to-day reality. The sense of both significance and efficacy is necessary.

- A mix of admiration for and realism about others in the organization (i.e., faculty, staff, and other administrators). As long as the admiration is not distancing or distorting, the AD can probably not err too far in this direction. This perspective helps to shrink the day-to-day operational irritations to a manageable size.

- Ability to derive genuine satisfaction from success of the whole unit. Without this ability, it will be difficult to configure the AD role in such a way as to both fulfill its central functions and experience job satisfaction.

Skills

The following skills are essential to, or at least positively correlated with, effectiveness and satisfaction.

- Capacity to manage several projects simultaneously while dealing with a variety of short-answer and short-term matters that occur in the normal flow of activity. This need is true of most administrative roles and contrasts with ideal faculty roles. Individual styles of accomplishing concurrent tasks will vary.

- Ability to separate opinion about the wisdom of an action from providing good information about how to do it, provided of course that the action is within legal and ethical boundaries. The AD has a responsibility both to give access to institutional policies and practices, as well as to participate in decision-making.

Actions

The following actions or practices are particularly important.

- To engage in the core work of the school (i.e., teaching, research, and/or practice, even if

the extent is necessarily limited). This activity grounds administrative work in the day-to-day reality of the school as a whole. It helps the AD focus on the fact that administrative activity serves and facilitates the core work of teaching and research, and it helps her or him to stay realistic about the demands on faculty (Rosovsky, 1990).

- Within the administrative role, some work must be done directly and some must be delegated. The mix of setting capacity and individual proclivity may lead to imbalance in either direction. At the least, there must be some clerical skill and capacity in the institution to receive and perform delegated work. At the other extreme, even if almost unlimited skill and capacity are available in the institution for work delegation (a truly hypothetical situation), some direct task involvement by the AD is necessary for effectiveness.

■ Qualifications for Associate Dean

When an associate dean is to come from within a school, both the candidate and the institution have considerable information beyond that provided in the typical search communication. When the position is to be filled by an external candidate, however, the challenge is to get self-selection to operate effectively by providing a full range of information about expectations, culture, and environment.

I believe there are really only two essential qualifications:

- ability to fulfill the functions of the role, and

- experience (academic preparation and academic and administrative experience) and presence necessary to create the initial expectation that the incumbent will be able to do the job.

Many would list several specifics in the second category, but I believe specifics are highly variable by time and place.

■ *The Future of the Associate Dean Role*

As higher education changes, the nature of the AD role also will change. In the near future, as long as pressure for both educated workers and more "efficient" education (i.e., same or more learning per learner unit of time and per payor cost) exist, there is every reason to believe that higher education will experience some of the same turbulence that health care is weathering at the present time. Indeed, higher education is widely cited as the last major sector of the economy ripe for restructuring (Munitz, 1995). However, when the supply–demand factors for educated workers change, higher education's recent past role will again be needed (i.e., keeping young adults productively busy, without increasing either the subjective sense or the statistical indicators of unemployment). This counterpressure will create a complicating undertow in the restructuring waves.

With health care as a model, what would "managed education" look like? I would expect to see middle roles such as the Associate Dean deleted and then reintroduced when the chaos of discoordination exceeds tolerable limits. Between abolition and reintroduction, there will be experiments with (a) allocating coordination of specific functions to noncentral roles (e.g., faculty members asked to coordinate), and (b) just not doing some things to see if they are really necessary (a consequence in any "rightsizing"). Experimenting with roles can be a good thing, as long as real outcomes are tracked, not just indicators that are available and reducible to numbers. Use of a particular title, or the organizational location of a person fulfilling a function, is not an issue provided that the organization remains effective.

In health care, some agile organizations are managing well in the turbulence, mostly in fortunate geographic or specialty niches. Other organizations are struggling but weathering the turbulence, though some have lost their names and identities in mergers. Still others in various ways have truly gone out of business because of past artificially stimulated capacity or current artificially shrunken demand. As the parallel process occurs in higher education, associate deans will experience rapid, unpredictable changes in role content and skill demands that the middle levels of nursing in health care agencies currently face.

With restructuring, the ratio of resources to work in higher education will be reduced overall. This conversion probably will take the form of a ratcheting down of funding ratios for institutions that are now partially state-supported, with spillover pressure on private institutions coming in a variety of ways. Agile schools therefore will spend increasing amounts of time hunting for money and dealing with obligations that are attached to what is found. Whether agile or not, schools will have fewer people (faculty, staff, and administrators) available to prepare more students and produce more research. This changed ratio will raise the level of conflict in organizations above current levels. Reduced resources will lead to increasingly urgent questions, such as "Do we really need to do X to have capable graduates?" and "Can we do essential X in a different, less expensive way?" Whether the end result of the restructuring is widely admired or deplored, the process will produce considerable uncertainty and longing for past relative stability.

Given all of this, what will the AD role look like in 15 years? Even if AD role functions fall into roughly unchanged categories, the institutional context in many organizations may be changed so substantially that it will be a qualitatively different role. For example, faculty membership may come to mean something quite different. The current usual arrangements—contiguous offices, expectation of participation in governance, and expectation of substantially full-time effort devoted to a single institution's work—may prevail to a more limited extent even in venerable schools with long traditions. Many faculty may become independent contractors who work in several institutions and perhaps intermittently in any one of them. For example, faculty may be hired primarily to design "learning packages," supervise prelicensure students in very limited experience with real patients (because of sophisticated simulations and lack of sufficient numbers of patients in one place), and do competency testing to supplement written tests. Schools then would consist of a skeleton force of faculty, administrators, clerical staff, technicians (to deliver the "learning packages" to students by whatever medium), and some supplemental short-term, part-time faculty. Funding for research in professional fields could be attached to the investigator's track record of implementation in one or more settings (health care, in the case of nursing), rather than the current tie solely to publication. As a consequence, a whole set of new relationships would become critical.

Academic leaders, both faculty and administrative, will be called on to project the long-term consequences of seemingly expedient, short-term decisions. These leaders also will be pressured to draw on collective wisdom about types of learning that can be mediated, in contrast to those that require direct interaction with faculty. In the context of turbulent change, schools will have to reclarify the essence of their core missions and single-mindedly fulfill these in order to preserve institutional integrity.

■ Concluding Statement

The Associate Dean role currently fulfills essential functions. As higher education changes, the balance among AD functions, and the specific activities within the role, will change considerably. In the transition, some units probably will experiment with deletion of the position and consequent redistribution of functions.

■ Notes

1. This discussion addresses the role that extends the overall administrative leadership capacity of the chief academic administrator of a nursing education unit, whether that title be Chair, Director, or Dean. Institutional custom will dictate the choice between "Associate" and "Assistant" titles. In systems where both exist, the Assistant Dean title usually denotes a narrower focus of responsibility. As I use "Associate Dean" in a somewhat generic sense, so do I also use "school," recognizing that the unit may be a college or a department.
2. These observations are shaped by my readings in organization studies and long experience, in two separate blocks of time, in the AD role in a single institution. No institution is "typical," but neither is any institution unique, as I have learned from conversations over time with others in such roles.

■ References

Balderston, F. E. (1995). *Managing today's university: Strategies for viability, change, and excellence* (2nd ed.). San Francisco: Jossey-Bass.

Eble, K. E. (1978). *The art of administration.* San Francisco: Jossey-Bass.

Fisher, R., & Ury, W. (1991). *Getting to yes* (2nd ed.). New York: Penguin Books.

Ginter, P. M., Swayne, L. M., & Duncan, W. J. (1998). *Strategic management of health care organizations* (3rd ed.). Malden, MA: Blackwell.

Hunt, J. G. (1991). *Leadership.* Newbury Park, CA: Sage.

Koerner, M., & Mindes, G. (1997, February). Leading from the middle. *Proceedings of the AACTE* (American Association of Colleges for Teacher Evaluation) *Meeting. 49th Annual AACTE Meeting.* (ERIC [Educational Resources Information Center] Document 406347). Phoenix, Arizona.

Munitz, B. (1995). *Managing transformation in an age of social triage.* In S. L. Johnson and S. C. Rush (Eds.), *Reinventing the university: Managing and financing institutions of higher education* (pp. 21–48). New York: Wiley.

Rosovsky, H. (1990). *The university: An owner's manual* (p. 257). New York: Norton.

Weeks, D. (1992). *The eight essential steps to conflict resolution.* New York: Putnam.

■ Editor's Questions for Discussion

What factors most influence the associate dean role? To what extent does the AD fulfill an "intermediary" type of role and with whom? What ethical issues and concerns arise about intermediary role relationships? How does Chaska's (Chapter 68) discussion regarding accountability apply to AD and dean roles?

To what extent should a "match" exist between AD and dean? Discuss Flood's suggestions for corresponding visions between dean and AD. How can the match best be assessed prior to appointment of an AD or dean? What negotiations and understandings between an AD and dean are critical? How may differences among responsibility, accountability, and authority be problematic? In addition to Flood's suggestion for an AD's positive working relationships with a dean, what characteristics and qualifications for both positions facilitates successful association?

What characteristics and qualifications are essential in AD candidates? What may or should be most satisfying for the AD in fulfilling the role? From Flood's discussion, what is most challenging in the AD role? What criteria may be used for measuring performance and success in the AD role? How would you characterize an effective AD?

Is the AD position most often a staff or line position? What difference does it make in fulfilling school functions and roles as to how the position is classified? When the dean focuses on external relations and the AD on internal operations, should the AD position be defined as a line function? Provide reasons and examples for your response. What factors should be considered for guiding decisions defining an administrative position as line or staff? How do Flood's relationship models with deans apply to line and staff positions? What issues may arise for faculty and a dean if the AD position is line or staff? Provide specific examples and indicate strategies to resolve those issues.

What risks are involved in "at will" type of appointments for ADs and deans? What "protection" should be negotiated prior to such administrative appointments? What is your prediction about how restructuring of the associate dean role may occur?

How do Flood's predictions regarding restructuring and the AD role compare with predictions by Fleming (Chapter 22), Lindeman (Chapter 63), Keating and Perry (Chapter 65), Biordi and McFarlane (Chapter 67), Lindell (Chapter 69), and Shaver (Chapter 76)?

67

Academic Roles and Faculty Development

Diana L. Biordi, PhD, RN, FAAN
Elizabeth A. McFarlane, DNSc, RN, FAAN

Contrary to the perceptions of many nonacademicians, academe does not exist in a social vacuum of ivory towers. Higher education is part of the social order of its time, and academicians reflect the placement of the university in time and space. Consequently, faculty development, both in the faculty role and in other academic roles, resonates to forces within the larger academic and social environment. Issues of supply and demand, economics, faculty research and teaching focus, employment and tenure status, ethics, governance, and intramural and extramural social and political relationships affect academic roles and their fulfillment. To help in understanding the impact of these factors, in this chapter we discuss higher education's historical, social, orga-

nizational, and administrative models to situate faculty, other academic roles, and their development. The relationship of these factors to nursing in academe is demonstrated following the initial exposition of more general features of higher education and academic roles. When the term *university* is used in this chapter, it refers to academe in general, unless stated otherwise.

■ *Historical and Organizational Models of Higher Education*

The Colonial College

Modern American higher education evolved from a colonial model, mainly British, grounded in a strong tradition of emphasis on character, religiosity, and leadership. Drawing on the prototypes of Cambridge and Oxford, the American colonial college welcomed "gentlemen" elite to prepare them for civic and religious leadership and commitment, with less emphasis on scholarship and, most certainly, on research (Brubacher & Rudy, 1997). If indeed research was conducted, it was largely outside the college, as conducted, for example, by Benjamin Franklin and Thomas Jefferson. For more than 200 years, the faculty role so focused on uplifting morality that becoming a teacher was close to being a clerical vocation (Boyer, 1991). To achieve proper morality, the colonial college greatly emphasized such institutions as residences, or what came to be known as the collegiate style of life. This style continues to this day in undergraduate programs, often illustrated by bucolic brochures that portray students in outdoor classes or in gothic buildings situated on green rolling hills.

University Development in the United States

Gradually, as the United States continued its westward expansion, needs of the great builders began to intrude on the earlier views of education as moral development. In the desire to build a nation, education captured the service needs of the community, and in doing so, changed the "product" of education to "serviceable men" (Boyer, 1991, p. 5). Not only had higher education begun to respond to the utilitarian needs of the time, but it drew larger numbers of students (primarily men) from the farmlands and prairies. In the democratization of education, these serviceable men also became "serviceable patriots" (Boyer, 1991, p. 5). This democratization coincided with development of land grant universities that supported not only liberal arts but, especially, the agricultural and mechanical skills needed for the new America. In turn, knowl-

edge that was generated in land grant universities came to be known as applied research for its utility and service (Brubacher & Rudy, 1997).

The German Research University

At about the same time as the westward American expansion, in Germany the concept of the university as an instrument dedicated to service of the state became the model, particularly for the natural and medical sciences. In contrast to earlier educational residential models, the essence of the German educational system was the freedom to pursue dispassionately truth through original investigation. This goal created a very different learning environment of independent nonresidential scholars, stratified into upper and lower divisions, who used newer methods of specialized lectures, seminars, and scientific investigation. Americans were impressed with the pragmatics of scientific practices as evidenced in the German system, which could be incorporated into the utilitarian education and service ideals then signifying American education. By the mid 19th century the American university was being organized into one of two major types: (a) the public state university, responding to democratization; and (b) the private university, responding to research imperatives. Both became centers of advanced learning and research (Boyer, 1991).

The American Research University

Still, change came slowly, and it was only in the late 19th and early 20th centuries that the German model came to be the dominant model of university education, leading to the PhD (Doctor of Philosophy) degree. Research had now taken a firm hold within the university, primarily at the graduate level. Nonetheless, land grant universities continued their emphasis on service, and, for a variety of reasons, the undergraduate model continued its colonial model of a residential study style (Boyer, 1991). Coexistence of the colonial and the German model within the same university created a certain schism of prestige, teaching methods, and research values among members of the faculty. The newer American university, unlike its European model, had diversified its faculties by virtue of diversifying its fields of study. Whereas the traditional European university had four great faculties—law, medicine, theology, and the arts—the American university had several divisional faculties (e.g., schools of journalism, business, education, pharmacy, nursing, engineering, library services, urban policy and public administration, fashion, and so forth) (Willis, 1960).

The Modern Academy: Government-Funded Research and Its Impact

During World War II (WWII) and thereafter, the government of the United States turned to the universities and their research traditions to seek answers to many questions posed by war effort and, later, peace. As the academy responded, a tight link developed between government funding and academic economics. Faculty stressed the doctorate, whose scholarship definition and emphasis were on research, not teaching. Almost simultaneously after WWII, a flood of returning veterans were rewarded with the GI bill and a subsidized college education. Higher education continued as a right, not a privilege, and became a ticket for upward social and occupational mobility. So, at the same time that education had become a nonelitist option for many potential students, emphasis on research had created a faculty elite, for whom "publish or perish" was the imperative. The emphasis on research was to the (a) detriment of undergrad-

uates, (b) hegemony of stratified specialized knowledge, and (c) ascendency of disciplinarian loyalty over campus loyalty for the professorate (Brubacher & Rudy, 1997).

■ Forces Having an Impact on Modern Academe

Corporate Thinking

The modern academy model has prevailed for almost 50 years. Only in the 1980s and 1990s did the American university and its professorate reexamined priorities, with a resultant slow change in academic posture. As university faculty and administration role changes created job mobility, power distribution became quite uneven, made more so by introduction of more broadly based boards of trustees. The newer trustee was drawn from outside the university, frequently a business and philanthropic leader of the community (Brubacher & Rudy, 1997). Using business norms and acumen, the newer trustees' aim was to manage (and frequently, to micromanage) the university more diligently. Because of the power changes and introduction of business norms, many academics have been exposed to what has been colloquially called the "corporate model." The term corporate model is a misnomer because most universities were incorporated under their initiating charter (Brubacher & Rudy, 1997). Rather, the corporate model should be called the corporate thinking model, in that power and office are delegated more clearly to trustees and university administration and expressed in business terms such as vice president (clearly, different from vice chancellor). Moreover, corporate business norms have been imported into the university, including more accountable fiscal management, capital investment and new construction, responses to faculty and unionized faculty demands, and the outsourcing of many in-house tasks. Like nursing's reluctant acceptance of secular models over more traditional sacred models of care, academics have had to come to terms with the inclusion of secularized, corporate ways of thinking and management. In the late 1990s, the modern university could be thought of as the "consumer university" because of the emphasis on short-term outcomes (e.g., occupational mobility for students), a contractor posture demanded by students, and because of the influence of many interest groups on the university and its position within the community.

Demographics

In keeping with the social world, public and university faculty reactions to the predominantly white, male-oriented faculty and their research resulted in an examination of the absence of women and minorities on faculty, in research studies, and in curricula. According to the Almanac Issue of the Chronicle of Higher Education (Almanac) (1998) even now, American faculties are largely composed of men (about 80%), with the fewest women being in the natural sciences (17%) and engineering (3%). Minorities are placed in universities unevenly, with more Asians as faculty in research organizations and more African Americans at liberal arts and community colleges. Both minorities and women are overrepresented at the entry levels of assistant professor. Salaries for minorities and women are also uneven and, typically, less than white male faculty.

Public Opinion: Critics of Curriculum and Faculty

In keeping with the times, public cynicism extended to close and critical evaluation of the focus and worth of the curricula in higher education, as well as to the faculty charged with developing and teaching the curricula. Students and faculty alike called for curricula to be expanded beyond that of "dead white European males" (i.e., Western Civilization). Elitist notions toppled and pluralistic curricula encompassing other cultures, women's studies, ethnic and black studies, and multiculturalism came into being. On the one hand, critics examined the faculty and its composition and charged that faculty were too male, too conservative, too slow to change, and out of touch with their disciplines, society, or student needs or all three. On the other hand, faculty also were charged with being too liberal, too trendy, desiring too much political correctness, and destroying important values of traditional study. Critics faulted faculty as being too selfish, lazy, or self-aggrandizing; they accused faculty of sacrificing teaching to research and of sacrificing community and students to the personal rewards of tenure. Faculty, upon obtaining tenure, were denounced as having sloughed off their work to (non-English–speaking) graduate assistants or to staff. Of those remaining (non-tenured) faculty, critics argued that such faculty were poor teachers who lacked clear thinking or writing skills, and that, despite their emphasis on research, actually conducted little research of high quality (Faculty Work, 1994). Although each of these complaints could be refuted, the important point was that faculty were no longer sacred icons of education but were as subject to bitter public scrutiny as any other worker in downsized corporate America. This shift in public sentiment, from the faculty as scholar to the faculty as employee or worker, was profound.

Changing Students, Changing Methods

Students other than the traditional young, able-bodied, white male are increasingly the norm: More women, minorities, and the disabled are college students, and as the population is aging, more "nontraditional" students (older than 18–22 years of age) are enrolled.

More than half the students are part-time enrollees (Almanac, 1998). Greater access to a college education has occurred through the establishment of (a) 2-year community-based colleges, (b) tighter articulation among educational programs from various educational institutions, (c) changing curricula, and (d) distance learning. Along with changing curricula and student bodies, new techniques of education, drawn from the technology, data, and entertainment industries came into being. Libraries and information management systems are increasingly being computerized, becoming more refined and expensive (Faculty Work, 1994). Distance learning (DL) across geographic boundaries is becoming a norm, addressing the solitary, independent student. Although distance learning techniques have been available for three decades, the advent of computerized DL has raised questions about privacy, university boundaries, tuition charges, professional licensure, freedom of speech and the intellectual property rights of the professorate, and university management. The mass distribution of high technology also has ushered in a new class of technocrats, along with questions about their proper place in the administrative and power elite.

Academic Funding and Partnerships

As universities—almost chronically underfunded—have established their niche in the United States, their economics and that of the country were not in good alignment. A few private universities were well endowed, but public universities were managed very differently by their state legislatures. Fiscal management required a focus on revenues and expenses, an emphasis made more important by business-oriented trustees. Gift getting and gift giving are now crucial to the survival of most universities, and many university presidents and deans must have, as a major criterion

of their performance, an ability to raise funds. To raise funds more easily, universities have drawn again on their long-standing service ideals—concretized into alliances with local and national "community partners" toward the good of the community or partner. In becoming active in their physical and social environments, university leaders have sought to conserve and improve those environments. Nature and environmental concerns are projects or curriculum areas that universities now undertake; these concerns also include investing endowments only in socially or environmentally acceptable funds.

International Partnerships

Another major initiative in partnerships has been undertaken by several universities—that of global partner. As never before, the world is seen to be "smaller," where similarities and needs override differences. American education is considered among the finest in the world, providing superior education to students from abroad, contributing to the science, economics, and health of other countries. By 1995, the most popular fields of studies for foreign-born students were, in ascending order, business, engineering, the natural sciences, mathematics, computer science, and the social sciences (*Barron's*, 1994). In nursing, international students are a major market for some programs. As students come to the United States for education, issues of brain drain, U.S. isolationism, economic subsidization, and alarm about foreign nationalism intruding on American business, health, or education systems now prevail.

Yet, despite the many questions raised by the breakdown of traditional, tightly held distinctions, popularization of education in the United States has produced commitment to education. In 1998, more than 4,000 institutions of higher education existed in the United States, enrolling more than 14 million students of whom, on average, 56% were women, 58% were full time, 27% were minority students, and 3% were foreign students. More than 36% of the students received some form of financial aid. Indeed, the United States had committed more than 2% of its gross national product (GNP) to education. In 1994–1995, 44,446 doctorate, 397,629 master's, 1,160, 134 baccalaureate, and 539,691 associate degrees were conferred by American institutions of higher education (Almanac, 1998). In applied research, the American ideal of utility and service has produced everything from vaccines, polymers, liquid crystal technology, to atomic physics and genetically engineered vegetables. In pure research, particularly of late, the American university is one of the few places that offers a secure job market and research subsidy. Similarly, although the body politic may be stingy with the arts, the arts thrive in academe (Brubacher & Rudy, 1997). Health and business professionals are educated well only in higher education, and the latest revitalization of vocational education has occurred in academe.

■ Nursing Units Within Higher Education

As we enter the 21st century, nursing is evolving from an education base that began early in the 20th century. During the first half of the 20th century, the "collegiate school of nursing" made "slow but continuous progress since its initiation at the University of Minnesota in 1909" (Williams & Stewart, 1950, p. 15). The 1950s brought continuing growth of programs offering baccalaureate degrees in nursing, as well as emergence of the community college and, with it, birth of the associate degree in nursing. Although introduced prior to 1950, since 1975 graduate education in nursing has experienced a rapid expansion of master's degree and doctoral programs. The same forces

influencing changes in the climate and organization of colleges and universities, in general, are affecting nursing education as well. Thus nursing education has examined its commitment to minority students, part-time students, multiculturalism in the curriculum, nurses in university administration, men in nursing, interdisciplinarity, and access to education.

However, particular to nursing and other health care disciplines are educational changes brought about by the changing health care system in the United States. Major forces in the health care system include the shift of the health care environment from hospital to community, a call for interdisciplinary models of health care practice, and the increasing complexity of health care technology. These factors have been the impetus to change not only in content and teaching methods, but also in the structure and organization of the nursing educational unit (O'Neil, 1993).

Structures

The structures and models of nursing education also are related intimately to the organization of the college or university within which they are located. Institutional characteristics to be considered include (a) institutional control (e.g., public versus private); (b) mission of the institution concerning emphasis on research, teaching, and service; (c) number of graduate programs; (d) size in terms of faculty and students (undergraduate and graduate); and (e) budget constraints. Characteristics of the nursing unit that can influence its structure include (a) nursing degrees offered (baccalaureate, master's, or doctorate); (b) number of nursing faculty (full-time and part-time tenured, tenure track, and non-tenure track); (c) numbers of nursing students in the various degree programs; (d) administration of the unit's budget; and (e) equity with similar units concerning faculty salaries and number of tenured and tenure track faculty. A combination of these characteristics can influence whether a unit is able to maintain itself autonomously or differently as an interdisciplinary unit in the organization. Organizational charts help locate a nursing unit and the degree of its independence in the organization.

Within community colleges (offering associate degree programs) and 4-year colleges (offering baccalaureate degrees), nursing and other units are often organized as departments or divisions. Heads of respective units report to the college's chief academic officer. Frequently, in 2- and 4-year colleges offering a variety of health related programs of study, a single structure may be designed to hold and unify the programs, for example, a Division of Health Sciences.

Within a university, independent academic units are named "schools" or "colleges"; these units are headed by deans who report to the chief academic administrator of the university (usually a provost or academic vice president). A school may focus on a particular discipline and a separate dean (e.g., the Dean of the School of Nursing or the Dean of the School of Pharmacy). Alternatively, a university may have a school or college with an interdisciplinary focus (e.g., a School of Health Sciences) that can include departments of nursing, medicine, and pharmacy, with each department headed by a chair, or director.

Interdisciplinary Schools

The budgetary constraints experienced by both public and private universities during the 1990s prompted many university administrators to reduce the number of independently budgeted units. This move resulted in some nursing programs being absorbed into interdisciplinary schools holding all the health programs of a campus. Nursing programs then became departments, divisions, or programs within a newly designated school. The former nursing deans assumed either the position of Dean of the new Health School or that of director or chairperson of the changed nursing department.

On the one hand, absorption of nursing programs into interdisciplinary schools prompted expressions of concern from nurses worried that nursing's visibility, autonomy, tenure reviews, or prestige would be compromised or reduced. On the other hand, such interdisciplinary absorption was applauded by those who believe that interdisciplinarity requires preparation for practitioners because it will be a major movement in the future in both health care and academe (Shugars, O'Neil, & Badar, 1991).

■ Career Ladders and Faculty Development

Forces on American higher education for the past 50 years have made their impact on the professorate and administrations in both subtle and large ways. The influence of hierarchy and research have dictated a career path for the professorate, which ranges in ascending order from lecturer, to instructor, assistant professor, associate professor, and professor. In turn, missions of the universities, particularly as expressed in faculty roles, are typically the triumvirate of research, teaching, and service, with research being the most important. Each level of faculty hierarchy must meet certain faculty-established criteria for status, which is often accompanied by a norm (formal or informal) of time-at-level (6 years) and a formal peer and administrative review process. Faculty evaluations differ from traditional career evaluations in terms of their formality and in their type, frequency, review system, and postreview action. Frequently wages or salaries are explicitly higher for each level. *Such a progressive, formal, evaluated structure is called a career ladder* in most types of organizations, but academics usually do not refer to their career hierarchy as a ladder.

In other types of organizations, career ladder *levels* often suggest differences in the nature or quality of work. The number of levels may vary, but they act as a guide or prescription whereby employees can assess themselves or others with regard to meeting important organizational objectives.

Benefits of a Career Ladder

The benefits to a career ladder are the careful explication of criteria against which a person will be assessed for mobility to the next level(s) and the incumbent's freedom to use the ladder for personal or career growth. Use of a career ladder can assist an individual in organizing career steps and content efficiently while helping the organization establish benchmarks of quality and quality control. In the case of an immobilized career-path workforce, a career ladder also can force organizational members to consider or develop alternative career paths or positions for the workforce. Such effects can increase job satisfaction for the individual while developing the organization functionally.

Barriers to a Career Ladder

The barriers to career ladders, particularly in profit-aware organizations, are (a) whether annual costs that can attach to the ladder can be controlled (i.e., who will use it this year and at what salary level?), (b) whether progression or competition is within personal and organizational norms, (c) whether the possibility of achieving the stated criteria is realistic, and (d) whether saturating upper levels of the ladder while closing entry levels will create an immobilized workforce.

Faculty Role Content and Job Mobility

Today, all university faculty have basically the same work—research, teaching, and service—although efforts differ in terms of emphasis, rank, mission, discipline, and personal preference (Faculty Work, 1994). Faculty governance is folded within faculty roles, and this reality can be a factor in promotion where university citizenship and service are important criteria.

Within the past century, faculty governance changed gradually as university administration changed from simple clerical responsibilities to broad-based management. As university presidents assumed broader powers, faculty power declined—delegated to other university functionaries (nonacademic staff roles) or folded into new structures called departments. As the department focus hardened and turfs developed, bridging mechanisms were developed in the form of new academic units, such as centers, institutes, and bureaus. Besides using departments or bridging mechanisms, faculty began to handle administrative concerns through committee structures, gradually yielding administrative details to councils. Eventually, faculty focused on instruction and investigation and left to others the judicial and executive functions of administration (Brubacher & Rudy, 1997).

All these structures—administration, departments, bridges, faculty, councils, and committees—brought a variety of roles, career visibility, and advancement or change opportunities that differed from traditional faculty career paths. As women and minorities came into academe but were kept in lower echelon faculty roles, these alternative roles offered administrative positions and mobility to them (Ost & Twale, 1988). The increased number and type of roles also opened the organization to more varied perspectives of role incumbents. Importantly, such roles were more likely to proliferate in larger or more flexible organizations that had resources to sustain them (Ost & Twale, 1988). The alternative governance structure and subsequent possibilities had implications for inclusion of other groups, acceptance of cutting edge thinking, and development of newer departments, such as nursing.

■ Nursing Challenges Within Universities

Acceptance of Nursing by Universities

Nursing has had to struggle to make its way onto campuses whose main interests were the arts, sciences, humanities, and the traditional professions of medicine, law, and theology. Professional education is costly, and mainstream academics believed that the professions drew much-needed resources away from core university foci. As a feminist profession, nursing faculty have had to displace notions of nonintellectualism and invisibility of nursing work. Only within the past three decades have nursing faculty conducted well-funded research; thus, nursing's earlier focus on teaching had only intensified and hardened the jealous husbanding of resources by competing departments. In the past two to three decades, nurses have found their place among university researchers. Acceptance evolved as nurses adapted to research norms while bringing in relevant findings and financial resources that offset the cost of nursing to the institution. Nursing's research and organizational placement had implications for the success of nursing faculty.

Roles

Particularly important to promotion and tenure of nurses was the nursing unit as an independent or interdisciplinary structure and its location in a public or private institution—

be its orientation a research, comprehensive, liberal arts university or a community college.

Because the mission of the university varies in terms of the emphasis placed on research, teaching, service, and subsequent expectations of faculty, nurse faculty going into an organization had to recognize their likelihood of success within that organization. For example, doctoral level universities emphasize the quantity and quality of research as important criteria for promotion and tenure, whereas universities founded as teachers' colleges may focus on innovative and creative teaching methods as their primary criteria. Early in the career path incoming nursing faculty, like others, need to determine the formal and informal promotion and tenure criteria of nursing and the university. Identifying mentors and having discussions with other faculty members who have successfully engaged in the promotion and tenure process especially can be helpful.

Tenure

As result of business-oriented trustees' assumptions and early faculty firings in the 1930s and 1940s, university faculties marshaled arguments for contracts and preservation of academic freedom; most particularly sought was lifelong tenure after a period of probation, which could be terminated only for adequate cause. On the one hand, tenure ensured faculty stability and freedom of political expression. On the other hand, tenure has come under attack from (a) disaffected junior faculty critical of academic "deadwood," (b) publics critical of lessened professorate accountability, (c) politicians critical of tenure's financial implications, and (d) activists concerned with tenure's exclusionary lock on positions—especially excluding minorities and women (Faculty Work, 1994).

Despite its criticisms, tenure is not granted cavalierly. Traditionally, tenure has been intended to permit faculty's freedom of inquiry to pursue thinking wherever it may lead, however unpopular or impolitic. Generally, the U.S. Supreme Court has upheld the role of academic freedom as an essential protection of free expression, particularly under the First Amendment protections of free speech. Tenure also has been determined to be a "property right" that requires due process under the Fourteenth Amendment. Academic freedom at public institutions comes under constitutional protection, whereas contract law is used to protect academic freedom at independent institutions (Faculty Work, 1994).

Although closely connected, academic freedom and tenure are not synonymous and indeed, in some universities, processes of tenure and promotion are separate. As assistant professors (normally non-tenured positions) apply for tenure, faculty carefully review credentials and support for the candidate, considering objective and subjective criteria of the university's faculty. Tenure reviews occur at several levels in the university, generally requiring final approval by the chief administrative officer and the board of trustees. Once tenure has been granted, the faculty member is assured that position for life, as long as the faculty line (budget position) remains intact or the incumbent does not violate certain university rules. Although there is much to be said for tenure, universities with a large proportion of tenured faculty usually have lessened program responsiveness, a larger proportion of its costs dedicated to faculty salaries, and constraints on new hiring.

The Influence of Ernest Boyer and the Carnegie Foundation

At about the time of (a) expanding and shifting paradigm boundaries, (b) criticisms of tenure, and (c) questions of rigid and distinct missions of research, teaching, and service, Ernest Boyer and the Carnegie Foundation presented a new model of scholarship. The Boyer model sought to reintegrate and make more capacious the meaning of scholarship. Rather than focusing on the rigid categories of (only) research, teaching, and service, Boyer offered four types of scholarship that faculty should pursue (Boyer, 1991). Two of these are the scholarship of discovery and of integration. *Discovery* is considered most like the traditional concept of research or the generation of knowledge. *Integration* connects the seemingly unconnected across disciplines, placing specialties within larger contexts, into what is most like interdisciplinarity. Discovery focuses on the nature of a phenomenon, whereas integration focuses on its meaning. Boyer also speaks to two other types of scholarship—application and teaching. *Application* is defined as the dynamic reciprocity of knowledge and problem, theory and practice, from which new intellectual understandings occur. The scholarship of *teaching* encompasses the active pursuit of teaching—transforming and extending knowledge, leading to lifelong learning and continuity between generations (Boyer, 1991; Wood et al., 1998).

Some faculties (in and outside nursing) have sought to build on Boyer's principles, asking newer questions that help align criteria for career ladders for faculty—on both the tenure and non-tenure tracks (Wood et al., 1998). Faculty were not trying to rearrange old nursing models into a new form but sought a new construction consistent with Boyer's more dynamic model of scholarship. This aim is critical if nursing is to come to terms with the inclusion of parallel non-tenure track faculty lines, or what also have been labeled variously as "part-time faculty," "term," "contract," and "clinical" faculty (Gosnell & Biordi, 1999).

Non-tenure track faculty always have been a bulwark of nursing faculties; they are now much more so within the general university. A 1998 study indicated that slightly more than two thirds of nursing faculty held short-term, non-tenure track status—an increase from 1985 when half of nursing faculty held term contracts (Gosnell & Biordi, 1999). In the general university, part-time faculty use increased from 30% in 1975 to 41% in 1995. Consequently, career ladders will have greater importance to both tenure and non-tenure track faculty as they attempt to cohabit in a dominant one-track tenure system (Rudy, Anderson, Dudjak, Kobert, & Miller, 1995).

Part-Time Faculty

Because of the forces impinging on the university, career ladders will be increasingly important in recruitment and retention of all faculty but, particularly in nursing, short-term, non-tenure track faculty. Satisfaction in nursing faculty is reported to be linked to length of faculty contracts (Moody, 1996). As universities require (a) greater flexibility and responsiveness to trends in their programs and schedules, (b) easier conservation of finances in meeting crises or short-term needs, and (c) reallocation of benefits financial pools, part-time faculty frequently serve a great purpose. On the contrary, part-time faculty in nursing and in the university have been criticized as (a) diluting the quality of a program; (b) having less commitment to the student, program, or institution; or (c) creating inequities in committee work between them and tenured faculty. In turn, part-time faculty complain of (a) not having benefits, (b) working more than one job to meet living needs, and (c) delays in research or obtaining research funding. The university must therefore strike a careful balance between demographics, technology, economics, teaching skills, research, and student access to excellent faculty, or, in the case of nursing, access to competent clinical practitioners. Despite the criticisms, a growing academic trend has been an increasing reliance on non-tenure track faculty, either part-time or under full-time short contracts.

■ Career Ladders and Developing the Administrator Role in Nursing Higher Education

As in the rest of the university, nursing has three general approaches to administration in higher education. The first is the most typical—moving through an established hierarchy of line positions within a norm of time-in-position. This approach means that an individual may choose to enter administration through positions beginning at the course or area coordinator level and subsequently move through such typical positions as Department Chair, Assistant or Associate Dean, and then, Dean. Beyond the dean position are several staff and line central administrative positions, such as Assistant or Associate Vice President, Vice President, Provost, President, and Chancellor. Typically, there are Vice Presidents for specific areas, such as Academic Affairs, Resource Management, Business and Finance, Development, and Alumni Relations. A Vice President for Academic Affairs may hold combined titles and positions of Vice President for Academic Affairs and Provost, denoting this position as chief academic officer. The chief university officer typically is the President or Chancellor, depending on the overall structure of the university (e.g., whether the university is part of a large state system with multiple campuses or a small private institution).

A second mobility path is that of taking on alternative roles, such as staff roles (e.g., Student Affairs) or of being in a position and executing it so well that a new position is created and named for the individual. A third, more distant and overlapping possibility, is being an individual imported from outside the university to develop or manage a unit using specialized skills developed elsewhere.

Criteria for selection of an effective administrator vary with the role and the institution's demands of the present and vision for the future. Administrative pathbreakers require a different set of skills than maintenance administrators. For these reasons, effective nurse administrators require not only career paths, but also sure acquaintance with the management skills and personality characteristics desired in the role and an understanding of the organization's evolutionary path.

In nursing, effective managers and leaders can be developed during the baccalaureate experience (Arolian, Meservey, & Crockett, 1996). First, students can be assisted in identifying goals, as well as the cognitive and interpersonal skills needed to support their goals. Second, the actual nursing care experience can guide students toward a choice in education or other nursing roles. If a nurse chooses education, practical successful nursing experiences in effective management of a unit or a group can be transferred to an academic role. Such experiences may lead the faculty-inclined nurse to expand goals to incorporate the role of academic administrator.

Preparation for Nursing Academic Administration

To prepare for the role of academic administrator, two graduate foci are necessary. For credibility and curriculum understanding, the graduate program must first ensure nursing expertise (i.e., a concentration in nursing science). The second focus is to provide expertise in educational administration. If master's and doctoral study included these two foci, the potential administrator would have a grasp of important programmatic and curriculum concerns for nursing as well as for other disciplines. Often, however, not until the faculty role has been realized do individuals desire to expand career goals to include that of the academic administrator.

Faculty members aspiring to deanships frequently assume an intermediate position of assistant dean or associate dean or entry positions such as course coordinator or department chair. Such positions provide opportunities to observe closely and experience the personal and professional skills required of a dean and to test a person's ability to apply a variety of management and leadership skills. But other characteristics are also important to the administrative role.

To determine the perceived importance of personal and professional characteristics for career development and advancement, deans and directors of nursing programs were surveyed. The results identified 24 "sources of influence." The top 10 ranked items were communication skills, interpersonal skills, creativity in thinking, ability to mobilize groups, intellectual activity, academic credentials, willingness to take risks, credibility within the profession, innovativeness, and collegial support (Short, 1997a). In another study, deans of top-ranked schools of nursing were surveyed to obtain self-reported leadership behaviors. Five thematic areas, related to transformational leadership areas, were assessed and analyzed. In this study, deans identified values as the most important theme followed by vision, people, motivation, and influence (Gevedon, 1992). Although perusal of the leadership and education administration literature can provide guidance in determining the characteristics most common to successful administrators, whether or how many of these characteristics can be developed or enhanced in every aspiring dean is questionable.

Career ladders for nursing deans or directors are useful in a self-evaluation of abilities and capacity for nursing educational leadership. Ladders also are a useful device in ascertaining the expectations of others at levels above and below that of dean or director, but who are important to that role. These expectations provide insights into the politics and needs of a developing organization, a plateauing organization, or a declining organization. At each rung of the ladder, aspirants should avail themselves of opportunities to assume successively responsible positions. Further, they should plan the length of time they want to spend at each level and consider potential sponsors or evaluators on whom they may need to rely to move to another position. Perceptions of each of the groups of evaluators can differ, and data from each provide valuable input (Rogers, 1989).

Mentors can provide needed support to the incumbent administrator. Mentoring, usually addressed for faculty and deans, is little discussed for mid-level administrators, yet it is critical for their growth (Kavoosi, Elman, & Mauch, 1995; Short, 1997b). Having at least one mentor who has been in the same or similar position and can offer practical administrative advice is helpful. If necessary, other mentors can help the administrator meet the scholarly and professional expectations of the role.

Career ladders lend credence and dignity to faculty development and job mobility. Many deans have recognized that a tenure of 7 to 10 years (often more) in the position is sufficient and have moved on. Not infrequently, successful academic administrators choose "to return to their first love—teaching and research" (Arden, 1997, p. 30). Conversely, deans of nursing are beginning to be tapped for mentoring other administrators, filling minority-short committees, and advancing to other university positions, such as graduate deans or president. Although career ladders seem to force an upward focus on the next rung, an incumbent may also discover a mid-level administrative role along the way to be fulfilling and rewarding in itself. In an age of ambition or downsizing, recognizing one's interests or limits can be gratifying, to both the incumbent and others.

■ Concluding Statement

Nursing faculty with sound political sensibilities and genuine substance can use a career ladder to help assess an organization and to plan for the future. Career ladders, properly used, can help both tenured and non-tenured nursing faculty achieve their potential—to their personal good and to that of academe. As the 21st century evolves, forces that have influenced change in the 1990s are likely to have further impacts on nursing education. Faculty and aspiring nursing academic administrators are well advised to prepare now for the beyond. The question remains—how?

■ References

Almanac issue. (1998, August 28). *The Chronicle of Higher Education, XLV*(1).

Arden, E. (1997). Is there life after administration? *Academe, 83*(4), 30–32.

Arolian, J., Meservey, P. M., & Crockett, J. G. (1996). Developing nurse leaders for today and tomorrow: Part 1, Foundations of leadership in practice. *JONA (Journal of Nursing Administration), 26*(9), 18–26.

Barron's Profile of American Colleges. (1994). Hauppauge, NY: Barron's Educational Series.

Boyer, E. L. (1991). *Scholarship reconsidered: Priorities of the professoriate* (special report). Princeton, NJ: The Carnegie Foundation for the Advancement of Teaching.

Brubacher, J. S., & Rudy, W. (1997). *Higher education in transition: A history of American colleges and universities* (4th ed.). New Brunswick, NJ: Transaction Publishers.

Faculty work: Briefing paper. (1994, March). *Information analyses.* Olympia: Washington State Higher Education Coordinating Board.

Gevedon, S. L. (1992). Leadership behaviors of deans of top-ranked schools of nursing. *Journal of Nursing Education, 31*(5), 221–224.

Gosnell, D. J., & Biordi, D. L. (1999). Personnel resource distribution for nursing programs in Carnegie-classified research I and II and doctoral I institutions. *Journal of Professional Nursing, 15*(1), 44–51.

Kavoosi, M. C., Elman, N. S., & Mauch, J. E. (1995). Faculty mentoring and administrative support in schools of nursing. *Journal of Nursing Education, 34*(9), 419–426.

Moody, N. B. (1996). Nurse faculty job satisfaction: A national survey. *Journal of Professional Nursing, 12*(5), 277–288.

O'Neil, E. H. (1993). *Health professions education for the future: Schools in service to the nation.* San Francisco: Pew Health Professions Commission.

Ost, D., & Twale, D. (1988, September). *An analysis of appointments of higher education administrators.* Washington, DC: U.S. Department of Education.

Rogers, M. A. (1989). Dimensions of leadership of assistant/associate deans in collegiate schools of nursing. *Journal of Nursing Education, 28*(9), 415–421.

Rudy, E. B., Anderson, N. A., Dudjak, L., Kobert, S. N., & Miller, R. A. (1995). Faculty practice: Creating a new culture. *Journal of Professional Nursing, 11*(2), 78–83.

Short, J. D. (1997a). Profile of administrators of schools of nursing, Part I: Resources for goal achievement. *Journal of Professional Nursing, 13*(1), 7–12.

Short, J. D. (1997b). Profile of administrators of schools of nursing, Part II: Mentoring relationships and influence activities. *Journal of Professional Nursing, 13*(1), 13–18.

Shugars, D. A., O'Neil, E. H., & Bader, J. D. (Eds.). (1991). *Healthy America: Practitioners for 2005, an agenda for action for U.S. health professional schools.* Durham, NC: The Pew Health Professions Commission.

Williams, D. R., & Stewart, I. M. (1950). *Administration of schools of nursing.* New York: Macmillan.

Willis, R. (1960). *The evolving liberal arts curriculum* (pp. 39–47). New York: Teachers' College, Columbia University.

Wood, S. O., Biordi, D. L., Miller, B. A., Poncar, P., Snelson, C. M., Banks, M. J., & Hemminger, S. A. (1998). Boyer's model of scholarship applied to a career ladder for non-tenured nursing faculty. *Nurse Educator, 23*(3), 33–40.

■ *Editor's Questions for Discussion*

Discuss the impact of different organizational models in higher education for nursing educational programs. What differences may exist in state, private, and medical center–based nursing programs? Are there differences in faculty and outcomes for nursing students? How have differences in university mission for the three types of structures affected nursing programs, nursing faculty, and nursing students? To what extent are challenges similar and dissimilar for professional disciplines based in universities? How has nursing as a profession benefited by university affiliation?

Discuss criticisms of curricula and faculty in higher education. How similar are expectations for nursing programs in higher education to other disciplines? To what extent do criticisms differ regarding nursing curricula and faculty? How have nursing programs responded to higher education critics? In university life to what extent are nursing programs inclusive? What initiatives may increase nursing program's innate value to universities?

Identify the advantages and disadvantages of nursing tenets being organizationally independent or as part of an interdisciplinary unit. What evidence indicates that university "career ladders" and faculty roles are changing? Discuss the impact of changing faculty roles as predicted by Lindeman (Chapter 63) and Hoffman (Chapter 64) for faculty and nursing programs. What impact might changes in faculty status from a tenure system to non-tenure system as discussed by Fleming (Chapter 22) have for nursing programs? How likely are faculty governance systems to change in the 21st century? Discuss the pros and cons of present faculty governance systems. What are the advantages and disadvantages of part-time faculty for nursing? How can nursing program quality and continuity for students be preserved when part-time faculty are utilized?

What has been the impact of Boyer's model of scholarship for university nursing programs? How has the model been implemented in state-supported and private universities with their differing mission emphases (i.e., research, teaching, and service)? What strategies are most effective in reconciling imbalances among the typical three-pronged mission of universities?

What effect does differing organizational structures (e.g., health science, state, and private) have on academic administration in nursing? How does Lindell's discussion (Chapter 69) about criteria for administrators apply to Biordi and McFarlane's discussion? What experiences are essential prior to assuming the role of academic administrator? How much in agreement are Lindeman (Chapter 63), Flood (Chapter 66), Keating and Perry (Chapter 65), Chaska (Chapter 68), Lindell (Chapter 69), Biordi and McFarlane (Chapter 67), and Shaver (76) regarding nursing academic administration roles, required characteristics, and personal and professional development for roles?

68

Avoiding the Fatal "By-Pass Operation" in Facilitating Accountability

Norma L. Chaska, PhD, RN, FAAN

W hile providing consultation at a university, I was presented concerns about accountability and communication in academic administration. The Dean of the Medical School raised questions about the frequency that designated channels for communication were being circumvented. The dean wondered about the effects in other universities of such detours. At the time, I recalled similar discussions with deans of various nursing programs. Additional university consultations and professional meetings convinced me that the problem was widespread. I have labeled this lack of accountability for communication the "fatal by-pass operation."

The purposes of this chapter are to (a) discuss the by-pass operation—what it is (process), factors involved, its typical substance (academic issues), examples of by-pass, its effects, and its management; (b) discuss ancillary considerations; and (c) explore solutions. My focus is on the dean's role (or person with final authority in the School of Nursing), with inference to other levels of administration as applicable. I conclude the chapter by identifying competency requisites of the dean and suggestions for research.

■ The By-Pass Operation

Definition

Two facets comprise the by-pass operation. First, the term refers to the tactic of circumventing the person who is directly accountable for specific issues, problems, or concerns. This type of action is commonly known as "going over the boss's head." Second, the maneuver includes conveying information to a person either above or below the designated line of authority. Managers see subordinate personnel as an important source of information and expect them to report on happenings within the manager's sphere of responsibility (Ellis & Arieli, 1999). However, if administrative boundaries are not clear or maintained, information gathering and processing creates complexity and turmoil.

Factors Involved

Chain-of-Command and Unity-of-Command Concepts: Outdated?

Fayol identified these principles of classical management theory in the early 1900s (Bateman & Snell, 1996; Ivancevich & Matteson, 1987). Although commonly associated with the military, both of these concepts were considered a cornerstone in the design of organizations 20 years ago. Even though far less important in organizational structures today (and the terminology considered passé by many), Robbins (1998) in his classic textbook series representing a sociological view of organizations emphasized that contemporary managers must "consider implications" of these principles when designing communication structures (p. 482). He went on to discuss these concepts further, as follows.

1. The chain-of-command is an "unbroken line of authority that extends from the top of the organization to the lowest echelon and clarifies who reports to whom."

2. The chain-of-command answers questions for employees as "to whom do I go if I have a problem" and "to whom am I responsible."

3. A chain-of-command requires complementary enforcement of authority and unity-of-command.

4. Authority in a managerial position connotes the right to "give orders and expect the orders to be obeyed."

5. Unity-of-command helps to preserve the concept of an unbroken line of authority, particularly when a person has "one and only one superior to whom she or he is directly responsible." (p. 482)

Kennedy (1998) noted that, in preserving the health of the academic community, boundaries must be respected. In particular, boundaries that facilitate channels of communication need to be honored. The academic administrator is in the key position to encourage appropriate use of channels.

Paths of Communication

Descriptions of the paths of communication referenced in this chapter follow (Bateman & Snell, 1996; Robbins, 1998).

1. *Vertical-upward.* Flows from lower to higher levels in the organization—ideally provides feedback to higher-ups on what's going on, informs them of progress toward goals, and relays current problems. Judgment and accountability—whose judgment and what accountability—are key to what should be communicated upward (Worthley, 1997).

2. *Vertical-downward.* Flows from higher to lower levels—updates persons regarding events, problems, policies, and procedures in organizations; provides instructions; points out problems; and offers feedback about performance.

3. *Lateral (horizontal).* Flows across functions (people, units, and departments) at the same hierarchical level in an organization—allows sharing of information and problem-solving in coordinating and integrating diverse functions. Such communication often is necessary to save time and facilitate coordination in organizations.

4. *Informal (the grapevine).* Unofficial channels short-circuit formal channels—may be positive (translating management's formal mes-

sages into employee language) or destructive (spreading irrelevant or erroneous gossip and rumors). May be a widespread activity when there are few official means of learning what is going on.

Accountability

The concept of accountability conveys being responsible for one's decisions, actions, and consequences. With regard to communication, Covey, Merrill, and Merrill (1995) perceive this responsibility to be most effective as self-accountability.

Line–Staff

Bateman and Snell (1996) make the following distinctions between line and staff authority.

- Line managers are responsible for operational activities; they deal directly with the institution's primary mission (also with faculty and students). Examples in a university are department chair, assistant and associate dean, dean, vice president, provost, president, vice chancellor, and chancellor.

- Staff people carry out procedures tangential to operational activities. Examples of staff are secretarial and support personnel (e.g., advising, recruiting, budgeting, and learning skills laboratory).

- Assistant and associate deans may be either staff or line, depending on their assigned functions. An example of staff assignments are the functions and processes of various committees—(e.g., curriculum and admissions). Line management of academic programs may be delegated by the dean.

- Research may be either a staff or line function, depending on the mission of the university. Faculty are accountable accordingly to functions of the designated manager.

Academic Issues

Numerous areas in academic administration are ripe for differences of opinion and

thus possible internal conflict. Itemized in Table 68.1 is a selection of typical issues of concern variously to hierarchical levels—from higher administration through support personnel—plus faculty and students.

Examples of By-Pass

For a variety of reasons, people do by-pass their "bosses." The motives are multiple and complex—stretching from fear of reprisal to sabotage. Part of the reason in this chapter for exploring the by-pass process is that its motivation is not always sinister. Some (e.g., faculty, students, or staff) may feel the need for someone to hear "their side." Others may be reacting to perceived inaction after attempting to bring their concerns through channels. Then too, some may confuse their *complaining* with *gossip*—making light of the fact that they are "sounding off" about something they should not be talking about to someone other than their line manager. However, labeling information passed out of appropriate channels as mere gossip avoids accountability for it. By-pass may occur in any direction—upward, downward, or horizontally. The following examples illustrate by-pass actions by various individuals and groups.

Students

Students who detour discussion that ordinarily should occur between their course instructor or faculty advisor are using by-pass. Course requirements and standards typically are the focus. Other aspects of by-pass include the student (a) complaining to another faculty member rather than the immediate instructor; (b) going over the head of the faculty advisor for program and curriculum planning; and (c) relating difficulties in clinical site experiences to other than appropriate persons responsible for clinical. Possibly the most dramatic by-pass maneuver is

TABLE 68.1   Issues in Academia

Academic workload—teaching, clinical supervision, research, committees, student advisement
- Sufficient full and part-time faculty
- Equitable distribution among faculty
- Competence in area of assignment
- Release time for research
- Financial compensation for special projects

Workload of support personnel
- Sufficient number of personnel available
- Appropriateness of tasks assigned
- Equitable distribution of workload
- Appropriate distribution of support among faculty

Curriculum
- Compatible with philosophy and goals of the institution and school
- Developed according to criteria and standards of the profession
- Congruent with expertise of faculty available
- Flexible in meeting student needs

Clinical sites
- Standards of practice congruent with curriculum objectives
- Appropriate opportunities for students
- Adequate and consistent supervision available

Performance appraisal
- Clear requirements and standards
  i.   program progression of students
  ii. staff and faculty salary increases
  iii. faculty appointment, reappointment, promotion, tenure, and post-tenure review
- Consistent evaluation procedures
- Realistic superior's expectations
  i.   faculty scholarship, service, and maintenance of clinical practice in university nursing programs

Committees (university, school, and faculty)
- Sufficient types (e.g., curriculum; program evaluation; faculty appointment, reappointment, promotion, tenure, and posttenure; admission; student progression; and grievance)
- Appropriate representation on committees (university and school)
- Consistent and orderly procedures for conduct of activity and reporting of results

Enrollment, personnel, and budgetary data
- Accurate compilation of status and needs
- Needs congruent with goals of the larger system (e.g., school and university)

Factors contributing to effective functioning of the organization
- Policies and procedures published and clearly communicated

Procedures established for handling irregularities

Channels established for communicating problems, dissatisfaction, plus ideas for improvement

the student who goes directly to higher administration (vice president or president)—skirting all school channels—for assistance when failing to meet program and progression standards.

Faculty

Complaining about other faculty to students represents downward vertical communication that should be handled horizontally or vertically upward. Expressing dissatisfaction to a department chair, without prior discussion with the faculty concerned, is horizontal by-pass. Reporting such matters directly to the dean may involve upward by-pass of several hierarchical levels.

Line Managers (Middle Management)

Department chairs voicing concerns to the dean that are the province of assistant or associate deans are examples of upward by-pass. Assistant or associate deans may be guilty of either horizontal or downward by-pass if, prior to conveying information to the dean, they fail to attempt to resolve issues with the person involved. Solid judgment is essential in determining whether situations warrant immediate notification of the dean, versus processing information through line management channels. At the department chair level, two chairs may collude (upward by-pass) to inflate faculty needs—presenting these data to the dean, but by-passing middle management (assistant or associate dean) who has the responsibility for meeting such needs.

Staff and Support Personnel

Offices of staff and support personnel frequently are located physically near the dean's office. However, for whatever reason, complaints of staff and support personnel often are directed to the dean for resolution. Except for the dean's secretary, such a referral most often is upward by-pass.

Dean's Office as a "Dumping Ground"

The dean of nursing may be confronted with one or all of issues cited in Table 68.1. Too often, the dean discovers that the appropriate person never was consulted regarding the dissatisfaction (upward by-pass) prior to an individual or group appearing at the dean's office.

Dean

A dean may be guilty of downward by-pass if directly apprising faculty, staff, or students about an issue—overlooking relevant administrators in the hierarchical order. Likewise, a dean may "blind-side" middle-management administrators by informing a department chair or faculty regarding a new policy that usually is developed or transmitted through the assistant or associate dean (or the department chair, in case of faculty). Or, a dean may attempt to pressure faculty directly (downward by-pass) to develop curricula in opposition to the beliefs of an associate dean charged to oversee curricula. An example of lateral and upward by-pass is the case where two deans, external to a College of Nursing, plan to have faculty from Nursing collaborate on a research project without negotiating with the dean of nursing and conferring with the appropriate vice president. Another example—this of upward by-pass—is deans, without knowledge of their vice president, presenting data to a budget office director about enrollment and faculty. In a competitive situation, that may be a subversive attempt to increase the budget allocation of individual schools, while undermining the more objective goals of the vice president and the university as a whole.

Whistle-Blowing

By-passing and whistle-blowing are not synonymous activities. Whistle-blowing deals with illegal or unethical behavior in an organization. Specifically, *whistle-blowing* is defined as "the disclosure by organization members (former or current) of illegal, immoral, or illegitimate practices under the control of their employees, to persons or organizations that may be able to effect action" (King III, 1999, p. 315). The significance of clear and proper channels for reporting such behavior is well documented in the literature (Clarke, 1999; Finn, 1998; Jubb, 1999; King III, 1997, 1999; Lewis, 1997; Lynn, 1998; Mills, 1998; Secretary, 1998; Seligman, 1999; Sims & Keenan, 1998; Stern, 1999; Worthley, 1997). In this chapter, I do not address behaviors that warrant whistle-blowing.

Effects of By-Pass

In general, the results of by-pass are dismal and negative for the individuals, programs, and institutions that foster such procedures. Individuals in a setting where by-pass is a mode of operation may experience strong internal conflict in personal integrity and solidarity of a school unit (Ellis & Arieli, 1999).

From a decision-maker's point of view, Falconi (1997) noted the need to be assured that a decision "is not always subject to second-guessing or being overturned" by someone at a higher level. Falconi likened being blind-sided by such an event to the experience of

> . . . being made to feel like a kid who gets caught making his little brother cry. . . . You should never hit your brother! Don't say you didn't. After all, he's crying. . . . I didn't hit him. He's crying because I took the lighter fluid away from him. He was going to barbecue the goldfish. (p. 14)

Too often, decision-makers in nursing education, detecting a need to take away "the lighter fluid," experience similar demoralized feelings when having their decisions circumvented or overturned.

A special type of problem is presented in the case of a by-pass that is enveloped in a promise of strict confidentiality. A scarce publication titled "Going Over Heads" emphasizes that if complaints are made in "strictest confidence . . . it is difficult to maintain that confidence

and take action at the same time" (Zetlin, 1991, p. 59).

One of the less blatant but more long-lasting effects of by-pass has to do with its repercussion on students. When faculty model the by-pass, it becomes a part of the students' professional socialization process. That is, such circumventive behavior may be perceived as appropriate for a professional and form the basis for its continuance in the profession.

Leob (1995) invited those contemplating by-pass to an examination of conscience that in the end warns of troublesome effects. Loeb's self-exam questions include (a) Am I totally clean . . . without blemish in any record? (b) If I confront the person involved, is the situation of concern likely to change? (c) Can the problem cause serious harm? (d) Will long-term benefits outweigh the harm . . . in circumventing a manager? and (e) Given the risk of being "labeled as a possible 'troublemaker' or 'backstabber,' am I prepared to suffer the consequences"? (p. 183).

Doubtless—whether upward, downward, or lateral—the by-pass maneuver is fraught with ill effects. To promote countertechniques that foster health in organizations, a clear understanding of by-pass is essential. Knowing when, in what type of situations, and how the by-pass comes into play, recognizing forces that contribute to its use, and developing strategies to prevent endorsing such subversive tactics are important.

Management of By-Pass

At whatever level by-pass occurs, immediate response is essential. Implied is that the by-pass behavior is recognized as such. Once evident, there are positive means for handling and resolving the situation. Because the dean is in a key position to do so, the following management process references that office. However, the principles apply to any line manager confronted with a by-pass situation.

Sequential steps toward management of the problem include: (a) recognize the immediate problem; (b) confront the person committing the offense; (c) address the problem versus shaming the offender; (d) help that individual to own the problem, reasons for it, and its resolution; and (e) negotiate or mediate the process, as applicable.

We in academic administration have had significant experience in deaning. Most important, we are learning more effective ways to deal with problems (e.g., it is better to confront than to avoid).

As to why issues concerning circuitous communication paths are not addressed directly may be related to complexity and uncertainty about how to resolve such concerns. Some administrators, trying to survive hostile dynamics may believe—mistakenly—that they are being politically astute in fostering information from deviant routes; those administrators overlook the negative effect of such behavior. Or, not addressing use of the by-pass technique in organizations simply may be an example of conflict between an administrator's belief and behavior. It is easy to know what is right, but difficult to do what is right.

Courage, energy, and sensitivity are required of administrators. Answerability for communication is essential to organizational health. Conquering "confrontophobia" enables an administrator to deal with conflict, miscommunication, inappropriate ventilation, power plays, and sabotage (Briles, 1999, p. 264; DeLucca, 1992; Emely, Power, Kennedy, & Cornish, 1995; Mayer, 1990; Rowland & Rowland, 1997). Suggestions for constructive confrontation include: (a) act affirmatively and immediately, and (b) speak diplomatically about circumvention—who should be the first to be informed. Such an approach puts others on notice that by-pass will not be tolerated. In contrast, avoidance enables negative behaviors to continue or escalate, and—worse—silence condones the offending behavior. Confronting

the "deviant" calls for the responsibility of leadership and holds the offender accountable.

The dean can set the climate for dialogue between the offender and the person offended (Hitt, 1993). Modeling acceptability of speaking up, being open, expressing both thoughts and feelings engenders trust that reprisal behavior is unacceptable. A dean who does so not only models effective problem solving but also becomes an antidote to the threat of reprisal. Developing the moral courage to resolve dilemmas has been best addressed by Kritek (1994). She stated that an administrator (the dean in this case) needs to help the person who circumvents to (a) recognize the problem, (b) "own" it in identifying reason(s) for the behavior, and (c) decide a way to resolve the difficulty. Deans cannot mandate conformance any more than someone can herd cats. According to Bennis (1997), neither humans nor cats will allow it. However, as cats may be "coaxed, cajoled, persuaded, adored, and gently led" . . . so too can humans (p. 197).

Zetlin (1997) recommends that higher administrators presented with a by-pass situation meet with the subordinate and line manager so that the three persons can discuss the problem. However, such involvement takes away the higher administrator's opportunity for objective review and evaluation. Kritek (personal communication, 1994) recommended instead that, in such a three-person meeting, the dean listen as the other two parties discuss the problem. Listening first and witnessing information as it is being shared, versus imposing logic, affords the ability to understand more fully what is being heard (Dorn & Marcus, 1997). This approach also gives the dean an opportunity to ascertain whether a threat of reprisal is there. The dean then can switch over to the mediation role in resolving the conflict. Deans who have not developed negotiator skills will need to develop them.

Table 68.2 presents an incremental process for dealing with the by-pass operation. The

TABLE 68.2   Guidelines for Management of the By-Pass Operation

1. If a person is concerned about something, he or she should first go directly and speak only to the individual(s) involved.

2. If the issue is one that may need to be addressed by someone else (as in a management chain-of-command), the person raising the issue should still go first to the individual(s) directly involved.

3. If the concern has to be referred to someone in administration, the concerned person should not circumvent the administrator next in the management line to avoid implementing a "by-pass operation."

4. If an issue has been referred to someone in the chain of command, that administrator always inquires about the extent to which the concern has been presented to the person(s) or administrator immediately below in the hierarchy.

5. If the issue has not been presented to the appropriate person(s) or administrator immediately below, the administrator at the higher level redirects it to the appropriate person(s) or administrator.

6. If the problem still cannot be resolved at the level immediately below, the administrator invites the parties to come together to be heard. The same strategy is advisable if two or more complainants or managers are involved.

7. The administrator listens to all parties simultaneously (never individually), asks for suggestions and recommendations, negotiates and asks for a decision. Examples of parties are (a) a student with an instructor in the presence of the student's advisor; (b) two faculty members in the presence of a Department Chairperson; (c) a faculty member with a Department Chairperson in the presence of an Assistant Dean; (d) a Department Chairperson with an Assistant Dean in the presence of an Associate Dean; or (e) an Assistant Dean with an Associate Dean in the presence of the Dean.

8. Only when the two initial parties could not resolve the disagreement should the group problem-solving session occur in the presence of the administrator next in the hierarchy. That person (who has been approached by one or more of the interested parties) is obligated to determine whether the first appropriate person in the line has been presented with the issue and the extent to which the issue has been addressed and resolved.

9. If one or more of the parties involved refuses to meet with the appropriate person lower in the hierarchy, the administrator should capitalize on "good will" for role modeling—as a health care professional—and render a decision to prevent further conflict and to provide leadership.

10. Every assurance must be given to the parties involved regarding fairness and openness in the negotiation process. Most often the party with the least power (e.g., a student having difficulty with an instructor) needs assurance that retaliation will not result and that follow-up of the situation will occur.

11. The administrator at the level where the issue is resolved should determine whether a pattern is occurring whereby one of the parties has previously presented complaints about others. If patterns are identified, the "pattern" should be addressed with the individual alone and aside from the issue being addressed in the group meeting.

steps outlined will be familiar to managers in a variety of situations as advice for dealing with conflict generally. I detailed the principles here because they so often are violated in dealing with by-pass. The lead-off statement—confront first the person involved—is of particular importance (Kritek, 1994).

■ Ancillary Considerations

More on Accountability

Accountability, when confronting management in higher education, ideally triggers responsive strategic planning. According to

Kennedy (1998), accountability is the word increasingly equated with alarm. No longer will the public, students, faculty, and staff be satisfied with reassuring statements about the struggles of higher education to meet challenges (Murphy & Louis, 1999). Multiplying expectations and demands for quality affect the roles of administrators daily. At every level, academic administrators in nursing are expected to be stretched in meeting responsibilities of the present and future (Birnbaum, 1992; Tucker, 1993).

True leaders realize that they are accountable for inaction as well as action (Hitt, 1993). This truism applies as well to communication processes inherent in the management role. Politics always is involved when it comes to implementing policies about reporting mechanisms, particularly when accountability may be an issue (Horwitt, 1998, Tournish & Hargie, 1998). Deans in their negotiator and mediator roles have a strategic opportunity to facilitate accountability on the part of all (Kritek, personnel communication, 1999).

Structure and Policies

When the roles and functions of managers and staff are not clear in institutions, chaos is apt to result. Faculty, students, and staff may not be certain to whom they should go for resolution of concerns. Clarity for all—regarding line authority and accountability—is important (Hall, 1996; Ivancevich, 1998). Each person in the institution bears responsibility for appropriate channeling of communication.

Open-Door Policy

Much has been written regarding open-door policies (Falconi, 1997; Mills, 1998). If the practice is to be effective, administrators must make clear to students, faculty, and staff publicly the nature of communication that will be considered appropriate. As a safeguard, a

screening process may be implemented. For example, the individual may be queried as to whether the subject is a personal matter or academic concern. If academic, the dean determines whether channels for such issues are being circumvented and takes appropriate action. However, with screening, the dean can only hope that the person will level as to the type of issue to be discussed. The dean may discover soon after the person begins talking about the "confidential personal" problem that the matter actually is an academic issue. The dean must then refer the person back along the appropriate channel.

Kritek (personal communication, 1999) has observed that administrators often have not been able to differentiate between confidentiality and being invited to participate in collusion. Instead of building credibility, a dean invites problems in listening to "back-biting." Rather, repositioning oneself as a dean regarding appropriate communication channels—a dean who cannot be manipulated—builds credibility.

Sabotage

Briles (1999) defined sabotage as "the act of undermining or destroying personal or professional integrity, creating mayhem in personal or professional lives, damaging personal or professional credibility, which can lead to the destruction or dismissal of self-worth" (p. 21). Mindful that individuals may be sabotaged as well as be saboteurs, Briles developed two instruments: (a) to determine whether a person is sabotage savvy; and (b) to determine if a person has ever sabotaged another.

Sabotage and the by-pass operation are evident in "six silent killers" of organizations, as identified by Fisher (1998). The specific behaviors he explored as deadly to institutional survival are (a) passive aggressive, (b) passive responsive, (c) passive defensive, (d) malicious obedience, (e) approach avoidance, and (f) obsessive compulsive actions. These behaviors are reflected in the circuitous communication of the by-pass technique.

In reporting results of her survey of work relationships, Briles (1999) noted that men rarely shared personal data, their inner selves, whereas women practice the "art of in-depth" sharing (p. 151). Perhaps more relevant is that women *confuse* friendliness at work with friendship. Friendliness shows as warmth, caring, compassion, and openness. Friendship is characterized by companionship, established mutual loyalty and commitment, and benevolent and confidant types of behaviors that evolve mutually after long-time association and sharing of common interests and goals. By not understanding the difference, women unknowingly may become victims of sabotage (with feelings of betrayal) or be the saboteurs (betray loyalty and trust of others).

King III (1997) has explored the linkage of close relationships (e.g., friendships between employees within organizations) to betrayal or subsequent sabotage. Barnum and Kerfoot (1995) in addressing the issue of friendships pointed out the need for open, honest, and direct relationships with clear systematic lines for communication and accountability.

Information Flow

Ideally, information should flow smoothly up the organization as well as down (Canadian Institute of Charted Accountants, 1998; Wheatley, 1994). Having regular and open meetings with faculty, staff, and students facilitates accurate sharing of information. Boxes for "questions and suggestions" are effective, but with a caveat: Responses must be timely and openly addressed. "Safe" forums for open discussion of sensitive issues with colleagues, with appropriate mutually agreed upon guidelines, also are helpful. Such intergroup sharing and problem solving is effective (Zander, 1994).

In sharing information, "dumping" is a potential problem (Sykes, 1999). Dumping may be defined as someone trying to shift his or her (the dumper) problems, rumors, or issues onto someone else (the dumpee) when these dissatisfactions should not be the concern of the person to whom the first person is ventilating. To avoid being victimized as a dumpee, the following self-examination assesses responsibility: (a) Did I cause the problem? (b) Do I control the things—resources—to correct it? (c) Will my action interfere with the rightful person's taking responsibility and being accountable as that individual should? and (d) Is this concern part of my function? If the concern borders on joint responsibility, then (a) What piece of the "action" is legitimately within my area of competence and responsibility? and (b) What is my authority? Confronting responsibility and accountability in this manner saves time and energy.

Organizational Culture

Assessment of the culture of an institution is an excellent predictor of its values, integrity, and trust (Reina & Reina, 1999; Shaw, 1997; Tetenbaum, 1999). Robbins (1998) defines organizational culture as a "system of shared meaning . . . organizational values" (p. 595). Robbins identifies seven variables that form the basis for (a) members' feelings of shared understanding, (b) how things are accomplished, and (c) the way personnel are supposed to behave. Determinants that mold organizational culture include (a) innovation and risk taking, (b) attention to detail, (c) outcome orientation and focus, (d) people orientation, (e) team orientation, (f) aggressiveness, and (g) stability.

Cultures and subcultures tend to develop and be in large institutions. Customs, tradition, and the socialization process within an institution have much to do with culture becoming an asset or liability. Pauchant and Mitroff (1992) noted that its culture can be a major factor in addictive, dysfunctional behaviors within an organization. Robbins (1998) pointed out that entry into an institution is the most critical time for socialization, adaptation, or change in its culture. He offers a "list of things" (p. 599) that include making queries regarding policies for information sharing and reporting of problems, which can help an applicant learn about an institution's culture. Assessment by and of applicants for administrative positions for "potential fit" with the desired culture of the institution thus is crucial.

Trust

Trust is essential for institutions to be successful and maintain integrity (Shaw, 1997). Shaw defines trust as the belief that those on whom we depend and those who depend on us will meet expectations. Perhaps no variable is more important as a factor in the by-pass problem.

Lack of trust in the person to whom an individual is directly responsible frequently accounts for detours higher. Briles (1999) writes about changing sabotage and betrayal to support and trust. In a similar vein, Dennis and Michelle Reina (1999) provide strategies for rebuilding trust when it has been lost. Of interest, these authors have developed instruments for measuring *capacity* for trust and trust *competence*. Approaches advocated by the Reinas (1999) and Shaw (1997) include (a) developing core operating values, (b) disclosing important information fully, (c) being willing to deal with reality, (d) having open agendas, and (e) insisting on consistency between words and action in various situations.

Shaw (1997) portrayed trust as a balancing act, in that administrators must deal with three often conflicting imperatives—achieve results, act with integrity, and demonstrate concern. "Enforcing accountability across all levels" may alleviate the dilemma effectively (p. 178).

Truth-telling is the "foundation for building trust" (Reina & Reina, 1999, p. 86). The Reinas also noted other essentials: (a) establishing and maintaining clear communication boundaries, (b) nurturing consistency in behavior, and (c) providing and receiving positive feedback as to how information is transmitted, received, and provided. Transactional trust—one that is created incrementally and reciprocal—is a thesis reflected in the Reinas' writings: a person has to give trust in order to get it. "An atmosphere of mutual confidence and trust between managers and their subordinates can facilitate communication" (Ivancevich & Matteson, 1987, p. 646).

Empowerment

Perhaps no leadership concept is more popular today (and into tomorrow) than *empowerment*. It means entrusting others to perform functions and then holding them accountable for the result. Barnum and Kerfoot (1995) contrasted the concept with power; empowerment is authority purposely shared with others, whereas power usually is conferred on oneself or authority granted by others. The theory is that sharing power with employees enhances their feelings of being worthwhile and influential contributors (Andrica, 1999; Bateman & Snell, 1996). Allowing real versus token participation in decision-making is one mark of an empowered environment. Another feature of empowerment is placing emphasis on pleasing the "customer" rather than focusing on the "boss."

In today's world, much work is being done on computers, is intellectual, and therefore is invisible. Thus former bureaucratic control systems—layers of hierarchy, standard operating procedures, rules, regulations, and close supervision—are no longer practical (Bateman and Snell, 1996). Frequently, there is no way to scrutinize what employees do every day, even if that were desirable. Hierarchical control and micromanagement are not options under these conditions. A positive alternative is to empower employees to make decisions and trust that they will act in the best interests of the organization. This approach implies that a positive organization climate has been nurtured.

Empowerment does not mean giving up control. Rather, it suggests making better use of clan control (Bateman & Snell, 1996). Clan control involves creating relationships among group members "built on mutual respect and encouraging each individual to take responsibility for his or her actions" (p. 483). The concept of empowerment subsumes close relationships among trust, accountability, and modern concepts of control. Governance models in academic institutions permit systematic and structural empowerment to be extended throughout an entire institution.

■ Exploring Solutions

Change is characteristic of management systems today; only more can be expected in the future. In the case of the Dean position in Nursing, no longer can it be a "rite of passage" due to length of service or renown in scholarship and research. Complexity of academic administration in this era demands different skills, such as mediation and management. Preparation *prior* to assuming the position mandates appropriate management credentials. Short-course remediation will not suffice.

Change in organizational structure is also probable, as currently shown needed in the health care industry. Questions to be asked include: Is the vertical bureaucratic structure too cumbersome for this age? Is there a relationship between that structure and the by-pass problem? Would a flatter structure be more effective?

Questions also related to current pressures in health care include: How much of the business model will be forced on higher education

administration? Factors such as profits and competition are likely to be critical issues in the future.

Management style warrants attention. May the by-pass problem in part be a symptom of rebellion to overcontrol or micromanagement? What potential is there for empowerment as an effective leadership style in academic administration?

Proliferation of on-line courses, distance and distributive learning programs, interdisciplinary team approaches, and advances in technology are certainties of the future. What change in organization structure, staffing, resources, management system, management style do these advancements foreshadow for the future?

In summary, dictating quick "fix-it" commandments for solving problems of higher education administration in nursing will not suffice. Serious research is needed.

■ Concluding Statement

Accountability in communication will be foremost in the minds of administrators in developing future academic programs. Administrators have become all too familiar with line managers being circumvented. Rather than become disillusioned about negative behaviors encountered, administrators must come to understand the factors related to the by-pass phenomenon, utilization of the by-pass procedure, and the likely outcomes of action or inaction.

With a thorough understanding of the negative ploy, deans of nursing are positioned to employ positive strategies to counteract by-pass and resolve conflicts in information processing. Most important, by functioning effectively in the role of dean they are positioned to prevent the phenomenon. Students, faculty, staff, line managers, and administrators of programs should increasingly be advised as to acceptable behaviors. Rather than pessimism, optimism for viable cultures in academic organizations may result and thrive.

Communication accountability will be the essence of effectiveness in administration for academic institutions. All will then be held accountable for how, to whom, and what information is processed in academic institutions—through appropriately defined channels—now and beyond tomorrow.

■ References

Andrica, D. C. (1999). Handling office politics. *Nursing Economics, 17*(13), 156.

Barnum, B. S., & Kerfoot, K. M. (1995). *The nurse as executive* (4th ed.). Gaithersburg, MD: Aspen.

Bateman, T. S., & Snell, S. A. (1996). *Management: Building competitive advantage* (3rd ed.). Chicago: Irwin.

Bennis, W. (1997). *Managing people is like herding cats.* Provo, UT: Executive Excellence.

Birnbaum, R. (1992). *How academic leadership works: Understanding success and failure in the college presidency.* San Francisco: Jossey-Bass.

Briles, J. (1999). *Woman to woman 2000: Becoming sabotage savvy in the new millennium.* Far Hills, NJ: New Horizon Press.

Canadian Institute of Chartered Accountants. (1998). Managers: How to walk the talk. *CA Magazine, 131*(3), 10.

Clarke, R. L. (1999). The ethics of whistle-blowing. *Healthcare Financial Management, 53*(1), 16–17.

Covey, S. R., Merrill, A. R., & Merrill, R. R. (1995). *First things first.* New York: Fireside, Simon & Schuster.

DeLuca, J. M. (1992). *Political savvy: Systemic approaches to leadership behind-the-scenes.* Horsham, PA: LRP Publications.

Dorn, B. C., & Marcus, L. J. (1997). Negotiating the bureaucracy: In search of options. *American Medical News, 40*(29), 23–28.

Ellis, S., & Arieli, S. (1999). Predicting intentions to report administrative and disciplinary infractions: Applying the reasoned action model. *Human Relations, 52*(17), 947.

Emely, M. A., Power, M., Kennedy, M. M., & Cornish, J. M. (1995). Is it ever OK to go over my boss's head? *Executive Female, 18*(3), 64–66.

Falconi, R. R. (1997). Where open-door policies fail. *Financial Executive, 13*(5), 14–15.

Finn, W. (1998). Don't shoot the messenger. *Director, 52*(2), 46–50.

Fisher, J. R., Jr. (1998). *Six silent killers: Management's greatest challenge.* Boca Raton, FL: St. Lucie Press.

Hall, R. H. (1996). *Organizations: Structures, processes, and outcomes* (6th ed.). Englewood Cliffs, NJ: Prentice-Hall.

Hitt, W. D. (1993). *The model leader: A fully functioning person.* Columbus, OH: Battelle Press.

Horwitt, E. (1998). The politics of policies. *Network World, 15*(41), 45–47.

Ivancevich, J. M. (1998). *Human resource management* (7th ed.). Boston: Irwin/ McGraw-Hill.

Ivancevich, J. M., & Matteson, M. T. (1987). *Organizational behavior and management.* Plano, TX: Business Publications.

Jubb, P. B. (1999). Whistleblowing: A restrictive definition and interpretation. *Journal of Business Ethics, 21*(1), 77–94.

Kennedy, D. (1998). *Academic duty.* Cambridge, MA: Harvard University Press.

King III, G. (1997). The effects of interpersonal closeness and issue seriousness on blowing the whistle. *The Journal of Business Communication, 34*(4), 419–436.

King III, G. (1999). The implications of an organization's structure on whistleblowing. *Journal of Business Ethics, 20*(4, Part 2), 315–326.

Kritek, P. B. (1994). *Negotiating at an uneven table: A practical approach to working with difference and diversity.* San Francisco: Jossey-Bass.

Leob, M. (1995). When to rat on the boss: The costs of snitching can be high. *Fortune, 132*(7), 183.

Lewis, D. (1997). Whistleblowing at work: Ingredients for an effective procedure. *Human Resource Management Journal, 7*(4), 5–11.

Lynn, M. (1998, October). The whistle blowers' dilemma. *Management Today,* 54–61.

Mayer, R. J. (1990). *Conflict management: The courage to confront.* Columbus, OH: Battelle Press.

Mills, D. (1998). Taking care of people. *Canadian Mining Journal, 119*(3) 23.

Murphy, J., & Louis, K. S. (Eds.). (1999). *Handbook of research on educational administration* (2nd ed.). San Francisco: Jossey-Bass.

Pauchant, T. C., & Mitroff, I. I. (1992). *Transforming the crisis-prone organization: Preventing individual, organizational, and environmental tragedies.* San Francisco: Jossey-Bass.

Reina, D. S., & Reina, M. L. (1999). *Trust & betrayal in the workplace: Building effective relationships in your organization.* San Francisco: Berrett-Koehler.

Robbins, S. (1998). *Organizational behavior: Concepts, controversies, application* (8th ed.). Englewood Cliffs, NJ: Prentice-Hall International.

Rowland, H. S., & Rowland, B. L. (1997). *Nursing administration handbook* (4th ed.). Gaithersburg, MD: Aspen.

Secretary whistleblower. (1998). *Government Executive, 30*(7), 12.

Seligman, D. (1999). Blowing whistles, blowing smoke. *Forbes, 164*(5), 158–162.

Shaw, R. B. (1997). *Trust in the balance: Building successful organizations on results, integrity, and concern.* San Francisco: Jossey-Bass.

Sims, R. L., & Keenan, J. P. (1998). Predictors of external whistleblowing: Organizational and intrapersonal variables. *Journal of Business Ethics, 17*(4), 411–421.

Stern, A. I. (1999). When you hear that whistle blowing. *Trustee, 52*(6), 6–9.

Sykes, T. A. (1999). Getting carried away. *Black Enterprise, 30*(1), 54.

Tetenbaum, T. J. (1999). Beating the odds of merger & acquisition failure: Seven key practices that improve the chance for expected integration and synergies. *Organizational Dynamics,* Autumn, 22–36.

Tourish, D., & Hargie, O. D. W. (1998). Communication between managers and staff in the NHS: Trends and prospects. *British Journal of Management, 9*(1), 53.

Tucker, A. (1993). *Chairing the academic department* (3rd ed.). Phoenix: American Council on Education/Oryx.

Wheatley, M. J. (1994). *Leadership and the new science.* San Francisco: Berrett-Koehler.

Worthley, J. A. (1997). Reporting unethical behavior. *Healthcare Executive, 12*(2), 44.

Zander, A. (1994). *Making groups effective* (2nd ed.). San Francisco: Jossey-Bass.

Zetlin, M. (1991). Going over heads. *Management Review, 80*(4), 59–60.

■ Editor's Questions for Discussion

Discuss strategies for development of accountability and responsibility. Provide examples of vertical and horizontal by-pass techniques. What alternative communication behavior could be utilized? How might administrators reinforce appropriate lines of communication? How is the discussion by S. Thomas (Chapter 60) reinforced through Chaska's Table 68.2? How might abuse of open-door policies for communication be prevented? Discuss examples of the "six silent killers" in organizations. How might these negative behaviors be discouraged?

Provide criteria for assessment of organizational culture. What other confrontation strategies may be employed in resolving the by-pass operation? How might administrators discern the validity and reliability of information provided? What options should be considered if the parties in a conflict situation refuse to engage in mutual disclosure and problem solving in the presence of an administrator?

Discuss mediation and the role of the dean as a mediator. How may trust be developed and reinforced in organizations? How may an administrator address situations of individuals attempting to disclose information on a "confidential" basis? How might potential administrators discern the level of trust required and the methods used in problem solving by an institution prior to accepting a management position?

69

Dynamics of Discernment in Administrative Team Development

Andrea R. Lindell, DNSc, RN

Today's nursing programs are more complex in nature and comprehensive in activities than at any time in the past. Nursing programs have always offered a variety of educational offerings leading to a formalized degree or certificate. However, current programs are vastly different and complex. Today's nursing program leader, administrator, and faculty have responsibilities that cover a much broader range in terms of mission and scope. These responsibilities include developing and managing academic and instructional technologies, distance learning, pedagogy with a globalization focus, national and international partnerships, interdisciplinary research, management of resource requirements, marketing and recruitment, community service, multidis-

ciplinary health care teamwork, nonprofit corporation management, outcome validation, fund raising and development, and nurse managed clinics. In addition, the advent of competition in health care, in both the private and public sectors, has increased the pressure on administrators to deal with threats to survival. One way of dealing effectively is through administrative teams.

■ The Administrative Team

Forces Having an Impact on Teams

Forces that will have an impact on an administrative team include (a) maintaining student enrollment, (b) designing innovative programs of learning to meet the needs of traditional and nontraditional students, and (c) ensuring a high-quality curriculum that meets the needs of students. As health care institutions consolidate services, the administrative team must enhance or maintain clinical teaching sites. Additionally, it must learn to respond effectively to changes in societal values and attitudes regarding health care and the rapidity of technological development. Further, administrative teams of the future will be faced with the difficult task of maintaining a stable, yet malleable, environment that allows for innovation and immediate change.

Is it possible to maintain internal standards and yet maximize the credibility of the academic unit? With all the intricacies of academic units' missions, is it possible for one individual or administrative team to be "all knowing"? Although attaining this status may seem impossible, administrative teams of the future can be successful and effective by adhering to a few simple principles. In this chapter I describe the characteristics of a model administrative team equipped to face the threats and forces that the future of nursing is certain to bring. I focus on discernment, intuition, and various managerial principles as a foundation for effective leadership.

Specific Issues Facing Administrative Teams of the Future

Many leaders have been engaged primarily in the dean's role to ensure that educational program outcomes meet standards for accreditation, state board approval, and board certification. To meet these standards, it was necessary to secure space and financial resources, assist in recruitment of faculty and students, promote nursing as a viable academic unit within the total educational institution, and promote the image of nurses and nursing. Tomorrow's educational leader must be con-

cerned with (a) continuation of cuts in financial and clinical resources; (b) maintenance of programmatic quality and efficiency by doing more with less; (c) validation of the achievement of programmatic outcomes; (d) creation of collaborative partnerships external to the program and institution; (e) design of new, flexible, nontraditional programs to meet consumer demands; (f) rapid changes in academic instructional technology; (g) oversight of entrepreneurial activities, as college or school nurse managed clinics; and (h) involvement in major fund development projects. Carol Aschenbrener (1998) believes that "the major skills essential to function effectively in these future roles are flexible thinking and the ability to change mental models" (p. 46). In addition she asserted that leaders of teams must be "change agents, with a deep understanding of people and the dynamics of change" (pp. 46–47). The leader must be a team builder who possesses leadership and management skills, genuinely understands issues, invites interactions or dialogue, demonstrates the attitudinal behavior of congruence, and takes and uses power wisely.

Discernment and Intuition

The changes in education and the resulting demands on administrators lend credence to a familiar cliche—"jack of all trades, master of none." It is not surprising that tomorrow's administrators, including deans, department heads, and assistant and associate deans, will need new ways to manage and lead people. Ask any successful administrator to identify the basis for success, and the one answer that consistently surfaces is having an administrative team that possesses a harmonious culture that enables it to work well together and with others.

How does the administrator establish an administrative team that functions well together and still is responsive to all the complex issues facing it every day? It is vital that tomorrow's administrator be well versed in *discernment*. *The Merriam-Webster New Collegiate Dictionary* (1998) defined *discernment* as the "quality of being able to grasp and comprehend what is obscure" (p. 330). Merriam-Webster further defines *discern* as the ability to "detect with other senses than vision," "recognize or identify as separate and distinct," and "see and understand the difference" (p. 330). As part of the discernment process, an administrator must be intuitive. *Intuition* is the perception of facts, truths, and relationships without reasoning.

Intuition is often dismissed or ignored because facts and logic point in another direction. However, some individuals believe that intuition is more than just a raw "gut feeling"—hidden or subconscious—that it involves the cognitive and analytical processes that legitimize it. Conversely, others claim that intuition is a fallacy of logic with no scientific basis or relation to any managerial principle. However, the administrator who couples intuition with learned principles of leadership and management, will be effective and successful. Adopting this process separates the excellent administrator from the good administrator. Administrators must allow for intuition to become part of their management style as they move toward the future of nursing education.

■ A Model—Tomorrow's Administrative Team

The literature abounds with many essential managerial principles and group dynamic skills that every leader of a working team must have to be effective in meeting its and the organization's mission and goals. Development of an administrative team model must adhere to the principle "function follows form," a concept first enunciated in architecture. Davidson (1996) advocated that members of the ideal team must be

- academically competent and have a broad range of skills that provide a firm foundation for organizational success;

- supported by modalities that foster effective communication styles, promoting a sense of trust and avoiding ambiguity;

- personally committed to continued self-improvement, which is paramount for mind development and organizational effectiveness; and

- able and skillful in flexibly functioning with uncertainty in an ever-changing organizational environment.

These competencies will enable the administrative team to empower others to accept responsibility for their actions and to act with professional authority. The main objective of a leader's role is to master and orchestrate change through the administrative team for the benefit of faculty, staff, and students. Aschenbrener (1998) maintained that leaders "must be able to foresee the need for change, develop a shared vision of change that is linked to the interests of constituents, and guide people through the process of transition" (p. 49). The success of change initiatives depends on the culture of the organization, and the culture of the organization depends on the ability of the administrative team and leader to manage change.

Leader as Conductor of Orchestra

In the development of an effective team, the leader's role can be perceived as analogous to the conductor of an orchestra. Throughout the audition process, the conductor assesses and validates. Expertise, sensitivity, and ability of the musician to read and interpret music are crucial when a musician auditions for, say, the woodwind section. Likewise, a dean assesses an individual interviewing for an administrative team position and assesses the person's knowledge, interpersonal skills, experience, and interest in teaching, research, and caring. The conductor seeks confirmation during the audition that the individual will be able to be an integral part of the woodwind section, but yet rise to the demands of solo performance. The administrative leader also seeks to confirm the ability of the individual to function as a team player, yet take the lead on assigned or self-appointed projects. The conductor has a vision for how the entire musical score comes together; however, it is essential that this vision be transmitted to the musicians through his conducting. The conductor, with a great deal of energy and motivation, leads the entire orchestra through the musical score. The individual players respond to his interpretation of movements as slow, fast, loud, soft, but he also is aware of individuals who are not synchronous with the others. Guided by musical principles and intuition—and intense rehearsals—the conductor leads the entire orchestra to a unified, electrifying performance.

As the conductor, the dean—leader of the administrative team—also must have vision and plans for achievement. It is vital that the vision be shared with the administrative team, as the conductor does with the orchestra. Each team member must know the part that he or she plays, as well as the part that the team plays within the organization. The leader delineates specific activities that come together into a total action plan. The team acts as a unified whole, but individual team members also are allowed to engage in solo activities. These solo actions must be evident in the plan and integrated with the overall team effort. Similar to the conductor, the dynamic leader of the future must use managerial principles, discernment, and intuition in leading the team to successful completion of an activity. The effective leader has a high energy level, motivates team members, takes risks, conveys sensitivity, and makes time for others. The leader must identify opportunities and open doors for team members and must never be afraid to admit mistakes. It is important that the leader be creative in conflict resolution and problem solving, shrewd in handling external forces, and skilled in guiding and leading others in team interactions.

Characteristics of Leaders

Frequently identified characteristics of leaders are honesty, being visionary and inspirational, being competent, and possessing integrity (Brooks & Smith, 1999). But what about intuition—the innate skill of being able to perceive (without reasoning) incongruity, untruth, and something being amiss in facts. It is this "gut feeling" that makes an interaction between individuals or an action seem comfortable and appropriate or foster a sense of discomfort and that something isn't quite right. The leader must be responsive to a "nagging sensation" that a team member might not be truthful when reporting on the status of a project. Although some may argue that intuition is not a supportable principle, credence must be given to that innate sense. To be effective, intuition must be used in conjunction with managerial principles, concepts of behavioral outcomes and interpersonal relationships, and communication strategies. Some individuals give examples of situations in which a successful outcome included reacting to intuition or in which a nonsuccessful result occurred when they chose to ignore intuition. The wise leader with an intuitive sense should always hear and listen to it and then apply managerial principles and skills as part of the assessment and evaluation process before taking action.

Key Elements of Discernment

Key elements in the discernment process affecting establishment of an effective administrative team are organizational culture and the team's power base. The organization's culture and power exert overall control of the team, its ability to motivate its members and others, and survive the politics involved in daily work life. Organizational culture defines acceptable behavior, who and what will be rewarded, and how information flows.

Organizational Culture and the Work Environment

The optimum organizational culture creates an environment wherein both individual and organizational objectives are fulfilled, healthy interpersonal relationships are supported, problem solving is facilitated, and appropriate risk-taking is encouraged (Manthey, 1993). Creating the optimum environment requires hard work, perseverance, political persuasion, and understanding. Arndt and Huckabay (1980) defined culture as "the component of the milieu that deals with the human element" (p. 118). The milieu is intangible but very real. Dealing with people is the most important variable of the work environment. Arndt and Huckabay believe that the administrative team must recognize that people seek personal satisfaction and responsibility, which is necessary for their growth, stability, and interaction. Furthermore, the administrative team must facilitate this achievement by establishing a climate that fosters cooperation, integration, communication, commitment, and reward. Perception and receptivity by the administrative team are an essential part of the work environment. Arndt and Huckabay (1980) maintain that, "if creative growth is to take place…[management] must foster a structure and climate that will produce security to overcome the anxiety…and must be enough motivation to recognize the need for work, change, growth and reform" (p. 118). They also asserted that the optimum work environment

1. fosters thinking and the freedom to make mistakes without negative recourse;

2. encourages individual initiative and insists on a high rate of innovations and effectiveness in operational activities;

3. allows for problem-solving and decision-making input by all individuals;

4. accepts flexibility and adaptability so that change can occur with relative ease;

5. facilitates positive interpersonal working relationships;

6. allows for upward career advancement;

7. favors creativity;

8. accepts that there is more than one way to achieve a goal;

9. encourages and allows individuals to achieve their highest level of self-actualization; and

10. fosters respect for others and promotes a feeling of belonging and a sense of identity and security. (p. 119)

The administrative leader must assess specific requirements for utility, amenity, and expression but also be responsive to inviting, intuitive feelings. These environmental variables significantly affect human functioning in any situation. The leader must question and sense whether sufficient space and resources have been provided for people to complete their tasks and whether the utility of space allows for easy communication between offices. Further, consideration must be given to the physical amenities, as in having adequate comfort levels in air temperature, humidity, noise level, and brightness. Is the space pleasant to look at? Does the décor promote a sense of belonging, caring, or warmth to each individual who works in or visits the organization? Does the individual perceive having access to privacy and relaxation as one of the amenities? Combination of the separate environmental variables facilitates the effective functioning and interplay of the administrative team, its leader, and other individuals in the organization.

Power Base

Team leaders become effective when they build on the richness of expertise, strengths, talents, skills, and abilities of their team members and work groups, and then effectively use power. Judith Sturnick (1988), in her writings about power, stated that real power is the ability to influence others to take effective action and that there is a link between power and leadership. The relation between power and leadership is the ability to facilitate process, movement, see beyond the present moment, empower others, clarify, remain open, and allow others to discover for them. Sturnick further suggested empowering others is an excellent way to change the course of events.

Leaders empower others by being truthful, sharing resources—which can be material or of themselves—articulating vision and goals clearly, serving as mentors, and making connecting actions to outcomes. Respecting and valuing others is essential. However, before leaders can respect and value others, they must respect and value themselves. Sturnick further advocates that effective leaders must give time, energy, and strength to face the challenges of change, but not lose themselves in the process. Wise leaders learn from their mistakes. Wise leaders also learn from others' successes and mistakes. The shrewd leader is able to discern a valuable lesson from each mistake or success and adjust accordingly for the future.

Control: Who Leads the Team

Administration is a poor choice for the person who likes predictability, a narrow focus, and control. Successful administrators, as leaders for tomorrow, must give up narrow focus to become generalists. They must enjoy unpredictability and be able to delegate control to others. The leader establishes the team to be an extension of herself or himself and willingly allows movement of control back and forth and among the entire team. Empowerment must be fluid to lead others to act in ways that are mutually satisfying (Tuchscherer, Bremer, Madden, McCain-Ruelle, 1998). The type and amount of control that leaders and administrative teams will be able to exercise in the future depend on the pace of change, scope of activity, roles and responsibilities; ability to work with and through people; and the power to get things done. Successful leaders must be clear about what is most important to themselves; in other words, they must know themselves.

Motivation

Merriam-Webster (1998) defines motivation as the thought or feeling that makes a person act (p. 759). Success in the future will rest on the leader's ability to allow and facilitate others to maximize personal achievements for the organization while getting the organization to heighten the satisfaction that individuals derive from their activities. People are motivated when their strengths, rather than limitations, are recognized and built on. The leader should be constantly attentive to achievements and then praise and reward them appropriately. The unchallenged or dissatisfied individual will seek or develop new opportunities that afford different but obtainable challenges. The future leader and team will facilitate challenge for the dissatisfied individual. They will seek formation of collaborative relationships with corporations, industry, and community agencies. They will facilitate development of a research project, nurse-managed clinic, or establishment of a nonprofit corporation to provide motivational opportunities for all team members. The era of paternalism is nearing its end.

Politics

The team leader must take into account and recognize the politics of the organization generally and the political aspects of the team specifically. Team members are unique and share equal but different strengths. Team strengths must be brought together to reflect the leader's competencies along with the unit's strategic plan and goals. Strengths that the leader must consider as essential for team success are (a) level of self-confidence, (b) ability to communicate, (c) ability to establish trust in others, and (d) willingness to take risks. Knowledge of each team member's strengths and limitations will create a more harmonious team. The astute leader will assess the strength of team members' abilities to develop and manage their skills, determine and set priorities, and create an environment conducive to change. Surrounding oneself with ineffective team members and a heavy workload is often motivated by the leader's need to retain tight control. Anderson (1992) stated that a strong, effective leader needs strong individuals to be part of the team—individuals who are capable of managing the chaos and complexity of change. The leader's effectiveness depends on the team's success.

Characteristics of the Team Member

Depending on the size of the academic unit, the administrative team will consist of one to four assistant or associate deans, administrative assistant to the dean, business administrator, department chairs and support staff. Members of the team will be innovative, able to generate ideas, and not afraid to act on those ideas.

The composition of the ideal team can be characterized as a group of people who are

- risk takers,
- unafraid to fail or make mistakes,
- flexible, and
- innovative, creative, and dedicated to self-improvement.

Ideal team members are able to

- inspire and motivate others,
- convey sensitivity,
- communicate honesty and genuineness in every interaction,
- convey acceptance and nonpossessive warmth to others,
- see beyond the present moment,
- empower others,
- remain open and allow others to discover for themselves, and
- perceive change as essential for survival.

The leader of the team has the responsibility to encourage the development of individual team members and the team as a unit. Resources must be available so that the team can continue to gain increased competencies necessary for successfully fulfilling its roles and responsibilities. In development and maintenance of a successful and effective team, the difference between a good versus an outstanding leader is one who does not ignore the element of intuition. The effect of using intuition wisely, when the situation demands, promotes the smooth and effective functioning of the team.

Discernment and Intuition as Survival Tools

Survival of the future administrator and team will depend on a few simple concepts: (a) coaxing an idea into existence, (b) fostering a creative climate, (c) accepting criticism (knowing how to take it), and (d) being indispensable.

Coaxing an Idea into Existence

Pollock (1971) believed that people's knowledge, experience, and observation must be reformulated into fresh ideas and solutions by shaking off mental shackles and not remaining prisoners of their own thinking. Status quo thinking must be given up if new ideas are to be generated. Taking the course of least resistance is a very comfortable and lazy way to do business for leaders and team members. Fear of ridicule must be conquered before any leadership action can be implemented. If the team leader intuitively suspects that something is amiss, he or she must logically analyze the situation and attempt to answer questions relative to its likely affects on the team and its tasks. Consideration must be given to questions such as (a) What made the plan too costly? (b) Why was it misunderstood? (c) What strategy was used in developing the plan?

When answers begin to emerge, the specific idea will begin to be coaxed into existence. Sudden formation and insight of the idea will occur, following mental analysis and putting aside the tenets of the idea—in other words, taking a break from the mental thought processes.

Creative Climate for an Idea

Pollock (1971) described the ideal climate for idea creation as needing "the incentive to produce ideas, the pressures to produce ideas and the willingness to accept ideas" (p. 63). The administrative team encourages creativity in individuals by providing incentives and rewards in the organization's culture.

Criticism and How to Take It

Utopia is a world without criticism. Pollock (1971) maintained that "we are free from criticism only on two occasions, the day of our birth and the day of our death" (p. 109). Criticism comes readily, steadily, and inevitably. It comes by surprise. It comes when a person fully expects it and when a person knows that it is deserved. Criticism should be viewed as a form of communication; the sender is sharing a thought with the receiver. Criticism can be a source of new knowledge or the start of a creative idea. However, criticism is often perceived as a personal attack against an idea, person, or action. For the administrative team to benefit from criticism, a personal perception of any attack must be discarded. Strategies that the administrative team might use to value criticism include: (a) tame one's temper, (b) do not become defensive or personalize the criticism, (c) listen carefully with objectivity, (d) keep an open mind, (e) do not let trigger words produce mental hysteria, (f) consider the source, or sender, of the message, and (g) always evaluate the comments. Use of these strategies will allow the administrative team to perceive criticism as constructive and having a positive outcome.

Being Indispensable

The final strategy for survival, according to Pollock, is to make the team and leader indispensable. The strategy can be as simple or complex as to look for trouble spots needing improvement. The administrative team must increase its knowledge and competencies and develop a special area of expertise. It must seek additional or different responsibilities, work hard and efficiently, and never settle for routine performance. Additionally, it is important to give recognition where it is due, always value individuals for their special uniqueness, and maintain an open, trusting, and caring environment. Aschenbrener (1998) believed that, to increase the likelihood of being perceived as essential to the organization, leaders must (a) set clear directions; (b) link directions to the interests of those involved; and (c) listen, hear, and give credence to feelings and emotions. Leaders and administrative teams must model behaviors and recognize similar behaviors in others. If these strategies are utilized, the successful team will be equipped to face future unknown challenges.

■ Concluding Statement

No one can predict with any certainty what tomorrow will bring. Equally, no one can accurately predict all the characteristics that a highly successful administrative team will need. Use of discernment and intuition along with established managerial principles to develop and maintain an effective administrative team will be the key to success. The leader and administrative team must keep in mind the unique values and attitudes of others through active participation and consistent recognition. Anything less will result in constant erosion of the administrative leader's and team's effectiveness in the 21st century.

■ References

Anderson, C. A. (1992). Developing an administrative team: Moving the organization forward by creating a healthy climate. In R. Booth (Ed.), *Executive development series II: The dean's role in organizational assessment and development* (pp. 65–77). Washington, DC: AACN (American Association of Colleges of Nursing).

Arndt, C., & Huckabay, L. M. D. (1980). *Nursing administration: Theory for practice with a systems approach.* St. Louis: Mosby.

Aschenbrener, C. A. (1998). Leadership, culture and change: Critical elements for transformation. In E. R. Rubin (Ed.), *Mission management: Vol. 2* (pp. 46–47). Washington, DC: Association of Academic Health Centers.

Brooks, A. M. T., & Smith, T. (1999). Managing across disciplines. In E. J. Sullivan (Ed.), *Creating nursing's future* (pp. 180–190). St. Louis: Mosby.

Davidson, R. J. (1996). A new health professions curriculum for a new delivery system. In M. Osterweis, C. J. McLaughlin, H. R. Manasse, Jr., & C. L. Hopper (Eds.), *The U.S. health workforce: Power, politics and policy* (pp. 175–186). Washington, DC: Association of Academic Health Centers.

Manthey, M. (1993). Empowering staff to create a professional practice environment. In *Nursing leadership: Preparing for the 21st century* (pp. 4–5). Chicago: AHA, American Hospital Publishing.

Merriam-Webster New Collegiate Dictionary, 10th ed. (1998). Springfield, Mass.: G. and C. Merriam Co.

Pollock, T. (1971). *Managing yourself creatively.* New York: Hawthorn.

Sturnick, J. (1988). Sea change in higher education offers women chances for power. *Women in Higher Education, 7*(11), 1–2.

Tuchscherer, B., Bremer, S., Madden, M., & McCain-Ruelle, L. (1998). Preview: The joys and jolts of becoming an administrator. *Women in Higher Education, 7*(11), 8.

■ *Editor's Questions for Discussion*

How does a leader ensure that internal standards are maintained in an academic unit? What strategies are most effective for the development and implementation of standards and ensuring adherence to them?

How important are discernment and intuition in management? Can discernment be taught? How does someone develop intuition? Provide examples of intuition being a part of (or lacking in) a person's management style. Identify the characteristics of an effective management team. How can potential management personnel be best assessed prior to employment? What clues may be provided by prospective managers concerning their ability to be an effective and harmonious team member? Provide examples of intuition being used with managerial principles in evaluation of behavior. How does a leader know who is a truth teller in complex situations? What group dynamics skills and competencies are critical not only for a leader, but also for members of a management team? What exceptional interpersonal skills and competencies are essential for the leader of a management team?

Discuss effective means of resolving conflict on a management team. How are competitive behaviors on a management team identified and addressed? What strategies are effective in developing a cohesive team? How does a management team influence the culture of a School of Nursing? What factors are relevant for altering organizational culture by a leader or management team? To what extent does organizational culture control a management team in a School of Nursing? Explicate relationships that exist between power and leadership. Provide examples of events being changed by the use of power.

How may healthy interpersonal relationships be developed in a school? What role does a dean, management team, faculty, and staff have in facilitating a positive climate and culture? What structure(s) and process(es) in Schools of Nursing may be most effective in promoting a harmonious atmosphere? To what extent do the 10 elements of an optimum environment, indicated by Lindell, exist in your institution? Apply Lindell's discussion regarding discernment and intuition as survival tools in your School of Nursing.

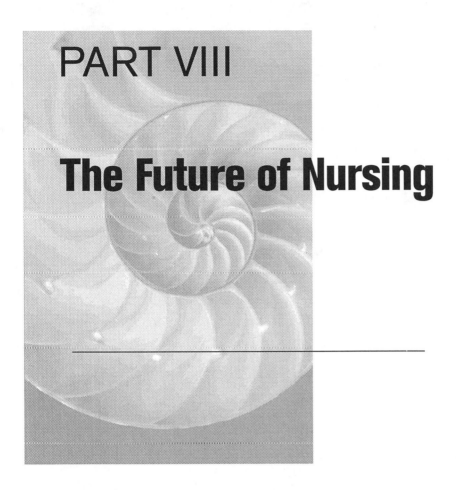

PART VIII

The Future of Nursing

" . . . I shall be telling this with a sigh
Somewhere ages and ages hence:
Two roads diverged in a wood, and I . . ."

Each of the previous Parts of this volume are highlighted in this Future of Nursing Part. The contributing authors show that each aspect of the profession is a critical link to each of the others. Many paths previously identified in other chapters are prominent. Demands are significant no matter which path the profession chooses; the authors yearn for the day when all will have been met effectively. Can you identify the challenges these writers recognize and pose others that would be of benefit to address? The authors concur in believing that most everything is possible through the action of all—personally and as a profession.

70

Healing into the Future

Re-Creating the Profession of Nursing Through Inner Work

Daniel J. Pesut, PhD, RN, CS, FAAN

The purpose of this chapter is to discuss the importance of therapeutic inner work for professional development. Intrapersonal inner work supports personal growth that in turn is manifested in outer work of social relevance. Service to others is enhanced when we ourselves are whole. As members of the nursing profession each of us is accountable for the inner work required to renew and re-create ourselves as we seek wholeness and healing. One way to seek wholeness is to explore the impact and influence that symbols, archetypes, and shadows play in our self and interpersonal relations.

■ Archetypes

Archetypes are manifestations of emotional states and stages we have reached in our growth and development (Arrien, 1993; Barry & Blanford, 1999; Gilligan, 1997; Myss, 1996; Wauters, 1997). Re-creating the profession of nursing requires attention to the influence of archetypes and shadows in the service of professional identity, mission, and vision. As the 20th century ended, there was increased interest in issues of consciousness, symbolism, energetics, and the role archetypes play in human growth, development, and health (Arrien,

1993; Gilligan, 1997; Myss, 1996; Pearson, 1986; Richo, 1999; Wauters, 1997).

Archetypes symbolically reveal psychological patterns and unveil self-care needs that each of us requires to maintain energy and vitality. Archetypes are about universal themes, images, and relational patterns. Archetypes contain both positive and negative shadows. Shadows are parts of ourselves that we have split off, repressed, denied, or are afraid to show even though they are part of our personalities. Archetypes and shadows are often played out in interpersonal dynamics and organizational politics. Both people and organizations can be related to archetypal images and shadows.

The shadow side of a business or enterprise deals with the covert undiscussable, the undiscussed (Egan, 1994). It includes arrangements not found in organizational manuals and company documents. Specifically the shadow side of an organization has three dimensions: (a) significant activities and arrangements that remain unidentified or undiscussed, (b) factors that fall outside of ordinary managerial interventions, and (c) activities and arrangements that affect productivity and quality of work life in a company or institution (Egan, 1994).

Egan (1994) defined five categories of shadows: (a) organizational culture, (b) personal styles, (c) social systems in the organization, (d) organizational politics, and (e) the informal or hidden organization within an institution. Egan suggested that the best ways to manage shadows in an organization are to bring issues out in the open. He offered the following strategies and suggestions: (a) be alert and inquisitive regarding hidden arrangements and activities; (b) become sensitive to the idea of unwritten rules; (c) become aware of blind spots by asking questions behind the question; (d) explore ways you have been surprised by behavior or events; (e) find out why you do not want to know certain shadow side activities; (f) move beyond defensiveness by identifying consequences of not discussing an issue; (g) deal with rather than avoid discomfort; and (h) challenge laziness, indifference, and cynicism. Turn embarrassment and disruption into learning. Such advice can be applied to issues of personal as well as organizational shadows.

Self-Leadership and Personal Change

The only real change is personal change (De Geus, 1997). Re-creating the profession of nursing requires each individual in the profession to assume responsibility for self-change in light of shadows and information that influence perceptions and action. Collectively, we are obliged to create and respect time, space, and opportunities for colleagues to engage in personal inner work that enriches professional public action. Such work is supported by ancient wisdom, symbolic frames of meaning, and contemporary innovations in psychotherapeutic methods.

Understanding the role of archetypes and shadows in our personal dynamics gives rise to a special type of self-leadership. Self-leadership involves understanding symbols and meanings, given the content and contexts of change. Frames are mental models that influence and guide our perception and behavior (Fairhurst & Sarr, 1996). Becoming aware of mental models in regard to inner work and professional development is crucial to development of self-leadership and intrapersonal change. For example, from an organizational perspective, traditional ways of framing process and outcomes have related to issues of structure, human resources, and politics (Bolman & Deal, 1997). In a structural frame, central concepts focus on rules, roles, goals, policies, technology, and the environment. In the human resource frame, central concepts are needs, skills, and relationships. The political frame is organized around concepts of power, conflict, competition, and organizational politics. A fourth frame proposed by Bolman and Deal (1997) is the symbolic frame. The 21st century is a time to examine and frame things in terms of symbols and meaning. I believe that we in the profession underestimate the power and influence of the symbolic frame in regard to inner work and self-leadership required to engage in such work.

Central concepts in the symbolic frame are culture, meaning, metaphor, ritual, ceremony, stories, energetics, archetypes, and shadows. Archetypes and shadows are symbolic energetic patterns of relating to oneself and others. Considering symbolic and energetic, rather than political or structural frames of reference, is more likely to lead to creation of health and wholeness. Framing issues symbolically highlights the need for inner work that complements our outer work. Guidance and personal growth strategies that promote such inner work is found in ageless wisdom texts and contemporary resources that interpret these texts for modern times. The combination of ancient wisdom and contemporary interpretation has resulted in principles and psychotherapeutic practices that promote personal growth and professional development.

Spiritual Politics and Principles

The 21st century is a time for expanding consciousness regarding the influence and effects of ancient wisdom and spiritual politics. Spiritual politics is informed by four levels of thinking: (a) level of information—facts and data about our human responses; (b) level of symbology—what symbols of names, place, and events tell us about inner forces and energies at work; (c) level of meaning—what events mean to us when seen through the eyes of a compassionate heart that understands the growth and development inherent in spiritual lessons; and (d) level of significance—how the event relates to outworking of purpose for a society, a community, or the planet (McLaughlin and Davidson, 1994).

Principles of ageless wisdom include (a) learning detachment and developing the stance of the observer, (b) developing compassion and a commitment to service, (c) trusting our own inner source of guidance, (d) appreciating the interconnectedness of all things, (e) appreciating the importance of learning gained through time, and (f) understanding how the inner worlds of individuals manifest themselves in the outer world of being and doing. The ageless wisdom meaning of the word spiritual is greater than a specific religious connotation. "Spiritual" applies to anything that relates to (a) expansion of consciousness; (b) drives an individual or society forward toward some form of development—physical, mental, emotional, intuitive; and (c) develops greater understanding, love, or beauty (McLaughlin & Davidson, 1994).

As the nursing profession pursues visions of the future, one of many tasks that confront each of us is the integration of symbolic information and levels of meaning with ancient wisdom and psychotherapeutic methods of personal growth and development. By analyzing, understanding, and considering meanings inherent in archetypal and shadow systems, we come to understand how we are influenced consciously and unconsciously. Such inner work is one path to a desired future.

Inner Work

Inner work refers to our soul-selves; outer work involves interaction outside ourselves (Fox, 1994). Soul, wrote Alan Briskin (1998),

> is a quality stirred into being through reflection on experience and action in the world. To care for soul within us and outside in the world, we need to recognize that soul is not our possession, but rather the points of overlap where inner experience and outer world are joined. In the workplace we have become polarized between

managing the outer organization—work processes, organizational objectives, managerial structures and the inner organization of people—emotions, attitude, mental processes, cooperative spirit. Following a path with soul suggests an approach that borders both worlds but is not contained by them. In attending to experiences and reflection on experience we develop heightened capacity to straddle these two worlds and discover something new. (p. xi)

Fox (1994) argues that when we lose our sense of an inner life we become alienated from ourselves and that this alienation is reflected in our outer work. Inner work is a remedy for this alienation. Reflecting on the nature of our outer work enables us to begin to do inner work that will support reinvention of what we do and how we go about our vocations. The Spirituality of Work Questionnaire was designed by Fox (1994) to stimulate reflection and inner work. Consider some of the questions contained in this tool.

1. When did I first feel drawn to the kind of work I am doing?

2. Do I experience joy in my work?

3. Do others experience joy as a result of my work?

4. How is my work a blessing to generations to come?

5. What inner work have I been involved in over the last five years?

6. What am I doing to reinvent the profession in which I work? (pp. 309–310)

Outer Work

A person's outer work is a manifestation of inner values, beliefs, ideologies, and identity. The relationship between outer work and inner work is reciprocal. The primal energetic source for outer work is core values derived from a soulful approach to work. David Whyte (1996) suggested that a soulful approach to work is probably the only way an individual can respond creatively to the high-temperature stress of modern work life without burning to a crisp in the heat. The soul's ability to elicit meaning from events, to meet fire with fire is at the center of it all. The 21st century will be a time for nursing to awaken its corporate soul. Soul holds the tension among opposing forces: individual and group, material, and spiritual. Soul is a place of meaningful paradox (McLaughlin & Davidson, 1994).

Soul Work

Soul work is the intrapersonal management of tension among opposites. Mind and emotions frequently function in polarities. One idea opposes another idea. With positive feelings, there are shadows of negative feelings. With negative feelings there are shadows of positive feelings. A person's spirit is the referee when it comes to managing the tensions among oppositions felt intrapersonally or interpersonally. When things do not make sense, the soul and spirit do the sorting out. Such sorting out depends on the degree to which someone has an awakened soul.

■ Paths to an Awakened Soul

There are four paths to awakening corporate soul (Klein & Izzo, 1998). The first path involves inner work and clarification of the person's passion; aspirations, values, and beliefs; sense of purpose; meaning; and mission. Sense of self influences soul. Klein and Izzo wrote:

> Soul awakens when people are aware of their own passion, in touch with their core values, and when they actively bring these alive in their daily work. Although this path is primarily about the individual discovery of vocation, leaders are

responsible for developing a climate that fosters the kind of self-discovery required to be sure people bring their values and passion into the workplace. (p. 23)

For some of us the sense of self is not clear.

Understanding archetypes and shadows can sometimes illuminate this sense of self. Sometimes we put others first in the name of service. But, on the one hand, unless we have a clear sense of self, boundaries, and values, self is fragmented. In place of service, resentment builds. On the other hand, too much of a self-path leads to narcissism, which dampens contributions of outer work.

The second path to awakening corporate soul is the path of contribution. In walking the path of contribution people discover the deeper reason for their work. They discover how work is a blessing to generations that will follow, and they are clear on the legacy they will leave that is derived from their contribution. As people recognize how their daily contributions serve something larger than themselves, they have greater understanding of the importance of a legacy. When people see the ultimate outcome of their work as valuable, especially when it is connected to a form of service to others, soul and commitment are evident and present. Understanding interplay among archetypes and shadow systems can influence the contributions they make in regard to their own personal development or organizational contributions.

The third path to awakening corporate soul is the path of craft. The path of craft is development of intense enjoyment in moment-to-moment action of work. Craft focuses on the ongoing process of learning. Inner work is not about problem solving but rather about learning. Markova (1994) notes that problem solving is about eliminating, discriminating, avoiding the unknown, and disconnecting from the finite. Problem solving is answer-oriented, appositional, and involves acquiring information. Problem solving is short-term, contracted, focused, linear, and reactive. In contrast, learning involves revealing, adding possibilities, entering the unknown, and connecting to the infinite. Learning is process-oriented, relational, and integrative. Learning is about developing abilities. The investment in learning is long-term, and expansive. Learning is about wondering. It is creative and proactive. The intention of inner work is to learn, not to solve problems. We tend to discount the moment-to-moment learning and healing that takes place in the intimacy of a caring nursing relationship. Balancing intra- and interpersonal dynamics and archetypal energies is a special craft that can be developed.

Finally, people find soul on the path of community when their connection to others goes deeper than their job description, touches the heart, and transcends traditional team building. Through the path of community, individuals join together to bring out the best in each other. People come alive when they are engaged in activities that call forth the highest level of skill and when they have capabilities that enable action necessary to support their values and beliefs. At this level, the symbolic assumes new meaning in terms of culture and community. In a true community, people see each others' limits without blaming and call forth each others' riches without demanding. The path of community is sometimes obstructed with jealousy and competition born of individual rather than group achievement. Community is about respect and the fact that gifts differ. On the path to community, inner work is required of everyone so that the balance of energy can be maintained and reinforced.

In summary, the path to an awakened soul involves attention to self, contribution, craft, and community. Attention to self becomes a key ingredient for full participation in a corporate community. Attending to self is where change is initiated and sustained. Attending to self requires reflection about the influence that energetic patterns have on self and others in a community. Inner work that supports discernment of a person's archetypes, shadows, and issues that implicitly and explicitly influence behavior is important for personal change.

■ The Inner Work of Personal Change: Archetypes and Shadows

Stephen Gilligan uses archetypes to foster insight and promote growth and understanding among clients in his self-relations psychotherapy. Gilligan (1997) suggested that the primary functions of archetypes are to help a person develop as a human being and that archetypes are especially active at times of identity change. Four major archetypes that have psychotherapeutic benefit in his system of therapy are (a) King or Queen, (b) Lover, (c) Warrior, and (d) Magician.

Archetype Dimensions and Shadows

The King or Queen archetypes are about giving blessing and creating a sense of place for people in a community. The Lover archetype is about acceptance and communion. The Warrior archetype is about agency, commitment, and boundaries. The Magician archetype is about transformation, healing, and enchantment. Each of these archetypes contributes an important concept and principle to healthy growth and development and psychotherapeutic healing. Each of these archetypes contributes to the balance of energy involved in interpersonal relationships. Each of these archetypes becomes a metaphor for gaining insight and understanding of an individual's sense of power and energy in relation to self and others.

Further, each of these archetypes has an unintegrated, dark or shadow side that mani-fests itself in terms of an imbalance of energy. The unintegrated forms of archetypes—be they positive or negative—are called shadows. The shadow, or unintegrated, aspect of the King or Queen is tyranny. The shadow, or unintegrated, side of the Lover is addiction. The shadow, or unintegrated, side of the Warrior is rage. The shadow, or unintegrated, aspect of the Magician is deception. Shadows are the repressed, denied, split off parts of people that they often project onto others. Shadows may be positive or negative. Shadow work generally involves exploring deep emotions of anger, sadness, fear, and joy, and the symbolic interactions that people have with their own perceptions and one another. Working through emotions in a safe container or space is often useful to foster healing and development of wholeness (Barry & Blanford, 1999).

Shadow Work

Barry and Blanford (1999) have designed a personal growth process called Shadow Work. Shadow Work provides a blueprint or model for engaging in inner work. Four major archetypal energies described by Barry and Blanford are Magician, Sovereign, Lover, and Warrior. Table 70.1 illustrates some of the dimensions of these archetypes and shadow issues involved with each. In addition, other characteristics of these archetypes are described. Each has a masculine and feminine valence. Each is associated with a particular family role. Emotions are associated with the archetypes. Animal instincts help explain and illustrate the energy and issues associated with the archetype. Of most interest is a specific psychological wound or an internalized shaming message connected to each. Finally, Barry and Blanford have identified specific psychotherapeutic tools that aid in the inner work related to balancing and healing issues associated with each archetype and its shadow manifestations.

TABLE 70.1   Dimensions of Archetypes and Their Shadow Issues

Category	Magician	Sovereign	Lover	Warrior
Purpose	Seeing options Guidance Detachment	Motivation through esteem	Connection through feeling	Power and service through boundaries
Masculine	Recipe	See vision	Spirit looking up	Offense
Feminine	Taste	Bless and support follow through	Soul looking down	Defense
Element	Air	Fire	Water	Earth
Family role	Clown Mascot Comedian	Hero Little parent Caretaker	Lost child Quiet but deep one	Rebel Scapegoat
Gateway emotion	Fear	Joy	Grief	Anger
Animal instinct	Predator	Alpha male or female	Bonding	Territorial
Shadows				
Too little	Dense/Rigid:"I don't know."	Shy: "I can't; it's too hard."	Dry/Stoic: "I can't get at it."	Flaky/Victim: "Please, no conflict."
Too much	Fragmented: "I'm confused."	Shining: "I can ace it!"	Overflowing: "It's getting me."	Savage/Defense: "You can't get me."
Deep wound	"I am bad."	"I'm not good enough."	"I don't love right."	"I don't exist apart from you."
The tool	Look from a split	Bring support from an ideal figure	Work in the body with a metaphor	Set a boundary

Note: Adapted from *Shadow Work,* by C. Barry and M. E. Blanford, 1999, Loveland, CO: Shadow Work Seminars.

As you examine these archetypes, consider the symbolic meaning of each in regard to yourself and your relationships with others. Use the following questions to facilitate your reflection.

1. To what degree do I possess this archetypal energetic pattern?

2. What archetypes am I least aware of?

3. What archetypes can I develop more?

4. How does thinking about this archetype represent critical issues of inner work for me?

5. How do the archetypes help me understand people with whom I work?

For example, the Magician archetype is about seeing options, providing guidance, and valuing detached observation. The masculine variation is best represented by analogy of cooking with a recipe versus the feminine variation of cooking by taste. The element associated with the Magician is air. Magician energies are derived from the family role of playing the clown, mascot, or comedian. Emotional access to the Magician is through the emotion of fear. The animal instinct linked with this energy is that of predator. Shadow manifestations of the Magician archetype are recognized as being too dense or fragmented. The deep psychological wound associated with the Magician archetype is "I am bad." The tool for helping to develop or modulate archetypal Magician energy is to look at a situation from split (or a variety of) frames of reference.

The purpose of the Sovereign archetype is motivation through esteem. The masculine variation is best represented by visions and blessing. The feminine variation involves support and encouragement. The element associated with the Sovereign is fire. Sovereign energies are likely derived from playing the family role of hero, little parent, or caretaker. Emotional access to the Sovereign is through the emotion of joy. The animal instinct linked with this energy is that of the lead or Alpha animal in a pack. Shadow manifestations of the Sovereign archetype are recognized in the following ways. Too much energy is characterized by shining and too little energy is manifested by shyness. The deep psychological wound associated with the Sovereign is "I am not good enough." The tool for helping to develop or modulate archetypal Sovereign energy is support from an ideal figure.

The purpose of the Lover archetype is connection through feelings. The masculine variation on this is best represented by the analogy of spirit looking up. The feminine variation involves the downward gaze of soul. The element associated with the Lover is air. Lover energies are likely derived from playing the family role of lost child or the quiet deep one in the family of origin. Emotional access to the Lover is the emotion of grief. The animal instinct linked with this energy is that of bonding. Shadow manifestations of the Lover archetype are recognized as stoicism in those that have too little and as overflowing emotionality in those that have too much. The deep psychological wound associated with the Lover is " I don't love right." Body work is especially helpful as the tool for developing or modifying archetypal Lover energy.

The purpose of the Warrior archetype is the exercise of power and service through defining and maintaining boundaries. The masculine variation is best described as defense. The feminine variation is about offense. The element associated with the Warrior is earth. Warrior energies are likely derived from playing the family role of rebel or scapegoat. Emotional access to the Warrior is through the emotion of anger. The animal instinct linked with this energy is that of territoriality. Shadow manifestations of the Warrior archetype are recognized as flakiness in those that have too little and as savage defensiveness in those that have too much. The deep psychological wound associated with the Warrior is "I don't exist apart from you." Setting boundaries is the tool that helps develop or modulate archetypal Warrior energy. Given the categories and associated issues, what inner work can be done to balance and modulate issues and energies associated with symbolic growth and developmental issues that are linked with archetypes and shadows?

■ Resources, Strategies, and Tools for Inner Work

It is surprising how much convergence is taking place among therapeutic modalities that use archetypes and energetic systems to stimulate insight, understanding, and therapeutic change. For example, several authors and therapists have developed systems and methods of therapeutic interventions around archetypes, shadows, and the energetic system of Chakras. Chakras are psychophysiological energy centers contained in the body. For example, therapist Ambika Wauters (1997) has linked the seven Chakras with both the positive and negative energies of major archetypes.

Linkage of Chakras with Archetypes

Wauters suggests that the first Chakra is linked with the positive archetype of Mother and the negative archetype of Victim. The emotional issue at this level is about being grounded. The second Chakra is linked with the positive archetype of Sovereign (Emperor or Empress) and the negative aspect of Martyr. The emotional issue at this level is organized around pleasure and well being. The third Chakra is linked with the positive archetype of Warrior and the negative archetype of Servant. The emotional issue at this level is organized around power and self-worth. The fourth Chakra is linked with the positive archetype of Lover and the negative archetype of Actor. Emotional issues at this level are organized around love. The fifth Chakra is linked with positive archetype of Communicator and the negative archetype of Silent Child. The issue linked with this level is effective communication. The sixth Chakra is linked with the positive archetype Intuition and the negative side of Intellectualization. The issues linked at this level are use of information for happiness and health. At the seventh Chakra level, Wauters suggested relationships among the archetype Guru and the negative valence of this archetype, Egotist. Through a series of exercises, meditations, affirmations, and suggested activities focused on developing self-responsibility, Wauters stimulates inner work and supports integration of issues of archetypes and shadows in a positive direction.

Linkage of Myss's Seven Truths with Chakras

Carolyne Myss, a popular speaker on healing and spiritual politics, has arrived at a similar set of conclusions about need for integration and understanding of archetypes and the energetic symbolic nature of Chakra systems. Based on her studies Myss has distilled seven truths across various religious traditions, scriptures, and ancient wisdom texts. Like Wauters, Myss associates these seven truths with the Chakras system of the body and belief that inner work is necessary to maintain personal power and health (Myss, 1996). These truths are:

1. *All is one.* This truth is related to the first Chakra and lessons related to the material world.

2. *Honor one another.* This truth is related to the second Chakra and lessons related to sexuality, work, and physical desire.

3. *Honor oneself.* This truth is related to the third Chakra and lessons related to the ego, personality, and self-esteem.

4. *Know that love is divine power.* This truth is related to the fourth Chakra and lessons related to love, forgiveness, and compassion.

5. *Surrender personal will to divine will.* This truth is related to the fifth Chakra and lessons related to will and self-expression.

6. *Seek only the truth.* This truth is related to the sixth Chakra and lessons related to mind, intuition, insight and wisdom.

7. *Live in the present moment.* This truth is related to the seventh Chakra and lessons related to spirituality.

Myss suggests a variety of meditations focused on these energetic Chakras systems and essential spiritual truths. The focus of

Myss's work is organized around the importance of forgiveness in light of spiritual understanding and learning.

Arrien's Principles and Archetypes

Cultural anthropologist Angeles Arrien (1993) has proposed four guiding principles of inner work that promote healing and understanding. Each principle is based on archetypes of the Visionary, Healer, Teacher, and Warrior. Arrien advocates a fourfold practice that includes the following guidelines.

1. Show up or choose to be present. Being present allows us to access the human resources or power, presence, and communication. This is the way of warrior.

2. Pay attention to what has heart and meaning. Paying attention opens us to the human resources of love, gratitude, acknowledgments, and validation. This is the way of the Healer.

3. Tell the truth without blame or judgment. Nonjudgmental truthfulness maintains our authenticity and develops our inner vision and intuition. This is the way of the Visionary.

4. Be open to outcomes, not attached to outcome. Openness and nonattachment help us to recover human resources of wisdom and objectivity. This is the way of the teacher.

Arrien believes that these four archetypes—Warrior, Healer, Visionary, and Teacher—provide guidelines and structure for understanding your own growth and developmental needs through the ancient wisdom of the past. Her book, *The Four-Fold Way*, provides experiences, meditations, resources, and suggestions that support inner work in service of integration of archetypes and shadows.

Arrien noted that archetypal work is midlife work. Midlife is a time for deep forgiveness and a time for reparation and rectification work. It's a time for making your life straight, a time of humility, a time of mercy, a time of grace. The second half of life is about integrating your shadows, fully actualizing energies of archetypes, and legacy leaving. Such inner work is about planting and nurturing seeds that generate a legacy of special wisdom for generations that follow.

■ Inner Work and Healing into the Future

Pritchett and Associates (1999) recently published 10 ground rules for job success in the next millennium.

1. *Think differently. See differently.* Career challenges of the future are likely to be more perceptual and psychological rather than technical and skills-based. The use and understanding of archetypes, shadows, and the symbolic way of thinking support ways of thinking and seeing differently. Thinking in symbolic terms and seeing relationships in terms of archetypes, energetic systems, and consequences of such information for inner work supports outer work.

2. *Migrate to the 4th level of change.* Level 1 change is problem-oriented and elicits coping responses from people. Level 2 change requires adjustment and elicits adaptive responses from people. Level 3 change frames problems as opportunities and fosters exploitation of opportunities. Level 4 change is about purpose, adventure, optimism, and faith. Level 4 change also is about creating the future based on symbolic and energetic frames of meaning.

3. *Manage your energy level.* Good energy management comes down to generating more, conserving it better, and channeling it with greater focus. What better way is there to manage energy than to begin to think in symbolic ways—understand the balance and importance of archetype and shadows and how these uni-

versal images drain or enhance a person's daily energetic output.

4. *Explore and innovate.* Exploration and innovation are linked with Magician and Visionary energy. They are about blessing and finding your unique place in the community—making your personal and professional contributions. Consider exploring archetypes and ways to manage these energetic ideas and structures in personal, professional, and organizational life; this may lead to new insights that generate different behaviors focused on learning rather than problem solving.

5. *Stay optimistic and opportunity minded.* Such a principle supports openness to need to pay attention to what has heart and meaning. Being open to outcomes is one of the principles of the fourfold way that is built on ancient wisdom and spiritual politics.

6. *Help create value.* Creating value for the profession depends on inner work made manifest in outer work. Such work is vital and relevant when it seeks to balance archetypal energies with personal and organizational shadow systems.

7. *Manage more of your own emotions.* Inner work is organized self-leadership associated with the self-regulation of emotions inherent in archetypal and shadow work.

8. *Make job changes judiciously.* If current situations are not contributing to development of your inner self or soul work, or if you are not deriving pleasure from your outer work, consider making a change. As you look for new job opportunities consider the energetic dynamics, symbolic frames, and shadow systems of such work.

9. *Practice self-leadership and a new kind of followership.* The sponsorship and self-relations required to thrive in the 21st century include the ability to invite and focus inner work in service of outer work.

10. *Balance yourself.* Energetically balancing the archetypes and shadows connected to your personal and professional dynamics is serious work that is required to renew the profession of nursing through individual efforts over time.

■ Concluding Statement

We can only wonder about the convergence and interest in archetypal patterns for therapeutic work at this moment in time. Archetypes generally manifest themselves in times of identity change. We could say that these patterns began emerging at end of the 20th century after a long time of incubation and professional development. Another frame is more future-oriented. Perhaps the appearance and use of ancient wisdom in contemporary contexts at the beginning of the 21st century provide a foundation for inner work and personal growth that is necessary for future outer work. Symbolically the message has many meanings. There are ways, means, and methods available to help people do inner work necessary for healing. Such inner work is universal and has been done through time in a variety of cultures. Inner work is focused at the level of symbol and meaning and has implications and consequences for re-creating the profession of nursing as we heal into the 21st century.

■ References

Arrien, A. (1993). *The four-fold way: Walking the paths of the warrior, teacher, healer and visionary.* New York: HarperCollins.

Barry, C., & Blanford, M. E. (1999). Shadow Work. Loveland, CO: *Shadow Work Seminars,* 13706 Buckhorn Rd., Loveland, Colorado, 80538. Telephone (970) 203-0400. [On-line]. Available: http://www.shadowwork.com.

Bolman, L., & Deal, T. (1997). *Reframing organizations: Artistry, choice, leadership* (2nd ed.). San Francisco: Jossey-Bass.

Briskin, A. (1998). *The stirring of soul in the workplace.* San Francisco: Berrett-Koehler.

De Geus, A. (1997). *The living company: Habits for survival in a turbulent business environment.* Boston: Harvard Business School Press.

Egan, G. (1994). *Working the shadow side: A guide to positive behind the scenes management.* San Francisco: Jossey-Bass.

Fairhurst, G., & Sarr, R. (1996). *The art of framing.* San Francisco: Jossey-Bass.

Fox, M. (1994). *The re-invention of work.* New York: HarperCollins.

Gilligan, S. (1997). *The courage to love: Principles and practices of self-relations psychotherapy.* New York: W. W. Norton.

Klein, E., & Izzo, J. (1998). *Awakening corporate soul.* New York: Mid-Point Trade Books.

Markova, D. (1994). *No enemies within: A creative process for discovering what's right about what's wrong.* Berkeley, CA: Conari Press.

McLaughlin, C., & Davidson, G. (1994). *Spiritual politics: Changing the world from the inside out.* New York: Ballantine Books.

Myss, C. (1996). *Anatomy of the spirit: The seven stages of power and healing.* New York: Harmony Books.

Pearson, C. (1986). *The hero within: Six archetypes we live by.* San Francisco: Harper.

Pritchett, P. (1999). *New work habits for the next millennium. Ten new ground rules for job success.* Dallas: Pritchett & Associates.

Richo, D. (1999). *Shadow dance: Liberating the power and creativity of your dark side.* Boston: Shambhala.

Wauters, A. (1997). *Chakras and their archetypes: Uniting energy awareness and spiritual growth.* Freedom, CA: Crossing Press.

Whyte, D. (1996). *The heart aroused: Poetry and the preservation of the soul in corporate America.* New York: Currency Doubleday.

■ Editor's Questions for Discussion

What specific content in Pesut's chapter may be applied to the discussions of Felton (Chapter 1), Snyder, Kreitzer, and Loen (Chapter 43), S. Thomas (Chapter 60), Disch (Chapter 61), Lindeman (Chapter 63), Keating and Perry (Chapter 65), Chaska (Chapter 68), Lindell (Chapter 69), Kritek (Chapter 74), Shaver (Chapter 76), and Sills and Anderson (Chapter 77)?

How are archetypes and shadows reflected in the culture of a School or College of Nursing? Provide specific examples of shadows in your organization. How much change is reasonable to expect in confronting shadows? How do leaders monitor such changes and evaluate their outcomes?

How may leaders motivate responsibility for self-change? How may symbolic frames be developed that promote a healthy environment? How may leaders facilitate bridging "inner work" of individuals with the "outer work" of a professional group? What role do leaders have and what role boundaries exist in spanning or connecting inner and outer work? How may leaders awaken, facilitate, or change the development of a corporate soul? What constraints may exist? How does a leader assess the extent, degree, or type of forces that exist, which inhibit inner and outer work? What strategies or options does a leader have if personnel resist development of a climate fostering self-discovery and inner work?

Provide specific examples of the four paths for awakening a corporate soul in your situation. To what extent are intra- and interpersonal dynamics and archetypal energies balanced in your School or College of Nursing? How may a balance of energy be maintained, reinforced, and by whom? Respond to Pesut's queries regarding symbolic meaning of archetypes in relation to self, others, and fostering culture in your school or college. Apply to your school Pesut's statement that "re-creating the profession of nursing requires attention to the influence of archetypes and shadows." What relationships exist between Felton's identification of nursing's bias (Chapter 1) and the inner work linked with archetypes and shadows?

What resources, strategies, and tools for inner work presented by Pesut are most applicable to yourself—relationships with others—and promotion of healthy environments in nursing education and practice? To what extent is the need for integration, understanding of archetypes, and symbolic energetic systems accepted in your school and the profession of nursing?

What strategies might you develop to increase acceptance, understanding, and utilization of tools for inner work in your school and the profession? What relationships exist between Arrien's archetypes and those delineated by Gilligan? What cultural environment may be more receptive than another for implementing the resources, strategies, and tools indicated by Pesut? How do variables such as faculty experience and seniority in education and practice influence the need for inner work? Suggest specific strategies and tools most appropriate for faculty and practitioners, given various personal and personnel variables. How ready are you—is the profession—to use archetypal patterns for therapeutic work? What are the implications and consequences for nursing should the profession choose or not choose to focus on symbol, meaning, and inner work?

71

The Future of Nursing Education

Helping to Determine If Nursing Is to Be or Not to Be

Donna L. Boland, PhD, RN

The future is always hard to discern. However, I believe that four major factors will play a significant role in helping shape the future of nursing education. One of the confounding factors to nurse educators is the lack of theoretical clarity about the work of nursing. This lack has an impact on the knowledge transmitted in nursing programs, the structure in which nursing knowledge is taught, and the capabilities of graduates upon completion of their programs. A second factor influencing the future of nursing education is the current atmosphere surrounding institutions of higher education, including but not limited to public scrutiny and financial constraints. A third factor facing nursing education is the need for programs to be responsive to continually changing topography of the health care industry. A fourth factor important to nursing education is the changing operationalization of learning and the changing face of the learner. If nursing education is to have a vital future, then we as educators must better understand the impact that these factors will have on our future. If history is a good teacher, our past is a good place to start.

■ Looking to the Past to Inform the Present

On the way to the future, it is important to ask: Where did we begin? Although we have William Shakespeare (1604/1998) to thank for the "to be or not to be" philosophy, it seems appropriate to use this similitude as we speculate on nursing education's role in shaping the preferred future of the profession as we move into the 21st century. Before we contemplate how to configure our preferred future, it is important to ask one critical question: "Do we have a future?" Do not assume that this is a rhetorical question. Our reflection must be taken seriously, as nursing exists within the context of a health care delivery system that is continually and rapidly being reconfigured. These ongoing reconfigurations have resulted in new categories of health care providers, repackaging of traditional health care providers, and substantially changed roles for others.

The future of nursing within such a volatile environment is best preserved if the discipline is able to clearly articulate nursing's unique contributions to health and the delivery of health care services. If nursing education is to remain viable we must determine how we will structure the academic setting and learning experiences that will prepare graduates with knowledge and skills to meet the needs of a health-conscious society in an out-of-control health care system. It is the prime responsibility of today's nurses to shape the future for tomorrow's nurses. A prime imperative for nurses and nurse educators is the clarification of the nature and work of nursing if nursing is to take its rightful place in the health care arena.

We are bombarded by pundits within and outside the discipline who are eager to share their visions of the future of nursing. Reflection on our past and on what Florence Nightingale wrote is appropriate. She is quoted as saying, "no system can endure that does not march" and asks us to determine if we are "walking to the future or the past. We [need to] remember that we have scarcely crossed the threshold of uncivilized civilization in nursing [we therefore can not afford to] stereotype

mediocrity" (Nightingale, 1839/1992, p. 11). Nightingale believed that nurses were to be independent practitioners who were intelligent, observant, and alert to changes in people and their environment.

Nightingale's thoughts are as powerful and provocative today as they were more than 100 years ago. We cannot afford to define our future as simply a remodeling of our past. We cannot be content to achieve and fight to retain mediocrity in our practice or educational settings. Nor can we be secure in believing that the profession of nursing has reached the level of maturity and sophistication necessary to move from an uncivilized to a civilized status. As a profession, nursing still struggles with development of a defined body of science and a common culture. We are faced with a number of difficult challenges if we are to move the profession to a new plateau of enlightenment.

Challenge for Theoretical Clarity

An immediate challenge is to determine the degree to which we, as nurse educators, can define the context of the discipline and prepare nurses for the journey toward greater clarity. Margaret Newman wrote in her reflections on Nightingale's *Notes on Nursing* (1839/1992) that Nightingale's vision "equated the knowledge of nursing with the knowledge of health" (p. 45). It is this proposition that continues to be central in most recognized nursing theories. Nightingale explicated that the work of nursing needed to focus on the principle of health and that the education of nurses needed to emphasize the ways of maintaining health (Nightingale, 1839/1992). For Nightingale, the work of nursing was different from the work of medicine. Although medical science and the biomedical model are critical to the work and learning of nurses, it is not quintessential to the science of health. In this aspect, Nightingale was clear that disease, illness, and health were different phenomena. An understanding of health and factors that contribute to the well-being of people and their communities must be the theoretical foundation providing the basis for "a body of knowledge specific to nursing—if nurses are to provide services consistent with a spacebound society [that] foretells the needs for a new reality and new ways of looking at people and their world" (Rogers, 1992, p. 60).

We in nursing have developed knowledge related to human nature and human responses to environmental stimuli, and the services that we have provided have at least partially focused on health. Educational programs talk about promoting, preserving, and restoring the health of individuals, families, and communities. The discipline of nursing also ascribes to caring as a social mandate, and we mentor students in this direction. What the profession of nursing has yet to do is raise society's consciousness of the intellectual demand attached to the work of caring, as it relates to the concept of health on individual and global levels. Additionally, nurses have yet to articulate plainly the outcomes of the work of caring, leaving many of the activities nurses do as invisible, undervalued, and nonreimbursable. With the exception of a few nursing entrepreneurs who have found creative ways to make nursing more visible and the work of nursing more valued, we do not appear to have made progress in promoting our unique abilities.

Concept of Health in Nursing Education

The education process is critical to the articulation of nursing as it is the educational process that is the means by which nursing knowledge is transmitted (Rogers, 1992). Education plays a fundamental role in the discipline's ability to develop new knowledge, to facilitate the organization and reorganization of this body of knowledge, and generate creative and innovative ways of making use of current knowledge to meet the needs of an ever-changing reality.

In discussing their view of modern nursing education, Bevis and Watson (1989) argued that "nursing curricula must be based in the lived human experience with nursing knowledge focused on phenomena associated with changing human conditions and life process" (p. 38). Dialogue, inquiry, and meaningful interactions are crucial to being able to understand the lived experience (Bevis & Murray, 1990) and use this knowledge in the promotion of health and well-being.

If we are to continue along the path forged by Florence Nightingale and shaped by such nursing leaders as Martha Rogers and Margaret Newman, we should be about development and use of knowledge to promote health in our practice and educational settings. However, it is not at all clear that there is universal buy-in to this premise. The 1995 American Nurses Association (ANA) Social Policy Statement, cited in Morgan and Marsh (1988) states that

> nursing involves practices that are restorative, supportive, and promotive in nature. . . . Promotive practices mobilize healthy patterns of living, foster personal and family development, and support self-defined goals of individuals, families, and communities. (p. 379)

The ANA statement is consistent with our working thesis, and many nursing programs in the United States have incorporated some or all of this statement into their missions, philosophies, and goals.

Concepts of health promotion, health restoration, and health maintenance are integrated into most nursing curricula. Nursing faculty generally define the practice population within the parameters of the individual, the family constellation, and the communities in which individuals and families live. It would be fair, therefore, to say that nurse educators build nursing curricula around the concept of health and teach the work of nursing from the perspectives of health promotion, health maintenance, and illness prevention. Even though the foundations for most curricula are constructed on the idea of health, it is the idea of pathological disease etiologies that have been taught in the classroom and experienced in most clinical practice settings.

The knowledge of nursing needs not only to reflect health from the aspects of the biomedical model (illness experiences that have a pathological basis) but, more important, from a humanistic model (illness experiences that may not have a pathological basis but are real for the individual). Lyon (1990) argued that nursing's unique health-related contribution to society is diagnosis and treatment of nondiseased-based etiologies of illness, defined as symptoms and functional problems. This is certainly not a direction that nursing education or practice has collectively embraced. The lack of clarity in what nursing is and what nurses should be about will become increasingly problematic in a health care system that rewards specific outcomes. It will also be problematic in an educational system that expects and rewards explicit professional outcomes. Our ability to educate nurses for the demands of an evolving health care system depends on the thought that we give to the nature of nursing knowledge and work and society's demand for our unique services.

Nursing Education Confusion

The lack of clarity about the discipline's unique contributions to society and health care has set nursing education on a path fraught with twists, turns, and potholes. This less than perfect path is reflected in our current educational system wherein nurse educators have chosen to create multiple variations in approaching the education of nurses. We have built an educational system of confusion for those who want to pursue nursing and those who want to employ the graduates. To complicate this educational muddle further, the users of nurses have adopted a "nurse is a nurse" stereotype for all nurses. Luther Christman (1998) in his article on "Who Is a Nurse?" argues that nursing education continues to generate confusion as we keep on educating nurses at different levels of preparation. He argues that this confusion has led to negative stereotyping, as the poorest prepared of nurses are the highest in number and that it is the poorest prepared among us that are role modeling professional nursing for patients, health care team members, and the public.

I would argue that the blending of nurse graduates into a uniform entity has devalued nursing knowledge and the educational experience. By creating the "generic nurse," the practice of nursing has regressed to a narrow set of performance expectations for all who are entering professional nursing. I believe that current educational practices lend themselves to professional mediocrity and the marginalization of the future of nursing practice. By breeding an atmosphere of mediocrity in nursing through conformity, nurses will find it difficult to meet future demands of the health care system that requires flexibility and diversity.

One known requirement of future nurses will be that of a knowledge worker. Such a worker is one who can manipulate and distill large, dynamic data sets and use them to effect positive care outcomes for diverse groups of people. To be an effective knowledge worker of the future, students will need skills quite different from those taught in today's nursing skills laboratories.

Lack of Differentiation in Nursing Practice

Nursing practice has made little attempt to differentiate the use of nurses in practice, and nurse educators have supported this lack of differentiation in the education of nurses. As nurse educators developed and defended different educational paths leading to the same outcomes, uniqueness of the learner and the learning process was diluted. I believe that this type of conformity supports mediocrity. Mediocrity does not mean that all nurses are educated by a uniform assembly system, nor does it mean that they function in the same practice capacity, nor does it ignore the increasing complexity of skills that nurses are called on to demonstrate. What mediocrity does mean is that, by not cultivating the differences in educational preparation of nursing graduates for the last 50 years, we have compromised our ability to break out of our stereotypic history and walk toward a future that embraces differences and encourages creativity and ingenuity.

In an attempt to homogenize the educational experience for entering nurses, we have been all too anxious to quiet or dismiss the few voices that have questioned the need for role delineation and functional differentiation. Many other health care disciplines have chosen educational and practice models that support role and function differentiation.

Without differentiation between and among undergraduate programs, students in all programs are expected to demonstrate increasing amounts and degrees of cognitive and psychomotor skills to keep pace with health care changes and expectations. Without differentiation, faculty and student frustration and stress levels are growing at a concomitant rate with the changing expectations from our practice partners. Faculty are faced with adding more and more to an already packed curricula.

Curriculum development and revision are being affected by the trickle-down phenomenon. For example, 2-year programs are adding concepts such as leadership, management, community, and families, and 4-year programs are emphasizing skills related to case management, policy setting, political activism,

and global visioning. Master's degree programs are trying to determine the meaning of "advanced practice," which in some cases has come to encompass medical diagnosis and medical therapeutics that were once reserved for physicians. Doctoral programs face the challenge of cementing the links among theory, practice, and research for students who come to their educational experience with different philosophies of nursing and nursing practice.

The reinventing of nursing programs by cannibalizing from other programs or disciplines brings little clarity to the discussion of what nursing knowledge is or when and how that nursing knowledge should be transmitted through the educational process. If nurses in the 21st century are to step forward and assume legitimate and viable leadership roles in a rapidly changing health care system, there can be no confusion about what they can bring to the table. We have to question whether an overburdened and often confused educational system can prepare nurses with a level of clarity to articulate nursing's contribution in a health care system of shifting values and desires.

■ Nursing Education Climate

The atmosphere of today's higher education climate has been under critical scrutiny, and this action has shaken both students' and faculties' respect for the educational process. This level of examination has specifically affected professional programs as public calls for change have focused on program accountability that is being driven by a market mentality. Institutions of higher education are being asked to adopt more of a customer orientation and are working to make the educational environment more user-friendly. Part of our commitment to becoming more user-friendly is to increase our reliance on costly technology and distributive learning methods that enhance accessibility and increase scheduling flexibility. However, the expense of technology is straining the shrinking fiscal resources of most institutions.

Another challenge is the growing chasm between the value of liberal education and professional education. As nursing education is housed in institutions of higher education, nurse educators will be involved in seeking ways to promote the value of liberal education on a career focused college bound population.

Push-Me-Pull-Me Phenomena

If we are to remain a viable profession full of potential, then we need to address what I call the push-me-pull-me phenomena within the education and health care systems. Current forces within and around the health care system are pushing and pulling nurses and nursing practice in directions we may not desire to go. Forces within and external to the educational system are also nudging nurse educators in directions that may not best suit their goals. As nurses we will need to take charge of our destiny, or we will increasingly feel the pushing and pulling from numerous stakeholders interested in the practice and education of future nurses.

Outcome Orientation

One major phenomenon facing today's nurse educators deals with the what, when, where, and how of learning (Mohr & Naylor, 1998; Skiba, 1997). We in education are being required to demonstrate our effectiveness in facilitating student learning. This outcome orientation is requiring faculty and administrators to underscore competencies in the preparation of new nurses who will be stepping into a dynamic health care system. Coupled with this outcome orientation is the need to identify efficient, effective ways of assessing student competence. This outcome focus emphasizes the ability "to do" rather than the ability "to think about doing" and is requiring nurse faculty to make a paradigm shift in their thinking about learning.

Our curricula have historically emphasized the process of teaching, assuming that teaching has a direct bearing on learning (i.e., the more effective you are as a teacher, the more students learn). Learning has been assessed primarily at the end of discrete courses, not at the completion of a program of study against specific outcomes. Although we taught students that the whole (in this case the curriculum) is greater than the sum of its parts (individual courses), we built curricula on the concept that the parts would equal the whole if we thoughtfully identified and linked all the parts. This philosophy carried into the learning environment where the learning focus was on the process of teaching that emphasized content and related skills.

Refocusing the learning lens on outcomes does not negate the importance of content and skills to the learning of nursing practice. However, it does allow faculty to structure content and skills under a professional performance umbrella, whereby competence is viewed as a dynamic entity anchored by the ability to perform (Curry & Wergin, 1997). New graduates are expected to possess (a) critical thinking and problem-solving skills, (b) quantitative reasoning skills, (c) communication skills, (d) information retrieval and management skills, (e) collaborative work skills, (f) delegation and supervisory skills, (g) management of resources skills, and (h) measurement and evaluation skills, among others. They must also be able to use research to inform practice, assume accountability and responsibility for practice of self and others, and collaborate in negotiating a complex and dynamic system (American Association of Colleges of Nursing [AACN], 1998; Skiba, 1997).

Preparation for Lifelong Learning Skills

Another push-me-pull-me phenomenon splitting educators is the need to prepare nurses for the next century with problem-solving skills that they can immediately apply in various care situations and practice settings while ensuring that these same nurses develop skills to be effective lifelong learners. The stress of addressing both the immediacy and long-term aspects of learning is further complicated by the reality that knowledge is growing much faster than students' ability to master it in any particular course or curriculum (Twigg, 1994). Given the fact that today's learners are struggling to keep up with yesterday's knowledge, it seems reasonable to assume that tomorrow's students need to focus on how to learn more than on what is important to learn.

Facilitating the student development of "lifelong" learning skills requires more than soaking up and regurgitating unprocessed information, but facilitating the learning process is challenging. Many of today's students come to institutions of higher education with different values about learning, with competing priorities, with passive acceptance of formalized classroom learning, and in some cases, with less than adequate academic skills. Additionally, many universities and colleges are experiencing large influxes of "new majority" students. The new majority student tends to be older, having taken time off between high school and college or changed career goals after preparing for one or more jobs. These students need to balance job with school, family responsibilities with studying, and aesthetic learning with practical job skills. A comprehensive review by Richardson and King (1998) concluded that these new majority students are capable of being as successful as their younger counterparts but that they have been struggling with a negative stereotype of themselves as less capable. Nurse educators are experienc-

ing challenges and opportunities posed by this new majority student. As the number of these students has increased, so has the average age of nursing students during the past decade (Division of Nursing, 1996).

Technology in Higher Education

Today's students, however, are coming to the learning environment having more comfort with technology than many educators. Technology has had a tremendous effect on higher education, as it has not only reformed the ways in which we can store, retrieve, analyze, and use information, but it has also triggered the creation of a whole new field of informatics that has become an evolving area of advanced study in nursing. There is no question that new and emerging technologies will continue to transform institutions of higher education in the years ahead (Dolence & Norris, 1995; Hall, 1995; Skiba, 1997). Privateer (1999) suggests that

> nothing has the power to shape the future of higher education as much as current strategies for deploying academic technologies, strategies that should begin to explore the real revolutionary nature of technology instead of restricting its role to simply automating the delivery instruction. (p. 68)

Currently, technology is being widely used to increase student access, giving students more flexibility in determining when to learn, what to learn and how to approach learning, and to engage students more fully in the learning process. Although students miss the personal connection between students and faculty that the classroom affords, students are satisfied with the learning experience and increased ease of learning from home or work (Billings et al., 1994). However, our understanding of how and when to use technology to maximize learning effectiveness is still quite limited.

Nursing Programs in the Changing Health Care Scene

Traditionally the nursing discipline has accepted the idea that undergraduate educational programs prepared generalists for entry into practice, whereas graduate programs focused on specialist preparation. Nurse educators are being asked to prepare entry-level nurses with knowledge and skills to care for a diverse population of people in a multiplicity of care settings, ranging from rural to global communities, from home to trauma settings, and from day care to hospice. New graduates are also expected to step into any one of a number of different settings and function safely, efficiently, and effectively despite a relatively lower level of educational preparation.

The current task of preparing students to function effectively within such diversity is stressing faculty, students, clinical practice settings, and patients. It is difficult to image the level of stress for students and faculty in the future as the level of patient acuity increases and health care interventions become increasingly complex. A few nursing programs have narrowed or built concentrated practice focuses into their undergraduate curricula, believing that students might be better prepared if they were able to be more focused in their scope of learning.

We need to rethink current curricular structures in light of the knowledge explosion in health care, as well as shifting demands for new graduates to bring to the workplace different and more exquisitely honed skills. In rethinking curricula, we need to consider the diverse talents of incoming students, determine the needs of a rapidly declining workforce, and resources available to prepare students.

The majority of nursing graduates enter the workforce wanting to practice with a specified population of individuals with specific needs in well-defined areas of practice. Many students new to nursing have already made up their minds about specialty practice and become frustrated when they cannot pursue these specialty areas at the start of their educational experience. All but gone are the general medical–surgical units where the majority of new graduates learned about the nuts and bolts of nursing practice. It might indeed be time to rethink what we mean by preparing a generalist for nursing practice when so little of the traditions of general practice are intact in today's health care system and may vanish from tomorrow's system.

■ Looking to the Future

Given our history and the current status of nursing, what does the future hold? I am greatly concerned about the viability of this profession. If the 20th century exemplified human creativity, then the 21st century promises to far exceed current attempts at visioning. Will the discipline of nursing be able to change to keep pace? What remains to be seen is whether our collective abilities will be adequate to respond to unforeseen challenges. The collective of nursing has not been able to coalesce for the good of the profession and the discipline to date. So far, there has been nothing in our past or present that has been strong enough to entice us to do so.

Changing Structure and Demographics

Given today's state of higher education, the future of nursing education will be determined by faculties' abilities to design austere educational programs that are effective in educating graduates with evolving skills for a dynamic work setting. Future success will require faculty and administrators in institutions of higher education to remain attentive to the changing demographics of the learner population, including how they learn, why they learn, what they need and are willing to learn, and where they choose to learn. Educators will need to be increasingly mindful of the context of learning, as lifelong learning skills are emphasized for the well-prepared nurse. Nurses will need to understand fully how advances in health care are being driven by technological innovation and how to use technology to our advantage. As a means to this end, nurses must become savvy in the areas of product development and assessment as ways of making important contributions to advances in technology and health care.

The traditional classroom will exist without walls—literally and figuratively. Learning will transcend all human-made boundaries with global asynchronous and synchronous technological communication tools. Within these highly interactive learning environments, faculty will be responsible for collaborating with students, to shape the context of the learning environment and facilitate learners in thinking and working with information to which they have been exposed. Faculty and students will jointly determine learning outcomes, and the learners will have the primary responsibility in directing their learning. The pace of learning will be individualized and based on learners' prior knowledge base and abilities. Individualization of the learning process will require faculty to create different pedagogical approaches to reflect the increasing diversity of the student learner population. Putting the responsibility for learning directly in the hands of the learner may address some of the current frustrations and tensions that faculties feel in trying to motivate and actively engage students in the learning process.

Virtual Classrooms and Patients

The virtual classroom and the virtual patient or client will be necessary teaching tools because the level of patient or client acu-ity and complexity of health care will continue to increase. Although students will need to function in many of these settings upon graduation, these settings do not foster experimental learning nor do they allow faculty much opportunity for mentoring. Learning best occurs in an environment where students can experiment, make mistakes, take risks, and be creative problem solvers. A high-stress environment provides little opportunity for this type of learning. However, a simulated environment with "real-time" information being exchanged between actual health care settings and virtual classrooms will allow students to access information related to current health status of simulated patients.

Students can then use this information to identify potential changes in health status, develop action plans, implement action plans, and assess outcomes of actions without placing themselves, those in their care, or faculty at risk. Students will be able to go back and examine errors in judgment or action and learn by having time to evaluate the appropriateness of their decision-making. Faculty will have the opportunity to facilitate learning by directing students' search and management of critical knowledge. Assessment of learning can occur quickly, and students can "rewind" the learning situation at any point and start over to reinforce their learning.

Problem-Based Learning

Student assessment will continue to be critical to the learning process. Assessment and evaluation will be built into all learning experiences, but students will step forward and take major responsibility for assessing their learning and those of their peers. Critique is a wonderful learning tool that has primarily been reserved for teaching. Outcomes are about evaluation, and student critique fosters responsibility in the learning process. A current learning approach being used in a number of health-related schools is problem-based learning. This approach encourages students to reflect on their actions and those of their peers (Curry & Wergin, 1997). Simulating actual care problems is costly, as technology is the main vehicle for creating these contrived learning situations. As technology costs grow, university and colleges will have to collaborate in building assessment centers that serve a large population of students from various disciplines. Collaboration will reduce costs, decrease duplication, and promote equability for students selecting campuses and programs that are not able to afford such elaborate high-tech learning environments.

Hall (1995) talked about the university as "a convergence of limitless exchange and interconnection" where knowledge is discovered and shared over these vast interconnections and where students will "engage with information and learn how to use it" (p. 3). Students of the future will have many choices to make about where to learn, how to learn, when to learn, and from whom to learn. This freedom will precipitate a real revolution in institutions of higher education (Hall, 1995).

Changing Face of the Learner

Today, we are facing a student population with different demographics and values than students of yesteryear. They are also coming to the learning environment with different ways of thinking about learning, and this trend is not expected to change in the future. This time is difficult for many educators who are not emotionally prepared to deal with such diversity and deviance from the traditional norms they were taught. There does not seem to be reverence for traditions of universities and colleges in the minds or attitudes of today's college-bound students. Students will continue to come focused on career specialization, not the

love of liberal learning (Boyer, 1987). This dichotomy is not a bad one, however, as it has forced residents of the academy into rich discussions about how to combine a professional orientation with a liberal arts focus. But higher education needs to continue to undergo a renaissance that will lead to new ways of stimulating the consciousness of learners and of providing them with values and skills to shape and reform their professional practice (Curry & Wergin, 1997).

Changing Scholarship

The push for institutions of higher education to focus on continuous quality improvement has generated new scholarship on what teaching excellence should be and how it should look now and into the future. According to Hutchings (1998), teaching excellence is being pursued by those who

> set out to inquire into their own practice, identifying key issues they want to pursue, posing questions for themselves and the field, exploring alternatives and taking risks, and doing all of this in the company of like-minded scholars who can offer critique and support. (p. 3)

Scholarship should be and is being revisited (Boyer, 1987). These activities have led to reinvestment in and refocus on the tripartite role, especially as it relates to promotion and tenure criteria, workloads, and systems of rewards. Research will continue to be valued, but funding will become increasingly competitive. Collaborative efforts will gain increasing attention, as problems being studied today across disciplines and currently defined areas of expertise.

Nursing scholarship needs to focus on two main areas in this century: (a) the scholarship of teaching and (b) the scholarship of informing practice. The scholarship of teaching needs to focus on student learning, assessment of student learning, and development of new teaching tools that expedite knowledge transmittal. The scholarship of practice needs to focus clearly on those phenomena of greatest concern to the work of nursing, with the belief that the work of nursing is to promote the health and well-being of the public with or without the presence of disease.

Levels of Nursing Practice and Education Preparation

For nursing to survive and prosper in the coming millennium, nursing must formally sanction different levels of nursing practice. Levels of practice should be defined around (a) the scope of practice for each level, (b) the functions that can be carried out by those at each level, and (c) the educational preparation necessary to prepare nurses to assume the roles ascribed to each level of practice. Professional nurses have been struggling with the idea of two levels of nursing practice for more than a quarter century, with no resolution, in part because we may not be asking the right questions to help us move forward. Our current system isn't preparing enough (and I would argue the right kinds of) nurses to meet the various demands of a health care system moving from the industrial age to the quantum age (Porter-O'Grady, 1999). Yet, the window for reform is small, considering the rapid and sweeping changes that we are experiencing and will continue to experience in the health care industry and in higher education. The decision to differentiate practice and education is critical, as our current multitier educational system leading to a single purpose practice outcome cannot advance either the practice of nursing or its accompanying knowledge requisites into the 21st century.

A recent editorial discussed the work of a Canadian nurse-futurist who researched how people learn about the future (Pesut, 1998).

Her findings suggest that we come to the future with (a) certain beliefs and values, (b) different perceptions of what the future will be, and (c) different feeling responses about those perceptions. To discuss the future of nursing takes courage, creativity, and insight for those committed to placing nursing in the best position for survival. I also believe that we need to continue to define what nursing is and what it is not (Nightingale, 1839/1992). In the words of Eleanor Roosevelt, "we face the future fortified only with lessons we have learned from the past. It is today that we must create the world of the future." (as cited in Bevis & Watson, 1989, p. 7). In a very real sense, tomorrow is now.

■ Concluding Statement

Although there is reason for concern about the future of nursing and nursing education, the discipline has the potential for being well positioned to meet the challenges of this millennium. It is up to us to decide whether this potential can be realized. Karen Kaiser Clark (1993) seemed to sum up life in general and nursing life in particular with the following thoughts.

> My Friend, within every relationship, in every experience, there are lessons to be learned, gifts that are given and seeds that are sown as results of our choices. Eventually stormy seasons challenge all of us and in time life asks each of us this question: WHAT DO YOU CHOOSE TO LEARN AND BELIEVE ESPECIALLY WHEN SEASONS ARE NOT OF YOUR CHOOSING? LIFE IS CHANGE—GROWTH IS OPTIONAL—WILL YOU CHOOSE TO GROW? (p. 241)

Nursing will certainly continue to exist and to experience change but it is our choice to make—as to whether we grow as a discipline and practice as we move to the future.

■ *References*

American Association of Colleges of Nursing. (1998). *The essentials of baccalaureate education for professional nursing practice.* Washington, DC: Author.

Bevis, E. O., & Murray, J. (1990). The essence of the curriculum revolution: Emancipatory teaching. *Journal of Nursing Education, 29*(7), 326–331.

Bevis, E. O., & Watson, J. (1989). *Toward a caring curriculum: A new pedagogy for nursing.* New York: National League for Nursing Press.

Billings, D., Durham, J. D., Finke, L., Boland, D., Manz, B., & Smith, S. (1994). Collaboration in distance education between nursing schools and hospitals. *Holistic Nursing Practice, 8*(3), 64–70.

Boyer, E. L. (1987). *College: The undergraduate experience in America.* New York: HarperCollins.

Christman, L. (1998). Who is a nurse? *IMAGE: Journal of Nursing Scholarship, 30*(3), 211–214.

Clark, K. K. (1993). *Life is change, growth is optional.* St. Paul, MN: Center for Executive Planning.

Curry, L., & Wergin, J. F. (1997). Professional education. In J. G. Gaff & J. L. Ratcliff (Eds.), *Handbook of the undergraduate curriculum* (pp. 341–358). San Francisco: Jossey-Bass.

Division of Nursing, Health Resources And Services Administration—Bureau of Health Professions. (1996). *National sample survey of registered nurses.* Washington, DC: Author.

Dolence, M., & Norris, D. (1995). *Transforming higher education: A vision for learning in the 21st century.* Ann Arbor, MI: Society for College and University Planning.

Hall, J. (1995). The revolution in electronic technology and the modern university: The convergence of means. *Educom Review 30*(4), 42–45.

Hutchings, P. (1998). Pursuing improvement. *About Campus,* July–August, 2–3.

Lyon, B. (1990). Getting back on track: Nursing's autonomous scope of practice. N. L. Chaska (Ed.), *The nursing profession: Turning points* (pp. 267–274). St. Louis: Mosby.

Mohr, W. K., & Naylor, M. D. (1998). Creating a curriculum for the 21st century. *Nursing Outlook, 46*(5), 206–212.

Morgan, I., & Marsh, G. (1998). Historic and future health promotion contexts for nursing. *IMAGE: Journal of Nursing Scholarship, 30*(4), 379–383.

Newman, M. (1992). Nightingale's vision of nursing theory and health. In D. P. Carroll (Ed.), *Notes on nursing: What it is, and what it is not* (pp. 44–47). Philadelphia: Lippincott. (Original work published 1839)

Nightingale, F. (1992). *Notes on nursing: What it is, and what it is not.* Philadelphia: Lippincott. (Original work published 1839)

Pesut, D. (1998). Matters of the mind, heart, and soul. *Nursing Outlook, 46*(4), 154.

Porter-O'Grady, P. (1999). Sustainable partnerships: The journey toward health care integration. In E. Cohen & V. DeBack (Eds.), *The outcomes mandate: Case management in health care today* (pp. 2–11). St. Louis: Mosby.

Privateer, P. M. (1999). Academic technology and the future of higher education: Strategic paths taken and not taken. *Journal of Higher Education, 70*(1), 60–79.

Richardson, J. T., & King, E. (1998). Adult students in higher education: Burden or boon? *Journal of Higher Education, 69*(1), 65–88.

Rogers, M. E. (1992) Nightingale's notes on nursing: Prelude to the 21st century. In D. P. Carroll (Ed.), *Notes on nursing: What it is, and what it is not* (pp. 58–62). Philadelphia: Lippincott. (Original work published 1839)

Shakespeare, W. (1998). In S. Barnet (Ed.), *The tragedy of Hamlet, prince of Denmark/William Shakespeare* (2nd rev. ed.) New York: Penguin. (Original work published 1604)

Skiba, D. (1997). Transforming nursing education to celebrate learning. *Nursing and Health Care Perspectives, 18*(3), 124–129.

Twigg, C. (1994). The need for a national learning infrastructure. *Educom Review, 29*(5), 7–12.

■ *Editor's Questions for Discussion*

To what extent do Felton (Chapter 1) and Boland agree regarding the essence of nursing? What crisis exists today for the future of the profession? What is the essential character of the nursing profession?

What implications does Donnelly's work (Chapter 28) have for Boland's statements concerning the need for and lack of theoretical clarity in nursing? How may a science of health contribute to a theoretical foundation for nursing? To what extent have nurse theorists been effective in utilizing a science of health to develop nursing knowledge? What has been the impact of the lack of theoretical clarity on nursing education and nursing practice?

How do current nursing educational practices encourage mediocrity in practice? What change(s) is (are) essential in education programs to prepare effective practitioners? What forces exist within nursing that deter such changes? How might constraints be diminished or altered to permit positive change? Why have role delineation and functional differentiation not occurred in education programs for practice? How likely is differentiation in nursing practice to occur? Who should determine the role and functions of nursing in practice? What forces exist in and around the health care system, as suggested by Boland, that are pushing nurses and practice in directions the profession may not want to go?

What factors contribute to limited and shrinking resources for nursing education programs? How might these constraints be addressed? What implications does A. Fisher and Habermann's discussion (Chapter 21) have for faculty resources? Discuss the impact of Boyer's model for scholarships in nursing education programs. Propose strategies for acceptance of this model in higher education and criteria for evaluation of faculty. What implications do the writings by Billings (Chapter 15) and Yeaworth et al. (Chapter 14) have for the technology needs discussed by Boland. What are the implications of Gaines' presentation (Chapter 12) for Boland's discussion regarding curricula for the future? How might all the needed changes recommended by Boland for nursing education programs be planned, coordinated, and implemented—and by whom?

What needs do nursing students have for the future that previously have not been addressed? How must the discipline of nursing change to meet future needs? Discuss the assumption that nursing education programs appear to go through cycles, such as emphasis on structure, process, or outcomes? Historically, how valid is that assumption? To what extent do nursing programs focus on all three aspects of nursing education simultaneously? Of the three elements, which is most critical? In nursing practice? Why? What is the likelihood that stability will occur in education regarding the elements (structure, process, and outcome) emphasized? What contributes to the demand for and supply of nurses in practice? What new influences affect the availability of professional nurses that previously have not existed? Recall the explication by C. Jones (Chapter 11).

72

From Fragmentation to Integration in the Discipline of Nursing

Situation-Specific Theories

Afaf I. Meleis, PhD,
Dr. PS (Hon.), RN, FAAN
Eun-Ok Im, PhD, MPH, CNS, RN

In the history of the discipline of nursing, fragmentation has manifested itself in many forms. Nursing scholars have tried to bring coherence and integrate nursing knowledge for further progress in the discipline, utilizing several different strategies. To continue integration of knowledge, several paradoxes must be addressed: (a) philosophical debates and substantive dialogues; (b) clinical stories and theories; (c) nursing phenomena and patient phenomena; (d) outcomes and process; (e) methods and substance; and (f) current and ideal phenomena. To transcend the enigma and integrate nursing knowledge, we suggest situation-specific theories for future general theory development and present two examples of the situation-specific theories.

■ Theoretical Progress

It is impossible to discuss knowledge development in any discipline without addressing its theoretical progress. In the nursing discipline, two patterns of responses to theoretical progress exist that may greatly constrain the rate of progress desired in developing and utilizing knowledge. One pattern of response is the growing skepticism about the significance and primacy of having a coherent framework for research and practice (Gortner, 1993). The second pattern is the lack of serious effort in integrating research findings into coherent theoretical proposals, models, or frameworks in ways that are cumulative and purposeful in driving continuity in research and theory building (Kirkevold, 1997). As a result of these patterns, opportunities to further develop these coherent and integrated thoughts become more limited (Schultz & Meleis, 1988).

Not having well-articulated, coherent, and integrated frameworks in the discipline of nursing constrains the quality of nursing care provided. In computer programs, default frameworks are automatically activated as commands unless they are overridden. In the discipline of nursing, the default framework has been the biomedical model, and unless we are sensitized and become conscious of our default program, nurses will continue to use it uncritically (Koch & Webb, 1996). Another, more contemporary, default framework is the economic model. Assumptions inherent in each of these two models tend to be somewhat incongruent with values and premises that we as nurses have consciously and deliberately constructed to guide our practices, such as holism, contextuality, health, and quality of interactions, among others.

We know that goals driven by different frameworks differ drastically and often conflict (Allan & Hall, 1988). As we pause to define assumptions inherent in each framework, including those in what have become our default frameworks, we may be surprised to find that we have selected frameworks for our study questions, care actions, and methods of interpretation of data that reflect goals and assumptions different from what we believe. We may discover that, instead of making contributions to the development of nursing knowledge that reflects our mission and assumptions, we may be adding to the existing fragmentation in nursing knowledge development.

Diversity

Furthermore, with increasing diversities in populations and with rising complexities in health care systems, variant perspectives and multiple methodologies are used prevalently in nursing knowledge and its theoretical foundations (Kim, 1993; Meleis, 1987). This diversity has been an asset to progress in the discipline of nursing, but it may also have resulted in increasing fragmentation in nursing knowledge, which is manifested in many forms (Meleis, 1998). For example, practice is still organized around developmental theories (pediatric nursing and geriatric nursing), biomedical models (medical and surgical units), system theories (outpatient and community health nursing), and organization theory (team nursing and task-oriented nursing). Recently, we have added to this collection of frameworks by organizing nursing around nursing theories and central concepts in nursing, including self-care, transition, family health, and symptom management. Structural divisions tend to drive the questions asked and the answers obtained. Answers tend to inform the frameworks that drive the questions and support existing fragmentation.

Fragmentation

There are other manifestations of fragmentation in nursing. Our research enterprise is driven by questions that reflect psychological, physiological, social, educational, and organizational theories (Meleis, 1997). Now, information and genetic theories are being incorporated in our discipline (Graveley & Murphy, 1995; Hays, Norris, Martin, & Androwich, 1994; Henry, 1995). Each of these theories reflects other disciplines and only one component of a human being. Additionally, much has been written and discussed about the separation between practice and theory and between clinicians and theorists (Fealy, 1997; Maeve, 1994; Reed, 1996). Similar discussions have addressed differences between theorists and researchers (Johnson, 1983). Each group accused the other of lacking in understanding of what others do. Theorists wondered why clinicians were not using their theories in practice. In contrast, clinicians could not understand the derivation of those theories because most of them did not reflect the clinicians' practice nor speak the language of their practice (Timpson, 1996). This fragmentation makes it difficult to determine our progress in knowledge development and to translate it to policy proposals.

Integrated Frameworks

Determining the status of knowledge development is a tricky matter. It certainly is not through review of single research findings, analysis of the credibility of a single research project, nor review of training programs. Each of these is important, but none of them alone gives a comprehensive framework of progress. We can analyze progress through a critical look at theoretical threads, themes, and frameworks that evolved to guide the practice of nursing (Meleis, 1997). Progress is depicted through existence of consistent patterns of findings that are connected and related. Progress is evidenced through programs of research that reflect an integrative conceptualization and include wisdom and understanding that go beyond research. We have been in search of ways to drive and analyze patterns of progress coherently.

We claim nursing to be a human science, we claim our mission to be an increasing sense of well-being in our patients, and we claim our patients as thinking, feeling, and perceiving human beings (Meleis, 1997). We claim that we have the right and capability to participate in and make decisions related to health and care of patients (Condon, 1992). We claim that we have more dialogues and interactional relationships with our patients than other health care professionals (Morse, Solber, Neander, Botroff, & Johnson, 1990). Does our progress in knowledge development reflect those claims? Coherent integrated frameworks

may help us answer such a question and may remind us to put evidence and outcomes within a context of process, relationships, and history. In this chapter, we discuss the paradoxes that may have contributed or resulted from this fragmentation and their influences on theoretical development of the discipline of nursing. Then, we propose future directions for theory development.

■ The Paradoxes

Continuing to develop an integrated and coherent knowledge base that will help direct nursing care is predicated on ways by which we will come to grip with several paradoxes. We will either continue to debate them, accept them as paradoxes, move forward to consciously resolve them, follow one side of the equation without totally resolving differences, or select to embrace paradoxes as a reflection of human sciences.

Philosophical Debates and Substantive Dialogues

One school of thought advocates that philosophical diversity be resolved before continuing with the business of developing knowledge that is coherent and integrated, knowledge that could influence health care and make a difference in patient care outcomes (Gortner, 1993; Moccia, 1988; Thompson, 1985). On the one hand, this school of thought has created many dialogues and debates focusing on processes in knowledge development. On the other hand, other dialogues in the literature are more substantive in nature, such as those that include strategies for managing symptoms (Bailey, 1995; Campbell, 1996; Harvey, 1996), definitions of health (Bruenjes, 1994; King, 1990), definitions of environments (Kleffel, 1991), predictors of quality care (Stone, Weissman, & Cleary, 1995), and patterns in care of clients during health–illness transitions (Ross, Rosenthal, & Dawson, 1997; Wilson, 1997). These dialogues have been instrumental in signaling a turning point in research and theory enterprises. Substantive debates focus on nursing phenomenon, processes of health and wellness, or outcomes of care. A question that must be continuously revisited is: Can we engage in substantive debates without philosophical debates? Substantive dialogues reflect nursing practice, nursing phenomenon, and nursing actions that may lead to maintaining and enhancing patients' well-being (Meleis, 1987, 1998). Philosophical debates not grounded in substance may tend to widen the gap between nursing practice and theoretical development of the discipline (Meleis, 1987). Progress is predicated on how thinkers in the discipline define the meaning of this paradox in relation to nursing knowledge and practice.

Clinical Stories and Theories

During the past decade, professional journals in the nursing discipline have contained numerous papers authored by nurse clinicians and nurse researchers describing the gaps that persist between research, theory, and clinical practice (Fawcett & Carino, 1989; Timpson, 1996). The nature of these gaps has been discussed and analyzed; clinicians were encouraged to consider utilization of evidence-based knowledge for practice and theoretical frameworks to guide their practice (Huth & Moore, 1998; Timpson, 1996). More recently, various middle-range theories were developed and used as theoretical frameworks for nursing practice and research (Good, 1998; Huth & Moore, 1998; Lenz, Pugh, Milligan, Gift, & Suppe, 1997). However, middle-range theories are still at a beginning stage in development; and the gaps between theory, research, and practice are still prevalent in nursing and continue to challenge clinicians.

Proponents of practice wisdom as the framework for practice argue that clinical practice and clinical wisdom, based on their expertise in practice, should become the bases for knowledge development (Benner & Wrubel, 1982; Fealy, 1997; Lauder, 1994; Maeve, 1994). Proponents of this approach to knowledge development believe that the basis for practice lies in collective "common-sense" understanding of practitioners who are engaged in clinical practice (Fealy, 1997). Questions related to this school of thought may include Could each clinician alone contribute to developing practice wisdom? Is practical wisdom based only on one nurse's experience, one nurse's story, one example of a phenomenon, one case, or one situation? Should collective wisdom in the form of integrative theories become the goal for practice-based knowledge? Practical wisdom that is based on experiences of one clinician is similar to research wisdom articulated and developed from one research encounter. Neither approach may provide sufficient rationale to provoke changes in policies. The power of wisdom generated from clinical practice may be in collective wisdom translated into coherent frameworks. Additionally, as Lauder (1994) asserted, the gap between theory and practice is perpetuated by separating thought and action. Linking thought with action and thinking with doing in articulated frameworks may fare better in grounding practice and driving a focused approach to knowledge development.

Nursing Phenomenon and Patient Phenomenon

Efforts in defining nursing and describing nursing phenomena resulted in the development of grand theories to answer questions about the nature, mission, and goals of nursing (Meleis, 1997). Rather than focusing on the patient care phenomenon, many efforts were diverted to exploring, describing, explaining, and understanding phenomenon related to nurses as agents of caregiving. By that, we mean the phenomenon related to nurses who provide care, their caregiving abilities, clinical judgments, presence during the care episode, satisfaction in the process of nursing care, and their transformation while providing nursing care. By patient care phenomenon, we mean the phenomenon related to patients' responses to health and illness, their experiences with a particular diagnosis or disease, and their abilities to live with a problem. Should or could we measure progress by the extent to which nurses are able to provide care, by the phenomenon reflecting who nurses are and what their experiences and achievements are, or by the extent to which nurses are able to explain patients' responses, reactions, and experiences? As trends in nursing practice began to emphasize patient-centered nursing care (Bickler, 1994; Dunst & Trivette, 1996), we needed to give equal, if not more, attention to the patient phenomenon over the nursing phenomenon.

Outcomes and Process

Developing theoretical knowledge in nursing is undoubtedly affected by the current tension between those who advocate outcomes research and evidence-based practice and those who think of nursing in terms of care processes. Nursing involves processes of interaction, healing, knowing the body, and awareness (Meleis, 1997). The current language of outcomes is unclear, hazy, and imprecise; it emphasizes results only, mostly driven by models that may not reflect assumptions nor the mission of nursing. Consequently, such models may focus less on the quality of nursing care and the context, structure, and processes inherent in providing care (Hogston, 1995; Smith, Atherly, & Kane, 1997). In human sciences such as nursing, context, structure, and process are significant in capturing illness and caring experiences as end results and outcomes. For example, when a nurse is providing nursing care to a person who is dying, the outcome is clear—the death of the person. However, the most important aspect of nursing care for a dying person and the significant others involved is the quality of the dying experience for the person and others in their immediate circle. Rather than the outcome of death, it is the sense of well-being of all involved during the process of dying that better reflects a nursing perspective and questions of interest to nurses. The nature of knowledge that could be developed in nursing is influenced profoundly by whether we are inclusive of processes and outcomes or exclusive in the kinds of theoretical and empirical questions asked.

Methods and Substance

A paradox similar to that of the philosophical and substance debates exists in relationships between substance and method. Certain nursing scholars define themselves in nursing from a methodological perspective (Kirkevold, 1997). They argue for, about, and against a particular research design or method (Kim, 1993). Some nursing scholars may vehemently support their positions as empiricists, phenomenologists, or interpretive phenomenologists (Allen, 1985; Dilthey, 1988; Gortner, 1993; Marshall, 1988). For the less experienced, a method advocated by their scientific gurus becomes the goal, defines what knowledge to develop, and prescribes how to develop the knowledge. Methodological debates without substance do not help the development of coherence in nursing knowledge (Acton, Irvin, Jensen, Hopkins, & Miller, 1997; Meleis, 1987, 1998). Is it possible that philosophical and methodological debates, without grounding them in substantive debates, may derail progress in answering significant fundamental questions about patient care? How do we reconcile the need for methodological expertise with the more urgent goal of developing coherent understanding of a phenomenon that may require a variety of methods to uncover the multiplicity of its dimensions? These are questions that reflect different sides of the paradox.

Current and Ideal Phenomena

A subtle tension may exist between extant theory and "ought to be" theories (Barnum, 1994). Should theories represent existing situations and truth, or should they create situations and truths (Reed, 1996)? What if the current situation is not conducive to providing optimal patient care? What if current situations are driven by default models of biomedicine and economics, based on the belief that theories should be developed from observations and experiences that nurses have with patients and from research findings? A theory may both serve a heuristic function to stimulate and provide rationale for studies and practice (Lenz, 1998). Theories can lead the research process with a theoretical formulation of the ideal nursing phenomenon; they can guide nursing practice with ideal standards that reflect visions of what quality nursing care should be.

Much criticism has been leveled at theoretical formulations that depicted ideal rather than existing nursing situations. The question is: Could we afford not to allow creativity of those who may be experts at envisioning new realities? What processes of evaluation could be used to establish credibility of theories that reflect practice realities, as well as "ought to be" realities?

■ Future Directions for Theory Development: Situation-Specific Theories

Studies and dialogues focusing on each of the paradoxes just discussed could shape processes inherent in development of knowledge for the future. What could make discussions more productive is discovery of shared goals for advancing knowledge and a thorough understanding of the nature and potential consequences of each paradox. Theories in a discipline reflect its level of sophistication, and progress in theory development is influenced profoundly by paradoxes. Progress in theory development may be constrained and or enhanced by these paradoxes. Throughout nursing's rich theoretical heritage, the goal for a sense of coherence was pursued through development of theories, concepts, and taxonomies. We are ready for a new stage in the theoretical progress of the discipline, which better reflects the discipline's history and nature, constraints of society, sophistication of methods, philosophical dialogues, and many turning points in the delivery of health care. As a future direction for theory development in nursing discipline, we propose situation-specific theories, which are more congruent with the nature of nursing knowledge, values, and assumptions that are integral to the mission of nursing. Such theories may help bridge gaps between theory, practice, research, and policy in ways that grand theories and middle-range theories could not do.

Definition

Situation-specific theories focus on specific nursing phenomena that reflect clinical practice and that are limited to specific populations or to particular fields of practice (Meleis, 1997). Compared with grand theories and middle-range theories, the situation-specific theories that we are proposing here are characterized by certain prominent descriptors.

First, situation-specific theories are grounded in a social and historical context (Im & Meleis, 1999a). Compared with situation-specific theories, grand theories and middle-range theories with their higher levels of abstraction rarely incorporate social and historical contexts in their conceptualization. Even middle-range theories, which are regarded as closely linking research and theory (Lenz, 1998), rarely consider the social and historical context of research encounters (Im & Meleis, 1999a).

Second, situation-specific theories reflect a specified time period as well as sociopolitical constraints on outcomes and the goals of nursing care. Situation-specific theories have limited scope, defined populations, limited situations, defined context, multiple and varied truths, and tentative interpretations in the context of time. Thus situation-specific theories are characterized by limited generalizability due to their specificity and dynamic evaluation.

Third, situation-specific theories are based on findings from a variety of sources that are empirical, interpretive, feminist, critical, ethical, or aesthetic research experiences. Multiple methodological perspectives within the nursing discipline have been argued, and the most appropriate paradigm for scientific inquiry in nursing has been debated (Acton et al., 1997). As Acton et al. (1997) asserted, we need to stop arguing for or against multiplicity and diversity in methodology, set aside methodological differences, and move to discover truths that will build the foundational base of nursing practice. Situation-specific theories incorporate various methodologies selected to complement and to be congruent with the type of phenomena observed.

Finally, situation-specific theories are congruent with the nature of nursing as a human science—friendlier to assumptions of holism, contextuality, and interactions (Meleis, 1997, 1998). These theories reflect diversities of clients, their voices, and silences. Situation-based theories rely on explanation of responses, meanings, interpretations, abilities, and goals by focusing on a phenomenon within a narrow scope of conditions. Those who are working on integrating knowledge by using multiple sources of philosophy, theory, and methodology may find situation-specific theories congruent with their goals. These type of theory may provide the means for both explaining and allowing multiple realities. Variables that are more contemporary, such as economic constraints and

other changes in social contexts, are better reflected in dynamic, evolving, and well-grounded situation-specific theories than in other types of theories. Therefore humanity in the nursing act, which has been the pride of nurse clinicians, may also be better incorporated in situation-specific theories. In sum, situation-specific theories may depict nursing realities in terms of history, voice, constraints, and strengths more than other types of theories do. The development of situation-specific theories may contribute to integration of nursing knowledge and bring coherence to our discipline.

Examples of Situation-Specific Theories

Although researchers in general tend not to identify and characterize their models or theories that may have been developed through research or practice as situation-specific theories, several examples of situation-specific theories exist in the nursing literature. For example, role integration theory resulted from research on women clerical workers in the United States (Hall, Stevens, & Meleis, 1992), as did the theory of menopausal transition of Korean immigrant women in the United States (Im & Meleis, 1999b).

Hall, Stevens, and Meleis (1992) examined ways by which women in low-income jobs tended to cope with the multiplicity of demands in their lives. These researchers developed a situation-specific theory of role integration to identify and relate aspects, processes, and patterns of women's multiple roles and to explain how these women experienced healthy resolution of the demands in their lives. The researchers presented structural aspects of roles—including focal role features, combinational role features, role depiction, evaluative processes of role integration, and patterns of role integration—to explain processes that women use to maintain or achieve a sense of coherence in life and a sense of well-being. The theory uncovered the context of women's multiple roles and how women in a specific situation integrated those roles in daily life. This theory explains women's responses as situated within socially, culturally, and politically constrained contexts.

Another example of a situation-specific theory is one developed to explain menopausal transition of low-income Korean immigrant women (Im & Meleis, 1999b). Although the research was based on an existing transition framework (Schumacher & Meleis, 1994), the unique situation of low-income Korean immigrant women was apparent in the requirement for consideration of context, timing, and other transitions that women were simultaneously experiencing. As a result, a situation-specific theory of the menopause experience of immigrant women was developed. Sources for the theoretical development included the researchers' previous experiences with immigrants and marginalized women—especially Korean immigrant women—the researchers' clinical experiences and wisdom with women in menopausal transition, a literature review, and a study of the menopausal transition of Korean immigrant women. Theoretical development included some modifications and additions of concepts more specific to particular patterns of immigrants from a Korean heritage, such as the number, seriousness, and priority of other transitions. This more focused theory helped explain why Korean immigrant women tended to neglect and ignore their menopausal transitions. Without understanding the multiple transitional situation, including immigration and work transitions, the menopausal transition experience of these women could not be understood fully. The newly developed situation-specific theory appears to give direction for clinical practice for the particular population of women by assessing their health care needs while considering other potential transitions that they may be undergoing.

■ Concluding Statement

Many examples of and reasons for fragmentation in nursing are evident; and many barriers exist toward developing a more coherent integrated knowledge base (Kirkevold, 1997; Meleis, 1998). Diverse models of biomedicine, sociology, psychology, education, administration, economics, and information led and continue to lead to developing nursing knowledge that lacks coherence (Meleis, 1997). Furthermore, diversities in nursing clients and increasing complexities in the health care system have been an impetus for members of the nursing discipline to use diverse perspectives and multiple methodologies for knowledge development (Kim, 1993; Meleis, 1998). Those trends have brought increasing fragmentation of nursing knowledge.

Integrating nursing knowledge and developing a coherent theoretical base are essential, pressing goals. To develop a more coherent knowledge base in nursing, we must consciously and deliberately enter into a dialogue about several existing tensions, which we presented in this chapter as paradoxes. The nature and progress of nursing knowledge can be analyzed, anticipated, and defined only when and if we proceed to examine the nature and outcome of each paradox. Further, we need to have a passion for giving our patients the best quality of nursing care; we need to integrate the way by which we understand our patients' experiences and plan our actions through situation-specific theories. In this chapter, we propose that development of situation-specific theories is more congruent with and integral to the nature and mission of nursing knowledge. Situation-specific theories may bridge gaps between theory, practice, research, and policy in the discipline of nursing. Situation-specific theories may be a means for transcending existing paradoxes.

■ References

Acton, G. J., Irvin, B. L., Jensen, B. A., Hopkins, B. A., & Miller, E. W. (1997). Explication of middle-range theory through methodological diversity. *Advances in Nursing Science, 19*(3), 78–95.

Allan, J. D., & Hall, B. A. (1988). Challenging the focus on technology: A critique of the medical model in a changing health care system. *Advances in Nursing Science, 10*(3), 22–34.

Allen, D. (1985). Nursing research and social control: Alternative models of science that emphasize understanding and emancipation. *IMAGE: Journal of Nursing Scholarship, 12*(2), 58–64.

Bailey, C. (1995). Nursing as therapy in the management of breathlessness in lung cancer. *European Journal of Cancer Care, 4*(4), 184–190.

Barnum, B. J. S. (1994). *Nursing theory: Analysis, application, and evaluation* (4th ed.). Philadelphia: Lippincott.

Benner, P., & Wrubel, J. (1982). Skilled clinical knowledge: The value of perceptual awareness, part I. *Journal of Nursing Administration, 12*(5), 11–14.

Bickler, B. (1994). Putting patient-focused care into practice. *Association of Operating Room Nurses Journal, 60*(2), 242–245.

Bruenjes, S. J. (1994). Orchestrating health: Middle-aged women's process of living health. *Holistic Nursing Practice, 8*(4), 22–32.

Campbell, M. L. (1996). Managing terminal dyspnea: Caring for the patient who refuses intubation or ventilation. *Dimensions of Critical Care Nursing, 15*(1), 4–12.

Condon, E. H. (1992). Nursing and the caring metaphor: Gender and political influences on an ethics of care. *Nursing Outlook, 40*(1), 14–9.

Dilthey, W. (1988). *Introduction to the human sciences. An attempt to lay a foundation for the study of society and history* (R. J. Betanzos, Trans.). Detroit: Wayne State University Press.

Dunst, C. J., & Trivette, C. M. (1996). Empowerment, effective help giving practices and family-centered care. *Pediatric Nursing, 22*(4), 334–337.

Fawcett, J., & Carino, C. (1989). Hallmarks of success in nursing practice. *Advances in Nursing Science, 11*(4), 1–8.

Fealy, G. M. (1997). The theory-practice relationship in nursing: An exploration of contemporary discourse. *Journal of Advanced Nursing, 25,* 1061–1069.

Good, M. (1998). A middle-range theory of acute pain management: Use in research. *Nursing Outlook, 46*(3), 120–124.

Gortner, S. R. (1993). Nursing's syntax revisited: A critique of philosophies said to influence nursing theory. *International Journal of Nursing Studies, 30*(6), 477–488.

Graveley, E. A., & Murphy, M. A. (1995). Nursing informatics. Making financial management come alive. *Computers in Nursing, 13*(5), 217–220.

Hall, J. M., Stevens, P. E., & Meleis, A. I. (1992). Developing the construct of role integration: A narrative analysis of women clerical workers' daily lives. *Research in Nursing and Health, 15,* 447–457.

Harvey, M. A. (1996). Managing agitation in critically ill patients. *American Journal of Critical Care, 5*(1), 7–16.

Hays, B. J., Norris, J., Martin, K. S., & Androwich, I. (1994). Informatics issues for nursing's future. *Advances in Nursing Science, 16*(4), 71–81.

Henry, S. B. (1995). Nursing informatics: State of the science. *Journal of Advanced Nursing, 22*(6), 1182–1192.

Hogston, R. (1995). Quality nursing care: A qualitative enquiry. *Journal of Advanced Nursing, 21*(1), 116–124.

Huth, M. M., & Moore, S. M. (1998). Prescriptive theory of acute pain management in infants and children. *Journal of the Society of Pediatric Nurses, 3*(1), 23–32.

Im, E., & Meleis, A. I. (1999a). Situation specific theories: Philosophical roots, properties, and approach. *Advances in Nursing Science, 22*(2), 11–24.

Im, E., & Meleis, A. I. (1999b). A situation specific theory of Korean immigrant women's menopausal transition. *IMAGE: Journal of Nursing Scholarship, 31*(4), 333–338.

Johnson, M. (1983). Some aspects of the relation between theory and research in nursing. *Journal of Advanced Nursing, 8,* 21–28.

Kim, H. S. (1993). Identifying alternative linkages among philosophy, theory and method in nursing science. *Journal of Advanced Nursing, 18*(5), 793–800.

King, I. M. (1990). Health as the goal for nursing. *Nursing Science Quarterly, 3*(3), 123–128.

Kirkevold, M. (1997). Integrative nursing research—An important strategy to further the development of nursing science and nursing practice. *Journal of Advanced Nursing, 25*(5), 977–984.

Kleffel, D. (1991). A ecofeminist analysis of nursing knowledge. *Nursing Forum, 26*(4), 5–18.

Koch, T., & Webb, C. (1996). The biomedical construction of ageing: Implications for nursing care of older people. *Journal of Advanced Nursing, 23*(5), 954–959.

Lauder, W. (1994). Beyond reflection: Practical wisdom and the practical syllogism. *Nurse Education Today, 14*(2), 91–98.

Lenz, E. R. (1998). Role of middle-range theory for nursing research and practice. *Nursing Leadership Forum, 3*(1), 24–32.

Lenz, E. R., Pugh, L. C., Milligan, R. A., Gift, A., & Suppe, F. (1997). The middle-range theory of unpleasant symptoms: An update. *Advances in Nursing Science, 19*(3), 14–27.

Maeve, M. K. (1994). The carrier bag theory of nursing practice. *Advances in Nursing Science, 16,* 9–22.

Marshall, B. L. (1988). Feminist theory and critical theory. *Canadian Review of Sociology and Anthropology, 25,* 208–230.

Meleis, A. I. (1987). ReVisions in knowledge development: A passion for substance. *Scholarly Inquiry for Nursing Practice: An International Journal, 1*(1), 5–19.

Meleis, A. I. (1997). *Theoretical nursing: Development and progress* (3rd ed.). Philadelphia: Lippincott.

Meleis, A. I. (1998). A passion for making a difference: ReVisions for empowerment. *Scholarly Inquiry for Nursing Practice: An International Journal, 12*(1), 87–94.

Moccia, P. (1988). A critique of compromise: Beyond the methods debate. *Advances in Nursing Science, 10,* 1–9.

Morse, J. M., Solber, S. M., Neander, W. L., Botroff, J. L., & Johnson, J. L. (1990). Concepts of caring and caring as a concept. *Advances in Nursing Science, 13,* 1–14.

Reed, P. G. (1996). Transforming practice knowledge into nursing knowledge—A revisionist analysis of Peplau. *IMAGE: Journal of Nursing Scholarship, 28*(1), 29–33.

Ross, M. M., Rosenthal, C. J., & Dawson, P. (1997). Patterns of caregiving following the institutionalization of elderly husbands. *Canadian Journal of Nursing Research, 29*(2), 79–98.

Schultz, P. R., & Meleis, A. I. (1988). Nursing epistemology: Traditions, insights, questions. *IMAGE: Journal of Nursing Scholarship, 20*(4), 217–221.

Schumacher, K. L., & Meleis, A. I. (1994). Transitions: A central concept in nursing. *IMAGE: Journal of Nursing Scholarship, 26*(2), 119–127.

Smith, M. A., Atherly, A. J., & Kane, R. L. (1997). Peer review of the quality of care: Inter-rater reliability and sources of systematic bias in outcome and process assessments. *Abstract Book Association for Health Services Research, 14,* 199–200.

Stone, V. E., Weissman, J. S., & Cleary, P. D. (1995). Satisfaction with ambulatory care of persons with AIDS: Predictors of patient ratings of quality. *Journal of General Internal Medicine, 10*(5), 239–245.

Timpson, J. (1996). Nursing theory: Everything the artist spits is art? *Journal of Advanced Nursing, 23*(5), 1030–1036.

Thompson, J. L. (1985). Practical discourse on nursing: Going beyond empiricism and historicism. *Advances in Nursing Science, 7,* 59–71.

Wilson, S. A. (1997). The transition to nursing home life: A comparison of planned and unplanned admissions. *Journal of Advanced Nursing, 26*(5), 864–871.

■ Editor's Questions for Discussion

How has diversity contributed to fragmentation in nursing knowledge? Provide examples of "integrative conceptualization" in research. Currently, what philosophical debates in nursing are grounded in substance? What is the difference between middle-range and grand theories in nursing? Provide examples.

Which is more important: to know that what nurses do in nursing practice makes a difference in patient outcome, or why a difference occurs? Which approach calls more attention to the patient phenomenon? Address each of the questions posed by Meleis and Im about theoretical formulations, methodologies, and evaluation.

How are situation-specific theories different from all other types of theories or conceptualizations? Of what value are they without generalizability? How may situation-specific theories contribute to integration of nursing knowledge?

How applicable is Donnelly's critique (Chapter 28) about nursing theory to situation-specific theories? Would situation-specific theories be equivalent to nursing practice theories? If not, what are the differences?

73

Nursing Research into the 21st Century

The Opportunities and the Challenges

Patricia A. Grady, PhD, RN, FAAN

A s we begin the 21st century, the need for nursing research, so evident today, will grow substantially during the next 100 years. Although a newly developing science, nursing research is already making significant contributions to the science base that informs health care practice and is emerging as a major force in patient-oriented research. Present and future challenges faced by nursing research are, in fact, opportunities to make a positive difference in the nation's health care—both immediately and at a time when national trends signal significant changes for the years ahead.

■ Characteristics of Nursing Research

The broad perspective of nursing research contributes an essential element to the nation's health research efforts. This research includes both basic and clinical investigations pertaining to the individual or patient. The approach addresses the whole person in his or her life's environment, including family, community, and home—all key influences on the course of health and illness. A major focus is on patient responses to effects of diagnosis, disease, or treatment. A special emphasis is on populations with particular health needs, including subpopulations of older people, women, minorities, residents of rural areas, and the economically disadvantaged (American Nurses Association [ANA], 1997).

Synergy between nursing research and nursing practice is critical to maintaining effective nursing science. Ongoing dialogue informs and enriches all components of the nursing discipline while ensuring that research addresses important health issues and that findings are both relevant and useful to healthcare practitioners.

Biomedical research on causes and cures of disease, although essential, must also embrace research on care issues, health promotion, and disease prevention (American Association of Colleges of Nursing [AACN], 1999). These are mainstays of nursing research. Recognition of the need for this type of research to be conducted in concert with biomedical research was a major factor in the formation and placement of a National Institute of Nursing Research (NINR) within the nation's foremost biomedical research organization, the National Institutes of Health (NIH).

■ *The National Institute of Nursing Research at the NIH*

In the 1980s, studies by the Institute of Medicine (IOM) (1983), and an NIH Task Force (U.S. Department of Health and Human Services [DHHS], 1984) found that nursing research should be in the mainstream of biomedical and behavioral science and that nursing research activities were relevant to the NIH mission. Following legislative action, the NINR began at NIH in 1986. Since then, nursing research has enriched research supported by NIH and other institutions through independent and multidisciplinary research efforts.

As NIH addresses the new century, reinvigoration of clinical research is emphasized so that patients and the public benefit from basic research applied to clinical practice. Clinically based, patient-oriented nursing research is well positioned to contribute to these "bench to bedside" efforts. Interrelationships of mind and body—between biological and behavioral—are increasingly under study at NIH, and nursing research has long been active in this area of inquiry. NIH scientific activities in prevention, including identification of those at risk for illness, also benefit from nursing research contributions; nursing studies are continually developing and testing strategies to predict and prevent illness. Rapid growth of technological advances in genetics and newly developed treatments demand the close attention of nursing research to help patients make choices about their health and adhere to and manage the side effects of treatment regimens. Together, NIH and NINR emphases coincide with national health concerns, such as prevention of low birthweight, reduction of cardiovascular disease and cancer, reduction of obesity, and issues surrounding end of life and palliative care.

■ *Responsiveness to Future Key Issues of Health Care*

Within the next several decades, health care as we currently know it will change substantially. Rapid progress of science is eliciting renewed enthusiasm for biomedical and behavioral research. Scientific breakthroughs are changing assumptions, generating new theories, and offering hope for cures and better health. Changing demographic and economic trends also influence new research directions, and nursing research is planning ahead to meet the new challenges. Although we cannot predict with precision the future course of the nation's health care, we can anticipate some general themes.

What follows are examples of key issues and opportunities that will shape the future of U.S. health and health care research. Examples of nursing research funded by the NINR also are cited to provide insights about contributions to the nursing scientific foundation at the beginning of the new century.

Anticipated Increase in Chronic Illness

Chronic conditions, which can occur at any age, are more prevalent in older adults and will continue to increase, as demographic trends project a marked rise in the older population. About 20% of the total U.S. population is expected to be 65 years of age or older by 2030, compared to the current 13%. In 2050, the fastest growing age group will be 85 years of age or older (Day, 1996). Implications of this age shift for patients, families, communities, the health care system, and the economy are tremendous. The issue, however, is not the increase in the older population, but an increase in those who are chronically disabled. Currently, chronic conditions are the leading cause of illness, disability, and death, affecting almost 100 million people. The cost to the U.S. economy is $470 billion (in 1990 dollars) in direct medical costs and more than $230 billion in lost productivity (The Robert Wood Johnson Foundation, 1996). Furthermore, at least one fourth of American households provide informal, unpaid care for an older relative or friend—a threefold increase over 10 years ago (Levine, 1997).

In addition to aging of the population, another factor in the rise of chronic illness is attributable to scientific advances. Improved therapies increasingly are converting acute illnesses to chronic illnesses that have a different and longer duration of complex care requirements. AIDS and heart disease are examples.

New nursing research opportunities that address chronic illness are plentiful, particularly those concerning management of chronic illness to avoid complications of disease and disability, including controlling pain and supporting family caregivers. NINR-funded investigators are active in these areas, but the challenge lies in obtaining resources for significant expansion of research necessary to meet demands of chronic illness in the 21st century.

The following are examples of current research in the area of chronic illness.

- *Managing symptoms.* Patient adherence to long-lasting and sometimes debilitating treatment regimens are often necessary to prolong life. Investigators are uncovering ways to optimize adherence to treatment—for example, by predicting which patients are likely to experience nausea during chemotherapy so that effective interventions can be provided to ward off unpleasant side effects and increase adherence (Morrow, 1991).

- *Preventing complications of disease and disability.* Most patients with Parkinson's disease experience significant sleep disturbances, although why that happens is not understood. Investigations are under way to determine effects of two different doses of melatonin on nocturnal sleep patterns of these patients, as part of an analysis of more effective physiologic therapies (Dowling, 1998).

- *Managing and controlling pain.* Understanding the biological and behavioral parameters of pain and their interrelationships is important in order to control this common symptom. New groundwork has been laid by nursing researchers who showed that certain pain relievers are more effective in women than in men. These findings point to new directions in pain research that explore such influential factors as gender and age (Gear et al., 1996).

- *Supporting family caregivers.* Lives of family caregivers are altered substantially by providing the care required by frail or ill relatives or friends. Typically, family caregivers are untrained, experience their own health problems, and lack confidence in their abilities to provide adequate care. Nurse investigators have shown that once patients have left the hospital for home, telephone calls by nurses to provide information and answer questions improved the health of both patient and caregiver, raised caregiver confidence, and cut in half phone calls to physicians' offices (Mishel, 1999).

Improving Quality of Life Despite Illness, Quality of Care, and Cost Effectiveness

The rise in chronic illness presents the need to design strategies that permit people to live their lives as normally as possible, even with illness. Shortened hospital stays have resulted in discharge of sicker patients, but their acute or chronic episodes do not end when they leave for home. Furthermore, improved therapeutics have made early discharge possible and, for certain groups of patients, even desirable. Home care therefore is assuming increasing importance as an essential ingredient of the U.S. health care system, whether the care is provided by professionals or family caregivers.

Nursing research has developed a transitional care model and tested it in various patient populations. These studies have shown that, when advanced practice nurses conduct carefully planned hospital early discharge programs with follow-up care in the home, the quality of patient care improves and health care costs are reduced significantly (Brooten, Roncoli et al., 1994; Brooten, Savitri et al., 1986). As indicated in Table 73.1, cost-effectiveness of the transitional care model is evident for a various patient groups, including very low birthweight infants, at-risk pregnant women, and older people with common cardiac conditions (DHHS, 1998a).

The model continues to be refined to include additional patient populations and geographic locations. These additions encompass patient groups that experience exacerbations of health problems, such as low birth-

weight infants in the first year of life and older adults with heart failure.

Research also shows that patients may be able to forestall progression of their diseases while enjoying fairly typical lifestyles. More nursing research studies are needed to determine the most effective methods to achieve these desired results, as illustrated by the following examples.

- An investigator has determined that coping-skills training helps teens who must live with diabetes. Whereas medication, exercise, and diet reduce complications of diabetes, another important factor is behavioral skills needed to control the disease. Young people have a harder time with control than adults. Teens may know what to do, but peer pressure to eat unwisely, for example, is hard to resist. Coping-skills training involves role-playing in difficult social situations. Scientists find that adding this training to other diabetes therapies consistently lowers glucose levels and increases teens' diabetes control as they participate in normal activities (Grey et al., 1998).

- Another investigator helps patients with multiple sclerosis (MS) maintain their narrow margin of health. These patients face uncertainty of the disease course while attempting to fulfil family and work obligations. Research includes determining proper exercise for these patients, who do not tolerate heat well, and techniques to promote good nutrition, stress reduction, and mobility. Results indicate that MS patients have a high interest in health promotion and self-care, and many indicate that the study intervention is helping them continue to live independently (Stuifbergen, 1998).

Increasing Importance of Health Promotion and Disease Prevention Research

Success based on health promotion and disease prevention research is expanding. Since 1900, improved health practices have been credited with increasing the American public's

TABLE 73.1   Transitional Care Model

Service	Patient Population	Savings
Initial hospitalizations	Very low birthweight babies	−11 days
	Cesarean births	−30 hours
Average charges for hospitalization	Pregnant diabetic group	−40%
	Cesarean group	−30%
	Very low birthweight group	−27%
	Hysterectomy group	−6%
Number of readmissions to hospital	Elderly cardiac medical group (6 weeks postdischarge)	−61%
Hospital charges for readmissions	Elderly cardiac medical group	−61%
Average cost of total health care services	Elderly cardiac medical group	−62%
Number of inpatient days for readmission	Elderly cardiac medical group	−70%

lifespan by 25 years (DHHS, 1999a). Better diet, exercise, and weight and blood pressure control, along with reduced smoking and infant mortality, have contributed to this statistic. Yet, special challenges also are associated with health promotion and disease prevention research. Lifestyle habits are difficult to change. Certain populations are difficult to reach. Positive results may be short-lived, or their benefits may not be evident for years. Advances have been realized, but people in the United States still demonstrate unacceptably high levels of obesity. This situation contributes to the prevalence of heart disease, cancer, and diabetes. Substance abuse and the spread of HIV continue. Toxic effects of the environment persist. Nonetheless, the importance of research in these areas is increasingly apparent to scientists and the public.

Many people today want to assume more responsibility for their own health. As it is likely that they will live longer, they want to live well—without impairments and with as much independence as possible. Health care consumers need advice based on scientifically sound evidence. They also need guidance in decision-making about complex issues, such as whether to take estrogen, undergo genetic testing, or write advanced directives. Nursing research addresses these questions and develops interventions directed toward maintaining or improving quality of life.

In promoting healthy lifestyles, it is important to begin early in life before risk-taking behavior takes hold. For example, an NINR-supported 8-week education and exercise intervention conducted in rural and urban elementary schools in the stroke-belt State of North Carolina significantly reduced risk factors for cardiovascular disease in preadolescents. Their cholesterol levels and body fat were lowered, aerobic power was increased, and diastolic blood pressure did not rise as much as in the control group. The investigator is now testing the intervention in rural, ethnically diverse middle-school students, while continuing to follow the younger children. Preliminary results from this expanded study indicate similar benefits, suggesting that additional research may validate the need for a national program, which, over time, could help decrease the high incidence of cardiovascular disease (Harrell et al., 1998).

In another health promotion study, nurses have made a significant impact. Nurses visiting homes of disadvantaged young pregnant mothers and continuing to provide them with assistance during the early childhood period produced significant physical and mental health improvements among both mothers and children. There were also reductions in child abuse and childhood injuries, fewer arrests of the mothers, and decreased dependence on welfare. These benefits are significant for local health and welfare programs and for criminal justice systems in high-crime neighborhoods (Kitzman et al., 1997; Olds et al., 1997).

Continual Improvement in the Management of Symptoms

A major emphasis of nursing research is managing symptoms of illness and treatment, such as pain, cognitive impairment, and chronic wounds. These symptoms accompany such problems as AIDS, cancer, and heart and Alzheimer's disease—symptoms that can profoundly affect quality of life, prolong hospital stays, and impede recovery. Examples of current symptom management studies include the following.

- *Pain.* The painful stress of surgery is potentially life threatening because it compromises immunity and may promote metastasis. Nursing research that used an animal model for the study of breast cancer indicates that providing morphine before and after surgery significantly decreases the metastatic-enhancing effects of surgery. Preoperative pain medication is particularly important; it promotes better pain management after surgery by preventing the cycle of pain from developing. These results demonstrate that management of pain is a physiologic necessity. If applicable to humans, pain relief could improve a person's resistance to metastasis following surgery (Page, McDonald, & Ben-Eliyaho, 1998). Other ongoing research is addressing (a) immunologic implications of

pain; (b) levels of pain in infants and others who cannot relate what they feel; (c) timing and dose of pain medication; (d) management of pain in children with sickle cell disease; and (e) ethnic, cultural, and gender differences in experiencing pain.

- *Cognitive impairment.* Agitation, frequently shown by Alzheimer's disease patients, is a typical symptom that is difficult for health care professionals and family members to manage. Because physical and chemical restraints are reserved for extreme circumstances, investigators are focusing on manipulating the patient environment to learn whether agitation can be reduced. Testing evening-light therapy is an approach to determine whether circadian rhythms and sleep patterns will improve and thereby lower agitation. Research also is being conducted to curtail wandering behavior, slow progression of cognitive impairment, and preserve everyday functions, such as dressing oneself, for as long as possible.

- *Chronic wounds.* Defined as venous stasis ulcers, pressure sores, and diabetic ulcers, these wounds are often associated with immobility, as when patients are confined to beds, and affect large numbers of people at large annual costs. At high risk are quadriplegic, older, and critical care patients. Pressure sores can develop within hours, but healing usually takes from 2 to 5 months. The total national cost of treating pressure ulcers has been estimated to be at least $1.3 billion (DHHS, 1994).

NINR-supported researchers have developed an evaluative scale to predict a patient's risk for pressure ulcers. Health care providers can then identify patients most likely to develop pressure ulcers within a few days of admission to a health care institution. Doing so permits immediate preventive action (Bergstrom, Braden, Kemp, Champagne, & Ruby, 1998). The assessment scale has been adapted for use in routine clinical practice and has been incorporated into the guidelines on *Pressure Ulcers in Adults: Prediction and Prevention* (DHHS, 1992), and *Treatment of Pressure*

Ulcers, developed by the Agency for Health Care Policy and Research (DHHS, 1994). Other promising areas of research include exploring cellular and biochemical characteristics of pressure ulcers. Also needed are investigations of the cellular, biochemical, and molecular mechanisms responsible for delayed healing in chronic wounds.

Easing the Transition in Adapting to New Technologies

The rapidly evolving field of genetics offers particular challenges and opportunities to nurse researchers. Soon people may be able to know their own health futures—which diseases are likely to develop and whether action may be taken to prevent them. Most mutated genes related to diseases indicate a predisposition that may be activated by environmental conditions or behavioral habits to produce the disease. Although genetic screening may reveal these mutations, little is known now about which lifestyle changes or environmental factors are influential and which modifications will produce the best results to maintain health. Many bioethical issues associated with genetics benefit from nursing research attention, including the informed consent process. People need help in making choices about undergoing genetic screening and coping with results that might indicate the likelihood of a fatal, presently untreatable disease.

Current NINR-supported research on the informed consent process includes testing for the BRCA1 gene that indicates a hereditary risk for breast cancer. One part of the study consists of a consumer survey of women at risk for breast cancer and their first-degree relatives and focus groups of physicians and nurse practitioners likely to be involved in the testing. Important discrepancies in expectations have been identified. For example, almost a quarter of physicians indicated informed consent is not important, but the investigator has determined that almost all the consumers and nurses disagreed with them.

Another area of inquiry examines the single and interactive influences of genetics, gender, and lifestyle changes on developing and reducing cardiovascular disease risks associated with obesity. Using a genetically obese animal model, an investigator is testing the effects of diet and exercise on risk-factor reduction.

Another technological advance is telehealth, which is gaining national attention. Use of this technology includes home-monitoring devices for electronic transmission of data to practitioners at a distance and computer-based instructional programs that can be used in universities or the home. Telehealth bridges the distance between patients and health care professionals in remote rural areas and enables clinical researchers to share patient records and diagnostic images.

NINR-supported investigators have identified and tested a telehealth technique that holds great promise for wide-ranging adaptations. A population of patients who received lung transplantations were followed in the home with spirometer-monitoring devices that recorded pulmonary function, vital signs, and symptoms daily. The patients also maintained an electronic diary about their condition. This diary was communicated weekly to health care professionals at a remote site, permitting early identification of problems and reducing emergency room use and hospitalization—with corresponding savings in health care costs (DHHS, 1998c).

Narrowing the Gap of Racial and Ethnic Disparities in Good Health and Health Care

Currently about 1 in 10 people in the United States is foreign born (Schmidley & Alvarado, 1997). Current demographic trends indicate that the fastest growing subpopulations in the United States are those of Hispanic and Asian origin, which together will account for 61% of the nation's population growth from 2000 to 2020 (Day, 1996). Because diversity is increasing continually, understanding why diseases affect some ethnic groups more than others is imperative. In some cases, there are wide disparities in health. For example, African Americans are almost twice as likely to die of heart failure as Caucasians (Dries et al., 1999), and their general life expectancy is almost 7 years less (Singh, Kochanek, & MacDorman, 1994). HIV is the fifth leading cause of death among those of Hispanic origin and the fourth leading cause among African Americans, but it is not among the top 10 leading causes of death for Caucasians (Peters, Kochanek, & Murphy, 1996). Prevalence of diabetes among Native Americans and Alaskan Natives is more than twice that of the U.S. population (DHHS, 1999b).

Multiculturalism in the United States dictates developing or fine-tuning interventions for maximum relevance and effectiveness if we are to reduce health disparities that persist in our society. The paucity of research in this area opens up additional opportunities for nursing research, which has long incorporated ethnic and cultural health particularities in designing projects and testing interventions. Many studies incorporate community leaders, health workers, and parish nurses in their programs.

An example of research that is applicable to many disorders, settings, and at-risk populations is a study to reduce high blood pressure of young, inner city African American men. These young men have the lowest rates of awareness, treatment, and control of this serious condition of any population group in the United States. Outreach was conducted, using community members to spread the word. A nurse practitioner, community health worker, and physician team provided an intense intervention that included free care and medica-

tion. Early results indicated that high blood pressure was controlled in two thirds of the men by the end of the project. An expanded study of a larger population has revealed major coexisting health problems, such as heart and kidney diseases. In addition, preliminary results in the larger study indicate that blood pressure control increased to 44%; and visits to the emergency room, which the young men typically use for primary care, decreased from 145 to 35 over a period of 12 months. Other researchers from around the world have expressed interest in this research—particularly its recruitment and retention aspects, which are so difficult to achieve in hard to reach populations (DHHS, 1998b).

Other NINR-supported research that focuses on specific ethnic groups includes obesity, low birthweight, HIV infection, diabetes, screening for cancer and other illnesses, parenting, caregiving, and self-management strategies for chronic diseases such as arthritis. Working to erase disparities in health and health care is one of the most challenging, but important and rewarding endeavors of nursing research.

Providing Effective Palliative Care at the End of Life

End of life is an important, but underaddressed area of health care. Several major studies by distinguished organizations, including the Robert Wood Johnson Foundation and the IOM, have issued reports capturing the public's attention. The IOM (1997) report, for example, defined a good death as "one that is free from avoidable distress and suffering for patients, families, and caregivers; in general accord with patients' and families' wishes; and reasonably consistent with clinical, cultural, and ethical standards" (p. 4). The IOM also determined that people fear they will either be technologically overtreated—leading to prolonged dying—or abandoned and untreated for physical distress. As a result, the IOM called for more research in palliative care.

The Robert Wood Johnson report also revealed problems with palliative care. It found that 40% of dying patients were treated aggressively in intensive care units and that pain was common to half of hospitalized patients during their last few days. Discrepancies between patient desires and actual treatment also existed. Furthermore, almost half the physicians in the study did not know that their patients' preference was not to be resuscitated (SUPPORT Principal Investigators, 1995).

A trans-NIH workshop convened by NINR, "Symptoms in Terminal Illness," which included multidisciplinary experts from throughout the United States, identified significant gaps in scientific knowledge. Many patients experience similar symptoms, regardless of their underlying medical condition. Pain is the most frequent, but others include dyspnea, cognitive disturbances and delirium, cachexia, nausea, fatigue, and depression. Clearly, this area presents current and future research opportunities for bringing together multidisciplinary teams of basic and clinical researchers to address ways to manage end-of-life symptoms better (Symptom Management Workshop, 1997).

The NINR has been designated as the lead institute at NIH for coordinating research on palliative care at the end of life. The NINR's research portfolio includes managing pain and other symptoms and decision-making related to health and illness—information needed by health care providers, as well as by patients and their families. Among its scientific interests are (a) the environment of critically ill patients, (b) family decision-making for incapacitated patients, (c) decisions that must be made in the absence of advanced directives,

and (d) studies of end-of-life caregiving practices. Additional concerns include how to enhance caregiving capacities of family members—how to help them manage stress, maintain their own health, and finally, deal with bereavement.

The following are examples of NINR-supported research.

- *Understanding what patients and families want and expect in end-of-life care.* Findings indicate family readiness to stop aggressive treatments in favor of high-quality comfort care if they understand that the condition is terminal; and physician and nurse behaviors, such as viewing death as a medical failure, greatly increase the family's grief and distress (Tilden, Tolle, Garland, & Nelson, 1995).

- *Analysis of dyspnea to shed light on appropriate treatments.* Findings show that people with chronic obstructive pulmonary disease can distinguish distress and anxiety caused by their perceived breathing difficulties from anxiety caused by worsening of disease (Carrieri-Kohlman, Gormley, Douglas, Paul, & Stulbarg, 1996).

Providing Research Training to Ensure a Sufficient Cadre of Future Nurse Researchers

Adequate numbers of nurse researchers are critical to meet future health care needs of the 21st century. This need has been recognized by the National Research Council (1994) of the National Academy of Science, which has called for an increase of researchers in the discipline of nursing. Nurses with advanced clinical skills bring important insights to the research arena. Their research training needs must be met.

The NINR is actively pursuing approaches to encourage growth in the number of future nurse researchers. Currently, it provides support for nearly the entire population of nurse postdoctoral students in schools of nursing. Other training support includes

- a highly successful Summer Nurse Scientist Training Program at NIH, cosponsored with the Clinical Center Nursing Department, to provide practical research skills and information on grantsmanship in order to produce successful future applicants for federally-funded research;

- a Summer Genetics Institute for Nurses, a new program to be supported through the NINR Intramural Research Program on the NIH campus, to develop much-needed expertise in genetics for nursing practice;

- new NIH training mechanisms for nurses to promote careers in patient-oriented research; and

- mentored research experiences through the NIH minority research career awards program.

Nursing research is a growing field. The challenge is to develop new, creative approaches to meet the array of training needs.

■ Concluding Statement

Health research, health care, and health choices are increasingly interdependent, and nurses and nurse researchers play a vital role in all three areas. The contributions that nursing research will make will enable future researchers to look back on the 21st century and marvel. As we go forward, scientifically validated methodologies, communication strategies, and effective interventions—coupled with a basic understanding of human nature and our nation's diverse populations—will make a significant difference in the health care and quality of life of the American people.

■ References

American Association of Colleges of Nursing. (1999). *Position statement on nursing research*. Washington, DC: Author.

American Nurses Association. (1997). *Directions for nursing research: Toward the twenty-first century*. Washington, DC. American Nurses Publishing.

Bergstrom, N., Braden, B., Kemp, M., Champagne, M., & Ruby, E. (1998). Predicting pressure ulcer risk: A multisite study of the predictive validity of the Braden scale. *Nursing Research 47*, 261–269.

Brooten, D., Roncoli, M., Finkler, S., Arnold, L., Cohen, A., & Mennuti, M. (1994). A randomized trial of early hospital discharge and home follow-up of women having cesarean birth. *Obstetrics & Gynecology, 84*, 832–838.

Brooten, D., Savitri, K., Brown, L. P., Butts, P., Finkler, S. A., Bakewell-Sachs, S., Gibbons, A., & Delivoria-Papadopoulos, M. (1986). A randomized clinical trial of early hospital discharge and home follow-up of very-low-birth-weight infants. *New England Journal of Medicine, 315*, 934–939.

Carrieri-Kohlman V., Gormley J. M., Douglas, M. K., Paul, S. M., & Stulbarg, M. S. (1996). Differentiation between dyspnea and its affective components. *Western Journal of Nursing Research, 18*, 626–642.

Day, J. C. (1996). *Population projections of the United States by age, sex, race, and Hispanic origin: 1995 to 2050*. (U.S. Bureau of the Census, Current Population Reports, P25-1130). Washington, DC: U.S. Government Printing Office.

Dowling, G. (1998). *Melatonin for sleep disorders in Parkinson's disease.* National Institutes of Health, National Institute of Nursing Research [On-line]. Available: http://www.commons.cit.nih.gov/crisp/.

Dries, D. L., Exner, D. V., Gersh, B. J., Cooper, H. A., Carson, P. E., & Domanski, M. J. (1999). Racial differences in the outcome of left ventricular dysfunction. *New England Journal of Medicine, 340*(8), 609–616.

Gear, R. W., Miaslowski, C., Gordon, N. C., Paul, S. M., Heller, P. H., & Levine, J. D. (1996). Kappa-opioids produce significantly greater analgesia in women than in men. *Nature Medicine, 2,* 1248–1250.

Grey, M., Boland, E. A., Davidson, M., Ma, C.Y., Sullivan-Bolyai, S., & Tamborlane, W. V. (1998). Short-term effects of coping skills training as adjunct to intensive therapy in adolescents. *Diabetes Care, 21,* 902–908.

Harrell, J. S., Gansky, S. A., McMurray, R. G., Bangdiwala, S. I., Frauman, A. C., & Bradley, C. B. (1998). School-based interventions improve heart health in children with multiple cardiovascular disease risk factors. *Pediatrics, 102,* 371–380.

Institute of Medicine. (1983). *Nursing and nursing education: Public policies and private actions.* Washington, DC: National Academy Press, 19.

Institute of Medicine. (1997). *Approaching death: Improving care at the end-of-life.* Washington, DC: National Academy Press.

Kitzman, H., Olds, D. L., Henderson, C. R., Jr., Hanks, C., Cole, R., Tatelbaum, R., McConnochie, K. M., Sidora, K., Luckey, D. W., Shaver, D., Engelhardt, K., James, D., & Barnard, K. (1997). Effect of prenatal and infancy home visitation by nurses on pregnancy outcomes, childhood injuries, and repeated childbearing. *Journal of the American Medical Association, 278*(8), 644–652.

Levine, S. (1997, March 24). One in four U.S. families cares for aging relatives. *Washington Post,* A13.

Mishel, M. (1999). Teaching cancer patients to be self-advocates. *Summary of the Capitol Hill breakfast briefing on symptom management for chronic neurological conditions.* National Institute of Nursing Research. [On-line]. Available: http://www.nih.gov/ninr/cancerbrief.htm.

Morrow, M. (1991). Predicting development of anticipatory nausea in cancer patients: Prospective examination of eight clinical characteristics. *Journal of Pain Symptom Management, 6*(4), 215–223.

National Research Council. (1994). *Meeting the nation's needs for biomedical and behavioral scientists.* Washington, DC: National Academy Press.

Olds, D. L., Eckenrode, J., Henderson, C. R., Jr., Kitzman, H., Powers, J., Cole, R., Sidora, K., Morris, P., Pettitt, L., & Luckey, D. (1997). Long-term effects of home visitation on maternal life course and child abuse and neglect: Fifteen-year follow-up of a randomized trial. *Journal of the American Medical Association, 278*(8), 637–643.

Page, G. G., McDonald, J. S., & Ben-Eliyaho, S. (1998). Pre- versus postoperative administration of morphine: Impact on the neuroendocrine, behavioral, and metastatic-enhancing effects of surgery. *British Journal of Anesthesia, 81,* 216–223.

Peters, K., Kochanek, K., & Murphy, S. (1996). *Deaths: Final data for 1996.* (National vital statistics report, 37, Vol. 47, No. 9, pp. 26–48.) Hyattsville, MD: National Center for Health Statistics.

Robert Wood Johnson Foundation. (1996, August). *Chronic care in America: A 21st century challenge.* Princeton, NJ: Hoffman.

Schmidley, D., & Alvarado, H. (1997). *Foreign born population in the United States: March 1997.* (U.S. Bureau of the Census, Current Population Reports, P20-507). Washington, DC: U.S. Government Printing Office.

Singh, G. K., Kochanek, K. D., & MacDorman, M. F. (1994). *Advance report of final mortality statistics, 1994.* (Monthly vital statistics report, Vol. 45, No. 3, Supp. p. 19) Hyattsville, MD: National Center for Health Statistics.

Stuifbergen, A. (1998). Health promotion and quality of life in chronic illness. *Summary of the Capitol Hill breakfast briefing on symptom management for chronic neurological conditions.* National Institute of Nursing Research. [On-line]. Available: http://www.nih.gov/ninr/fninr-may98.htm.

SUPPORT Principal Investigators. (1995). A controlled trial to improve care for seriously ill hospitalized patients: The study to understand prognoses and preferences for outcomes and risks of treatments (SUPPORT). *Journal of the American Medical Association, 274,* 1591–1598.

Symptom Management Workshop. (1997, September). National Institute of Nursing Research. [On-line]. Available: http://www.nih.gov/ninr/end-of-life.htm.

Tilden, V. P., Tolle, S. W., Garland, M. J., & Nelson, C. A. (1995). Decisions about life-sustaining treatment: Impact of physicians' behavior on the family. *Archives of Internal Medicine, 155*(6), 633–638.

U.S. Department of Health and Human Services. (1984). *Task force on nursing research: Report to the director, 1984* (National Institutes of Health), (pp. 17, 42). Bethesda, MD: Author.

U.S. Department of Health and Human Services. (1992). *Pressure ulcers in adults: prediction and prevention* (Clinical Practice Guidelines Number 3, AHCPR Publication Number 92-0047) Rockville, MD: Author.

U.S. Department of Health and Human Services. (1994). *Treatment of pressure ulcers* (Clinical Guideline Number 15, AHCPR Publication Number 95-0652) Rockville, MD: Author.

U.S. Department of Health and Human Services (1998a). *Making a difference series: Early discharge from hospital to home—Transitional care can improve patients' health and lower costs to the health care system* (p. 6). National Institutes of Health, National Institute of Nursing Research. [On-line]. Available: http://www.nih.gov/ninr/makingadifference.pdf.

U.S. Department of Health and Human Services (1998b). *Making a difference series: High blood pressure reduced in young urban African-American men.* National Institutes of Health, National Institute of Nursing Research. [On-line]. Available: http://www.nih.gov/ninr/makingadifference.pdf.

U.S. Department of Health and Human Services. (1998c). *Research on nursing telehealth interventions supported by the National Institutes of Health* (p. 8). National Institute of Nursing Research. Bethesda, MD: Author.

U.S. Department of Health and Human Services. (1999a). *Ten great public health achievements—United States, 1900–1999.* (Morbidity and Mortality Weekly Report Synopsis, April 2, 1999). Atlanta: Author.

U.S. Department of Health and Human Services. (1999b, June). *Minority burden of chronic disease.* National Center for Chronic Disease Prevention and Health Promotion. [On-line]. Available: http://www.cdc.gov/nccdphp/.

■ Editor's Questions for Discussion

Develop research questions for investigation by nurse researchers pertaining to areas of need identified by Grady. What aspects of the research needs identified by Grady would best benefit from the interdisciplinary research approaches suggested by Lindsey (Chapter 29)? How might measurement concerns presented by Froman and Owen (Chapter 33) be resolved via interdisciplinary approaches? What research preparation is essential for nurse researchers to conduct studies in the suggested subjects? How might an investigator best plan and develop a program of nursing research?

How might nursing research findings be applied in nursing practice settings and nursing education programs? What mechanisms could facilitate such application? What relationships are essential for linking faculty practice, knowledge development, and curricula content? Should faculty be required to link developing research programs, applying findings in practice, and teaching in education programs? Realistically, how might such linkages be achieved? Or should faculty focus predominantly on one aspect of their role? How might postdoctoral students best be facilitated in developing research programs? What obligations and responsibilities exist for mentoring postdoctoral students? Should they be mentored to link research and practice? If so, by whom?

Identify researchable questions prompted by Grady, particularly those that may be developed from the 18 nursing practice chapters in this volume. Which researchable queries are inherent in the discussions of Kopala (Chapter 5), Davis (Chapter 6), and Lane and Paterson (Chapter 7)? What researchable questions may be suggested in each chapter of other Parts of this textbook?

74

Toward a Philosophy of Healing Practices in Nursing

Phyllis Beck Kritek, PhD, RN, FAAN

All right. Once more. It is not abstract versus concrete.
If you try to force that rule on Ruanja, you'll make consistent errors.
It is spatial versus unseen or nonvisual.

Emilio in *The Sparrow* by Mary Doria Russell (1996, p. 246)

When asked, most practicing nurses acknowledge that they indeed engage in practices that support healing processes in human beings. Asked, however, if they are healers, the answers become a bit more varied. Beneath this dissonance hovers myriad philosophical issues that shape any given nurse's perceptions of the concept of healing as expressed in nursing practice. This chapter is a written reflection about these philosophical issues.

■ A Point of Departure

The past 30 years of cognitive and linguistic sciences have fostered a new respect for the power of naming. Naming alone contributes mightily to the social realities we elect to create. Hence my point of departure in this chapter starts with its name. I am discussing motion *toward* something because I have reason to believe that I have not yet arrived—perhaps in the spirit of the truism that success is more about the journey than the destination. I am discussing a *philosophy* because my focus is primarily on the ontology and epistemology of healing practices in nursing, the "what we know and how we know it" of such practices. I find it increasingly compelling to recognize that the undone business of nursing scholarship in the United States is its philosophical assumptions, a melange of diverse, sometimes incompatible ideas that we nurses too often nervously fail to scrutinize.

My reflections are on the healing practices that nurses engage in—those activities and behaviors designed to further healing in the patients we serve. It appears that these behaviors encompass just about everything we do, and that is why the discussion is of merit. Knowing what we do and why we do it seems germane and warrants reflection. A simple dictionary definition of *healing* (Webster, 1985, p. 558) emphasizes the concept of wholeness: a desired wholeness, a progression toward that desired wholeness, and the interactions that lead to that desired wholeness.

Finally, these reflections emerge not from some unique intellectual foray into the land of "healing practices" but from the lived experience of my clinical practice and that of nurse colleagues observed. More immediately, my reflections have been honed and refined during the creative process of developing, implementing and directing a doctoral program focused on "healing" as a central nursing construct (Kritek, 1997). In 1994, the school of nursing faculty at the University of Texas Medical Branch at Galveston voted to create this focus in its proposed doctoral program.

Five years, three admitted classes, and myriad dialogs later, we collectively know more than we knew at the outset of the journey. Hence my observations are largely the outcome of a reflective "lived experience" with patients, nurse colleagues, and a group of pioneer doctoral students and faculty exploring

this context—a group of people as concerned about the realities of clinical nursing as they are about the realities of intellectual discourse. In this chapter, I attempt to describe some insights that have emerged from this shared journey.

■ Concerning Philosophy

Deliberative development of a philosophy of nursing lurks as unfinished business in our discipline, particularly here in the United States. Our colleagues in other parts of planet Earth seem to have moved into this realm with greater comfort and far less imitative behavior. When I reflect on the development of scholarship in nursing in the United States, I imagine it as a process of traveling in reverse. Rather than moving from philosophy to construct delineation to theory construction to theory testing through research, we have followed the reverse process. We had a sizable research enterprise before we noted that we lacked nursing theory. Indeed, we are still a bit confused and ambivalent about nursing theory. We dismiss it, often with a bias toward concrete thinking and sometimes frank anti-intellectualism, as if it were a gawky, unkempt, country cousin. Conversely, we often have been prescriptive in our use of theories, seeing them as imposed blueprints for preferred actions.

We engaged in a frenzied effort toward theory development for about 10 years, acted as if somehow we had completed the task, and moved on. More recently our impulse has been to solve this dilemma with greater interest in additional derivative theories, often calling them middle-range theories. We are still stumbling with construct delineation, despite good-faith efforts of persons involved in the enterprise, such as the dogged workers in the North American Nursing Diagnosis Association (NANDA), Nursing Intervention Classification (NIC) System, and Nursing Outcomes Classification (NOC) System (Documenting Conference, 1999). Needless to say, we have not yet, in the United States, fully attended to philosophy, more often simply assuming that it is a given, derivative or not.

We do, however, teach philosophy courses in our doctoral programs. Interestingly, this philosophy often is not ours, but like all other phases of our knowledge development enterprise, is acquired from others—an essentially derivative philosophy. In the United States this philosophy is most notably that of European and European American males. It is often absorbed somewhat unreflectively as if somehow whatever they came up with as their idea of the "what we know and how we know what we know" would readily fit the reality of the practicing nurse. We have tended to take the worldview of others and impose it on nursing, rather than attempting to ascertain the worldview of nurses and articulate its underlying philosophy. This pattern of derivative scholarship warrants scrutiny.

Carol Christ (1980) noted that

> even the most seemingly objective scholarship in every field reflects an implicit interest in preserving the patriarchal status quo, including certain notions of canon, authority, and tradition from which the contributions of women and others have been excluded [observing that] because these concerns are usually unstated, they often go unrecognized. (p. xi)

It would seem that a discipline still excessively and persistently gender structured would be wise to attend to this observation.

Unreflective adoption of established philosophies implicitly sustains worldviews that may or may not be compatible with realities experienced by the practicing nurse. Any discipline still well over 90% female will bear the stamp of that gender structuring. Not the least of subtle emergent problems is the unexam-

ined tendency to further those very "patriarchal status quo" ideas so harmful to nurses in their day-to-day existence. Thus it would seem wise to study the effect of this gender structuring; there are few places left where we can discover how a worldview—created and sustained largely by women—might differ from that of men. It is not my intent to posit that this would be a better worldview, merely that it might be different and therefore informative.

As is perhaps evident, I am describing this gender-aware backdrop to my observations with some degree of care. It is the task of the philosopher to observe and reflect, to be a thoughtful mirror of sorts. Gender-structuring has been a persistent issue in nursing. Our willingness to examine this reality and its implications often has been unequal to the challenge, too often expressed in self-indulgent victim-think or equally thoughtless rages. Nurses always have known that they "know" things about patients that it seems no one else knows. Most nurses view these things as quite important and powerful. So do most patients. These things seem to speak to an unexamined ontology. We know some things that we have neither named nor studied. Interestingly, we often associate these things that we know with being women. We chalk up this unique, sometimes ineffable knowing to intuition or a sixth sense or a deep connection with the patient, but only rarely do we choose to claim it, study it, and perhaps most important, champion it.

Managed care is instructive in this regard. We currently tend to measure our worth and value by the degree of creative adaptation we have made to a health care delivery system that we often disdain. We secretly hope that we are still giving nursing care in the shadows, knowing full well that the entire process of corporatization, downsizing, reengineering, and withholding of services has dramatically altered the amount and quality of care possible. Nurses, the group of health professionals who "know" something about the destructive nature of this entire process, have had little to say other than either secretly lamenting the losses, sometimes even with shame, or perkily adapting to the costumes and customs of the new order.

The ontology and epistemology of a discipline, neglected or denied, will out. Nature, abhorring a vacuum, with fill it with something. In our case, I believe that it has been filled in the main by the very philosophical systems that have proven most negligent of nurses and nursing. That we unthinkingly follow this path only furthers the problem. Hence moving toward a philosophy more in keeping with the values and traditions of nursing seems to me to be in our self-interest. It is in this spirit that the following reflections are recorded.

A Side-Bar on Creativity

Angeles Arrien, speaking at the 1999 Conference of the Institute of Noetic Sciences, posited that the two purposes of human life are to learn about and express love and to create (Arrien, 1999). The former, though often not named such in nursing, characterizes much of what is best about expert nursing practice. The latter is less overtly claimed. At that moment when we might best create, we turn derivative. It often seems that the desire to gain academic approval, and the fear of academic disapproval, makes us willing to accept socially credible ideas and view them as preferred to our own deep creativity.

Creativity theorists consistently posit that creating involves taking disparate "parts" never before related and making new wholes (Myers, 1999). One of the earliest discipline-level examples was the merger of sociology and psychology to create a whole new discipline: social psychology—a discipline bearing the mark of both but distinctively different from each. More recently, psychoneuroimmunology demonstrates a complex variant on this theme. Such acts of creativity are not purely derivative

because the bringing together of the "parts" alters the nature of each. Derivative practices merely take a given pattern, replicate it, and make it fit, even cram it into a second reality. It is my contention that we have been more derivative than creative in our scholarship, purchasing acceptability at the price of authenticity.

Albert Einstein once observed that one cannot solve a problem at the same level of consciousness that created it (1950/1993). Creating our own scholarship initiative would not only call us to move beyond the derivative script, but ask us to stretch ourselves to new levels of scholarship that would implicitly expand our consciousness. Interestingly, this is Newman's picture of health! (Newman, 1994).

I have taken time to describe the importance of creativity to our intellectual authenticity and health because repeatedly I believe that the capacity to differentiate between derivative and creative practices eludes us. It is my intent in this chapter to support the creative initiative. I prefer to err on the side of making something new in our philosophy of healing practices—something that really fits us—rather than wear the mental costumes of western science—a science already found wanting in many ways.

I cannot in this brief space develop a full-scale philosophical narrative, and will not try. I can, however, provide exemplars that reveal a pattern that might better serve us as we craft new ontological and epistemological practices.

■ A Metaparadigm in Process

Nursing's metaparadigm, described by Flaskerud and Halloran (1980) and significantly expanded upon by Fawcett (1984), includes four components: nurse, patient, health, and environment. For purposes of this discussion, I use these four dimensions as a framework. In each, I examine a single substantive change that serves as a precursor and invitation to creativity in evolving an emergent philosophy of healing practices in nursing. This structure admittedly is a bit artificial. All dimensions continuously are experiencing multiple rapid interactive changes. That is indeed a central point in my presentation. The focus on one change is useful, however, in providing an exemplar and a sense of orderliness, even if both are a bit illusional. I acknowledge this at the outset, noting too that writing itself is a rather linear process and not at all like the thinking and doing we are all about.

Nurse

In looking at the nurse, and more particularly the discipline of nursing, focusing on the increased sophistication of nursing's conceptual enterprise will best serve my purposes. Our burgeoning world of scholarship has altered profoundly our intellectual grasp of what we are about. We have new tools to better know our work, and we have new knowledge skills that demonstrate at least to us that we can function competently as scholars and researchers. And we have generated an amazing amount of useful and influential knowledge.

We have also, however, elected primarily to use extant ways of knowing and knowledge generation practices; indeed, we have demanded that of one another. We are slow to welcome the innovative thinker. This provides an initial clue about our collective fog about philosophy. We have elected to perpetuate a set of philosophical assumptions about reality as received from other sciences, and in most cases, the most traditional of their technologies.

A second change of focus for me involves the current state of science. Although the historic canons of Western science (followed systematically) generate useful information, emergent sciences tell a somewhat different story. Interestingly, the most striking and relevant for our purposes is that from the biological sciences. While there is no effort here to imitate these emergent ideas, they serve notice that alternatives are evolving outside nursing. We are not the only ones who may have noticed that the science we embraced in the past may be too restrictive and therefore not meet our needs.

Willis Harman (1991) aptly describes this condition. He notes four causality-related anomalies that merit scrutiny. The first emerges from current work in theoretical physics and indicates that "the search for the ultimate reductionist explanation seems to point to a wholeness" (p. iii). The second notes that there is a "fundamental self-organizing force in living systems [that] remains unexplained." The third involves our scientific knowledge about the universe as incomplete because it does not accommodate or account for the "consciousness of the observer" or any of the attributes of consciousness, such as volition. The fourth is that we have no scientific way of dealing with nonlocal causality, exemplified in quantum physics and "meaningful coincidences" (p. iii).

Harman's analysis of these "problems" concludes with a proposal of a "wholeness" science in contrast to the current "separateness" science (pp. 100–101). Among the desirable outcomes of such a science, he notes, is that it would "tend to stimulate research in the entire spectrum of states of consciousness" and "foster a worldview supportive of the highest values of all societies" (p. 99). Implicit in Harman's discussion is the contention that "value-free" science does not exist, that we would be wise to note this fact and get on with the task of dealing with the values in our science more deliberatively.

Harman's observations have a promising fit with the challenges facing nursing and indicate that we may not be alone in our need for a more robust philosophy to inform our theories and hence direct our science. While we need not repeat our patterns of using derivative ideas and imitate Harman's starting point, he does unveil a science of the future at odds with that of the present. At the root of this contrast between traditional Western science and Harman's description of a "wholeness" science is a set of differing philosophical assumptions about what is real and how we might best go about studying these real things. This distinction is of particular interest in the study of healing because healing as a concept refers to a desired state of wholeness. Hence a philosophy of healing practices in nursing appropriately would focus on wholeness of the patient and how nurses attempt to further the patient's journey toward greater wholeness.

The nurse conceptualist would, perforce, need to scrutinize her or his beliefs about what is real in order to begin to understand that the nurse studying nursing practices, by selecting some and declaring others nonexistent or of little worth and value, perpetuates patterns of practice that shape the care that patients receive. A very good example is the gradual disappearance of comfort measures once so integral to nursing practice in hospital settings. What was once a comfort measure called a back rub is now a million dollar business called massage therapy. Nurses, having eliminated a reality or accepted its elimination over time, find now that patients—for whom this comfort measure was a healing practice—have gone elsewhere to find what they need.

It is obviously not enough to become skillful conceptualists. Disciplined reason and reflection about what the real world of healing practices in nursing encompasses and what resources are available is essential. To study these practices systematically will require, I believe, whole new approaches to the entire enterprise: the constructs that we acknowledge as existent, the theories that we create, and the methods that we use to investigate these phenomena of concern. Our nursing reality is a unique one, and having failed to see that, we often find ourselves recycling the worldviews of others while neglecting to articulate our own.

Then, when asked to describe our unique contribution to healing, we are unable to protect central dimensions of nursing practice because we cannot name, describe, explain, or study them. The result, of course, is that patients who might have benefited from these healing practices find that they are simply not available.

Patient

Which brings us to changes in the patients we serve. Demographic projections in the United States posit rapid ethnic shifts already manifest in urban centers. Simply stated, European Americans—74% of the population in 1995—will by 2050 be only 53%. The U.S. Bureau of the Census predicts that by 2050 our population will be "24% Hispanic, 14% African American, 8% Asian American, and 1% Native American" (Morganthau, 1997, p. 59). This distribution means that the groups of citizens whom we now call minorities will, combined, be 47% of the population. The health care delivery system that we created and the health care practices that we engage were largely shaped by the philosophical stance of the present majority. So too were the sciences that we developed.

This shift is underscored by a further shift, one toward globalization. National boundaries are increasingly permeable, if for no other reason than the dialog of the Internet. Worldwide social, political, and economic structures are quickly replacing the nation state, and the historic "other" is increasingly part of a much more complex and diverse "us." Adding further complexity, we are witnessing steady democratization of the planet, with self-determination a worldwide value rather than a unique trait here "at home." Healing practices that once fit a majority in a more insular United States will perforce shift to attend to this patchwork quilt of differences in the self-determining patients whom we serve.

As is apparent, "old" philosophical systems will strain, indeed are straining, under this burden. Definitions of wholeness vary and abound, and few are consonant with those of the prevailing European American community. An example is the current strange debate about violence. While the National Rifle Association (NRA) continues its impassioned monologue about the constitutional right to bear arms (a uniquely early American value of European immigrants), a sobering alternative analysis is happening as subtext.

In a special report titled "America Under the Gun," *Newsweek* (1999) published a two-page spread of the last 14 shooting-spree suspects. The article described the violence of the suspects and showed pictures of their guns, yet managed not to observe that all 14 were white males. Excluding a 70-year-old schizophrenic male, the mean age of the remaining 13 suspects was 19; 10 suspects were 21 or younger. All either wanted to assert themselves or felt that they had been disadvantaged in some respect, some very specifically as white males.

Nursing attends to violence and its sequelae. What are the healing practices that respond to this crisis? Is the European American community ready to cope with ethnic distribution shifts, with global communities, with a loss of dominance of assumed privilege. What philosophical system will respond to this dilemma? In discussing the possibilities of nonviolent resistance, Beck (1996) noted that the philosophical assumption about conflict that has dominated this country, as exemplified in the ever-popular books of Louis L'Amour, is justifiable violence. That assumption is also the basis of our wars. This system of philosophy assumes dominance as a right. That assumption also prevails in our current Western science and our provider-driven health care systems.

Conversely, we might ask whether the philosophical systems that have guided Chinese medicine, African American herbal practices, Aruvedic health care in India, or even the healing practices of our own native peoples in the United States might posit different philosophical options than the ones that we currently embrace, albeit often mindlessly. The diversification of our patient populations may accelerate the urgency of that question. Serious consideration of these systems has already emerged and is rapidly reframing our prior understanding of the meaning of health.

Health

This third dimension of nursing's metaparadigm has always been a construct that has eluded us in the United States, largely because we have framed it (a philosophical decision) in terms of the absence of disease. Using the prevailing metaphor for our country—competition—health care workers often translate absence of disease as a "victory"; as in we sponsored a "war" on AIDS. Our health care system has been a disease care system with excellence most apparent when illness or trauma was most "deadly" or life threatening. One of the most interesting changes emerging about our understanding of health, however, is actually occurring in spite of traditional practices of the health care community and its fondness for Western science.

This change is the rapid expansion and use of what are euphemistically called alternative or complementary therapies. The language alone is instructive. What is alternative to us in the United States is often traditional practice elsewhere (e.g., acupuncture in China). The word *complementary* has an interesting undertone of patronization in it, as if we can only count on such practices to augment the central and most valuable of practices, those of Western medicine. Perhaps most sobering of all, these therapies are increasingly those focused upon in discussions of "healing"—as if they were expressions of healing practices in contrast to those of Western health care, which implicitly are not healing.

Many of these "new" practices emerge from philosophical systems that are neither European nor European American. Many are from philosophical systems viewed as "not dominant," the distinction itself being instructive. All are critiqued, however, using the measuring stick of Western science, a science increasingly recognized as decontexted, fragmented, isolationist, and materialistic. Although this science is a wonderful resource that has given us much useful information, it is only one way of knowing and, at least in some cases, clearly unequal to the task. An easy example helps. Someone does not "know" Monet's *Waterlilies* only by doing a laboratory analysis of the chemical composition of his paints and canvas, although that is one option.

Apparently many people in the United States have a new definition of healing and health, one quite different from that posited by the philosophical assumptions of Western science and medicine. Eisenberg, Kessler et al. (1993) reported in the *New England Journal of Medicine* on a study conducted in the United States in 1990. They reported that 34% of the population had used alternative therapies that year, resulting in 425 million visits, or substantially more than the 388 visits to allopathic practitioners. Average cost of a visit was $27.60; three fourths of all expenditures were paid out-of-pocket.

In 1997 Eisenberg, with a different team, did a follow-up study and reported in 1998 that 42% of the population had used alternative therapies (Davis et al., 1998). The number of visits was even more startling. There were now 629 million, or more than 200 million more than in 1990. Concurrently, the number of allopathic visits dropped to 386 million. The average cost had gone up to $33.00, while percentage of users paying completely out-of-pocket had not changed significantly. No matter what we in allopathic practice believe or cherish, our patients are making a decision.

Astin reported in JAMA (1998) a study in which he attempted to ascertain the major reason why this shift is happening on such a large scale; that is, why so many people are using alternative therapies. He found the major predictor to be the degree to which these alternative practices were congruent with the patients' beliefs, philosophical orientations, and values about health and life. Almost all the alternative practices were based on a philosophical system different from that of traditional medicine, almost all now bearing the social construction of "healing practices." Clearly, the meaning of health and healing are changing, and these circumstances appear to be more and more remote from the philosophical roots of Western health care. We are working in a new environment.

Environment

Edgar Mitchell, the astronaut who returned from the moon enlivened by a new sense of mission about planet Earth, aptly describes the new scientific environment we inhabit. He summarizes this "new science" as one that views the universe as learning, self-organizing, adaptive, creative, trial and error, intelligent, aware, evolving, unpredictable and expanding (Mitchell, 1998). He is influenced by emergent theories of chaos, dissipative structures, complexity, cognition, and molecular biology. He embraces a science of consciousness where the role of the observer counts, knowing that consciousness is ever capable of expansion. He is, in effect, a man living in a postmodern era.

Walter Truett Anderson (1995) observed that we have no obligation to embrace the philosophy of postmodernism, articulated largely by European men such as Foucault (1970) and Derrida (1981). Anderson did note, however, that we really have no choice about living in the environment of postmodernity. It is the nature of the times; the limits of modernity, and its failures are now evident. Knowing this, we find ourselves searching about, sometimes in the dark, for some philosophical system that will replace the one we have—one that, here in the United States, has shaped our thinking, learning, and living since the birth of the nation. The assumptions of modernity are in our roots: They informed the minds and lives of our immigrant founders, a group of visionaries that created the first viable democracy yet concurrently refused the vote to women, practiced slavery, and abided Native American genocide emergent from a sense of birthright and privilege.

Contending with postmodernity draws us to back to our creativity. If we as nurses were to imagine philosophical systems that addressed both the historic strengths of traditional allopathic care and the emergent insights from alternative care, might we not find ourselves ensconced in the postmodern world? If we as nurses were to imagine philosophical systems that honored the numerous philosophies of the world, stretched beyond the boundaries of our European roots, might we not begin to move toward more comprehensive narratives and dialogs about the nature of healing? If we as nurses were to embrace the deep roots of Nightingale (1860/1946), who, among other things, advised us to dare to stand alone, might we not evolve philosophical systems that begin to discuss the most elusive dimension of healing: the mystery of the human spirit, the force that informs all else? Might we not elect to break the shackles of a derivative, and too often ineffectual and confining philosophical system? Are we capable of creating this kind of environment, as nurses facing patients dealing with health and their desired healing?

■ Concluding Statement

As the new millennium begins and we look in the rearview mirror, we have a better sense of from whence we came than of where we are going. We know that our new environments will differ dramatically from the ones we knew. We as nurses have become expert scholars. We serve patients from a global community with differences that are more numerous than the list of variables in our health assessment forms. We are watching the rapid emergence of new sciences and new philosophies, with new definitions of health and healing. Einstein (1950/1993) observed that imagination is more important than knowledge. It seems a time for some new imaginings.

And it seems fitting to give the last word to a popular contemporary philosopher, Jimmy Buffett:

Some people love to lead, and some refuse to dance.
Some play it safely, others take a chance.
Still it's all a mystery, this place we call the world
Where most live as oysters while some become pearls.
(Buffett & McAnally, 1999)

I'm looking forward to the pearls.

■ References

America under the gun. (1999, August 23). *Newsweek: Special Report, CXXXIV* (8), 20–51.

Anderson, W. T. (Ed.). (1995). *The truth about the truth: De-confusing and reconstructing the postmodern world.* New York: G. P. Putnam's Sons.

Arrien, A. (1999, July). *The braided way: Universal practices of wisdom.* Paper presented at The Institute of Noetic Sciences' 8th Annual Conference, Lake Buena Vista, Florida.

Astin, J. A. (1998). Why patients use alternative medicine: Results of a national survey. *The Journal of the American Medical Association, 279*(19), 1548–1553.

Beck, R. R. (1996). *Nonviolent story: Narrative conflict resolution in the Gospel of Mark.* Maryknoll, NY: Orbis Books.

Buffett, J., & McAnally, M. (1999). Oysters and Pearls [Recorded by J. Buffett]. *On beach house on the moon* [CD]. Key West, FL: Margaritaville Records.

Christ, C. P. (1980). *Diving deep and surfacing: Women writers on spiritual quest* (2nd ed.). Boston: Beacon Press.

Derrida, J. (1981). *Positions* (A. Bass, Trans.). London: Athlone Press.

Documenting nursing effectiveness by using nursing informatics. (1999, April). The Second Conference on Nursing Diagnoses, Interventions, & Outcomes, New Orleans. Philadelphia: Nursecom, Inc.

Einstein, A. (1993). *Einstein on humanism.* New York: Carol Publishing Group. (Original work published 1950)

Eisenberg, D. M., Davis, R. B., Ettner, S. L., Appel, S., Wilkey, S., Van Rompay, M., & Kessler, R. C. (1998). Trends in alternative medicine use in the United States, 1990–1997: Results of a follow-up national survey. *Journal of the American Medical Association, 280*(18), 1569–1575.

Eisenberg, D. M., Kessler, R. C., Foster, C., Norlack, F. E., Calkins, D. R., & Delbanco, T. L. (1993). Unconventional medicine in the United States: Prevalence, costs, and patterns of use. *New England Journal of Medicine, 328*(4), 246–252.

Fawcett, J. (1984). *Analysis and evaluation of conceptual models of nursing.* Philadelphia: F. A. Davis.

Flaskerud, J. H., & Halloran, E. J. (1980). Areas of agreement in nursing theory development. *Advances in Nursing Science, 3*(1), 1–7.

Foucault, M. (1970). *Archeology of the human sciences* (A. Sheridan-Smith, Trans.). New York: Random House.

Harman, W. W. (1991). *A re-examination of the metaphysical foundations of modern science.* (Causality Issues in Contemporary Science Research Report CP-1). Sausalito, CA: Institute of Noetic Sciences.

Kritek, P. B. (Ed.). (1997). *Reflections on healing: A central nursing construct.* New York: National League for Nursing Press.

Mitchell, E. (1998, July). *Frontier developments in consciousness studies produce new medical advances.* Paper presented at The Institute of Noetic Sciences' 7th Annual Conference, Kansas City, Missouri.

Morganthau, T. (1997, January). The face of the future. *Newsweek,* 58–86.

Myers, T. P. (Ed.). 1999. *The soul of creativity: Insights into the creative process.* Novato, CA: New World Library.

Newman, M. A. (1994). *Health as expanding consciousness* (2nd ed.). New York: National League for Nursing Press.

Nightingale, F. (1946). *Notes on nursing: What it is and what it is not.* New York: Appleton (Original work published 1860)

Russell, M. D. (1996). *The sparrow.* New York: Fawcett Columbine.

Webster's Ninth New Collegiate Dictionary. (1985). Springfield, MA: Merriam-Webster, Inc.

■ *Editor's Questions for Discussion*

What relationship exists between the current status of nursing theory and a philosophy of nursing? What has impeded development of a specific philosophy of nursing? Provide examples of derivative philosophy in nursing. How has derivative philosophy affected nursing scholarship and practice? What examples are available of nursing scholarship being more derivative than creative? Are there examples of nursing combining derivation with creativeness? Suggest creative initiatives for nursing's philosophy of healing practices.

How has gender structuring influenced leadership in nursing? Provide examples other than managed care where gender structuring has had an impact on the role of nursing. As described by Kritek, how are Harman's observations about the science of the future at odds with the science of the present?

What values may engender development of nursing as a science? How important is explication of values in advancing scholarship? What is the difference between postmodernism and postmodernity? What dilemma is evident in nursing regarding postmodernism? Is postmodernism evident in Kritek's explication of the nurse? How might nursing address the questions raised by Kritek about evolving philosophical systems in terms of dimensions of healing? How does Kritek's chapter pertain to those by authors in the Nursing Theory Part of this volume, particularly, with regard to the discussions about philosophical assumptions and reality? How may nursing philosophical systems of nursing be explicated? How do differing philosophical assumptions about reality have an impact on healing and wholeness?

How could the "compact measure called a back rub" have been secured as a nursing healing practice? Provide examples of other healing practices and strategy for establishing them as parts of the nursing domain.

Discuss the impact of globalization and resulting need to address philosophical options in health care. How does Kritek's discussion regarding the patient and health pertain to those of Purnell (Chapter 37) and Snyder, Kreitzer, and Loen (Chapter 43)? How can the philosophical beliefs systems and meaning of health by patients best be ascertained? How may those different belief systems become part of nursing practice? To what extent may it be desirable to quantify varying beliefs for broad consideration and applications in nursing practice?

75

Nursing in the New World of Health Care

A Vision or an Illusion?

Karlene M. Kerfoot,
PhD, RN, CNAA, FAAN

T he future of the profession of nursing cannot be certain. Forces are constantly at work to erode or build up what has been. We sometimes have control over these forces, and sometimes we do not. The only thing certain is that the future holds great change. Nothing will be static. Nursing as we know it today will not exist in the future. To be a viable entity in the years ahead, nursing will need to reinvent itself several times over in order to survive.

■ Nursing History

History shows that the nursing profession has already reinvented itself many times. The pro-

fession started with nurses who were self-employed, working in homes while students provided care in hospitals. With the advent of World War II, nurses moved into hospitals. Then a need for advanced practice nurses resulted in specialist training in administration and clinical nurse specialties. And finally the current movement to prepare nurse practitioners and nurses at the doctoral level has taken nursing in yet another direction. Each of these metamorphoses has not been without conflict. Historically, there was resistance to nurses learning to take blood pressures because it was believed by some not to be within the practice of nursing. Many highly positioned nurses initially resisted the movement to train nurses in physical assessment skills, by claiming that assessment was the domain of medicine and not a part of nursing. As nurses, we have all learned certain mental models (Senge, 1990) or paradigms (Barker, 1993) through which we view our world.

There will always be resistance to change. The history of nursing has been written by valiant nurses who could see a reinvented vision of nursing that they were able to turn into reality. If nursing had stayed in just the arena of home care, other health care workers would have moved into hospitals to fill the void and then on into advanced practice roles. Nurse futurists (although they certainly weren't recognized as futurists at the time) saw a pathway for nursing that was a definite deviation from what was the norm and probably saved nursing from extinction on several occasions.

We face the same danger of extinction today. If the profession of nursing is unable to anticipate future health needs of the population and move in new ways to meet those needs, nursing as we know it will not survive. Other groups will move into the void created by our inability to analyze and meet the needs of our society. Our future as nurses depends on our profession's collective ability to predict the future and to develop continually evolving models that will fit the ever-changing landscape of health care. It will be necessary to consider the essence of our profession in the future and to evolve better ways of serving our constituents (Beckhard & Pritchard, 1992).

■ Predicting the Future

Futurists are people who study the future and develop tools and techniques to aid them in their studies (Bell, 1997; Cornish, 1997). A large part of being a successful leader is possessing the ability to do the kind of long-range thinking and planning that is needed to move to the next level of development. Organizations

that are successful also have this collective ability. If nursing endures as a profession in the future, it will be because of the collective ability of nurses and nursing organizations to develop a view and vision of the future that meshes with the needs of society. The next step is to operationalize that vision, making it a reality.

Futurists cannot always predict the future. In fact, futurists now shy away from linear predictions of the future based on the present. Instead, futurists now are more prone to develop propositions, concepts, and scenarios that articulate a vast array of competing vignettes to prepare people for a future that is essentially unpredictable. Futurists now conceptualize a set of probable and possible scenarios that can become a reality and plan actions around each of these scenarios (Schwartz, 1991). With potential scenarios to consider, a person or organization will not be surprised and blindsided by future events. Scenario planning, as it is called, is done after much research and analysis of trends and also creative brainstorming whereby a person is forced to think "out of the box." Potential scenarios are based on this analysis. Next these scenarios are rated in terms of their probability of happening. Extensive planning activity is then devoted to the most likely scenarios and less planning to the least likely.

For linear thinkers, the temptation is to focus on one of the most plausible scenarios and to plan the future around that one. However, successful companies and leaders pursue many paths at once. They are willing to be wrong because they see inability to guess right as a learning experience. And the more unsettled the situation is, the faster it changes into unpredictable ways. The advantage of planning for several scenarios, even those that seem somewhat ridiculous at the time, is that the planner is not surprised about the future because so many possible scenarios have been considered. With this kind of planning, there are fewer surprises and the future can be addressed in an orderly manner.

Unfortunately, we as nurses are often taught the reductionist method of thinking, which has been the basis of medicine for years. The scientific method and hypothesis testing has ingrained in our thinking the need to find the one best solution, as opposed to several, and to pursue that one solution relentlessly. We also hate to admit failure, and we hate to go back continually and review previous decisions. However, chaos theory, which has been promulgated and popularized by Margaret Wheatly (1992) and others, has drawn our attention to the fact that the world is not necessarily linear. In fact, many things are evolving at once out of what appears to be chaos and volatility but is in reality evolution to different levels of organization.

■ The Tools and Techniques of Futurists

Many corporations invest in extensive research and development activities to ensure viability in the future. Large planning departments are charged with the responsibility of helping their organizations move into the future. Brainstorming possibilities, even those that are totally ridiculous, open thinking and break the box of ordinary considerations of the future. Transprofessional scanning teams look for trends and innovations that might affect the future and often are used to gather information about possibilities. "Fringe" activities also are assessed to determine trends that might become part of the mainstream of human activity. For example, many activities of the 1960s and 1970s "hippies" are now part of the mainstream. Vegetarianism, herbal therapies, yoga, acupuncture, and other activities once promulgated by "flower children" are now validated under the umbrella of complementary or alternative medicine. A futurist doing environmental scanning in the 1970s would have picked up these practices and developed a possible scenario of future acceptance.

We in the profession of nursing have the opportunity to avail ourselves of the tools and techniques of futurists to build our future. We need to develop processes that will help build possible future scenarios for us to consider.

■ Building Scenarios for the Future: The Drivers of Health Care

There are multiple scenarios for our future that we can consider, and there are multiple forces that will drive these scenarios. The drivers of change are many, and the possible scenarios are endless. The drivers of change are not single-focus factors. Multiple drivers can interact to create a mosaic of the future. If we think about many plausible scenarios and then narrow these down to the most likely to occur, we can be prepared for the most probable outcomes and never be really surprised. The following are examples of scenarios that the profession could consider as drivers of future change.

Biotechnology Will Drive Future Change in Health Care

Technology has been the driver of much change in nursing. For example, critical care nursing evolved because of innovations in cardiac and respiratory support that necessitated a nurse with special training to monitor patients and intervene in critical situations. Other specialized areas of nursing such as oncology also have grown because of advanced treatments made possible by advances in technology. That kind of change will be minor compared to the revolutionary changes that will come about with mapping of the human genome. Customized treatments and medicines with genomics as a basis will become the norm.

The science of cloning can potentially create duplication of needed body parts in the future. Growing of a human heart valve is potentially achievable, as is the ability to grow bone and skin grafts. Human aging is likely to be dramatically altered as enzyme breakthroughs and other innovations retard the aging process. Robotic surgery, bio glue that replaces sutures, islet cell transplants, and use of pig organs for transplant are all potentially feasible alternatives. Information technology can provide diagnostic patches and continuous monitoring. The world of telemedicine will bring the most remote place within direct access of the greatest minds in medicine. The list of technological innovations is endless.

If we build a scenario in which technology drives change, what does that mean for the profession of nursing and the individual nurse? Obviously, with this scenario, the education of nurses will need to change drastically to meet the future demand for technologically able nurses. Coursework in genetics and mathematics will be required along with sophisticated information technology competencies. When diagnostic and treatment options of the future are based on the ability to do genetic assessments and manipulations, nursing will have a great opportunity to become prepared to work in these areas. If, in contrast, nurses and nursing organizations do not conceptualize future revolutionary change driven by technological change, people in other disciplines will recognize and fill the void created by nurses' failure to become prepared.

The Political Process Will Drive Health Care

If we track major changes in health care, we find that the political process drives many of them. For example, federal government funding of advanced education for nurses in spe-

cialty areas dramatically changed the landscape of nursing. Medicare opened a whole new world of health care with many subsequent reiterations that changed the way hospitals organized themselves and carried out patient care. The prospective payment system, managed care, and for-profit hospitals all resulted from legislation that was passed by people elected to Congress who believed that they were representing interests of their constituents in legislating these programs.

Many opportunities exist for nurses to be involved in the political process and affect health care and social policy. Many nurses have accepted this responsibility and worked individually with legislators and through professional nursing organizations. Many thousands of other nurses have not and thus have missed opportunities to improve health care. However, if nurses have little interest in and experience with the political process, it is difficult to build scenarios around what can potentially change through governmental influence.

The Republican and Democratic parties have differing views on health care and pass different kinds of legislation when one party or the other is in power. Nurses who are prepared to work in the arena of social policy will be able to help create the desired future for nursing. If nurses are not prepared to work in this area, the profession will be the victim of forces stronger than nursing, which will determine nursing's future.

Costs Will Drive Health Care

The cost of funding health care for employees of companies has become a major issue as profits have eroded and costs of insurance premiums have increased. Businesses in major cities have formed coalitions to negotiate the purchase of health care and to demand that information on quality data be published so that a better informed choice can be made for their employees. With the perceived threat of bankruptcy of the Medicare system, many new programs were initiated to head it off, such as Medicare HMOs. Intense scrutiny of practice patterns of physicians and hospitals has been initiated to eliminate waste and fraud.

If costs are felt to be a significant factor for driving health care, nurses are poorly prepared for this reality. Few curricula require courses in the business side of nursing and health care. Thus many nurses are unprepared to operate in this arena. Many advanced practice nurses have met their demise in health care organizations because they could not speak the language of finance to articulate desired changes and innovations to decision makers. Finance must be seen in the same light as learning the language of medicine or statistics. It is a necessary skill for any level of nurse in the sophisticated future of health care and health care financing.

Information Technologies Will Drive Health Care

The Internet in a very few years has revolutionized the way we do business and how we interact with others. People now have instant access to information about health care. They not only search the Web for information about how to choose their health care professional, but also come armed with volumes of information downloaded from the Internet. The Internet is becoming an electronic web around the earth, with nodes being formed that might in time look almost like the information processing functions of the brain. This electronic web is emerging much like an ecosystem evolves. In time, we might see a complex web of the earth's activity linked with many inputs and outputs that potentially function as the human system does, to warn of danger and to take action automatically. If quantum computers that can escape the rule-based activity of present computers become a reality, we also will see the advent of artificial intelligence. And then, if nanotechnology (science of things smaller than billionths of

a meter) becomes a reality, the possibilities for miniaturized machines that can perform in an artificial intelligence mode are endless.

With this scenario, we can begin to see how information technology may become the central infrastructure around which almost all our activity in health care and outside health care could be handled. If we in nursing ignore this scenario, implications for the future of the profession are enormous. It begins to beg the question about what is appropriate preparation for the beginning nurse and the advanced nurse. It is very difficult to teach entry-level competencies to ensure that the new nurse will be a safe practitioner in 2 years. With the overlay of information technology, it will become even more difficult to prepare the new nurse in 2 years. Other implications also revolve around this scenario, such as preparation of nurses to be leaders in the information technology evolution and building this technology around needs of the patient.

Other Scenarios

Many other scenarios might be considered. The following are just a few.

- Democratization of leadership will occur with loss of the leader as superhero and the necessity to move to brighter and more courageous self-managed teams (Bennis, 1989; DePree, 1997).

- Spirituality will evolve into new forms that take on intimate meaning for people on the journey of the soul. The workplace will be expected to be a place where the soul can grow.

- Consumers of health care will demand to be given quality data about their health care provider and will demand public disclosure of outcomes in order to make informed choices about health care.

- Accountability in medicine and nursing will be elevated to new heights and "zero defects" in the delivery of care will be expected.

The list of scenarios is endless. This brief discussion of scenarios is meant only to introduce the process of scenario planning, as used by futurists to anticipate the future and prepare for it. Scenarios provide possible "stories" of the future that we as nurses need to consider. Germane to all these scenarios is the infrastructure of the nursing profession that must be capable of coping with a future that is uncertain and essentially unpredictable.

■ *The Profession of Nursing: Vision or Illusion in the New World of Health Care*

A strong, well-articulated infrastructure for considering the future and consequent decision-making is essential. Many organizations visualize their preferred futures through the strategic planning process, which often includes the use of scenarios and other mechanisms that we have discussed. As we consider scenarios for nursing's future, we must address issues that must be resolved if we are to be successful in coping with whatever challenges nursing will be called upon to face.

Shared Vision

No organization can survive if there is no consensus about a shared vision for that organization. Without a shared vision, activity takes place in many disconnected forms that waste energy and create disillusionment among staff. It is impossible to believe in the organization unless you can believe in the values and direction that it is taking.

There are some very fine examples of shared vision for several nursing organizations. The American Association of Critical-Care Nursing (AACN) has a strongly shared vision that is totally supported by the membership. This vision drives strategic and tactical efforts of the organization and has created a successful organization that produces worthy outcomes. Sigma Theta Tau is another example of excellence in this area, and we could add several more to the list. But where is the shared vision for the profession of nursing?

Unfortunately, the vision for nursing is fragmented among approximately 80 nursing organizations that have their own perspectives of nursing. No overall vision has been articulated and agreed upon as a guiding light for the new millennium. As a result, all too often there is lack of synergy between organizations and lack of clear direction for the future of nursing. To survive as a viable entity in the future, connectedness within nursing is essential. The following topics are offered as "food for thought" for considering the infrastructure that we need to develop to deal with various scenarios of the future.

■ *Is There a Future for Nursing Administration and Leadership?*

Leadership, either negative or positive, formal or informal is perhaps the strongest variable in predicting the future of an organization. Nursing leadership at the executive level is undergoing great change in many health care organizations. Many nurses are moving on to chief executive officer (CEO) positions in health care organizations, but others are still hoping to be admitted to the executive's strategic planning meetings. Nurses have not been always supportive of nursing leaders who step out of the mold and leave the bedside for other positions. Often these people are said to have "left nursing," when in reality they have the potential to do more for nursing in their broadened position of influence.

Factors

A critical success factor for nursing's future will be our ability to maintain unity among nurses and between nurses and nurse leaders. Unfortunately, with the advent of nurses joining unions, an adversarial relationship between nurses and their leaders has become common. Nursing leadership must take responsibility for the gulf between nurses that has occurred—but so must nurses. We cannot go forward productively when our allegiances are not to each other and to a vision of synergy and excellence.

Role Variations

Will nursing leaders lead nursing in health care facilities, or will these positions be taken over by nonnurses? The future role of the nurse executive is not clear at this time. In some organizations, the nurse executive does not have line authority but serves as a staff person to others in the organization to whom nursing reports. In a product-line organization, the nursing staff will report to the administrator of that product line, a specialized area of practice such as neuroscience or orthopedics, for example. That product-line administrator may or may not be a nurse and most often is not. In other organizations, the bulk of nurses will report to the nurse executive, but nurses in certain departments, such as radiology, may not.

Is there an ideal structure for the future nursing leader in an organization? There really is no an ideal. A few years ago the nurse executive was responsible only for nursing. Now that person commonly also has responsibility for other patient care areas. The successful nursing leader of the future who is reading this chapter now is beginning to think of the many possible scenarios that will exist and the many ways of becoming prepared to serve in the reengineered roles of the future. The traditional role of leader in a specific position is certainly a possibility. But leadership opportunities exist throughout health care in nontraditional roles where the influence of a nursing leader can be felt and valued.

Preparation

What will be the necessary preparation for nursing leaders in the future? The scenarios presented, if they are viable, begin to delineate the preparation that these leaders will need. Financial management, sophisticated knowledge of quality, and customer relations will be among the additional tools that the nursing leader will need to manage effectively in the future.

Will nursing leaders be influential in the arena of health care in the future? Nurses are particularly well positioned to take a leadership role because of their broad education and varied experiences in health care. But many scenarios of the future are already being played out wherein nurses are not involved. Boards of companies that own managed care organizations, health care system boards, pharmaceutical companies, and political processes at the federal, state, and local levels need the expertise of nurses. Advocacy groups such as the American Association of Retired Persons (AARP) would be enriched by the leadership of nurses.

■ Systems Thinking and Synergy

Systems thinking makes us aware that the whole is greater than the parts and that a change in one part of the system creates reactions elsewhere in the organism. If we think of the nursing profession as an organism that operates as a system, we can start to conceptualize the profession as an entity that has a shared vision and does the work of the system effortlessly. For example, a cow operates as a system, rather than as individual, compartmentalized parts. No one part is more important than another to the working of the cow. We cannot think of cutting off the tail without also realizing dramatic consequences for the cow's ability to keep insects at bay. And the cow does not need to get permission from the leg to send blood to the stomach to accomplish digestion when that becomes a priority for the cow's survival.

For the profession of nursing to be successful in the future, systems thinking is essential. Needs of nurse practitioners are different from those of nurses working in home care. However, if the profession were synergized around nursing's strategic direction as it relates to society, the profession could easily determine a strategic direction and operate as a system— not a collection of independent parts. Our present system of operating as independent organizations will be a detriment to our future.

Synergy within nursing is mandatory if we are to meet the needs of society and the community. Synergy does not come naturally. It must be adopted as a value of all nurses and all nursing organizations. Synergy can and must be taught. Unfortunately "nurse autonomy" has been in vogue the past few years. We can only wonder how different our profession would be if concepts of systems thinking and synergy were taught in schools of nursing.

Merger mania has been the watchword of many organizations and corporations in the past decade. Merging has been heralded as the way for organizations to save costs, focus on strategic direction, and operate efficiently and effectively. That movement has not yet struck nursing's professional organizations. We have increased rather than decreased the number of organizations and potentially increased inefficiency of operations while having to pass that cost along to dues-paying members. We need connective leaders for the future. As Lipman-Blumen (1996) describes in *The Connective Edge,* we need leaders who can build bridges between disparate groups and help organizations achieve synergism around a shared vision.

Synergizing with Other Health Care Providers

Nursing cannot survive as an independent entity in the complexity of health care in the future, and neither can other disciplines. Professions in health care work fairly well together at the bedside, but dialogue and synergistic planning are not there on the national level. For the good of society, synergistic operating models must be developed not only at the point of service to the consumer of health care, but also at the national level.

We are not as prepared to work with other professions as we might be. We have been surpassed educationally by almost all other professions, and we are earning the dubious distinction of being the least educated profession in health care. Creating peer relationships and synergistic models is difficult when we are the only profession that has reduced the amount of time required for entry into practice. We have moved from a 3-year diploma program to a 2-year Associate Degree requirement for entry into practice. While we have been doing that, pharmacists have moved to a PharmD degree for entry into practice; physical therapists to a 5-year program; social workers to a master's degree, and the list goes on. Creating synergy and peer relations with other organizations that require a college degree plus extra requirements is difficult when we do not. If we want peer relationships, we have to address the fact that other professions have raised their levels for entry into practice, but we have not.

Becoming Customer-Driven

We as a profession have done fairly well organizing care around the needs and demands of our patients and their families. However, we could serve other customers better if we had the organization to do so. Payors, employers, and other health care professionals are all consumers of health care, but we have given little thought to organizing care around demands of these customers. We have very successful models of nurse entrepreneurs who have identified needs, filled these voids, and built businesses on their discoveries. However, there is much left to do as a profession to truly organize around needs of many stakeholders and consumers of health care.

■ Demanding Excellence and Accountability for the Quality of Nursing Outcomes

The profession of medicine has come under much scrutiny and criticism for the variance between the number of physicians, the types of medicine they practice, and the geographic distribution of their practice (Millenson, 1997). Only a short time will transpire before that same scrutiny is focused on nurses. In the meantime we have the opportunity to address variability among nurses in practice and to demand excellence from each and every one. Profiling of outcomes of physicians is now common practice, but we have not yet determined how to profile outcomes of nurses. However, we must do so to guarantee the best outcomes to our constituency. We must be willing to settle only for evidence-based practice and to develop measurement systems that can provide data about variability of outcomes among nurses. We must insist that the educational level and preparation of our profession is such that it can rise to this challenge and guarantee our constituents only the best care that is grounded in research. Each nurse must be practicing in a "best practice" modality at all times to fulfill a commitment of excellence to our constituents.

■ Addressing the "Brain Drain" in Nursing

"Where have all the nurses gone?" is a frequent cry as we enter yet another cycle of nursing shortages. However, predictions for this shortage are more dire than that for others, as the aging workforce in practice and education moves on to different pastures. The lack of interest in nursing as a profession and an inability to recruit the best and brightest should be of monumental concern to our nation and to each one of us. If this problem is not solved, we can assume that nursing will not exist in the future as it has in the past and the health care of the nation will suffer.

Brain drain and the nursing shortage are beyond what nursing alone can fix. We as a profession certainly can do our part by raising educational requirements and building programs that compete with other professions for desirability. However, that is not enough. We need to work with a variety of stakeholders to determine long-term solutions for the future. For example, the American Hospital Association, American Medical Association, and nursing leaders need to address quality of life in hospitals as an issue of recruitment and retention. Fatigue and stress in pilots and long-distance truck drivers have been cited as causes of accidents. Consequently, specified limits for flying or driving are mandated. However, nurses and other health care professionals are rewarded for working excessive amounts of overtime when patient safety could be at stake. Governmental and health care leaders also can address the problem of a rapidly aging population that faces care provided by a cadre of fewer and less highly educated nurses. Planning to avoid shortages in nursing must be seen as an ongoing task and not something that happens only when a critical shortage occurs. We in nursing cannot solve this brain drain alone.

The issue remains though, "Who is nursing?" Who speaks for the approximately 80 nursing organizations that have no mechanism of consensus building? Who speaks for thousands of nurses who reject the responsibilities of belonging to and working within a professional organization? We must have one strong voice for nursing that represents all of nursing as we enter this millennium. Who will be that strong voice that will sit at the table with other entities to make the future of health care what it needs to be?

■ Concluding Statement

As the health care futurist Leland Kaiser (1999) has said, "The future is between our ears." In his view, we have created everything that troubles our society today. In his view, we have created crime, pollution, and hunger and only we, by coming together in communities, can overcome them and create healthy communities. Rather than being a victim of the future, Kaiser believes that, intentionally, we can create our own realities and our own futures. What we pay attention to determines our future.

We have a great opportunity through "intention-ality" to create a future for the profession of nursing that will beget a healthy, fulfilled future for our society and for those we serve in sickness and in health. However, this future won't happen without systems thinking, planning, and synergizing with those whom we serve. We cannot serve our constituents when we as a profession are divided into many isolated organizations that lack connectedness of purpose and an ability to act together for the good of society. Nor can we serve our constituencies without being synergizing with our peers in other professions. "Nurse autonomy" is an outmoded idea that needs to be replaced with concepts of synergy and accountability. We are at a crossroads now, and we need to demand nothing less than excellence from ourselves and those with whom we work. We must be willing to stand for a new level of practitioner and more sophisticated levels of accountability to create the desired future for our society.

We can imagine many scenarios for our future and, through "intention-ality," make the most desirable ones happen. However, we cannot do it alone. We need full support of all nurses in all nursing organizations, connectedness with other professions that will create synergy, and a mandate to synergize with our constituents. The future is ours for the making.

■ References

Barker, J. (1993). *Discovering the future: The business of paradigms*. New York: Harper Business.

Beckhard, R., & Pritchard, W. (1992). *Changing the essence: The art of creating and leading fundamental change in organizations*. San Francisco: Jossey-Bass.

Bell, W. (1997). *Foundation of futures studies: Human science for a new era*. New Brunswick, NJ: Transaction.

Bennis, W. (1989). *On becoming a leader*. Reading, MA: Addison-Wesley.

Cornish, E. (1997). *The study of the future*. Washington, DC: World Future Society.

DePree, M. (1997). *Leading without power*. San Francisco: Jossey-Bass.

Kaiser, L. (1999). *Lecture*. Houston, TX: Hermann Hospital/Memorial Hermann Healthcare System.

Lipman-Blumen, J. (1996). *The connective edge, leading in an interdependent world*. San Francisco: Jossey-Bass.

Millenson, M. (1997). *Demanding medical excellence*. Chicago: University of Illinois Press.

Schwartz, P. (1991). *The art of the long view*. New York: Doubleday.

Senge, P. (1990). *The fifth discipline: The art and practice of the learning organization*. New York: Doubleday/Currency.

Wheatley, M. (1992). *Leadership and the new science*. San Francisco: Berrett-Koehler.

■ Editor's Questions for Discussion

Define forces that erode nursing as a profession. What interventions may diminish those forces? How might "scenario planning" for the future prepare the profession for change and survival? By whom and how may scenario planning be done? Project scenarios about the nursing profession with regard to nursing education and practice. Provide examples of the impact of biotechnology on future nursing practice and nursing education. How may nursing best prepare for future scenarios such as those presented by Kerfoot? What specific implications for nursing education exist in the scenarios? What evidence is available regarding plausibility of the scenarios?

What forces bring a political process into being? Provide examples of how nursing could have intervened politically in issues but has not. How might you as a professional become involved in the political process to affect the future of health care?

Define shared vision as it is held by individual nursing organizations. How may nursing develop a shared vision for the profession? What role can nursing organizations as a whole play in promoting a shared vision for the profession? How can systems thinking and synergy, as presented by Kerfoot, be applied to professional associations, as discussed by Thompson and Lavandero (Chapter 9)? How does Kerfoot reinforce issues identified by Sills and Anderson (Chapter 77)?

Discuss strategies for improving relationships between nurses and their leaders. What factors influence role variation for nursing executives? How might nurse executives shape their role? What relationships are there between the ideas presented by Kerfoot and those of McClure (Chapter 62)? Discuss essential preparation for nursing leaders of the future.

76

Looking to the Future of Academic Administrative Leadership

Joan L. F. Shaver, PhD, RN, FAAN

Leadership is on the tip of many tongues in American culture and particularly those associated with health care. The collective voice calls for more effective leadership, but why such an emphasis at this point in time? The answer is "speed of change." Leaders who could provoke and sustain gradual forward movement in relatively stable or slow growth periods often seem diminished in the context of rapidly evolving interconnected systems. Nowhere is change more evident than in health care. For a clinical practice discipline such as nursing, orchestrating productivity in concert with the changing face of health care delivery presents a major challenge to academic leaders.

Health care delivery venues are shifting to integrated health systems, away from fragmented and disconnected health care institutions; and to home and community sites, away from tertiary hospitals. The shift in nurse practitioner and physician practices is to group and multidisciplinary practices aligned with health care systems, away from individual, unaligned practices. The shift in health care financing is toward managed care for large groups of people on a prospective per person pay rate, away from individual fee-for-service payments. The shift in financing is toward providing incentives for preventing disease and promoting health—values long held by nursing but only minimally actualized historically—away from tertiary care and curing of disease. Generated by these changes, windows of opportunities have opened for the expansion of nursing practice into venues more autonomous than institutional bureaucracy and into care domains beyond disease care. Encompassed are practice opportunities that allow advanced practice nurses to sustain relationships better with clients or patients. The benefits of sustained health care include making superb nursing practice more recognizable by clients and patients and more satisfying for clinicians.

Although the preceding changes represent the current context of health care, even more sweeping changes are likely to ensue. Although the nature of future changes is difficult to foresee in detail, the onus is on academic nursing leaders to align education and research endeavors to fit emerging environments and to shape future practice realities. In this chapter, I outline my views pertaining to the short-run and longer-run potential changes affecting academic administration. I discuss (a) currently evolving environments, (b) features of new-age environments as the context for academic nursing leadership, (c) personal capabilities that make for generative leaders, and (d) skills required for leading-edge leadership in possible courses of change. Intuitively, it seems that effective leader capabilities for the future, regardless of whether practiced in academia or other settings, will be those that are effective today. Futuristic aspects of leadership pertain to (a) predicting and shaping the environments in which leaders engage those capabilities and (b) determining which leadership skills to utilize at various points in time.

■ Evolving Environments: Trends Affecting Academic Leadership

The paradigm shift in health care delivery to more primary and less tertiary care, with a resurgence of nurse practitioner focus and an aging nursing workforce, underlie important contemporary changes needed in academia. Certainly, explosion of information technologies and the societal pressures for more productivity and accountability from academia in general also are remodeling the landscape for academic nursing leaders. These features create both opportunities and demands to conduct academic endeavors more creatively than in the past.

Primary Care—The Nurse Practitioner Emphasis

The shift to more primary-based from tertiary-based care rapidly has reinforced the nurse practitioner type of practice (Marion, 1996), with opportunities for nurses to deliver primary care and practice outside traditional institutional and community venues. Graduate educational institutions have met this market demand through rapid expansion of nurse practitioner (NP) programs. Expanded NP education has placed greater demands on accessing primary care sites for education and has increased the clinical practice hours in many graduate education programs. Alternatively, the preceptor model of education has been strengthened, fostering more and closer connections between academia and the direct practice community.

The shift to NP education has provoked radical change in the "faculty mix" within academic nursing. Quickly, the complement of faculty in schools and colleges with master's degree programs seemed mismatched to the learning needs of NP graduate students; thus hiring NP faculty or retooling faculty for NP practice became an intense activity. In research-intensive institutions, the need for practice-intensive faculty in teaching programs competed with the need for research-intensive faculty. In the process, marketplace salaries for NPs put pressure on academia to elevate the salaries for those teaching clinical practica.

The surge in NP education and practice has accelerated the movement within academia to develop model practice sites whereby nursing values could reign and nursing faculty could integrate teaching, practice, and research. The fostering of such sites has led many academic nursing leaders to concentrate on expanding the "direct" clinical practice enterprise of the school or college and to obtain a new revenue source in some cases. Putting infrastructure in place for the delivery of care services in a rapidly changing health care system is a major challenge for administrators. That infrastructure includes the capacity to (a) find sites, (b) assess risk, (c) plan clinical services, (d) create quality control and resources utilization processes, (e) bill for services, (f) document care, (g) develop and evaluate practice models or protocols, (h) partner with community agencies, and (i) enter into solid contractual agreements based on mutual benefits. Clearly, a huge window of opportunity has opened for innovative academic administrators to envision, implement, and test new nursing and multidisciplinary practice models (Marion, 1997). At the same time, these dynamics have necessitated deeper understanding of the business elements of practice on the part of academic leaders.

Although trends have created opportunities to practice nursing more autonomously from physicians and institutions, evidence indicates that the majority of advanced practice nurses have retained an alignment with them. Physician-led groups and clinics are increasingly cognizant of the potential for NPs to expand practice in cost-effective ways, but NPs are predominantly hired into practices as employees. Nurses apparently either are not successful at or do not desire to negotiate "partner" status within clinical practices. To do so would require creating a cost-effective practice with an opportunity for sharing in profits—but also risk sharing in liability for deficits. Avoiding these challenges prevents nurses from creating delivery mechanisms that allow more "say in" or control over practice. Perhaps too little education regarding health care financing and practice management is given to NPs to motivate their engaging in partnered practice. It behooves academic leaders to incorporate dimensions of these aspects of health care into professional practice education.

Education for Practice

Education at the entry level has been affected by health care system delivery changes as well. Conventionally, the major site for experiential clinical learning for entry-level students has been hospitals, accessed mostly through direct alignment or contractual agreements with academic institutions. Community-based sites are complementary to hospital-based sites. Pressure to shift care from the most costly form (i.e., hospital tertiary care) and the closing and size reductions of hospitals has reduced clinical teaching capacity. Reengineering of tertiary care and the doing more-with-less phenomenon has reduced the motivation to facilitate education. The expansion of ambulatory and home care creates potential clinical education sites, but capacity varies. These practice domains are subject to economic pressures that lead to the avoidance of accepting educational responsibilities (American Association of Colleges of Nursing [AACN], 1999).

The trends just enumerated compel academic administrative leaders to develop novel ways of maintaining or expanding access to clinical practice sites, either for entry or advanced practice levels. Doing so means forming partnerships with newly merged organizations and in new and different ways than in the past or creating faculty practice sites. Opportunities to access practice sites in integrated health systems abound, but the task of persuading agencies to connect with educational institutions for value added is a challenge. Faculty practice sites allow new models to be envisioned and tested. This process promotes integration of nursing education, practice, and research, although it requires an infusion of energy to conduct academic programs as a business and assume the inherent risks. Clinical practice in community-based domains (e.g., health centers and schools) means accommodating fewer students at single sites and generating creative ways to provide faculty guidance over dispersed sites.

Nurses—An Aging Workforce

Statistics reveal that the current mean age of employed registered nurses is 42.3 years and that in the next 10 to 15 years, more than half the nursing workforce will be eligible to retire (Buerhaus & Staiger, 1999). At the same time, the U.S. population is getting older. Chronic illness care and functional status retention will expand the areas for which nurses are crucial. Movement to better salaries in practice and more options for practice already are luring individuals away from an academic nursing career and the study of nursing science. Further, academic nursing leaders currently are being challenged in recruiting research-intensive faculty.

Within the next decade, nursing leaders must market the profession as a career with wide-ranging, lifelong professional opportunities and satisfactions. In a statewide Illinois event called *The Power of Nursing Leadership,* we profile the extraordinary ways in which nurses are helping shape the health care system, citing leadership roles in health systems, academia, public health, corporations, professional associations, and entrepreneurship. The notion thus is conveyed that nurses practice across a surprisingly wide range of venues and that nursing represents one of the most versatile professions in health care. Academic nursing leaders need to engage in motivational recruitment for those choosing a career—to urge that nursing be considered for its true,

although mostly unrecognized, potential and to overcome stereotypical views of nursing as practice only at the bedside in a hospital. Although this latter view is an image not to be discounted, it represents only where about half of all nurses practice and less than that for where nurses with higher education degrees practice. Students who have selected nursing as their major deserve to see the nursing practice of tomorrow. The practice of tomorrow stands poised to go beyond the face-to-face and even the one-on-one patient and client encounters of today.

Information Technologies

One profound dynamic of today that will influence nursing practice and education of tomorrow clearly is the explosion of information technology. Current satellite and digital technologies allow information to be transmitted rapidly across boundless distances. On the practice side, informational technologies are allowing care delivery through telehealth. Many of today's disease management companies (e.g., for congestive heart failure) have sites where nurses are providing monitoring, surveillance, coaching, and guidance services to patients at home over the telephone.

Development of more convenient computer-based imaging and camera devices will allow video diagnosis and monitoring of health status in the home, as well as enhance coaching from a distance for adherence to treatment regimens. For example, patients placed on nasal continuous positive airway pressure (CPAP) ventilator breathing for sleep apnea could be monitored at home by cameras that allow nurse coaching by video for proper self-administration of the CPAP over the course of adapting to the therapy. Physiological monitoring devices are being tested for certain measures (e.g., body weight or blood pressure). They are capable of transducing analog to digital data and are fitted for modem transmission of data into health providers' (usually nurses') offices. Nurses long have been found to be proficient in case management of patient groups for effective use of resources in health systems, but the mechanisms and modalities through which this will be done will change dramatically with rapidly evolving information technologies.

On the education side, Internet-based technologies allow learning encounters to occur at will between teachers and students. Virtual educational institutions that deliver education to vast numbers of students without ever seeing them in traditional classrooms now exist. Such types of education are threatening to eclipse the traditional bricks and mortar institutions of higher learning in providing education to the masses—anywhere, anytime. The concept of virtual nursing degrees granted entirely through distance learning may seem remote—but is it? Distance learning also can solve some access issues in clinical field experiences.

Intuition would dictate that, in a professional practice discipline, active field work is required for at least part of the curriculum. Although it is difficult to envision nursing practica done by teacher guidance from afar, health care is being delivered in such a manner and the same modalities are applicable for education. Ability to televise student practice would eliminate on-site faculty oversight. Furthermore, greater dispersion of student learning sites demands futuristic ways of helping students prepare for practica (e.g., creative simulations in learning laboratories via virtual reality).

Beyond teaching and learning, the information technology explosion is changing the face of other academic work by highlighting data repositories. The creation and linking of large health-related databases are allowing scientists to mine vast amounts of data regarding groups of individuals and understand more about their health and the context of their lives in relation to health. Design of health care records, as documentation of health care encounters, has been dominated by medical practice values and less by nursing practice values. The importance of understanding the context in which patients are sick or well is increasing, and nursing professionals bear responsibility for expanding health information models to embrace a broader view. Integrating taxonomies within emergent health care documentation is essential. Examples of such taxonomies include the Nursing Interventions Classification (NIC) or Nursing Outcomes Classification (NOC) (McCloskey & Bulechek, 1996), Community Health Classifications Systems (Martin & Scheet, 1992; Saba, 1997), or an agreed upon minimum nursing data set with multidisciplinary data sets (Simpson, 1996).

In the future, academic administrators will have to reengineer educational programs to accommodate and extend the use of information technologies to nursing education and practice. Creation of infrastructure to provide increasingly more capacity for computer-based and distance learning and provision of experiential learning in the realm of telehealth are pertinent goals. Such development would give the concept of learning centers or skill centers a whole new meaning. These areas should provide access to learning modalities that represent the most advanced stages of knowledge linkage, clinical simulation, and real-system mimicry. Thus students can avoid being placebound and can learn anytime, anyplace. The necessity to educate nursing generalists or specialists remains important, including generation and manipulation of standardized data elements (including financial ones) relevant to nursing practice and health care systems by means of state-of-the-art information technologies.

Demands for Accountability

Societal demands for more productivity accountability is affecting academia in general. Greater proportions of budgets for nursing institutions come from special projects, federal, state, and foundation grants, and individual or corporate gifts; leaders in many of these institutions thus consider their universities to be state-assisted rather than state-subsidized. Even though the proportion of education paid by tuition or government subsidy has been dropping steadily, those who provide revenues to higher education, especially legislators, students, and financial backers, are increasingly watchful and critical of faculty productivity. The public now expects higher education to prepare individuals for productive economic lives. Academic administrators increasingly are being held accountable for fiscal health and discipline practicality.

In some universities, models with labels such as responsibility-center or value-center management or budgeting have been adopted to encourage efficient and entrepreneurial fiscal management (Whalen, 1991). These management models for academic units generally have involved clearer attributions of income (i.e., tuition), as well as costs, by individual academic unit. The amount of subsidy to various programs then is revealed. Academic administrators of the future will experience continuing pressures to be financial and business managers. The high cost of nursing education as a professional practice discipline has spawned movement toward generation of new income streams (e.g., outreach professional development education, consultation, and direct practice). Generating venture capital for growth will come from the creativity of shifting resources from less efficient or obsolete endeavors to seeking new income sources.

■ Environments: New-Age Systems

That the health care enterprise will continue to represent a solid percentage of our gross domestic product, at least in the near future, seems evident. However, in a new age, various contextual factors can be envisioned that may change the landscape for academic administration. Examples of salient factors include (a) demographics of the population, (b) growth of biomedical science, (c) organizational and professional convergence and merging, and (d) intrapreneurship within organizations. Academic leaders need to monitor these factors and make academic endeavors synchronous with or enhance these factors.

■ Population Demographics

In the foreseeable future, the U.S. population will reflect a rapidly growing number of older adults, making chronic illness care and enhancement of functional status more prominent. Moreover, evolving ethnocultural diversity of faculty, students, patients, and clients will continue to exert pressures for developing learning and health care delivery climates that are multicultural in nature. The near future of academic administrative leadership will have to involve integrating programs of teaching, research, and practice around chronic illness management and geriatric therapeutics for ethnoculturally diverse groups. However, with a longer time frame, it is conceivable that genetic engineering and molecular biological advances will (a) halt or slow the aging process, (b) all but eradicate chronic illness, and (c) put more health care emphases on health and growth versus disease and aging. Further, while we now emphasize and seek culturally relevant care delivery, various global economic trends could diminish the emphasis on diversity over time. Although highly speculative, worldwide information access, government and religious reforms, common language, and currency adoptions might modify the trend toward more cultural differences. These processes may move us in the direction of more cultural homogeneity and thus reform care delivery yet again.

Biomedical Science Growth

The contemporary expansion of biomedical science in the direction of genetics molecular biology and advances in immune manipulation have begun to affect practice, education, and research. Outcomes include major transplant technology applications and transplant specialty nursing. Developing genetic counseling and specialists in gene therapy and ethicists in the field of genetics has begun and is worthy of further considerations for academia. Perhaps the future holds that human beings will be engineered genetically and that the role of nurses might be to coach parents on design of their offspring or to help people adapt to newly engineered bodies, minds, or brains. If so, harvesting cells and providing protective growth environments for transplanted tissues will be necessary activities. The ethical impact of such science could spawn a whole new realm of practice for controlling exploitation.

Corollary to today's biomedical advances is the expansion of complementary and alternative therapies. In the short run, nurses are, and in greater numbers should be, developing expertise in natural therapies (i.e., noninvasive and nonpharmacological), such as deep relaxation, exercise, massage, music, nutritional, herbal, and multisensory therapies. Stress-related illness is common and behavioral intervention fits with the root values of nursing. In the long run, genetically driven therapeutics and health-enhancing behaviors might ameliorate the consequences of certain diseases, but, additionally, modifications to home and work environments so that they become less "toxic" and more growth-enhancing will cause many illnesses and diseases to disappear. Future therapies might be more focused on environmental modifications rather than on person modifications in health therapeutics. As these therapies evolve, so should health care curricula in order to reflect emerging practice trends.

Converging and Merging Institutions

On today's horizon, the growth of health care and nursing education in whatever form will not take place in isolation but increasingly will be accomplished through organizational and professional collaborations and mergers. Multi- and interdisciplinary initiatives will be established firmly as the norm. Pooling of intellectual, spiritual, and financial capital through connecting people and organizations is a powerful way to create change. Presently, the convergence and merging of organizations is most striking among health systems, and though evident, it promises to become an increasing eventuality in education. Over time, we will see the melding of hospital-based, community college–based and university-based nursing education entities. Costs of higher education and reductions in resources (including the threat of not having enough star faculty) mandate the need for mergers.

A longer horizon might reflect the eventual obliteration of institutions and disciplines, as we now know them, with a matched reform of education. Picture the following reengineering of current health care activities. Primary care advanced practice nurses are incorporated into a single health care generalist practitioner role that is a merger of positions now labeled NP, primary care physician, physicians assistant, and perhaps others. Primary care encompasses cradle-to-grave health monitoring and promotion with surveillance for disease or illness in individuals. This approach marries the knowledge related to the mind to that of the body and generates an altered scientific research emphasis. It also encompasses interventions that shape health behavior for optimizing functional status, be it physical, emotional, social, or spiritual. Personal health care generalists deliver such care with referrals to health care specialists for extraordinary health challenges. Health care specialties are derived according to realms of therapies such as pharmacological, surgical, genetic, nutritional, herbal, stress management, body manipulation, mind manipulation, touch, exercise, and other lifestyle therapies, rather than by body organ systems or diseases. Additionally, population-based health care specialists would work to assess challenges to health emanating within or from environmental (system) contexts such as workplaces, climates, or biospheres. Probably systems-level interventions such as temperature or sensory input controlled environments would be prescribed or integrative care sites would be developed that offer the various realms of therapies.

Eventually, we might see well-integrated health care delivery systems, well-integrated health educational systems, and well-integrated health care disciplines—perhaps integrated across all three domains (i.e., education, practice, and research). Regardless of whether these are the directions of change or how fast they might be accomplished if they are, leaders who can promote integration and determine how to achieve distinction among leading organizations will excel. Irrespective of the categories of health care providers who are to be educated in the future, to-date unimagined technologies will allow learning to be accessed from anywhere—perhaps even outer space, under the sea, or in derived biospheres—and data will be linked from a vast array of sources. The creation of education that is fluid and flexible in time, place, and expectations and that is technologically current has now and will become increasingly imperative. The ability to create a niche and market flexible programs that have a high potential fit with what consumers want will expand in importance, as a basis for new system and provider success.

Intrapreneurship

The spirit of change is most definitely seen in highly imaginative individuals. Creating infrastructure (e.g., think tanks, coaching groups, and creativity circles) that gives inno-

vators the freedom to create and test ideas is rudimentary for organizational achievement. Encouraging intrapreneurship within organizations, be it multi- or interdisciplinary or completely different from what exists, will maximize successful academic leadership. Small entrepreneurial companies are said to produce about 20 times as many innovations per research and development dollar as do large corporations (Ferris, 1987). Leaders in large organizations, including academia, must assess and reduce the barriers to capitalizing on entrepreneurial bents. Generating environments in which individuals feel free to experiment and innovate is a mark of generative leadership.

■ Personal Capabilities of Generative Leaders

Leadership excellence in any field is predicated on universal general capabilities (style and skills) that will likely endure through time. In a general sense, academic nursing leaders are accountable for positioning their organizations to influence health care systems through academic pursuits. Fundamentally, the capabilities for doing so encompass having a vision based on analytical environmental scanning and deciding strategically on direction, ends, and means to the ends. Masterminding innovations then is necessary, using skills to enable individuals and groups to create action plans for moving in novel directions or ways (strategic implementation). Leadership is not about power—it is about having influence or perhaps the power of influence. Therefore how a leader engages with people to shape and enable behavioral change is what really creates influence. A recently suggested definition of leadership is: "Leadership is the art of engaging with people to envision and enable the creation of desired futures." (N. Langston & J. Shaver, coauthors, in personal communication with each other, 1999). We can expect that change will drive an urgency to develop leaders and understand the essence of effective leadership.

Developing Leaders

The current hype about leadership is evident in an expanding array of leadership development opportunities sponsored by professional organizations of all types. In one initiative, sponsored by the American Nurses Foundation and Academy of Nursing with the American Nurses Association, several interesting elements about nursing leadership emanated from a set of activities completed under subcontract to the University of Illinois at Chicago (UIC) College of Nursing (American Academy of Nursing/American Nurses Foundation [AAN/ANF], 1998). As part of this effort, staff at Health Care Resources of Rochester, New York, asked health care executives who work with or hire nurses how they perceived nurses as leaders (AAN/ANF, 1998, Appendix II). The UIC nursing faculty also convened an expert panel with leaders from both inside and outside nursing to discuss leadership.

Many of the surveyed health care executives believed nursing education to be more like training than education and that more emphasis on developing analytical ability, critical thinking, and judgment should be incorporated into nursing education. Although nurses were thought to have developed leadership skills, they were not perceived to apply them outside clinical nursing practice. Most executives revealed that their own personal style was directive but saw nurses as focused on process. These executives saw nurses as insular, wanting to have their value noticed without having to advocate on their own behalf, rigid, lacking flexibility in communication and leadership styles, averse to risk, and overly hierarchical.

The panel of experts convened as part of the project were leaders representative of academia (emeritus business school dean), health and law, philanthropy, a physician women's organization, government (nurse and a congresswoman), and health systems (nurse). These experts categorized the highest leadership characteristics in a set as having a defined sense of purpose and vision, a broad perspective beyond the individual's own organization, and being able to take risks. According to the panel, this last concept implied doing things differently or trying new things, but it also connoted the potential for tolerating unacceptable negative outcomes, especially if the outcomes involved a high financial impact (AAN/ANF, 1998). In my view, most people are likely to think of a course of action as a risk mainly if there is fear of failure. Helping people avoid a fear of failure and see a course of action as a test or a trial could help them deal with change. Most courses of action can be corrected while being tested. When that test or trial is truly creative, it is an innovation. In this vein, strong leadership means experimenting or innovating as the corollary to risk-taking.

Even when conceptualizing a course of action as a trial or test, development of that course of action must be strategic. Strategic planning became buzz words in the 1990s, but some pitfalls to effective outcomes of strategic planning often are evident. The basis for strategy is environmental or contextual analyses. Inability to see important elements or trends retards innovation. Sometimes, a plan is not strategic by virtue of failure to articulate it in sufficiently actionable terms, often due to global or complex planning. Additionally, when a course of action is implemented, leadership may be inadequate to keep it on track or fail to evaluate it in an ongoing sense—using meaningful indicators of progress—and thereby preventing timely course corrections.

Leadership Essence

Features of excellent leaders have been articulated by John Maxwell, in a book called *Developing the Leader Within You* (1993). Maxwell said that success is the progressive realization of predetermined goals predicated on vision. I define vision as a mental image of a strategic direction, path, or outcome that can be put into words. Envisioning inspires people to think differently and then to think through ways that they can contribute to achieving the vision. It is impossible to create a satisfactory vision without having a broad perspective about how the world works and without creating innovative solutions for expansion or growth of organizational productivity. I think that evoking a vision, articulating the vision, persuading others to be on track in working toward the vision, and clarifying expected milestones and outcomes are activities that create influence. An especially powerful way to be influential is to model expected behaviors. The best leaders are innovators by nature, but, more important, leaders can inspire others to innovate.

A number of features of effective now-and-beyond leaders are outlined in *The 10 Commitments of Leadership* by Kouzes and Posner (1995). They define strong leaders to be those who (a) challenge the status quo, (b) inspire a collective vision, (c) enable others to act, (d) model the way, and (e) encourage the heart. A leader who is skillful in communication, collaboration, coaching, and guiding rather than directing, and who can put in place the infrastructure needed for a productive organization, stands to be successful in contemporary contexts. Those same skills will hold a leader in good stead in new-age organizations.

■ Leading Edge Skills for New-Age Leadership

As we move into the 21st century, all signs point to change continuing at a rapid pace. Effective new-age leaders, above all, will need well-honed skills for optimizing change and forging new connections. The style of leadership required to accelerate such change will build on today's trend toward a more feminine style, although likely will evolve into a blended style that could be termed humanistic.

Optimizing Change

Optimizing change is predicated on analyzing trends, envisioning the preferred position within the environment, amassing resources (people, time, technology, and money) needed to move toward the preferred position, and inspiring and enabling productivity. Innovative solutions or evolution are promoted by continual questioning of existing traditions as the best way to achieve ends while building on existing strengths. A standard question should be: Is this the only or most effective or innovative way to do this? What new thinking or technologies apply to this realm and how can I test it or them? Who is doing the best job of handling this particular issue? How do I replicate or adapt ways to achieve a set of ends (a process called benchmarking)? Coaching people to map trends, do strengths, weaknesses, opportunities, and threats (SWOT) analyses, create action plans, and instigate innovative ways to move agendas will be paramount tasks for the leader.

The mix of talent and skills required ultimately might become the basis for new disciplines. For nursing, the research enterprise presently is leveraged by having a critical mass of faculty well grounded in a variety of research methodologies and with the expertise to produce focused and funded programs of research. The practice enterprise is enlarged by having scholarly faculty clinicians who want to push the boundaries of new practice models by testing applications of the latest scientific discoveries. These research and practice scholars are not necessarily one and the same but in the future might be more so as practice and research become better integrated. The best source for a variety of educational innovations in academia likely will be faculty who most strongly integrate research and practice. Futuristic leaders of the preeminent health professions will increasingly push the boundaries of lifelong education that are in synchrony with discovery of new knowledge and practice trends.

Forging Connections

The future likely will reveal continuing evolution of systems and organizations. Thus navigating the partnerships, collaborations, and mergers that constitute the evolution of new organizations will be an enduring activity. Skills of negotiation, conflict resolution, consensus building, and management of human motivation will be necessary. Collaborative efforts are and will continue to be fostered by top leader commitment, support of human resources, seeing a goal beyond financial, and recognizing enhanced community as a rewarding outcome, among other aspects (Sullivan, 1998). Within enduring or new organizations, future leaders in academia increasingly will find themselves in need of more business savvy and a mentality for seeking venture capital and maximizing return on investment.

Leadership Style

Currently, U.S. businesses, including health care organizations, tend to be hierarchical and authoritarian, but a feminine style of leadership stands to emerge as dominant. Women, in general, and nurses, in particular, stand to gain in leadership status as this trend continues. Pat Heim in *Hardball for Women* (1993), a guide for women on how to succeed in business, reflected on females and males and how they learn about leadership as they mature. In her view, American boys are more likely than girls to learn to compete because more of them play sports. In sports, they learn about winning and losing and following a leader (e.g., the coach). American girls play dolls, which doesn't involve competition or winning or losing. Therefore

girls learn to be collaborative rather than directive. The differences in how boys and girls grow up and what their play is like influence how they will lead and respond to leadership. In the case of males, a strong leader is valued and direct approaches are accepted—so boys learn to give and take orders. In the case of females, direction is negotiated and girls learn to accomplish goals only if relationships are kept intact.

Therefore men may feel more comfortable with directive leaders, and women may prefer working with coaching or supporting managers. Women can feel uncomfortable taking a leadership role if men are present. Neither is seen as right or wrong. Depending on composition of the group to be led, effective leaders choose the appropriate leadership style based on competence, commitment level, and composition of the work group. In some circumstances, supporting and coaching might be successful; in others, directing and delegating might be most productive. Perhaps a humanistic style that is a blend of these approaches will dominate in the future.

■ Concluding Statement

Trends in information technologies and science development are provoking a continually changing face of nursing practice and education. Determining how we will be educating for that future and practicing in the future is the challenge. The foundation for leadership in the future will be the ability to optimize change. Frontrunner leaders are both trend-getters and trend-setters. Learning to seek and interpret trends and thinking creatively about how to both capitalize on them and shape them is essential to new-age leadership. Influence is best applied by enabling and empowering others to set their sights high and develop skills to advance productivity. Collective productivity allows organizations to excel.

We can expect that today's and tomorrow's information technologies will expand our capacities for teaching, practice, and research and will provoke closer scrutiny of academic productivity. Perhaps the nurses of today will evolve into a workforce of tomorrow that represents an integration of a set of professions that function separately today. Health care workers of tomorrow likely will be knowledge workers, but the knowledge that they utilize to shape the behavior of people with regard to their health will continue to evolve. Perhaps they will be genetic engineers and ecology or environmental counselors.

Helping people (clients or patients) shape behaviors to promote the fit of person to environment, within the confines of how we have learned to harness the latest technologies, is still likely to be the essence of nursing or whatever nursing has encompassed as it has evolved over time. The age-old necessity of providing education in synchrony with the evolution of new-age practice will continue to be the challenge for leaders in health care professional education. Thinking about the specific form that it is taking and will take constitutes the excitement of standing on the horizon and contemplating the future.

■ *References*

American Academy of Nursing/American Nurses Foundation. (1998). W. Young, J. Shaver, S. Feetham, B. McElmurray, R. Richards, M. Albrecht, J. Cooksey, W. Panko, K. Curtis, & J. Syer (Report authors). *Leadership excellence to advance performance (LEAP) in health care* (Report to AAN/ANF Leadership Development in Nursing Initiative).Washington, DC: Author.

American Association of Colleges of Nursing. (1999). B. Durand, J. Broad, M. Miller, J. Shaver, E. Stullenbarger, E. Zungalo, M. Broome, & J. Stanley (Report authors). *Essential clinical resources for nursing's academic mission* (Task Force Report). Washington, DC: Author.

Buerhaus, P. I., & Staiger, D. O. (1999). Trouble in the nurse labor market? Recent trends and future outlook. *Health Affairs, 18*(1), 214–222.

Ferris, R. J. (1987, January). Capturing corporate creativity. [Editorial Opinion]. *United Magazine,* p. 7.

Heim, P. (1993). *Hardball for women: Winning at the game of business.* New York: Plume.

Kouzes, J., & Posner, B. (1995). *The leadership challenge: How to keep getting extraordinary things done in organizations.* San Francisco: Jossey Bass.

Marion, L. N. (Ed.). (1996). *Nursing's vision for primary health care in the 21st century.* Washington, DC: American Nurses Association.

Marion, L. N. (1997). *Faculty practice: Applying the models.* Washington, DC: National Organization of Nurse Practitioner Faculties.

Martin, K., & Scheet, N. (1992). *The Omaha system: Applications for community health nursing.* Philadelphia: W. B. Saunders.

Maxwell, J. C. (1993). *Developing the leader within you.* Nashville: Thomas Nelson.

McCloskey, J. C., & Bulechek, G. M. (1996). *Nursing interventions classification (NIC); Iowa Intervention Project* (2nd ed.). St. Louis: Mosby.

Saba, V. K. (1997). Why the home health care classification is a recognized nursing nomenclature. *Computer Nursing, 15* (Suppl. 2), S69–76.

Simpson, R. L. (1996). The 21st century nurse executive. *Nursing Informatics, 20*(2), 85–88.
Sullivan, T. J. (1998). *Collaboration: A health care imperative.* New York: McGraw-Hill.
Whalen, E. L. (1991). *Responsibility center budgeting.* Indianapolis: Indiana University Press.

■ Editor's Questions for Discussion

What factors contributed to the demand for nurse practitioners and the consequent development of nurse practitioner graduate programs in nursing? How may academic nursing administration resolve issues concerning the need for nurse practitioner practice-intensive faculty versus need for research-intensive faculty? What new challenges exist for administration in developing practice sites? To what extent does Barger (Chapter 52) open options? How do Keating and Perry (Chapter 65) address issues regarding competition for resources?

How does Shaver's presentation of "state-assisted" institutions and responsibility-centered management relate to Keating and Perry's (Chapter 65) views? How does C. Jones (Chapter 11) contribute to understanding of the nursing workforce? What evidence is provided by Buerhaus (Chapter 10) and C. Jones (Chapter 11) regarding the aging workforce? What suggestions do Buerhaus (Chapter 10), C. Jones (Chapter 11), and Shaver offer to address this issue?

How do the Yeaworth et al. (Chapter 14), Billings (Chapter 15), and Schroeder and Long (47) discussions about information technology pertain to Shaver's call for reengineering educational programs? Indicate specific strategies for positioning schools of nursing. What suggestions are offered by Hoffman (Chapter 64)? Compare Shaver's approach to future academic leadership and needs with the presentations by Lindeman (Chapter 63), Hoffman (Chapter 64), and Lindell (Chapter 69). What characterizes "feminine" leadership? What is the difference between transformational leadership and what is advocated by Shaver?

How may increased demand for faculty productivity and responsibility-centered management as presented by Shaver affect tenure issues? Would Fleming (Chapter 22) agree with your response? How may faculty further develop as entrepreneurs? What effect might faculty intrapreneurship and entrepreneurship have on administration of nursing programs? How do Duffy's (Chapter 53) views on entrepreneurship apply to nursing programs? Should emphasis on research be balanced with practice expertise in academia? If so, how?

How do Jenkins' (Chapter 54) discussion of genetics and Snyder, Kreitzer, and Loen's (Chapter 43) emphasis on healing practices reinforce Shaver's predictions about biomedical science's "impact on nursing curricula and practice"? How do the presentations by Porter-O'Grady (Chapter 55) and Pinkerton (Chapter 56) apply to Shaver's discourse about integrated health delivery systems?

77

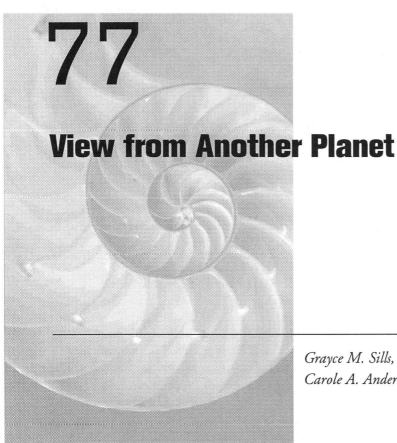

View from Another Planet

Grayce M. Sills, PhD, RN, FAAN
Carole A. Anderson, PhD, RN, FAAN

The preceding chapters have woven an enthusiastic and positive scenario for the profession of nursing as we enter a new millennium. Yet, despite all our progress and promise, some basic challenges that have faced the profession for many years still need to be addressed if nursing as a profession is to realize its full potential. Although not new, these are enduring issues that the profession has been unwilling or unable to confront and resolve in any significant way.

Our basic premise in this chapter is that unless such confrontation occurs, the wonderful future and vision that could be ours as nurses will in fact elude us and never allow nursing to reach its full potential. Relevant issues as we define them are (a) the struggle between dependence and independence; (b) resistance to rigorous self-scrutiny and quality control measures; (c) the dynamics of gender on the profession; (d) the separation of education from practice; (e) dissipation created by the existence of multiple, often conflicting professional organizations; and (f) the language we speak. In this chapter, we discuss the ways in which these factors have influenced nursing's past and are apt to limit its future.

■ Dependence–Independence–Interdependence

In the latter half of the 1990s, the health care system in the United States underwent rapid transition. This major paradigm shift, driven by massive economic and social forces, reflects a health care system where there is major emphasis on managing costs by ostensibly managing care. Nursing is hampered by the profession's own paradigm in its collective response to the challenges of this new era.

Nursing's paradigm has its foundation in the historical structure that frames initial socialization into nursing. This hierarchical structure has two main roots: military traditions (Knight's Hospitaliers) and the religious tradition (nuns and sisters). These two traditions markedly influenced the nature and character of hierarchical structures of the hospitals in which many in the profession received most or all their training and now do their work. Moreover, a third and deeper root is present—the gender root. The gender root arises from the reality that in American society, as in most societies, the female gender has always been, to a greater or lesser extent, oppressed by the larger society. These three roots—the militaristic tradition, the religious tradition, and the female gender—created the nursing paradigm for viewing the world. Most in the profession were socialized with this paradigm, which created a way of looking at the world that has made many changes more difficult than they would be otherwise. To illustrate, the hierarchical structure of the hospital continues to this day despite numerous efforts over time to introduce different models and different patterns of care. The same structure insidiously seeped into the structure of schools and colleges of nursing around the nation. Many of these institutions are so hierarchically organized that they seem very little different from the hospital, despite the competing paradigm of the traditional college or university as a "community of scholars."

The views and values that arise from nursing's socialization paradigm are several: (a) a deep sense of distinctions based on rank and not necessarily on competence; (b) a long experience with deference to authority, particularly male-dominated, physician-based authority; and (c) the deeply embedded notion that in this society being a woman means being something less. When that idea is so entrenched in the consciousness, the way to success then becomes one of competing for the attention, affection, and favor of the people with the power—typically males.

Paradigm Consequences

The consequences of this paradigm are many. First, movement of the nursing profession from a posture of dependence to independence to interdependence becomes very difficult. In fact, to push the analogy from personality growth and development to the collective level, we could say that nursing collectively seems to be in its adolescence and very much focused on its independence. That seems unfortunate when what seems to be required in the present environment is interdependence. It seems that we have few, if any, engendered skills in, predilections for, or comfort in interdependent relationships, which has meaning for the work in our field. Research makes it clear that collaborative work with patients or consumers and their families is one key to successful programs of care. Yet most in the profession were trained in a paradigm that considered the patient and the family to be in a "down one" position, irrelevant, not to be worked with—as individuals to be done to and for rather than to be done with! Until we can acknowledge that working in collaboration with each other is the model for the future, it will be difficult for us to move on. This deficiency makes for great difficulty in our working relationships and in our abilities to work collaboratively with patients and families.

This same notion can be applied to nursing's interprofessional relationships, which typically are with social workers, pharmacists, x-ray technicians, psychologists, physicians, and physical and occupational therapists. These relationships have been fraught with tension and there are few, if any, case studies of productive outcomes. More often than not, we face attitudes of distrust, mistrust, and competition, rather than of collaboration. Most efforts toward interprofessional collaboration to resolve self-centered issues take place after basic professional training. To resolve these issues after initial professional socialization has taken place is much more difficult than if they were addressed during that process. The task for the future is to learn together, actively, and early in professional training. Yet, to date, attempts at interdisciplinary education have been largely unsustainable.

Perhaps the most devastating feature of the nursing paradigm is related to gender and the difficulty that we as women have in valuing our differences, rewarding differences, and allowing differences. At each stage of the discussion and debate surrounding the issue of entry into practice, we find that this root of the paradigm rears its ugly head. For example, early clinical nurse specialists—after master's-level preparation—go into practice settings and literally are "done in" by colleagues who seemingly could not understand their difference, did not want to see them as different, and did not want to value their difference. This discomfort with differences sometimes may go the other way—often the well-educated, well-prepared nurse is dismissive of the competencies and value of the less well–credentialed nurse.

Nursing has existed almost 100 years in a professional association that often appears conflicted about whether it represents individuals, as in collective bargaining arrangements, or collectively, as in professional standards and credentialing. The American Nurses Association continues to try to represent both aims and finds that, very often, they are at odds. It is natural that they should be at odds. However, the lowest common denominator comes into play in the politics of the organization and makes it increasingly difficult for the direction of the organization to be clear and distinct.

Need for Model Change

A major shift—a genuine paradigm shift—must take place in nursing education so that a new paradigm is taught. Values must be demonstrated in the educational settings where initial preparation for the nursing role occurs. Much emphasis must be given to interpersonal skills training—to collaborative work, interdependence, peer review, and peer supervision as integral to professional competence. All these things must be reflected in a commitment to support one another for a greater common good. We can be prisoners of the paradigm wittingly or unwittingly. If wittingly, we can recognize these issues and take steps to move up and away from the old paradigm. The ability to move out of the old paradigm will allow the profession to flow into new structures when the right time comes. The right time is here.

■ Quality Control

Nursing is intensely committed to being independent of constraint and hence free to innovate—to be novel and unique. For nursing education, this commitment has resulted in a lack of standardized curriculum at any level of nursing education. For nursing practice, it has meant the lack of a set of gold standards. In both instances, these deficiencies make it impossible to "benchmark" with other academic and health care practice institutions in order to make qualitative distinctions among them. It is not even clear that we want to make qualitative distinctions, given our strong value of egalitarianism—of equating distinction with elitism. Yet, we live in a world that values high quality, and benchmarking has become commonplace.

Nursing Programs

Nursing education fought passionately to maintain diversity in its offerings, curricular design, and multiple entry levels into the profession. As a profession we have been unable to form (a) a unified bond to support common educational preparation for the profession, (b) standardized curriculum at any level, and (c) not even standard nomenclature for program offerings. The result: Nurses are the least educated of all the health professions.

Nursing's educational programs consist of curricula that vary considerably from institution to institution, making it virtually impossible, for example, for students to transfer from one program to another. Master's degree programs lack consistent titling to enable potential students to compare programs realistically and make the best choice for them. This diversity, which is so strongly supported, has made it virtually impossible to develop benchmarking standards—a practice that has become routine in higher education.

Not until the mid 1990s were standards published for both undergraduate and graduate programs (American Association of Colleges of Nursing [AACN], 1994, 1999). Even after being developed, these standards were selectively adopted or given parochial definitions. How else, for example, could the number of doctoral programs in nursing have grown from 59 to 70 in just 6 years while enrollment remained virtually constant (AACN, 1999)? How else could small colleges, with a primary mission for teaching undergraduates, develop graduate programs when accepted standards dictate that graduate programs be limited to comprehensive or research universities taught by faculty who are active scholars?

As we enter the new millennium, approximately 50% of nursing faculty in colleges and universities possess the doctorate (AACN, 1997–1998, 1998–1999). A well-accepted and standard quality indicator in higher education is the percentage of faculty who possess that terminal degree. In this regard, nursing falls far short of academic colleges. But, in recent years, we have seen progress to increase that percentage stalled, and in fact, many programs are hiring more faculty without the doctorate to provide clinical teaching in advanced practice programs.

Nursing leaders have long criticized the continuation and proliferation of diploma and associate degree programs. Yet, 4-year colleges and universities also have been accommodating, making their undergraduate and graduate programs easily available to these graduates. No other profession does this! In so doing, nursing education essentially is defining its basic preparation at the associate degree level and then adding general education courses for obtaining the baccalaureate, thereby making these graduates eligible for entry into graduate programs. A close look at the registered nurse (RN) "completion" programs and the so-called bridge programs at the graduate level bear witness to this reality. RN completion programs are baccalaureate completion programs for registered nurses who received their basic preparation in a diploma hospital-based program or an associate degree in a 2-year program. Bridge programs leading to a master's degree enroll RNs who earned a diploma in nursing or an associate degree.

Quality of Students

The quality of students entering an educational program is a major indicator of quality in higher education. Yet, for nursing, that quality has varied significantly at all levels. Nowhere is the quality of the students in nursing programs published. Schools are not compared on, for example, the average American College Test (ACT), Scholastic Aptitude Test (SAT) or Graduate Record Examination (GRE) scores of the entering class. Nor are they compared on the basis of standardized outcome measures, such as graduation rates, percentage of graduate students who successfully pass the credentialing exam or go on for further study, or National Council Licensure Examination (NCLEX) scores. In fact, tremendous resistance likely would be met to even suggesting such comparisons. But that is precisely what needs to happen for nursing to become more selective and hence more professional and attractive to the brightest students interested in careers.

Preparation for Practice

Nursing practice never has focused long enough on creating a professional workplace where education is valued, rewarded, and used to differentiate roles. Rather, despite our general criticism of others for doing so, nurse administrators regard all nurses, regardless of educational preparation, equally qualified. Actually, a license rather than an educational degree is the requisite preparation for practice. This reality sets us apart from all other health professions who have at least postbaccalaureate educational preparation for entry into professional practice. Yet, despite of this wide gap in educational preparation, we expect other health professionals to treat us as equals and involve us in decision-making at all levels. Clinging to the very lowest of standards seals our fate of marginalization in organizations that are dominated by well-educated professionals.

■ Gender Issues

Although nursing has made some progress in attracting men to the profession, it remains predominately female. That fact and its impact on both daily lives and the profession as a whole rarely have been discussed and debated.

Since the 1960s, women have made tremendous strides in gaining entry into fields that previously had been closed to them. Prior to that time, nursing, education, and social work were among the few fields open to bright, ambitious, and career-oriented women. The number of women recipients of PhDs is growing in many fields at unprecedented rates. Early in this century, their numbers will equal and may well surpass those of men. What has that done to nursing?

We do not know because we do not ask the question, and since our demographics are well-guarded secrets, we cannot tell whether or how much the quality of our applicants may have eroded. Has nursing, in fact, suffered a "brain drain"? We know for sure that, although the number of men entering nursing has increased, their numbers do not correspond to the numbers of women now entering predominately male fields such as business, medicine, and law. So, it may well be that our talent pool has suffered.

This lack of information presents a serious issue for the profession and is one that we must confront. We have to examine honestly the quality of our students and compare it to the quality of students in competing fields; if quality has decreased, we must determine how to attract a higher quality student to ensure our place in the professional world of health care. Unless we do so, we run the risk of being relegated to being considered nonprofessionals.

The last 25 years or so have witnessed the development of a new academic discipline—women's studies. The women's movement gave birth to this field and it has mushroomed. As a result of this scholarship, we now know that men and women differ significantly from one another in (a) psychological development; (b) how they function interpersonally and in small groups; (c) how they reason, think, and make decisions; and (d) most important, how their bodies function and respond to stimuli.

Although some nursing literature has been devoted to the "feminist" perspective, a robust body of science has not developed in such areas as the ways in which women function in a female- (as contrasted to male-) dominated work environment, how women interact with women leaders, and how women become socialized by other women.

Yet there is much informal dialogue about these topics. Many believe, for example, that women differ in the way they interact with women peers, that women students respond differently to women teachers, that women workers differ in how they respond to women managers, and so on. But, we do not really *know* whether such differences exist. At this point, differences, both positive and negative, are only *thought* to exist. The need is for systematic study of women who function in predominately female (as opposed to male) environments and whether there are differences that affect performance and progress toward goal achievement.

■ *The Separation of Nursing Education and Nursing Service*

At one time, nursing education and nursing service were blended and united. Nursing education was embedded in hospitals, and teachers were nurses who provided and supervised nursing care. Strong allegiances to these models developed, but they were sustained far too long. As nursing education programs moved out of hospitals and into educational institutions, the faculty moved with them, and in so doing, moved away from clinical practice. Over time, this created a *schism* between the two. One result of that schism was that (a) clinicians came to believe that students were not being adequately prepared for the real world of practice; and (b) educators believed that the real world of practice did not utilize the cognitive skills of new graduates and that

clinical sites were not good learning environments without those skills.

Eventually, the negative implications of this schism became visible enough to cause nursing leaders to call for reform in ways that would enable clinicians to teach and educators to practice. Yet, after many years of advocacy for this change—the purpose of which was to ensure quality education for students and achievement of excellence in clinical practice—the reality falls quite short of the ideal.

For the most part, the majority of faculty are not engaged in clinical practice in any regular way; and, with few exceptions, full-time nursing staff are not heavily involved in nursing education. There are reasons for this situation. Faculty, especially those in research institutions, also must be engaged in research and scholarship. The changing emphasis in undergraduate education from process to outcomes has placed new demands on faculty to make qualitative changes in their approach to teaching. Faculty roles have become increasingly demanding as the "bar" for success continues to be raised.

Impact of Health Care Reform

Health care reform has increased pressures on the clinical enterprise to become more efficient, economical, and productive. These pressures leave little room for nonclinical activities such as teaching.

Nowhere are these pressures more apparent or dramatic than in academic health centers. These centers (N = 86 with nursing programs) produce a disproportionately large number of all new graduates (AACN, 1997–1998). Health care reform has created special challenges as academic interests attempt to compete with hospitals and ambulatory enterprises whose missions include neither education nor indigent care. Academic physicians, confronted with significant reductions in reimbursement rates, scramble to keep both their clinical and research activities vital and productive. In so doing, these physicians are apt to be less collegial and collaborative than in previous "good" times. They are under great pressure to be more productive, and nurses in these systems, whether staff or advanced practice, are subject to the same influences.

Nursing faculty in academic health centers are being subjected to tougher requirements for retention and promotion while their educational commitments are remaining the same or even intensifying, particularly at the graduate level in the preparation of advanced practice nurses. In these institutions, nursing is the only health science profession with (typically large) undergraduate programs. Moreover, undergraduate clinical teaching is labor intensive, creating additional challenges for faculty.

Concomitantly, academic health centers always have placed value on clinical care—the highest quality clinical care. In these settings, nursing faculty are finding it increasingly difficult to engage in clinical practice because of other demands, which isolate them from a major mission of the academic health center. Continuing down this path will no doubt erode both the education and research missions of the institutions, as faculty find themselves "shut out" of the clinical world.

New models are desperately needed if nursing is to garner the clear mutual benefits derived from faculty who practice and clinicians who teach. A faculty member who also practices can look forward to that practice enhancing both teaching and research. An expert clinician knows what to teach and students respond favorably to relevant instruction thereby heightening the teacher's success and satisfaction. Gaining the cooperation of clinical personnel is infinitely more doable for faculty who are active clinicians. Faculty who are directly involved in clinical care will also have a voice in those settings and therefore can play a major role in creating a quality clinical labora-

tory in which to educate students. And finally, faculty research is augmented because it is easier to identify significant and researchable clinical problems when individuals are practicing on a regular basis. Also, knowing contemporary care and practices helps to not only shape the research question but also to identify relevant variables.

Clinicians and the clinical setting benefit from the involvement of teachers and their students because they bring contemporary thinking, research findings, and innovations to the clinical setting. With the current emphasis on evidence-based practice, there is a major benefit to the clinical setting when it fully engages faculty and students in developing protocols and practices that reflect state-of-the-art clinical care. The combination of faculty, students, and clinicians can produce stimulating and rewarding interactions. Importantly, clinicians have the opportunity of teaching and modeling professional practice for the next generation—a time honored tradition in the professions.

■ Nursing Organizations and Associations

Fifty years ago, there were two major national nursing organizations: The American Nurses Association (ANA) and the National League for Nursing (NLN). Nurses who belonged to an association typically were members of one or the other, often both (Carter, Peplau, & Sills, 1997). In 1966, the ANA formed five clinical divisions, and many practicing nurses believed that their practice concerns and needs were being handled by the work of these divisions. Exceptions were nurse anesthetists and the operating room nurses.

Nurse anesthetists and operating room nurses were two of the earliest groups to organize in the interest of their specialty practices. The American Association of Nurse Anesthetists was founded in 1931, and 96% of nurse anesthetists belong to their association. The Association of Operating Room Nurses began in 1949 and incorporated in 1957. The history of both groups suggests failed efforts to develop relationships with the ANA, which foundered somewhere on the political shoals of the times (Carter et al., 1997).

In 1994, there were 94 types of nursing organizations. Fifty-two are classified as organizations with a delineated clinical focus. Proliferation of the ever-smaller pieces of the clinical nursing pie can be viewed as part of the societal response to the increasing complexity of the world of the 1980s and 1990s. Conventional wisdom suggests that in more complex societies, individuals seek to participate in ever-smaller segments of the social arena, as that appears to be one way of reducing tensions created by ever-increasing complexity. Participation in these ever-smaller groups permits their members to find a comfortable place where a sense of affinity, a common purpose, and often a shared identity can be perceived. Thus the growth in the number and types of nursing organizations is not surprising. What is less clearly understood are the reactions and responses of the ANA to the evolution and expansion of specialty practice associations.

Issues for the Future

More complex issues have produced greater challenges for the whole of nursing. In 1972, efforts to bring the specialty nursing organizations together in some kind of an arrangement with each other and the ANA elicited some interest. These initiatives were less than successful, and hence two major nursing coalitions emerged. The National Federation of Specialty Nursing Organizations was formed and is supported by dues from its constituents. The Nursing Organization Liaison Forum was founded under the aegis of the ANA.

The total number of nurses in specialty nursing organizations now exceeds the number of members of the ANA's constituent associations. However, this total does not account for the possibility of one nurse holding multiple memberships in several organizations. Thus it is difficult to know with precision the number of unduplicated memberships in the nursing organizations combined. What seems likely is that the total number of nurses in the state nurses associations and the specialty nursing associations is less than 20% of the practicing nurses in the United States.

American Nurses Association

One issue from this account concerns the capacity of the ANA to keep a multipurpose mission. Clearly, by the name itself—the American Nurses Association—one of its missions is an advocacy focus on the needs of its members, nurses—that is, their economic, workplace, and general well-being.

The ANA's second mission is concern for the phenomenological focus of the work of nurses, that is, nursing. It is to this purpose, the clinical practice of nursing, that the specialty nursing organizations have addressed their activities. The expansion of the number and types of nursing organizations raises two questions. First, should there be an umbrella association that could be flexible, expandable, and contractible, and thus better serve the profession and society in the next millennium? Second, are the organizational structures and forms that could be developed in the service of nurses and nursing the right, best, and most desirable models to fulfill nursing's contract with the world it serves?

■ Nursing's Language

If we accept the postulate that "language influences thought," rather than the other way around, it seems useful to consider the language of nurses and nursing. That language reflects all too well the socialization paradigm referred to earlier. There is the language of the hierarchy of the hospital: head nurse, charge nurse, and so forth—implying that orders come only from above and thereby disputing the claim of professional expertise. There is the language reflecting gender differences: "the girls on nights," "the girls in my office."

There also is the heavily loaded phrase "doctors' orders and nurses' orders." What seems preferable is that physicians and nurses prescribe courses of action, medications, treatments, and so forth, aimed at helping the patient or client or consumer to have a better result, a result that is obtained by collaboration rather than by "following orders."

The ANA focuses its efforts on workplace advocacy and uses collective bargaining as the primary method for working with employers on behalf of nurses. Collective bargaining is industrial language and is most useful in industries involved in the production of goods (e.g., cars, refrigerators, etc.). This language crystallizes and solidifies the nurse's status as an employee of the hospital or agency and thus, by contract language, the nurse now sits in a relationship of secondary, rather than primary, accountability to the patient.

Recently, the profession has used the term "advanced practice nurse" to encompass a large group of nurses under one rubric. Nurse practitioners, nurse midwives, nurse anesthetists, and clinical specialists were all lumped together in that inclusive term. Although perhaps useful for political reasons, the language reflected a "leveling" of educational disparities.

Notable also in perusing the literature in nursing, we found much emphasis given to caring, empowering, and unity—concepts that often signify the inability of nurses to speak of what they know and how that knowledge is used to produce desired outcomes in giving care.

Notable also is nursing's proclivity to use equivocal language, that is, language that has more than one meaning or denotes uncertainty as to direction. We are socialized into this language by being taught to make observations that do not diagnose. For example, "it appears as if the patient is bleeding" rather than "the patient is hemorrhaging." Patients "appear" to have or be a lot of things, but nurses are taught to hedge. This tendency extends likewise to the assessment of others' work. Rather than being analytical and judgmental, evaluations are laden with descriptions. With students, faculty are prone to load the front end of the evaluation with positives and save the "fatal flaws" to the end. Often, this type of assessment is confusing to students who then do not address weaknesses in the areas in which they need to improve.

Heightened awareness exists in our culture of the importance of language and what words convey. We have seen the disappearance of chair*men,* paper*boy,* the terms *girl* or *boy* referring to adult women or minority men, and the indiscriminate use of *he* in organizational documents. We in nursing need to develop linguistic self-consciousness—in the words we use and how these words influence both our own thinking and the image we portray to others.

■ Concluding Statement

In many respects, we can feel a great deal of optimism regarding opportunities for nursing in the future. We will be able to build on the successes of the century just concluded to move the profession forward. But, throughout this chapter, we have issued this caution: Unless the profession unites to resolve some fundamental, thorny, and potentially damaging issues that have plagued it for most of the century, its full potential may never be realized. Coming to terms with the need to move to a stage of interdependence; developing and enforcing the highest standards to maintain quality control of our programs and practices;

looking objectively at how gender influences our interactions with each other and the world; uniting our professional organizations to create a greater voice; reducing the education and practice schism; and scrutinizing our language are the challenges before us. These issues are significant and require more than tinkering at the margin. To resolve them finally will take the undaunting commitment of all of us.

■ References

American Association of Colleges of Nursing. (1994, 1999). *Enrollment and graduation in baccalaureate and graduate programs in nursing.* Washington, DC: Author.

American Association of Colleges of Nursing. (1998–1999). *Salaries of instructional and administrative nursing faculty in baccalaureate and graduate programs in nursing, 1998–1999.* Washington, DC: Author.

American Association of Colleges of Nursing. (1997–1998). *Institutional data systems, 1997–1998.* Washington, DC: Author.

Carter, E., Peplau, H. E., & Sills, G. M. (1997). The ins and outs of psychiatric nursing and the ANA. *Journal of the American Psychiatric Nurses Association, 3*(1), 10–16.

■ Editor's Questions for Discussion

Discuss the six concerns cited by Sills and Anderson as being unresolved by the nursing profession. To what extent do you agree or disagree that these six issues may prevent nursing from achieving its potential? What efforts, if any, have been made to resolve each issue? Why have these six troublesome areas persisted? Suggest strategies for resolving them. How can faculty and nursing students facilitate addressing those six points for positive outcomes? Identify other challenges that have endured and handicapped nursing. How has "language" contributed to difficulties for nursing as a profession and consumers' understanding of nursing roles and functions? How does Kerfoot's (Chapter 75) discussion reinforce the concerns identified by Sills and Anderson?

How can a collaborative model evolve for the profession? What implications exist for nursing programs and practice in Sills and Anderson's plea for collaboration? How does Fitzpatrick's (Chapter 18) discussion about interdisciplinary education address issues raised by Sills and Anderson?

What forces must come into play for nursing to agree regarding the type of educational preparation for entry into professional practice? What factors will influence quality control concerns being sufficiently addressed? How may strategies offered by Nichols and Renwanz-Boyle (Chapter 16), Lenz and Hardin (Chapter 20), Boland (Chapter 71), Lindeman (Chapter 63), Keating and Perry (Chapter 65), and Shaver (Chapter 76) relate to concerns about quality? What data are needed to address the gender issues raised by Sills and Anderson?

How are faculty attempting to bridge the gap between education and service? Propose new models for blending clinical practice and nursing education? What content or suggestions offered by Felton (Chapter 1), Carter (Chapter 39), McCausland and McCauley (Chapter 40), Gray (Chapter 42), Barger (Chapter 52), Pinkerton (Chapter 56), McClure (Chapter 62), and Shaver (Chapter 76) facilitate unification between education and practice?

How is Thompson and Lavandero's (Chapter 9) discussion about nursing organizations helpful in addressing the concerns raised by Sills and Anderson? What factors keep all nursing organizations from being united under one umbrella? How important is it for nursing as a profession to have one overall organization or association? Address the specific questions posed by Sills and Anderson.

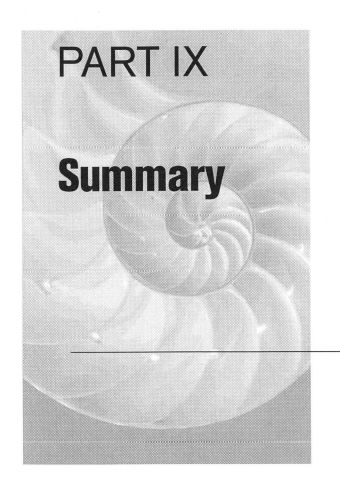

PART IX

Summary

*" . . . I took the one less traveled by,
And that has made all the difference."*

For nursing to continue to thrive and realize its goals, critical paths identified in Parts I–VIII of this book must be addressed. Individual nurses and the nursing profession have choices to be made about directions for the future. For a whole view of the profession, the dimensions of nursing and the predominant themes of the contributing authors are addressed. "One less traveled" path may well be a distinctive road never before chosen by practitioners and the profession for a united whole. Can you project what that might be to make "all the difference" for nursing as a profession?

78

Paths to Make a Difference

Norma L. Chaska, PhD, RN, FAAN

Robert Frost in his poem "The Road Not Taken" refers to being a traveler and having to choose between two roads that diverged in a woods. He goes on to say that choosing the one less traveled made all the difference (1916/1993). Nursing has taken many roads in its travels as a profession, some less worn than others, ever struggling to look ahead as far as possible for paths leading to fulfillment of its mission and goals. Perhaps never before in the history of nursing have so many directions been available. As we have the opportunity to choose the best for our profession and the consumers we serve, our journey continues into this new century.

Embarking on the road, once again, we—the profession of nursing—must foresee the possible outcomes of divergent paths. For nursing, choosing "the one less traveled" may mean selecting a path once started but never followed to conclusion. Or it may mean venturing into completely unknown terrain. Still, it may mean focusing so totally on the mission and goals of the profession that outside forces are not permitted to divert nursing from them. Even perhaps all three methods may be used as the profession decides which paths or directions to follow in continuing our journey.

My goal in this summary chapter is to put forth various "paths" presented by the numerous contributing authors for this book that may make a difference. It is up to you, the practitioner—the professional—and the profession to reflect, choose, promote, and develop the path(s) nursing must follow for a future. First, however, I will share an event that may help you understand the basis for my approach.

Many years ago, having enrolled in a particular theology course, my classmates and I learned a valuable lesson. Whereas course assignments were grueling, the final exam was known to be a "breeze." Previous students passed on the secret that there always was only one query at the end—the same one—each year: "Trace Saint Paul's travels!" Fearlessly, we filed into the classroom. Our confidence, however, quickly dissolved into horror as the professor wrote on the blackboard: "Critique the Sermon on the Mount."

Stunned—we looked at each other, put down our pens, quietly left our seats, and exited—all except one fellow. Looking back, we saw this young man without hesitation start to write—and write—and write! Shocked, some of us wondered, "How did this guy know the switched final exam question?" We waited for him with suspense outside the door, determined to ask him. Finally, he came out, completely at peace with himself. He explained, "When I saw that question—'Critique the Sermon on the Mount'—I thought to myself, 'Who am I to criticize God?, so I went ahead and traced Saint Paul's travels!'" Thus, being privileged to work with the most renowned in the nursing profession as contributing authors, no way could I critique their writings! Rather, while "traveling" through their chapters, I decided to trace patterns in their thoughts to identify salient points. Therefore I present particular "paths," in comparing chapter content within each Part. In addition, I trace some patterns between Parts.

I posed questions for reflection in Introductions to the nine Parts of this book. In addition, I offered extensive Editor's Questions for Discussion at the end of each chapter. These questions further enable you to identify common themes among the contributing authors' writings.

I pose additional comments in this Summary in my capacity as editor of this text and consultant for Academic Administration in Universities. I condense predominant patterns detected throughout the chapters in a concluding statement. Through all these means, I hope directions will become visible for paths that make a difference in nursing's future as a profession.

■ Part I: Professionalization

In Part I, Professionalization, all elements critical to the profession are emphasized. These chapters form the basis for many patterns enlarged upon throughout the remaining eight Parts.

Geraldene Felton (Chapter 1) sets the tone by emphasizing altruism as the heart of nursing. Selflessness is difficult in a profit-driven system and managed care environment, which threatens interactions essential to nursing. Felton addresses numerous challenges related to collective bargaining among professionals, health and income inequality, managed care, and differentiated practice. Keys for future direction of nursing, such as (a) opportunism for lifelong learning; (b) self-assessment of talents; (c) personal competence; and (d) combinations of diverse abilities, talents, and skills of many professionals are offered. Following the blueprint for inner work and self-assessment provided by Pesut (Chapter 70), building the profession in this century as suggested by Felton can occur. She touches on some issues, such as collective bargaining, which are increasingly becoming consequential.

A significant change has occurred with the American Nurses Association (ANA) (1999) creating a separate national labor entity—United American Nurses (UAN)—to support state nurses associations in their collective bargaining efforts. Although labor leaders concede that nurses are not yet in a position to effect major change in the hospital industry, registered nurses (RNs) are rethinking their ideas about organized labor (Breda, 1997; Cleeland & Bernstein, *San Francisco Examiner,* 1999). Barbara Tone (1999), author of a lead article in *NurseWeek,* suggests caution in evaluating "whether unionization ultimately is in the best interests of the profession and its patients" (p. 31). The desire to obtain voice and power is evident. However, given the continuing upheaval in health care, splintering of organizations and associations in nursing, unionization is a questionable and uncertain path for the future.

JoEllen Koerner (Chapter 2) introduces the need to redefine the meaning of health and the role of healing disciplines in light of the transformation traced to Florence Nightingale. Transformation, according to Koerner, includes emphases on preventive care and wellness and utilization of complementary or alternative therapies in health care. These same elements are themes in many of the chapters in Part V, Nursing Practice.

Nursing regulation and competency concerns are distinctive patterns addressed. Initially, Carolyn Yocom and Katherine Thomas (Chapter 3) address the topic in presenting strong and clear explanations of the Mutual Recognition Model and Interstate Compacts. All states have not yet endorsed the Interstate Compact for Mutual Recognition, but all are expected to comply soon. Legal recognition of advanced practice registered nurses (APRNs) is anticipated in the Mutual Recognition Model, but actual application of the model to APRNs is on a different time line (American Association of Colleges of Nursing [AACN], 1999b). Many implications exist for registered nurses who live in one state and practice or teach in one or more other states. Rosalee Yeaworth and colleagues (Chapter 14) discuss implications of the Mutual Recognition Model in distributive learning programs. Essentially, the registered nurse must be licensed in the state of residence.

However, they must follow the Nurse Practice Acts governing practice in each state in which the nurse may practice.

Given the leadership of the National Council of State Boards of Nursing (NCSBN) in developing the Mutual Recognition Model, the question remains, "Could that Board not develop licensure levels to facilitate differentiation of practice in nursing?" This question comes to mind again in both Part II, Nursing Education, and Part V, Nursing Practice. A further point, in which the NCSBN could provide leadership, needs to be noted: Licensure does not ensure continued competence!

Charlie Jones-Dickson (Chapter 4) presents strong arguments for state boards of nursing to provide leadership. At present, no system exists to measure continued competence, although some states have initiated varying models (Eichelberger & Hewlett, 1999). According to Jones-Dickson, most professionals believe that continuing education does not confirm competency; what effect credentialing programs have on ensuring competency is open to question. Ideally, the responsibility for competency rests on the individual, with less left to regulation. However, some method is needed to validate safe practice. Jones-Dickson advocates valid, reliable, and legally defensible standards. To that end, she offers questions essential for regulatory boards to consider and presents legal principles for regulatory boards to follow in developing models for examining competency. She asserts that legally defensible standards are critical for the future. Given the recommendations of the Pew Health Professions Commission (Bellack & O'Neil, 2000), Jones-Dickson's suggestions for ensuring competencies are well advised.

Such clarity and legally defensible guidelines in nursing education are essential for professional programs. Legal concerns are further discussed by Lane and Paterson (Chapter 7).

Beverly Kopala (Chapter 5) addresses common ethical issues in (a) the classroom (e.g., academic dishonesty), (b) teaching and writing letters of reference, (c) research (e.g., minimizing risks to participants), (d) practice and decision-making in the best interests of the patient, and (e) nursing service administration. The importance of challenges such as ensuring the safety of nurses and recognizing difficulties that new graduates have in their first position are considered. Because of the increasing concern in nursing practice about assisted suicide and end-of-life care, you are well advised to review additional publications (Ketefian, 1999a, 1999b; O'Brien & Renner, 2000; Tilden, 1999; White, 1999; White & Zimbelman, 1999; Zimbelman, 1999; Zimbelman & White, 1999).

Ethical concerns as they pertain to cultural diversity constitute another pattern that permeates a number of additional chapters. Particularly, Anne Davis (Chapter 6) and two chapters of Part V, Nursing Practice—those by Larry Purnell (Chapter 37) and Jean Jenkins (Chapter 54)—focus on cultural diversity.

Davis explicates the importance of nursing's values in ethics and presents an in-depth discussion of cultural relativism as an increasing challenge to the idea of universal ethics. She raises many critical questions, such as whose ethics establishes universal ethics. Further, Davis points out the numerous complexities and difficulties involved in advocating universal ethics even when all countries value virtuous, ethically principled, and caring nurses. Purnell's discussion (Chapter 37) explores the four levels of cultural competence, which also apply to the content presented by Davis in resolving challenges inherent in concepts of cultural relativism and universal ethics. Jenkins (Chapter 54) touches on ethical issues in relation to genetics and counseling services.

Academia and health care delivery are the environments of nursing practice and education that are the focus of nursing programs, faculty, and students. Lois Lane and Craig Paterson (Chapter 7) identify some of the

major legal issues that universities and nursing education programs must be prepared to address. Legal concerns pertaining to faculty and nursing students are discussed in relation to the internal forum of the university and external environment of clinical agencies and the community. Through Lane's and Paterson's presentation, students, faculty, and academic administrators are provided valuable information regarding their legal responsibilities and rights and are offered helpful suggestions in the prevention of legal problems.

The pathway of health policies and legislation is presented clearly by Janet Heinrich and Mary Wakefield (Chapter 8). They identify nursing's role in developing health policies and legislation that has implications for nursing education, research, and the future of nursing practice. Wakefield (1999) gives further suggestions as to how nurses should track activity at both the state and federal levels. Peter Buerhaus (Chapter 10) reinforces the need for involvement by nursing and nurses in policy making as he describes forces affecting Medicare and implications of the Balanced Budget Act of 1997 for reimbursement. His concerns are followed up in salient points by Karen Robinson, Hurdis Griffith, and Eileen Sullivan-Marx (Chapter 41) and by Mikel Gray (Chapter 42). Buerhaus further identifies issues that he initiated in a previous publication related to Medicare (Buerhaus, 1998): (a) the need for education programs that address aging, geriatrics, and chronic disease; and (b) relevance of the aging registered nurse workforce. In addition, new vistas are open for nurses to participate in development of health policy (Pulcini, Mason, Cohen, Kovner, & Leavitt, 2000).

The problem of splintering organizations and associations within the profession comes to mind as Patricia Thompson and Ramon Lavandero (Chapter 9) discuss associations that are thriving as the new century begins. These authors present quality indicators for associations. Need for communication among organizations is obvious. The question of an "umbrella" organization for nursing also surfaces and is addressed in other chapters, particularly those by Karleen Kerfoot (Chapter 75) and Grayce Sills and Carole Anderson (Chapter 77).

Significant patterns further emerge regarding the nursing workforce and in other issues are addressed by Cheryl Jones (Chapter 11). She explicates thoroughly the relationships among supply, wages, and demand in presenting critical factors pertaining to the aging and future nursing workforce and nursing shortage. Nursing shortage data are further substantiated in a study report by the University of California at San Francisco (UCSF) Center for California Health Workforce Studies (Russell, 1999). Another study reveals slow growth in the number of minorities in the RN workforce (Buerhaus & Auerbach, 1999). Attracting, educating, and retaining minorities in nursing education and practice could be positive strategies for increasing the workforce.

Cheryl Jones raises pertinent questions regarding the substitution of unlicensed personnel for registered nurses and nurse practitioners for physicians. Clinical practice policies that influence the workforce are clearly presented. Jones notes that Medicare funds are being assigned to hospitals with diploma programs, whereas only Title VIII funds go to nursing education programs directly—indicating a potential negative result for nursing. Consequently, she raises questions as to whether nurses' human capital (in terms of productivity output, competencies, and quality in performance and delivery of care) is sufficient to meet market demands.

Jones also raises the critical and thorny question of *interchangeableness* in one-for-one substitution of nurses prepared at the baccalaureate, associate degree, and diploma levels. Such practices encourage purchasers of nursing services to view nursing as a *commodity*, not as a profession! Recent studies show how

marginalization reduces individuals to commodities (David, 1999; Harrison, 1999). By citing data based on scientific studies and the reality of nurses demonstrating their clinical and economic value to purchasers and providers, these authors observe that barriers to professional practice will begin to fall.

The foundation offered by Cheryl Jones provides a solid basis for understanding workforce issues. Concerns regarding employment and utilization of professionals are evident in numerous other chapters and are identified later in this Summary.

■ Part II: Nursing Education

Many themes are shared by various authors in the chapters of Part II, Nursing Education. The clear consensus is that the entry into practice debate must be resolved. Emphasis on outcomes and quality are addressed from many aspects. Partnerships and interdisciplinary approaches for education programs are advocated. Innovative types of nursing programs are supported that will revolutionize the faculty role and expectations regarding tenure. The potential for use of technology—now, and as the wave of the future—is pervasive throughout the chapters.

Program Development and Evaluation

Specific points made by the authors in Part II have implications for suggestions in later Parts. Barbara Gaines (Chapter 12) lays the foundation for curriculum content and outcomes connected to practice and accountability in curriculum planning. Indeed, outcome is the dominant focus in numerous chapters. Development of cognitive skills, learning experiences to reinforce partnerships, and active learning strategies are advocated. Gaines suggests (personal communication, November

1999) that our responsibility is to "teach the edges not boundaries." Boundaries are viewed as being too firm for our time—change being so constant. Gaines further believes that it is critical to ask about the level(s) at which are we preparing students for entry into practice: Are we to prepare a generalist or, instead, a specialist who has sufficient generalist knowledge to pass the licensure examination? Her questions are supported further by other authors (Acord, 1999a; Rambur, 1999).

Long advocated, curriculum transformation is being realized (Kupperschmidt & Burns, 1997). With the advent of genetics in the mainstream of health care, integration of genetics content in undergraduate nursing programs is a mandate. Preparation of faculty to incorporate genetics into curricula also is a must, as emphasized by Jean Jenkins (Chapter 54) and other authors (Lashley, 1999; Monsen et al., 2000; Prows et al., 1999). Gaines supports a seamless process for curriculum and program development. Such a process is based on the principle that there should be no barriers between segments of the educational system. This path also is advocated by others (Lindeman, Chapter 63; McCahon, Niles, George, & Stricklin, 1999).

Flexible program evaluation environments are urged by Shirley Dooling and Barbara Gaines (Chapter 13). They present three models for evaluation frameworks and raise the potential of market forces for determining success of accrediting agencies. Outcomes assessment clearly has become a prime criteria for accreditation. Helpful guidelines for nurse educators are available (Thompson & Bartels, 1999). Evaluation of critical thinking long has been a challenging concern (Dexter et al., 1997). Various means of program evaluation are employed, including use of innovative residencies for programs (Howell & Coates, 1997). Possibilities of evaluation bodies, such as credentialing centers (i.e., state or regional bodies having a substantial role in accredita-

tion) are suggested. Rethinking accreditation processes and practices offer distinctive opportunities to evaluate how nursing helps learners become the best professional practitioners.

Delivery and Approaches

Distributive learning with a focus on student-centeredness is a dominant theme of Rosalee Yeaworth, Lani Zimmerman, Bevely Hays, and Carol Pullen (Chapter 14). Advances in technology have altered teaching, learning environments, practice opportunities, and expectations—to make possible many types of distance and distributive learning undertakings. The infrastructure needed for learning and human resources, particularly in developing on-line education communities, is clearly defined and explored by Diane Billings (Chapter 15). Connectedness in distributive learning programs is essential. In addition to suggestions provided by Yeaworth et al., other models are available (Hoagberg, Vellenga, Miller, & Li, 1999).

Problem-based learning as presented by Amy Nichols and Andrea Renwanz-Boyle (Chapter 16) and Mary Fisher (Chapter 17) changes the focus from teacher to student. Further, this method utilizes service-learning and requires teamwork so that students are more likely to link theory with practice experience. Institutionalizing service-learning is exemplified in a project described White and Henry (1999).

Fisher (Chapter 17) views the problem-based approach as a significant opportunity for strong curricula in Nursing Administration programs. Unification of clinical skills and business proficiency, which is more likely to occur in problem-based approaches, is essential for nursing leadership education.

As a result of the shift to community-based practice, teaching, and service-learning, Joyce Fitzpatrick (Chapter 18) sees opportunities for developing interprofessional teams through interdisciplinary education programs. One of the main reasons is that managed care has emphasized interprofessional care. Thus identification of core content across disciplines would facilitate increased team approaches in education, delivery of care, and evaluation of outcomes.

Learning and partnerships are expounded upon by Diane Billings (Chapter 15), Amy Nichols and Andrea Renwanz-Boyle (Chapter 16), Mary Fisher (Chapter 17), Joyce Fitzpatrick (Chapter 18), Shake Ketefian and Richard Redman (Chapter 19), and Elizabeth Lenz and Sally Hardin (Chapter 20). Partnerships in nursing education have offered clear paths in the past (Keating, 1997), but promise more now and for the future (Heller, Oros, & Durney-Crowley, 2000). These partnerships are also illustrated by numerous authors in chapters of Part V, Nursing Practice (Alexander, Chapter 44; Hollinger-Smith, Chapter 45; Pullen, Chapter 50; Todero, Chapter 51; and Barger, Chapter 52).

Graduate Programs

In master's programs curricula, the three most important topics identified for nurse practitioners were primary care, health promotion and disease prevention, and effective patient–provider relationships and communication (Bellack, Graber, O'Neil, Musham, & Lancaster, 1999). Further, business management preceptorships are advocated for nurse practitioners because they must have a competent understanding of basic business functions, including accounting, finance, economics, marketing, and reimbursement in their primary care practices (Wing, 1998). Knowledge and experiences in these areas are advocated by Mary Fisher (Chapter 17), particularly for graduate students majoring in nursing administration.

Graduate education in nursing at the master's and doctoral levels has advanced globally

and continues to develop rapidly (Shake Ketefian and Richard Redman in Chapter 19). Diverse approaches characterize state-of-nursing development in various countries and regions. Cited issues that must be addressed are similar for both international programs and graduate programs in the United States.

The predominant concern in international programs is quality. Collaboration and consultation services to develop explicit criteria for evaluation of graduate education programs are direly needed. A common basis for interpreting international education systems is lacking. Unfortunately, AACN indicators do not provide guidance that is universally relevant. To further compound the problem, diverse roles are assumed by graduates of international programs.

Quality is the all-encompassing concern for doctoral programs also in the United States, as pointed out by Elizabeth Lenz and Sally Hardin (Chapter 20). Aspects for ensuring quality are addressed in depth—considering resources (faculty, students, and technology), curriculum content, and structure of programs. Lenz and Hardin make an important point regarding the AACN Quality Indicators: Quality Indicators are normative recommendations for what should be present and done to achieve quality, with an emphasis on structure and process—not on outcomes. Interestingly, that distinction differs from the focus on outcomes, as advocated by accreditation bodies in their evaluations of curricula and programs. A serious question remains as to how quality is approached, if doctoral programs are not in sync with master's degree and undergraduate nursing programs. The question needs to be phrased—as: What implications might this difference have in building from one education level to another or in identifying outcomes for practice and roles graduates assume?

Only limited agreement exists regarding substantive content of nursing science and specifics of that content for curricula. Most often, doctoral curriculum are based on the expertise of faculty. Describing differences between the academic and professional doctoral programs, Lenz and Hardin indicate that a small but growing number of schools offer the professional doctorate to provide scholarly clinical leadership and innovation in practice. Given the difficulties in attempts to attain consensus with regard to content for the discipline as a whole, Lenz and Hardin suggest that the focus might better be directed to content pertinent to particular clinical populations. At present, no explicit trends or agreement exists as to the type and content of doctoral programs in nursing. However, Lenz and Hardin predict that increasing efforts will be made to differentiate professional and academic program curricula.

Lenz and Hardin also stress that doctoral education must be in a state of continuing evolution. They draw attention to the need for flexible administrative structures of doctoral programs that fit the overall philosophical structure of the university and school of nursing. Collaborative programs, which may be intra-institutional, inter-institutional, or joint endeavors, are described as ways to enhance quality. Lenz and Hardin predict trends in programs such as postbaccalaureate entry by students and increased utilization of information technology.

Faculty Transitions

Perhaps more disconcerting are the challenges faced by new graduates of doctoral programs in making the transition to an academic career. Inherent in this transition is conflict between teaching and research expectations. Workload issues have long been problematic, particularly when clinical teaching is part of assignments (Schuster, Fitzgerald, McCarthy, & McDougal, 1997). Larson (1997) offered some initial suggestions to resolve the balanc-

ing of roles. Anastasia Fisher and Barbara Habermann (Chapter 21) explicate the dilemma and offer viable strategies for prevention of problems and their solution when they do occur. Their recommendations warrant support.

Liaschenko and A. Fisher (1999) presented an example of how faculty apply their knowledge in teaching and practice in conducting empirical research regarding requisite knowledge for nursing work. Building and integrating roles is one way to approach balance. Another is support of doctoral faculty, which is increasing (Acord, 2000).

Most often newly prepared doctoral faculty are called on for leadership roles for which they have had insufficient preparation (Triolo, Pozehl, & Mahaffey, 1997). Such assignments carry unreasonable expectations and can greatly inhibit development of their scholarship. Norbeck (1998) proposes options for balancing multiple role expectations. Although the sacred triad of teaching, research, and service is unlikely to continue its reign as universally as in the past, change in expectations is uncertain.

The extent that Boyer's model for scholarship, described by Juanita Fleming (Chapter 22), will become a pattern in meeting criteria for tenure remains to be seen. The AACN developed the *Position Statement: Defining Scholarship for the Discipline of Nursing,* which was approved by the membership on March 15, 1999 (AACN, 1999a). Those standards, although intended to differ in application by institution, provide a framework that may be utilized in tenure reviews by the academic nursing community.

However, relevance of tenure and the emerging trend of post-tenure reviews in some universities will continue to raise thorny questions. Given Fleming's discussion and the changes predicted in faculty roles by numerous other authors, dramatic reconceptualization and alteration in expectations for faculty and tenure are on the horizon. For example, Sharon Hoffman (Chapter 64); Diana Biordi and Elizabeth McFarlane (Chapter 67); Sarah Keating and Shannon Perry (Chapter 65); Joan Shaver (Chapter 76); and particularly Carole Lindeman (Chapter 63) offer critical insight into changes that we can expect which will affect faculty making transitions, faculty roles, and tenure.

■ Part III: Nursing Theory

Writings in Part III present an intriguing challenge. The chapters reflect the postmodernism dilemma: How do we determine which is the best truth? If all truth is relative, what anchors us as professionals and a profession? To which values do we subscribe? Postmodernism is characterized by competing versions of reality in the absence of agreed-upon criteria for truth. Postmodern approaches "challenge the view that it is possible to represent reality, speak for others, make truth claims and attain universal essential understandings" (Cheek, 2000, p. 5). In some respects, the totality of the chapters on nursing theory show a postmodern approach for theory development in nursing. Multiple voices, views, and methods for analyzing realities are evident. For nursing to draw on numerous realities offers diversity in the development of knowledge. But postmodern approaches also may result in confusion, particularly in the practice arena. The disparity of views expressed in these chapters, however, may indicate nursing's ability to deal with varying beliefs and opinions and to convey a willingness to dialogue.

Hesook Suzie Kim (Chapter 23) calls for some "order" in knowledge development . She emphasizes pulling pluralism in philosophies together to guide future theory development and shows linkages between frameworks from a philosophy of science perspective. She identifies and describes specific orientations for nursing science: inferential, referential, transformative, and desiderative. She concludes that nursing knowledge for the future needs development in all four spheres.

Peggy Chinn (Chapter 24) presents a philosophic theory that offers a conceptual definition of the art of nursing from an aesthetic rather than an empirical perspective, stressing that nursing as a healing art assumes that empirical theory does not provide insight on how to carry out nursing actions. Chinn describes what it means to be a nurse—to experience the practice of nursing. She shows how nursing practice is derived from four patterns of knowing, with art transforming experience.

The postmodern approach to development of nursing knowledge is explored by Jean Watson (Chapter 25). She counters the deconstruction postmodern debate with what she labels "reflective reconstruction"—seeking to sustain nursing's covenant of caring practices with the public. Watson demonstrates reconstruction by sharing a personal experience. She invites nurses as individuals to deal first with their own caring–healing needs. Then, as a result of reflection and reconstruction—integrating and embracing what has come before—Watson believes that nurses will be able to become mature, caring–healing practitioners.

Four fundamental premises for advancing nursing knowledge are detailed by Jacqueline Fawcett and Mary Bourbonniere (Chapter 26). These postulates are: (a) nursing is a distinct discipline; (b) knowledge is formalized through conceptual models and grand and middle-range theories; (c) distinctive nursing research and practice methodologies are used to develop, test, and apply knowledge; and (d) new knowledge must be associated with existing formal nursing knowledge. Fawcett and Bourbonniere offer challenges to the four premises. Further, they warn that Advanced Practice

Nursing (APN) programs divert attention from development of nursing knowledge to medical knowledge. These authors urge that APN programs be built on the foundation of nursing.

An overview and application of the conceptual model for nursing—the Neuman Systems Model (NSM)—is explained by Betty Neuman (Chapter 27). She describes the NSM as an international guide for nursing research, education, administration, and practice and posits that wholistic concepts in a constantly changing environment are needed in health and illness care. The NSM markers as an aid to professionals in providing holistic care are further exemplified as a true practice model in this chapter and another recent publication (Neuman, Newman, & Holder, 2000).

A comprehensive analysis of nursing theories is offered by Eleanor Donnelly (Chapter 28). She labels such theories frameworks for conceptualizing the practice of nursing within a science of nursing. Donnelly evidences belief in scientific theory and scientific investigation. She presumes objective reality and that this reality is knowable. She demonstrates that scientific theories are about actual states, not desirable states.

Donnelly clearly traces the origins of conceptualizing nursing. She reviews early arguments about theory development, testing reported in nursing's empirical research literature, and the resulting confusion. She reconsiders Jan Beckstrand's critical examination of nursing theories, recalling that Beckstrand was the first nurse scholar to do so from the standpoint of a philosophy of science. Donnelly also addresses the further arguments and questions raised by Carol Deets. Donnelly concludes that insufficient understanding exists as to what scientific inquiry entails. Although acknowledging efforts to date, she sees the results not as scientific theories but as normative frameworks for conceptualizing practice. As to where we go from here, see the discussion offered by Afaf

Meleis and Eun-Ok Im (Chapter 72) in Part VIII, The Future of Nursing.

■ Part IV: Nursing Research

Part IV might be described as having four foci: (a) clinical nursing research, (b) methodology and instrumentation, (c) outcomes and quality, and (d) preparation for research. Those areas are addressed extensively, with some of the chapters including all four aspects of nursing research.

Clinical Nursing Research

Clinical research pertaining to cancer nursing is the focus of Ada Lindsey (Chapter 29). She urges integration of nursing research with that of other sciences for testing of interventions and interdisciplinary collaboration. Lindsey uses cancer nursing research to illustrate her points. She stresses significant research areas that need to be addressed: (a) genetics; (b) confidence in the quality of nursing research regarding framework, instrumentation, intervention, and analysis; and (c) evidence of building on previous research.

Responses of different individuals to exercise under varying conditions and states of mobility is reported by Christine Kasper (Chapter 30). She urges further investigation to determine appropriate exercise for the aged and during recovery from various conditions; also noted is the need for research on the use of electrical stimulation of skeletal muscle (EMS) to increase skeletal muscle size and strength. Kasper demonstrates the need for incorporating clinical research content in nursing education.

Methodology and Instrumentation Concerns

Nursing language and its relationship to knowledge development in nursing is explored by Dorothy Jones (Chapter 31). She details the value of (a) standardized nursing language, (b) ongoing development for nursing practice, and (c) documentation of cost-effective, quality services with implications for reimbursement of professional services. Standardization of nursing language makes capturing the patient experience from a nursing perspective possible. Various data sets for classification systems and nomenclatures are shown and described.

A pattern for nursing research—focusing on evidence-based research and outcomes—is portrayed by Ida Androwich and Sheila Haas (Chapter 32). They discuss identification of research questions, methodology, design, measurement and instrumentation, and data analysis by means of integrated systematic reviews of the literature. The need for a common language, as demonstrated by Jones (Chapter 31), is substantiated.

With cultural diversity and pluralism increasing in the United States, according to numerous authors and chapters (Davis, Chapter 6; Jones, Chapter 11; Lenz & Hardin, Chapter 20; Purnell, Chapter 37; and Jenkins, Chapter 54), valid and reliable instrumentation and measurement are challenges that must be met in nursing research. Robin Froman and Steven Owen (Chapter 33) present valuable information regarding scale development, instrumentation, and translation of alternative language forms. They also discuss response considerations and empirical assessment of translated instruments. They insist that scale development and translation require as much art as statistical expertise.

Theory-based interventions are the focus of a meta-analysis conducted by Carol Deets and Euisoo Choi (Chapter 34). Purpose, value, process, and procedures in developing evidence tables are demonstrated. First, evidence tables were initiated through an extensive review of the literature. Deets and Choi found inadequate reporting of critical information, particularly by journals focused on practice. Only 24 studies were found that appeared to test theory-based interventions. One intervention only—therapeutic touch (TT)—had been studied sufficiently to include in the project. Deets and Choi present a six-category system to assess study quality and evidence that supported interventions. They deduced that theory-based interventions have not been studied sufficiently to justify use in practice. In the case of evidence tables, they concluded that this method allows easy documentation of an article's content and summarization of evidence from any number of research articles. Importantly, Deets and Choi illustrate the methodology for future use of evidence tables.

Another approach in research, different from evidence tables but supported by theory, is that of typologies for grading evidence-based practice. Evidence-based practice is not necessarily derived from theory. Marita Titler (Chapter 35) focuses on development of evidence-based practice guidelines, typologies, and the science of moving evidence to use in practice. In promotion of research-based practice, she offers strategies to persuade health care workers to adopt evidence-based practice guidelines and typologies. In so doing, she presents the Iowa Model of Research-Based Practice to Promote Quality Care as an exemplar. Providing options for quality in nursing practice is helpful. Another model for changing practice to being evidence-based was recently described by Rosswurm and Larrabee (1999).

Outcomes research is again the theme, this time presented in terms of needs for doctoral preparation, of Kenneth Miller (Chapter 36). He proposes blending the content of an academic Doctor of Philosophy (PhD) research degree with the enhanced clinical component in Doctor of Nursing Science (DNS) professional degree program. He advocates outcomes research similar to that presented by Titler (Chapter 35). In addition, Miller urges research aimed at new models for delivery of care and translating research findings into health policy.

■ Part V: Nursing Practice

In Part V, threads and strands provided in previous chapters are beginning to be woven into patterns for directions in nursing practice. Major paths regarding cultural competency, technology, reimbursement, preparation of advanced practitioners, healing practices, partnerships, outcomes, and variations in sites and modes of practice become obvious. The routes for future nursing practice depend on clear understanding, courage, communication, integration, and collaboration to reach goals and fulfill nursing's public mandate.

Essentials for Nursing Practice

Cultural Competence

Although the theme of cultural diversity is apparent in numerous previous chapters, Larry Purnell (Chapter 37) offers a comprehensive foundation for understanding the importance of culture globally. Appropriately, culture is inherent in every aspect of nursing practice, including skill competency; wellness, illness, and healing care practices—and particularly in values and ethics. Diverse venues in practice demand knowledge, understanding, and effective communication for cultural competence.

Informatics

The importance and role of information technology is a theme explored previously by Yeaworth et al. (Chapter 14) and by Billings (Chapter 15). Building on that content, the merger of technology and clinical nursing practice can be understood as an all-encompassing specialty called nursing informatics, clearly presented by Kathleen Stevens and Elizabeth

Weiner (Chapter 38). Role preparation at the undergraduate and graduate levels, consumer access to telehealth sites, linkage of standard nursing language with health information systems, and conversion of technology are shown to be changing the face of nursing practice.

Practice by Educators and in Integrated Partnerships

Faculty Practice

Faculty increasingly are using their expertise in providing direct care. Faculty who practice clinically further benefit by maintaining their knowledge base and skills, making use of opportunities to develop research and clinical innovation, and possibly, through producing additional revenue. Michael Carter (Chapter 39) succinctly describes four models of faculty practice, points out possible collision between practice and education cultures—particularly when practice is part of faculty role expectations—and identifies new issues for resolution. A sampling of the complex challenges faced by university-based nursing programs attempting to implement a clinical track is presented by Barger (1999). Carter enlarges on factors involved in faculty practice, considering (a) promotion and tenure, (b) distribution of income, (c) liability, (d) funding of nursing units, and (e) potential shifting of education costs. A number of Carter's points are further developed in Lindeman's predictions (Chapter 63) regarding the changing faculty role.

Integrated Partnerships

A key pathway in nursing practice—an effective means for providing health and illness care—is that of integrated partnerships. Tracing the history of combined endeavors between nursing education and nursing practice, a distinctive partnership model is explicated by Maureen McCausland and Kathleen

McCauley (Chapter 40). The model at The University of Pennsylvania Health System is unique. Excellent examples of the integrated system, with educators, clinicians, and administrators using the professional practice model, are provided. McCausland and McCauley also offer recommendations for concentrated further development of partnerships.

Elements of Nursing Practice

Remuneration

Reimbursement is obviously part of the blueprint for future nursing practice. Compensation for services provided is discussed in some previous chapters and most chapters in this Nursing Practice Part; it is also commented on in the remaining Parts of the book. A cry for more acceptable reimbursement is understandable, as compensation is interrelated with many concerns of nursing as noted by Karen Robinson, Hurdis Griffith, and Eileen Sullivan-Marx (Chapter 41).

They present findings of studies wherein Current Procedural Terminology (CPT) Codes identified as billable activities were those performed by nurses. Although direct reimbursement to some advanced practice nurses became possible with signing of the Balanced Budget Act of 1997, this method is not available to all practicing nurses. Robinson et al. predict that evidence-based practice is likely to be the criterion for future reimbursement. Problems in reimbursement are identified, such as (a) lack of uniform educational requirements (i.e., entry for professional practice); (b) lack of practice-based data; (c) inconsistencies in state and national legal and regulatory provisions for nursing practice; and (d) lack of unity within the profession. These same authors suggest extensive strategies for facilitating improved reimbursement; they also provide specific directions for future research on the unsatisfactory reimbursement situation.

Advanced Practice Roles

The positive impact of the Balanced Budget Act of 1997 for nursing services is further explored by Mikel Gray (Chapter 42). He presents the evolution of advanced practice nursing (APN), focusing on the APN roles of nurse anesthetist, nurse midwife, clinical nurse specialist, and nurse practitioner. Gray makes distinctions between advanced nursing practice, specialty practice, and expert nursing practice. Although conceptualized differently, his delineation of differences among the three types of practice is somewhat similar to the levels of practice for the future workforce depicted for consideration by Cheryl Jones (Chapter 11).

Gray addresses shared and unique aspects of each APN role and its requisite educational preparation. Debate continues regarding blending content of the clinical nurse specialist (CNS) and nurse practitioner (NP) roles into one graduate program. Regardless of how the debate is resolved, APN programs and the profession are urged to heed the advice offered in 1974 by Barbara Bates, MD (as cited in Catlin & McAuliffe, 1999). Bates, speaking at one of the first NP graduations, is quoted in part as follows:

> By expanding into medicine, you will need—more than ever before—to increase your consciousness of what nursing is all about. The values of nursing must not get lost in the dominant medical culture. If [they] do, you justly risk the epithet of junior doctor. Our patients do not need junior doctors. They need the knowledge and skills of both medicine and nursing. (p. 177)

Perhaps those words are even more relevant today, particularly in the present collaborative practice climate (Moser & Armer, 2000). With the emphasis on integration in health care, it seems reasonable to predict that graduate nursing programs, to achieve their goals, need to become more integrated in structure, content, and roles.

Gray predicts that the Health Care Financing Administration (HCFA) by 2002 will require nurse practitioners to hold a master's degree plus certification from a nationally recognized board. Implications are many—if Gray's prediction becomes reality—for nursing education programs and nurse practitioners who were prepared through certificate type, not master's degree programs. The rapid pace of change in reimbursement legislation (Lindeke & Chesney, 1999) suggests the wisdom in considering and planning master's degree education programs for such certified nurse practitioners.

Gray also makes a plea for collaboration and increased communication among disciplines. His plea is similar to that urged by other contributing authors—for example, Cheryl Jones (Chapter 11), Joyce Fitzpatrick (Chapter 18), and Ada Lindsey (Chapter 29).

Therapies

Complementary therapies in integrating care through holistic philosophy—regarding the patient as healer, caring, physical presence, and active listening have long been part of nursing practice. Regulation, reimbursement, and research issues pertaining to alternative therapies are presented by Mariah Snyder, Mary Jo Kreitzer, and Marilyn Loen (Chapter 43). Measurement of caring in relation to outcomes must be assessed. Given the findings of Deets and Choi (Chapter 34), scientific evidence for effectiveness of therapeutic touch is warranted. The increasing use of complementary and alternative therapies portends a future path in nursing practice.

The Community in Nursing Practice and Partnerships

The community offers an enlarged blueprint of nursing services and care for the future. Community health is aptly described by Judith Alexander (Chapter 44), as is her projection for the 21st century. Population assessment is presented as being distinctive in "community-focused care," and different from "community-based care." Examining the technological and structural variables, Alexander presents a model for community health services delivery. Leadership skills and competencies of practitioners in the community are viewed as the appropriate fit between technology and structure. Alternative and complementary forms of health care, outcome measurement, and partnerships again are themes—identified previously in other chapters and explored further by Alexander.

The partnership pattern shifts from professionals as individuals to providers as a community of partners in the extensive explication by Linda Hollinger-Smith (Chapter 45). She describes models of community empowerment and services offered—with shared responsibilities being at the core of collaboration and health promotion. Hollinger-Smith shows the need for changes in how education is provided, programs are evaluated, and research is conducted (i.e., population-focused and action-oriented).

Settings for Nursing Practice

Significant variation exists in patterns of community and health care services. Modalities in providing care also are diverse. The remaining chapters in this Nursing Practice Part focus on form, location, and methods of health care delivery, and types of services offered in the community and larger public arena. Appropriately, this Part concludes with a focus on genetics—a major variable that is just beginning to have a significant impact on health, illness, and the practice of nursing.

Transition

A link between acute and chronic care is being defined more clearly. Inclusion and unity of palliative care with acute and chronic care modalities is illustrated by Inge Corless (Chapter 46). Palliative care is described as not necessarily implying terminal illness, end-of-life, or hospice care. Rather, emphasis is on total care of patients whose disease is not responsive to curative treatment. Making the transition from aggressive to comfort care is a challenge. The appropriate time to initiate such care is debatable, particularly in regard to reimbursement. Palliative care at present is practiced essentially by the medical profession. However, Corless indicates that restructuring for the provision of better palliative care to include nursing practice is underway. She also stresses the need for education of nursing students and all health care practitioners in palliative care.

Home Care

The natural site for palliative care is the patient's home, an increasingly used component in the continuum of care. Transition of care to places of residence, the types of home care, and classification systems for such care are described by Mary Ann Schroeder and Carol Long (Chapter 47). Although fraudulent and abusive practices are being exposed (Tahan, 1999), Schroeder and Long are optimistic that the financial and reimbursement challenges will rectify the types of improprieties uncovered. They emphasize the need for the HCFA to develop a case-mix adjuster that reflects cost of providing services to various types of patients. Leaders in nursing are advocating new models for developing nursing student experiences in home care nursing (Pinkerton, 1998). Schroeder and Long enlarge on home care opportunities for nursing students and define competencies and skills that must be developed through nursing education programs and experiences for adequate provision of that type of care.

Consumer Choice

With options increasing for primary care, health care, and prevention of illness, the question becomes: How does a consumer choose? Models for consumer decision-making are presented by Elizabeth Sefcik and Rebecca Patronis Jones (Chapter 48). They offer a scenario that illustrates application of the models.

Parish Nursing

A unique expansion of the community, parish nursing entwines health and faith. The focus of practice is the faith community and its health history. Roots of parish nursing are based in early church history. In presenting current practice, Mary Ann McDermott (Chapter 49) describes the parish nurse role in relation to integration of health and faith and seven diverse functions (e.g., referral agent and developer of support groups). Education of the parish nurse, accountability, credentialing, and infrastructure support are examples of challenges McDermott explores. As an integrator of health and faith, parish nursing is rapidly becoming a distinctive specialty.

Rural Nursing

Community nursing practice is being extended to rural settings. Carol Pullen (Chapter 50) discusses various definitions of rural—centering on population and economic factors—and the challenge of making health care available, affordable, and accessible to people in rural areas. The focus is on ambulatory care and community-based clinics. Opportunities for nurse practitioners are abundant; however, attracting and retaining them are challenges. Rural case managers in clinical practice can play a key role in integrating care in rural communities (Anderson-Loftin, 1999). Pullen outlines needs and strategies for developing nursing education programs in rural areas. Recent advances in technology and telehealth and interdisciplinary health care models promise to be paths for care and health in rural communities.

Mobile Nursing Centers

Nursing practice can exist without walls, although space and place often define its characteristics. Mobility, flexibility, and connection to the communities served are features of mobile nursing centers explored by Catherine Todero (Chapter 51). Most often, mobile centers are designed to target needy groups and vulnerable populations, such as children, the elderly, and the homeless. Showcasing the University of Nebraska College of Nursing Mobile Nursing Center (MNC), Todero outlines the establishment of a mobile center and its advantages, opportunities, services, and challenges. As a distinctive partnership model, the MNC provides excellent learning opportunities for students and offers opportunities for integration of service, education, and research. Survival in the future is perceived to depend on (a) innovative technology, (b) greater emphasis on business and negotiation skills, and (c) a shift in thinking of nursing and academic models. Funding, reimbursement, measurement of outcomes, and proof of cost-effectiveness are issues of importance for all nursing centers whether mobile or fixed in location.

Nursing Centers

Retaining the core values of nursing centers while learning new survival strategies as keys to the future is the message of Sara Barger (Chapter 52). She details the history of nursing centers and addresses five challenges suggested by the Pew Health Professions Commission: (a) balancing interests of the individual and society, (b) demanding accountability, (c) truly managing care, (d) making consolidation work, and (e) responding to demands of the emerging health care market.

Barger urges positioning for a preferred future in relation to those challenges. She identifies nine trends as (a) continued increases in health care costs; (b) oversupply of resources—

hospitals, providers, and technology; (c) aging population; (d) consumer use of information technology; (e) advances in disease treatment; (f) improved measurements of quality; (g) informed consumer decision-making; (h) increasing disparities in population affecting the nation's health; and (i) expansion of preventive care. She explores these trends and offers strategies for the success of nursing centers.

Entrepreneurship

Changes in the health care system and the practice of nursing have spurred emergence of nursing entrepreneurship. Nursing practice clearly has become deinstitutionalized, thereby opening new frontiers and modes of practice for nurses as independent practitioners. Virginia Duffy (Chapter 53) presents possibilities and barriers, how to overcome obstacles, and describes the world of marketing. She reveals entrepreneurship as a clear path for nursing through "stories" of three successful entrepreneurs, including herself. Nurses on-line is another excellent example of opportunity for entrepreneurship (O'Brien & Renner, 2000). Duffy ends with a strong note of optimism for the future.

Knowledge Factor's Effect on Future Practice

Jean Jenkins (Chapter 54) depicts knowledge of genetics as a critical variable in developing directions for nursing and health care. She elaborates on aspects of health care practice expected to be affected by the rapidly expanding knowledge of genetics. Elements identified include infrastructure, economics, models of care, and ethical dilemmas in health care and nursing practice. Jenkins addresses specific consequences for nursing practice, such as scope of practice, nursing education (preparing faculty, developing curricula, and educating nursing students), and opportunities for nursing research.

In presenting new opportunities and markets for service in nursing, Jenkins outlines the role of the nurse in genetics education, use of methods and tools in genetics, and obligations. Clearly, genetics knowledge will need to be integrated into every aspect of nursing practice in the future.

■ Part VI: Nursing Administration– Service

Integrated delivery systems is the predominant pattern in structuring organizations and care for nursing services. Integration increasingly is used as an approach to process in (a) reducing costs, (b) collaborating for continuity in providing care, (c) reducing risk factors in providing care, and (d) creating healthy environments. Working cooperatively and providing executive leadership—inherent in nursing service endeavors—are the themes evident in the chapters for Part VI, Nursing Administration—Service.

Structures for Health Care Delivery

New structures and models for health care systems are proposed by Timothy Porter-O'Grady (Chapter 55). Emphases on cost control, information flow management, impact of technology, consumer awareness and options, and management in chronic care are some of the factors influencing reconfigurations of institutions as systems. Development of new models is based essentially on integration of services along a continuum of life services for defined patient populations. Porter-O'Grady advocates (a) aligning service pathways, (b) building on technology and information infrastructure for portability of services, and (c) transferring sets of skills to facilitate nurse mobility. The future depends on structures for service being integrated, fluid, and flexible.

The integrated delivery system (IDS) is the structure of choice delineated by SueEllen Pinkerton (Chapter 56). She identifies vertical integration as being separate departments organized with products that are inputs to other services (e.g., physician practices (inputs) to patients in ambulatory care (outputs)). Pinkerton envisions horizontal integration as multihospital systems (i.e., hospital, hospice, nursing home, and physician practice groups). Nursing care delivery is proposed to be structured to connect all points in an integrated system. Through shared governance, organizations need to look at their organizational cultures in terms of a continuum of care. IDS may best be developed by looking at how nursing components are connected along that continuum of care.

Case management, as a specialty for nursing practice innate to integration of services and care, is addressed by Rose Gerber (Chapter 57). She outlines state-of-the-art practice of the specialty, requisite education and its integration into academic programs, and roles for patient advocacy, accountability, and research. The need for case management is evident in the integration of a continuum of care in diverse settings, as previously suggested in rural health care. The future of case management depends on partnerships and flexible delivery of quality care.

The structure and environment of managed care are the foci of Margaret Conger (Chapter 58). She depicts managed care as a means for concentrating services for groups of persons. Models of managed care are described in terms of (a) staff—where providers are employed by health maintenance organizations (HMOs); (b) groups—through contracts to provide care on capitation basis; (c) networks—contracts with HMOs and groups of physicians; (d) independent practice associations (IPAs)—whereby individual physicians contract with an HMO to provide services; and (e) preferred provider organizations (PPOs)—through insurance company contracts at discounted rates for health care providers.

Nursing's role in managed care is emphasized—health promotion, coordination of care, developing outcome measures, and primary providers of care. Nurses increasingly are viewed as a key resource in managed care because they have competencies beyond technical skills. Cognitive, integrative, and leadership skills are essential for effective performance in managed care environments (Valanis, 2000).

Environmental Health

Environmental risk factors involved in nursing practice are aptly addressed by Jacqueline Dienemann, Jacquelyn Campbell, and Jacqueline Agnew (Chapter 59). Identification of hazards and control of the environment in providing health care are discussed. They show how separation of health, social, and environmental services affects delivery of care.

Inherent as a threat for healthy environments is conflict. Sandra Thomas (Chapter 60) traces the genesis of conflict; stresses the importance of addressing, not ignoring, conflict; and emphasizes promotion of healing dialogues. Creating a culture of cooperation as a means for solving problems is key in conflict prevention and resolution. Realistic suggestions are offered for managers and staff for improving relationships with each other. Thomas projects a positive nursing future through empowerment of nurses—enhancing nursing's ability to take action and resolve problems—and formation of coalitions for addressing issues such as unsafe working conditions, inadequate resources, and ill-conceived policies. She advocates building on strong collegial relationships and replacing destructive conflict in nursing's environments.

Healthy environments, workplace aggression, and the syndrome of traumatic stress are discussed by Joanne Disch (Chapter 61). Verbal abuse is the most common form of aggression in health care environments. Disch describes elements common to healthy work environments: (a) administrative commitment, (b) opportunities for open communication, (c) employee involvement, and (d) training and education programs. Opportunities for developing healthy work environments are available, which Disch aptly demonstrates by means of a case study concerning the merger of the University of Minnesota Hospital and Clinic (UMHC) with Fairview Riverside Medical Center (FRMC).

Preparing for Administration of Services in the Future

Projecting the future for administrators of nursing services elicits anxiousness in the most experienced. But not for Margaret McClure (Chapter 62), who confidently confronts the challenges. She presents the shifts in focus for care and in nursing executives from the individual and institution to macro systems. As a result, emphasizing prior integrator experiences, most nursing executives have expanded chief operating officer types of roles. Changed roles for nurse administrators and education preparation are affirmed by Krejci (1999). McClure emphasizes that titles in corporations need to reflect leadership for the practice of nursing. She portrays the corporate role for nurse executives as being in its formative stages. Consequently, McClure declares the need for developing strategies to prepare nursing administrators (including executives) for organizational leadership roles, such as enabling some APNs to perform at that level.

Two among a number of major points made by McClure stand out. The first concerns her proposal for two levels of nursing workers: professional nurses prepared at the baccalaureate or higher degree level and unlicensed assistive personnel (UAPs) prepared in on-the-job training programs. The second reflects the great need to prepare new graduates for the marketplace. McClure's description of a one-year residency program for new graduates at New York University Medical Center is helpful. She suggests that this program be a national model.

A further point needs to be considered regarding the potential for two levels of practice. Shirley Dooling (personal communication, January 10, 2000) offers a relevant, but different, perspective. Conceivably, master's degree education as the entry for professional practice provides a good science basis for critical thinking. However, Dooling believes that, rather than individuals being able to move from one level to another, there should be an interface between two levels of practice.

Noteworthy, Margaret McClure is credited for being the nursing leader who first advocated strongly the baccalaureate degree as minimal educational preparation for entry into the profession. Her original writing was first published in 1976 and later in the first book of the series titled: *The Nursing Profession* (1978). The subtitle of that book, "Views Through the Mist," was an unforeseen forecast of the future anathema for discussions about "entry into practice." We can only hope that McClure's suggestions for final resolution of the issue and for additional preparation regarding new graduates will not encounter similar resistance.

■ *Part VII: Nursing Administration– Academic*

Creating healthy environments in which students are willing, wanting, and able to learn and qualified faculty can guide, mentor, and demonstrate scholarship are essential to effective administration of academic nursing programs. Such environments, in which students and faculty and staff want to belong, also require visionary leadership as described by Robert Dilts (1996, 2000). Environments that

are creative also have structure, utilize processes, and produce relevant outcomes.

Themes of structure, process, and outcomes of higher education and patterns for effective leadership are woven into the chapters of Part VII, Nursing Administration—Academic. Differences in organizational structure are delineated according to variables such as type or category of institution, size (personnel and type and number of programs offered), resources, and enrollment. For example, significant differences in structure exist among public and private institutions and academic health centers. Organizational structures, titles, roles, and functions vary for the chief executive officers (CEOs) of nursing programs and other associate management personnel according to type of institution. Cautious optimism is evident as the authors in this Part examine current challenges in the constant changing environment and predict dramatic future changes.

Environment and Changing Roles

The higher education environment is traced by Carol Lindeman (Chapter 63) from the post–World War II period beginning in the late 1940s to the present day, showing a strong foundation for the major changes predicted for tomorrow. Funding demands, pressures for quality, and competition in the marketplace of higher education are evident. One of many responses is to develop a seamless education system. Pressure is increasing to remove barriers for students between education levels and segments. Custom-designed programs are predicted for survival of higher education in the marketplace. Accountability and technology will be increasingly emphasized. Such programs will inherently have an impact on faculty roles. Lindeman details those factors that are influencing major changes in expectations of faculty and also of the dean.

Lindeman demonstrates keen insight in explaining the changing role of the dean. She presents a true and real vision of the role and its relationships with faculty, challenges that are inherent (and increasing) in the role, and changes in the role that are expected. Importantly, Lindeman asserts the need for discernment on the part of the dean (i.e., the ability to see clearly is not only essential for sanity but also for success in the role). Strategies and suggestions for success are offered. Reorientation of one's values, courage, and confidence and trusting one's own intuition are requisite.

Academic Administration: Structure and Chief Nursing Officer Role

Academic Health Centers

Various organization models, goals, and responsibilities of the Dean of a School of Nursing in an Academic Health Center (AHC) are presented and explored by Sharon Hoffman (Chapter 64). She emphasizes the need for strategies, focusing particularly on positioning. Recognizing the AHCs are basically different, but share some similarities with other types of higher education institutions, Hoffman predicts increasing generalized stress in AHCs and in the role of the dean of nursing. These ill effects are related to (a) conflict among the three missions of AHCs (research, education, and service), (b) clash in values, (c) decreased funding, (d) increased oversight and responsibilities, and (e) changes in the delivery of health care. Collaborative initiatives in strategic planning, goal setting, and resource allocation are suggested as necessary for AHCs to survive and thrive.

Public and Private Sectors

Titles (e.g., dean, director, chair) of the chief academic officer for administration of nursing programs vary not only with the type of institution (AHC, public, or private) where nursing programs are offered, but also according to the mission and goals of institutions. Although the leadership functions of deans are classical for both public and private institutions, differences in mission and goals, faculty governance, and challenges vary. The funding arena of distance learning programs is more competitive for private than public institutions. Crumbling infrastructures may affect success—for private schools more than for public institutions—especially when survival depends more on tuition.

Keating and Perry point out commonalities between organizations in public and private higher education and assert that opportunities for collaboration to influence policy abound. They echo a critical issue, previously cited, that must be resolved: level of education appropriate for licensure (i.e., entry into professional practice). Although the onus is on the boards of nursing licensure and legislation, Keating and Perry insist that leadership and collaboration are requisites for total resolution of the issue. They assert that the benefits of additional education at whatever level must be recognized.

Keating and Perry advocate partnerships (again, a theme in previous chapters), consortia, and new types of organizational structures . They assert that new structures are needed to address increasing complexity, such as generic master's degree programs for individuals holding a nonnursing baccalaureate degree entering nursing—all requiring some type of collaboration. Additionally, they emphasize that curricula must be responsive to constant change, and they urge that rigid criteria be avoided in evaluation. In essence, Keating and Perry capture patterns revealed in previous chapters—importance of outcomes, regulation, and global collaboration—while providing depth. At the same time they clearly make distinctions between public and private institutions in terms of how organizational structures affect the process of education.

Academic Administration: Administrative and Faculty Roles

Associate Dean

Associate dean (AD) role and functions are delineated by Marilyn Flood (Chapter 66). She offers a valuable description of the role in terms of extending the overall administrative leadership of the chief academic administrator. The discussion presented is relevant to all associate types of administrators. Substantive application is possible regardless of the title of the "chief" role or the type of institution—AHC, public, or private. Flood herself is positioned in an AHC. Factors influencing the role, initiatives, coordinating processes, and activities are detailed.

Flood explores the relationship between the AD role and dean role. She portrays the AD role as one negotiated over time but offers three generalizations to characterize the relationship: (a) corresponding positive and negative visions; (b) contributions of energy, ethics, moral engagement, and aptitude by both parties; and (c) service of the AD at the pleasure of the dean. Essential characteristics, attitudes, skills, and practices for holding the position are addressed. Qualifications are outlined, with Flood emphasizing ability and experience. She predicts extensive change in the nature of the AD role as higher education is forced to restructure.

Essential for effectiveness in institutions where the associate dean (or similar) position is employed are criteria that I often have advised as a consultant: (a) clear and explicit boundaries for decision-making established between the associate dean and dean; and (b) a reporting and accountability process established for the associate dean. For an AD to "screen" information that should be provided "unedited" to the dean is unacceptable. Such screening diminishes the dean's capability for making effective decisions on the basis of complete and accurate knowledge and facts.

Academic Administration: Processes

Administrative roles, such as associate dean, historically vary according to the structures of higher education institutions. Diana Biordi and Elizabeth McFarlane (Chapter 67), who are positioned in public and private universities, respectively, portray the influence of public and private organizational structures on roles and faculty. Focus is directed toward career paths and ladders for preparation and development of roles in administration, such as the associate dean and those in the professoriate. Communication skills and credibility—regarding aptitude in curriculum development and processes—are among the characteristics that Biordi and McFarlane emphasize.

They present a comprehensive picture of how changes in higher education are affecting nursing units. The influence of Ernest Boyer on a newer model of scholarship is discussed. Advantages and disadvantages of tenure and questions regarding changing requirements for tenure surface. Both the tenure theme and that of increased reliance on nontenure track faculty are evidenced, similar to those identified in previous chapters.

Resolving a Common Problem

Deans are learning more effective ways of dealing with problems and challenges; it is better to confront than avoid. In so doing, deans are finding that they need to develop mediation skills and apply them in performing their role. Research (Valentine, Richardson, Wood, & Godkin, 1998) and my own experience as a consultant for administration in universities, indicate that nurse educators and administrators may have distinctive approaches to conflict management. A maneuver in academia that is increasingly of concern—going over the head of someone in line authority to impart information to someone higher up—is addressed by Norma Chaska (Chapter 68). Causes, examples, and outcomes of the phenomenon—labeled by Chaska as the "by-pass operation"—and deployment of strategies for effective mutual resolution are explicated. Her focus is on the role of dean, with an emphasis on prevention of the by-pass phenomenon. She stresses that research concerning organizational culture and the work environment of nursing in academic institutions is a necessity.

Dynamics, Teams, and the Role of the Dean

Complexity is inherent in nursing programs and is best addressed through effective teamwork. Forces, such as demands for program quality, financial cuts, and changes in technology are factors that require team action. Andrea Lindell (Chapter 69) addresses the team approach, focusing on the dean as leader. She argues that discernment is the characteristic essential in leadership to be provided by the dean—the key to survival of both the team and the person's position as dean.

Lindell depicts visionary leadership for the dean role but recognizes the importance of 10 elements of the work environment. Development of a power base (because political aspects of the job are inevitable) and the need for leaders to be generalists (not narrowly focused) are requisites. Lindell also identifies relevant characteristics that are valuable for team members to possess.

■ Part VIII: The Future of Nursing

In this Part, the chapters highlight factors that are critical to the future of the nursing profession. Presented in the same sequence as the preceding Parts of the book, these fundamental elements of the profession are: professionaliza-

tion, education, theory, research, practice, administration of service and administration in academia. A concluding chapter offers an overview of the profession for the future.

Professionalization

Inner work for professional development is the key for success, as urged by Daniel Pesut (Chapter 70). He outlines means and methods as a blueprint to recreate the profession of nursing. Archetypes, shadows, and awakening of the corporate soul are all part of the framework that he offers.

The socialization process in nursing programs may well serve as the basis for understanding commitment, healing, and the need for renewal (Waugaman & Lohrer, 2000). Values that are the essence and heritage of the nursing profession must be the foundation for renewal. Caring, courage, inclusion, reflective thinking, and social responsibility are values that are its mainstay (Salmon, 1999). Therein—values and inner work—lies the profession's future.

Nursing Education

In discussing nursing education's future, patterns similar to those in previous chapters, are captured by Donna Boland (Chapter 71). She addresses confounding factors for the future. She further reinforces themes previously addressed, including (a) lack of theoretical clarity about the work of nursing, (b) lack of differentiation in the education of nurses, (c) insufficient recognition of the need for role delineation and functional differentiation in practice, and (d) implications for changes in faculty scholarship and role. Differentiation for practice begs the question: How can such recognition occur without differentiation in education programs for expected outcomes and roles? Boland's approach to themes differs from those of the authors of previous chapters.

For example, Boland emphatically embraces the concept of health in nursing education.

Much of what Boland advises, particularly in relation to health, education, and preparation for practice, is also advocated also by others (Acord, 1999b; Bowen, Lyons, & Young, 2000; Chaffee, 2000; Jacobs, DiMattio, Bishop, & Fields, 1998; Lindeman, 2000; McBride, 1999; Reutter & Williamson, 2000; Vinson, 2000).

Previous chapters by Gaines (Chapter 12), Dooling and Gaines (Chapter 13), and a speech by Lindeman (cited by Gaines) suggest that accreditation as we now know it may be a thing of the past. Carol Lindeman (personal communication, August 19, 1999) envisions accreditation (or certification) of faculty in the future. That prediction is based on belief that faculty members—as individuals—will be the key to quality. Faculty will be expected to guide the student through an individualized program of studies and will work for more than one educational institution. According to Lindeman, "competition in higher education will drive universities to seek out the best talent and use that in whatever way fits the university's programming" (personal communication, August 19, 1999). The challenge is: How can nursing education best prepare for such a transition?

Nursing Theory

Diversity, reflected in previous chapters on knowledge development, may be countered with integration, as described by Afaf Meleis and Eun-Ok Im (Chapter 72). Whereas prior chapters focus predominantly on process and methods in theory development, Meleis and Im argue for inclusiveness of process and outcomes. Care of the dying patient is presented as an illustration of the benefits of that approach. Rather than focusing entirely on death as an outcome, the quality of the dying experience and the sense of well-being of all during the process of dying also may be outcomes.

Thus situation-specific theories, focusing on specific nursing phenomenon reflected in clinical practice and limited to specific populations or fields of nursing practice, are advocated. Most important, empirically developed situation-specific theories will help bridge gaps among theory, practice, research, and health policy.

Nursing Research

Themes concerning research in Chapters 11, 29–36, 42, 43, 44, 45, and 54 pervades the comprehensive presentation by Patricia Grady (Chapter 73). Patterns of health promotion, quality of life and management of chronic conditions, focus on the whole patient, and adaptation to new technologies as a result of evolving genetics knowledge are some of the themes that she encapsulates. Although careful analysis regarding schools' readiness to conduct research is essential (Deets, 1999), Grady cites extensive support and continued commitment for nursing research through federal funding. Funding in the future from the National Institute of Nursing Research (NINR) is expected to increase.

Nursing Practice

A method and process for developing a philosophy of healing practices in nursing is expressed clearly and effectively by Phyllis Beck Kritek (Chapter 74). Reflection on ontology and epistemology of healing practices in nursing through "lived experience" is the method that Kritek demonstrates. Throughout her explication of nursing's metaparadigm (nurse, patient, health, and environment) Kritek illustrates creativity in espousing initiative for a philosophy of nursing practice. In searching for a philosophical system that may embrace the roots of Nightingale, Kritek advocates starting by considering the elusive dimension of healing—the mystery of the human spirit.

Nursing Administration– Service

To be a viable entity, according to the comprehensive explication provided by Karlene Kerfoot (Chapter 75), nursing needs to reinvent itself significantly. The blueprint for renewal suggested by Pesut (Chapter 70) may further enable nursing to achieve the goals suggested by Kerfoot. Leadership in administration of services, including the expanded role of nurse executives, is addressed extensively. Executive coaching for leadership is to be used with caution, as shown also in a recent study (Hall, Otazo, & Hollenbeck, 1999).

With the emphasis on integrated systems (Porter-O'Grady, Chapter 55, and Pinkerton, Chapter 56), the question becomes: How do we manage both differentiation and integration? The dilemmas encountered in grouping people, processes, and operating units for their uniqueness and at the same time linking them to the larger organization needs further consideration (Nadler & Tushman, 1999). Somewhat similar to the ideas of McClure (Chapter 62), but different in approach, Kerfoot emphasizes a shared vision in maintaining unity between nursing staff and management. Further, the concepts of synergy and accountability are advocated as a replacement for the concept of autonomy.

Predicting the future, particularly regarding leadership by the profession as a whole, is a major focus. Kerfoot points out the need for "one strong voice" in the profession. She further draws attention to the approximate 95 nursing organizations (see Sills and Anderson, Chapter 77) that have no mechanism for consensus building and the "thousands" of nurses who reject belonging to any professional organization. That theme—the need for unity— is repeated one way or another in Chapters 4, 9, 65, 71, and 77. When, how, and by whom will the questions concerning "unity" and a "spokespersons organization" for the profession be addressed? Who has the professional base and criteria needed to accomplish that goal? Is not the time now?

Nursing Administration– Academic

Leadership for new-age environments in academia are strongly advocated (Langston, Cowling, & McCain, 1999; Starck, Warner, & Kotarba, 1999). That need is aptly addressed by Joan Shaver (Chapter 76). Reengineering education programs to accommodate environmental forces positively is a major challenge. The trends identified are similar to many shown in previous chapters. However, emphases and responses conveyed by Shaver are different. For example, the shifting to (a) preparation of NPs in graduate programs, (b) emphasis on primary-based care and away from tertiary-based care, (c) development of model practice and community-based sites, and (d) explosion of information technologies is noted.

Shaver highlights merger of positions, such as the advanced practice nurse (APN) role into one health care generalist. In so doing, she reinforces the need for an articulated health care delivery system. Further, the need for integrated systems in academia is stressed. For example, the coordinating of programs of teaching, research, and practice around management of chronic illness, geriatric therapeutics, and culturally diverse groups is advocated. Emphasized also is that the need for integrated systems in academia includes consolidation of basic structures and programs. Clearly, a foundation for leadership rests in ability to optimize change.

The Future of Nursing

However superfluous it may seem, concluding Part VIII, The Future of Nursing, with a chapter that presents an overview is far from redundant. Weaving through the entire profession, Grayce Sills and Carole Anderson (Chapter 77) identify distinct challenges that nursing must address. Examples of direction for change in the future lie in (a) moving toward interdependence and collaboration in nursing programs and interprofessional relationships, (b) increasing quality control in education, and (c) garnering new models of education and service. The most complex challenge among those identified for the larger whole of nursing is that of uniting its professional organizations.

Leadership for this new millennium will require increased creativity for nursing to survive and thrive as a serving profession. A piece of wisdom exists in every person. Verification is suggested in the book *Jesus CEO: Using Ancient Wisdom for Visionary Leadership,* by Laurie Beth Jones (1995); true leaders will find ways to unleash wisdom for the sake of nursing's mission.

■ Concluding Statement

I have addressed the linkages, connections, themes, and patterns that are evident in the writings of the various contributors to this book. Predominant patterns include (a) values, cultural relativism versus universal ethics, competency and regulation concerns, and implications of the aging nursing workforce; (b) preparation for entry practice, technological

innovation, and collaboration; (c) education outcomes and evaluation, distributive learning, faculty role changes, and global education; (d) diversification in knowledge development; (e) high-quality, evidence-based nursing research; (f) influence of culture, partnerships and innovative practice models, and community-focused and community-based practices; (g) integration in administration of service and academic programs, building healthy environments, and management roles and leadership; and (h) unification of the profession.

A summary of the dominant themes presented encompasses (a) values; (b) integration, outcomes, and technology throughout every aspect of the profession (education, theory, research, practice, and administration)—for high-quality service by the profession for the public served; and (c) unification of the profession. The linkages between the Parts and chapters illuminate a complete picture—a blueprint—of the profession as a whole for the future.

The first in this series of books, *The Nursing Profession,* was subtitled: "Views Through the Mist" (1978). This fourth and latest work could easily have been subtitled "Paths Through the Mist." I am hopeful and optimistic that the paths presented by the contributing authors will direct and carry the profession through to make "all the difference" for tomorrow and beyond.

■ References

Acord, L. (1999a). The baccalaureate revolution. *Journal of Professional Nursing, 15*(1), 5.

Acord, L. (1999b). The case for differentiated practice. *Journal of Professional Nursing, 15*(5), 264.

Acord, L. (2000). Help wanted—Faculty. *Journal of Professional Nursing, 16*(1), 3.

American Association of Colleges of Nursing. (1999a, March 15). *Position statement: Defining scholarship for the discipline of nursing.* Washington, DC: Author.

American Association of Colleges of Nursing. (1999b). Certification and regulation of advanced practice nurses. *Journal of Professional Nursing, 15*(2), 130–132.

American Nurses Association. (1999). ANA creates new "house" for all nurses. *The American Nurse, 31*(4), 1, 8.

Anderson-Loftin, W. (1999). Nursing case managers in rural hospitals. *JONA (Journal of Nursing Administration), 29*(2), 42–49.

Balanced Budget Act of 1997. (P.L. 105–33), August 1997, HR 3426–Medicare and Medicaid Health Insurance Act. *U.S. Statutes at Large.* (Vol. III, pp. 251–788). Washington, DC: U.S. Government Printing Office.

Barger, S. (1999). Establishing a clinical track for faculty–Feat or folly? *Journal of Professional Nursing, 15*(2), 71.

Bellack, J. P., & O'Neil, E. H. (2000). Recreating nursing practice for a new century: Recommendations and implications of the Pew Health Professions Commission's final report. *Nursing and Health Care Perspectives, 21*(1), 14–21.

Bellack, J. P., Graber, D. R., O'Neil, E. H., Musham, C., & Lancaster, C. (1999). Curriculum trends in nurse practitioner programs: Current and ideal. *Journal of Professional Nursing, 15*(1), 15–27.

Bowen, M., Lyons, K. J., & Young, B. (2000). Nursing and health care reform: Implications for curriculum development. *Journal of Nursing Education, 39*(1), 27–33.

Breda, K. L. (1997). Professional nurses in unions: Working together pays off. *Journal of Professional Nursing, 13*(2), 99–109.

Buerhaus, P. (1998). Op-Ed: Medicare payment for advanced practice nurses: What are the research questions? *Nursing Outlook, 46*(4), 151–153.

Buerhaus, P., & Auerbach, D. (1999). Slow growth in the United States of the number of minorities in the RN workforce. *IMAGE: Journal of Nursing Scholarship, 31*(2), 179–183.

Catlin, A., & McAuliffe, M. (1999). Proliferation of non-physician providers as reported in the Journal of the American Medical Association (JAMA), 1998. *IMAGE: Journal of Nursing Scholarship, 31*(2), 175–177.

Chaffee, M. (2000). Health communications: Nursing education for increased visibility and effectiveness. *Journal of Professional Nursing, 16*(1), 31–38.

Cheek, J. (2000). *Postmodern and poststructural approaches to nursing research.* Thousand Oaks, CA: Sage.

Cleeland, N., & Bernstein, S. (1999, October 24). Nurses across U.S. increasingly turn to unions. *San Francisco Examiner,* pp. A-6–A-7.

David, B. A. (1999). Nurses conflicting values in competitively managed health care. *IMAGE: Journal of Nursing Scholarship, 31*(2), 188.

Deets, C. (1999). Impact of federal funding increase for research. *Journal of Professional Nursing, 15*(2), 70.

Dexter, P., Applegate, M., Backer, J., Claytor, K., Keffer, J., Norton, B., & Ross, B. (1997). A proposed framework for teaching and evaluating critical thinking in nursing. *Journal of Professional Nursing, 13*(3), 160–167.

Dilts, R. (1996, 2000). Visionary leadership skills: Creating a world to which people want to belong. Capitola, CA: Meta Publications. [On-line, 2000]. Available: http://www.nlpu.com/.

Eichelberger, L. W., & Hewlett, P. O. (1999). Competency model 101: The process of developing core competencies. *Nursing and Health Care Perspectives, 20*(4), 204–208.

Frost, R. (1916/1993). The road not taken. In Robert Frost, *The road not taken and other poems* (p. 1). New York: Dover Publications, Inc. (1993) and New York: Henry Holt & Co. (1916).

Hall, D. T., Otazo, K. L., & Hollenbeck, G. P. (1999). What really happens in executive coaching. *Organizational Dynamics, 27*(3), 39–52.

Harrison, J. K. (1999). Influence of managed care on professional nursing practice. *IMAGE: Journal of Nursing Scholarship, 31*(2), 167–173.

Heller, B. R., Oros, M. T., & Durney-Crowley, J. (2000). The future of nursing education: Ten trends to watch. *Nursing and Health Care Perspectives, 21*(1), 9–13.

Hoagberg, B. L., Vellenga, B., Miller, M., & Li, T. Y. (1999). A partnership model of distance education: Students' perceptions of connectedness and professionalization. *Journal of Professional Nursing, 15*(2), 116–122.

Howell, S. L., & Coates, C. J. (1997). Utilizing narrative inquiry to evaluate a nursing doctorate program professional residency. *Journal of Professional Nursing, 13*(2), 110–123.

Jacobs, L. A., DiMattio, M. J. K., Bishop, T. L., & Fields, S. D. (1998). The baccalaureate degree in nursing as an entry-level requirement for professional nursing practice. *Journal of Professional Nursing, 14*(4), 225–233.

Jones, L. B. (1995). *Jesus CEO: Using ancient wisdom for visionary leadership.* New York: Hyperion.

Keating, S. (1997). Education and practice partnerships in California. *Journal of Professional Nursing, 13*(4), 211–216.

Ketefian, S. (1999a). Knowing good and doing good—Is there a difference? *Journal of Professional Nursing, 15*(1), 4.

Ketefian, S. (1999b). Ethics content in nursing education. *Journal of Professional Nursing, 15*(1), 4.

Krejci, J. W. (1999). Changing roles in nursing: Perceptions of nurse administrators. *JONA (Journal of Nursing Administration), 29*(3), 21–29.

Kupperschmidt, B. R., & Burns, P. (1997). Curriculum revision isn't just change: It's transition. *Journal of Professional Nursing, 13*(2), 98–99.

Langston, N. F., Cowling, W. R., & McCain, N. L. (1999). Transforming academic nursing: From balance through integration to coherence. *Journal of Professional Nursing, 15*(1), 28–32.

Larson, E. (1997). Academia freedom amidst competing demands. *Journal of Professional Nursing, 13*(4), 211–216.

Lashley, R. R. (1999). Integrating genetics content in undergraduate nursing programs. *Biological Research in Nursing, 1*(2), 113–118.

Liaschenko, J., & Fisher, A. (1999). Theorizing the knowledge that nurses use in the conduct of their work. *Scholarly Inquiry for Nursing Practice: An International Journal, 13*(1), 29–41.

Lindeke, L. L., & Chesney, M. L. (1999). Reimbursement realities of advanced nursing practice. *Nursing Outlook, 47*(6), 248–256.

Lindeman, C. A. (2000). The future of nursing education. *Journal of Nursing Education, 39*(1), 5–12.

McBride, A. B. (1999). Breakthroughs in nursing education: Looking back, looking forward. *Nursing Outlook, 47*(3), 114–119.

McCahon, C. P., Niles, S. A., George, V. D., & Stricklin, M. L. (1999). A model to restructure nursing education: Vision on 22nd Street. *Nursing and Health Care Perspectives, 20*(6), 296–301.

McClure, M. L. (1978). Entry into professional practice: The New York proposal. In N. L. Chaska (Ed.), *The nursing profession: Views through the mist* (pp. 93–99). New York: McGraw-Hill.

Monsen, R. B., Anderson, G., New, F., Ledbetter, S., Frazier, L. G., Smith, M. E., & Wilson, M. (2000). Nursing education and genetics: Miles to go before we sleep. *Nursing and Health Care Perspectives, 21*(1), 34–37.

Moser, S. S., & Armer, J. M. (2000). An inside view: NP/MD perceptions of collaborative practice. *Nursing and Health Care Perspectives, 21*(1), 29–33.

Murphy, C. P., Sweeney, M. A., & Chiriboga, D. (2000). An educational intervention for advance directives. *Journal of Professional Nursing, 16*(1), 21–30.

Nadler, D. A., & Tushman, M. L. (1999). Strategic imperatives and core competencies for the 21st century. *Organizational Dynamics, 28*(1), 45–60.

Neuman, B., Newman, D. M. L., & Holder, P. (2000). Leadership–scholarship integration: Using the Neuman systems model for 21st-century professional nursing practice. *Nursing Science Quarterly, 13*(1), 60–63.

Norbeck, J. S. (1998). Teaching, research, and service: Striking the balance in doctoral education. *Journal of Professional Nursing, 14*(4), 197–205.

O'Brien, B. S., & Renner, A. (2000). Nurses on-line: Career mobility for registered nurses. *Journal of Professional Nursing, 16*(1), 13–20.

Pinkerton, S. (1998). Home care nursing—Needs for the future. *Journal of Professional Nursing, 14*(4), 193.

Prows, C., Latta, K. K., Hetteberg, C., Williams, J. K., Kenner, C., & Monsen, R. B. (1999). Preparation of undergraduate nursing faculty to incorporate genetics content into curricula. *Biological Research for Nursing, 1*(2), 108–112.

Pulcini, J., Mason, D. J., Cohen, S. S., Kovner, C., & Leavitt, J. (2000). Health policy and the private sector: New vistas for nursing. *Nursing and Health Care Perspectives, 21*(1), 22–28.

Rambur, B. (1999). Fostering evidence-based practice in nursing education. *Journal of Professional Nursing, 15*(5), 270–274.

Reuter, L., & Williamson, D. (2000). Advocating healthy public policy: Implications for baccalaureate nursing education. *Journal of Nursing Education, 39*(1), 21–26.

Rosswurm, M. A., & Larrabee, J. H. (1999). A model for change to evidence-based practice. *IMAGE: Journal of Nursing Scholarship, 31*(4), 317–326.

Russell, S. (1999, December 10). Severe nursing shortage ahead in California, report says. *San Francisco Chronicle*, p. A-7.

Salmon, M. (1999). Thoughts on nursing: Where it has been and where it is going. *Nursing and Health Care Perspectives, 20*(1), 20–25.

Schuster, P., Fitzgerald, D. C., McCarthy, P. A., & McDougal, D. (1997). Work load issues in clinical nursing education. *Journal of Professional Nursing, 13*(3), 154–159.

Starck, P. L., Warner, A., & Kotarba, J. (1999). 21st century leadership in nursing education: The need for trifocals. *Journal of Professional Nursing, 15*(5), 265–269.

Tahan, H. (1999). Home health care under fire: Fraud and abuse. *JONA's Healthcare Law, Ethics, and Regulation, 1*(1), 16–24.

Thompson, C., & Bartels, J. E. (1999). Outcomes assessment: Implications for nursing education. *Journal of Professional Nursing, 15*(3), 170–178.

Tilden, V. (1999). Ethics perspectives in end-of-life care. *Nursing Outlook, 47*(4), 162–167.

Tone, B. (1999). Pulled apart: Does unionizing serve the profession? *NurseWeek, 12*(16), 1, 30–31.

Triolo, P. K., Pozehl, B. J., & Mahaffey, T. L. (1997). Development of leadership within the university and beyond: Challenges to faculty and their development. *Journal of Professional Nursing, 13*(3), 149–153.

Valanis, B. (2000). Professional nursing practice in an HMO: The future is now. *Journal of Nursing Education, 39*(1), 13–20.

Valentine, P. E. B., Richardson, S., Wood, M. J., & Godkin, M. D. (1998). Nurse educators'/administrators' ways of handling conflict. *Journal of Professional Nursing, 14*(5), 288–297.

Vinson, J. A. (2000). Nursing's epistemology revisited in relation to professional education competencies. *Journal of Professional Nursing, 16*(1), 39–45.

Wakefield, M. (1999). State and federal health priorities. *Journal of Professional Nursing, 15*(2), 72.

Waugaman, W. R., & Lohrer, D. J. (2000). From nurse to nurse anesthetist: The influence of age and gender on professional socialization and career commitment of advanced practice nurses. *Journal of Professional Nursing, 16*(1), 47–56.

White, B. C. (1999). Assisted suicide and nursing: Possibly compatible? *Journal of Professional Nursing, 15*(3), 151–159.

White, S. G., & Henry, J. K. (1999). Incorporation of service-learning into a baccalaureate nursing education curriculum. *Nursing Outlook, 47*(6), 257–261.

White, B. C., & Zimbelman, J. (1999). Why nurses must actively participate in the debate on assisted suicide: A symposium. *Journal of Professional Nursing, 15*(3), 139–141.

Wing, D. M. (1998). The business management preceptorship within the nurse practitioner program. *Journal of Professional Nursing, 14*(3), 150–156.

Zimbelman, J. (1999). Legal decisions and public opinion informing the debate on assisted suicide. *Journal of Professional Nursing, 15*(3), 146–150.

Zimbelman, J., & White, B. C. (1999). The moral appeal of assisted suicide in end-of-life decisions. *Journal of Professional Nursing, 15*(3), 142–145.

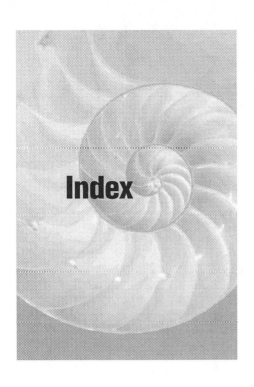

Index